UNIVERSITY OF GLAMORGAN
LEARNING RESOURCES CENTRE

Pontypridd, Mid Glamorgan, CF37 1DL
Telephone: Pontypridd (01443) 482626

Books are to be returned on or before the last date below

Conservative Management of Sports Injuries

Conservative Management of Sports Injuries

Editors

Thomas E. Hyde, D.C., D.A.C.B.S.P.

Fellow of the International College of Chiropractors
Postgraduate Faculty
New York College of Chiropractic
Seneca Falls, New York

Logan College of Chiropractic
Chesterfield, Missouri

Palmer College of Chiropractic
Davenport, Iowa

Northwestern College of Chiropractic
Bloomington, Minnesota

Private Practice
Miami, Florida

Marianne S. Gengenbach, D.C., D.A.C.B.S.P.

Fellow of the International College of Chiropractors
Postgraduate Faculty
Logan College of Chiropractic
Chesterfield, Missouri

Northwestern College of Chiropractic
Bloomington, Minnesota

Texas College of Chiropractic
Pasadena, Texas

Private Consultant
Crawfordville, Florida

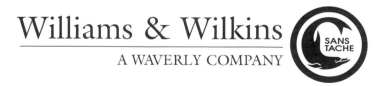

Williams & Wilkins
A WAVERLY COMPANY

BALTIMORE • PHILADELPHIA • LONDON • PARIS • BANGKOK
BUENOS AIRES • HONG KONG • MUNICH • SYDNEY • TOKYO • WROCLAW

Editor: John P. Butler
Managing Editor: Linda S. Napora
Production Coordinator: Raymond E. Reter
Copy Editor: Christiane Odyniec
Designer: Wilma Rosenberger
Illustration Planner: Lorraine Wrzosek
Cover Designer: Wilma Rosenberger
Typesetter: Graphic World, Inc., St. Louis, Missouri
Printer & Binder: Maple-Vail Book Mfg. Group, Binghamton, New York
Digitized Illustrations: Publicity Engravers, Inc., Baltimore, Maryland

Original illustrations drawn by Felix Fu.

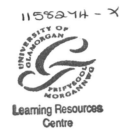

Copyright © 1997 Williams & Wilkins

351 West Camden Street
Baltimore, Maryland 21201-2436 USA

Rose Tree Corporate Center
1400 North Providence Road
Building II, Suite 5025
Media, Pennsylvania 19063-2043 USA

Accurate indications, adverse reactions, and dosage schedules for drugs are provided in this book, but it is possible that they may change. The reader is urged to review the package information data of the manufacturers of the medications mentioned.

Printed in the United States of America

Library of Congress Cataloging-in-Publication Data

Conservative management of sports injuries / editors, Thomas E. Hyde,
   Marianne S. Gengenbach.
      p.   cm.
   Includes bibliographical references and index.
   ISBN 0-683-03944-X
   1. Sports injuries—Chiropractic treatment.   I. Hyde, Thomas E.
II. Gengenbach, Marianne S.
   [DNLM: 1. Athletic Injuries—therapy.   2. Chiropractic—methods.
QT 261 C755 1196]
RZ275.S65C66 1996
617.1'027—dc20
DNLM/DLC
for Library of Congress   96-5025
                                                                     CIP

The publishers have made every effort to trace the copyright holders for borrowed material. If they have inadvertently overlooked any, they will be pleased to make the necessary arrangements at the first opportunity.

To purchase additional copies of this book, call our customer service department at **(800) 638-0672** or fax orders to **(800) 447-8438**. For other book services, including chapter reprints and large-quantity sales, ask for the Special Sales department.

Canadian customers should call **(800) 268-4178,** or fax **(905) 470-6780**. For all other calls originating outside of the United States, please call **(410) 528-4223** or fax us at **(410) 528-8550**.

Visit Williams & Wilkins on the Internet: **http://www.wwilkins.com** or contact our customer service department at **custserv@wwilkins.com**. Williams & Wilkins customer service representatives are available from 8:30 am to 6:00 pm, EST, Monday through Friday, for telephone access.

96 97 98 99 00
1 2 3 4 5 6 7 8 9 10

This text is dedicated to all the chiropractic pioneers who saw the natural relationship between chiropractic and sports injury management and dared to further its use in the treatment of athletes. Their commitment to the provision of care to athletes, both on the field and in the office, and their vision in establishing specialty certification in sports injury management have led the way to the publication of this work.

In particular, we dedicate this text to the memory of Vivian Santiago, D.C., D.A.C.B.S.P., and Joseph Santiago, Sr., D.C., D.A.C.B.S.P. In the spirit of true pioneers, they remained committed to their profession, and its application to athletics, for a lifetime. While continuing to care for patients, and continuing to offer their experience to new chiropractors through teaching, they also exhibited an endless thirst for new learning that led them to pursue specialty certification and new research late in their careers. May their exemplary dedication to the profession that they loved provide an inspiration to us all.

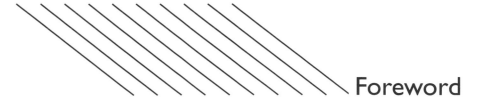

Foreword

It is an honor to have been invited to write a foreword for this textbook. This work has been edited by two accomplished sports physicians within the chiropractic profession, Drs. Marianne S. Gengenbach and Thomas E. Hyde, and has an impressive list of contributing authors who cover the various disciplines and expertise in the area of sports injuries. Most impressive are the unique chapters dealing with issues that are considered peripherally related to sports medicine, such as medicolegal issues, exercise physiology, basic concepts of rehabilitation, and principles of manipulation in sports medicine. The chapters on female, senior, and young athletes are unique in their thoroughness and depth of evaluation of these patient populations. Thorough evaluations of the various regions of the body beginning with the head and including the spine and upper and lower extremities are offered. Each author has excelled in providing an in-depth, yet clinically practical assessment of each area.

As long as I can remember, I have been very active and have competed in many sports. Upon my arrival at Logan College of Chiropractic, I met John Danchik, D.C., who was very instrumental in guiding me toward building my practice around the treatment of athletes. He provided inspiration, motivation, and education. A few years after beginning practice, Mr. Mike Stein and Richard Herrick, M.D., provided the next opportunities that set the stage for later achievements. Finally, Coach Don Soldinger opened many doors that gave me the opportunities to provide chiro-

practic care to athletes with all levels of skill. These are the people that are responsible for the success I enjoy today in Sports Chiropractic.

I was pleased to see a chapter dedicated to diagnostic imaging of sports injuries that assists the clinician in establishing the role of imaging in the overall evaluation of the athlete. Special chapters concerning nutrition and strength and conditioning provide significant augmentation to an already thorough and impressive textbook.

I believe this work will fill a significant void in the library of those who are interested in the overall assessment and treatment of sports-related injuries. On a more personal note, it pleases me to see two ex-students of mine from Logan College of Chiropractic, Drs. Marianne S. Gengenbach and Thomas E. Hyde, as the editors of this textbook. I fully understand the amount of effort it takes to publish a work of this magnitude and I am extremely proud of their efforts. They are to be commended for creating this textbook.

Terry R. Yochum, D.C., D.A.C.B.R.
Adjunct Professor of Radiology
Los Angeles College of Chiropractic
Whittier, California

Director
Rocky Mountain Chiropractic Radiological Center
Denver, Colorado

Instructor, Skeletal Radiology
Department of Radiology
University of Colorado School of Medicine
Denver, Colorado

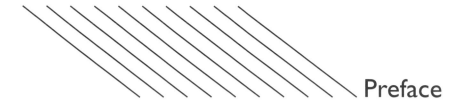
There is no doubt that the field of sports injury management has enjoyed increasing recognition as a legitimate subspecialty in the health-care professions. The past 15 years have brought great advances in our understanding of injury mechanisms and sports biomechanics, as well as in treatment technologies for the athlete and exercising individual. An increasing percentage of individuals in the various health professions have sought advanced knowledge in the area of sports injuries, and certification programs and fellowships have gained popularity. Along with this burgeoning field of knowledge has come a proliferation of texts that cover a range of issues in sports injuries and their management, from the general overview to highly specific discussions of one joint of the body or one sport. This text is intended to bridge the information gap that often exists in these works, between the evaluation of the injury and the initiation of surgical intervention. Many of the injuries we see in daily practice, once they have been designated as nonsurgical, are traditionally managed in a somewhat passive fashion. In emphasizing the concept of active conservative care, this text represents an approach that we believe gives it a special place among the many.

Athletes have traditionally demanded treatment by conservative means whenever possible, with surgical approaches considered as a last resort. The exception to this has been those emergencies that require immediate medical intervention. This text is designed to provide the opportunity for any health-care practitioner, regardless of specialty, to explore the possible use of conservative management in the treatment and rehabilitation of injured athletes. We also recognize that highly sophisticated rehabilitation may not be available to everyone and may not always represent the most cost-effective road to recovery. To that end, we have included "low-tech" methods of providing rehabilitation that are easily accomplished in a small office space, are inexpensive, and in many cases can be performed by the athlete at home.

We have attempted to cover the human body from the top down. We have given attention to female, young, and senior athletes. As our knowledge of the human body continues to increase on a daily basis, so will our knowledge of optimum treatment of injuries. In this never-ending search, it is our goal to provide information that fosters a multidisciplinary "team" approach to the treatment and rehabilitation of athletic injuries. The gaps between the various health-care professions are being bridged, as we have discovered that we each offer unique and important components to the specialty of sports injuries management. We believe that the future will bring a comprehensive delivery of care to the athlete, in which delineations of health-care specialty will become less important than the concerted efforts to address all aspects of injury diagnosis, treatment, and rehabilitation as a team. When health-care team members work together, the athlete will be the ultimate winner.

As chiropractic physicians, our interest in the conservative care of injuries is particularly keen. The role of chiropractors in the conservative management of athletic injuries began with the birth of the profession in 1895. Dr. Earle Painter, who treated Babe Ruth and other members of the New York Yankees, was one of the early recognized pioneers in the field. With chiropractic's growth as a science, it became increasingly important to provide an avenue of additional education for those who wanted to treat athletes. In 1972, Dr. Leonard Schroeder and several other chiropractors formed the American Chiropractic Association's Sports Council and established a postgraduate sports medicine subspecialty certification for chiropractors. This program has grown along with interest in the field. It now includes extensive classroom hours as well as practicum and publication requirements. With the acceptance of chiropractic care as an often integral component of musculoskeletal medicine, our need to add to our profession's knowledge in the area of sports injuries management has become increasingly clear. Therefore, although this text may certainly be useful to any health-care practitioner interested in conservative care, we hope that it is especially useful to our chiropractic colleagues, and offer it to our profession with that goal in mind.

Acknowledgments

This undertaking was in danger of dying when I became involved. I had developed a strong belief in the project's merits and embarked on my job with great enthusiasm. The universe, on the other hand, was in the process of trying to teach me about limitations, patience, and the perils of overcommitment. Bringing this book to print has been a constant confrontation between the universe and me. As with many ventures of this nature, the initial size of the project was grossly underestimated, calendars for completion came and went, and one problem after another seemed to raise its head. Nonetheless, the project went forward, albeit slowly. It became, for all of those involved, a challenge to be met and a labor of love. Luckily, our time commitments, enthusiasm, and energy waxed and waned at different paces, and somehow, with the help and patience of many of our authors and our publisher, the project has come to fruition. It is my hope that the perspective of this text will bring something of value to the everyday practices of our profession and to the athletes whom we treat.

I would like to thank Bob Hazel, D.C., for being courageous or crazy enough to launch this project and allow me to be a part of it. I would also like to thank Tom Hyde, D.C., for his constant efforts and energy throughout the endeavor. His willingness to stay the course and to trust in our combined abilities to "pull this off" was integral to making this book a reality.

I also owe my husband, William Treichel, D.C., a great deal of gratitude for his patience and understanding during the countless instances when "that book" took my time and attention and kept me from catching the wind and sailing away with him.

Finally, I would like to thank Linda Napora, our managing editor at Williams & Wilkins, for her steadfast support through all the moments of doubt, crisis, and panic. Her ability to find the positive in any situation, her willingness to let me vent as necessary, and her calm delivery of motivation kept me going on many occasions when I would have preferred to throw up my hands in despair and quit. It is through her faith in us, and the faith and commitment of others at Williams & Wilkins, that this book has finally been published.

—*Marianne S. Gengenbach, D.C.*

A task of this magnitude cannot be completed without the aid and assistance of many individuals. I would like to thank Mr. John Butler of Williams & Wilkins who stuck with this project and provided encouragement even when we ran several years behind the original projected date of publication. Without a doubt, my wife and daughter suffered on many occasions when I failed to do something with them in favor of this book. A great deal of gratitude goes to my wife, Susan, and my daughter, Jennifer.

On more than one occasion I, and others, thought this text would never see publication. Murphy's law seemed to prevail at every turn. We lost authors who provided text in the early stages, but refused to rewrite and update as time elapsed. Others stuck with us and made all revisions requested. To those who stayed with us, I owe respect and a thank you. To those who began the project with us and dropped out, I still would like to say thank you for making the attempt to get us going. I also would like to thank all the others at Williams & Wilkins who did not give up on us.

Finally, I would like to thank Marianne Gengenbach, D.C., for helping to save the book. Without her help and assistance, the text would never have been published. She became the final glue needed to make the project complete. Through this ordeal, I have learned much about personalities, those who are friends, those who were friends, and most of all, more about who I am.

—*Thomas Hyde, D.C.*

Contributors

Donald D. Aspegren, D.C.
Postgraduate Faculty
National College of Chiropractic
Lombard, Illinois
New York Chiropractic College
Seneca Falls, New York
Biology Department
Red Rocks Community College
Lakewood, Colorado

Scott D. Banks, D.C.
Postgraduate Faculty
Logan College of Chiropractic
Chesterfield, Missouri
Private Practice
Virginia Beach, Virginia

Michael S. Barry, D.C., D.A.C.B.R.
Staff Radiologist
Rocky Mountain Chiropractic Radiological Center
Denver, Colorado
Postgraduate Faculty
Logan College of Chiropractic
Chesterfield, Missouri

David J. BenEliyahu, D.C., D.A.C.B.S.P.
Private Practice
Selden, New York

Thomas F. Bergmann, D.C.
Editor, *Chiropractic Techniques*
Private Practice
Minneapolis, Minnesota

Joel P. Carmichael, D.C.
Private Practice
South Denver Neck and Back Pain Clinic
Denver, Colorado
Adjunct Clinical Faculty
Postgraduate Education
Los Angeles College of Chiropractic
Whittier, California

Thomas R. Daly, Esq.
Odin, Feldene & Pittleman, PC
Fairfax, Virginia

John J. Danchik, M.S., D.C., C.C.S.P.
Fellow of the International College of Chiropractors
Postgraduate Faculty
Logan Chiropractic College
Chesterfield, Missouri
New York Chiropractic College
Seneca Falls, New York
Palmer Chiropractic College
Davenport, Iowa
Northwestern Chiropractic College
Bloomington, Minnesota
Private Practice
Boston, Massachusetts

Mauro G. Di Pasquale, B.Sc., M.D.
Medical Consultant on Drug Use in Sports
Associate Professor of Sports Medicine
School of Physical and Health Education
University of Toronto
Warkworth, Ontario
Canada

Dante M. Filetti, Esq.
Wright, Robinson, McCammon, Osthimer & Tatum
Virginia Beach, Virginia

Ted L. Forcum, D.C.
Private Practice
Beaverton, Oregon

Marianne S. Gengenbach, D.C., D.A.C.B.S.P.
Fellow of the International College of Chiropractors
Postgraduate Faculty
Logan College of Chiropractic
Chesterfield, Missouri
Northwestern College of Chiropractic
Bloomington, Minnesota
Texas College of Chiropractic
Pasadena, Texas
Private Consultant
Crawfordville, Florida

James M. Gerber, D.C.
Associate Professor of Clinical Sciences
Western State Chiropractic College
Portland, Oregon

Joseph P. Hornberger, M.S., D.C., C.C.R.D.
Private Practice
Sarasota, Florida

Robin A. Hunter, D.C., D.A.C.B.S.P.
Postgraduate Faculty
Logan College of Chiropractic
Chesterfield, Missouri
Private Practice
Columbus, Ohio

Thomas E. Hyde, D.C., D.A.C.B.S.P.
Fellow of the International College of Chiropractors
Postgraduate Faculty
New York College of Chiropractic
Seneca Falls, New York
Logan College of Chiropractic
Chesterfield, Missouri
Palmer College of Chiropractic
Davenport, Iowa
Northwestern College of Chiropractic
Bloomington, Minnesota
Private Practice
North Miami, Florida

Abigail A. Irwin, D.C., C.C.S.P.
Life Chiropractic College
San Lorenzo, California

Dale K. Johns, M.D.
Chief, Division of Neurosurgery
Palmetto General Hospital
Hialeah, Florida

Margaret E. Karg, M.S., D.C., D.A.C.B.S.P.
Postgraduate Faculty
Logan College of Chiropractic
Chesterfield, Missouri
Private Practive
Boston, Massachusetts

Norman W. Kettner, D.C., D.A.C.B.R.
Chairman and Associate Professor
Department of Radiology
Logan College of Chiropractic
Chesterfield, Missouri

Larry J. Kinter, D.C., C.C.S.P.
Private Practice
Harlan, Iowa

D.A. Lawson, D.C.
Private Practice
Columbia, Missouri

Michael Leahy, D.C., C.C.S.P.
Private Practice
Colorado Springs, Colorado

Thomas C. Michaud, D.C.
Private Practice
Newton, Massachusetts

William J. Moreau, D.C., D.A.C.B.S.P., C.S.C.S.
Fellow of the International College of Chiropractors
Assistant Professor
Northwestern College of Chiropractic
Bloomington, Minnesota

Stephen M. Perle, D.C., C.C.S.P.
College of Chiropractic
University of Bridgeport
Bridgeport, Connecticut

Gerry G. Provance, D.C., C.C.S.P.
Private Practice
Metairie, Louisiana

Edward J. Ryan III, M.S., A.T.C.
Athletic Trainer, Permanent Staff
U.S. Olympic Training Center
Colorado Springs, Colorado

Rick S. Saluga, D.C., D.A.B.C.O.
Fellow of the International College of Chiropractors
Chiropractic and Rehabilitation Center
Metairie, Louisiana

Steven M. Skurow, D.C., D.A.B.C.O.
Private Practice
Cincinnati, Ohio

Thomas A. Souza, D.C.
Associate Clinical Professor
Palmer College of Chiropractic—West
Sunnyvale, California

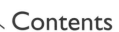

Contents

Section I   *A CONSERVATIVE APPROACH TO SPORTS-RELATED INJURIES*

Section II   *SITE-SPECIFIC SPORTS INJURIES*

Section 1

CONSERVATIVE APPROACH TO SPORTS-RELATED INJURIES

I

Overview of Sports Injuries Management

Stephen M. Perle

HISTORY

It has been said that a proper history is often more valuable in making a diagnosis than physical examination or laboratory tests (1). When diagnosing athletic injuries, this is an understatement; an accurate knowledge of the mechanism of injury can often lead to a presumptive diagnosis.

The significance of the answers to the following questions will be explained in other chapters that are related to the regions injured.

Age

In a sports medicine practice, the age of the patient is important in three ways. First, there are a few injuries that are seen only in certain age-groups. Second, there are many diseases that are not actually sports injuries but may present as such. The patients associate the symptoms with either a previous sports injury or a sports injury they have read or heard about. If the condition is of insidious onset, they may be unable to discern a cause other than their physical activity. Some of these conditions are associated with certain ages. Third, age is a determinant in prognosis. Routinely, humans repair at a slower rate as they age (2). Motivation to comply with a rehabilitation program may vary with age and be lower at both ends of the spectrum (3).

Gender

With the enactment of Title IX, which has brought more women into sports (4), there has been an increase in the number of female athletic injuries (5). In the 1970s, after Title IX was enacted, women did appear to be at increased risk for sports injury (6). This is believed to be due in part to lack of conditioning and preseason conditioning (7). Experience with first-year, female midshipmen at the U.S. Naval Academy also sug-

gests that women, for societal reasons, are more apt to complain of minor problems such as blisters, sprains, and strains than men, who will "grin and bear it." By the second year in the Academy, after becoming aware of the "grin and bear it" attitude, women also ignore minor complaints as do their male counterparts (6).

One might also assume that women are injured more often because it is generally accepted that women are the weaker sex. Studies done by Wilmore (8) have shown that with respect to the lower extremity, women have on average 73.4% of the absolute leg press strength of men. However, when comparing leg press strength relative to body weight, women perform at 92.4% of men; when women's leg press strength is compared with men's relative to fat-free weight, the women's strength is 106% of men's. This shows that women are the weaker sex only in an absolute sense because they are, generally, the smaller sex, and that women could really be considered the stronger sex (8).

Lack of adequate strength is not a reason for any increased incidence of female athletic injuries. In reality, women today tend, in comparable sports, to become injured at a rate that is statistically no different from the male injury rate (9–11).

With children, boys do tend to have a higher rate of injury due to increased participation in higher-risk sports (9).

UNDERSTANDING THE COMPLAINT

Onset

Was the onset insidious, which suggests an "osis" (e.g., tendinosis (12) and arthrosis), or acute, which suggests fracture, sprain, dislocation, and muscle or tendon rupture? Was there any noise associated with the occurrence of the injury, such as a loud snap or crack heard with muscle, tendon, or ligament rupture? Are the symptoms the same, better, worse, or different from when the injury occurred (13)? What position was the body in at the time of the injury? What is the athlete's habitual pattern (timing, duration, biomechanics, technique duration, or number of repetitions) of training and/or competition? This is termed the mechanism of injury and is the most crucial part of a sports medicine history.

Palliative and Provocative

Has the athlete undergone any treatment? Was it effective? Was it done by a professional? Did anyone administer any first aid? Minor acute injuries will often be treated improperly with heat and be made worse. Has the athlete been able to compete or train since the injury (13)?

Quality

Does it burn, stab, or throb? Does the joint lock (13)?

Radiation

Does the pain radiate? If so, a pain diagram is helpful. If the pain is referred, there are only four sources: visceral, myogenic (myofascial trigger points), sclerogenic (joint or bone), and neurogenic (disc herniation or peripheral entrapment or neuropathy) (13).

Site

Where are the location of initial injury and location of present symptoms? Is injury localized (13)? Do not, however, let the patient's localization of the injury blind you to other sources of the symptoms or to other concurrent conditions. A good example of this is the child with a slipped femoral capital epiphysis who presents without hip pain but with knee pain (14). Lewit has said, "The doctor that treats the site of pain is lost" (15).

Timing

With relation to training, is the pain felt only after a period of training, during training, as soon as activity is started, or is the pain constant (Table 1.1) (13, 16)?

CLINICAL FINDINGS

The material that follows is appropriate only for those conditions for which conservative management is suitable. It is assumed, therefore,

that conditions such as fractures, dislocations, and muscle ruptures have been ruled out before undertaking the following methods of evaluation.

Ranges of Motion

A decreased active range of motion due to pain, with a normal passive range of motion, suggests a dysfunction in the prime mover in the restricted range. Pain in the opposite direction of passive range of motion is confirmation. Pain on isometric contraction of the prime mover is further confirmation of a muscular dysfunction, either an acute or chronic strain or tear, or a myofascial trigger point of the prime mover (17, 18). Remember that loss of bilateral symmetry can be the cause or the result of the patient's complaint.

Joint Dysfunction

Joint dysfunction is a loss of joint play. Joint play is a very small motion in a joint that cannot be created by voluntary action of muscles crossing the joint. These fine joint play motions are required for painless voluntary motion of a joint. Joint play movements cannot be produced by the action of voluntary muscles. The loss of joint play (i.e., joint dysfunction) results in joint pain and loss of voluntary range of motion (19).

MECHANISM OF INJURIES

Joints may be injured by intrinsic or extrinsic trauma. Intrinsic trauma is the unguarded motion of the joint. Extrinsic trauma is an injury from forces applied to the joint from outside the body. These injuries to a joint cause inflammation that results in fibrosis. Fibrosis develops into scar formation that restricts joint motion and/or joint play. Joint dysfunction is also a common sequela of immobilization of a joint (19).

CLINICAL FEATURES

Symptoms of joint dysfunction usually arise suddenly. Joint dysfunction is the likely diagnosis for sudden pain after a traumatic insult that is not associated with swelling. Joint dysfunction

Table 1.1 Grading of Overuse Syndromes

Grade	Timing of Symptoms
First degree	Pain at the start or end of athletic activity
Second degree	Pain during and after activity, with no significant functional disability
Third degree	Pain during and after activity with significant functional disability
Fourth degree	Pain all the time, with significant functional disability

is also a likely cause of pain that appears with the restoration of function after immobilization. Keep in mind that athletes often sustain injuries during competition but do not recall the injuries happening (19).

Pain from joint dysfunction is usually sharp and often intermittent. The patient will often complain that the pain occurs when performing one particular motion and is easily reproducible. The pain usually abates, at least significantly, by rest or the cessation of the motion that initiated the pain (19). Janda has suggested that joint dysfunction without concomitant muscle dysfunction is painless (20).

Muscle Strain

It is generally accepted that muscle strain is a stretching or tearing of fibers within the musculotendinous unit (21, 22) and that these are the most frequent injuries in sports (23). Injuries to muscles are more common during eccentric (lengthening) contraction (22, 24–28). Muscles that cross two joints are more prone to injury. Athletes whose sport requires a burst of speed are more prone to injury (23).

Experimental evidence (29), clinical evidence (30), computed tomography (CT) scanning (31), and magnetic resonance imaging (MRI) (32) have shown that most of these injuries occur at the muscle-tendon junction or tendon-bone junction (23). Both CT (22) and MRI (31) confirm that a majority of these injuries result in edema and not bleeding. When bleeding does occur, the hematoma collects between the muscle tissue and the fascial compartment. This is in contrast to bleeding from contusion that occurs within the muscle substance (23). The injury tends to involve smaller volumes of muscle in trained athletes compared with occasional athletes (32).

Prevention of muscle strains has generally centered on stretching and warm-up. Adequate studies have not yet proved conclusively that stretching and warm-up prevent muscle strains, but experiments with animals do support this. There is also some evidence that fatigue and previous incomplete injury predispose muscle to injury, but these also are not conclusively proven (23).

General treatment of muscle strains in the acute stage includes rest, ice, and compression (23). Strains are graded as follows.

- First degree—minimal stretching without permanent injury.
- Second degree—partial tearing without permanent injury.
- Third degree—complete disruption of a portion of the musculotendinous unit with swelling, bleeding, and localized discomfort that may produce temporary disability (22).

First-degree strains should be treated with early stretching as often as every hour (33). More details about treatment are presented with specific injuries in other chapters of this text.

CLINICAL ENTITIES THAT CAN CAUSE OTHER PROBLEMS

Muscle Tightness

Janda has written extensively about the concept of muscle tightness or shortening (34–51). This is a pathophysiologic condition wherein the noncontractile elements of a muscle have shortened, the muscle spindle adapts to this new length, and the muscle is hyperexcitable.

The increased tension in the muscle and its hyperexcitability result in a pseudoparesis of its antagonist. It causes the tight muscle to fire at unusual times (e.g., during contraction of its antagonist) (34, 36). In the early stages of muscle shortening, the muscle is strengthened; in extreme and/or long-standing cases, the shortened muscles become weakened as noncontractile tissue replaces the active muscle fibers (34). This results in altered muscle firing orders (34, 36), which are discussed in the next section.

The adaptation of the muscle spindle results in the muscle being hyperexcitable and not responsive to any lasting degree to any of the usual stretching techniques. Any attempt to stretch the muscle statically results in stimulation of the myotatic reflex, and the muscle contracts against the stretching force with minimal improvement in resting length. The preferred method for treating this condition has been termed postfacilitation stretch (34).

Postfacilitation stretching is accomplished by having the athlete perform a maximal effort contraction of the affected muscle for 10 seconds while held in its midrange of motion by a second individual. This results in fatigue of the muscle spindle. During the muscle spindle's refractory period, a rapid stretch is applied to the muscle and held for 10 seconds. This stretches the noncontractile elements of the muscle during the refractory period so that the myotatic reflex cannot interfere. The muscle is then returned to its midrange and rested for 20 seconds. Janda suggests repeating the procedure three to five times per visit and for three to five visits with a day's rest in between. In the author's experience with elite athletes, this procedure does not usually need to be repeated for more than two visits. However, athletes at a less competitive level are likely to require three to five visits.

Joint dysfunction and muscle tightness have a chicken-or-the-egg type of relationship. It is unclear which is the cause and which is the effect (34, 35, 50). Nevertheless, muscle tightness is also believed to be caused by overuse of postural muscles, by prolonged sitting or standing or other repetitive actions (41, 45) as seen in sports (49, 50).

The author has found that in athletes the best diagnostic criterion for muscle tightness is not the range of motion of the joint crossed by the muscle tested (as described by Janda (35)). Instead, one should examine for the endfeel when attempting to stretch the muscle. When stretched, normal muscles have a rubbery feel. As one continues to stretch a normal muscle, the athlete may complain of some discomfort. However, while stretching a shortened muscle, the endfeel is abrupt, like trying to stretch a steel cable. In this case, the athlete will complain of extreme pain. Athletes with shortened muscles will probably tell the doctor that they have always been "tight" or that they became so after an injury. They will also relate that they do not like to stretch because it is quite uncomfortable or painful. Generally, they have found that if they stop stretching regularly for a few days, they lose all the gains in range of motion and must start stretching from scratch.

Muscle Dyssynergy (Bad Firing Order)

Janda has also described the concept of dyssynergy (i.e., aberrant muscle firing orders). As a result of muscle dysfunction (e.g., muscle tightness, myofascial trigger point) or joint dysfunction, the normal firing order of muscles to create a particular action is altered. A muscle with muscle tightness often will predominate or fire prematurely. Correction of firing order is accomplished by first correcting the causative dysfunction (35). If the order does not spontaneously return to normal, proprioceptive reeducation methods must be used (51, 52).

Muscle firing orders are examined by a very light palpation of the muscles involved. For example, the normal muscle firing order during hip abduction is as follows.

1. Glutei.
2. Tensor fascia lata.
3. Quadratus lumborum (36).

However, one might find the following order in a patient with dyssynergy.

1. Quadratus lumborum.
2. Glutei.
3. Tensor fascia lata.

Too much tactile stimulation to the skin overlying the muscles being palpated can lead to a temporary restoration of firing orders to normal. These firing orders can also be evaluated by observation of the motion. A muscle that fires prematurely will alter the appearance of the motion. In the example given above, the chronically tight quadratus lumborum can make the patient lift the pelvis superiorly before abducting the hip.

Myofascial Trigger Points

MECHANISM OF INJURIES

Myofascial trigger points are localized hyperirritable foci within a muscle that refer pain in a characteristic pattern depending on the muscle involved. Trigger points are the result of either acute overuse of a muscle or chronic overuse fatigue (18). Both acute and chronic causes are seen regularly in athletic populations. Myofascial trigger points are common causes of pain in athletes (53, 54).

CLINICAL FEATURES

Pain from trigger points tends to come and go with periods of acute exacerbation (active). Trigger points cause the affected muscle to become shortened and weakened. An athlete with asymptomatic (latent) trigger points may notice weakness, incoordination, or restricted range of motion.

CLINICAL EVALUATION

Athletes with myofascial pain syndromes will relate a history of sudden onset during or shortly after acute overload stress, or of gradual onset with chronic overload of the affected muscle. Pain is increased when the affected muscle is strongly contracted against fixed resistance. Myofascial trigger points have characteristic patterns of pain that are specific to individual muscles (18). Due to their overall better body sense, athletes often feel trigger points before they are active enough to cause pain; their only complaint is tightness, that the joint or muscle does not "feel right," or there is a vague sensation.

There will be a weakness and restriction in the stretch range of motion of the affected muscle. When active trigger points are present, passive or active stretching of the affected muscle increases pain. The maximum contractile force of an affected muscle is weakened. A joint stabilized by the affected muscle may "give way" (18) or, in the author's opinion, is more likely to be traumatized or have a greater degree of trauma from a particular injury.

A taut band can be palpated within the affected muscle. The trigger point is found in a palpable band as a sharply circumscribed spot of exquisite tenderness. A trigger point feels like a BB in a bass guitar string and is within the afflicted muscle. Moderate, sustained pressure on a sufficiently irritable trigger point causes or intensifies pain in the reference zone of that trigger point. If the trigger point is causing much pain at the time of examination, there may not be any change in symptoms on palpation. A trigger point that is not very irritable may elicit only local pain on palpation. Generally, the further the referral, the worse the trigger point (18).

Digital pressure applied on an active trigger point usually elicits a "jump sign"; that is, the patient jumps from the pain. Muscles in the immediate vicinity of a trigger point feel tense to palpation. A local twitch response can be elicited through snapping palpation (similar to plucking a guitar string) or needling, with a hypodermic needle, of the tender spot (trigger point) (18).

The patient's pain complaint is reproduced by pressure on, or needling of, the tender spot (trigger point). The trigger point has been found when the patient says, "Doctor, that's my pain" (18).

The last criterion for diagnosis of myofascial trigger point pain syndrome is the elimination of symptoms by therapy directed specifically to the affected muscles (18).

Myofascial trigger points do not show up on radiographs, CT scans, or MRI but can be found on thermographic imaging. In the acute stages, trigger points will appear as a hot spot within the belly of the muscle. Notwithstanding, in the chronic case the trigger point will appear as a cold spot (18).

TREATMENT

Appropriate treatment for myofascial trigger points includes the following.

A. Stretch and spray.
B. Injection.
C. Ischemic compression.
D. Postisometric relaxation/Lewit stretch technique (similar to contract and relax—proprioceptive neuromuscular facilitation).
E. Hot packs and/or massage.
F. Electrical stimulation of trigger points (intermittent is better).
G. Ultrasound of trigger points (intermittent is better) (18).

Manipulation of joint dysfunction in the region of the involved muscle may help in the treatment of myofascial trigger points (35, 54–56).

Muscles prone to muscle tightness and their pseudoparalyzed antagonists are prone to trigger points; therefore, muscle tightness must be properly addressed to treat trigger points effectively (52).

For a detailed explanation of all aspects of the myofascial trigger point phenomenon, the reader is referred to Travell and Simons (18, 55).

References

1. Wilkins RW. Clinical internal medicine. In: Wilkins RW, Levinsky NE, eds. Medicine essentials of clinical practice. 2nd ed. Boston: Little, Brown & Co., 1978:3.
2. Marti B, Vader JP, Minder CE, et al. On the epidemiology of running injuries: the 984 Bern Grand-Prix study. Am J Sports Med 1988;16:285–294.
3. Shepard JG, Pacelli LC. Why your patients shouldn't take aging sitting down. Phys Sportsmed 1990;18:83–84, 89–90.
4. Wilkerson LA. The female athlete. Am Fam Physician 1984;29:233–237.
5. Cox JS, Lenz HW. Women in sports: the Naval Academy experience. Am J Sports Med 1979;7:355–360.
6. Kowal DM. Nature and causes of injuries in women resulting from an endurance training program. Am J Sports Med 1980;8:265–269.
7. Haycock CE. The female athlete: past and present. J Am Med Wom Assoc 1976;31:350–352.
8. Wilmore JH. Alterations in strength, body composition and anthropometric measurements consequent to a 10-week weight training program. Med Sci Sports Exerc 1974;6:133–138.
9. Watson AWS. Sports injuries during one academic year in 6799 Irish school children. Am J Sports Med 1984;12:65–71.
10. Protzman RR. Physiologic performance of women compared to men: observations of cadets at the United States Military Academy. Am J Sports Med 1979;7:191–194.
11. Whiteside PA. Men's and women's injuries in comparable sports. Phys Sportsmed 1980;8:130–140.
12. Nirschl R. Elbow tendinosis/tennis elbow. Clin Sports Med 1992;11:851–870.
13. Cyriax J. Textbook of orthopaedic medicine. Diagnosis of soft tissue lesions. 8th ed. London: Balliere-Tindall, 1982;1:43–69.
14. Collins HR. Epiphyseal injuries in athletes. Cleve Clin Q 1979;42:285–295.
15. Lewit K. Manipulation, pain and the locomotor system. Seminar notes, 1990.
16. Roy S, Irvin R. Sports medicine prevention, evaluation, management, and rehabilitation. Englewood Cliffs, NJ: Prentice-Hall, 1983:128.
17. Magee DJ. Orthopedic physical assessment. Philadelphia: WB Saunders, 1987:8–13.
18. Travell JG, Simons DG. Myofascial pain and dysfunction: the trigger point manual. Baltimore: Williams & Wilkins, 1983:5–44, 52, 648–649.
19. Mennell JM. Joint pain: diagnosis and treatment using manipulative techniques. Boston: Little, Brown & Co., 1964:12–16.
20. Janda V. Muscles and cervicogenic pain syndromes. In: Grant R, ed. Physiotherapy of the cervical and thoracic spine. New York: Churchill Livingstone, 1988:153–166.

21. American Academy of Orthopaedic Surgeons. Athletic training and sports medicine. 2nd ed. Park Ridge, IL: American Academy of Orthopaedic Surgeons, 1991:209–210.
22. Baker BE. Current concepts in the diagnosis and treatment of musculotendinous injuries. Med Sci Sports Exerc 1984;16:323–327.
23. Garrett WE Jr. Muscle strain injuries: clinical and basic aspects. Med Sci Sports Exerc 1990;22:436–443.
24. Charpentier J. Observation and reflection concerning a musculoarticular study of the dorso-lumbar and pelvic regions in a group of professional soccer players. Eur J Chir 1984;32:150–159.
25. Stauber WT. Eccentric action of muscles: physiology, injury and adaptation. In: Pandolf KB, ed. Exercise and sports sciences review. Baltimore: Williams & Wilkins, 1989;17:157–185.
26. Torg JS, Vegso JJ, Torg E. Rehabilitation of athletic injuries: an atlas of therapeutic exercise. Chicago: Year Book, 1987:107–110.
27. Hammer WI. The thigh and hip. In: Hammer WI, ed. Functional soft tissue examination and treatment by manual methods: the extremities. Gaithersburg, MD: Aspen Publishers, 1990:117.
28. Injeyan HS, Fraser IH, Peel WD. Pathology of musculoskeletal soft tissues. In: Hammer WI, ed. Functional soft tissue examination and treatment by manual methods: the extremities. Gaithersburg, MD: Aspen Publishers, 1990:18.
29. Garrett WE Jr, Safran MR, Seaber AV, et al. Biomechanical comparison of stimulated and nonstimulated skeletal muscle pulled to failure. Am J Sports Med 1987;15:448–454.
30. Safran MR, Garrett WE Jr, Seaber AV, et al. The role of warm-up in muscular injury prevention. Am J Sports Med 1988;16:123–129.
31. Garrett WE Jr, Rich FR, Nikolaou PK, et al. Computed tomography of hamstring muscle strains. Med Sci Sport Exerc 1989;21:506–514.
32. Fleckenstein JL, Weatherall PT, Parkey RW, et al. Sports-related muscle injuries: evaluation with MR imaging. Radiology 1989;172:793–798.
33. Ryan JB, Wheeler JH, Hopkinson WJ, et al. Quadriceps contusions: West Point update. Am J Sports Med 1991;19:299–304.
34. Janda V. Pain in the locomotor system: a broad approach. In: Glasgow EF, Twomey LT, Scull ER, et al., eds. Aspects of manipulative therapy. 2nd ed. New York: Churchill Livingstone, 1985:148–151.
35. Jull GA, Janda V. Muscles and motor control in low back pain: assessment and management. In: Twomey LT, Taylor JR, eds. Physical therapy of the low back. New York: Churchill Livingstone, 1987:253–278.
36. Janda V. Muscle weakness and inhibition (pseudoparesis) in back pain syndromes. In: Grieve GP, ed. Modern manual therapy of the vertebral column. New York: Churchill Livingstone, 1986:197–201.
37. Janda V. Muscles as a pathogenic factor in back pain. Proceedings of the IFOMT Conference, Christ Church, New Zealand. 1980:1–20.
38. Janda V. Rational therapeutic approach of chronic back pain syndromes. Proceedings of the Symposium on Chronic Back Pain, Rehabilitation and Self Help, Turku, Finland. 1985:69–74.
39. Janda V. The relationship of hip joint musculature to the pathogenesis of low back pain. Proceedings of International Conference of Manipulative Therapy, Perth, Western Australia. 1983:28–31.
40. Janda V. Muscle spasm: a proposed procedure for differential diagnosis. J Manual Med 1991;6:136–139.
41. Máckova J, Janda V, Máckova M, et al. Impaired muscle function in children and adolescents. J Manual Med 1989;4:157–160.
42. Berger M, Janda V, Sachse J. Methods for objective assessment of muscular spasms. In: Emre M, Mathies H, eds. Muscle spasms and pain. Lancaster, PA: Parthenon Publishing Group, 1988:55–66.
43. Janda V. On the concept of postural muscles and posture in man. Aust J Physiother 1963;29:83–84.
44. Janda V. Introduction to functional pathology of the motor system. In: Howell ML, Bullock MI, eds. Proceeding of the VII Commonwealth and International Conference on Sport, Physical Education Recreation and Dance. Physiotherapy in Sports, University of Queensland, 1982;3:35–42.
45. Janda V. Muscles, central nervous motor regulation and back problems. In: Korr IM, ed. Neurobiologic mechanisms in manipulative therapy. New York: Plenum, 1978:27–41.
46. Janda V. Comparison of spastic syndromes of cerebral origin with the distribution of muscular tightness in postural defects. In: Rehabilitacia-suplementum 14-15. Proceedings of the 5th International Symposium of Rehabilitation in Neurology. 1977:87–88.
47. Janda V. Muscle and joint correlations. In: Rehabilitacia-suplementum 10-11. Proceedings of the 4th Congress Fédération Internationale de Médecine Manuelle, Prague. 1975:154–158.
48. Janda V, Stara V. The role of thigh adductors in movement patterns of the hip and knee joint. Courier 1965;15:563–565.
49. Janda V. Sport, exercise and back pain. Proceedings of the 4th European Congress of Sports Medicine, Prague, 1985. Prague: AVICENUM, Czechoslovak Medical Press, 1986:231–235.
50. Janda V. Prevention of injuries and their late sequelae. In: Howell ML, Bullock MI, eds. Proceeding of the VII Commonwealth and International Conference on Sport, Physical Education Recreation and Dance. Physiotherapy in Sports, University of Queensland, 1982; 3:35–38.
51. Janda V. Rehabilitation in chronic low back disorders. In: Second Annual Interdisciplinary Symposium (Published Symposium Notes), Los Angeles College of Chiropractic Postgraduate Division. 1988.
52. Lewit K. Manipulative therapy in rehabilitation of the motor system. London: Butterworth, 1985.
53. Perle SM. Runner's pelvis. Chiropractic J 1989;3:13.
54. DeFranca GG. The snapping hip syndrome: a case study. Chiro Sports Med 1988;2:8–11.
55. Travell JG, Simons DG. Myofascial pain and dysfunction: the trigger point manual. Lower extremities. Baltimore: Williams & Wilkins, 1992:16–18, 193.
56. Liebenson C. Active muscular relaxation techniques: part II. clinical application. J Manipulative Phys Ther 1990;13:2–9.

Medicolegal Issues in Sports Medicine (with Special Considerations for the Chiropractor)

Thomas R. Daly and Dante M. Filetti

The increasing involvement of chiropractic medicine in the area of sports medicine is evidence of its increasing visibility and acceptance. The unique nature of the sports medicine practice holds special liability considerations for the doctor of chiropractic.

In sports medicine, the application of the medical arts and sciences is combined to both preserve the health of athletes and improve performance. The dimensions of sports medicine have been described as the following.

- Sports biotypology, aiming to establish the athlete's biotype in each sports discipline.
- Sports physiopathology, i.e., the study of human adaptation to physical effort during athletic training.
- Sport-medical evaluation, i.e., to establish the athlete's conditioning to the effort required.
- Sports traumatology, examining sports injuries, their treatment, and possible prevention through the study of biomechanics of each sports discipline.
- Hygiene of sports, dealing with the hygienic behavior of the athlete and the conditions under which the sport is conducted (1).

A team doctor or sports physician will generally be a medical or chiropractic physician who renders professional care to athletes or students or both. Such providers may hold themselves out to specialize in sports medicine or sports chiropractic and may be compensated for services rendered.

Although the professional scope of practice for physicians varies from state to state (2), all physicians—including chiropractors—are authorized and required to perform certain fundamental procedures including the diagnosis of a patient's medical condition, the treatment of such a condition, and if appropriate, the referral of a patient to another health-care provider (3). This basic responsibility and authority enable the physician to fulfill the functions of a team doctor or sports physician within the scope of professional practice outlined by state law. The critical questions become what duty of care and what standard of care does the physician assume while practicing under his or her state license in the field of sports medicine?

DUTY OF CARE

In any malpractice or negligence action, liability will flow from the demonstration by an injured party that, among other things, a physician owed a particular duty of care to the injured party and that the physician breached such a duty by performing to a standard less than the required standard of care for such a physician. The duty of care can be viewed as "an obligation, to which the law will give recognition and effect, to conform to a particular standard of conduct toward another" (4). Ordinarily, the duty of care owed to a patient by a physician is established through the existence of the doctor-patient relationship. This is done by direct, consensual agreement between the parties when the patient enters the physician's office and the physician agrees to treat the patient. This direct relationship between the parties becomes somewhat clouded when a physician functions as a team doctor or is otherwise retained by an institution (such as a school or other entity) to perform physical examinations or other health-care services for athletes. In this situation, the question concerns to whom the duty is owed; and if the duty is owed to the athlete, what is the extent of such duty? The answer to these questions will have a critical impact on the potential liability of the physician.

DOCTOR-PATIENT RELATIONSHIP AND THE TEAM CHIROPRACTOR

There is a minimal duty owed by a chiropractor to any individual regardless of whether a doctor-patient relationship has been established. The chiropractor owes an affirmative minimal duty not to injure the patient in the course of examination or treatment. Therefore, regardless of a chiropractor's arrangement with a team, the chiropractor has the minimal duty not to inflict injury on the athlete during the course of examination or treatment (5).

However, there is a broader duty that requires the chiropractor to take steps and exercise reasonable care to prevent harm to the athlete that is triggered by the doctor-patient relationship (6). The existence of a doctor-patient relationship is not wholly dependent on who hired the team chiropractor or if the team chiropractor is serving with or without compensation. Rather, what is essential in the establishment of this relationship is the expectation of the patient and the action of the chiropractor. The fact that the team chiropractor undertakes to provide professional services to an athlete and the athlete recognizes the chiropractor as doing so for his or her benefit is sufficient to establish a doctor-patient relationship and the concomitant broader duty to prevent potential harm to the athlete within the scope of the chiropractor's undertaking.

Liability may result from substandard care when one undertakes to render services that he or she recognizes are necessary to protect the safety of another, and his or her failure to exercise due care increases the other's risk of harm or harm is suffered because the other relied on the undertaking (7). One who takes charge of another who is helpless may be liable for bodily harm caused by failure to exercise reasonable care to secure the other's safety while in the chiropractor's charge by leaving the other in a worse position than before by discontinuing aid (8).

The primary example of the limited duty of care of the team chiropractor arises in the situation of a physical examination to determine the fitness of an individual to participate in sports. Although the chiropractor may be retained by a team, school, or other entity, a limited duty is owed to the athlete to determine whether the athlete is physically capable to perform a particular sport. The reasonable expectation of both the athlete and the team is that the team chiropractor will properly conduct the examination to identify, within the scope of the physical examination, any impairment that might exist. A limited duty

based on a doctor-patient relationship has been established by this expectation and by the chiropractor's voluntary rendering of professional care (9). If in a subsequent action against the chiropractor, negligence is alleged by the athlete, the issue will not be the existence of a duty of care but the scope of the duty of care based on the nature of the physical examination and the standard of care exercised by the chiropractor.

SCOPE OF THE DUTY OF CARE

As discussed previously, a broader duty of care will be recognized with the establishment of the doctor-patient relationship, and such a relationship may be created in the course of a team physician's function. The scope of such duty is limited by the scope of medical service provided to the athlete. For example, in the previously described situation of a team physical that may be done in a matter of minutes, a team physician cannot reasonably be expected to perform the battery of diagnostic tests and evaluations that he or she would perform in the office. The scope of the duty in these situations is limited by the scope of the undertaking itself. In addition, such scope of legal duty may be limited by the terms of the agreement by which the physician performs his or her services (10).

A chiropractor, because of his or her specialized training and particular scope of practice, may decide to limit his or her services to the treatment of particular sports ailments or to the evaluation of certain physical conditions related to physical performance. The scope of the duty of care to the athlete can be defined through an arrangement that reflects the voluntary limitation of the scope of undertaking. The chiropractor will be responsible for those physical conditions and ailments within the defined scope of duty. Chiropractors should not be held responsible for the variety of medical conditions that may otherwise be identified and diagnosed in the normal general practice of chiropractic. However, chiropractors will remain responsible for conditions or ailments that otherwise may be outside their predefined scope of undertaking when they know of or should reasonably know of such conditions or ailments while functioning within their scope of service (11).

For example, if the agreed scope of a team chiropractor's function is to diagnose and treat lower back injuries, and in the process of examining an injured athlete the chiropractor detects a condition or reasonably should have detected a condition outside his or her predetermined scope of service, the chiropractor nevertheless has the duty to either treat the condition or to refer the athlete for additional medical care. In other words, while a chiropractor may elect to limit his or her scope of services to a particular area, he or she will be responsible for any condition or ailment he or she detects or should reasonably be expected to detect while operating within that limited scope of services.

A concise agreement and related waivers of liability (if authorized), drafted with the advice of legal counsel, can be a valuable safeguard for the team physician to identify the scope of the physician's professional undertaking. Such an agreement serves to disclose to potential examiners and athletes when and how a professional doctor-patient relationship will come into being. An arrangement of this type should be executed with the team, school, or other entity; most importantly, the details of the physician's scope of duty should be communicated to the athlete.

The fact that a physician may render services to an athlete on the sidelines of a sporting event does not diminish the need to keep and maintain adequate records. At a minimum, such record-keeping should include the athlete's name, sport, nature of the injury or illness, date, immediate treatment, and rehabilitation recommended (12). The doctor should establish a regular procedure of writing or tape-recording notes on the sidelines. Such record-keeping can be invaluable in the defense of a malpractice action.

The team physician should also inform the athlete as to medical information concerning the athlete's physical condition. Failure to inform the athlete can result in liability if the athlete can demonstrate that he or she was damaged as a result of a failure to inform. This duty to inform flows from the fiduciary responsibility inherent in the doctor-patient relationship and should include the following.

1. The risk to the athlete of continued participation in the sporting activity.
2. Conditions, ailments, or diseases detected in the scope of the physician's services.
3. Any specific adverse test results.

The responsibility to disclose this type of information may at times be troublesome for the team physician because of potential conflicts between team interests and athlete interests. Pressure to return the athlete to the playing field as soon as possible will undoubtedly exist. The athlete must be informed of the reasonable risks of playing injured as opposed to not playing. Informed consent procedures in which the physician discloses all alternative approaches to the treatment of a condition or injury, as well as the prognosis for each treatment, should be followed with the athlete as with any other patient. The importance of the responsibility to disclose and to follow regular informed consent procedures in the sports medicine field was illustrated by a malpractice action brought in Canada. In *Wilson Vancouver Hockey Club*, 5 D.L.R. 4th 282 (1983), a professional hockey player brought action against his hockey team, contending that the team physician failed to diagnose and treat properly a cancerous mole on his left arm. The physician suspected that the mole might be cancerous, but advised the player that it could wait until after the end of the hockey season to be treated. The delay resulted in more radical surgery to treat the condition. The player argued that if he had been adequately informed of the options for treatment, he would have spent considerably less time recuperating from surgery and suffered less loss of income. The Court ruled that the doctor was negligent for not immediately informing the player of the suspected cancer and the risks involved in waiting for treatment.

The *Wilson* case demonstrates the view of most courts that consent is informed when the patient is advised of all the available alternatives and the prognosis for each. If the team doctor does not advise an injured athlete in this manner, negligence or the basis of lack of informed consent will most likely be found if it is demonstrated that the failure to disclose information affected the patient's treatment decision.

The team physician should also obtain the consent of the patient to release medical information. Unauthorized release of confidential medical information obtained in the course of an examination or the course of medical treatment may be a basis for liability in a tort action (13). Such an authorization should be in writing whenever possible.

STANDARD OF CARE

In addition to the establishment of a duty of care and the defining of the scope of such duty of care, there must be evidence that a physician breached such duty for liability to attach. The evidence must demonstrate the physician's negligence in treatment or other "wrongful" conduct. Malpractice actions are usually based on allegations of negligence in the performance of professional services. Negligence has been defined as "conduct which falls below the standard established by law for the protection of others against unreasonable risk of harm" (14).

The standard of care will be established by expert testimony before a court. Once this standard of care is established, there must be additional evidence that the physician has departed from the established standard (15).

The standard of care for a team physician or sports physician can be generally described as a standard requiring that the physician should perform with the level of knowledge, skill, and care that is expected of a reasonably competent physician under similar circumstances, taking into consideration reasonable limits that have been placed on the scope of the physician's undertaking (16).

A higher standard of care is applied to physicians certified as medical/chiropractic sports physicians or otherwise certified as a diplomate in a particular clinical area of medicine/chiropractic that relates to sports medicine/chiropractic. In such cases, a higher standard of care is applied and the professional conduct of these chiropractors is judged by a standard of care applicable to the specialty (17). This higher standard of care for an individual holding himself or herself out as a medical/chiropractic sport specialist will mean that the physician may be liable for misdiagnosis or mistreatment of sports-related injuries for which a general medical/chiropractic practitioner may not be liable. The higher standard of care is established by expert testimony relative to the practice of the chiropractic sports specialty on a national level.

ECONOMIC CONSIDERATIONS

To recover losses in a medical malpractice action, a potential plaintiff must demonstrate a loss or damage as a result of the physician's action. This type of loss is ordinarily a physical harm. However, the functions of a team physician may result in harm to an athlete that is economic rather than physical. For example, liability for economic loss can result when a physician negligently certifies an athlete as unable to participate in a professional sport, and as a result the athlete's career is shortened. Or it can result when information about an athlete's condition is wrongfully communicated to a third party (18).

As is the case with physical harm, a determination of economic harm will center on the question of duty. Ordinarily, there is no liability for strictly economic harm resulting from negligent interference with an athlete's contract or potential contract with a professional team (or with a scholarship or potential scholarship with a college). However, when a legal duty of care has been established (through the doctor-patient relationship or otherwise), such an action for negligence, to include economic loss, can be maintained against the physician by the athlete (19). Therefore, a physician who misdiagnoses an athlete's condition, in the course of a physical examination in which the athlete reasonably perceives the physician to be acting within the doctor-patient relationship, may be subject to liability for the economic opportunities that the athlete can prove were lost.

A professional athlete may, because of economic considerations, want to assume and accept a certain degree of risk of participation despite being fully informed by the team physician or other provider of the risks involved. All sports and indeed any physical endeavor contain a degree of risk-taking. Arguably, the degree of risk-taking should be left up to the individual athlete on the basis of informed consent regarding the potential hazards of continued athlete participation. Clearly, for a professional athlete such informed choice may have a significant economic impact. This, however, may conflict with the physician's ethical duty to practice for "the greatest good of the patient" (20). It has been suggested that athletes who are legally capable of assuming a particular risk should not be authorized to continue to participate in a contraindicated sports activity when the following criteria are met.

1. There are significant risks of injury and harm from continued participation.
2. There is a question concerning the athlete's lucidity or capacity for sound judgment, such as a so-called "ding" injury involving head trauma but no loss of consciousness or when certain medication may mask the seriousness of an injury.
3. The informed decision is to be made during the "heat of battle" of an athlete's competition.
4. The authorization to participate may be beyond generally accepted and broadly defined standards of acceptable professional practice (21).

"GUARANTEE" OF RESULT OR PERFORMANCE

Perhaps in no other field of health care is the problem of guaranteeing a particular treatment or procedure result more apparent. The tendency among sports physicians to claim that a particular procedure or treatment will have a particular result is a natural outgrowth of the competitive nature of sports. However, the sports physician should exercise caution not to make assurances as to the effect of a particular procedure or treatment. To do so may involve an express warranty, in which case the physician will be liable if the promised results do not materialize.

An action for breach of warranty, unlike a negligence claim, does not require proof of negligence on the part of the physician. It is essentially a contract issue in which the athlete must simply show that the physician promised a specific result, that the athlete relied on this assurance and underwent treatment, and that the promised result did not occur. Statements such as "I guarantee" or "I promise" can create this contractual warranty of results. Any statement given by a physician in the pretreatment stage that clearly and unmistakably makes positive assurances of a particular result will act to create an enforceable warranty at law (in *Scarzella v Saxon*, 436 A2d 358 [D.C.App. 1981], an assurance that a procedure was "safe and without complications" was adequate to constitute express warranties).

The unique nature of the sports physician practice brings with it a variety of new legal concerns for the physician. Careful attention should be paid by any practicing doctor to assure that the special relationship with athletes meets the various requirements of the law. In this way, doctors can render their professional services to athletes while simultaneously assuring their own protection.

References

1. La Cava: What is sports medicine: definition and tasks. J Sports Med Phys Fitness 1977;17:1.
2. 1992/93 Official Digest, Federation of State Chiropractic Licensing Boards.
3. Fanelli. The duty and authority of a chiropractor to diagnose and refer their patients. American Chiropractic Association, 1980.
4. Prosser, Keeton. The law of torts. 5th ed. 1984:356.
5. Prosser, Keeton. *supra*, note 19 at 358.
6. *Restatement (Second) of Torts.* Note 23 at § 323.
7. *Restatement (Second) of Torts. supra*, at § 323.
8. *Restatement (Second) of Torts. supra*, at § 324.
9. *Rule v Cheeseman*, 317 P. 2d 472 (1957).
10. Holder A. Medical malpractice law. 2nd ed. 1975:34–35.
11. *Restatement (Second) of Torts. supra*, Note 23 at § 12.
12. Gallup. Sports medicine law: staying in bounds and out of court (Editorial). Physician Sports Med 1991;19.
13. *Hammonds v Aetna Casualty and Surety Co.*, 243 F.Supp 793 (1965, ND. Ohio).
14. *Restatement (Second) of Torts. supra*, Note 23 at § 282.
15. Prosser, Keeton. *supra*, Note 1 at 235.
16. King. The duty and standard of care for team physicians. 18 Houston Law Review 657, 692 (1981).
17. *Restatement (Second) of Torts. supra*, Note 23 at § 289A.
18. *Chuy v Philadelphia Eagles Football Club*, 595 F.2d 1265 (1979).
19. *Restatement (Second) of Torts. supra*, Note 35 at § 766(c). Comment e.
20. King. ACA code of ethics. American Chiropractic Association, 1992.
21. King. *supra*, at 699-700.

The Physiology of Exercise, Physical Fitness, and Cardiovascular Endurance Training

Joseph P. Hornberger

Understanding the physiologic response to exercise requires a conceptual understanding of how energy is produced in the body, beginning with the breakdown of foods, then progressing to energy delivery and use in the metabolic and physiologic systems. Several components of the physiology of exercise are related to endurance training and physical fitness. These components are metabolism (the production of energy for work), circulation and respiration (i.e., the oxygen transport system), the muscular system, the performance of mechanical work, proper nutrition and weight control, evaluation of exercise capabilities, and prescription of safe and effective training techniques.

This chapter delineates the exercise physiology principles related to the development of cardiovascular fitness for the adult population. The information is drawn from empiric knowledge of the author and research literature in physical education, physiology, metabolism, health, and nutrition.

PRODUCTION OF ENERGY

Metabolism is the production of energy for work that is ultimately powered by food. Energy and work cannot be considered separate entities because energy is defined as the capacity to perform work, and work is defined as the application of a force through a distance. This combination of energy and work can be demonstrated by an individual who performs any physical function, for example, an activity as simple as walking across a room. This activity requires a certain amount of energy to achieve a certain amount of work, i.e., getting to the other side of the room.

Adenosine triphosphate (ATP) is the basic unit of energy and chemically consists of one adenosine and three phosphate groups (Fig. 3.1). After ATP is broken down and converted through anaerobic and aerobic metabolic pathways, it is hydrolyzed to form ATP and heat (1), which leads to muscle contraction and the generation of force expressed as newtons or kilograms (2).

Between 7 and 10 kilocalories (kcal) of energy are released when ATP is broken down to adenosine diphosphate (ADP) and an inorganic phosphate (P_i). The more ATP that is broken down, the more energy that is available for work.

$$ATP \rightarrow ADP + P_i + \textbf{ENERGY}$$

ATP can be broken down and resynthesized by three different series of reactions within the cells of the body. Two series of reactions do not require oxygen and are, therefore, anaerobic. The third series of reactions operates only when oxygen is present and is, therefore, referred to as aerobic metabolism. During exercise, both anaerobic and aerobic reactions are important sources of ATP breakdown and resynthesis for the production of energy.

The two anaerobic metabolic processes are referred to as the phosphagen system (3), also called the phosphocreatine (PC) system (4), and anaerobic glycolysis. The third system, which is aerobic, is known as oxidative phosphorylation. These systems are discussed in the following sections.

ENERGY-PRODUCING SYSTEMS

Phosphagen System

When ATP in the muscle cells breaks down, it produces approximately 8000 calories (8 kcal) of energy and becomes the end products creatine (C) and inorganic phosphate (P_i) (5). When ATP is broken down during muscle contraction, it is continuously resynthesized from ADP and P_i by the energy liberated during the breakdown of the stored phosphocreatine (PC). This process is a coupled reaction because the energy released is coupled with the energy needs of the reaction that resynthesizes ATP.

$$PC \rightleftharpoons P_i + C + ENERGY \rightarrow P_i + ADP \rightarrow ATP$$

DeVries (5) refers to the energetics of muscle contraction, from a chemical standpoint, as a four-level process (Fig. 3.2). Three of these levels are common to aerobic and anaerobic contraction. The first three reactions are reversible in that some molecules of ATP are broken down to provide energy for muscle contraction, and other molecules of ADP and P_i are regenerated. However, this process occurs at an energy cost provided by the next reaction ($CP \rightarrow C + P$). Each reaction shown depends on the energy supply from below to remain in balance while supplying energy to the reaction above. The rate of breakdown balances the rate of regeneration; otherwise, muscle fatigue occurs; that is, each succeeding reaction supplies energy for the reverse of the preceding reaction.

Since stores of ATP and PC in the muscle are relatively small, the amount of energy available from the phosphagen system is limited. In fact, these stores in a working muscle would be depleted after an all-out sprint lasting approximately 10 seconds (1). This rapid depletion may not be important at rest, but it is extremely important for physical activities. Activities such as jumping, kicking, throwing, and swinging, requiring less than 10 seconds to perform and a maximum amount of power in a short period, rely heavily on the phosphagen energy system.

This system provides quick energy, which is important for of explosive power and speed. It does not, however, provide enough energy for endurance activities. Of the three energy systems, the phosphagen system provides the fastest source of energy but the shortest duration.

ANAEROBIC GLYCOLYSIS

After the phosphagen stores are depleted, which takes approximately 10 seconds, the body must produce energy from another source. Anaerobic glycolysis provides the next source of energy. As with the phosphagen system, glycoly-

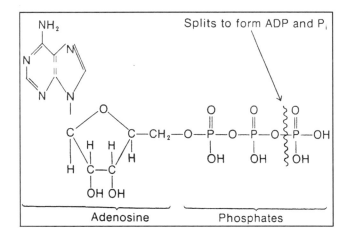

Figure 3.1. Adenosine triphosphate (ATP). (From Strauss R. Sports medicine and physiology. Philadelphia: WB Saunders, 1979:382.)

Figure 3.2. Process of muscle contraction. (From deVries HA. Physiology of exercise for physical education and athletics. 2nd ed. Dubuque: Wm. C. Brown Company, 1974:19.)

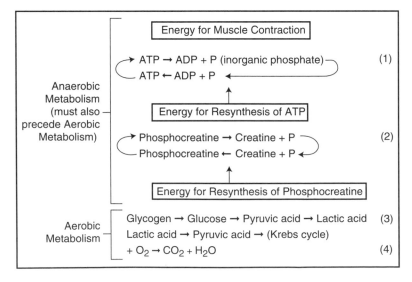

Aerobic Breakdown of Glycogen

$$(C_6H_{12}O_6)_n + 6O_2 \rightarrow 6CO_2 + 6H_2O + Energy \rightarrow + 39P_i + 39ADP \rightarrow 39ATP$$
(glycogen)

Anaerobic Breakdown of Glycogen

$$(C_6H_{12}O_6)_n \rightarrow 2C_3H_6O_3 + Energy \rightarrow + 3P_i + 3ADP \rightarrow 3ATP$$
(glycogen)

Figure 3.3. Energy yield from glycolysis. If 180 g of glycogen is broken down, approximately 3 moles of ATP can be resynthesized as compared with 39 moles of ATP when the oxygen system is used.

sis involves the breakdown of glycogen to glucose. Research by Bloomfield et al. (6) and the American College of Sports Medicine (ACSM) (2) indicates that lactate is produced by anaerobic glycolysis. It is often claimed that lactic acid is produced (1, 3, 5, 7), and that its subsequent dissociation is responsible for the accumulation of hydrogen ions during vigorous exercise. However, it is probably actually lactate that is produced because the major cellular source of hydrogen ions is the breakdown of ATP. As hydrogen production begins to exceed oxidation down the respiratory chain, excess hydrogen ions accumulate, leading first to the production of lactate in the cells and blood (6), then muscle fatigue.

The energy generated by hydrogen oxidation provides the ATP for muscle contraction. During light to moderate exercise, any lactate produced is rapidly oxidized and the blood lactate levels remain fairly stable although oxygen consumption increases; that is the removal or maintenance of lactate levels is a function of the aerobic system.

During exercise, if the energy demands are adequately met by reactions that use oxygen, the exercise is said to be aerobic. If the oxygen system allows the buildup of lactate to exceed its elimination, the exercise is said to be anaerobic. This concept is elaborated in the section on oxidative phosphorylation when the aerobic system is discussed.

Lactic acid or lactate starts to accumulate at approximately 50 to 55% of maximal aerobic capacity when untrained people attempt to perform endurance activities (8). In trained atheletes, this anaerobic threshold occurs at a higher percentage of their aerobic capacity (9). This adaptation to exercise is attributed to genetic makeup and specific adaptations to training. The anaerobic threshold is the level of exertion at which the aerobic source of metabolism is unable to provide for the necessary energy because lactate accumulation exceeds the rate of removal via the Krebs metabolic cycle. Here again, hydrogen production begins to exceed its oxidation down the respiratory chain; the excess hydrogen is converted to pyruvic acid, leading to the accumulation of lactate. As exercise intensity increases, the muscle cells cannot meet the additional energy demands aerobically.

However, under aerobic conditions, lactate removal is equal to lactate formation, so the concentration of blood lactate levels remains relatively stable. If lactate accumulates in the blood and muscles after moderate to intense exercise, temporary muscle fatigue sets in and results in "muscle burn." This accumulation of lactate in the blood and muscles slows down and eventually stops the muscle contraction process (2, 10).

Åstrand et al. refer to the accumulation of lactate as cell poisoning by the body's own metabolic products (1). In contrast, during aerobic metabolism the number of hydrogen ions required for the resynthesis of ATP is equivalent to the number released in its breakdown; therefore, no fatiguing by-products are formed (6). The energy yield from glycolysis is relatively small compared with the yield from oxygen (Fig. 3.3).

The blood can tolerate the accumulation of approximately 60 to 70 g of lactate before fatigue sets in (3). Bloomfield et al. (6) state that exercise involving absolutely maximal rates of anaerobic glycolysis can usually be maintained for only 30 to 90 seconds. Therefore, from a practical standpoint, only a small amount of ATP can be broken down and resynthesized using both anaerobic systems during intense exercise; with further exercise, lactate in the blood and muscles reaches the point of exhaustion.

The phosphagen system provides explosive power and speed for the first 10 seconds of activities such as the 220- or 440- meter run. Anaerobic glycolysis provides energy from 10 seconds to approximately 3 minutes. The limitations of this energy system are obvious. This system of metabolism provides the second quickest source of energy for activities lasting up to 3 minutes. The production of lactate in the blood and muscles causes muscle fatigue which prevents effective performance. Lactate is valuable in weight-lifting, sprint-running, gymnastics, golf, football, swinging, jumping, or other activities lasting less than 3 minutes but requiring speed and explosive power. However, anaerobic sources of metabolism are of limited value when participating in events such as a 3-mile run.

In summary, if exercise intensity is so high that exhaustion ensues within 3 minutes, the energy must be supplied largely by anaerobic processes, that is, through the phosphagen system and anaerobic glycolysis. The oxygen system of metabolism cannot provide oxygen to the tissues fast enough (5).

OXIDATIVE PHOSPHORYLATION (AEROBIC SYSTEM)

Ordinarily, oxygen can provide the energy for muscle contraction as long as the exercise intensity is low enough. If the intensity of muscle contraction is high, the body is unable to supply or break down oxygen quickly enough to provide for the immediate energy demands, thus the need to draw on anaerobic sources. Studies indicate that lactate is formed continuously at rest or during mild exercise. However, under aerobic conditions, lactate is removed as fast as it is formed, thus stabilizing blood lactate levels.

Anaerobic sources of energy are able to release only approximately 5% of the energy within the glucose molecule (8). When pyruvic acid is converted to a form of acetic acid (acetyl CoA), it enters the second stage of carbohydrate breakdown, the Krebs or citric acid cycle. This second stage offers another way for the remaining energy from carbohydrate sources to be released from the incomplete breakdown that occurred during anaerobic metabolism.

The oxygen system of metabolism produces the most efficient source of energy. For example, the same 180 g of glycogen can yield up to 39 moles of ATP compared with approximately 3 moles yielded from anaerobic sources (see Fig. 3.3).

Aerobic metabolism for energy production is not used for quick energy, but rather for endurance activities. Energy is released more rapidly during anaerobic glycolysis than during aerobic metabolism. However, relatively little ATP is resynthesized in this manner; therefore, the potential is for high explosive power of short duration. When using aerobic metabolism for energy production, much more ATP is available, but it is unable to meet the rapid energy requirements needed in activities such as jumping, swinging, and sprinting. For endurance activities exceeding 2 to 3 minutes, aerobic metabolism is valuable for the final stage of energy transfer.

Because aerobic metabolism uses oxygen from the air, the aerobic system resynthesizes ATP, leaving no fatiguing by-products, and allowing sustained exercise. The carbon dioxide produced diffuses freely from the muscle cells into the blood, where it is carried to the lungs and exhaled; the water produced by the reactions is used on the cellular level and excreted through the pores to cool the body during exercise.

ENERGY SUBSTRATE USE

Carbohydrates, proteins, and fats are foods that can be broken down to provide the energy for muscle contraction. The breakdown of each of these foods requires different amounts of oxygen, and they are eventually oxidized to their end products, carbon dioxide and water. The ratio between the amount of carbon dioxide produced to the amount of oxygen consumed is the respiratory quotient, which is used to determine the nutrients being used for energy production (2).

Table 3.1 demonstrates this substrate use process during exercise (2). Carbohydrates are a source of quick energy. Fat stores have a higher caloric density and are a good source of stored energy, primarily because more oxygen is required for their oxidation. However, less energy is released than when carbohydrates are metabolized.

Amino acids from proteins can also enter the Krebs cycle and be oxidized to provide the necessary energy for exercise. However, because protein use is extremely low during exercise, this food source is generally disregarded. During submaximal exercise, both carbohydrates and fats are used to varying degrees depending on the demands of the exercise. Although a combination of fats and carbohydrates is used during prolonged exercise at a steady rate, the percentage of fat use increases over time. However, as the exercise intensity increases, more carbohydrates are used.

Aerobic Metabolism: Using Fat Stores

Fat represents the body's greatest source of energy, with an almost unlimited supply, considering the amount of fat versus carbohydrate stored as muscle and liver glycogen. Fat cells

Table 3.1. Substrate Use During Exercise

Fuel	Energy Content (Kcal · g^{-1})	Oxygen Equivalent (Kcal · L^{-1})	Respiratory Quotient
Carbohydrate	4.1	5.0	1.00
Fat	9.3	4.7	0.70
Protein	4.3	4.4	0.80

From American College of Sports Medicine. Guidelines for exercise testing and prescription. 4th ed. Philadelphia: Lea & Febiger, 1991:14.

Aerobic Breakdown of Fat

$$C_{16}H_{32}O_2 + 23O_2 \rightarrow 16CO_2 + 16H_2O + Energy \rightarrow + 130P_i + 130ADP \rightarrow 130ATP$$
(palmitic acid)

Aerobic Breakdown of Glycogen

$$(C_6H_{12}O_6)_n + 6O_2 \rightarrow 6CO_2 + 6H_2O + Energy \rightarrow + 39P_i + 39ADP \rightarrow 39ATP$$
(glycogen)

Figure 3.4. Equations for aerobic breakdown of fat versus glycogen.

(adipocytes) are the most abundant, which suppliers of fatty acids; which diffuse into the circulation, where they are metabolized for energy. From 30 to 80% of the energy used for biologic work is derived from intracellular and extracellular fat molecules, depending on a person's state of nutrition, exercise intensity level, and duration of physical activity (8). The equation in Figure 3.4 depicts the breakdown of 1 mole of fat, i.e., palmitic acid, into carbon dioxide and water in the presence of oxygen. This comparison between the aerobic breakdown of fat and glycogen helps to illustrate the efficiency of fat as an energy source.

During rest and submaximal endurance-type exercise, such as marathon running and cross-country skiing, the body prefers to use the oxygen system of metabolism because of the high yield of ATP available from fat stores.

SLOW TWITCH AND FAST TWITCH MUSCLES

For years muscle tissue was considered to be of two major fiber types, red and white. The red fibers were said to contain increased myoglobin good for increased oxidation and therefore good for endurance exercise. White fibers were con-sidered to be glycolytic fibers; which had high power-producing capabilities but were not good for endurance activities. Bergstrom (11) pioneered muscle fiber classification by using biopsy techniques to determine muscle-fiber types. He classified human skeletal muscle fibers into slow twitch oxidative (type I), fast twitch oxidative-glycolytic (type IIa), and fast twitch glycolytic (type IIb) motor units. Table 3.2 shows the specific functional characteristics of each type. Type I motor units are preferred for endurance activities such as walking or jogging. Type II motor units are used for the strength and power needed in activities such as weight training and sprinting. Athletes who sprint have a preponderance of type II fibers, whereas endurance athletes typically have a preponderance of type I fibers (9).

Almost all muscles contain all fiber types, although weighted in a particular direction (fast or slow). Athletes usually gravitate toward the athletic event in which they do well; that is, they end up performing in a sport through natural selection. However, various sophisticated methods using muscle biopsy analyses can determine fiber type. In some cases, these analyses can match athletes to the best sport that capitalizes on the preponderance of a certain muscle fiber type. For years, this technique has been used in the former Soviet Union with young children, who are channeled into the sports for which they show the most promise.

It is generally believed that fiber type is largely genetically determined and that the relative proportions of type I and II fibers do not change with training, although muscle hypertrophy does occur (12). However, ongoing research shows conflicting results in terms of whether muscle hypertrophy response to exercise training results from individual muscle fiber growth or from muscle hyperplasia, the formation of new, increased numbers of muscle fibers (13–17). With such conflicting evidence, it is impossible to state the exact mechanisms of hypertrophy; therefore, the research continues in this area.

ENERGY SYSTEMS VERSUS ACTIVITY DEMANDS

The use of different energy systems during specific activities depends on the predominance

Table 3.2. Characteristics of Motor Units Comprising Human Skeletal Muscle

Characteristics	Type I	Type IIa	Type IIb
Contraction time	Slow	Fast	Fast
Oxidative capacity	High	Moderate	Low
Myofibrillar ATPase activity	Low	High	High
Stored phosphagens	Low	High	High
Glycolytic capacity	Low	Moderate	High
Fatigability	Low	Low	High

From American College of Sports Medicine. Guidelines for exercise testing and prescription. 4th ed. Philadelphia: Lea & Febiger, 1991:14.
ATPase, adenosinetriphosphatase.

of the energy system challenged. For example, if performing a short-term, high-intensity activity such as the 100-meter dash, the majority of ATP is supplied by the phosphagen system; a long-term, low-intensity activity such as marathon racing is supported almost exclusively by the aerobic system. It is logical that anaerobic glycolysis can support activities such as the 400- and 800-meter dash. However, the 1500-meter requires a blend of both anaerobic and aerobic metabolism.

Getting the proper amount of ATP or energy for different activities is similar to driving a manual-shift transmission in which different terrains and types of driving govern gear shifting to move the vehicle optimally. Shifting into first gear provides power and quickness when at slower speeds, whereas fifth gear is good for long-distance treks. Similarly, there is constant interaction among the different types of metabolic systems, depending on the type of demands placed on the body.

In the wide array of athletic events, although both aerobic and anaerobic energy systems contribute ATP during the performance of various sports, one system usually contributes more (18). Therefore, the training of a particular metabolic system should be specific to the energy demands of that particular event for optimum levels of ATP production and thus performance.

Dave Waddle, a 1974 Olympic track and field competitor noted for wearing his sun visor when he competed, won several gold medals as a result of training all three metabolic systems. He would sprint from last to first place on the bell lap of his races, then downshift into a lower gear to pass his competitors for the gold, using anaerobic stores to boost his performance on the final lap. Specific training of anaerobic metabolic sources enabled him to draw on reserve glycogen for that final lap. If the predominant energy system of any given activity is developed more than the other systems, performance in that particular activity also improves (3). Conversely, training of the anaerobic systems would not help a marathon runner very much because the energy to perform the 2.5- to 3-hour race is supplied predominantly by the aerobic system.

Fox (3) sums it up nicely when he categorizes various sports activities on an "energy continuum" and defines the relationship among the different energy systems and the performance times of different activities. Table 3.3 categorizes activities requiring performance times equal to or less than 30 seconds (i.e., those activities using the phosphagen system) in area 1. Area 2 includes those activities requiring between 30 seconds

and 1.5 minutes to perform. In this case, the training of the phosphagen system and anaerobic glycolysis would enhance the performance of these activities. Area 3 of activities lasting from approximately 1.5 to 3 minutes to perform, would have to involve the training of anaerobic glycolysis and, to a lesser degree, oxidative phosphorylation to result in improved performance. Area 4 includes those activities that take more than 3 minutes to complete. The training for these activities is best served by enhanced oxidative phosphorylation function. However, an athlete can focus on training any of these systems to enhance performance in a particular category. An example would be an athlete who wants to develop a "kick" during the last lap of an endurance running event, as Dave Waddle did in the 1974 Olympic Games, by training anaerobic systems.

Each of these energy systems is cumulative in production of energy to do work, although one system usually contributes more due to specific demands.

PHYSIOLOGIC ADAPTATIONS FOLLOWING AEROBIC ENDURANCE TRAINING

Exercise physiologists have been searching for decades for better training techniques and methods to create the fastest and strongest gold medal winners. When considering training for the aerobic system of metabolism, one critical component in attaining optimal performance is the ability of the body to deliver oxygen to the tissue cells and

Table 3.3. Four Work/Effort Areas with Performance Times, Major Energy System(s) Involved, and Examples of the Type of Activity

Area	Performance Time	Major Energy System(s) Involved	Examples of Type of Activity
1	Less than 30 seconds	ATP-PC	Shot put, 100-yard sprint, base stealing, golf, and tennis swings
2	30 seconds to 1.5 minutes	ATP-PC-LA	220- to 440-yard sprints, halfbacks, fullbacks, speed skating, 100-yard swim
3	1.5 to 3 minutes	LA and O_2	880-yard dash, gymnastics events, boxing (3-minute rounds), wrestling (2-minute periods)
4	More than 3 minutes	O_2	Soccer and lacrosse (except goalies), cross-country skiing, marathon run, jogging

From Fox EL, Mathews DK. Interval training: conditioning for sports and general fitness. Philadelphia: WB Saunders, 1974.
ATP, adenosine triphosphate; PC, phosphocreatine; LA, lactic acid.

maximize oxygen metabolism, that is, optimizing the oxygen transport system by improving cardiorespiratory function. Various components are necessary for an efficient cardiorespiratory system, such as adequate blood components (e.g., red blood cell count, hemoglobin, hematocrit, blood volume, and other cellular components that facilitate oxygen use during exercise (1, 8)); however, the most important aspect of oxygen transport is the heart, circulation, and cellular function (7).

It is important to maintain and improve pulmonary functions such as total lung volume, vital capacity, pulmonary diffusion capacity, ventilation, breathing rate, and maximum breathing capacity. However, these entities generally do not limit cardiovascular endurance performance unless the athlete has a disease or is training at high altitudes (1, 19). The following tests are important for assessing the function of the pulmonary system.

1. Vital capacity (VC). VC is the maximum amount of air in the lungs that can be expired after a maximum inspiration. VC plus residual volume (air left in the lungs after maximal expiration) constitute the total lung capacity.
2. Forced vital capacity (FVC). FVC is similar to VC, but the expiratory phase is completed as rapidly as possible. A decreased FVC is common to restrictive diseases such as obesity and pulmonary fibrosis and obstructive diseases such as emphysema and asthma.
3. Forced expiratory volume in 1 second (FEV 1.0). FEV 1.0 measures the volume of air expired during the first second of the FVC test and further aids in determining the severity of obstructive and restrictive diseases.
4. The percentage of FVC expired during the first second of the FVC test should be between 75 and 85%. Again, this test aids in determining the severity of obstructive and restrictive diseases.

Under most conditions, arterial blood leaving the heart is approximately 97% saturated with oxygen. Most limitations to endurance performance, as stated previously, depend on the capacity of the heart, circulation, and cellular function (7), i.e., the oxygen transport system.

The oxygen transport system spans several physiologic processes discussed later in this chapter. The process begins with ventilation, air passing in and out of the lungs. Subsequently, oxygen must diffuse from the lungs to the blood, which must then combine with hemoglobin, the oxygen-carrying component of the red blood cell. The blood is then transported by the pumping action of the heart through the vascular system (arteries, arterioles, and capillaries) to the tissues.

When the oxygen-rich red blood cells reach the muscle tissue, important energy-yielding chemical reactions must take place in the muscle cell mitochondria to ensure energy production for work. The end products of cellular metabolism are then transported back through the venous system to the heart for reoxygenation and carbon dioxide elimination via the lungs. Buffering and biochemical reactions also take place in the liver, kidney, and the body's cells, which help maintain homeostasis and replenish energy supplies for continued work. However, despite the importance of these other processes, the heart is most important and is the key to the oxygen transport system because it must continuously pump blood to the tissues of the body.

Two major blood flow changes are necessary to meet the oxygen transport demands during exercise: (1) there must be a redistribution of blood flow from inactive organs to the active skeletal muscles, and (2) there must be an increase in cardiac output, i.e., the amount of blood pumped by the heart per minute (3).

Cardiac Output

Cardiac output, the product of stroke volume (the amount of blood pumped per heartbeat), is the amount of blood pumped by the heart and is measured in liters per minute. Increasing exercise intensity brings a linear increase in cardiac output. Maximum oxygen uptake, or aerobic capacity, is the largest amount of oxygen used for the most strenuous exercise (20, 21). Maximum oxygen uptake correlates highly with cardiac output because it reflects what is happening in the oxygen transport system during maximal exercise (1, 7, 22).

When measuring cardiorespiratory fitness levels during exercise, untrained individuals have lower maximal cardiac outputs (approximately 20 to 25 L/min) than trained individuals, who have higher work and aerobic capacities (up to 40 L/min) (23). In general, the higher the maximal cardiac output, the higher the maximal aerobic power and vice versa. The highest aerobic capacities are found in those athletes who excel in endurance events such as cross-country skiing or marathon running.

When comparing men and women, changes in cardiac output described previously for men and women are similar (24, 25). However, women tend to have a slightly lower cardiac output when performing work at the same level of oxygen consumption (24, 26). Women have a lower oxygen-carrying capacity due to lower levels of hemoglobin in the blood. In addition, trained or untrained men generally tend to have higher cardiac output than their female counterparts.

The increase in cardiac output during exercise reflects the increase in stroke volume, which is the amount of blood pumped by the heart per beat, multiplied by the heart rate (HR).

Cardiac Output (liters per minute) =
Stroke Volume (liters per beat) ×
Heart Rate (beats per minute)

Stroke Volume

Figure 3.5 shows the relationship between stroke volume and exercise. As indicated in the progression from rest to moderate work, stroke volume increases; however, there is little or no increase in stroke volume when progressing from moderate to maximal work. In most cases, in trained and untrained men or women, stroke volume becomes maximal at a submaximal workload when oxygen consumption is only approximately 40% of maximum (3). For women in general, values for stroke volume are generally lower than those for men under all conditions, which can be explained by the smaller heart volume of women.

Starling's law of the heart states that stroke volume increases in response to an increase in the volume of blood filling the ventricle during the resting phase of the heartbeat. This increase in volume stretches the heart muscle and promotes a more forceful ventricular contraction, resulting in more blood ejected at a higher systolic pressure. This relationship was described by two physiologists, Frank and Starling, in the early 1900s, and for many years was widely accepted as the reason for all increases in stroke volume (8). However, it has been shown that increased stroke volume during exercise does not occur in that manner (8, 27, 28).

Two physiologic mechanisms are responsible for the regulation of stroke volume. The first requires enhanced cardiac filling followed by a more forceful contraction of the heart. The second and most important mechanism is the mediation of stroke volume through neurohormonal influences. Increased stroke volume results from a forceful systolic contraction accompanied by

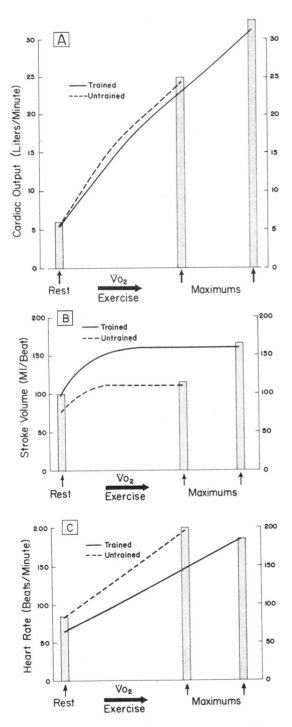

Figure 3.5. (A) Cardiac output, **(B)** stroke volume, and **(C)** heart rate during exercise in trained and untrained subjects. Cardiac output and heart rate are closely related to oxygen consumption over the entire range from rest to maximal exercise; maximal stroke volume is usually reached at submaximal exercise. (From Fox E. The physiological basis for exercise and sport. 5th ed. Dubuque: Times Mirror Higher Education Group, 1993:252.

normal filling of the heart, thereby resulting in a greater emptying capacity (8). The former is found to be more significant as a person moves from the upright to the recumbent position and is seen in supine activities such as swimming.

At rest, approximately half of the total diastolic volume is emptied during each ventricular contraction, which means that without increasing diastolic volume, a stronger contraction could double the stroke volume due to efficient emptying of the ventricles. This situation occurs mainly due to neurohormonal influences (29, 30); the myocardial strength increase occurs due to the hormonal action of epinephrine and norepinephrine. In addition, increased stroke power develops from the increased contractile state of the myocardium due to endurance training (8). In any case, it is now believed that the neurohormonally induced increase in stroke volume is responsible for improved cardiac output in trained athletes.

Oxygen Transport

Understanding the components of oxygen transport and their interrelations clarifies the increase in cardiac output and the reallocation of blood flow that is seen during exercise (3). These components are as follows:

$$\text{Oxygen Transport (VO}_2) =$$
$$\text{Stroke Volume (SV)} \times \text{Heart Rate (HR)} \times$$
$$\text{Arterial–Mixed Venous}$$
$$\text{Oxygen Difference (a VO}_2)$$

Because the oxygen-carrying capability of blood is approximately 20 mL of oxygen per 100 mL of blood (4), the a–VO$_2$ difference represents the amount of oxygen that is used by the cells from oxygenated blood and reflects how much oxygen is extracted by the tissues. This difference in oxygen content between the blood entering and the blood leaving the pulmonary capillaries is the difference in oxygen content of the arterial blood and mixed venous blood. Overall, a–VO$_2$ represents the extraction of oxygen from the blood by the peripheral tissues. As submaximal exercise increases to a maximal level, a linear relationship exists as a–VO$_2$ increases to maximum values.

With maximal exercise, approximately 85% of all oxygen in the blood is removed, although some oxygen in the mixed venous blood always returns to the heart (4). Table 3.4 shows components of the oxygen transport system at rest and during maximal exercise for trained and untrained individuals and endurance athletes. Note how each component reflects increased oxygen transport to the muscles.

The oxygen transported and consumed during maximal exercise is approximately 10 times that found during rest, when comparing untrained with trained individuals. This increase includes an increase in stroke volume, HR, and a–VO$_2$ difference. Also notice, when comparing untrained and trained athletes, that the largest difference is in the magnitude of the stroke volume. It is evident that the stroke volume is the most important component of the oxygen transport system.

Most changes that occur in the body during exercise are related to the increase in energy metabolism that occurs within the contracting skeletal muscles. During intense exercise, total energy expenditure may be up to 25 times that of resting metabolic rate. This expenditure is mostly used to provide energy for the exercising muscles. This exercise may increase energy use by a factor of up to 200 times the resting levels (31). Fox has summarized well those long-term physiologic changes that result from endurance training. Table 3.5 shows different physiologic changes at rest and during submaximal and maximal endurance exercise following physical training in men and women.

Table 3.4. Components of the Oxygen Transport System at Rest and During Maximal Exercise for Trained and Untrained Subjects and Endurance Athletics

Condition	$\dot{V}O_2$ (mL/min)	=	Stroke Volume (L/beat)	×	Heart Rate (beats/min)	×	a-$\bar{v}O_2$ Diff. (mL/L)
Untrained							
Rest	300	=	0.075	×	82	×	48.8
Maximal exercise	3100	=	0.112	×	200	×	138.0
Trained							
Rest	300	=	0.105	×	58	×	49.3
Maximal exercise	3440	=	0.126	×	192	×	140.5
Endurance athletes							
Maximal exercise	5570	=	0.189	×	190	×	155.0

Data for untrained and trained subjects from Ekblom B, et al. J Appl Physiol 1968; 24:518. Data for endurance athletes from Ekblom B, Hermansen L. J Appl Physiol 1968; 25:619. Reprinted in Fox E. The physiological basis for exercise and sport. 5th ed. Dubuque: Times Mirror Higher Education Group, 1993:259.

Table 3.5. Physiologic Changes at Rest and During Submaximal and Maximal Exercise Following Physical Training in Men and Women

| Rest | Exercise | |
	Submaximal[a]	Maximal
Cardiac hypertrophy	No change or slight decrease in $\dot{V}O_2$	$\uparrow$ed max $\dot{V}O_2$
$\uparrow$ed ventricular cavity (endurance athletes)	$\downarrow$ed muscle glycogen depletion and lactic acid production	$\uparrow$ed cardiac output
$\uparrow$ed myocardial thickness (nonendurance athletes)	$\uparrow$ed number and size of mitochondria	$\uparrow$ed O_2 extraction by muscles
$\downarrow$ed heart rate	No change or slight decrease in cardiac output	$\uparrow$ed lactic acid production
$\uparrow$ed vagal tone		$\uparrow$ed glycolytic capacity
		$\uparrow$ed cardiac output
$\uparrow$ed stroke volume cardiac hypertrophy	$\uparrow$ed stroke volume cardiac hypertrophy	$\uparrow$ed stroke volume
$\uparrow$ed myocardial contractility	$\uparrow$ed myocardial contractility	$\uparrow$ed stroke volume cardiac hypertrophy
	$\downarrow$ed heart rate	$\uparrow$ed myocardial contractility
		No change or slight decrease in heart rate
$\uparrow$ed blood volume and Hb	$\downarrow$ed sympathetic drive	$\uparrow$ed heart volume
$\uparrow$ed skeletal muscle hypertrophy and capillary density	$\downarrow$ed blood flow per kg muscle	$\downarrow$ed sympathetic drive
	$\uparrow$ed O_2 extraction by muscles	No change in blood flow per kg working muscle
		$\uparrow$ed O_2 extraction by muscle blood flow distributed over larger muscle mass

From Fox E. Physical training: methods and effects. Orthop Clin North Am 1977;8:543.
$\uparrow$ed, increased; $\downarrow$ed, decreased; $\dot{V}O_2$, average volume of oxygen consumed.
[a]Same amount of work before and after training.

Cardiorespiratory Changes

Morganroth et al. have shown that heart size increases with endurance training and that this increase is characterized by an increase in the size of the ventricular cavity with normal thickness of the ventricular wall. Conversely, cardiac hypertrophy in the nonendurance athlete, such as shotputters and wrestlers, consists of a thickening of the ventricular wall and a normal-size ventricular cavity (32). It has been shown that long training sessions with a sustained high-level cardiac output, such as aerobic endurance events, result in increased ventricular volume. However, those events that require intermittent, brief, but powerful activities, such as wrestling, result in increased ventricular hypertrophy without an increase in ventricular volume.

Metabolic Change

Other metabolic changes that occur with cardiovascular training include the decrease in glycogen depletion and lactate production during steady-rate or steady-state submaximal workload due to mechanisms not totally known. These changes are believed to result from the increase in the number and size of mitochondria located in the muscle tissue. This, combined with the fact that steady-state exercise can be attained at lower levels of phosphagens resulting from the anaerobic breakdown of ATP (33, 34), results in a glycogen-sparing effect. This sparing effect also occurs with increased fat oxidation in trained muscle during prolonged submaximal exercise, which also contributes to increased endurance.

Oxygen Uptake

Oxygen uptake, also known as aerobic capacity, is the amount of oxygen used by the tissues per kilogram of body weight per minute (mL/kg/min). Oxygen uptake increases with aerobic training. The increased ability of the body to deliver oxygen to tissues shows a high correlation with cardiac output. Oxygen uptake summarizes what is happening in the oxygen transport system at all levels and correlates well with cardiovascular fitness. However, it is important to understand the mechanism of oxygen consumption during exercise and the increased oxygen uptake resulting from regular aerobic exercise, which is discussed later in this section.

In Figure 3.6A, the curve shows the amount of oxygen consumed during an exercise session continued at a steady pace during the first 4 minutes of light to moderate exercise, such as experienced when jogging or bicycling. Oxygen consumption rises rapidly during the first minutes of exercise;

however, by the fourth minute a plateau is reached, and the oxygen consumed during the rest of the exercise session remains stable. This plateau of the oxygen consumption curve represents a steady state, a balance between the energy required by the working muscles and the rate of ATP production using aerobic metabolism (8).

As indicated previously, during light to moderate exercise, the ATP for muscular contraction is made available mainly through energy generated by hydrogen oxidation. Therefore, any lactate formed is rapidly oxidized, and the blood lactate levels remain fairly stable although oxygen consumption increases. The energy demands are adequately met by reactions that use oxygen. Under aerobic conditions, or steady-state/steady-rate conditions, lactate removal is equal to the rate of formation, so the concentration of blood lactate levels remains relatively stable with few fatiguing by-products. One might think that if the energy demands of exercise were met by the oxygen system of metabolism, an exercise session could continue indefinitely, as there would be no fatiguing by-products.

However, other factors to consider include electrolyte depletion, fluid loss, and adequate fuel reserves (i.e., blood glucose for central nervous system function and glycogen stores in the liver and exercising muscles). The body can adapt to a regular, effective exercise routine that enhances the oxygen transport system and thereby increases the body's ability to perform, by increasing the ability to deliver and use oxygen at the cellular level.

Steady-state levels are relative to individual adaptation to exercise and are largely attributed to a combination of genetic makeup and specific adaptations to effective training methods. The spectrum of steady states might range from a person lying in bed to a triathlete who maintains a steady state of aerobic metabolism throughout an entire race.

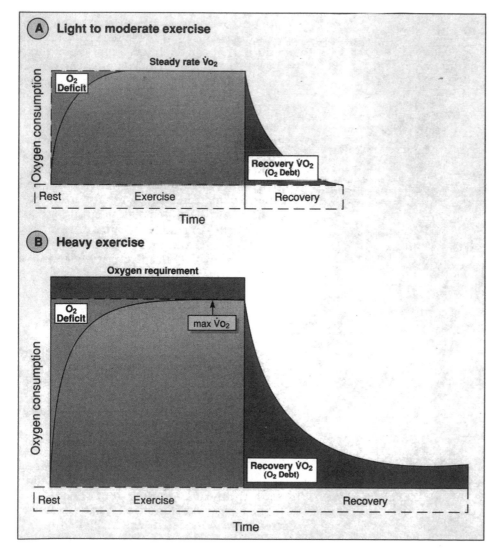

Figure 3.6. Oxygen consumption during and In recovery from light to moderate steady-rate exercise **(A)**, and heavy exercise with the resulting buildup of lactic acid **(B)**. (From Katch FL, McArdle WD. Nutrition, weight control, and exercise. Copyright 1977 by Houghton Mifflin Company.)

Oxygen Deficit

Referring back to Figure 3.6A, the curve of oxygen consumption increases gradually to a steady-state level. In the beginning of the exercise session, the oxygen uptake is below the steady-state level, although the energy required to perform the exercise presumably remains unchanged throughout the work period. Because the oxygen system of metabolism is unable to provide the ATP quickly enough to meet the oxygen demands during the first few minutes of exercise, it must rely on anaerobic metabolism during this "deficit" phase.

The anaerobic metabolic systems provide energy from stored phosphates and from glycolysis until a steady-rate or steady-state condition is reached between oxygen consumption and the energy demands of exercise. Oxygen becomes important only when it serves as an electron acceptor and combines with the hydrogens generated during glycolysis, beta oxidation of fatty acids, or the reactions of the Krebs cycle (8).

The oxygen deficit that occurs during the initial phases of exercise can be seen as the difference between the total oxygen consumed during exercise and the total that would have been consumed had a steady rate of aerobic metabolism been reached immediately.

Maximum Oxygen Consumption (VO$_2$ max)

When exercising at a steady-rate or steady-state level, a point comes when an individual's capacity to resynthesize ATP and consume oxygen does not increase with an additional workload. This condition is called maximum oxygen uptake (Vo$_2$ max) and is a state in which the body must use anaerobic sources for energy to perform more work. Additional work is accomplished by the energy transfer reactions of glycolysis with the resulting formation of lactate. An example of this situation is an athlete attempting to sprint during the last few minutes of a marathon. Under these circumstances an endurance athlete soon becomes exhausted and unable to continue.

Figure 3.6B shows that the oxygen system cannot provide for the energy needs of heavy exercise, thus incurring a continuing oxygen deficit. It is at this level of exertion that the aerobic source of metabolism is unable to provide the energy needs, and hydrogen production begins to exceed its oxidation down the respiratory chain, which results in excess hydrogens passing to pyruvic acid, leading to the accumulation of lactate. This lactate accumulation exceeds its rate of removal via the Krebs metabolic cycle. As exercise intensity increases, the muscle cells cannot meet the additional energy demands aerobically, which leads to muscle exhaustion. Under maximal exercise conditions, it is impossible to exercise longer than 4 or 5 minutes.

Oxygen Debt

During the initial phases of submaximal exercise, the oxygen system of metabolism is unable to provide the energy quickly enough to meet the energy demands. Therefore, during the first few minutes an oxygen deficit is incurred; then a steady-state condition occurs, and oxygen metabolism can meet the energy requirements. This concept was discussed previously. The difference between the oxygen requirement and the actual oxygen consumed is called the oxygen debt.

The anaerobic sources (phosphagen system and glycolysis) provide the immediate energy needs during that initial 2- to 3-minute phase of exercise until the oxygen system takes over. After the exercise session, cardiopulmonary functions remain elevated to replace the oxygen deficit incurred during the initial phase of exercise and support physiologic functions during recovery.

Oxygen consumption during the recovery phase of exercise is termed (repayment of) oxygen debt (8). Immediately after exercise, the bodily processes remain at an elevated level, and recovery from both moderate and strenuous exercise is associated largely with the specific metabolic and physiologic processes resulting from the type of exercise performed. During this time immediately after exercise oxygen consumption and cardiopulmonary functions remain elevated to replenish some of the original carbohydrate stores depleted during the initial stages of exercise; this replenishing occurs by the resynthesis of some of the lactate back to glycogen in the liver. Oxygen consumption also remains elevated to fuel the reactions that replace phosphagen energy stores (phosphocreatine). The remaining lactate is catabolized via the pyruvic acid–Krebs cycle pathway powered by the ATP generated in this process. In addition, other physiologic functions are supported during exercise recovery. However, it is believed that most of the glycogen "burned" during the initial phases of exercise is replaced by carbohydrates consumed (35) and not converted from lactate as once believed.

Oxygen consumed during exercise and recovery from moderate and strenuous work is relative to the overall intensity of exercise. During light exercise (when the deficit is small), the quantity of oxygen consumed in recovery is also small, and preexercise metabolic rate is achieved rapidly. During exhaustive exercise, the opposite situation occurs. Postexercise recovery takes a considerable amount of time, and excessive amounts of lactate accumulate. During exercise recovery, when the oxygen consumed is in excess of the resting value, oxygen debt is present and is calculated as the total oxygen consumed in recovery minus the total oxygen theoretically consumed at rest during the recovery period (8).

Heart Rate

Heart rate, measured in beats per minute (bpm), decreases proportionately with the increase in stroke volume during submaximal exercise. The heart becomes more efficient and needs less oxygen to function. Figure 3.7 shows HR response to oxygen consumption during upright exercise in endurance athletes and sedentary college students before and after 55 days of aerobic training. Although HR increases with oxygen consumption in all categories, the HR of the untrained group accelerates rapidly as exercise intensity increases compared with less acceleration in trained individuals. The trained group achieves a higher oxygen consumption before reaching a particular submaximal HR.

In each instance, the cardiac output is approximately the same. Consequently, a trained individual does more work, achieving a higher oxygen consumption before reaching a particular submaximal HR than a sedentary individual, although the cardiac output is approximately the same (8). Therefore, the difference is in the increased stroke volume that occurs with training. The heart is able to pump a greater amount of blood with fewer "heartbeats." The decrease in resting HR as a result of endurance training, approximately 10 to 15 beats/min, is attributed to enhanced parasympathetic tone, decreased sympathetic discharge, and decreased intrinsic firing rate of the SA node of the heart (2).

Blood Pressure

Blood pressure is the product of cardiac output and peripheral vascular resistance. During exercise, systolic pressure rises to accommodate an increased oxygen demand. Diastolic pressure normally drops or stays the same due to the vasodilation of the blood vessels, thus decreasing the resistance to blood flow. Pulse pressure (systolic blood pressure minus diastolic blood pressure) widens and mean blood pressure rises with increasing exercise intensity. Research indicates that long-term aerobic exercise results in a lower

systolic blood pressure for a given submaximal workload due to increased efficiency of the heart and vascular system (2).

Glycogen Loading

It has been shown that endurance training under a heavy aerobic workload is determined largely by the level of glycogen storage in the muscle cells. Therefore, the rate or intensity for such work is set by oxygen transport capacity. However, the duration or total work performed is set by the level of glycogen stored within the cell. In addition, further research shows that when a muscle is worked hard enough to bring about glycogen depletion, it develops the ability to store more than normal amounts of glycogen. However, diet plays an important role in this process. A particular combination of diet and exercise results in a significant "overstoring" of depleted glycogen stores. This process is called carbohydrate loading and is used almost exclusively by endurance athletes, especially marathon runners.

After depleting glycogen stores from muscles used to complete a particular athletic event, a carbohydrate-rich diet has been found to replenish these stores within 24 hours. On a carbohydrate-free diet of the same caloric content, resynthesis becomes complete after 8 to 10 days. This description is true for muscle and liver glycogen stores. If carbohydrates are not supplied in the diet, liver glycogen can decrease to values that cannot support work for more than approximately 1 hour.

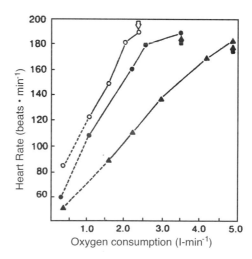

Figure 3.7. Heart rate in relation to oxygen consumption during upright exercise in endurance athletes (▲) and sedentary college students before (○) and after (●) 55 days of aerobic training: (↑ = maximal values). (From Saltin B. Physiological effects of physical conditioning. Med Sci Sports 1969;1:50. Copyright 1969 by The American College of Sports Medicine.)

The procedure for achieving a glycogen loading effect is to deplete muscle glycogen stores with prolonged steady-state exercise approximately 6 days before competition. It is important that the athlete use those muscles required to complete the athletic event because depletion occurs only in those specific muscles exercised. McArdle et al. (8) indicate that this process occurs in two stages. Stage 1 is the glycogen depletion stage in which day 1 would include exhausting exercise. For example, a marathon runner would run 15 to 20 miles. Then for the next 3 days, in addition to continuing a moderate training regimen, the athlete would maintain a low-carbohydrate diet (between 60 and 100 g/day) to deplete glycogen stores further. Two days before competition, the athlete would switch to a high-carbohydrate diet and maintain it up to and including the pre-event meal. However, adequate daily protein, minerals, and vitamins as well as lots of water must also be a part of the daily diet. Glycogen loading may be potentially hazardous to individuals with a predisposition to health problems such as diabetes or hypoglycemia. Training also has a glycogen-sparing effect in that the better trained individual can supply more free fatty acids that provide the bulk of the energy for resting and low-level, long-duration exercise. It is recommended that glycogen loading be used sparingly throughout an athletic season.

Other Training Effects

Although many physiologic and biochemical training effects have been presented, this list is by no means complete. Table 3.6 shows other physiologic changes resulting from exercise

Table 3.6. Other Physiological Changes Induced by Physical Training*

Respiratory changes
  ↑ed maximal minute ventilation†
    ↑ed tidal volume
    ↑ed breathing frequency
  ↑ed ventilatory efficiency
  ↑ed static lung volumes
  ↑ed pulmonary diffusion capacity
Other changes
  Changes in body composition
    ↓ed total body fat
    no change or slight increase in lean body weight
    ↓ed total body weight
  ↓ed blood cholesterol and triglyceride levels
  ↓ed exercise and resting blood pressures
  ↑ed heart acclimatization

*From Fox, E.: Physical training: Methods and effects. Orthop. Clin. North Am., 8(3):545, 1977.
†↑ed = increased; ↓ed = decreased

Table 3.7.   Health Classification Categories by the American College of Sports Medicine

When entering an exercise program there are three major categories
  Apparently healthy individuals
    Those individuals who are asymptomatic and apparently healthy and have no more than one major coronary risk factor (see below)
  Individuals at higher risk
    Those who have symptoms suggestive of possible cardiopulmonary or metabolic disease (Table 3.8) and/or two or more major coronary risk factors (see below)
  Individuals with disease
    Those with known cardiac, pulmonary, or metabolic disease

Major coronary risk factors
Diagnosed hypertension or systolic blood pressure greater than or equal to 160 mm Hg or diastolic blood pressure greater than or equal to 90 mm Hg on at least two separate occasions, or patient taking antihypertensive medication
Serum cholesterol greater than or equal to 6.20 mmol/L (greater than or equal to 240 mg/dL)
Cigarette smoking
Diabetes mellitus*
Family history of coronary or other atherosclerotic disease in parents or siblings before age 55

*Persons with insulin-dependent diabetes mellitus (IDDM) who are older than 30 years of age, or have had IDDM for more than 15 years, and persons with non–insulin-dependent diabetes mellitus who are older than 35 years of age should be classified as patients with disease and treated according to the guidelines in Table 3.10.

training. The effects of training on hormonal output and regulation, connective tissue chemistry, and motor unit recruitment patterns are a few of many changes now receiving proper experimental attention by many research teams (3).

HEALTH SCREENING AND MEDICAL CLEARANCE

Before any exercise test, participation, or rehabilitation program, a careful evaluation of the individual is important for a number of reasons (2). Individuals with medical contraindications to exercise should be identified and excluded from participation. Persons with clinically significant diseases should be identified and referred for a medically supervised exercise program. Individuals with disease symptoms and risk factors for disease development should receive further medical evaluation before starting an exercise program. Finally, it is important to identify those individuals with special needs, such as the elderly and pregnant women, for safe exercise participation.

Therefore, individuals participating in any exercise program or testing procedure, as outlined in this section, should be categorized as apparently healthy individuals as described by the ACSM Guidelines for Exercise Testing and Prescription (Table 3.7) (2). This includes being free from any signs and symptoms suggestive of cardiopulmonary or metabolic disease (Table 3.8), or from any contraindications or relative contraindications to exercise testing (Table 3.9). If the patient falls into the "higher risk" or "with disease" category (Table 3.7), a medical release should be required before exercise testing, participation, or rehabilitation to identify any contraindications, limitations, or precautions. Table 3.10 lists guidelines for exercise testing or participation.

GUIDELINES FOR ATTAINING AN AEROBIC TRAINING EFFECT

There is a linear relationship between oxygen uptake and HR. Therefore, when monitoring HR, functional capacity (oxygen uptake) can be estimated because it highly correlates with energy expenditure. Golding et al. (36) state that an exercise workload should elicit an HR response over 50% of the heart's maximum rate if it is to have a training effect. The ACSM (2) lists the following cardiorespiratory fitness guidelines.

1. The activity must use large muscle groups for a prolonged period and must be rhythmic, as would be seen in jogging, bicycling, walking, cross-country skiing, swimming, and rowing.
2. The recommended intensity of exercise should be between 55 and 90% of maximum HR. The lower intensity may provide important health benefits to those who have health problems or are at a low fitness level.
3. Recommended duration of exercise is 15 to 60 minutes of continuous or discontinuous aerobic exercise.
4. Recommended frequency of exercise is 3 to 5 days per week. The conditioning effect allows individuals to increase the total work per session. In continuous exercise this result occurs by increasing the intensity, duration, or some combination of the two.

Table 3.8. Major Symptoms and Signs Suggestive of Cardiopulmonary or Metabolic Disease[a]

Pain or discomfort in the chest or surrounding areas that appears to be ischemic
Unaccustomed shortness of breath or shortness of breath with mild exertion
Dizziness or syncope
Orthopnea/paroxysmal nocturnal dyspnea
Ankle edema
Palpitations of tachycardia
Claudication
Known heart murmur

From American College of Sports Medicine. Guidelines for exercise testing and prescription. 4th ed. Philadelphia: Lea & Febiger, 1991:6.
[a]These symptoms must be interpreted in the clinical context in which they appear because they are not all specific for cardiopulmonary or metabolic disease.

Table 3.9. Contraindications for Exercise Testing

Absolute contraindications
　Recent significant change in the resting ECG suggesting infarction or other acute cardiac events
　Recent complicated myocardial infarction
　Unstable angina
　Uncontrolled ventricular dysrhythmia
　Uncontrolled atrial dysrhythmia that compromises cardiac function
　Third-degree A-V block
　Acute congestive heart failure
　Severe aortic stenosis
　Suspected or known dissecting aneurysm
　Active or suspected myocarditis or pericarditis
　Thrombophlebitis or intracardiac thrombi
　Recent systemic or pulmonary embolus
　Acute infection
　Significant emotional distress (psychosis)
Relative contraindications
　Resting diastolic blood pressure over 120 mm Hg or resting systolic blood pressure over 200 mm Hg
　Moderate valvular heart disease
　Known electrolyte abnormalities (hypokalemia, hypomagnesemia)
　Fixed-rate pacemaker (rarely used)
　Frequent or complex ventricular ectopy
　Ventricular aneurysm
　Cardiomyopathy including hypertrophic cardiomyopathy
　Uncontrolled metabolic disease (diabetes, thyrotoxicosis, myxedema, etc.)
　Chronic infectious disease (e.g., mononucleosis, hepatitis, AIDS)
　Neuromuscular, musculoskeletal, or rheumatoid disorders that are exacerbated by exercise
　Advanced or complicated pregnancy

American College of Surgeons. Guidelines for exercise testing and prescription. 4th ed. Philadelphia: Lea & Febiger, 1991:59.

Most training effects occur during the first 6 to 8 weeks of an exercise program. The more deconditioned an individual is before starting an exercise program, the faster and more dramatic the adaptations are. The exercise prescription should be adjusted as these conditioning effects occur. It is recommended that for adult aerobic fitness programs, the topic of this section, exercising for 20 to 30 minutes, three times per week, working at 80% of maximum HR, is optimal (7). Exercising for the purpose of optimal body fat reduction requires longer periods (40 to 45 minutes), working at a lower intensity (50 to 70% of maximal HR), four to five times per week. Usually, the best low-intensity exercise includes walking.

For the first 8 weeks of an exercise program, it is recommended that individuals use group 1 activities, for which the exercise intensity is easily sustained with little variability in HR, e.g., jogging, walking, or swimming. Participants can readily monitor HR to stay within their HR training ranges. After a few weeks of exercise, individuals also learn to "listen to their body," perceiving exertion levels and adjusting their workout

Table 3.10.   Guidelines for Exercise Testing and Participation

	Apparently Healthy		Higher Risk[a]		
	Younger (less than 41 yr [men]) (less than 51 yr [women])	Older	No symptoms	Symptoms	With disease[b]
Medical examination and diagnostic exercise test recommended before					
Moderate exercise[c]	No[d]	No	No	Yes	Yes
Vigorous exercise[e]	No	Yes[f]	Yes	Yes	Yes
Physician supervision recommended during exercise test					
Submaximal	No	No	No	Yes	Yes
Maximal testing	No	Yes	Yes	Yes	Yes

American College of Sports Medicine. Guidelines for exercise testing and prescription. 4th ed. Philadelphia: Lea & Febiger, 1991:8.
[a]Persons with two or more risk factors (Table 3.1) or symptoms (Table 3.2).
[b]Persons with known cardiac, pulmonary, or metabolic disease.
[c]Moderate exercise (exercise intensity 40 to 60% of $\dot{V}O_2$max): exercise intensity well within the individuals, current capacity and can be comfortably sustained for a prolonged period, i.e., 60 minutes, slow progression, and generally noncompetitive.
[d]The "no" responses in this table means that an item is "not necesssary." The "no" response does not mean that the item should not be done.
[e]Vigorous exercise (exercise intensity greater than 60% $\dot{V}O_2$max) Exercise intense enough to represent a substantial challenge and which would ordinarily result in fatigue within 20 minutes.
[f]A "yes" response means that an item is recommended.

accordingly. Those who are uncomfortable during exercise should slow down or stop if necessary. After 8 weeks of training, group 2 activities of varied intensity can be used, e.g., dancing or game-type activities (2).

Cardiovascular fitness levels can be assessed by various testing procedures. A few of the fitness tests used by the YMCA include the PWC 170, bicycle ergometer test developed by Sjostrand, and the estimation of maximal oxygen uptake by Åstrand and Rhyming (36, 37). Both tests use HR to determine oxygen uptake based on response to steady-state exercise. The YMCA also uses a 3-minute step test developed by Dr. Fred W. Katch of San Diego State College. This test is especially good because it can be used for mass or individual testing.

The step test requires a minimal amount of equipment, is simple to administer and interpret, and, most important, clearly reflects cardiorespiratory fitness changes. The drawbacks of using a step test are obvious, especially for those who are very obese or have balance or lower extremity problems. Another testing method would be appropriate in these situations. In any case, the step test can be used for most adult fitness programs.

Equipment needed for this test includes a 12-inch high bench, a metronome, and a watch with a second hand. The bench should be sturdy with a large enough platform to accommodate a large person. A 12-inch high by 1-inch thick plank is ideal to form a 24 × 24 × 12-inch step. It is advisable to place the bench against a wall so it does not move during the step testing procedure. The metronome should be set at 96 clicks/min. Four clicks of the metronome equal one step cycle, i.e., up-1 (right foot), up-2 (left foot), down-3 (right foot), down-4 (left foot). It is

important that the participant step to the beat of the click.

Before performing the step test, resting HR and blood pressure should be measured. The participant should then practice stepping for a moment. Start the test when the participant is comfortable with stepping in time with the metronome. Observe participant appearance and presence or absence of distressing symptoms. Stop the test if the participant is feeling undue discomfort or displaying undue distress.

At the end of the 3-minute test, instruct the participant to sit for a full 1-minute. The test administrator can use an HR meter or manually palpate the carotid or radial pulse to assess HR. This postexercise HR is then used to arrive at a performance score. Use the YMCA nomogram (Table 3.11) to find the fitness score—very high, high, above average, average, below average, low, or very low.

After a score is known, follow the ACSM guidelines for exercise prescription as referenced previously. For example, if the participant is a 40-year-old man with a recovery HR of 105, his score is average. To review, the ACSM (2) uses 55 to 90% of maximal HR as the training range and assigns different training percentages to different levels of fitness: 50 to 70% for low fitness; 70 to 80% for average fitness; and 80 to 90% for high fitness. Thus, the individual with an average score should train between 70 and 80% of age-adjusted HR. After a score is known, use the Karvonen formula or consult the Karvonen table (Table 3.12) to find the appropriate exercise training HR range.

The Karvonen formula is one widely accepted method of determining the proper exercise HR intensity. The formula encompasses taking a percentage of the difference between the maximal and the resting HR (HR range or reserve), and is stated as follows: (Maximum HR) − (Resting HR) × (Exercise percentage) + (Resting HR) = training HR. For example, calculating the training HR of a 20-year-old with a resting HR of 70 beats/min, training at 60% of age-adjusted HR, can be described as follows:

$$[\text{Max HR} - (\text{RHR})] \times \text{Exercise Percentage} + \text{RHR} = \text{Training Heart Rate (THR)}$$

$$(220 - \text{Age}) - 70 \times 60\% + 70 \text{ bpm} = \text{THR}$$

$$200 - 70 \times .60 + 70 \text{ bpm} = 148 \text{ bpm}$$

Implementing an Aerobic Exercise Session for the Adult Fitness Population (38)

An aerobic exercise program for the adult population should be started as follows but differs from competitive athletic training. To avoid strains, sprains, or other more serious in-

Table 3.11.   Cardiovascular Rating (3-Min Step Test) (YMCA 1989)

	Age (yr)					
	18–25	26–35	36–45	46–55	56–65	>65
Men						
Very high	70	73	72	78	72	72
	72	76	74	81	74	74
	78	79	81	84	82	86
High	82	83	86	89	89	89
	85	85	90	93	93	92
	88	88	94	96	97	95
Above average	91	91	98	99	98	97
	94	94	100	101	100	100
	97	97	102	103	101	102
Average	101	101	105	109	105	104
	102	103	108	113	109	109
	104	106	111	115	111	113
Below average	107	109	113	118	113	114
	110	113	116	120	116	116
	114	116	118	121	118	119
Low	118	119	120	124	122	122
	121	122	124	126	125	126
	126	126	128	130	128	128
Very low	131	130	132	135	131	133
	137	140	142	145	136	140
	164	164	168	158	150	152
Women						
Very high	72	72	74	76	74	73
	79	80	80	88	83	83
	83	86	87	93	92	86
High	88	91	93	96	97	93
	93	93	97	100	99	97
	97	97	101	102	103	100
Above average	100	103	104	106	106	104
	103	106	106	111	109	108
	106	110	109	113	111	114
Average	110	112	111	117	113	117
	112	116	114	118	116	120
	116	118	117	120	117	121
Below average	118	121	120	121	119	123
	122	124	122	124	123	126
	124	127	127	126	127	127
Low	128	129	130	127	129	129
	133	131	135	131	132	132
	137	135	138	133	136	134
Very low	142	141	143	138	142	135
	149	148	146	147	148	149
	155	154	152	152	151	151

From Golding LA, Myers CR, Sinning WE. Y's way to physical fitness. 3rd ed. Champaign, IL: Human Kinetics Publishers, 1989.

Table 3.12. Karvonen Method of Determining Training Heart Rate

Instructions: Use this chart to determine training heart rate, using the Karvonen formula, for 60%, 70%, and 80% of age adjusted heart rate. If you need to find any other heart rate percentage, use the Karvonen formula as follows: $220 - age = \underline{\hspace{1cm}} - $ resting heart rate $= \underline{\hspace{1cm}} \times$ heart rate $\% = \underline{\hspace{1cm}} + $ resting heart rate $= \underline{\hspace{1cm}}$ training heart rate. Do this formula twice to determine an upper and lower heart rate range. As your fitness improves, you will notice a decrease in the resting heart rate for a given workload. You will have to retake your fitness test to determine your new fitness level. Use this chart, or re-calculate using Karvonen's formula to determine your new training heart rate.

Part A

Resting Heart Rate

Age (yr)	40			42			44			46			48			50			52			54			56			58		
	60%	70%	80%	60%	70%	80%	60%	70%	80%	60%	70%	80%	60%	70%	80%	60%	70%	80%	60%	70%	80%	60%	70%	80%	60%	70%	80%	60%	70%	80%
18	137	153	170	138	154	170	139	155	170	140	155	171	140	156	171	141	156	172	142	157	172	143	158	172	144	158	173	144	159	173
20	136	152	168	137	153	168	138	153	169	138	154	169	139	154	170	140	155	170	141	156	170	142	156	171	142	157	171	143	157	172
22	135	151	166	136	151	167	136	152	167	137	152	168	138	153	168	139	154	168	140	154	169	140	155	169	141	155	170	142	156	170
24	134	149	165	134	150	165	135	150	166	136	151	166	137	152	166	138	152	167	138	153	167	139	153	168	140	154	168	141	155	168
26	132	148	163	133	148	164	134	149	164	135	150	164	136	150	165	136	151	165	137	151	166	138	152	166	139	153	166	140	153	167
28	131	146	162	132	147	162	133	148	162	134	148	163	134	149	163	135	149	164	136	150	164	137	151	164	138	151	165	138	152	165
30	130	145	160	131	146	160	132	146	161	132	147	161	133	147	162	134	148	162	135	149	162	136	149	163	136	150	163	137	150	164
32	129	144	158	130	144	159	130	145	159	131	145	160	132	146	160	133	147	160	134	147	161	134	148	161	135	148	162	136	149	162
34	128	142	157	128	143	157	129	143	158	130	144	158	131	145	158	132	145	159	132	146	159	133	146	160	134	147	160	135	148	160
36	126	141	155	127	141	156	128	142	156	129	143	156	130	143	157	130	144	157	131	144	158	132	145	158	133	146	158	134	146	159
38	125	139	154	126	140	154	127	141	154	128	141	155	128	142	155	129	142	156	130	143	156	131	144	156	132	144	157	132	145	157
40	124	138	152	125	139	152	126	139	153	126	140	153	127	140	154	128	141	154	129	142	154	130	142	155	130	143	155	131	143	156
42	123	137	150	124	137	151	124	138	151	125	138	152	126	139	152	127	140	152	128	140	153	128	141	153	129	141	154	130	142	154
44	122	135	149	122	136	149	123	136	150	124	137	150	125	138	150	126	138	151	126	139	151	127	139	152	128	140	152	129	141	152
46	120	134	147	121	134	148	122	135	148	123	136	148	124	136	149	124	137	149	125	137	150	126	138	150	127	139	150	128	139	151
48	119	132	146	120	133	146	121	134	146	122	134	147	122	135	147	123	135	148	124	136	148	125	137	148	126	137	149	126	138	149
50	118	131	144	119	132	144	120	132	145	120	133	145	121	133	146	122	134	146	123	135	146	124	135	147	124	136	147	125	136	148
52	117	130	142	118	130	143	118	131	143	119	131	144	120	132	144	121	133	144	122	133	145	122	134	145	123	134	146	124	135	146
54	116	128	141	116	129	141	117	129	142	118	130	142	119	131	142	120	131	143	120	132	143	121	132	144	122	133	144	123	134	144
56	114	127	139	115	127	140	116	128	140	117	129	140	118	129	141	118	130	141	119	130	142	120	131	142	121	132	142	122	132	143
58	113	125	138	114	126	138	115	127	138	116	127	139	116	128	139	117	128	140	118	129	140	119	130	140	120	130	141	120	131	141
60	112	124	136	113	125	136	114	125	137	114	126	137	115	126	138	116	127	138	117	128	138	118	128	139	118	129	139	119	129	140
62	111	123	134	112	123	135	112	124	135	113	124	136	114	125	136	115	126	136	116	126	137	116	127	137	117	127	138	118	128	138
64	110	121	133	110	122	133	111	122	134	112	123	134	113	124	134	114	124	135	114	125	135	115	125	136	116	126	136	117	127	136
66	108	120	131	109	120	132	110	121	132	111	122	132	112	122	133	112	123	133	113	123	134	114	124	134	115	125	134	116	125	135
68	107	118	130	108	119	130	109	120	130	110	120	131	110	121	131	111	121	132	112	122	132	113	123	132	114	123	133	114	124	133
70	106	117	128	107	118	128	108	118	129	108	119	129	109	119	130	110	120	130	111	121	130	112	121	131	112	122	131	113	122	132

Table 3.12. Karvonen Method of Determining Training Heart Rate—continued

Part B

Resting Heart Rate

Age (yr)	60			62			64			66			68			70			72			74			76			78		
	60%	70%	80%	60%	70%	80%	60%	70%	80%	60%	70%	80%	60%	70%	80%	60%	70%	80%	60%	70%	80%	60%	70%	80%	60%	70%	80%	60%	70%	80%
18	145	159	174	146	160	174	147	161	174	148	161	175	148	162	175	149	162	176	150	163	176	151	164	176	152	164	177	152	165	177
20	144	158	172	145	159	172	146	159	173	146	160	173	147	160	174	148	161	174	149	162	174	150	162	175	150	163	175	151	163	176
22	143	157	170	144	157	171	144	158	171	145	158	172	146	159	172	147	160	172	148	160	173	148	161	173	149	161	174	150	162	174
24	142	155	169	142	156	169	143	156	170	144	157	170	145	158	170	146	158	171	146	159	171	147	159	172	148	160	172	149	161	172
26	140	154	167	141	154	168	142	155	168	143	156	168	144	156	169	144	157	169	145	157	170	146	158	170	147	159	170	148	159	171
28	139	152	166	140	153	166	141	154	166	142	154	167	142	155	167	143	155	168	144	156	168	145	157	168	146	157	169	146	158	169
30	138	151	164	139	152	164	140	152	165	140	153	165	141	153	166	142	154	166	143	155	166	144	155	167	144	156	167	145	156	168
32	137	150	162	138	150	163	138	151	163	139	151	164	140	152	164	141	153	164	142	153	165	142	154	165	143	154	166	144	155	166
34	136	148	161	136	149	161	137	149	162	138	150	162	139	151	162	140	151	163	140	152	163	141	152	164	142	153	164	143	154	164
36	134	147	159	135	147	160	136	148	160	137	149	160	138	149	161	138	150	161	139	150	162	140	151	162	141	152	162	142	152	163
38	133	145	158	134	146	158	135	147	158	136	147	159	136	148	159	137	148	160	138	149	160	139	150	160	140	150	161	140	151	161
40	132	144	156	133	145	156	134	145	157	134	146	157	135	146	158	136	147	158	137	148	158	138	148	159	138	149	159	139	149	160
42	131	143	154	132	143	155	132	144	155	133	144	156	134	145	156	135	146	156	136	146	157	136	147	157	137	147	158	138	148	158
44	130	141	153	130	142	153	131	142	154	132	143	154	133	144	154	134	144	155	134	145	155	135	145	156	136	146	156	137	147	156
46	128	140	151	129	140	152	130	141	152	131	142	152	132	142	153	132	143	153	133	143	154	134	144	154	135	145	154	136	145	155
48	127	138	150	128	139	150	129	140	150	130	140	151	130	141	151	131	141	152	132	142	152	133	143	152	134	143	153	134	144	153
50	126	137	148	127	138	148	128	138	149	128	139	149	129	139	150	130	140	150	131	141	150	132	141	151	132	142	151	133	142	152
52	125	136	146	126	136	147	126	137	147	127	137	148	128	138	148	129	139	148	130	139	149	130	140	149	131	140	150	132	141	150
54	124	134	145	124	135	145	125	135	146	126	136	146	127	137	146	128	137	147	128	138	147	129	138	148	130	139	148	131	140	148
56	122	133	143	123	133	144	124	134	144	125	135	144	126	135	145	126	136	145	127	136	146	128	137	146	129	138	146	130	138	147
58	121	131	142	122	132	142	123	133	142	124	133	143	124	134	143	125	134	144	126	135	144	127	136	144	128	136	145	128	137	145
60	120	130	140	121	131	140	122	131	141	122	132	141	123	132	142	124	133	142	125	134	142	126	134	143	126	135	143	127	135	144
62	119	129	138	120	129	139	120	130	139	121	130	140	122	131	140	123	132	140	124	132	141	124	133	141	125	133	142	126	134	142
64	118	127	137	118	128	137	119	128	138	120	129	138	121	130	138	122	130	139	122	131	139	123	131	140	124	132	140	125	133	140
66	116	126	135	117	126	136	118	127	136	119	128	136	120	128	137	120	129	137	121	129	138	122	130	138	123	131	138	124	131	139
68	115	124	134	116	125	134	117	126	134	118	126	135	118	127	135	119	127	136	120	128	136	121	129	136	122	129	137	122	130	137
70	114	123	132	115	124	132	116	124	133	116	125	133	117	125	134	118	126	134	119	127	134	120	127	135	120	128	135	121	128	136

continued

Table 3.12. Karvonen Method of Determining Training Heart Rate—continued

Part C

Resting Heart Rate

Age (yr)	80 60%	80 70%	80 80%	82 60%	82 70%	82 80%	84 60%	84 70%	84 80%	86 60%	86 70%	86 80%	88 60%	88 70%	88 80%	90 60%	90 70%	90 80%	92 60%	92 70%	92 80%	94 60%	94 70%	94 80%	96 60%	96 70%	96 80%	98 60%	98 70%	98 80%
18	153	165	178	154	166	178	155	167	178	156	167	179	156	168	179	157	168	180	158	169	180	159	170	180	160	170	181	160	171	181
20	152	164	176	153	165	176	154	165	177	154	166	177	155	166	178	156	167	178	157	168	178	158	168	179	158	169	179	159	169	180
22	151	163	174	152	163	175	152	164	175	153	164	176	154	165	176	155	166	176	156	166	177	156	167	177	157	167	178	158	168	178
24	150	161	173	150	162	173	151	162	174	152	163	174	153	164	174	154	164	175	154	165	175	155	165	176	156	166	176	157	167	176
26	148	160	171	149	160	172	150	161	172	151	162	172	152	162	173	152	163	173	153	163	174	154	164	174	155	165	174	156	165	175
28	147	158	170	148	159	170	149	160	170	150	160	171	150	161	171	151	161	172	152	162	172	153	163	172	154	163	173	154	164	173
30	146	157	168	147	158	168	148	158	169	148	159	169	149	159	170	150	160	170	151	161	170	152	161	171	152	162	171	153	162	172
32	145	156	166	146	156	167	146	157	167	147	157	168	148	158	168	149	159	168	150	159	169	150	160	169	151	160	170	152	161	170
34	144	154	165	144	155	165	145	155	166	146	156	166	147	157	166	148	157	167	148	158	167	149	158	168	150	159	168	151	160	168
36	142	153	163	143	153	164	144	154	164	145	155	164	146	155	165	146	156	165	147	156	166	148	157	166	149	158	166	150	158	167
38	141	151	162	142	152	162	143	153	162	144	153	163	144	154	163	145	154	164	146	155	164	147	156	164	148	156	165	148	157	165
40	140	150	160	141	151	160	142	151	161	142	152	161	143	152	162	144	153	162	145	154	162	146	154	163	146	155	163	147	155	164
42	139	149	158	140	149	159	140	150	159	141	150	160	142	151	160	143	152	160	144	152	161	144	153	161	145	153	162	146	154	162
44	138	147	157	138	148	157	139	148	158	140	149	158	141	150	158	142	150	159	142	151	159	143	151	160	144	152	160	145	153	160
46	136	146	155	137	146	156	138	147	156	139	148	156	140	148	157	140	149	157	141	149	158	142	150	158	143	151	158	144	151	159
48	135	144	154	136	145	154	137	146	154	138	146	155	138	147	155	139	147	156	140	148	156	141	149	156	142	149	157	142	150	157
50	134	143	152	135	144	152	136	144	153	136	145	153	137	145	154	138	146	154	139	147	154	140	147	155	140	148	155	141	148	156
52	133	142	150	134	142	151	134	143	151	135	143	152	136	144	152	137	145	152	138	145	153	138	146	153	139	146	154	140	147	154
54	132	140	149	132	141	149	133	141	150	134	142	150	135	143	150	136	143	151	136	144	151	137	144	152	138	145	152	139	146	152
56	130	139	147	131	139	148	132	140	148	133	141	148	134	141	149	134	142	149	135	142	150	136	143	150	137	144	150	138	144	151
58	129	137	146	130	138	146	131	139	146	132	139	147	132	140	147	133	140	148	134	141	148	135	142	148	136	142	149	136	143	149
60	128	136	144	129	137	144	130	137	145	130	138	145	131	138	146	132	139	146	133	140	146	134	140	147	134	141	147	135	141	148
62	127	135	142	128	135	143	128	136	143	129	136	144	130	137	144	131	138	144	132	138	145	132	139	145	133	139	146	134	140	146
64	126	133	141	126	134	141	127	134	142	128	135	142	129	136	142	130	136	143	130	137	143	131	137	144	132	138	144	133	139	144
66	124	132	139	125	132	140	126	133	140	127	134	140	128	134	141	128	135	141	129	135	142	130	136	142	131	137	142	132	137	143
68	123	130	138	124	131	138	125	132	138	126	132	139	126	133	139	127	133	140	128	134	140	129	135	140	130	135	141	130	136	141
70	122	129	136	123	130	136	124	130	137	124	131	137	125	131	138	126	132	138	127	133	138	128	133	139	128	134	139	129	134	140

juries, each exercise session should include the following:

1. General warm-up (5 minutes)
2. Stretching (5–10 minutes)
3. Aerobic warm-up (2–3 minutes)
4. Aerobic exercise (15–60 minutes)
5. Cool down (2–10 minutes)
6. Strength training, rehabilitation, or therapeutic exercise
7. Cool-down stretching (5–30 minutes)

GENERAL WARM-UP

Before any type of physical exercise, a warm-up for approximately 5 minutes should be performed with moderate continuous movement using activities such as walking, slow jogging, or bicycling to increase circulation and prepare muscles for stretching. Stretching before a warm-up period increases chances of injury.

PREEXERCISE STRETCHING

Gently stretching out the muscles using gradual static (nonballistic) movements for approximately 5 to 10 minutes is recommended to prepare muscles and joints for more vigorous activity and to avoid injuries. One should consult a fitness specialist for stretching techniques for a specific sports activity.

AEROBIC WARM-UP

The goals and needs of athletes, elementary school children, elderly men and women, and cardiac patients clearly differ. For example, many safeguards concerning intensity and progression of exercise are not as closely followed when an athlete trains as they are when a nonathletic adult trains for fitness gains. An intense, abrupt training approach to adult fitness can result in injury, discouraging future motivation for participation in endurance or other activities. Therefore, the initial experience with exercise training should be of low to moderate intensity and slow to moderate progression that allows for gradual adaptation (39–44).

Warming up to vigorous activity should include a slow start, approximately 50% of maximum HR (7, 36, 38), for approximately 2 to 3 minutes. Cooper and Cooper (41) indicate that intensity should then gradually increase to the target HR for 15 to 60 minutes. As indicated previously, for adult exercise programs, exercising aerobically for at least 20 to 30 minutes every other day, 3 to 4 days per week, is recommended to improve cardiovascular endurance, increase

energy levels, and decrease body fat (7). However, exercising for shorter periods, such as 10-minute "pain-free" exercise bouts, two to three times per day, 3 to 5 days per week, is appropriate for those who are just starting an exercise program and are not in the habit of regular exercise, or who do not have the time to for those longer periods for exercise. Initially, exercising this way encourages the habit of exercising regularly and lifestyle change. As benefits of this "short bout" program are realized, it becomes more natural to continue longer without discomfort and realize more cardiovascular results. The author believes that as adaptation to exercise occurs, one should exercise aerobically at light to moderate intensity (55 to 70% of age-adjusted maximum HR), 20 to 30 minutes, 5 days per week, for best physiologic and psychological benefit.

During an exercise session, exercise intensity should be adjusted by monitoring HR or by perceiving pain (fatigue) levels (1–3, 5, 7, 36, 38, 39). If training for cardiovascular endurance, loss of body fat, or both, it is imperative that an individual not feel any pain from "muscle fatigue" during exercise. If steady state HR is above or below recommended levels, workout intensity should be adjusted accordingly. If using perceived exertion, the individual should slow down or stop if uncomfortable.

AEROBIC EXERCISE

Exercise HR should not be taken until at least 3 minutes into the aerobic exercise session (Fig. 3.8). By then HR has reached a steady/state level, in which energy demands are provided by the oxygen system of metabolism (see section on the production of energy). HR taken at this time represents a working exercise intensity and determines if exercising is in a training HR zone (1–3, 5, 7, 36, 38, 39). If exercise HR is above the recommended level, exercise intensity should be decreased. If it is below the recommended level, speeding up to increase exercise intensity is advised. A good rule of thumb to remember is to slow down if pain occurs. To trigger a training effect, exercise should continue (within a training HR range) for the recommended period.

TAKING HR—PALPATION TECHNIQUE

To measure exercise HR, HR count should begin within 5 seconds after stopping, if using palpation technique, for an accurate exercise HR reading. The full HR count must be completed within 15 seconds after stopping aerobic exercise to get an accurate working HR (7). Exercise

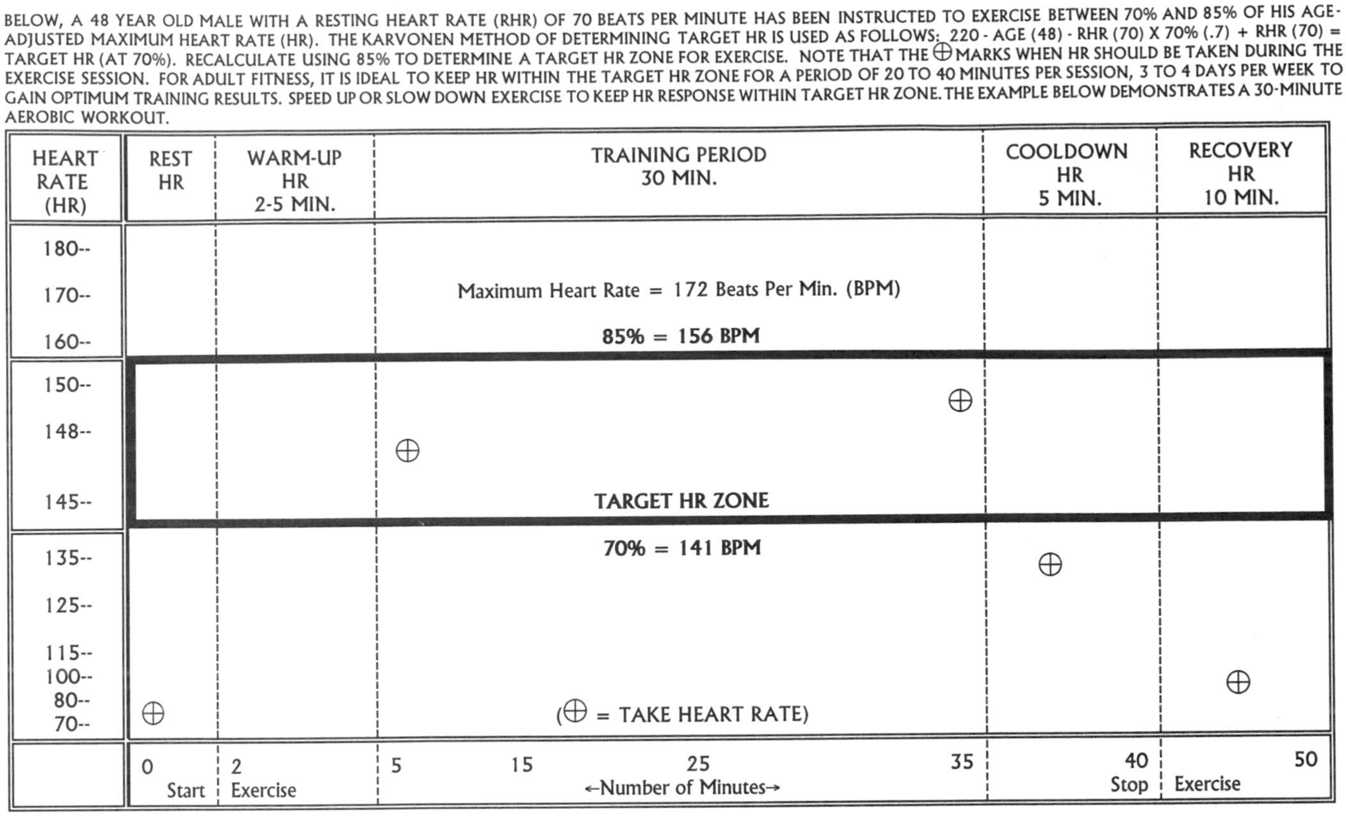

BELOW, A 48 YEAR OLD MALE WITH A RESTING HEART RATE (RHR) OF 70 BEATS PER MINUTE HAS BEEN INSTRUCTED TO EXERCISE BETWEEN 70% AND 85% OF HIS AGE-ADJUSTED MAXIMUM HEART RATE (HR). THE KARVONEN METHOD OF DETERMINING TARGET HR IS USED AS FOLLOWS: 220 - AGE (48) - RHR (70) X 70% (.7) + RHR (70) = TARGET HR (AT 70%). RECALCULATE USING 85% TO DETERMINE A TARGET HR ZONE FOR EXERCISE. NOTE THAT THE ⊕ MARKS WHEN HR SHOULD BE TAKEN DURING THE EXERCISE SESSION. FOR ADULT FITNESS, IT IS IDEAL TO KEEP HR WITHIN THE TARGET HR ZONE FOR A PERIOD OF 20 TO 40 MINUTES PER SESSION, 3 TO 4 DAYS PER WEEK TO GAIN OPTIMUM TRAINING RESULTS. SPEED UP OR SLOW DOWN EXERCISE TO KEEP HR RESPONSE WITHIN TARGET HR ZONE. THE EXAMPLE BELOW DEMONSTRATES A 30-MINUTE AEROBIC WORKOUT.

HEART RATE (HR)	REST HR	WARM-UP HR 2-5 MIN.	TRAINING PERIOD 30 MIN.	COOLDOWN HR 5 MIN.	RECOVERY HR 10 MIN.
180--					
170--			Maximum Heart Rate = 172 Beats Per Min. (BPM)		
160--			85% = 156 BPM		
150--				⊕	
148--		⊕			
145--			TARGET HR ZONE		
135--			70% = 141 BPM	⊕	
125--					
115--					
100--					
80--					⊕
70--	⊕		(⊕ = TAKE HEART RATE)		
	0	2	5 15 25 35	40	50
	Start	Exercise	←Number of Minutes→	Stop	Exercise

Taken from, Hornberger, Joseph P.: Protocol Manual. Exercise Testing, Prescription, Therapeutic Exercise, Rehabilitation Guidelines for a Chiropractic and Rehab Facility...A Practical Approach. 5646 Beneva Woods Circle, Sarasota, Florida. Hornberger Publications, 1995. (941) 366-2440, Fax: (941) 921-9140.

Figure 3.8. A sample aerobic training session. How long the person stays in the target heart rate zone is crucial when developing cardiovascular endurance. A 48-year-old man with a resting heart rate (HR) of 70 beats per minute has been instructed to train between 70% and 85% of maximum age-adjusted HR. Note that HR is monitored throughout the exercise session. It is most important to keep HR in the target HR zone for a period of 20 to 60 minutes to gain optimum training results. Speed up or slow down exercise to keep HR response in training HR zone.

should be performed within a training HR range for optimal results.

Because it is difficult to count HR while exercising, unless monitored by an HR monitor, counting pulse rate manually requires momentarily stopping in most cases. A pulse beat should be found at the carotid or radial artery, and the HR counted within 5 seconds of stopping. The HR count is completed within 10 seconds; otherwise, HR starts to decrease to preexercise levels (2, 7). It is important to monitor HR during the aerobic phase or steady-state phase of an exercise session. After temporarily stopping, the fingertips of one hand are placed on the carotid artery (adjacent to voice box) with just enough pressure to feel the heart. After establishing the HR rhythm, within 5 seconds after stopping exercise, the HR count is started on a full beat with the first count being zero. The HR is counted for 10 seconds, then multiplied by 6 for heartbeat per minute.

COOLING DOWN

After vigorous activity it is important to cool down before stopping. If jogging, the individual should slow down to a slow trot. After vigorous bicycling, the athlete should slow to one-half to one-quarter speed for a few minutes. This practice gives the body time to reallocate blood and adjust to preexercise levels. It may also prevent dizziness, fainting, increased heartbeats, and nausea due to inadequate blood supply to the brain, heart, and intestines. This cooldown is especially important in the elderly.

STRENGTH TRAINING, REHABILITATION, THERAPEUTIC EXERCISE

If any participation in strength training, rehabilitation, ortherapeutic exercise is recommended, it should be implemented after the aerobic phase of exercise. Performing strength training before the aerobic portion of a workout is not recommended due to the increased peripheral blood flow to the muscles and surrounding surface area. Starting an aerobic workout after strength training may result in decreased venous return to the heart. Doing the aerobic workout first is especially recommended for fitness training of the elderly or persons with other health problems, because decreased venous return is more likely to cause fainting in such individuals.

COOL DOWN STRETCHING

After cooling down, stretching is recommended to help prevent muscle soreness and tightening and aid in the development and maintenance of muscle and joint flexibility. If a person is not flexible or tends to have frequent musculoskeletal aches and pains or postural problems, a stretching and therapeutic exercise program is very important. Stretching should be continued as long as needed for flexibility.

RATE OF EXERCISE PROGRESSION

Cooper and Cooper (41) have developed the aerobic point system to quantify aerobics. Because every aerobic activity has different oxygen demands, each exerciser's oxygen quantity and energy cost are converted into points. Therefore, the exercises that require more oxygen and energy merit more points. For example, a cyclist exercising at a low speed takes longer to process the same amount of oxygen then someone cycling faster. Because elevating HR and using more oxygen are major goals of aerobic training, a low-intensity cyclist has to bike longer and cover more ground than a high-intensity cyclist to use the same amount of oxygen or merit the same number of aerobic points.

Cooper and Cooper (41) compare the energy expenditure of a runner to a singles tennis match. This situation is quite different in that tennis play requires stop-and-go maneuvers, with frequent bouts of standing around. The action is temporary and more or less depends on skill level. HR is elevated to a training range temporarily, but this rise is short-lived. Therefore, the average elevated HR during a singles tennis match is lower than the HR with nonstop aerobic activities such as running, jogging, or cycling. Although there is an aerobic benefit to an aggressive tennis game, it is certainly lower than that attained during nonstop aerobic activities such as running, swimming, or cycling and falls somewhere between running and walking. Singles tennis must be played far longer to match the aerobic benefit and to earn more

Cooper points compared with running or cycling, which have higher aerobic metabolic costs.

Cooper's point system is based on the FIT formula (41). The acronym FIT represents frequency (how often to exercise), intensity (how much exercise to exert), and time (how long each aerobic session lasts, which ultimately dependend on the frequency and intensity of a particular exercise because there is an inverse relationship; that is, the person who exercises at a low intensity must exercise longer, and vice versa.

The points earned depend on (1) the type of aerobic exercise and the demands it makes on the heart and lungs, (2) the duration of activity, and (3) the intensity with which it is performed (41). It is a goal-oriented, motivation program that allows specific points for different activities based on aerobic development. It is a numeric standard against which people can judge their exercise effort and is good for those individuals who have exorbitant demands on their time and whose lives are often ruled by change. Being able to adapt an aerobic program to fluid circumstances has definite advantages.

As indicated previously, it has been widely accepted that before healthy people participate in an aerobic exercise program, a cardiorespiratory fitness test is very helpful to assess the initial level of fitness and to aid in choosing the correct program. Pollock et al. (7) suggest that in healthy people, the exercise prescription has three levels of progression (Fig. 3.9). The initial level is classified as a starter program (in which intensity is low) that includes stretching and light calisthenics followed by aerobic exercise of low to moderate intensity. This phase, lasting approximately

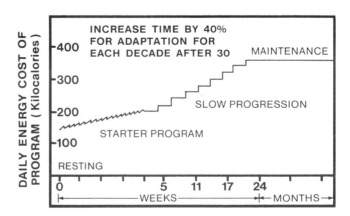

Figure 3.9. Progression for average participants in an aerobic training program. (From Pollock ML, Wilmore JH, Fox SM. Exercise in health and disease: evaluation and prescription for prevention and rehabilitation. Philadelphia: WB Saunders, 1984:261.)

2 to 6 weeks, depending on how quickly an individual adapts to the exercise program, introduces exercise at a low level. In addition, it allows time to adapt to the initial weeks of training, allows a period for minimal muscle soreness, and helps the person circumvent the usual injuries associated with starting an exercise program.

For example, a participant who is classified at a poor or fair fitness level, as determined by the fitness test, may spend as many as 4 to 6 weeks in the starter program. For a participant scoring in the good or excellent categories, a starter program may not be necessary. Those in the starter program should participate in group 1 activities. As mentioned previously, with these activities a participant can be steady because there is little variation of exercise intensity. HR and perceived exertion methods will aid the participant in performing the exercise at the proper intensity range. Game-type activities are not recommended in the early stages of training.

In the next stage of training, known as slow progression, the participant progresses at a faster rate, as the intensity and duration of exercise are increased every 1 to 3 weeks, depending on how well an individual adapts to training. Generally, the older the patient and the lower the fitness level, the longer it takes to adapt and progress in a training regimen. Pollock (7) estimates that the adaptation to a training load takes approximately 40% longer for each decade in life after age 30 (7, 44). For example, if the progression to increase workout loads in bicycling is every 2 weeks for men between 30 and 39 years of age, the interval may be 3 weeks for those who are 40 to 49 years and 4 weeks for those who are 50 to 59 years.

After approximately 6 to 12 months, the maintenance stage of prescription occurs (44, 45). It is at this stage that further improvement in cardiorespiratory fitness is minimal, because the participant has reached a satisfactory level of fitness and may no longer be interested in increasing the training load, but rather wants to continue the same workout schedule. Retesting should occur in approximately 6 to 8 weeks. If the principles described are followed, cardiovascular fitness levels improve steadily. Exercise sessions easier and it takes a higher exercise intensity to get HR to a target HR zone. Resting HR decreases and recovery rate returns more quickly to preexercise levels as the cardiovascular system becomes more efficient. Energy levels increase; it is easier to sleep. When a workout is missed, the participant misses that invigorating feeling resulting from exercise.

If cardiovascular efficiency is to increase, an increase in exercise frequency, intensity, or duration must occur. For example, it may take 35 minutes to jog 3 miles working at 70% of maximum HR. At the end of an 8-week training program, a participant may be jogging a longer distance or at a higher intensity due to increased cardiovascular fitness levels without experiencing any increased distress levels. Again, monitoring progress using a cardiovascular step or bicycle ergometer test every 6 to 8 weeks is helpful in updating training HR ranges and assures that effective and efficient workouts can be maintained. After a desired level of cardiovascular fitness is achieved, it is imperative that workouts continue at least two times per week to maintain these levels. Exercising three times per week is more desirable if continued fat weight loss is desired.

Cardiovascular exercising should be a lifelong endeavor, because it improves quality of life and increases energy levels. Sporadic workouts should be avoided. Consistency is of utmost importance if cardiovascular fitness is to be maintained. All fitness gains can be lost within 5 weeks of inactivity, and half of the gains can be lost exercising one time per week in a period of 10 weeks. If certain situations that make regular exercise impossible, exercise should be started slowly when it is resumed. Overanxiousness may cause injuries and lead to other unproductive exercise habits. The goal is to return to a productive exercise lifestyle. This transition may be difficult if caution is not used when resuming an exercise program. Even if an exercise program is followed closely, certain situations may indicate that a participant is overdoing it. Changes in weather, humidity, and altitude may cause HR to increase. Therefore, it is important to listen to the body, use common sense, and not overdo it!

This chapter has made clear that different physical activities have varying durations and intensities that require interaction between different energy-producing systems, each of which shares anaerobic and aerobic metabolic pathways. It would be difficult to place a certain activity in any one particular system, as all three energy transfer systems—phosphagen, glycolysis, and oxidation phosphorylation—operate interdependently. In this energy continuum is directly related to the length of time and intensity (power output) of the specific activity performed.

However, the major objective in achieving a training effect to those specific metabolic pathways, whether aerobic or anaerobic, is to cause biologic adaptations by stressing the systems in a planned manner so that changes on the cellular level can occur for improved performance. Attention to such factors as length of workouts, frequency, type of training, speed intensity, duration, and repetition of the activity should be carefully coordinated for a predictable result.

To enhance physiologic improvements effectively and to bring about a training change, a specific overload must be applied. Exercising in this manner results in a variety of training adaptations that cause the body to function more efficiently. The appropriate overload can be achieved by manipulating frequency, duration, and intensity of exercise. This concept of individualizing an exercise program applies to sedentary individuals wanting general fitness gains, athletes, obese individuals who want to lose weight, or many clinical conditions including the rehabilitation of cardiac patients, patients with metabolic disease, those managing chronic obstructive pulmonary disease, cardiac rehabilitation patients, or patients rehabilitating musculoskeletal injuries. Research continues in this area, because of strong interest in the effects of exercise on health and physiologic performance.

References

1. Åstrand O, Rodahl K. Textbook of work physiology: physiological bases of exercise. 2nd ed. New York: McGraw-Hill, 1977:16.
2. American College of Sports Medicine. Guidelines for exercise testing and prescription. 4th ed. Philadelphia: Lea & Febiger, 1991:11, 14, 16, 20, 22, 36, 95, 96.
3. Strauss RH, ed. Sports medicine. Philadelphia: WB Saunders, 1984:383, 384, 386, 401, 427.
4. Blair SN, Painter P, Pate RR, et al., eds. ACSM resource manual for guidelines for exercise testing and prescription. Philadelphia: Lea & Febiger, 1988:37, 52.
5. deVries HA. Physiology of exercise for physical education and athletics. 2nd ed. Dubuque: Wm. C. Brown Company, 1974:18, 19.
6. Bloomfield J, Fricker PA, Fitch KD. The textbook of science and medicine in sport. Champaign, IL: Human Kinetics, 1992:72.
7. Pollock ML, Wilmore JH, Fox SM. Exercise in health and disease: evaluation and prescription for prevention and rehabilitation. WB Saunders, 1984:261.
8. McArdle WD, Katch FI, Katch VL. Exercise physiology, energy, nutrition, and human performance. Philadelphia: Lea & Febiger, 1981:71, 74, 81, 83, 87–91, 223–225, 316.
9. Costill DL. A scientific approach to distance running. Los Altos, CA: Track and Field News, 1979:251.
10. Walsh ML, Banister EW. Possible mechanisms of the anaerobic threshold: a review. South Med J 1988; 5:269–302.
11. Bergstrom J. Muscle electrolytes in man. Scand J Clin Lab Invest 1962;68:11–13.
12. Komi PV, Karlsson J. Physical performance, skeletal muscle enzyme activities, and fibre types in monozygous and dizygous twins of both sexes. Acta Physiol Scand Suppl 1979:462.
13. Goldberg AL, Etlinger JD, Goldspink DF, et al. Mechanism of work-induced hypertrophy of skeletal muscle. Med Sci Sports 1975;7:248–261.
14. Goldspink G. The proliferation of myofibrils during muscle fibre growth. J Cell Sci 1970;6:593–604.
15. Gollnick PD, Timson BF, Moore RL, et al. Muscular enlargement and number of fibers in skeletal muscles of rats. J Appl Physiol 1981;5:936–943.
16. Gonyea WJ. Role of exercise in inducing increases in skeletal muscle fiber number. J Appl Physiol 1980;48: 421–426.
17. Edgerton VR. Exercise and the growth and development of muscle tissue. In: Rarick GL, ed. Physical activity: human growth and development. New York: Academic Press, 1973.
18. Fox E. Sports physiology. Philadelphia: WB Saunders College Publishing, 1979:24.
19. Taylor HL, Rowell LD. Exercise and metabolism. In: Johnson W, Buskirk ER, eds. Science and medicine of exercise and sport. 2nd ed. New York: Harper & Row, 1974:84–111.
20. Mitchell JH, Sproule BJ, Chapman C. The physiological meaning of the maximal oxygen intake test. J Clin Invest 1958;37:538–547.
21. Taylor HL, Buskirk ER, Henschel A. Maximal oxygen intake as an objective measure of cardiorespiratory performance. J Appl Physiol 1955;8:73–78.
22. Wilmore JH. Training for sport and activity: the physiological basis of the condition process. 2nd ed. Boston: Allyn and Bacon, 1982.
23. Ekblom B, Hermansen L. Cardiac output in athletes. J Appl Physiol 1968;25:619.
24. Åstrand P, Cuddy T, Saltin B, et al. Cardiac output during submaximal and maximal work. J Appl Physiol 1964;19:268.
25. Kilbom A, Åstrand I. Physical training with submaximal intensities in women: part II. effect on cardiac output. Scand J Clin Lab Invest 1971;28:163.
26. Freedson P, Katch VL, Sady S, et al. Cardiac output differences in males and females during mild cycle ergometer exercise. Med Sci Sports 1979;11:16.
27. Braunwald E, Goldblatt AK, Harrison DL, et al. Studies on cardiac dimensions in intact unanesthetized man: part III. effects of muscular exercise. Circ Res 1963;13:448.
28. Simon G, Dickhuth HH, Starger JL, et al. The value of echocardiography during physical exercise. Int Sport Sci 1980;1:900. Abstract.
29. Michielli DW, Stein RA, Krasnow NL, et al. Effects of exercise training on ventricular dimensions at rest and during exercise. Med Sci Sports 1979;11:82.
30. Slutsky R, Karliner J, Ricci D, et al. Response of left ventricular volume to exercise in man assessed by radionuclide equilibrium angiography. Circulation 1979;60:565.
31. Armstrong R. Biochemistry: energy liberation and uses. In: Strauss RS, ed. Sports medicine and physiology. Philadelphia: WB Saunders, 1979.
32. Morganroth J, Maron B, Henery W, et al. Comparative left ventricular dimensions in trained athletes. Ann Intern Med 1975;82:521.
33. Holloszy J, Booth F. Biochemical adaptations to endurance exercise in muscle. Ann Rev Physiol 1976; 38:273.
34. Holloszy J, Oscai L, Mole P, et al. Biochemical adaptations to endurance exercise in skeletal muscle. In: Pernow B, Saltin B, eds. Muscle metabolism during exercise. New York: Plenum, 1971:51–66.
35. Stainsby WN, Barclay JK. Exercise metabolism: oxygen deficit, steady level oxygen uptake and oxygen uptake in recovery. Med Sci Sports 1970;2:177.
36. Golding LA, Myers CR, Sinning WE. Y's way to physical fitness. 3rd ed. Champaign, IL: Human Kinetics Publishers, 1989:35, 90.
37. Åstrand PO, Rhyming I. A nomogram for calculation of aerobic capacity from pulse rate during submaximal work. J Appl Physiol 1954;7:218–221.
38. Hornberger JP. Protocol manual: exercise screening, testing, prescription, therapeutic exercise, rehabilitation guidelines for a chiropractic and rehab facility. a practical approach. Sarasota, FL: Hornberger Publications, 1993.

39. Cureton TK. The physiological effects of exercise programs upon adults. Springfield, IL: Charles C. Thomas, 1969.
40. Cooper KH. The new aerobics. New York: JB Lippincott, 1970.
41. Cooper KH, Cooper M. The new aerobics for women. New York: Bantam Books, 1988:27, 29, 115.
42. Wilmore J. Individual exercise prescription. Am J Cardiol 1974:33:757–759.
43. Balke B. Prescribing physical activity. In: Larson L, ed. Sports medicine. New York: Academic Press, 1974: 505–523.
44. Pollock ML, Wilmore JH, Fox SM. Health and fitness through physical activity. New York: John Wiley & Sons, 1978.
45. Cooper KH. The aerobics way. New York: M. Evans and Company, 1977.

Bibliography

American College of Sports Medicine. The recommended quantity and quality of exercise for developing and maintaining fitness in healthy adults. Med Sci Sports 1978;10:vii.

American College of Sports Medicine. Guidelines for exercise testing and prescription. 3rd ed. Philadelphia: Lea & Febiger, 1986.

American Heart Association, The Committee on Exercise. Exercise testing and training of apparently healthy individuals: a handbook for physicians. New York: American Heart Association, 1972.

Andersen P, Henriksson J. Capillary supply of quadriceps femoris muscle of man: adaptive response to exercise. J Physiol (Lond) 1977;270:677–690.

Åstrand I. Aerobic work capacity in men and women with special reference to age. Acta Physiol Scand Suppl 1960;49:1.

Åstrand P, Cuddy T, Saltin B, et al. Cardiac output during submaximal and maximal work. J Appl Physiol 1964; 19:268.

Åstrand PO. Diet and athletic performance. Nutr Today 1968;3:9.

Bourne GH. Nutrition and exercise. In: Falls HB, ed. Exercise physiology. New York: Academic Press, 1968:155–171.

Brooks GA. Anaerobic threshold: review of the concept and directions for future research. Med Sci Sports 1985;17:22–31.

Burke F, Cerny F, Costill D, et al. Characteristics of skeletal muscle in competitive cyclists. Med Sci Sports 1977;9:109.

Callow M, Morton A, Guppy M. Marathon fatigue: the role of plasma fatty acids, muscle glycogen and blood glucose. Eur J Appl Physiol 1986;55:654–661.

Carlsson LA, Ekelund LG, Froberg SO. Concentrations of triglycerides, phospholipids and glycogen in skeletal muscle and free fatty acids and B-hydrocybutyric acid in blood in man in response to exercise. Eur J Clin Invest 1971; 1:248–254.

Clausen J. Effects of physical conditioning: a hypothesis concerning circulatory adjustment to exercise. Scand J Clin Lab Invest 1969;24:305.

Conconi F, Ferrari M, Ziglio PG, et al. Determination of the anaerobic threshold by a non-invasive field test in runners. J Appl Physiol 1982;52:869–873.

Costill D, Daniels J, Evans W, et al. Skeletal muscle enzymes and fiber composition in male and female track athletes. J Appl Physiol 1976;40:149.

Costill DL, Coyle E, Dalsky G, et al. Effects of elevated FFA and insulin on muscle glycogen usage during exercise. J Appl Physiol 1977;43:695–699.

Costill DL, Coyle EF, Fink WF, et al. Adaptations in skeletal muscle following strength training. J Appl Physiol 1979; 46:96.

Costill DL. Metabolic responses during distance running. J Appl Physiol 1970;28.

Coyle EF, Martin WH, Sinacore DR, et al. Time course of loss of adaptations after stopping prolonged intense endurance training. J Appl Physiol 1984;57:1857–1864.

Coyle EF, Hemmert MK, Coggan AR. Effects of detraining on cardiovascular responses to exercise: role of blood volume. J Appl Physiol 1986;60:95–99.

DeJours P. Respiration. New York: Oxford University Press, 1966.

Delorme T, Watkins, A. Techniques of progressive resistance exercise. Arch Phys Med Rehabil 1948;29:263.

Delorme T, Watkins A. Progressive resistance exercise. New York: Appleton-Century-Crofts, 1951.

Dons B, Bollerup K, Bonde-Petersen F, et al. The effects of weight-lifting exercise related to muscle fiber composition and muscle cross-sectional area in humans. Eur J Appl Physiol 1979;40:95.

Droghetti P, Borsetto C, Casoni I, et al. Non-invasive determination of the anaerobic threshold in canoeing, cross-country skiing, cycling, roller and ice-skating, rowing, and walking. Eur J Appl Physiol 1985;53:299–303.

Ekblom B, Åstrand P, Saltin B, et al. Effect of training on circulatory response to exercise. J Appl Physiol 1968;24:518.

Ekblom B. Effect of physical training on oxygen transport system in man. Acta Physiol Scand 1969;(Suppl 328):1–45.

Foster C, Costill DL, Fink WJ. Effects of pre-exercise feedings on endurance performance. Med Sci Sports 1979;11:1.

Fox E. A simple accurate technique for predicting maximal aerobic power. J Appl Physiol 1973;35:914.

Fox E, Bartels R, Billings C, et al. Intensity and distance of interval training programs and changes in aerobic power. Med Sci Sports 1973;5:18.

Fox E, Mathews D. Interval training: conditioning for sports and general fitness. Philadelphia: WB Saunders, 1974.

Fox E. Differences in metabolic alterations with sprint versus endurance interval training. In: Howald H, Poortmans J, eds. Metabolic adaptation to prolonged physical exercise. Basel: Birkhauser Verlag, 1975:119–126.

Fox E, Bartels R, Billings C, et al. Frequency and duration of interval training programs and changes in aerobic power. J Appl Physiol 1975;38:481.

Fox E, McKenzie D, Cohen K. Specificity of training: metabolic and circulatory responses. Med Sci Sports 1975;7:83.

Fox E. Physical training: methods and effects. Orthop Clin North Am 1977;8:543.

Fox E. The physiological basis for physical education and athletics. 3rd ed. Philadelphia: WB Saunders College Publishing, 1981.

Freedson P, Katch VL, Sady S, et al. Cardiac output differences in males and females during mild cycle ergometer exercise. Med Sci Sports 1979;11:16.

Frost HM. Orthopedic biomechanics. Springfield, IL: Charles C. Thomas, 1973.

Gaesser GA, Brooks GA. Metabolic base of excess post-exercise oxygen consumption: a review. Med Sci Sports 1984;16:29–43.

Giese AC. Cell physiology. Philadelphia: WB Saunders, 1979.

Gollnick P, Armstrong R, Saubert C, et al. Enzyme activity and fiber composition in skeletal muscle of untrained and trained men. J Appl Physiol 1972;33:312.

Gollnick P, Hermansen L. Biochemical adaptations to exercise: anaerobic metabolism. In: Wilmore J, ed. Exercise and sports sciences reviews. New York: Academic Press, 1973:1–43.

Gollnick PD, Armstrong RB, Saltin B, et al. Effect of training on enzyme activity and fiber composition of human skeletal muscle. J Appl Physiol 1973;34:107–111.

Goodhart RS, Shils ME. Modern nutrition in health and disease. 6th ed. Philadelphia: Lea & Febiger, 1980.

Hanson J, Tabakin B, Levy A, et al. Long-term physical training and cardiovascular dynamics in middle-aged men. Circulation 1968;38:783.

Hemmingsen E. Enhancement of oxygen transport by myoglobin. Comp Biochem Physiol 1963;10:239.

Hermansen L, Saltin B. Oxygen uptake during maximal treadmill and bicycle exercise. J Appl Physiol 1969;26:31.

Ho K, Roy R, Taylor J, et al. Muscle fiber splitting with weight-lifting exercise. Med Sci Sports 1977;9:65.

Holloszy J. Biochemical adaptations to exercise: aerobic metabolism. In: Wilmore J, ed. Exercise and sports sciences reviews. New York: Academic Press, 1973:45–71.

Holloszy J. Adaptation of skeletal muscles to endurance exercise. Med Sci Sports 1975;7:155.

Holloszy J, Booth F, Winder W, et al. Biochemical adaptation of skeletal muscle to prolonged physical exercise. In: Howald H, Poortmans J, eds. Metabolic adaptation to prolonged physical exercise. Basel: Birkhauser Verlag, 1975:438–447.

Hornberger JP. A prescriptive exercise program: chiropractic assistant's training manual. Sarasota, FL: Hornberger Publications, 1993.

Hornberger JP. A prescriptive exercise program: patient's manual. Sarasota, FL: Hornberger Publications, 1993.

Houston ME, Bentzen H, Larsen H. Inter-relationships between skeletal muscle adaptations and performance as studied by detraining and retraining. Acta Physiol Scand 1979;105:163–170.

Ivy JL, Costill DL, Fink WJ, et al. Influence of caffeine and carbohydrate feedings on endurance performance. Med Sci Sports 1979;11:6.

Jacobs I. Blood lactate and the evaluation of endurance fitness. In: Sports-science periodical on research and technology in sports. Ottawa, Ontario: The Coaching Association of Canada, 1983.

Jacobs I, Tesch PA, Bar-Or O, et al. Lactate in human skeletal muscle after 10 and 30 s of supramaximal exercise. J Appl Physiol 1983;55:365–367.

Katch FI, McArdle WD. Nutrition, weight control and exercise. Philadelphia: Lea & Febiger, 1983.

Katch FI, McArdle WD. Nutrition, weight control and exercise. Boston: Houghton Mifflin, 1977.

Kaufmann D, Swenson E, Fencl J, et al. Pulmonary function of marathon runners. Med Sci Sports 1974;6:114.

Kilbom A. Physical training in women. Scand J Clin Lab Invest 1971;28(Suppl 119):1–34.

Klausen K, Rasmussen B, Clausen J, et al. Blood lactate from exercising extremities before and after arm or leg training. Am J Physiol 1974;227:67.

Komi P, Rusko H, Vos J, et al. Anaerobic performance capacity in athletes. Acta Physiol Scand 1977;100:107.

Lehninger AL. Biochemistry. New York: Worth Publishers, 1975.

MacDougall JD, Ward GR, Sale DG, et al. Biochemical adaptation of human skeletal muscle to heavy resistance training and immobilization. J Appl Physiol 1977;43:700.

Magaria R, Aghemo I, Rovelli E. Measurement of muscular power (anaerobic) in man. J Appl Physiol 1966;21:1662.

Martin BJ, Sparks KE, Zwillich CW, et al. Low exercise ventilation in endurance athletes. Med Sci Sports 1979;11:181.

McArdle W, Magel J. Physical work capacity and maximum oxygen uptake in treadmill and bicycle exercise. Med Sci Sports 1970;2:118.

McArdle W, Katch F, Pechar G. Comparison of continuous and discontinuous treadmill and bicycle tests for max V_{O_2} Med Sci Sports 1973;5:156.

Medbo JI, Mohn A-C, Tabata I, et al. Anaerobic capacity determined by maximal accumulated oxygen deficit. J Appl Physiol 1988;64:50–60.

Merriam-Webster. Webster's new collegiate dictionary. Springfield, MA: G. & C. Merriam Company, 1975

Meyer RA, Kushmerick MJ, Dillon PF, et al. Different effects of decreased intracellular pH on contractions in fast versus slow twitch muscle. Med Sci Sports 1983;15:116.

Morgan T, Short F, Cobb L. Effect of long-term exercise on skeletal muscle lipid composition. Am J Physiol 1969; 216:82.

Morgan T, Cobb L, Short F, et al. Effects of long-term exercise on human muscle mitochondria. In: Pernow B, Saltin B, eds. Muscle metabolism during exercise. New York: Plenum, 1971:87–95.

Parkhouse WS, McKenzie DC. Possible contribution of skeletal muscle buffers to enhanced anaerobic performance: a brief review. Med Sci Sports 1984;16:328–338.

Parkhouse WS, McKenzie DC, Hochachka PW, et al. Buffering capacity of deproteinized human vastus lateralis muscle. J Appl Physiol 1985;58:14–17.

Pechar G, McArdle W, Katch K, et al. Specificity of cardiorespiratory adaptation to bicycle and treadmill training. J Appl Physiol 1974;36:753.

Pitstick MR. Balanced living: realizing your fullest potentials. Lake City, FL: Rainbow Books, 1992.

Pollock ML, Wilmore JH, Fox SM. Health and fitness through physical activity. New York: John Wiley & Sons, 1978.

Richter EA, Galbo H. High glycogen levels enhance glycogen breakdown in isolated contracting skeletal muscle. J Appl Physiol 1986;61:827–831.

Roy S, Irvin R. Sports medicine prevention, evaluation, management, and rehabilitation. Englewood Cliffs, NJ: Prentice-Hall, 1983.

Sahlin K, Henriksson J, Juhlin-Dannfelt A. Intracellular pH and electrolytes in human skeletal muscle during adrenaline and insulin infusions. Clin Sci 1984;67: 461–464.

Saltin B, Blomqvist G, Mitchell J, et al. Response to exercise after bed rest and after training. Circulation 1968;38 (Suppl 7):1–78.

Saltin B, Karlsson J. Muscle glycogen utilization during work of different intensities. In: Pernow B, Saltin B, eds. Muscle metabolism during exercise. New York: Plenum, 1971: 289–299.

Saltin B, Karlsson J. Muscle ATP, CP and lactate during exercise after physical conditioning. In: Pernow B, Saltin B, eds. Muscle metabolism during exercise. New York: Plenum, 1971:395–399.

Sapega AA, Sokolow DP, Graham TJ, et al. Phosphorous nuclear magnetic resonance: a non-invasive technique for the study of muscular bioenergetics during exercise. Med Sci Sports 1987;19:410–420.

Sawka MN, Knowlton RG, Critz JB. Thermal and circulatory responses to repeated bouts of prolonged running. Med Sci Sports 1979;11:177.

Stegmann H, Kindermann W. Comparison of prolonged exercise tests at the individual anaerobic threshold and the fixed anaerobic threshold of 4 mmol 1^{-1} lactate. Int J Sports Med 1982;3:105–110.

Stryer L. Biochemistry. San Francisco: WH Freeman and Co., 1975.

Sutton JR, Jones NL. Control of pulmonary ventilation during exercise and mediators in the blood CO_2 and hydrogen ion. Med Sci Sports 1979;11:198.

Tabakin B, Hanson J, Levy, A. Effects of physical training on the cardiovascular and respiratory response to graded upright exercise in distance runners. Br Heart J 1965;27:205, 1965.

Taylor A. The effects of exercise and training on the activities of human skeletal muscle glycogen cycle enzymes. In: Howald H, Poortmans J, eds. Metabolic adaptation to prolonged physical exercise. Basel: Birkhauser Verlag, 1975: 451–462.

Tipton CM, Matthes RD, Maynard JA, et al. The influence of physical activity on ligaments and tendons. Med Sci Sports 1975;7:165.

Tokmakidis SP, Leger LA, Fotis AV, et al. The Conconi's heart rate and lactate "anaerobic threshold." Med Sci Sports 1987;19:S17.

Urhausen A, Kullmer T, Kindermann W. A 7-week follow-up study of the behaviour of testosterone and cortisol during the competition period in rowers. Eur J Appl Physiol 1987;56:528–533.

Vander AJ, et al. Human physiology: the mechanisms of body function. New York: McGraw-Hill, 1975.

Vandewalle H, Peres G, Monod H. Standard anaerobic exercise tests. South Med J 1987;4:268–289.

Witzmann FA, Fink WJ, Foster CC, et al. Changes in muscle lipid metabolism during endurance training. Med Sci Sports 1978;10:41.

4

Conservative Rehabilitation of Athletic Injuries

William J. Moreau, Larry Kintner, and Edward J. Ryan III

To be effective and efficient in addressing athletic injuries, rehabilitation must play a fundamental role in the care of the injured athlete. Proper rehabilitation will facilitate the safe return of athletes to athletic participation. Each program must be specific for the individual, the specific injury, and the demands of the athlete's sport. To develop a rehabilitation program, the physician must perform a comprehensive analysis of the treatment requirements of the specific injury in terms of the specific requirements of the sporting activity. Considering this philosophy, the most accurate gauge of when athletes are able to return to full participation is their functional ability to perform the specific skills required by their sport. This is in contrast to showing only increases in strength and range of motion or reductions in pain and edema.

Conducting a rehabilitation program does not necessarily require a high-tech clinic, weight room, or training room. The effectiveness and appropriateness of low-tech rehabilitation have been reported (1). Using a low-tech approach also enables the patient to exercise at home instead of traveling to perform exercises.

The physician should plan the program so the injured athlete can have easy access to any equipment that may be needed. Successful programs are achieved by being creative in applying conditioning principles and keeping a positive progressive functional outcome in mind when planning the athlete's rehabilitation program. A complete rehabilitative program can be structured by setting up and striving to attain goals (Fig. 4.1). The exact method of accomplishing these goals is not critical; however, the proper application of reconditioning principles is critical. The physician must use realistic time frames when dealing with sports injuries. Athletes are highly motivated individuals, and prematurely returning them to athletics can lead to reinjury and chronic problems. Alternatives to the regular athletic activities should be provided once it is decided that the athlete must stop participating in the sport. Serious athletes will be more responsive to the treatment plan that is outlined if it leads them to alternative methods of improving their game while they get rehabilitation for their injury. For example, a tennis player with an elbow injury that prohibits playing tennis can be directed to perform a lower extremity exercise program or another cross-training activity that will enhance the player's game on return to the sport.

In determining the criteria for return to play, one must consider the preinjury level of fitness and sport ability of the athlete. The physician determines if the athlete has had an examination that will provide information about baseline physical condition. Returning the athlete's functional level to a level one higher than the preinjury status is essential in many situations, because the athlete's preinjury level may not have been sufficient to prevent injury. To reduce the chance of reinjury, the athlete must achieve a higher level of performance. The means of achieving this goal is through a progressive exercise rehabilitation prescription. The exercise progression will use sport-specific exercises that are modified according to the athlete's skill level and the severity of the injury. There are five basic components to include in this prescription (Fig. 4.2).

The athlete must also have confidence in the treating doctor. This can be attained by carefully explaining the athlete's diagnosis and by outlining the rehabilitation program in detail. Explaining the need for the program is esasential; and how following the plan will return the athlete to the sport in the quickest and safest manner. It is

1. Preserve structural integrity
2. Provide an environment conductive to tissue healing
3. Restore joint range of motion
4. Increase muscular strength
5. Restore proprioception
6. Maintain and increase cardiovascular aerobic capacity
7. Enhance coordinated movement and agility in sport-specific tasks

Figure 4.1. Goals for rehabilitation.

also essential to describe how each component will reestablish flexibility, strength, and skills needed to return to play as quickly as possible.

FOUR PHASES OF REHABILITATION

This section presents a general rehabilitation program for injuries. Each athlete is unique, and the physician must design a program to rehabilitate the athlete according to that person's specific needs (2). The key to rehabilitation is to find those activities that will safely accomplish established goals in the minimum amount of time, while still keeping the athlete's interest throughout the program. The athlete's rehabilitation program should be set up according to the injury's phase or stage of healing. Typically, there are four phases of treatment through which the athlete will progress. Each phase will address specific goals in the rehabilitation process (Fig. 4.3). Not all athletes present in the acute phase of injury; many present with chronic complaints that may require placement in a phase other than phase I initially.

There are three important physiologic principles in the establishment of a rehabilitation program. The first of these is the overload principle. It states that the athlete must subject muscle and connective tissue to a load greater than that of the usual stresses of daily activity if muscle hypertrophy is to occur (3, 4). The second principle is the principle of specific adaptation, which states that the athlete must specifically exercise the muscles for the task at hand, so they will adapt in very specific ways. This is known as the specific adaptations to imposed demands (SAID) principle. It is important to remember that the more specific the exercise that the athlete is to perform, the more specific the resultant muscle adaptation is (5). The third principle is the overtraining principle, which is very important in athletic rehabilitation and training. With exercise, muscle breakdown occurs, and the body requires adequate rest to repair and strengthen itself.

With too much training and too little rest, the body cannot make repairs and rehabilitation will cause injury (6).

Phase I

Rehabilitation should begin as soon as an athletic injury occurs. The physician must properly treat the athlete in the acute stage to control collateral damage by limiting swelling, soft tissue injury, and atrophy (7, 8). Supportive taping and bracing are important components of this phase. Bracing will enable the athlete to begin exercises earlier and allow for regaining lost function, while still allowing the injury to subside and heal with as little additional damage as possible.

In phase I, the exercises should include isometric strengthening exercises and static muscle stretches. The goal of these exercises is to create a flexible and strong scar tissue that is oriented in the connective tissue lines of stress. There should never be pain during this phase secondary to performing these activities. Pain is a warning that further damage is occurring.

The athlete should perform isometric exercises as soon as possible in the rehabilitation process. Isometric exercises are, by definition, muscle contractions during which the length of the muscle remains the same (8). This type of muscle contraction allows for localized muscle exercise without joint movement. The athlete should perform the exercises for multiple sets at multiple joint angles (9). There is a 20° crossover from isometric activities that creates a strength gain on each side of the position of contraction (10). To recruit as many muscle fibers as possible, the athlete should perform pain-free isometric contractions as close to a maximal level as possible (11). At first the athlete will probably perform at a submaximal level, which should be expected in the acute phase of a more severe injury. Typically, the athlete should perform two to three sets of 10-second contractions using 10 repetitions at each joint position, with repetition of the series two to three times daily. A good point to remember is that performing exercises twice daily will yield a greater improvement than performing ex-

1. Type of exercise
2. Intensity of exercise
3. Duration of exercise
4. Frequency of exercise
5. Progression of exercise

Figure 4.2. Components of the exercise prescription.

Phase I	Isometric Exercise
	Static Stretching
	Pain-Free ROM
Phase II	Isometric Exercise
	Open-Chain Activities
	Therapeutic Muscle Stretching
	Aerobic Activity
	Proprioceptive Drills
Phase III	Eccentric Exercise
	Closed-Chain Activities
	Aerobic Activity
	Running or Throwing Drills
Phase IV	Dynamic Flexibility Exercise
	Sport-Specific Strengthening Exercise
	Agility Drills
	Plyometric Training

Figure 4.3. Phases of rehabilitation.

ercises once a day, especially in the early phases of rehabilitation (12).

Isometric exercises can take place in the frontal, sagittal, or coronal planes or a combination of all three planes. An example of this would be isometric hip flexion. The athlete can perform hip flexion with the foot in a neutral position and the hip in various angles of hip flexion. This same activity of hip flexion can then recruit different muscles by placing the hip into abduction at different angles and continuing to change the hip angle from full extension to full flexion. Internally rotating or externally rotating the hip in any of these angles will again recruit different muscle fibers. Finally, flexing the knee creates yet more variables for this one exercise. The physician can use this same concept for all musculoskeletal injuries.

The athlete needs to maintain flexibility and pain-free range of motion using exercises in the same way. Initially, the physician should prescribe static stretches because the athlete will be able to control these maneuvers easily (Fig. 4.4) (13–16). The same thought process that went into isometric muscle contraction should go into static stretch positions. Using an example of a hamstring strain, initially the athlete will be able to stretch the hamstring in a supine straight leg position only. As the injury resolves, the athlete will be able to add additional positions such as the seated and standing leg positions. Additional changes of internal or external hip rotation in all three body positions will incorporate different muscle involvement. It is important to teach the athlete to use this knowledge in performing all lower extremity muscle stretches.

Phase II

In most cases, the initiation of phase II activity is signaled by the athlete's ability to perform isotonic strengthening exercises. Isotonic exercises should be started when there is a full range of motion and the athlete can perform these exercises in a pain-free state (17). Isotonic muscle contractions occur when the length of the muscle changes while the tension on the muscle remains essentially the same. Concentric isotonic contractions are said to perform positive work and result in a contraction in which the individual muscle fibers shorten as the origin and insertion of the muscle approximate. Eccentric isotonic contractions are negative work (18). The working muscle fibers go through a lengthening process as the origin and insertion move apart. Isotonic exercises are a common form of strength training. They typically relate more closely to sporting activities than isometric exercise does.

Initially, concentric activities are the most important. The athlete will perform a combination of open- and closed-chain activities. Open-chain exercises are those exercises performed with the terminal component of the kinetic chain relatively free or not fixed. For example, when an athlete performs knee extensions while seated with the foot not in contact with the ground or another supporting structure, that athlete is performing open-chain exercises of the quadriceps. Open-chain exercises have the advantage of being easier for the athlete to perform. They can also be used to isolate the injured muscle.

In contrast, closed-chain exercises are those in which the terminal point of the kinetic chain is in contact with the ground or a supporting structure. An example of a closed-chain exercise for the quadriceps is the squat. There are multiple advantages to performing closed-chain activities during rehabilitation, the first of which is that closed-chain exercise can produce a force localized precisely at the joint, instead of distal to the joint, thereby reducing the joint reaction forces. Closed-chain exercises are more sports-specific and their muscular movement is a functional movement. With the lower extremity muscles working in uni-

1. Athlete is relaxed
2. Enter stretch position slowly
3. Stretch should not be painful
4. Maintain stretch for 10–30 seconds for 10 or more repetitions

Figure 4.4. Static stretching and range-of-motion guidelines.

son, the motion occurs in all three planes and the activity requires balance and coordination. Athletes may use their body weight or tubing to perform the concentric exercise when starting. Later, they may progress to more traditional exercises as their strength increases (19).

The athlete should also perform isotonic exercises at multiple joint angles. An example of this is a straight-leg raise, which can be performed in a variety of ways. Traditionally, the athlete is supine with the opposite leg bent, while keeping the injured leg straight and raising it to an angle where that side is level with the opposite leg. The athlete can then either hold the leg isometrically or perform multiple repetitions. There are many variations of this open-chain activity, such as rising up, resting on the elbows, or sitting. The exercise becomes more difficult with greater amounts of upper body angle. As with isometrics or flexibility exercises, the physician can augment the standard position by adding internal or external hip rotation to recruit different muscle fibers. Adding weights, rubber bands, or tubing to increase the resistance provides another helpful option. These modification concepts may be used with as many of the exercises as possible.

Bilateral mini-squats will probably be the first closed chain activity attempted with lower extremity injuries (20), with a progression from bilateral to unilateral mini-squats. Step-ups are the next closed chain activity the athlete will often include in the program. The athlete can perform step-ups in the sagittal plane (forward step-up) or in the transverse plane (lateral step-up). To help eliminate pushing off with the noninvolved leg, the step-up should be started with the heel of the noninvolved foot on the floor (20).

In a hamstring strain, for example, the strengthening exercises to be performed would include hip extensor, flexor, adductor, and abductor exercises. Mini-squats and step-ups should concentrate on the lowering phase to fire the hamstring muscles. The athlete should also be performing multiple sets of hamstring curls in the prone and sitting positions.

Dynamic flexibility or therapeutic muscle-stretching exercises should also be initiated in phase II. There are many proprioceptive neuromuscular facilitation patterns and techniques available (21). These include a variety of therapeutic stretching exercises. These active stretching techniques use the concepts of postisometric relaxation, motor learning, and reciprocal inhibition. These and other techniques increase flexibility and are to be initiated during this phase.

The last part of phase II is aerobic activity (7, 22). Athletes will prolong their return to competition if they do not continue aerobic activities during the rehabilitation process (18). The aerobic activities must be pain-free and should be as close to the athlete's sporting activity as possible. Aerobic exercise can be achieved by activities such as running or by use of many different types of equipment (stationary bike, stepper machine, tracked ski machine, slide board, activities in a pool, upper body ergometer, or treadmill). Most cases require the use of a combination of many aerobic activities to allow the athlete to exercise for longer periods without aggravation or reinjury.

One more exercise that may be included in phase II is retro (backward) walking. The athlete performs this exercise using a treadmill for walking up a slight to moderate incline. This exercise shifts the emphasis during stance phase from concentric quadriceps activity to concentric hamstring activity.

Phase III

The exercises and activities during phase III will continue to prepare the athlete for return to play in the next phase. This phase should continue strengthening exercises and initiate eccentric activities, which are introduced as the final set of a three- or four-set exercise. Later as the athlete's strength improves, three to four sets of eccentric exercises may be performed.

In the example of a hamstring strain, the athlete performs eccentric exercise by slowly extending the leg from a flexed position during a prone hamstring curl. This results in muscle activity of the hamstring while it is undergoing lengthening. The hamstring injury often occurs during a hurdling maneuver, in which the knee is fully extended and the hip is flexed. Before sending the athlete back to competition, reproduce this position during a strengthening exercise. This allows the doctor to control the amount of work the muscle is required to perform while in a position similar to the one in which the injury initially occurred. The athlete can also perform this exercise using rubber tubing to achieve an eccentric contraction of the hamstrings.

The athlete will now perform functional activities before returning to competition. This allows for gradual increases of activity in a controlled environment. The first activity attempted is jumping (20). Jumping drills are initiated by having the athlete jump forward and backward over a line taped on the floor. Emphasis is placed on landing on each side of the line as rapidly as possible. Once the athlete can tolerate front-to-back jumping, side-to-side and then diagonal jumping can begin. The athlete can perform diagonal jumping drills using two lines of tape in the shape of a plus sign, jumping diagonally between the quadrants. Initially, the jumping drill should emphasize technique that minimizes jump height. As performance improves, the height of the jump should increase. The jumping drill should also progress from bilateral maneuvers to unilateral activities.

The next stage of functional activities should include figure-eight and cutting drills. With figure eights, the change of direction is initially more gradual, thus allowing the athlete to build slowly to more strenuous cutting activities. Figure-eight patterns are initiated over a distance of 40 yards, with performance of 10 repetitions at half speed (jogging), then 10 repetitions at three-quarter speed (running), and finally 10 repetitions at full speed. This procedure is repeated at 20- and 10-yard distances. These cutting drills should be performed with the participant approaching a predetermined spot at which to make the cut. The athlete first jogs to the spot and performs the cut, followed by cutting at a three-quarter speed sprint, and finally at a full-speed sprint. Initial cutting angles of 45° are used, progressing to 60°, and finally to 90°.

Phase IV

In phase IV the ultimate goal is the return of the athlete to play and the maintenance of strength and flexibility gains. The athlete should continue to perform dynamic flexibility exercises. The athlete should perform specific strengthening exercises designed to continue to increase and maintain strength. These exercises could include concentric and eccentric strengthening activities such as curls, lunges, squats, and running.

REHABILITATION OF SPECIFIC INJURIES

Hamstring Strains

Injuries to the hamstring muscles most often occur during eccentric muscle contractions associated with running or jumping (23). During rehabilitation exercises it is important, if possible, to place the muscle into the position in which it was injured. Hamstring injuries tend to heal with moderate amounts of scar tissue. It is common for an athlete to reinjure the hamstring muscle; therefore, a rapid progression of agility drills should be avoided (24, 25). It is important to completely rehabilitate this injury to prevent its recurrence. Eccentric muscle work should provide an important component of the program, and these exercises can be achieved by isokinetic equipment, leg curls, or manual resistance. Placement of the patient in the prone position while exercising will provide the muscle length to tension ratio closest to that of running.

Adductor Strains

Adductor muscle strains are common (26). They tend to heal well, but often require a long time before the athlete feels comfortable and secure coming back to competition. During phase I and phase II exercises, bilateral isometric adduction is important. The athlete can use a volleyball for resistance during this exercise and should perform the exercise at multiple joint angles. The slide board is a fine rehabilitation tool for adductor strains. The exercise is begun with the bumpers close together, increasing the distance between the bumpers as the athlete becomes stronger (27). A mixture of endurance and interval activities can be used on the slide board. Endurance sets on the slide board can be performed by placing the bumpers wide apart and using long steady slides for longer periods. The interval sets can begin with 20 seconds and progress to 2 or more minutes. During interval sets, the athlete should concentrate on very brisk and deliberate slides. Adequate recovery time should be provided between intervals by having the athlete slow the slide pace.

Iliotibial Band Friction Syndrome

The iliotibial-band friction syndrome is primarily an overuse injury that presents in long- distance runners and cyclists (28, 29). Training errors are often the cause, especially sudden increases in mileage or intensity. Other causes are downhill running, excessive stride length, overpronation, and angular surfaces (30). In the cyclist, a common cause is equipment that does not fit properly. The bulk of rehabilitation is aimed at increasing the flexibility of the iliotibial band (Fig. 4.5).

Knee Rehabilitation

Rehabilitation of injuries of the knee is dependent on whether the injury was nontraumatic or traumatic. Rehabilitation of each is different because traumatic knee injuries treated by surgical intervention often include severe soft tissue damage and atrophy. Rehabilitation after surgery may be coordinated with the surgeon.

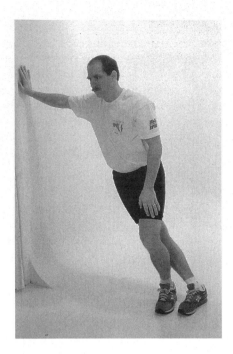

Figure 4.5. Standing iliotibial band stretch.

Nontraumatic injuries include patellar-femoral tracking problems, proximal and distal patellar tendinitis, distal hamstring tendinitis, and iliotibial band friction syndrome localized to the lateral knee.

GENERAL REHABILITATION OF KNEE INJURIES

Phase I

The athlete should perform isometrics and static flexibility exercises during phase I. These should concentrate on using various joint angles and achieving a full range of motion. The athlete may be instructed to swim, using a kickboard if needed. Patellar mobilization has also been helpful.

Phase II

Isotonic exercises and active stretches should be initiated. There should be a good balance between open-chain exercises (straight leg raises, leg extensions, and leg curls) and closed-chain exercises (short arc quadriceps extensions, mini-squats, lateral and frontal step-ups, and lunges) (31). Use of therapeutic stretching protocols for all lower extremity muscles is helpful, as is having the athlete run in place while wearing a personal flotation device in deeper water.

Phase III

This phase should concentrate on eccentric activities and increasing aerobic capacity. Many activities that cause nontraumatic knee injuries are due to a large aerobic component associated with the athlete's activity (32). The previously described jumping and cutting drills should be included here.

Phase IV

The key to return to play for these conditions is to ensure proper patellar tracking, mobility, adequate knee flexibility, and proper quadriceps strengthening, especially of the muscle's eccentric ability (33).

PATELLAR-FEMORAL TRACKING PROBLEMS

There are many factors associated with patellar-femoral tracking problems. The key to successful rehabilitation of these problems is first to assess any biomechanical problems associated with the condition (34). Failure to treat these problems first will often result in failure of rehabilitation.

Patellar tracking requires a balance between the strength of the medial-knee soft tissue and the flexibility of the lateral-knee soft tissue. Atrophy of the vastus medialis oblique muscle may be associated with tracking problems (35). This muscle may be strengthened using many exercises, but one that is especially effective is maximal isometric quadriceps contraction in a semilunge position (36). It is very important for the athlete to concentrate on the task to exercise the vastus medialis oblique selectively. The soft tissue of the lateral knee includes the lateral retinaculum and the distal iliotibial band. The athlete can stretch these structures using the distal iliotibial band stretch shown previously for iliotibial band syndrome treatment (37).

The hip abductors and lateral rotators may also be weak in the athlete with patellofemoral pain (38). The athlete can isolate these muscles for exercise by performing side-lying hip abduction with the hip in a neutral position. The athlete must be careful to avoid substitution by the tensor fascia lata (TFL) during hip abduction. This is achieved by keeping the foot and hip in the neutral position.

Anatomically, the vastus medialis oblique arises from the adductor magnus tendon. Therefore, it is important that adductor muscle exercises be included in patella-femoral rehabilitation (39). Initially the athlete should perform isometric adduction exercises, which facilitate vastus medialis oblique contraction. This exercise also helps to de-emphasize the role of vastus lateralis and rectus femoris muscles in initiating the contraction. Later bilateral isometric and isotonic activities may be added.

Ankle Sprain Rehabilitation

Ankle injuries in the general sporting population are very common (40, 41). The majority of isolated ankle sprains are of the lateral ligaments (42). Rehabilitation should concentrate on strengthening the lateral ankle-supporting structures and enhancing and restoring proprioception (43, 44).

PHASE I

As mentioned previously, rehabilitation should start at the onset of injury. This is especially true with ankle sprains. If the physician can limit swelling, through an open taping technique or compressive bracing, the athlete will be able to initiate earlier rehabilitation of the ankle at an accelerated pace.

Phase I of ankle rehabilitation begins with reestablishing range of motion and using pain-free isometric contractions of the ankle in all planes of motion. Later, as ankle range improves, "alphabet" range-of-motion exercises are added (43). These exercises can be performed by having the athlete get in a whirlpool use the first toe as a pointer and repeatedly go through the motions of writing the alphabet with the toe and ankle. The whirlpool temperature should be 105°F, and the duration of these drills should be 20 minutes. If swelling is encountered after whirlpool treatment, ice may be applied with compression for an additional 20 minutes. Weight-bearing should be encouraged as tolerated.

PHASE II

Phase II goals include the following:

1. Full range of motion,
2. Initiation of isotonic exercises,
3. Beginning proprioceptive activities, and
4. Pain-free aerobic activities.

The athlete should continue range of motion exercises as initiated in phase I. It is extremely important in the rehabilitation of ankle injuries to obtain the full range of motion, and this should be stressed to the athlete. Dorsiflexion is one of the more difficult motions to recover. The athlete can be instructed to walk up stairs backward, while using a handrail for support, to facilitate the recovery of this motion.

Isotonic exercises are begun using band tubing, with bands selected by their degree of resistance. The ankle joint in inversion and eversion has a small range of motion, so it is important to use a tubing form that does not stretch far. The athlete is asked to perform exercises including ankle eversion, inversion, dorsiflexion, and plantar flexion. Different resistance bands will often be required for the different muscle groups. Multiple positions are accomplished by changing the degree of dorsiflexion or plantar flexion, internally or externally rotating the foot, or bending the knee. The athlete should perform these exercises to fatigue, and then should start heel raises to strengthen the ankle plantar flexor.

Pain-free aerobic activities, which could include cycling, ski machines, pool activities, or stair climbers, are initiated in this phase.

PHASE III

The athlete should perform maximum exercise, which includes maximal-effort surgical tubing exercise, during this phase to prepare for the return to play. Complex proprioceptive activities and increased aerobic activities should also be stressed. The athlete should begin jumping rope, if possible, to simulate athletic activities. Other aerobic activities from phase II should be continued, and treadmill walking should be initiated. The physician should have the athlete walk forward, uphill, and retro. The athlete who can perform in the lateral position, should also attempt side walking drills.

PHASE IV

On return to play, the athlete should continue a maintenance program that may include balance exercises, rubber tubing exercises (Fig. 4.6), and slide-board activities.

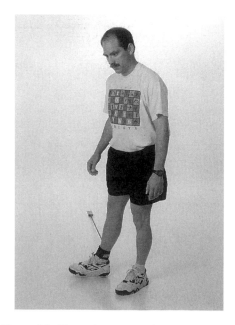

Figure 4.6. Using tubing to train for the soccer kick.

Upper Extremity Rehabilitation of Rotator Cuff Injuries in the Overhand Athlete

Repetitive overhand activities such as throwing, tennis, or volleyball place the athlete at risk for overuse injuries (45). The glenohumeral joint is inherently unstable because capsular, ligamentous, cartilaginous, and muscular structures provide most of the stability. There is little static stabilization at the glenohumeral joint.

The repetitive, high-velocity nature of throwing can lead to microtrauma and resultant impingement on the musculotendinous stabilizers. If the diagnosis of impingement is made, then scapulothoracic stabilization and strengthening must be accomplished before aggressive rotator cuff strengthening is initiated (46). The mode of failure is almost always eccentric. This leads to decreased or asynchronous firing of the injured muscles and, consequently, less dynamic joint stability. This places a larger burden on the static stabilizers to maintain stability. In time, these static restraints may also fail, leading to subtle or frank glenohumeral instability. Altered biomechanics due to instability can lead to secondary impingement in the coracoacromial arch as the humeral head rides anteriorly and superiorly. It is common for overhand athletes to present with instability and secondary impingement injury.

The goal of rehabilitation of the overhand athlete is to stabilize the humeral head functionally. The athlete can accomplish this by improving the function of the rotator cuff and the scapulothoracic stabilizers, restoring scapulohumeral rhythm and shoulder proprioception, and increasing flexibility of the shoulders' internal rotators and posterior capsule (47).

There are basic rules in shoulder rehabilitation that should result in a successful outcome.

1. Rehabilitate the shoulder in functional planes of motion. Perform exercises anterior to the scapular plane or in the scapular plane, which is generally a pain-free range.
2. Use short lever arms to strengthen the shoulder. Initiate passive and active movements with the elbow flexed to decrease torque about the shoulder. This is important early in the rehabilitation program, particularly in the athlete who is experiencing pain.
3. Gain muscular control of the arm in the deceleration phase of throwing. In this phase, the stresses occur, making the shoulder more prone to injury. Because most injury appears to occur during eccentric loading of the muscle, it is important to strengthen ec-

centrically the external rotators of the cuff, biceps brachii, and latissimus dorsi.
4. Obtain a stable scapular platform, which is essential for success in any shoulder rehabilitation or conditioning program (45).
5. The exercise program in the overhand athlete should attempt to reproduce forces and loading rates that will approach the athlete's functional demands.
6. Start rehabilitation with the muscles closest to the midline and work distally. Start with scapular protraction and retraction.

Hydrotherapy has been found to be very effective in treating athletes with difficult shoulder problems that are not responding to the standard treatment regimen (47). The basic exercises include shoulder flexion and extension in the sagittal and scapular planes while the arms are kept completely submerged. The athlete can also work through proprioceptive neuromuscular facilitation (PNF) patterns while using the water for buoyancy and resistance. The athlete can use paddles or water baffles for increased resistance while regaining function and strength. Athletes should be cautioned not to push themselves too hard during this exercise program; many patients feel overly secure in this environment.

PHASE I

This phase begins with early motion exercises, which are performed with a T-bar in pain-free shoulder flexion, external rotation, and internal rotation. During flexion motion, the athlete should lead with the thumb to clear the greater tuberosity from under the coracoacromial arch. Shoulder external and internal rotations are initiated at 0° abduction, progress to 45°, and finally to 90° of abduction. Capsular stretches for the posterior and inferior capsule begin with a static stretch avoiding further impingement. The posterior capsule stretch can be achieved by having the athlete adduct the arm across the body toward the opposite shoulder. The inferior capsule stretch is performed by flexing the shoulder maximally forward and modifying the triceps stretch, then pulling the involved elbow across the back instead of straight posterior (45).

Isometrics are the initial muscle contraction performed (48). The shoulder exercises should include:

1. Abduction at 30° and 60°,
2. External rotation at 0° and 30° abduction,
3. Internal rotation at 0° and 30° abduction,
4. Elbow flexion at various angles, and

5. Scapular protraction and retraction at 30° and 60° of arm flexion.

Isometric muscle contractions are performed to reinitiate rotator cuff function while preventing excessive uncontrollable humeral head migration (49). The athlete performs the contractions submaximally, at multiple joint angles in a pain-free fashion. At the end of this phase, the muscle contractions will be closer to maximal effort.

The final step in phase I is weight-bearing co-contractions (48), which are performed in side-to-side, forward-to-backward, and diagonal movements. These weight-bearing exercises are performed with the athlete standing or kneeling, placing a proportionate amount of body weight through the hands. The athlete is instructed to shift his weight in the appropriate direction. As the athlete improves, this exercise progresses to using manual resistance, then a large ball, and finally a smaller ball to provide an unstable platform for closed-chain loading. Hand placement can progress in this exercise from the sides of the ball, to the top of the ball, then to one hand on top of the other.

Criteria for initiation of phase II include full pain-free range of motion, minimal tenderness and pain, and good strength of the rotator cuff (grade 4 muscle strength on a scale of 1–5, with 5 being the strongest).

PHASE II

Phase II strengthening exercises progress from maximal isometric muscular contractions to submaximal isotonic contractions. The goals of this phase are to improve muscular strength, endurance, and neuromuscular control of the shoulder complex.

Codmans pendular exercises are begun in rotation and linear movements. It is important to use a device attached to the athlete's wrist so that stabilizing muscular activity is not produced in the shoulder, minimizing the desired effect. The athlete must recognize that arm movement is like a pendulum, passive and secondary to trunk movement.

The isotonic contractions should be performed in concentric fashion. Those exercises to perform are:

1. Abduction from 30° to 90°,
2. Supraspinatus isolation from 30° to 90°,
3. Flexion from 30° to 90°,
4. Extension from 0° to 30°,
5. External rotation at 30° with a rolled towel under arm,

6. Internal rotation also at 30° with the rolled towel under the arm,
7. Biceps curls at 35° of shoulder flexion,
8. Diagonal (D2) pattern flexion, if pain-free, with isometric holds at 30°, 60°, 90°, and 120°.

Isometric holds of 2 seconds are added as soon as possible at two to three points of the isotonic exercise. This type of hold emphasizes cocontraction and glenohumeral steering and the effect of the biceps brachii long head and shoulder extensors as strong humeral depressors.

Strengthening of the scapulothoracic musculature is imperative for normal glenohumeral joint function. The scapulothoracic articulation must provide a stable base and proximal stability to allow distal mobility of the arm (50). The stabilization should start at the proximal aspect of the kinetic chain. The serratus anterior is important in fixing the scapula to the chest wall. Those exercises to perform should include:

1. Rowing activities,
2. Upright rows,
3. Latissimus pull-downs,
4. Push-up with exaggerated movement at the end of the push-up to strengthen the subscapularis muscle (51, 52),
5. Push-offs, and
6. Press-ups.

The last new exercises to be performed during phase II are doctor-assisted neuromuscular control exercises. The athlete is lying on the contralateral side. The involved hand is placed on the table with the shoulder abducted to 90° and internally rotated. The drill is for the athlete to slowly elevate and depress the scapula, then retract and protract the scapula against the doctor's manual resistance. The goal of this activity is the isolation of scapular movements (53), with the physician using progressive manual resistance as the athlete masters the movement.

PHASE III

The emphasis of exercise for this stage is high-speed, high-energy strengthening drills, eccentric muscular contraction, and diagonal movements in functional positions (48). To begin this stage, the athlete must exhibit full nonpainful range of motion, no pain or tenderness, and strength equal to 70% of the contralateral shoulder.

The athlete should continue isotonic muscular exercises with progressive increases in the arc of motion and add eccentric contractions. The exercises to perform are:

1. Flexion from 0° to 60° with isometric holds of 2 seconds at two points,
2. Flexion from 60° to 120° with isometric holds again at two points,
3. External rotation at 90° abduction and 90° elbow flexion,
4. Internal rotation also in the 90°/90° position,
5. Biceps curls through a full range of motion,
6. Diagonal (D2) flexion pattern with isometric holds at various places, and
7. Diagonal (D2) extension pattern also with isometric holds at various positions.

If equipment is available, plyometric activities should begin at this point. The athlete can perform medicine ball throws with a 4-lb plyoball and plyobay. The exercises to be performed include:

1. Soccer throw,
2. Chest pass,
3. Step and pass,
4. Side throw, and
5. One arm throw and catch.

The athlete should perform four sets of eight repetitions of each exercise. These activities allow the athlete to overload the shoulder with a heavy object to throw and then to create eccentric activity when catching the plyoball. Two other exercises used for balance and strength include the plyometric push-up and the same push-up on a balance board.

PHASE IV

When athletes are able to return to competition, they should continue to maintain the strength developed in rehabilitation to remain injury-free. They should continue progressive isotonic weight-training, performing three to five sets of 10 to 15 repetitions 3 days per week. The exercises to perform are:

1. Supraspinatus position with a 5-lb dumbbell,
2. External rotation at 90° of abduction of the shoulder with tubing,
3. Internal rotation at 90° of abduction of the shoulder with tubing,
4. Diagonal (D2) pattern for shoulder flexion and extension with exercise tubing,
5. Dumbbell lateral raises with external rotation,
6. Elbow flexion and extension exercise,
7. Dips with terminal shoulder depression,
8. Shoulder shrugs,
9. Latissimus pull-downs,
10. Seated rowing,
11. Bench press with a focus on the terminal range to elicit the serratus anterior, and
12. Lower body (trunk) stabilization exercises, which would be appropriate to round out this routine as most throwing activities require a stable lower body.

Elbow Rehabilitation

PHASE I

In the first phase of elbow rehabilitation, the goals are to reestablish nonpainful range of motion, decrease pain and inflammation, and retard muscular atrophy. The exercise prescription should be designed to minimize the effects of immobilization in all instances while respecting the healing constraints of the tissues involved (54).

When bracing athletes with lateral epicondylitis, it is important to make sure that the athlete positions the counterbalance brace correctly over the proximal extensor carpi radialis brevis muscle belly. If the brace is placed correctly, the athlete should be able to contract the fist with decreased lateral elbow pain.

The athlete's pain level is used as a guide for initiating and increasing the exercise program (55). Active-assisted and passive range-of-motion exercise in all planes of elbow and wrist motion prevents the formation of scar tissue and occurrence of adhesions. The reestablishment of full elbow extension is a primary goal during this initial phase of the rehabilitation process. By obtaining full elbow extension, the organization and alignment of collagen fibers will be improved, preventing elbow flexion contracture.

An effective exercise designed to obtain full elbow extension is passive elbow extension using a handheld weight to produce a passive overpressure extension stretch. Place a towel roll posterior to the elbow joint to effect a greater extension movement during this activity. This stretch is performed for 5 to 7 minutes with a light weight (2 to 4 lb), thus using a long-duration, low-intensity stretch.

An additional focus in the early phase of rehabilitation is retarding the muscular atrophy of the elbow and wrist musculature. The athlete is instructed to perform submaximal isometric exercises for elbow flexion and extension as well as for wrist flexion, extension, pronation, and supination. The athlete should perform three to five sets of 10 isometric repetitions at multiple joint angles.

PHASE II

Stretching exercises are continued to maintain elbow extension, flexion, pronation, and supination. The muscles are placed in their lengthened state for stretching. In addition, the athlete should perform stretches for the wrist flexor and extensors and shoulder muscles. This will help prepare the athlete for the eventual return to sporting activities.

The athlete should perform dumbbell or tubing progressive resistive exercises for the biceps, triceps, pronator, supinator, and wrist flexor and extensors. In addition, the athlete should strengthen the shoulder complex late in this phase of the rehabilitation program. The shoulder program emphasizes proximal stability for distal mobility to ensure adequate neuromuscular performance as well as muscular strength and power in the performance of all upper extremity activities.

Finally in this phase, the athlete should perform neuromuscular control exercises for the elbow and shoulder muscular complexes to enhance the ability of the muscles to control the elbow joint during functional activities. These exercises include proprioceptive neuromuscular facilitation exercises such as diagonal patterns with dynamic stabilization and proprioceptive activities such as push-up on a wobble board or gym ball.

PHASE III

The exercises to perform in this phase include plyometric exercise, high-speed and high-energy strengthening, and eccentric muscular contractions performed in functional positions.

The elbow flexors are exercised by using elastic exercise tubing and emphasizing slow and fast muscular contractions in a concentric and eccentric fashion. The athlete can perform plyometric exercise for the biceps using exercise tubing (54). The athlete initiates this plyometric exercise with the elbow fully flexed, the shoulder flexed to 60°, and the exercise tubing held in the hand. The athlete then releases this isometric hold, allowing the elbow to extend rapidly (eccentric phase). When the athlete reaches full elbow extension, the elbow is quickly reversed to full flexion to complete the plyometric activity (concentric phase).

Advanced exercises using a weighted medicine ball should start in phase III. Other forms of plyometric or proprioceptive exercises begin at this time, including box push-ups progressing to plyo–push-ups, balance board push-ups, or Swiss ball exercises.

PHASE IV

The goal of this phase is to assure that athletes achieve adequate motion, strength, and functional capabilities before return to competitive participation. Athletes continue to progress with functional drills that prepare them to return to their specific sport (Fig. 4.7).

Conservative Rehabilitation of the Wrist

The treatment of the wrist, as well as other injuries, must be initiated with an accurate diagnosis. Several serious injuries, including fracture, can present with minimal associated complaints. The diagnosis of a wrist sprain can be made only as a diagnosis of exclusion. Wrist injuries after fracture and immobilization must initially focus on regaining active range of motion while preserving the patient's pain-free state. Instabilities of the wrist will provide a clinical challenge for even the most experienced clinicians.

The primary focus should be on regaining active motion and then progressing to restoring strength, power, and endurance. It is especially important to make sure that the patient with wrist and hand complaints does not increase the pain during rehabilitation. Reflex sympathetic dystrophy may follow nerve injury or even minor trauma; this condition must be avoided at all costs. Athletes who do not show steady positive progress should be reassessed or referred for further evaluation.

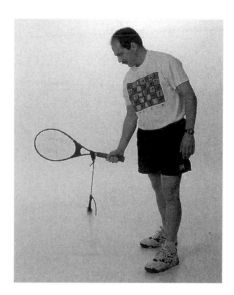

Figure 4.7. Using tubing to train for tennis strokes.

PHASE I

Marked edema is rarely encountered in wrist injuries unless significant trauma has occurred. The edema can be controlled by applying ice and compressive wraps or by using tubular compression stocking materials. When there is significant pain associated with the injury, splinting is indicated to allow for early tissue healing.

PHASE II

The use of an extremity whirlpool is very helpful in the rehabilitation of wrist and hand injuries (Fig. 4.8). Range of motion will be facilitated while the injured tissue has increased temperature and elasticity in the whirlpool. The typical treatment will last 15 to 20 minutes at 105° F. Benefit from the massaging effect of the whirlpool is also significant. An active and active-assisted range-of-motion program can be carried out in the whirlpool. Stretching exercises are applied to the pain-free end of the range of motion in all planes of motion, including flexion, extension, ulnar and radial deviation, supination, and pronation. The endpoint of motion should be held for 3 seconds before returning to the starting point, with use of as large a tendon excursion as possible by incorporating wrist and finger flexion and extension.

PHASE III

Tubing exercises are incorporated while maintaining and increasing wrist flexibility. High repetition exercises with low resistance are initially used with exercises in the previously described planes of wrist motion. When performing wrist flexion, it is important for the patient to place the tube at the distal interphalangeal joint before beginning wrist flexion; this ensures that the muscles are placed at the end of their lengthened state before muscle contraction is initiated. Proprioceptive exercises begin at this time, for example, box push-ups, progressing to plyo–push-ups, and balance board or Swiss ball push-ups. Push-ups may also be performed on a stair-climbing machine. Use of a dumbbell for continued recovery of muscle function is also necessary, with emphasis on stabilization of the athlete's forearm by positioning it on a table or the patient's thigh. The patient should be encouraged to use full range of motion.

PHASE IV

In this phase, the athlete should advance to specific progressive resistance exercises using tubing attached to equipment that the athlete would use in the sport. Equipment that has been manufactured specifically for this purpose can be purchased, or designed and man-

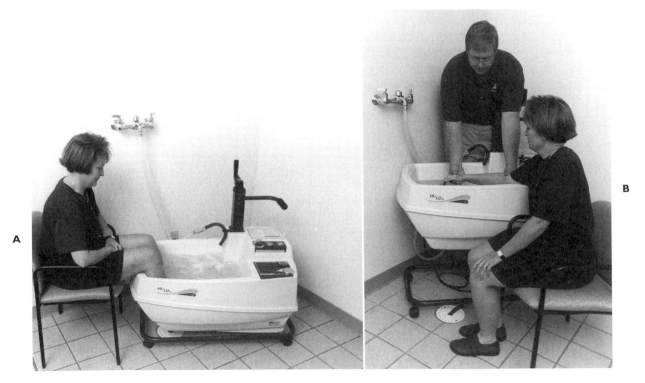

Figure 4.8. Extremity whirlpool.

ufactured at minimal expense (Figs. 4.6 and 4.7). Advanced exercises using a weighted medicine ball or gel ball should be emphasized, and plyometric exercises should also be continued.

Hand and Finger Rehabilitation

The rehabilitation of injuries to the hand and fingers is unfortunately often ignored because the athlete can typically continue to participate with the injury. If these injuries are not accurately diagnosed early and treated with appropriate rehabilitation, a permanent loss of function may result and affect not only athletic activities, but also everyday skills (56).

PHASE I

Edema is commonly encountered in finger and wrist injuries when trauma has occurred. The edema of an injured finger may persist for several months. The edema can be controlled through the application of ice and compressive wraps or tape such as Elasticon (Johnson & Johnson Medical, Arlington, TX) or Coban (Andover Coated Products, Salisbury, MA). When there is significant pain, ligamentous laxity, or effusion associated with the injury, splinting is indicated to allow for early tissue healing. The boutonniere and mallet finger injuries are commonly encountered. The mallet finger injury requires the uninterrupted splinting of the distal interphalangeal joint with a stack splint in terminal extension for 6 weeks. After sizing the splint initially, be sure to recheck the athlete to evaluate for wounds secondary to the pressure from the splint and to change to a smaller splint as the swelling resolves. The boutonniere injury to the central slip of the extensor tendon at the proximal interphalangeal joint is the second most common closed tendon injury in athletes (56). The boutonniere deformity should be splinted with the proximal interphalangeal joint in terminal extension and the distal interphalangeal joint left to move freely. The splint should be applied for 6 to 8 weeks.

PHASE II

Simultaneous use of the extremity whirlpool and active range of motion exercises will provide for the return of lost motion. Early active motion will enhance functional recovery. The athlete should begin gripping exercises with therapeutic putty or other similar materials to restore the intrinsic hand and finger strength and endurance. The throwing athlete should perform isometric gripping exercise throughout the throwing motion, stopping at several joint angles for several repetitions. Previously described proprioceptive activities should also be implemented at this stage.

PHASE III

The athlete should be instructed to continue the previously described gripping activities. The inclusion of resistance against rubber band for the fingers and gripping exercises for the hand are initiated. The use of heavy resistance is not usually needed in the rehabilitation of the athlete unless the sport requires it.

PHASE IV

Hand grips and free weights are continued with high repetitions and low resistance to perpetuate strength developement. Sport-specific strengthening activities are implemented. For example, if the patient is a running back, a mesh harness with a trailing rope can be applied around a football. The patient then attempts to run and to continue to secure possession of the ball, while another person pulls on the rope. This same theme can be adapted for a variety of sports.

Conservative Rehabilitation of Lumbar and Thoracic Injuries

The goal of injury rehabilitation must be to return the athlete to the highest level of performance possible (57). In the athlete with a spinal injury, this is especially important because the spine acts as the link between the upper and lower extremities. Injuries to the extremities will affect the spine, and injuries to the spine affect the extremities. The athlete with a back injury often will experience muscular deconditioning. This will create joint contracture muscle atrophy, ligament weakening, and cartilage degeneration (58). The muscle atrophy that occurs after injury will primarily be of the Type I slow twitch endurance fibers. This makes it necessary to concentrate on high-repetition, low-intensity spinal exercises in the initial phases of spinal rehabilitation. The physician can prevent deconditioning in the athlete by initiating aggressive spinal rehabilitation as early as possible.

PHASE I

The goal of this stage is general preparation of the lumbar spine for stabilization activities that will come later. The exercises the athlete will perform in this stage include isometric strengthening, stretching, and proprioception activities. The physician will also work with the athlete to ensure that proper motor patterns are used with muscular activity.

The isometric exercises include pelvic tilts and prone pelvic presses. The athlete can perform the pelvic tilt in multiple positions including supine, sitting, and standing. To perform the prone pelvic press, the athlete tightens the gluteal muscles and presses the pelvis to the floor.

Flexibility exercises should be tailored to the athlete's flexibility inadequacies. Initially, the athlete performs stretching exercises concentrating on muscles directly affecting the lumbar spine. In phase II, the athlete will perform a whole-body flexibility program.

A general flexibility program for phase I will include one knee to chest, both knees to chest, piriformis stretch, supine hamstring stretch, prone lumbar extensor stretch, and hip flexor stretch.

It is common for the physician to include proprioceptive activities in the treatment of ankle injuries but they are unfortunately usually ignored in low back rehabilitation (57, 58). Initial proprioception activities should include a single plane rocking board. The athlete stands first with both feet on the board, and later on only one foot. The athlete attempts to rock in a smooth, rhythmic fashion with the body positioned in different ways (59). The lumbar spinal muscles will learn to fire systematically and properly to stabilize the athlete in this controlled environment. The athlete can then carry this technique over to other activities. Other balance activities to be attempted include a wobble board and a balance beam. In phase III, the athlete will use the Swiss ball for both strengthening and proprioceptive exercises.

PHASE II

This phase will concentrate on the athlete increasing both general fitness and intensity of lumbar exercises. The athlete will perform isotonic strengthening exercises, concentrating on full range of motion and including crossed motor activity exercises. These crossed motor activity exercises help to improve proper motor muscle firing patterns. Flexibility exercises should now include the entire lower extremity and lumbar spine. The athlete will continue proprioceptive activities and should also be encouraged to begin a general fitness program. This may include any aerobic activity the athlete can perform without aggravating the symptoms.

A general strengthening program for phase II will include pelvic lifts, abdominal crunches, prone active lumbar extension, prone opposite arm and leg lift, all-four exercises, wall squats, and lunges. When performing prone active lumbar extension, the athlete should have a pillow under the abdomen (60, 61). The athlete can make progress in these strengthening exercises by using the effects of gravity. Initially the hands are at the sides, followed by the hands behind the head, and finally with the hands straight out in front. Finally, the athlete can load the lumbar spine by raising both the arms and legs. The athlete should begin the all-four quadruped exercise by lifting one arm. Then the athlete should lift one leg and finally lift the opposite arm and leg simultaneously. The athlete can often initiate the wall squat early in rehabilitation (62). The wall supports the back and protects it from strain. This exercise primarily strengthens the quadriceps and the gluteal muscles. Lunges will allow the athlete to use a more complete and functional range of motion. They also help to work with the proprioceptive system.

As the athlete becomes comfortable with the above exercises, Swiss ball exercises can be added. The Swiss ball exercises improve strength, balance, and mobility. The athlete can perform a variety of activities on the ball.

The athlete continues the flexibility exercises initiated in phase I. Stretches of the following muscles should also be added: gastrocnemius, quadriceps, abductor, adductor, quadratus lumborum, iliotibial band, and latissimus dorsi.

PHASE III

The athlete who reaches this stage should be able to perform all phase II activities without discomfort. The range of motion should be full, and the athlete should have good core strength. The athlete is then ready to begin weight-training exercises that maximize core strength.

A general strengthening program for phase III includes back squats, dead lift, back extensions, and power cleans. The athlete should begin all exercises with light weights and concentrate on perfect lifting form. The exercises should be halted as soon as the patient breaks form. Later, as the athlete perfects technique and realizes increases in strength, the weights can be heavier. The athlete should continue to stress abdominal exercises because a strong abdomen is very important in lumbar spine stability. The athlete also needs exercises to strengthen the upper and lower rectus abdominis as well as the oblique muscles. The athlete should also continue Swiss ball activities. The proprioceptive balance the athlete regains while exercising on the ball will be very important on return to competition.

PHASE IV

On return to activity, the athlete should continue to maintain strength and flexibility of the lumbar spine. The athlete should continue to stretch before and after practice and should perform the preceding strengthening activities two to three times per week.

Cervical Spine Rehabilitation

The rehabilitation of the spine will need to be customized depending on the injury sustained. Injuries for which therapeutic exercise is indicated include cervical sprains, brachial plexus axonotmesis, vertebral body end plate fractures, wedge compression and other stable fractures, and peripheral nerve injuries (63). This discussion will focus on sprain and strain injuries to the cervical spine. It is assumed that the patient has a stable spine before the rehabilitation program described is initiated.

PHASE I

The initial treatment goal is to prevent further injury and control pain while maintaining as much motion and flexibility as possible. It may be necessary to place the more severely injured athlete in a soft cervical collar initially. Remember that these soft collars do not stabilize the spine; they merely provide support to the injured soft tissues. The soft collar should be removed for 1 hour out of every 3 within 3 days. Initial applications of ice are indicated. The patient should be encouraged to maintain pain-free motion by performing cervical range-of-motion exercises several times daily. Pain-free isometric exercises should be performed at multiple cervical spine positions several times daily. Gentle static stretches can be performed at the point of tension. Gentle manual distraction of the cervical spine may also provide pain relief. Manual resistance may be applied to the cervical spine at several angles along the planes of motion, if tolerated.

PHASE II

The range-of-motion exercises are continued. It may prove helpful to precede the exercise with moist heat treatments. The stretches will be more effective if the patient relaxes and the stretches are performed slowly. Additional exercises to be included are shoulder shrugs, shoulder presses, upright rows, and behind the neck presses (64). Therapeutic muscle stretching and myofascial release techniques are also prescribed.

PHASE III

The exercise intensity and frequency should be increased to build muscular endurance and strength. It is important to ensure that aerobic activities are also being performed. Stabilization exercises using the therapeutic ball are recommended (Fig. 4.9). Isotonic exercise can be performed by using a four-way neck machine.

PHASE IV

Continued flexibility and strengthening exercises are recommended, as preperation for the athlete's sport. Whole body exercise and agility drills should be included along with plyometric training.

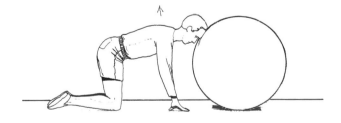

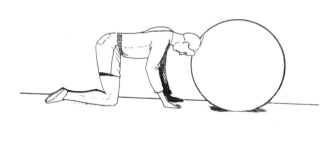

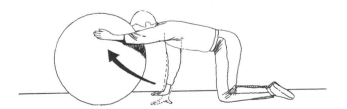

Figure 4.9. Cervical spine stabilization drills.

References

1. Timm KE. A randomized-control study of active and passive treatments for chronic low back pain following L5 laminectomy. J Orthop Sports Phys 1994;20:276–286.
2. Walsh WH, Huurman WW, Shelton GL. Overuse injuries of the knee and spine in girls gymnastics. Clin Sports Med 1984;3:829.
3. DeLorme TL, Watkins AL. Techniques of progressive resistance exercise. Arch Phys Med 1948;29:263–273.
4. Sanders M, Sanders B. Mobility: active-resistive training. In: Gould JA, Davies GJ, eds. Orthopedic and sports physical therapy. St. Louis: CV Mosby, 1985.
5. Baechle TR. Essentials of strength training and conditioning. Champaign, IL: Human Kinetics, 1994:406.
6. Stone MH, O'Bryant HS, Garhammer JG. A hypothetical model for strength training. J Sports Med Phys Fitness 1981;21:342–351.
7. Kellett J. Acute soft tissue injuries: a review of the literature. Med Sci Sports Exerc 1986;18:489.
8. Shelton GL. Principles of musculoskeletal rehabilitation. In: Mellion MB, ed. Sports injuries and athletic problems. St. Louis: CV Mosby, 1988.
9. Davies GL. A compendium of isokinetics in clinical usage. 2nd ed. LaCross, WI: S&S Publishers, 1984.
10. Knapik JJ, Mawdsley RH, Ramos MU. Angular specificity and test mode specificity of isometric and isokinetic strength training. J Orthop Sports Phys Ther 1983; 5:58–65.
11. Rasch P, Morehouse L. Effect of static and dynamic exercises on muscular strength and hypertrophy. J Appl Physiol 1957;11:29–34.
12. Dickinson A, Bennet K. Therapeutic exercises. Clin Sports Med 1985;4:417–429.
13. Vegso JJ, Torg E, Torg JS. Rehabilitation of cervical spine, brachial plexus, and peripheral nerve injuries. Clin Sports Med 1987;6:136.
14. Anderson B. Stretching. Bolinas, California Shelter Publication, 1980.
15. Stone WJ, Kroll WA. Sports conditioning and weight training. Boston: Allyn and Bacon, 1986.
16. Alter MJ. Sport stretch. Champaign, IL: Leisure Press, 1990.
17. Gould JA, Davies GJ. Orthopaedic and sports rehabilitation concepts. In: Gould JA, Davies GJ. Orthopedic and sports physical therapy. St. Louis: CV Mosby, 1985.
18. Fox EL, Mathews DK. The physiologic basis of physical education and athletics. Philadelphia: WB Saunders College Publishing, 1981.
19. Prentice WE. Rehabilitation techniques in sports medicine. St. Louis: CV Mosby, 1994:98–101.
20. Tippett SR, Voight ML. Functional progressions for sport rehabilitation. Champaign, IL: Human Kinetics, 1995.
21. Voss DE, Ionta MK, Myers BJ. Proprioceptive neuromuscular facilitation. Philadelphia: Harper & Row, 1985:307–311.
22. Sady SP, Wortman M, Blanke D. Flexibility training: ballistic, static or proprioceptive neuromuscular facilitation. Arch Phys Med Rehab 1982;63:261–263.
23. Coole WG, Gieck JH. An analysis of hamstring strains and their rehabilitation. J Orthop Sports Phys Ther 1987;9:77–85.
24. Worrell TW, Perrin DH. Hamstring muscle injury: the influence of strength, flexibility, warm-up and fatigue. J Orthop Sports Phys Ther 1992;16:12–18.
25. Tyson A. Hamstring injuries: rehabilitation and prevention, strength and conditioning. 1995;17:30–32.
26. Karlsson J, Sward L, Kalebo P, et al. Chronic groin injuries in athletes. Sports Med 1994;17:141–148.
27. Williford HN, Wang N, Olson MS, et al. Energy expenditure of slideboard exercise training. Med Sci Sports Exerc 1993;25:621.
28. Barber FA, Sutker AN. Iliotibial band syndrome. Sports Med 1992;14:144–148.
29. Holmes JC, Pruitt AL, Whalen NJ. Iliotibial band syndrome in cyclists. Am J Sports Med 1993;21:419–424.
30. Hooper M. Iliotibial band friction syndrome: a common injury. Practitioner (London) 1989;233:948–951.
31. Hughston JC. Patellar subluxation. Clin Sports Med 1989;8:153–161.
32. LaBrier K, O'Neill DB. Patellofemoral stress syndrome current concepts. Sports Med 1993;16:449–459.
33. Shelton GL, Thigpen LK. Rehabilitation of patellofemoral dysfunction: a review of the literature. J Orthop Sports Phys Ther 1991;14:243–249.
34. Arno S. The a angle: a quantitative measurement of patella alignment and realignment. J Orthop Sports Phys Ther 1990;12:237–242.
35. Linsheng WU. Evaluation and manipulative therapy of patellar malalignment: a clinical review and preliminary report. J Manipulative Physiol Ther 1991;14:428–435.
36. McConnell JS. The management of chondromalacia patellae: a long term solution. Aust J Phys 1986;32: 215–233.
37. Sahrmann SA, Dixon KK. Measurement of medial glide of the patella. Presented at the annual conference of the American Physical Therapy Association, Las Vegas, NV, June 12–16, 1988.
38. Beckman M, Craig R, Lehman RC. Rehabilitation of patellofemoral dysfunction in athletes. Clin Sports Med 1989;8:841–860.
39. Hanten WP, Schulthies SS. Exercise effect on electomyographic activity of the vastus medialis oblique and vastus lateralis muscles. Phys Ther 1990;70:561–566.
40. Boruta PM, Bishop JO, Braly G, et al. Acute lateral ankle ligament injuries: a literature review. Foot and Ankle 1990;11:107–113.
41. O'Donoghue DH. Treatment of injuries to athletes. Philadelphia: WB Saunders, 1976:707.
42. Reid DC. Sports injury assessment and rehabilitation. New York: Churchill Livingstone, 1992:222.
43. Birrer RB, Cartwright TJ, Denton JR. Primary treatment of ankle trauma. Phys Sports Med 1994;22:33–42.
44. Hoffman M, Payne VG. The effects of ankle disk training on healthy subjects. J Orthop Sports Phys Ther 1995; 21:90–93.
45. Litchfield R, Hawkins R, Dillman CJ, et al. Rehabilitation for the overhead athlete. J Orthop Sports Phys Ther 1993;18:433–441.
46. Kamkar A, Irrgang JJ, Whitney SL. Nonoperative management of secondary shoulder impingement syndrome. Orthop Sports Phys Ther 1993;17:212–224.
47. Speer KP, Cavanaugh JT, Warren RF, et al. A role for hydrotherapy in shoulder rehabilitation. Am J Sports Med 1993;21:850–853.
48. Wilk KE, Arrigo CJ. Current concepts in the rehabilitation of the shoulder. J Orthop Sports Phys Ther 1993;18:365–378.
49. Howell SM, Galinat BJ, Renze AJ, et al. Normal and abnormal mechanics of the glenohumeral joint in the horizontal plane. J Bone Joint Surg 1988;70A:227–232.
50. Butters KP. The scapula. In: Rockwood CA, Matsen FA, eds. The shoulder. Philadelphia: WB Saunders, 1990: 335–366.
51. Nuber GW, Jobe FW, Perry J, et al. Fine wire electromyography analysis of the shoulder during swimming. Am J Sports Med 1986;14:7–11.
52. Ryu RK, McCormick J, Jobe FW, et al. An electromyographic analysis of shoulder function in tennis players. Am J Sports Med 1988;16:481–485.
53. Wilke KE, Arrigo CA. An integrated approach to upper extremity exercises. Orthop Phys Ther Clin North Am 1992;9:337–360.
54. Wilke KE, Arrigo MS, Andrews JR. Rehabilitation of the elbow in the throwing athlete. J Orthop Sports Phys Ther 1993;17:305–317.
55. Warhold LG, Osterman AL, Skirven T. Lateral epicondylitis: how to treat it and prevent reoccurrence. J Musculoskeletal Med 1993;10:55–70.
56. McCue FC, Mayer V. Rehabilitation of common hand injuries of the hand and wrist. Clin Sports Med 1989;8:731.

57. Saal JA. Lumbar injuries in gymnastics. In: Hochschuler SH, ed. The spine in sports. St. Louis: CV Mosby, 1990: 192–206.

58. Glisan B, Hochschuler SH. General fitness in the treatment and prevention of athletic low back injuries. In: Hochschuler SH, ed. The spine in sports. St. Louis: CV Mosby, 1990:31–42.

59. Hubka MJ, Hubka MA. Conservative management of idiopathic hypermobility and early lumbar instability using proprioceptive rehabilitation: a report of two cases. Chiro Tech 1989;1:88–93.

60. Janda V. Treatment of chronic low backpain. J Man Med 1992;6:166–168.

61. Moffroid MT, Haugh LD, Haig AJ, et al. Endurance training of trunk extensor muscles. Phys Ther 1993;73:3–17.

62. Aspegren DD. Treating the athlete's back: the ultimate challenge. Chiro Sports Med 1992;6:49–55.

63. Torg JS. Athletic injuries to the head, neck, and face. St. Louis: CV Mosby, 1991:556.

64. Baechle TR. Essentials of strength training and conditioning. Champaign, IL: Human Kinetics, 1994:345–401.

Principles of Manipulation in Sports Medicine

5A/ *Manipulating the Spine*

Thomas F. Bergmann

INTRODUCTION

Chiropractic care generally and spinal manipulative therapy specifically are growing in popularity and in acceptance. This acceptance of spinal manipulation by other health-care professions, industry, and the general population continues to grow despite controversies in clinical practice and lack of appropriate validation. This chapter presents general concepts regarding manipulative therapy, including a rationale for use of manipulation, joint assessment procedures, characteristics of the chiropractic adjustive thrust, and complications and contraindications to manipulative therapy.

History

Although there appears to be no single origin of the art of manipulation, vague accounts of manual therapy usage may be attributed to the ancient Chinese (1) and were used in the eastern Mediterranean region approximately 5000 years ago (2). However, since the time of Hippocrates, who described and illustrated the use of joint manipulation and spinal traction, considerable controversy and debate have concerned the clinical efficacy and purpose. Despite these ancient roots, and despite the efforts of the likes of Mennell, Cyriax, Stoddard, and Maigne, very few medical physicians practice joint manipulation. In the early 1900s, osteopathy and chiropractic developed along similar paths, with both professions emphasizing the use of manipulative therapy. However, the curricula in osteopathic schools began to de-emphasize the use of manipulation and have ascribed to medical practice, stressing the use of pharmaceuticals and surgery. Chiropractic has maintained that the most specialized and significant therapy involves the adjustment of the articulations of the human body, especially the spinal column. This may be done manually or mechanically, actively or passively, with the purpose of restoring normal articular relationship and function as well as restoring neurologic integrity and influencing physiologic processes.

ROLE OF MANIPULATIVE THERAPY IN SPORTS INJURIES

More than half of the body's mass comes from the musculoskeletal system, although it remains the most clinically neglected system in the body. The mechanical principles that determine what functions the body is able to perform are the same regardless of the activity, be it athletic, recreational, occupational, or everyday tasks.

Manipulative or manual therapeutic procedures have been the mainstay of coaches, trainers, sports physicians, and therapists since the beginning of competitive sports (3). An increasing interest in spinal manipulation by those associated with sporting activities comes from the fairly frequent incidence of spinal pain syndromes among athletes. Injuries to the lower back and neck become incapacitating and can lead to loss of performance and eventual permanent disability if not corrected. Moreover, elite athletes are claiming that regular manipulative treatment has led to improved performance and this undoubtedly has stimulated increased interest in manipulative therapy.

RATIONALE FOR MANIPULATIVE THERAPY

The assessment and treatment of mechanical joint problems should have a biomechanical basis. Knowledge of normal biomechanics and the ability to detect changes in joint mechanics are essential for the successful management of mechanical joint dysfunction. The use of manipulative therapy emphasizes the restoration of free movement between articular surfaces as well as affecting the contiguous soft tissues. Because manipulative techniques may not be indicated in all cases, a thorough clinical investigation is necessary to clarify the nature and extent of the clinically important lesion(s). Once this is done and joint manipulation is deemed appropriate, suitable techniques must be selected and skillfully applied based on the direction and extent of restrictions of joint movement and the nature of the soft tissue involvement.

Movement of the body's articulations occurs in three planes (Fig. 5A.1). The types of movement a joint can perform consist of movement around an axis (rotation), motion through a plane (translation), or a combination of the two. The rotational movements in the sagittal plane are flexion and extension, whereas translational movements in the sagittal plane consist of anterior to posterior

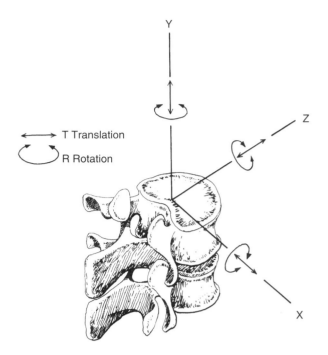

Figure 5A.2. Rotational and translational movements of the vertebral functional unit demonstrating the six degrees of freedom. (Adapted from White AA, Panjabi MM. Clinical biomechanics of the spine. Spine Philadelphia: JB Lippincott, 1978.)

and posterior to anterior glide. Rotational movement in the transverse plane is axial rotation, whereas translational movements in the transverse plane consist of axial compression and distraction. Rotational movements in the coronal plane are lateral flexion movements; translational movements in the coronal plane consist of lateral glide (Fig. 5A.2).

Biomechanics is the application of mechanical laws to living structures, specifically to the locomotor system of the human body. Clinical biomechanics involves the study of the interrelationship of the bones, muscles, and joints. In mechanics, a lever is used to its advantage when a force moves it about a pivot point or fulcrum. In the body, muscles provide the forces to move the bony levers around the joint that forms a pivotal hinge. The efficiency of this musculoskeletal mechanical unit is dependent on the integrity of the joint and the surrounding soft tissues. Knowledge and understanding of how the joint movement, muscular action, and osseous lever systems work together to produce the composite activity in the joints of the spine and extremities are necessary to identify abnormalities and to apply corrective manipulative therapy. With this knowledge the health-care provider is better able to evaluate the numerous neuromusculoskeletal disorders and to understand the anatomic and physiologic basis of their conservative management.

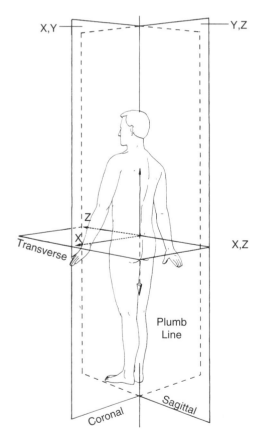

Figure 5A.1. The three planes and axes of the body illustrating their interrelationships. The sagittal plane is defined by the Y,Z axis and rotates around the X axis. The transverse plane is defined by the X,Z axis and rotates around the Y axis. The coronal plane is defined by the X,Y axis and rotates around the Z axis. (Adapted from White AA, Panjabi MM. Clinical biomechanics of the spine. Philadelphia: JB Lippincott, 1978.)

The Manipulable Lesion

It has long been a basic premise of chiropractic that a relationship exists between dysfunction of the nervous system and disease (4–11). It is also fundamental that some aberration within the spinal column produces the nerve dysfunction. It is doubtful if a more debatable, opinionated, or emotive subject exists in the chiropractic profession than that of subluxation, including its definition, mechanism, and significance (12). It is certainly hoped that some consensus of educated opinion, not embellished in dogma, will soon be reached. The definition ratified by the American Chiropractic Association in 1987 states:

Subluxation is an aberrant relationship between two adjacent articular structures that may have functional or pathological sequelae, causing an alteration in the biomechanical and/or neurophysiologic reflections of these articular structures, their proximal structures, and/or other body systems that may be directly or indirectly affected by them (13).

D.D. Palmer defined subluxation as:

A partial or incomplete separation; one in which the articulating surfaces remain in partial contact (14).

This concept was most appropriate for the body of knowledge available at the time. However, contemporary thought places significance on the functional component, and while alignment—or lack thereof—is indeed important for proper functioning of an articulation, it is by no means the only factor that should be considered in defining or identifying the subluxation. Moreover, the nervous system reacts to external and internal irritations so as to establish certain patterned responses leading to physiologic and structural alterations. These internal sources of sensory stimulation may then cause motor responses that give rise to functional and morphologic alterations. Therefore, it is hypothesized that the subluxation leads to pathophysiologic changes that in turn lead to pathologic changes and tissue damage. The subluxation can be viewed as a clinical entity whose complexity is established by any of the following:

1. Neurologic changes that may include evidence of irritation, or compression, or both;
2. Kinesiologic changes including evidence of hypomobility, hypermobility, aberrant motion, and loss of joint play or;
3. Myologic changes including evidence of hypertonicity, hypotonicity, or both;
4. Histologic changes including evidence of edema and products of the inflammatory process;

5. Biochemical changes including the effects of histamines, kinins, prostaglandins, and substance P (15).

D.D. Palmer's original concept for determining causes of disease (subluxation) was, "traumatism, poison, and autosuggestion" (14). Translated into contemporary language, the causes are mechanical, chemical, and mental. Generally, it can be said that subluxations are caused by irritation from the stresses and strains to which the body is subjected. Environment, hereditary, developmental anomalies, and posture all play a role in the production of subluxation.

Specifically, extrinsic and intrinsic factors can be identified. The extrinsic causes include trauma, the effects of gravity and posture, occupation, and the microtrauma of daily living. Intrinsic causes include fatigue, psychosomatic influences, unequal or asymmetric muscle pull due to trauma, postural compensation, biochemical changes, psychological stresses, primary disease, and reflex mechanisms. Structural alterations of supporting tissue due to developmental abnormalities, acquired disease processes, and resolution of trauma may also occur intrinsically.

To bring about a subluxation, a force of some kind must be applied on the osseous or supporting structures. If the force is of a severe nature or is allowed to continue over a period of time, the effect on the articulation is subluxation. The result of a subluxation is the presence of any of the following signs and symptoms: misalignment, segmental mobility changes, pain and tenderness, changes in spinal musculature, temperature changes, and findings referable to certain organ systems or other parts of the body (somatovisceral, somatosomatic reflexes) (16–21a).

The primary concern is that a disorder in structure contributes to disturbed physiology, which promotes a breakdown in body processes (pathology). According to Kirkaldy-Willis, the initial cause of spinal dysfunction and pain is found in the abnormal function of the intervertebral joints (22). An intervertebral joint is the articulation between the component parts of a functional unit of the spine. The functional unit (or motion segment) is composed of two vertebrae, the disc between them, and the contiguous soft tissues, including intrinsic ligaments and muscles. The functional unit has an anterior and posterior portion, each with its own characteristics. The anterior portion is formed by the two vertebral bodies, the intervertebral disc, the cartilaginous end plates, and the anterior and posterior longitudinal ligaments. The function of the anterior portion is to provide support, bear weight, and disseminate axial compression forces. This joint is classified as an amphiarthrodial (symphysis) articulation and, by definition, allows movement through the intrinsic property of the discal material. The posterior portion is composed of the neural arch and foramen, pedicles, lamina, transverse processes with apophyseal articulations, capsular ligaments, interspinous ligaments, and ligamentum flava. The function of the posterior portion of the motion unit is to allow movement in a specific direction. The apophyseal joints contain capsular ligaments (joint capsule), synovial membranes, and synovial

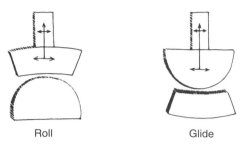

Roll   Glide

Figure 5A.4. Movements possible in a synovial joint and the therapeutic procedures that will influence them. (From Bergmann TF, Peterson DH, Lawrence D. Chiropractic Technique Principles and Procedures. 1993.)

fluid. Therefore, they are true diarthrodial (synovial) articulations. The movement of the facet articulations of the posterior portion of the functional unit is determined primarily by the plane of the facets. Each region is different and, therefore, has different characteristic movements. The cervical facets allow movement in all directions, the thoracic facets allow rotation (although the rib cage limits that movement), and the lumbar facets allow mainly forward flexion and extension movements (Fig 5A.3). The motion segment is subject to biomechanical derangements, including internal derangements of the synovial joints and disc, that may alter the normal dynamics of the spine, leading to joint dysfunction and subluxation (23–32).

At any functional unit of the spine, the intervertebral joint is made up of three parts; hence, a three-joint complex. The only exceptions are the atlanto-occipital articulation as it is composed of two synovial joints only and the atlanto-axial articulation that is composed of three synovial joints. The three-joint complex in the rest of the spine is formed by the two posterior synovial joints and anterior body-disc joint. Changes affecting the posterior joint also affect the disc and vice versa. Kirkaldy-Willis describes a continuum of pathomechanic change in the intervertebral joint complex that can be divided into three phases: that of dysfunction leading to instability and ending in restabilization (Fig. 5A.4) (22).

Paris proposed a mechanism for intervertebral joint dysfunction that begins with an episode of rotational or compressive trauma to the three-joint complex, leading to posterior joint strain and a strain to the annular fibers (22). This causes a minor facet subluxation characterized by synovitis and pain. This process stimulates sustained segmental hypertonicity of muscle, which itself becomes ischemic and painful through altered muscle metabolism. The muscle contraction results in a splinting of the posterior joint, which

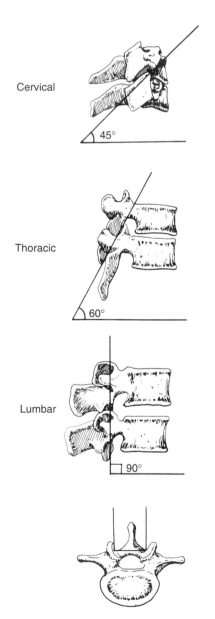

Cervical   45°

Thoracic   60°

Lumbar   90°

Figure 5A.3. The planes of the articular facets in the spine. (Adapted from White AA, Panjabi MM. Clinical biomechanics of the spine. Philadelphia: JB Lippincott, 1978.)

maintains the subluxation and perpetuates the posterior joint strain.

The changes that occur in the posterior joints are the same as those characteristic of any synovial joint. They consist first of synovitis, which may then proceed to the formation of a synovial fold that projects into the joint between the articular surfaces. These changes lead to fibrosis. The three-joint complex then becomes dysfunctional. With continued stress or further trauma, progressive changes are seen in the facet joints and the disc. Articular cartilage begins degenerating and the joint capsule attenuates, leading to laxity of the capsule and the potential for hypermobility of the posterior joints. Meanwhile, within the disc, small circumferential tears in the annulus later become larger and coalesce to form radial tears. These tears increase in size until the disc becomes completely disrupted internally. Disc resorption then takes place, resulting in a reduction in disc height and further formation of osteophytes and spondylophytes. The end result is increased abnormal movement of the three-joint complex leading to segmental instability (22).

As time passes, the posterior joints stiffen because of the destruction of articular cartilage, fibrosis within the joint, enlargement and locking of the facets, and periarticular fibrosis. Similar changes take place within the disc. Loss of nuclear material, approximation of vertebral bodies, fibrosis within the disc, destruction of the cartilaginous end plates, and osteophytes and spondylophyte formation around the periphery of the disc are occurring. The three-joint complex is restabilizing, but there is a price to pay. This process invariably decreases the size of the central canal and intervertebral foramen, often causing entrapment of spinal nerves and possible cord compression (cauda equina). Further, there is a decrease in range of motion of the intervertebral joints (22).

The dysfunction phase is most readily responsive to manipulative therapy (25). Restoration of the facet joint to normal juxtaposition and normal motion is thought to prevent further damage and progression (22,25). If damage and progression have exceeded the capacity of repair, the condition may pass into the unstable phase. Manipulative therapy applied to an unstable joint serves only as a further irritant (22).

Although the extremity joints do not share the same kind of three-joint complex makeup, they may follow the same progression as the posterior joints of the spine. When exposed to trauma, the extremity joints can move from a normal functioning state into a dysfunctional process and eventually become unstable if no intervention occurs.

Pathology and thus disease should not be viewed as a single entity but as an abnormal functional process with an alteration of morphology out of sync with environmental need—physiology gone awry.

JOINT ASSESSMENT PROCEDURES

The most important step in the management of musculoskeletal disorders is a comprehensive examination. The role of the assessment process is first to identify appropriate case management, i.e., to determine whether the problem lies within the practitioner's scope of practice or whether a consultation with, or referral to, another healthcare professional is necessary. The next goal for assessment is to localize the site of the lesion and identify the extent of the involved tissue (localize the subluxation). Because of significant variance among the types and applications of manipulative therapy, the assessment procedure should also be used to help identify what type of manipulative procedure should be used. For example, if the assessment procedure can identify a patient who is exhibiting characteristics of Type A behavior most likely due to hypersympathetic involvement, techniques including massage and low-force procedures may be more appropriate. For a person who is more lethargic and is in a hyperparasympathetic state, techniques using dynamic cavitation-type thrusts may be indicated. Finally, the assessment procedure should be used in an ongoing fashion to monitor the effects of care. Although it appears that the assessment and treatment process is directed at the specific joint lesion itself, it must not be forgotten that the purpose of treatment is the rehabilitation of the patient and the eventual return to an optimal level of functioning.

As a primary health-care provider, the doctor of chiropractic uses findings derived from the case history, physical examination, clinical laboratory tests, and special testing procedures to assess the patient's state of health and to determine the nature and cause of any ailments. However, it is the chiropractic spinal examination and joint assessment that set chiropractic apart from other areas of the healing arts. Knowing how complex the human body is and, specifically, the neuromusculoskeletal system, it would seem inappropriate to use a single evaluative procedure to decide on the presence of a manipulable lesion. Furthermore, reliability studies on single evaluative tools have demonstrated less than desirable statistical significance (33–77). No one evaluative tool should be used or relied on to make clinical decisions.

Structured evaluation of the integrity of the joint systems of the body should be viewed in terms of a multidimensional index of abnormality. The examination of the musculoskeletal system should never be done in isolation, but should be done within the confines of the rest of the clinical evaluation.

The methods used in identifying the presence of joint dysfunction (subluxation) include the usual physical examination processes of observation, palpation, percussion, and auscultation. The acronym PARTS is used to identify the five diagnostic criteria for identification of joint dysfunction (78, 79).

P—Pain/tenderness: The location, quality, and intensity of the patient's perception of pain and reported tenderness must be evaluated. Because a painful response is quite characteristic of most primary musculoskeletal disorders, the patient's description and location are essential. Eliciting pain responses from bony and soft tissue structures by palpation should also be noted.

A—Asymmetry: Sectional or segmental asymmetric qualities should be identified. This includes the static palpation procedures for misalignment of vertebral segments and observation for changes in posture and gait. Static x-ray is also used to identify segmental misalignments, sectional changes in curves, and structural asymmetries.

R—Range of motion abnormality: Increases or decreases in the active, passive, and accessory joint motions should be noted through the use of motion palpation and stress x-ray. A decrease in segmental motion is a common component of joint dysfunction. An increase in segmental motion is thought to be a nonindication for manipulative therapy.

T—Tissue texture, tone, temperature abnormality: Identification of changes in the characteristics of the associated soft tissues including skin, fascia, muscle, and ligament must be noted. These findings can be identified through the use of observation, palpation, instrumentation, and tests for length and strength.

S—Special tests: They include the use of procedures that are unique to a specific manipulative technique system.

The total management of the patient must include diagnosis, treatment, and education. The most difficult task of collecting and processing clinical data into usable information to make judgments as to how to solve the patient's problem is a part of clinical practice. It is important to record the various aspects of this process. It is imperative that the clinical notations of the physician's personal record be complete and translatable. If it is not written down, it is not done! A systematic and adequate record of evaluation facilitates quick reference to salient findings, which should be noted. By recording clinical data in the form of history, examination findings, and treatment progress, this information can be collected for subsequent needs, including publication in journals for intraprofessional and interprofessional scrutiny.

CHARACTERISTICS OF THE ADJUSTIVE THRUST

Sandoz (23, 80) has defined the chiropractic adjustment as a passive manual maneuver during which the three-joint complex is suddenly carried beyond the normal physiologic range of movement without exceeding the boundaries of anatomic integrity. Characteristics of an adjustment include a specific contact on a bony structure via the overlying soft tissues; a single dynamic thrust in a specific direction, amplitude, and speed; use of a lever mechanism to affect a minimum of three vertebrae (two functional units); usual association with an audible articular release, although this is not necessary to make an alignment change; a motion correction; and a neurologic stimulation.

Various forms of manipulation affect different aspects of joint function. In most joint positions, a joint has some "play" because joint surfaces do not fit tightly and because the capsule and ligaments remain somewhat lax (81, 82). This joint play is essential for normal joint function (15). Movement at a joint cannot occur around a rigid axis because the joint surfaces are of varying radii (Fig 5A.5). The joint capsule must allow some play for full movement to occur. The joint demonstrates joint play in the neutral position, followed by a range of active movement that is under the control of the musculature. A small degree of passive movement then occurs, which is followed by an elastic barrier of resistance called endfeel. Joint play in the neutral joint position and endfeel at the end point of joint movement are both accessory movements that are necessary for normal joint function. A loss of either movement can result in a restriction of motion, pain, or both. Active movements can be influenced through exercise, whereas passive movement can be influenced with traction and mobilization. Joint play and endfeel movements are affected when the joint is taken beyond the elastic barrier into the paraphysiologic space, creating a sudden yielding and frequently a cracking noise. Moving the joint beyond the paraphysiologic space would take the joint beyond its limit of anatomic integrity and into a pathologic zone of movement. Should a joint go into the pathologic zone, there would be damage to the joint structures and injury to the ligaments and capsule (23, 79).

The therapeutic emphasis is not on forcing a particular anatomic movement of a joint, but on restoring normal joint mechanics. Range of motion can therefore be restored to the joint with less risk of damaging the joint due to compression of the articular cartilage. Moreover, pain and

muscle guarding from overstretching capsuloligamentous structures can be prevented.

EFFECTS OF MANIPULATION ON NORMAL AND ABNORMAL JOINTS

The goals of manipulation include a combination of mechanical, soft tissue, neurologic, and psychological effects.

Mechanical Effects

The mechanical effects of an adjustment include changes in alignment, dysfunction of motion, and spinal curvature dynamics. Studies done by Roston and Wheeler Haines (83) and Unsworth et al. (84) demonstrate that as tension is applied causing a separation of the joint, at one point the joint surfaces separate quickly coinciding with a cracking noise. Once the tension is removed from the joint, the surfaces approximate themselves once again but at a distance

Figure 5A.5. Joint surfaces with varying radii necessitating some "play" within the joint to allow for rotational and translational movements—roll and glide. (After Kaltenborn FM. Mobilization of the extremity joints. 3rd ed. Oslo: Olaf-Norlis-Bokhandel, 1980.)

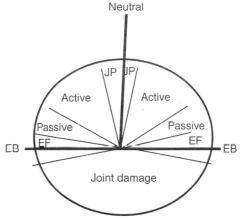

JP = Joint play; EF = End feel; EB = Elastic barrier

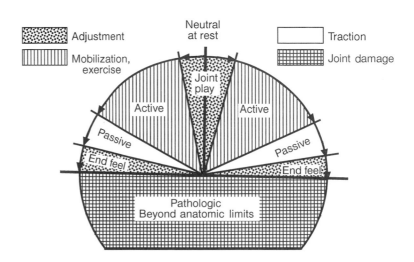

slightly more apart. A correlation of these studies with intervertebral joint adjustment is seen in Figure 5A.6.

As the elastic barrier is passed and the articular surfaces separate suddenly, a cracking noise can be heard, and a radiolucent space appears within the joint space (85). The explanation of the radiolucent space rests with the fact that normally a small negative pressure is present in a synovial joint. Its purpose is to maintain the cartilage surfaces in apposition, which helps to maintain the stability of the joint. Separation of the joint surfaces beyond the elastic barrier creates a drop in the interarticular pressure, and gas is suddenly liberated from the synovial fluid to form a bubble in the joint space. The bubble bursts almost immediately with an audible crack. The gas produced by synovial fluid cavitation was shown to be more than 80% carbon dioxide (84).

A synovial joint may become dysfunctional through entrapment or extrapment of a synovial fold (26–32). The application of an adjustive thrust that separates the articular surfaces may release the entrapped or extrapped synovial fold.

Soft Tissue Effects

Soft tissue effects include changes in the tone and strength of supporting musculature and in-fluences on the dynamics of supportive capsuloligamentous connective tissue (viscoelastic properties of collagen). Connective tissue elements lose their extensibility when their related joints are immobilized (86). With immobilization, water is released from the proteoglycan molecule allowing connective tissue fibers to contact one another, encouraging abnormal cross-linking and resulting in a loss of extensibility (87). It is hypothesized that manipulation can break the cross-linking and any intra-articular capsular fiber fatty adhesions, thereby providing more freedom of motion and allowing water inhibition. Furthermore, action of the adjustment can stretch segmental muscles, stimulating spindle reflexes that may decrease the state of hypertonicity (88).

Neurologic Effects

Neurologic effects include reduction in pain, influencing spinal and peripheral nerve conduction, thereby altering motor and sensory function and influencing autonomic nervous system regulation. Wyke (89) theorizes that manipulative procedures may stimulate the mechanoreceptors associated with synovial joints and thereby affect joint pain. He has identified four types of receptors. The first three (Types I, II, and III) are cor-

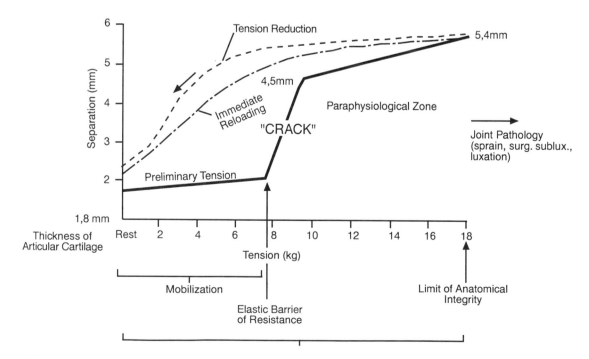

Figure 5A.6. Correlation of experiments (83, 84) demonstrating the effects of manipulation on a normal joint. With joint separation with 9 kg of tension, a cracking noise is heard. After the tension is released, the neutral resting joint separation is slightly more than it was before the tension was applied (dotted line). On immediate reloading of the joint, no cracking noise is heard (dashed lined). (After Sandoz R. The significance of the manipulative crack and other articular noises. Ann Swiss Chiro Assoc 1969;4:47 (85).)

Table 5A.1.   Characteristics of Articular Receptor System[a]

Type	Morphology	Location	Parent Nerve Fibers	Behavioral Characteristics
I	Thinly encapsulated globular corpuscles (100 μm $\times$ 40 μm), in tridimensional clusters of 3–8 corpuscles	Fibrous corpuscles of joints (in superficial layers)	Small myelinated (6–9 μm)	Static and dynamic mechanoreceptors: low-threshold, slowly adapting
II	Thickly encapsulated conical corpuscles (280 μm $\times$ 120 μm), individual or in clusters of 2–4 corpuscles	Fibrous capsules of joints (in deeper subsynovial layers); articular fat pads	Medium myelinated (9–12 μm)	Dynamic mechanoreceptors: low-threshold, rapidly adapting
III	Thinly encapsulated fusiform corpuscles (600 μm $\times$ 100 μm), individual or in clusters of 2–3 corpuscles	Applied to surfaces of joint ligaments (collateral and intrinsic)	Large myelinated (13–17 μm)	Dynamic mechanoreceptors: high-threshold, slowly adapting
IV	(a) Tridimensional plexuses of unmyelinated nerve fibres	Fibrous capsules of joints; articular fat pads; adventitial sheaths of articular blood vessels	Very small myelinated (2–5 μm) and unmyelinated (<2 μm)	Nociceptive mechanoreceptors: very high-threshold, nonadapting; chemosensitive (to abnormal tissue metabolites); nociceptive receptors
	(b) Free unmyelinated nerve ending	Joint ligaments (collateral and intrinsic)		

[a]From Wyjke BD. Articular neurology and manipulative therapy. In: Glasgow EF, Twomey LT, Shcull ER, Kleynhans AM, eds. Aspects of manipulative therapy. New York: Churchill-Livingston, 1985:133.

puscular mechanoreceptors that detect static position, acceleration and deceleration, direction of movement, and overdisplacement of the joint. The fourth receptor, Type IV, is a network of free nerve endings that have nociceptive capabilities. Type IV receptors are usually inactive under normal conditions; however, if noxious mechanical or chemical stimulation or if Type I-III receptors are not able to function, Type IV receptors become active and pain results. If manipulative therapy can restore normal function to the joint—allowing Types I-III receptors to function—the Type IV pain receptors should be inhibited, thereby decreasing the patient's pain. The structures most sensitive to noxious stimulation are the periosteum and joint capsule. Characteristics of the articular receptor system are shown in Table 5A.1>.

Additionally, current research provides evidence supporting spinal adjustments playing a role in decreasing pain, increasing range of motion, increasing pain tolerance in the skin and deeper muscle structures, raising beta-endorphin levels in the blood plasma, and having an impact on the nerve pathways between the soma and viscera that regulate general health (90–99).

Psychological Effects

The psychological effect of the laying on of hands cannot be denied or overlooked. Paris (100) states that with the addition of a skilled evaluation involving palpation for soft tissue changes and altered joint mechanics, the patient becomes convinced of the interest, concern, and manual skills of the clinician. If at the conclusion of the examination, a manipulation is performed resulting in an audible pop or snap, the placebo factor is undeniably high. It is no wonder that some patients report total relief within a second or two following manipulation—far too short a time for any genuine benefit to be appreciated. The astute clinician accepts and reinforces this report, recognizing that the patient is in need of all possible assistance.

TYPES OF ADJUSTIVE THRUSTS

Whereas manipulation is a term broadly used to define the therapeutic application of a manual force, chiropractors emphasize the application of specific adjustive techniques. The chiropractic adjustment is a unique form of manipulation and is characterized by a specific high-velocity, short-amplitude thrust (79, 101).

It is necessary to understand that a wide variety of methods exists so that the assumption that all manipulations are equivalent can be avoided (3). Factors that influence the selection of manipulative procedures include the following:

- Age of the patient
- Acuteness or chronicity of the problem
- General physical condition of the patient
- Clinician's size and ability
- Effectiveness of previous therapy, present therapy, or both (21)

The adjustive thrust is characterized by a transmission force using a combination of muscle power and the body weight of the practitioner. The force is delivered with controlled speed, depth, and magnitude through a specific contact on a particular structure such as the transverse or spinous process of a vertebra (102).

The specific high-velocity, low-amplitude manipulation is performed in one of two ways. Both require a sudden impulse delivered to the joint. In the first instance, the joint is maintained in a neutral position while specific contacts are taken over appropriate bony elements and a thrust given in a specific direction. Neutral joint slack and tissue elasticity are taken out before deliver-

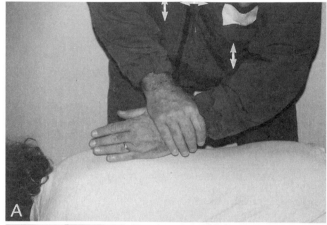

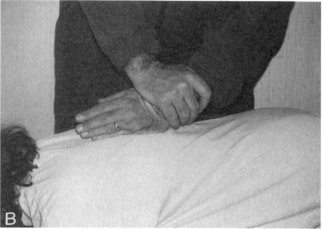

Figure 5A.9. Demonstration of an impulse thrust requiring extension of the elbows through isolated contraction of the triceps and anconeus muscle group while isolated contraction of the pectoralis major muscles stabilizes the shoulder.

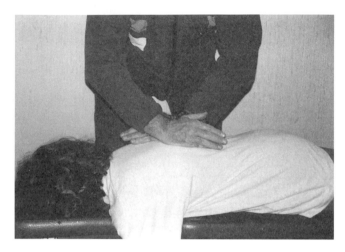

Figure 5A.7A. Typical example of an impulse thrust applied to the thoracic spine in neutral joint position affecting the paraphysiologic space of joint play.

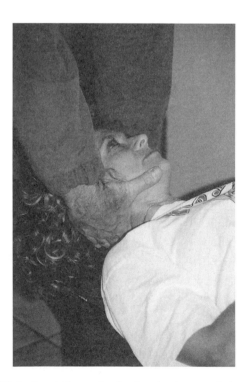

Figure 5A.8. A typical example of an impulse thrust applied to the cervical spine at the end point of joint movement affecting the paraphysiologic space of endfeel.

ing the thrust. A typical example of this type of procedure is correction of thoracic spine dysfunction using a posterior-to-anterior vector of force on the transverse processes with the patient lying in the prone position (Fig. 5A.7).

The second approach moves the joint through its active and passive range of motion in the specific direction of the adjustment. The thrust is given at the end point of movement, beyond the elastic barrier and into the paraphysiologic space (Fig. 5A.8).

The typical method of delivery of an impulse thrust is created by the controlled extension of the clinician's elbows done with a sustained action through the isolated contraction of the triceps and anconeus muscle groups combined with a contraction from the pectoralis major muscle to stabilize the shoulder (Fig. 5A.9). However, a body-drop thrust or a recoil thrust may also be used. The clinician locks the elbows and shoulders while using body weight to deliver the impulse thrust (Fig. 5A.10). The recoil thrust uses a controlled extension movement of the elbow but is followed by a quick release and elbow flexion. It is quite commonly associated with a mechanical drop-section of the adjusting table (Fig. 5A.11). Impulse thrusts can be developed using pulling maneuvers as well.

Another form of manual therapy is termed mobilization, which is applied within the physiologic passive range of joint motion and is characterized by a nonthrust, passive joint movement. By taking the joint to its barrier and repetitively moving along or beside it, the barrier may be encouraged to recede (20). Characteristics of a mobilization include a general contact on a number of bony structures with a single movement; a specific contact on a single bony structure with a multiple, repetitive movement action; or a general contact on a number of bony structures with a multiple repetitive movement action. Mobilization procedures help to loosen and break adhesions and fixations, allowing the adjustment to be more effective.

Manual traction is yet another form of manual therapy in which joint surfaces are held in sustained separation for a period of time. Traction may be solely through contacts made by the clinician or may be aided by a mechanized table or other devices. These forces may be applied manually or mechanically. Traction techniques serve to aid adjustments by first allowing physiologic

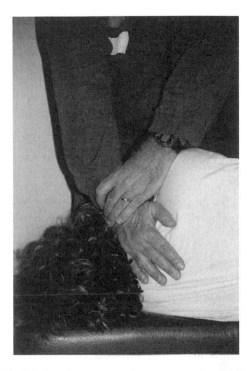

Figure 5A.11A. Recoil thrust uses elbow extension but is followed by a quick release and elbow flexion. A mechanical drop-section is frequently used. This procedure is commonly adapted to the extremities for adjustment of the carpal and tarsal bones.

rest to the area, relieving compressive pressure due to weight bearing, applying an imbibing action to the synovial joints and discs, and opening the intervertebral foramen to allow a break in reflex neurologic cycles. Many of these procedures are also quite useful for the elderly patient when a thrust procedure may not be indicated.

Manual therapy procedures can also be specifically directed to the soft tissues. Common to all techniques, whether an adjustment, a mobilization, or traction, is movement of the soft tissues. The justification for a separate classification is to draw attention to the prime importance of including techniques that have the specific purpose of improving the vascularity and extensibility of the soft tissues (21a). If one of the primary goals of manipulative therapy is the restoration of normal painless joint motion, it would be essential that treatment include measures to relax muscle and restore its normal vascularity and extensibility to the soft tissues. Soft tissue manipulations include massage (stroking or effleurage, kneading or pétrissage, vibration or tapotement, transverse friction massage), trigger point therapy, connective tissue massage, body-wall reflex techniques (Chapman lymphatic reflexes, Bennett vascular reflexes, acupressure point stimulation, etc.), and muscle energy techniques. Soft tissue manipulation tends to relax

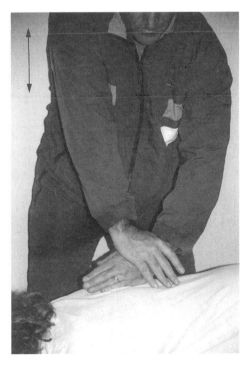

Figure 5A.10. Body-drop thrust is done with elbows locked and the doctor's body weight used to deliver the impulse.

hypertonic muscles so that when the adjustment is given, equal tensions are exerted across the joint.

Basic rules for the application of effective manipulative technique are as follows (79).

1. It is better not to adjust than to adjust incorrectly.
2. It is more important to know when not to adjust than when to adjust.
3. Be careful not to overadjust.
4. Select the most specific technique for the primary problem.
5. Position the patient for comfort and biomechanics.
6. The doctor should be relaxed and comfortable and maintain proper balance.
7. The contact should be taken correctly and specifically.
8. Articular and tissue slack should be taken up before the thrust is applied.
9. The doctor should visualize the structures contacted, the correct line of drive, and the exact thrust that is to be given.
10. The doctor's center of gravity should be as close as possible to the contact point.
11. The thrust must be given with optimum speed and minimal force necessary to make the correction.
12. *Primo non nocerum*—first do no harm.

Points of contact on the hand are as follows:

1. Pisiform
2. Hypothenar
3. Fifth metacarpal (knife edge)
4. Digital
5. Distal interphalangeal (DIP)
6. Proximal interphalangeal (PIP)
7. Metacarpophalangeal (MP or index)
8. Web
9. Thumb
10. Thenar
11. Calcaneal
12. Palmar (Fig. 5A.12)

ROLE OF ADJUNCTIVE PROCEDURES

Variable degrees of muscular and ligamentous involvement are associated with joint dysfunction. Unequal tensions are exerted across the joint and these must be overcome for an effective correction. The adjustment cannot always stand alone. In many cases it can be enhanced through adjunctive therapies. Whereas the most specialized and significant therapy used by the chiropractor involves adjustment of the articulations of the human body, adjunctive therapeutic procedures are used for their preparatory and complementary influence on adjustment effectiveness and their support of innate healing processes, thereby promoting wellness and preventing illness. Although every accredited chiropractic college teaches the use of various modalities and supportive appliances, it is ultimately individual state laws that govern their use.

Immobilizing procedures including tape, collars, supports, braces, slings, and casts can be used to facilitate and preserve joint realignment and tissue apposition.

Radiant heat, moist heat, short-wave diathermy, microwave diathermy, diapulse, ice, vasocoolant spray, interferential therapy, ultrasound, trans-

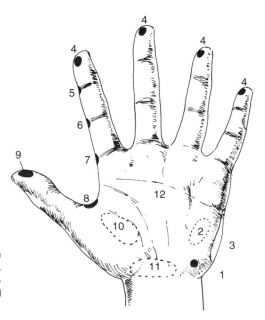

1. Pisiform
2. Hypothenar
3. Fifth metacarpal (knife edge)
4. Digital
5. Distal interphalangeal (DIP)
6. Proximal interphalangeal (PIP)
7. Metacarpophalangeal (MP or index)
8. Web
9. Thumb
10. Thenar
11. Calcaneal
12. Palmar

Figure 5A.12. Points of contact on the hand. (Redrawn from Kirk CR, et al., eds. States manual of spinal, pelvic and extravertebral technics. 2nd ed. Lombard, IL: National College of Chiropractic, 1985.)

cutaneous electrical nerve stimulation (TENS), electrical muscle stimulation, iontophoresis, mechanical vibrators, high-volt galvanic, and low-volt galvanic have all been prescribed for achieving a preadjustment relaxatory state, facilitating repair of injured or diseased tissue, and reducing pain and inflammation. If one had to be restricted to a single method of adjunctive treatment allied to techniques of passive and active movement, it would probably be ultrasound (21a, 103).

Nutritional hygiene including dietetics and supplementation for correction of faulty nutritional habits, elimination of deficiency, and restoration of optimum nutrient balance may also be used to augment therapeutic intervention.

Postural training, therapeutic exercise, environmental hygiene, principles of ergonomics, and structured rehabilitation are used for restoring and maintaining body functions compromised by faulty posture, restoring and/or preserving joint alignment and function, and facilitating general physiologic processes.

It is disconcerting, however, to encounter practitioners who are not comfortable unless their patients are hooked up to an electrical appliance or a new device, or they want their patients to leave with a shopping bag full of vitamin supplements, when between their ears and at the end of their forearms lie the most advanced technologies in the world—wit and hand (104). In the treatment of joint problems, adjunctive physical methods should remain as secondary modalities. These procedures should not assume the importance of primary treatment although they may be used very appropriately at the initiation of treatment as in the case of acute trauma or inflammation.

COMPLICATIONS AND CONTRAINDICATIONS TO MANIPULATIVE THERAPY

The primary purpose of manipulative therapy is to restore function and to relieve pain. This goal is achieved by a combination of mechanical, soft tissue, neurologic, and psychological effects. Most therapeutic procedures that demonstrate benefit also carry some risks and dangers. Many hold that one of the great advantages of manipulative therapy is that it is harmless. Why is this statement often repeated when it is known to be false? Because the severe dangers, sometimes fatal ones, that accompany manipulations are rare, and can nearly always be avoided (104). Manipulation is an effective therapeutic procedure with few complications provided high standards of

manipulative therapy are applied (105). Suitable manipulative procedures are less frequently associated with complications than is almost any other treatment. It is of utmost importance, however, that they be recognized because, although rare, complications can be serious (20).

An understanding of the causes of reported complications from manipulative therapy, awareness of the contraindications to manipulative therapy, and use of a diagnostic assessment before manipulative therapy are all necessary for preventing of complications.

Causes of Complications

Kleynhans and Terrett identify a number of both practitioner-related and patient-related factors (106). Diagnostic error can be responsible for or contribute to complications from manipulative therapy. It is simply unacceptable to apply manipulative therapy indiscriminately and without attempting to understand the nature and extent of the patient's condition.

A practitioner who lacks skill and training in the application of manipulative therapy poses just as great a threat to the patient as does the application of manipulative therapy by practitioners untrained in diagnosis. If brute force is used as a substitute for experience and skill, damage and even death can be the consequence. Health-care personnel should either study manipulative therapy thoroughly or avoid it (107).

A lack of rational attitude manifested as delays in reevaluation and referral, along with a lack of interprofessional cooperation and excessive use of manipulative therapy contribute greatly to the possibility of complication. A significant criticism of practitioners using manipulative therapy is that a patient may be delayed or prevented from seeking proper advice and care. This is unacceptable.

Patient intolerances such as excessive pain, fear of pain, and emotional instability must not be ignored to prevent complications.

Pathologic and Structural Factors

Contraindications to manipulative therapy include the presence of frank bone or joint disease that precludes the use of the dynamic adjustive thrust. Pathologic conditions that contraindicate manipulative therapy are listed in Table 5A.2.

Critics of manipulative therapy in general, and chiropractic specifically, emphasize the possibility of serious injury from cervical manipulation. Only the rare occurrence of manipulative-related

Table 5A.2. Contraindications to Spinal Manipulative Therapy

Absolute Contraindications	Relative Contraindications (Restricted indications for SMT)
Articular derangements	Articular derangements
Arthritides	Ankylosing spondylitis after
Acute arthritis of any type	acute stage
Rheumatoid arthritis	Articular deformity
Acute ankylosing spondylitis	Basilar impression
Cervical spondylosis with ver-	Congenital anomalies
tebrobasilar ischemia	Hypertrophic spondyloarthritis
Dislocation	Osteoarthritis
Hypermobility	Osteochondrosis with de-
Ruptured ligaments	fertive "holding apparatus"
Trauma of recent occur-	Rheumatoid arthritis
rence—whiplash	Torticollis
Bone weakening and destructive	Whiplash
disease	Bone weakening and modifying
Calvé's disease	disease
Fracture	Hemangioma
Malignancy (primary or sec-	Paget's disease
ondary)	Spondylolisthesis/spondylolysis
Osteomalacia	Disc lesions
Osteoporosis	Posterolateral and posterome-
Osteomyelitis	dial disc protrusions
Tuberculosis (Pott's disease)	Degenerative disease
Circulatory disturbances	Neurological dysfunction
Aneurysm	Brachial pain (longer than
Anticoagulant therapy	2 months' duration
Vascular insufficiency of verte-	Migraine (true migraine)
brobasilar area of vertebral	Myelopathy
artery disease	Nonvertebragenous pain
Disc lesions	Pyramidal tract involvement
Prolapse with serious neuro-	Radicular pain from disc lesion
logic changes (including	Viscerosomatic reflex pain
cauda equina syndrome)	Unclassified
Neurologic dysfunction	Abdominal hernia
Micturition with sacral root	Asthma
involvement	Basilar ischemia
Painful movement in all	Dysmenorrhea
directions	Epicondylitis
Vertigo	Operations—postspinal
Unclassified	Peptic ulcer
Infectious disease	Pregnancy
Patient intolerances	Scoliosis

Modified from Kleynhans AM, Terrett AGJ. The prevention of complications from spinal manipulative therapy. In: Aspects of manipulative therapy. New York: Churchill-Livingston, 1985:110.
SMT, spinal manipulative therapy.

accidents is needed to malign a therapeutic procedure that, in experienced hands, gives beneficial results with few side effects (108). Although an evaluative procedure to identify patients at risk has been developed (109) and factors that need to be considered warning signs are known (110), it is not apparent that any of these factors or tests, alone or in combination, specifically increase the chance of identifying the patient who is more susceptible to vascular injury. However, it would be imprudent to ignore significant factors that point to a predisposition to accidents from manipulative therapy (110).

Vertebrobasilar accidents resulting in paralysis and even death comprise the most severe complication of spinal manipulative therapy. The use of combined rotation and extension during the adjustive thrust is considered an etiologic mechanism for either the production and release of a thrombus or spontaneous dissection within the vertebrobasilar system.

The vertebral arteries are inevitably linked with cervical spine syndromes because of their unusually tortuous course, close relationship to the cervical nerves and vertebrae, and their potential for causing bizarre and often dramatic clinical manifestations (111). Hypotheses have been put forth to explain how vascular accidents may occur following manipulative procedures. The mechanism of injury is brain-stem ischemia, which may be due to trauma to the arterial wall producing vasospasm, frank damage to the arterial wall, or both. In most cases, the pathophysiologic process is vascular stasis or turbulence that then precipitates thrombus formation. The result is obstruction, embolus formation leading to infarction, intramural hematoma formation, or all three. The use of combined rotation and hyperextension of the cervical spine during the adjustment is often suggested as a common etiologic factor (112–115).

Although rotational head movements can cause vertebral artery compression, the clinical significance of compression must be suspect. Furthermore, it appears to be impossible to determine which patients possess a vertebral artery that may be attenuated (116).

It has been previously reported that the most common age for vascular accidents is approximately 30 to 50 years (112). However, this may be a reflection of the age-group most likely to seek the services of the practitioner using manipulative therapy (108).

Historical factors should always be the initial consideration. Terrett reviewed the major presenting complaints of patients who subsequently suffered manipulation-induced vertebrobasilar accidents (113). However, most patients presented with typical musculoskeletal complaints that revealed little to alert the practitioner to the impending accident. Moreover, even the symptom of dizziness is known to have a possible cervical spine origin responsive to manipulative therapy. It is still highly recommended that an inventory of systems, history, familial history, and drug history be part of the initial evaluative process coupled with evaluation of the chief complaint.

Physical examination of the patient should include a blood pressure and heart rate evaluation.

It is suggested that it be taken bilaterally. If elevation is bilateral, it indicates hypertension, a warning sign. If there is a difference of 10 mm or more between the left and right systolic pressures and the radial pulse is feeble on the side of decreased systole, a subclavian artery stenosis or occlusion is suggested (109). However, the victims of vascular accidents are usually fairly young and neither hypertensive nor hypotensive.

Auscultation of the carotid bifurcation of the subclavian fossa to rule out the presence of a bruit is also widely recommended. If a bruit is found, it represents an important finding related to the future health of the patient and must not be ignored. The reliability of a bruit in predicting susceptibility to vascular accidents is very low. However, it is a useful sign for myocardial infarction. Kleynhans and Terrett warn that if positive findings are encountered with any of the blood pressure evaluations, heart rate, or auscultation, the next step—provocational position testing—should not be performed (106, 110).

Provocational position testing includes variations of the same basic principles of placing the patient's head in rotation and extension. George et al. (109) state that the position be held for only 10 seconds, whereas Kleynhans (112) recommends up to 40 seconds unless positive findings occur sooner. Common to all tests are the important warning signs of vertigo, dizziness, nystagmus, nausea, vomiting, headache, tinnitus, and sensory disturbances. If any of these ischemic symptoms appear, the test should be considered positive, the patient's head should be quickly returned to a neutral position, and any attempt to manipulate using that position should be abandoned.

Maigne's Test

The patient is seated as the examiner brings the patient's head into extension and rotation. The patient's eyes are kept open and the examiner looks for the presence of nystagmus and the usual warning signs.

De Kleyn's Test

The patient lies supine with the head over the edge of the table, so as to obtain maximum cervical extension. The examiner holds the patient's head and rotates it to each side, observing the patient's eyes for the presence of nystagmus and the usual warning signs.

Hautant's Test

The patient is seated with both arms stretched out forward with the forearms supinated, palms up. The patient is then asked to close the eyes while the head is passively moved into extension and rotation. In addition to the identified warning signs, an arm may drop into pronation with ischemia.

Underberger's Test

The patient stands with eyes closed and arms outstretched forward, then is asked to march in place. The feet must completely leave the ground. The patient's head is then placed in extension and rotation. A positive ischemic response is swaying or staggering and the identified warning signs. The examiner should stand close to the patient to be able to help in case of a fall.

There are two major problems with the reliability of these positional tests as predictors of vascular injury and ischemia. First, although a test may be negative, an accident may still occur. Furthermore, the tests produce only some of the stresses of an adjustment, not the actual thrust. Second, there is a problem with false-positive results. However, vertigo and nystagmus of cervical origin are well documented and other conditions may be responsible for these same symptoms (113).

Despite these precautionary steps, a few patients still suffer from brain-stem injuries from iatrogenic stress forcibly applied to the head and neck. For the competent physician to provide proper management for a patient who has suffered a vascular accident after a cervical adjustment, it is absolutely essential to recognize the problem in its earliest stages.

Should a patient report adverse effects from a cervical adjustment consistent with a vascular etiology, some simple steps should be taken to provide the best possible care (117).

1. Do not administer another cervical adjustment.
2. Do not allow the patient to ambulate.
3. Keep the patient as comfortable as possible.
4. Note all physical and vital signs (pallor, sweating, vomiting, heart and respiratory rate, blood pressure, body temperature, etc.).
5. Check the pupils for size, shape, and equality as well as light and accommodation reflexes.
6. Test the lower cranial nerves (facial numbness or paresis, swallowing, gag reflex, slurred speech, palatal elevation, etc.).
7. Test cerebellar function (dysmetria of extremities, nystagmus on ocular motility, tremor, etc.).

8. Test the strength and tone of somatic musculature.
9. Test the somatic sensation to pinprick.
10. Test for muscle stretch and pathologic reflexes.

Documentation of this information clearly identifies that the clinician understands what to do in case of a vascular accident. Many times the effects of a vascular phenomenon are temporary and initial monitoring is the appropriate clinical action. Should the patient's condition worsen, referral for crisis care is warranted.

Other complications from cervical spine manipulation include dislocation of atlas on axis due to agenesis of the transverse ligament (commonly in Down's syndrome), rupture of the transverse ligament (common in the inflammatory arthropathies), and agenesis of the odontoid process (112).

Thoracic Spine

The main complication from manipulative therapy in the thoracic spine is rib fracture. Sprain to the costovertebral joints, strain to the intercostal muscles or both may also occur. Transverse process fracture and hematomelia have also been identified in rare instances (112). These problems are usually due to excessive or forceful manipulative therapy. They can be avoided by appropriate technique and adequate evaluation.

Lumbar Spine

The most frequently described complication from spinal manipulative therapy in the lumbar spine is compression of the cauda equina by a midline disc herniation at the level of the third, fourth, or fifth intervertebral disc (112). The resultant cauda equina syndrome is characterized by paralysis, weakness, pain, reflex change, and bowel and bladder disturbances. Although there is a risk of precipitating cauda equina compression syndrome through manipulative therapy, there is evidence that an uncomplicated herniated disc can be treated effectively and conservatively with manipulative therapy (118).

Furthermore, it has been postulated that rotary manipulations apply a torsional stress throughout the lumbar spine, creating undue forces in a relatively weakened area of the intervertebral disc, the posterolateral region (119, 120). Furthermore, Cassidy (25) and others (121, 122) claim that the torsional stress produced by rotary manipulations exerts a centripetal force, reducing the prolapsed or bulging disc material.

Bilateral radiculopathies with distal paralysis of the lower limbs, sensory loss in the sacral distribution, and sphincter paralysis should be considered surgical emergencies (123).

In 1973, the New Zealand Commission on Chiropractic reported, "chiropractors are the only health care practitioners who are necessarily equipped by their education and training to carry out spinal manual therapy" (124). Practitioners of manipulative therapy need to continue to develop skills and knowledge, not only in learning more about the area of therapeutics, but also in recognizing potential patients at risk. Studies to collect the facts should serve to quell fears in the minds of practitioners and disarm the opponents of manipulative therapy who aim to denigrate by alarming the public with information that is distorted and overstated and implanting in the public mind a fear of a genuinely safe and effective form of health care (108). Even though the disastrous complication of permanent neurologic damage is a very rare event, the term acceptable risk is suitable when applied to manipulative therapy (125).

However, the studies cited to draw these conclusions were done on cadavers with the posterior elements removed. If the posterior elements are intact, the facet joints limit the amount of rotation that could be damaging to the disc.

References

1. Shafer RC. Chiropractic health care. 3rd ed. Des Moines: Foundation for Chiropractic Education and Research, 1979:10–17.
2. Anderson R. Spinal manipulation before chiropractic. In: Haldeman S, ed. Principles and practice of chiropractic. 2nd ed. East Norwalk, CT: Appleton-Lange, 1992:3–13.
3. Haldeman S. Spinal manipulative therapy and sports medicine. Clin Sports Med 1986;5:2.
4. Strasser A. The chiropractic model of health: a personal perspective. Dig Chiro Econ 1988;31:12.
5. Strasser A. The dynamics of human structure in the chiropractic model of health. Dig Chiro Econ 1990;32:14.
6. Jamison JR. Chiropractic and medical models of health care: a contemporary perspective. J Manipulative Physiol Ther 1985;8:17.
7. Hildebrandt RW. The scope of chiropractic as a clinical science and art: an introductory review of concepts. J Manipulative Physiol Ther 1978;1:7.
8. Lantz CA. The vertebral subluxation complex. ICA Rev 1989;45:37.
9. Leach RA. The chiropractic theories: a synopsis of scientific research. 2nd ed. Baltimore: Williams & Wilkins, 1986.
10. Homewood AE. The neurodynamics of the vertebral subluxation. St. Petersburg: Valkyrie Press, 1979.
11. Herbst R. Gonstead chiropractic science and art: the chiropractic methodology of Clarence S. Gonstead, D.C. Mt. Horeb, WI: SCI-CHI Publications, 1980.
12. Vear HJ. An introduction to the science of chiropractic. Portland, OR: Western States Chiropractic College, 1981:138.
13. American Chiropractic Association membership directory. Indexed synopsis of ACA policies on public health

and related matters. Arlington: American Chiropractic Association, 1992–1993:C-22.

14. Palmer DD. The chiropractor's adjustor: the science, art, and philosophy of chiropractic. Portland, OR: Portland Printing, 1910.

15. Schafer RC, Faye LJ. Motion palpation and chiropractic technic: principles of dynamic chiropractic. Huntington Beach, CA: ACAP and MPI, 1989.

16. Brantingham JW. A survey of literature regarding the behavior, pathology, etiology, and nomenclature of the chiropractic lesion. J Am Chiro Assoc 1985;19:65–70.

17. Cassidy DJ, Potter GE. Motion examination of the lumbar spine. J Manipulative Physiol Ther 1979;2:151–158.

18. Faucret B, Mao W, et al. Determination of body subluxations by clinical, neurological and chiropractic procedures. J Manipulative Physiol Ther 1980;3:165–176.

19. Sandoz R. The choice of appropriate clinical criteria for assessing the progress of a chiropractic case. Ann Swiss Chiro Assoc 1985;8:53–73.

20. Bourdillon JF, Day EA. Spinal manipulation. 4th ed. London: William Heinemann Medical Books, 1987.

21. Greenman PE. Principles of manual medicine. Baltimore: Williams & Wilkins, 1989.

21a. Grieve GP. Common vertebral joint problems. 2nd ed. Edinburgh: Churchill Livingstone, 1988.

22. Kirkaldy-Willis WH, ed. Managing low back pain. 2nd ed. New York: Churchill Livingstone, 1988:118.

23. Sandoz R. Some physical mechanisms and effects of spinal adjustments. Ann Swiss Chiro Assoc 1976;6:91–141.

24. Sandoz R. Newer trends in the pathogenesis of spinal disorders. Ann Swiss Chiro Assoc 1971;5:93–179.

25. Cassidy JD. Manipulation. In: Kirkaldy-Willis WH, ed. Managing low back pain. 2nd ed. New York: Churchill Livingstone, 1988.

26. Giles LGF. Anatomical basis of low back pain. Baltimore: Williams & Wilkins, 1989.

27. Giles LGF, Taylor JR. Intra-articular synovial protrusions in the lower lumbar apophyseal joints. Bull Hosp Jt Dis Orthop Inst 1982;42:248–255.

28. Giles LGF, Taylor JR, Cockson A. Human zygapophyseal joint synovial folds. Acta Anat 1986;126:110–114.

29. Giles LGF, Taylor JR. Innervation of lumbar zygapophyseal joint synovial folds. Acta Orthop Scand 1987;58:43–46.

30. Giles LGF. Lumbar apophyseal joint arthrography. J Manipulative Physiol Ther 1984;7:21–24.

31. Giles LGF. Lumbo-sacral and cervical zygapophyseal joint inclusions. Manual Med 1986;2:89–92.

32. Bogduk N. Clinical anatomy of the lumbar spine. New York: Churchill Livingstone, 1990.

33. Russell R. Diagnostic palpation of the spine: a review of procedures and assessment of their reliability. J Manipulative Physiol Ther 1983;6:181–183.

34. Haas M. The reliability of reliability. J Manipulative Physiol Ther 1991;14:199–208.

35. Keating J. Several strategies for evaluating the objectivity of measurements in clinical research and practice. J Can Chiro Assoc 1988;32:133–138.

36. Keating J. Inter-examiner reliability of motion palpation of the lumbar spine: a review of quantitative literature. Am J Chiro Med 1989;2:107–110.

37. Keating JC, Bergmann TF, et al. Interexaminer reliability of eight evaluative dimensions of lumbar segmental abnormality. J Manipulative Physiol Ther 1990;13:463–470.

38. Boline P, Keating J, et al. Interexaminer reliability of palpatory evaluations of the lumbar spine. Am J Chiro Med 1988;1:5–11.

39. Panzer DM. Lumbar motion palpation: a literature review. Proceedings of the Sixth Annual Conference on Research and Education. Monterey, CA. 1991:171–184.

40. Johnston W, Allan BR, et al. Interexaminer study of palpation in detecting location of spinal segmental dysfunction. J Am Osteopathic Assoc 1983;82:839–845.

41. Deboer KF, Harmon R, et al. Reliability study of detection of somatic dysfunctions in the cervical spine. J Manipulative Physiol Ther 1985;8:9–16.

42. Zachman Z, Traina AD, et al. Interexaminer reliability and concurrent validity of two instruments for the measurement of cervical ranges of motion. J Manipulative Physiol Ther 1989;12:205–210.

43. Keeley J, Mayer TG, et al. Quantification of lumbar function: part 5. reliability of range-of-motion measures in the sagittal plane and an in vivo torso rotation measurement technique. Spine 1968;11:31–35.

44. Cooperstein R, Gardner R, Nansel D. Procedure-specific concordance of two methods of motion palpation with goniometrically-assessed cervical lateral flexion asymmetry. Proceedings of the 1991 World Chiropractic Congress, Toronto. 1991:45.

45. Tucci S, Hicks J, et al. Cervical motion assessment: a new, simple and accurate method. Arch Phys Med Rehabil 1985;67:225–230.

46. Liebenson C, Phillips R. The reliability of range of motion measurements for lumbar spine flexion: a review. J Chiro Tech 1989;1:69–78.

47. Johnston W, Elkiss ML, et al. Passive gross motion testing: part II. a study of interexaminer agreement. J Am Osteopathic Assoc 1982;8:304–308.

48. Fitzgerald GK, Wynvcen K, et al. Objective assessment with establishment of normal values for lumbar spinal range of motion. Phys Ther 1983;63:1776–1781.

49. Boone D, Azen S. Reliability of goniometric measurements. Phys Ther 1978;58:1355–1359.

50. Mayer TG, Tencer AF, et al. Use of noninvasive techniques for quantification of spinal range-of-motion in normal subjects and chronic low-back dysfunction patients. Spine 1984;9:588–595.

51. Vernon H. An assessment of the intra- and inter-reliability of the posturometer. J Manipulative Physiol Ther 1983;6:57–60.

52. Adams AA. Intra- and inter-examiner reliability of plumb line posture analysis measurements using a three dimensional electrogoniometer. Res Forum 1988;4:60–72.

53. D'Angelo MD, Grieve DW. A description of normal relaxed standing postures. Clin Biomechanics 1987;2:140–144.

54. Nanzel DD, Peneff AL, et al. Interexaminer concordance in detecting joint-play asymmetries in the cervical spines of otherwise asymptomatic subjects. J Manipulative Physiol Ther 1989;12:428–433.

55. Mootz RD, Keating JC, Kontz HP. Intra- and inter-examiner reliability of passive motion palpation of the lumbar spine. J Manipulative Physiol Ther 1989;12:440–445.

56. Herzog W, Read LJ, et al. Reliability of motion palpation to detect sacroiliac joint fixations. J Manipulative Physiol Ther 1989;12:86–92.

57. Love RM, Brodeur RR. Inter- and intraexaminer reliability of motion palpation for the thoracolumbar spine. J Manipulative Physiol Ther 1987;10:1–4.

58. Carmichael JP. Inter- and intraexaminer reliability of palpation for sacroiliac joint dysfunction. J Manipulative Physiol Ther 1987;10:164–171.

59. Bergstrom E, Courtis G. An inter- and intra-examiner reliability study of motion palpation of the lumbar spine in lateral flexion in the seated position. Eur J Chiro 1986;34:121–141.

60. Mior SA, King RS, et al. Intra- and interexaminer reliability of motion palpation in the cervical spine. J Can Chiro Assoc 1985;29:195–198.

61. Wiles MR. Reproducibility and interexaminer correlation of motion palpation findings of the sacroiliac joints. J Can Chiro Assoc 1980;24:59–69.

62. Leboeuf C, Gardner V, et al. Chiropractic examination procedures: a reliability and consistency study. J Aust Chiro Assoc 1989;19:101–104.

63. Johnston W, Hill JL, et al. Palpatory findings in the cervicothoracic region: variations in normotensive and hy-

pertensive subjects. a preliminary report. J Am Osteopathic Assoc 1980;79:300–308.

64. Gonnella C, Paris SV, Kutner M. Reliability in evaluating passive intervertebral motion. Phys Ther 1982;62:436–444.

65. DeBoer KF, Harmon RO, et al. Inter- and intra-examiner reliability of leg length differential measurement: a preliminary study. J Manipulative Physiol Ther 1983;6:61–66.

66. Fuhr Aw, Osterbauer PJ. Interexaminer reliability of relative leg-length evaluation in the prone, extended position. J Chiro Tech 1989;1:13–18.

67. Venn EK, Wakefield KA, Thompson PR. A comparative study of leg-length checks. Eur J Chiro 1983;31:68–80.

68. Shambaugh MS, Sclafani L, Fanselow D. Reliability of the Derifield-Thomas test for leg length inequality, and use of the test to determine cervical adjusting efficacy. J Manipulative Physiol Ther 1988;11:396–399.

69. Rhudy TR, Burk JM. Inter-examiner reliability of functional leg-length assessment. Am J Chiro Med 1990;3:63–66.

70. Haas M. Interexaminer reliability for multiple diagnostic test regimens. J Manipulative Physiol Ther 1991;14:95–103.

71. Brunarski DJ. Chiropractic biomechanical evaluations: validity in myofascial low back pain. J Manipulative Physiol Ther 1982;5:155–161.

72. Jull G, Bogduk N, Marsland A. The accuracy of manual diagnosis for cervical zygapophyseal joint pain syndromes. Med J Australia 1988;148:233–236.

73. Falltrick D, Pierson SD. Precise measurement of functional leg length inequality and changes due to cervical spine rotation in pain-free students. J Manipulative Physiol Ther 1989;12:364–368.

74. Koran LM. The reliability of clinical methods, data and judgements. N Engl J Med 1975;293:642–646.

75. Nelson MA, Allen P, et al. Reliability and reproducibility of clinical findings in low back pain. Spine 1979;4:97–101.

76. Alley RJ. The clinical value of motion palpation as a diagnostic tool. J Can Chiro Assoc 1983;27:91–100.

77. Waddell G, Main CJ, et al. Normality and reliability in the clinical assessment of backache. Br Med J 1982;284:1519–1523.

78. Bergmann TF. Chiropractic spinal examination. In: Ferezy JS, ed. The chiropractic neurological examination. Gaithersburg, MD: Aspen Publications, 1992.

79. Bergmann TF, Peterson DH, Lawrence D. Chiropractic technique: principles and procedures. New York: Churchill Livingstone, 1993:51–122.

80. Sandoz R. Some reflex phenomena associated with spinal derangements and adjustments. Ann Swiss Chiro Assoc 1981;7:45.

81. Hertling D, Kessler RM. Management of common musculoskeletal disorders: physical therapy principles and methods. 2nd ed. Philadelphia: JB Lippincott, 1990.

82. Kaltenborn FM. Mobilization of the extremity joints: examination and basic treatment principles. 3rd ed. Oslo: Olaf-Norlis-Bokhandel, 1980.

83. Roston JB, Wheeler Haines RW. Cracking in the metacarpophalangeal joint. J Anat 1947;81:165.

84. Unsworth A, Dowson D, Wright V. Cracking joints, a bioengineering study of cavitation in the metacarpophalangeal joint. Ann Rheum Dis 1971;30:348.

85. Sandoz R. The significance of the manipulative crack and other articular noises. Ann Swiss Chiro Assoc 1969;4:47.

86. Akeson WH, Amiel D, Woo S. Immobility affects of synovial joints: the pathomechanics of joint contracture. Biorheology 1980;17:95.

87. Akeson WH, Amiel D, Mechanic GL, et al. Collagen cross linking alterations in joint contractures: changes in reducible cross links in periarticular connective tissue collagen after 9 weeks of immobilization. Connect Tissue Res 1977;5:5.

88. Burger AA. Experimental neuromuscular models of spinal manual techniques. Manual Med 1983;1:10.

89. Wyke BD. Articular neurology and manipulative therapy. In: Glasgow EF, Twomey LT, Schull ER, et al., eds. Aspects of manipulative therapy. New York: Churchill Livingstone, 1985:72–80.

90. Terret ACJ, Vernon H. Manipulation and pain tolerance: a controlled study of the effect of spinal manipulation on paraspinal cutaneous pain levels. Am J Phys Med 1984;63:217–225.

91. Cassidy JD, Quon J, LaFrance L. Effect of manipulation on pain and range of motion in the cervical spine. In press. 1988.

92. LaFrance L, Cassidy JD. The effects of manipulation on the range of motion of the cervical spine. In press.

93. Vernon HT, Dhami MSI, et al. Spinal manipulation and beta-endorphin: a controlled study of the effect of a spinal manipulation on plasma beta-endorphin levels in normal males. J Manipulative Physiol Ther 1986; 9:115–123.

94. Vernon HT. Pressure pain threshold evaluation of the effect of spinal manipulation on chronic neck pain: a single case study. JCCA 1988;32:191–194.

95. Hood RP. Blood pressure results in 75 abnormal cases. Dig Chiro Econ 1974;16:36–38.

96. Tran TA, Kirby JD. The effectiveness of upper cervical adjustment upon the normal physiology of the heart. ACA J Chiro 1977;58–62.

97. Sato A, Swenson RS. Sympathetic nervous system response to mechanical stress of the spinal column in rats. J Manipulative Physiol Ther 1984;7:141–147.

98. Briggs L, Boone WR. Effects of a chiropractic adjustment on changes in pupillary diameter: a model for evaluating somatovisceral response. J Manipulative Physiol Ther 1988;11:181–189.

99. Dhami MSI, Coyle BA, et al. Evidence for sympathetic neuron stimulation by cervicospinal manipulation. Proceedings of the First Annual Conference on Research and Education of Specific Consortium for Chiropractic Research, California Chiropractic Association, Sacramento. 1986:A51–55.

100. Paris SV. Spinal manipulative therapy. In: Clinical Orthopedics and Related Research, October 1983;179.

101. Peterson DH. Western States Chiropractic College adjustive technique manual. Portland, OR: Western States Chiropractic College, 1988.

102. Grice AS. Biomechanical approach to cervical and dorsal adjusting. In: Haldeman S, ed. Modern developments in the principles and practice of chiropractic. New York: Appleton-Century-Croft, 1980.

103. Clarke GR, Stenner L. Use of therapeutic ultrasound. Physiotherapy 1976;62:185.

104. Lescure R. Incidents, accidents, contraindications. Med Hyg (Geneva) 1954;12:456.

105. Lewit K. Complications following chiropractic manipulation. Dtsch Med Wochenschr 1972;97:784.

106. Kleynhans AM, Terrett AGJ. The prevention of complications from spinal manipulative therapy. In: Aspects of manipulative therapy. New York: Churchill Livingstone, 1985.

107. Livingston M. Spinal manipulation causing injury. British Columbia Med J 1971;14:78–81.

108. Terrett AGJ. Vascular accidents from cervical spine manipulation: a report on 107 cases. J Aust Chiro Assoc 1987;17:1.

109. George PE, et al. Identification of high risk, prestroke patient. J Chiropractic 1981;15(suppl):26–28.

110. Terrett AGJ. Importance and interpretation of tests designed to predict susceptibility to neurocirculatory accidents from manipulation. JACA 1983;13:2.

111. Bland JH. Disorders of the cervical spine. Philadelphia: WB Saunders, 1987.

112. Kleynhans AM. Complications and contraindications of spinal manipulative therapy. In: Haldeman S, ed. Modern

developments in the principles and practice of chiropractic. New York: Appleton-Century-Croft, 1979.

113. Terrett AGJ. Vascular accidents from cervical spinal manipulation: the mechanisms. J Aust Chiro Assoc 1987;17:131–144.

114. Gatterman M. Contraindications and complications of spinal manipulative therapy. ACA J Chiro 1981; 18(suppl):75–86.

115. Gatterman MI. Chiropractic management of spine related disorders. Baltimore: Williams & Wilkins, 1990:55.

116. Bolton PS, Stick PE, Lord RSA. Failure of clinical tests to predict cerebral ischemia before neck manipulation. J Manipulative Physiol Ther 1989;12:304–307.

117. Ferezy JS. The chiropractic neurological examination. Gaithersburg, MD: Aspen Publishers, 1992:123–140.

118. Matthews JA, Yates DAH. Reduction of lumbar disc prolapse by manipulation. Br Med J 1969;3:696–697.

119. Fisher ED. Report of a case of ruptured intervertebral disc following chiropractic manipulation. Kentucky Med J 1943;41:14.

120. Poppen JL The herniated intervertebral disc: an analysis of 400 verified cases. N Engl J Med 1945;232:211.

121. Cyriax J. Correspondence. Br Med J 1956;4:173.

122. Hooper J. Low back pain and manipulation: paraparesis after treatment of low back pain by physical methods. Med J Australia 1973;1:549–551.

123. Jennet WB. A study of 25 cases of compression of the cauda equina by prolapsed IVD. J Neurol Neurosurg Psychiatry 1956;19:109.

124. Chiropractic in New Zealand: report of the Commission of Inquiry 1979. Presented to the House of Representatives by Command of His Excellency the Governor-General, Government printer, Wellington, New Zealand, 1979.

125. Ferezy JS. Neuroischemia and cervical manipulation: an acceptable risk. ACA J Chiro 1988;22:61–63.

5B/ Extraspinal Joint Manipulation

Gerry G. Provance

This chapter presents a basic understanding of the evaluation and manipulation of the extraspinal joints.

All joints are capable of physiologic movement. For muscles, tendons, ligaments, and other soft tissue structures to remain healthy it is imperative that joint function be optimal, thereby allowing athletes to reach their peak athletic performance and potential.

Athletes traditionally have been treated for sprains, strains, etc., with less than adequate results. These results are not due to a lack of understanding of active and passive movement, but are instead due to being unaware of the third movement—joint play.

Joint play is that degree of end movement (paraphysiologic space) beyond active and passive motion that cannot be achieved through voluntary movement. However, total joint mobility is the sum of the voluntary range of movement plus or minus the joint play. Loss of joint play cannot be restored by any exercise program.

Joints have or should have this very small but precise joint play movement that is not controlled by muscles. This movement is important for normal articular cartilage nutrition, for pain-free range of motion, for muscles to work through their full range, and for overall optimal joint function. Dysfunction will develop if these small joint play movements are decreased (hypomobile), increased (hypermobile), or lost.

This joint dysfunction is mechanical, and to correct a mechanical fault it is logical to seek a mechanical form of treatment. Hence, the chiropractor and joint manipulation.

The prerequisite for successful treatment in any field of health care is an accurate diagnosis. It is therefore necessary to perform a comprehensive examination, including complete history, physical examination, x-rays when available, special tests, and biomechanical analysis. This exam is very important in the management of an athlete's musculoskeletal structure. However, it is most important to determine if the joint play movement is normal, hypomobile, or hypermobile. Normal joint play movement needs no manipulation, whereas hypomobility requires specific manipulation in the direction of that restriction. Hypermobility also needs no manipulation. However, to slow this increased mobility it is imperative to increase any restricted joint motion within that joint or in nearby joints, thereby allowing optimal joint function.

The rules for joint play examination and manipulation are as follows.

1. The athlete must be relaxed.
2. The doctor's grasp must be firm and supportive but not uncomfortable.
3. One joint must be examined at a time.
4. One movement at each joint is examined at a time.
5. In the examination of each joint, one hand will usually stabilize while the other hand performs the movement.
6. The extent of normal joint play movement in the capsule of any synovial joint is never more than $\frac{1}{8}$ inch in any plane. It can usually be ascertained by examining the same joint on the unaffected side of the body.
7. The joint play endfeel should be normal. Normal can be a soft endfeel, such as in glenohumeral posterior shear, or a hard endfeel (bone-to-bone), such as in ulnohumeral (elbow) extension.
8. In the presence of obvious clinical signs of inflammation, fracture, or disease process, no examining movements need to be or should be undertaken.
9. Forceful or abnormal movement must never be used.
10. The examining movement must be stopped at any point at which pain is elicited.
11. The manipulative thrust is a controlled short, sharp, push or pull with speed and accuracy.
12. Before applying a manipulative thrust, always remove the soft tissue slack surrounding the joint structure.
13. Reevaluation should be performed after the manipulation to determine if a correction has been made and the progress of that restriction.

Contradictions to manipulation are as follows:

1. Congenital anomalies (e.g., joint fusion);
2. Recent fracture;
3. Disease processes such as primary bone tumors and metastases; and
4. Manipulation in the direction of normal or hypermobile joint play movement.

THE SHOULDER

The shoulder is not a single joint but a complexity of three joints and one articulation: the sternoclavicular joint, the acromioclavicular (A-C) joint, the glenohumeral joint, and the scapulothoracic articulation.

It is a finely tuned structure that works in synchronous function. However, the intricacy of combined versatile movement makes this multiple joint structure vulnerable to injury. During motion, there is a constant compromise occurring within the shoulder joint complex to balance the competing demands of stability and mobility.

Glenohumeral Joint

The shoulder (glenohumeral) joint is a synovial joint of the ball-and-socket variety in which the humeral head is three times larger than the shallow glenoid cavity where it articulates.

The humeral head slides in the opposite direction of the humerus. When the humerus is abducted, the humeral head slides in the inferior direction; when the humerus is adducted, the humeral head slides in the superior direction.

This joint, due to its laxity, is the most common site of dislocation and dysfunction involving the extremities.

EXAMINATION/MANIPULATION

Lateral Distraction (Fig. 5B.1)

Athlete: Supine with involved upper arm relaxed on the table, elbow flexed.

Doctor: Standing inferior to and facing toward the involved shoulder. The medial hand is placed on the medial surface of the humerus, high in the axillary region, palm facing outward, and the forearm is placed across the athlete's chest. The lateral hand grips the elbow with the palm facing inward.

Action: To test the lateral distraction of the humeral head going away from the glenoid cavity, the lateral hand applies a pressure on the elbow going toward the athlete's rib cage while the medial hand simultaneously removes the soft tissue slack going laterally and testing joint play. Correction of the restriction is the test plus an added impulse.

Anterior Glide (Fig. 5B.2)

Athlete: Supine with the involved upper arm relaxed on the table, elbow flexed.

Doctor: Standing inferior to and facing toward the involved shoulder. The medial hand (palm upward) grasps the posterior proximal humerus high in the axillary region. The thumb web of the lateral hand (palm downward) is placed in the antecubital space (between the athlete's forearm and upper arm) for stabilization.

Action: Apply a downward pressure with the stabilization hand while simultaneously removing the soft tissue slack, and then test the anterior glide of the humeral head in the glenoid cavity for joint play. Correction of restriction is the test plus an impulse.

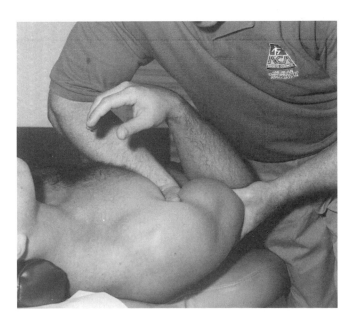

Figure 5B.1. Lateral distraction.

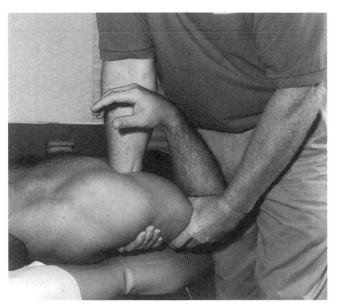

Figure 5B.2. Anterior glide.

Posterior Shear (10°–90°) (Fig. 5B.3)

Athlete: Supine with involved shoulder near the side of the table and the elbow flexed.

Doctor: The lateral hand cups the athlete's posterior shoulder, palm upward. The medial hand cups the elbow, and the doctor's upper chest is placed over the medial hand for support.

Action: Place the athlete's upper arm in 10° flexion with the elbow slightly adducted while removing the soft tissue slack going posteriorly and stretching the posterior capsule. Proceed upward, testing posterior joint play without go-

ing beyond 90°. Correct any restriction from 10°–90° by adding an impulse. Do not jam the humeral head into the acromial process, glenoid cavity, or table. This manipulation can also be done with the athlete in the sitting position using the alternate method of manipulation for the posterior and superior glide of the A-C joint.

Lateral-Posterior Glide (Fig. 5B.4)

Athlete: Supine with the involved upper arm flexed at 90° with the hand resting on the chest.

Doctor: Same as above with the exception of placing the doctor's body lateral to the involved shoulder and placing the doctor's inferior shoulder on the humerus.

Action: Pull the humeral head lateral and downward toward the floor. Correction of a restriction is the test plus an impulse.

Posterior-Inferior Glide (Fig. 5B.5)

Athlete: Same as above.

Doctor: In a crouched position with the body at the inferior aspect of the involved shoulder. The fingers of both hands are interlaced on the most proximal aspect of the humerus. The athlete's humerus is placed on the doctor's medial shoulder, which is used as a fulcrum and for support.

Action: First apply pressure on the humeral head going in a lateral and posterior direction, and then in an inferior direction testing the joint play. Correction of a restriction is the test plus an impulse.

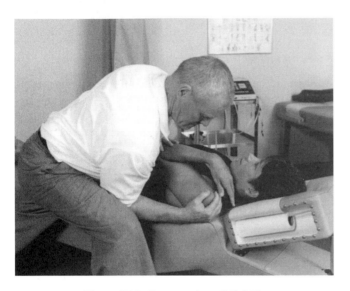

Figure 5B.3. Posterior shear (10°–90°).

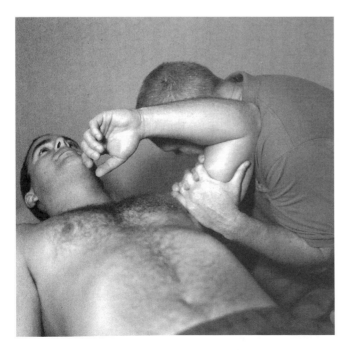

Figure 5B.4. Lateral-posterior glide.

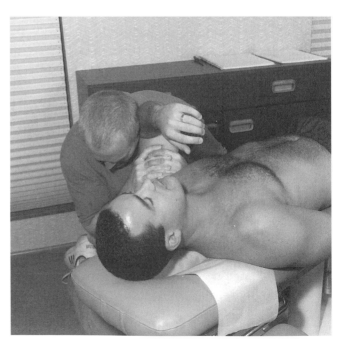

Figure 5B.5. Posterior-inferior glide.

External Rotation (Fig. 5B.6)

Athlete: Supine with the involved arm abducted and externally rotated (hold up position) at a comfortable range.

Doctor: Facing perpendicular to the patient, the doctor grasps, with both hands, the proximal humeral shaft with the thumbs on the anterior shaft and the fingers on the posterior aspect. The athlete's forearm is supported by placing the doctor's superior forearm on theirs, also for leverage.

Action: Remove the soft tissue slack going toward external rotation with both hands and forearm testing for a springy endfeel. Correction of a restriction is the test plus an impulse.

Internal Rotation (Fig. 5B.7)

Athlete: Supine with involved arm abducted and internally rotated (palm downward) at a comfortable range.

Doctor: Same as above with the exception of placing the thumbs on the posterior humeral shaft and the fingers on the anterior aspect.

Action: Remove the soft tissue slack going toward internal rotation and test for the springy endfeel. Correction of a restriction is the test plus an impulse.

Inferior Glide (Fig. 5B.8)

Athlete: Sitting with the involved shoulder and elbow at 90°, palm facing downward.

Doctor: Facing perpendicular to the involved shoulder. The athlete's distal humerus is placed over the doctor's trapezius area. The most proximal portion of the humerus is grasped with both hands, being sure not to contact the acromion process.

Action: Apply a downward (inferior) glide on the most proximal humerus with both hands. The humeral head should glide downward in the glenoid cavity. The correction of restriction is the test plus a light impulse thrust.

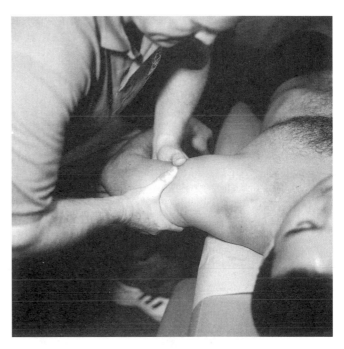

Figure 5B.7. Internal rotation.

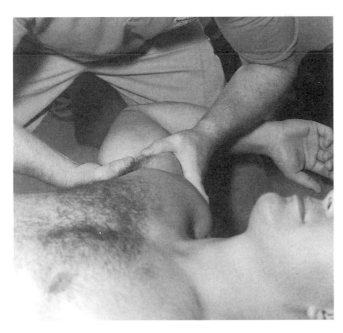

Figure 5B.6. External rotation.

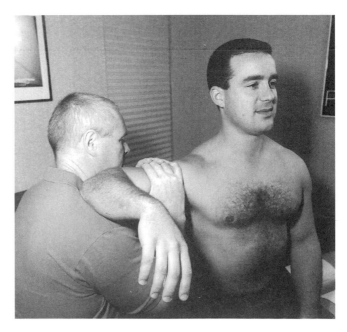

Figure 5B.8. Inferior glide.

Circumduction (Fig. 5B.9)

Athlete: Prone with the involved shoulder and elbow at approximately 90°, palm facing caudally.

Doctor: Facing perpendicular with the lower humeral shaft or forearm between the lower thighs for stabilization. The proximal humerus is grasped with both hands.

Action: Circumduct the head of the humerus in the glenoid cavity, first going in a counterclockwise direction and then in a clockwise direction applying a wide range of motion testing for any restrictions within the socket. At any time a fixation is noted, add a quick impulse into the direction of restriction.

Long-Axis Distraction (Fig. 5B.10)

Athlete: Supine with the involved arm slightly abducted in a neutral position.

Doctor: Kneeling on the medial knee and positioned at the inferior aspect of, and between, the involved shoulder and the athlete's trunk. The lateral hand grasps the distal humerus, while the distal forearm is placed between the doctor's chest and upper arm for support and distraction. The thumb web of the medial hand is placed (thumb up) into the axilla to stabilize the scapula.

Action: Apply a long-axis traction by leaning backward. A separation (distraction) should occur at the glenohumeral joint . Correction of a restriction is the test plus an impulse.

Sternoclavicular Joint

This synovial joint is stabilized by ligaments and often contains a fibrocartilaginous meniscus. It is extremely important because it is the only bony attachment between the upper limb and the axial skeleton. It is actually a pivot point about which movements of the shoulder as a whole occur.

This joint is commonly hypermobile in athletes who perform a large amount of throwing or play racket sports. This is due to the repetitive over-accentuating movement in the cocking phase.

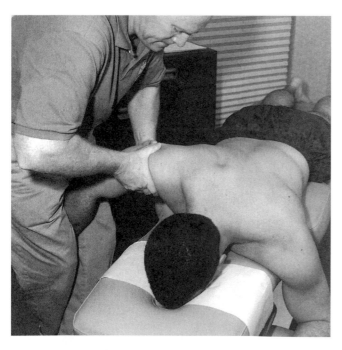

Figure 5B.9. Circumduction.

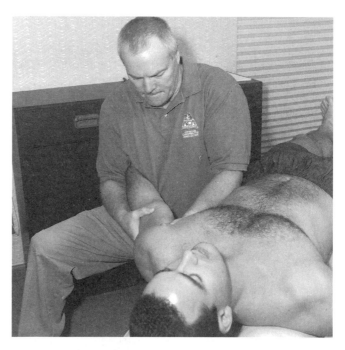

Figure 5B.10. Long-axis distraction.

EXAMINATION/MANIPULATION

Posterior, Superior, Anterior, and Inferior Glide (Fig. 5B.11)

Athlete: Supine with the head slightly elevated and both hands on the abdomen.

Doctor: On the side of involvement, facing toward the sternoclavicular (S-C) joint. A pinch-grip is placed with the medial hand (single hand contact), or both hands are used to apply a double hand pinch-grip on the proximal clavicle near the sternum.

Action: Apply a push (posterior and superior) and pull one direction at a time (anterior and inferior) on the clavicle to test the joint play of the clavicle on the sternum. Correction of a restriction is the test plus an impulse.

Alternative Method of Manipulation (Fig. 5B.12). The correction of a superior or posterior restriction can also be made using a double thumb contact or the pisiform of the medial hand.

Acromioclavicular Joint

The A-C joint is a satellite joint of the shoulder that moves throughout shoulder abduction, especially during the initial and late stages of this motion. Its stability is primarily due to the deltoid and trapezius origins that surround it; additional reinforcement is given by the A-C ligaments and by the coracoclavicular ligaments. This joint is commonly hypomobile in athletes who perform a large amount of throwing or play racket sports.

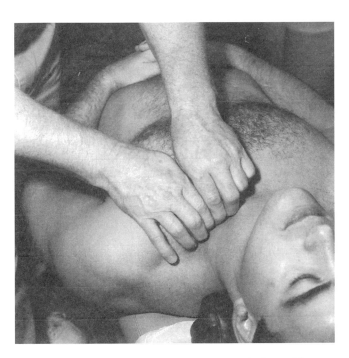

Figure 5B.11. Posterior, superior, anterior, and inferior glide.

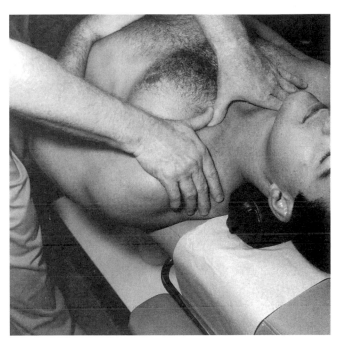

Figure 5B.12. Alternative method of manipulation.

EXAMINATION/MANIPULATION

Posterior and Superior Glide (Fig. 5B.13)

Athlete: Supine with the head slightly elevated and hands on the abdomen.

Doctor: On the side of involvement, facing toward the A-C joint. The acromion is grasped, with the fingers on the posterior surface and the thumb on the anterior surface, with the lateral (stabilization) hand. The thumb, index, and middle fingers of the contact hand grasp the distal third of the clavicle.

Action: Apply a push-pull movement with the fingers on the clavicle going in an anterior and superior direction and then in a posterior and inferior direction. Correction of a restriction is the test plus an impulse.

Alternative Method of Manipulation (Fig. 5B.14)

Athlete: Sitting with the elbow in flexion.

Doctor: Standing behind the athlete. The doctor reaches around in front of the athlete and cups the elbow with both hands. The elbow is lifted, removing the soft tissue slack.

Action: Apply an impulse thrust with the hand contact on the elbow in a posterior and superior direction to separate the fixated A-C joint.

Scapulothoracic Articulation

There is no "true joint" between the scapula and the thoracic cage. It is a bone-muscle-bone articulation. The scapula slides along the thoracic cage where there is considerable soft tissue flexibility that allows the scapula to participate in all upper extremity motions.

Scapulohumeral motion should be smooth and coordinated. For every 30° that the arm is elevated, the humerus moves 20° and the scapula 10°.

Dysfunction at this articulation is primarily due to muscle shortening within the shoulder girdle or adhesions between the scapula and the underlying ribs.

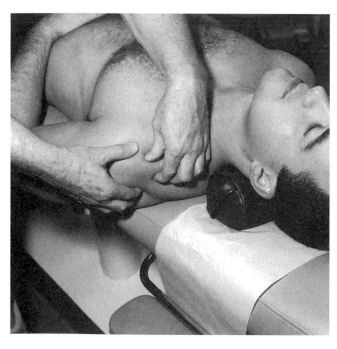

Figure 5B.13. Posterior and superior glide.

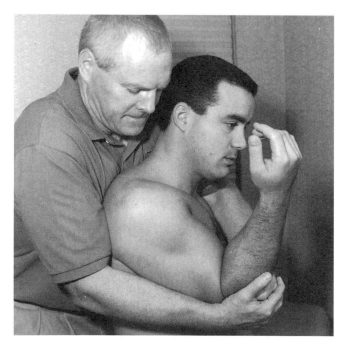

Figure 5B.14. Alternative method of manipulation.

EXAMINATION/MANIPULATION

Distraction With Combined Mobilization (Fig. 5B.15A and B)

Athlete: Prone or lying on side.

Doctor: On the side of the involved shoulder, facing perpendicular. The patient's arm is abducted to 90° and placed between the doctor's thighs for stabilization. The superior indifferent hand cups and slightly elevates the shoulder in an anterior-posterior direction. The fingers of the active hand grasp the medial, inferior border (underneath) of the scapula.

Action: Move the scapula through the desired direction by lifting with both the active and indifferent hands. Begin testing scapular mobility first with the posterior distraction maneuver, followed by (any order) superior, inferior, lateral, medial, clockwise, and counterclockwise movements. The correction of a restriction is made with several impulse thrusts in the direction of restriction to break up and stretch the adhesive connective tissue.

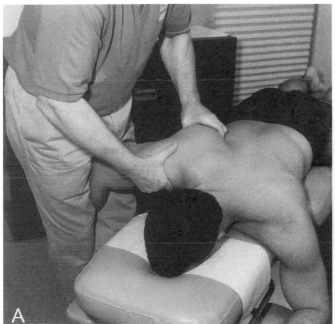
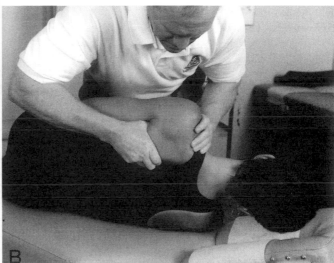

Figure 5B.15. Distraction with combined mobilization.

THE ELBOW

The elbow consists of three joints: the proximal radioulnar, ulnohumeral, and radiohumeral.

The elbow is a key link in the kinetic chain of the upper extremity and adds mobility to the hand as well as flexion, extension, pronation, and supination to the forearm.

Proximal Radioulnar Joint

This joint is a uniaxial pivot joint with the distal radioulnar joint. The distal radioulnar joint moves the proximal radioulnar joint as a functional unit in rotation, that is, pronation and supination.

EXAMINATION/MANIPULATION

Upward Glide of the Radial Head on the Ulna (Fig. 5B.16)

Athlete: Standing with the elbow flexed 90° and the wrist extended.

Doctor: Standing on the lateral side and facing the involved elbow. The doctor's thenar eminence is placed over the athlete's thenar eminence. The elbow is stabilized with the doctor's other hand, while the thumb contacts the superior aspect of the radial head for palpation.

Action: Apply a combination of extension and supination on the athlete's wrist. The radial head should glide in an upward direction. Correction of a restriction is the test, plus an impulse through the long axis of the radius.

Downward Glide of the Radial Head on the Ulna (Fig. 5B.17)

Athlete: Standing with the elbow in approximately 45° flexion and wrist slightly flexed.

Doctor: Standing on the lateral side of the involved arm and toward the front of the athlete. The distal radius and thenar area are grasped with the doctor's medial hand. The other hand is placed on the elbow with a thumb contact on the radial head.

Action: Apply a combination of flexion and pronation on the athlete's distal radius and hand. The radial head should glide in a downward direction. Correction of a restriction is the test, plus thumb pressure on the radial head going downward in alignment with the radial shaft, plus an impulse.

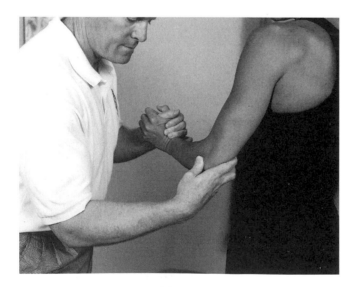

Figure 5B.16. Upward glide of the radial head on the ulna.

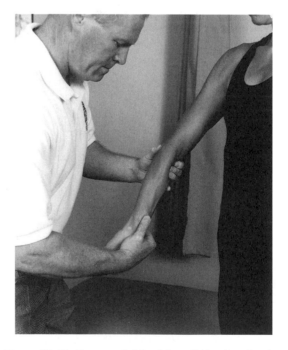

Figure 5B.17. Downward glide of the radial head on the ulna.

Anterior Glide of the Radial Head on the Ulna (Fig. 5B.18)

Athlete: Standing with elbow toward the anterior (approximately 45°) in a nearly extended position, palm facing outward.

Doctor: Standing on the lateral side of the involved elbow. The doctor's anterior hand is placed on the athlete's distal radius and ulna just above the wrist. The active hand grasps the elbow, with the fingers on the medial epicondyle area and the thumb on the posterior aspect of the radial head.

Action: Apply pressure with the thumb on the radial head going in an anterior direction. The radial head should have a springy endfeel. Correction of a restriction is with a sharp quick thrust in the direction of the restriction.

Posterior Glide of the Radial Head on the Ulna

Athlete: Sitting with the elbow in flexion and the forearm in pronation.

Doctor: Standing in front of the involved elbow with a foot on the table. The athlete's elbow is placed on the doctor's knee. The distal forearm is grasped with the doctor's medial hand, and the radial head is pinch-gripped with the other hand.

Action: Pull the radial head in the posterior direction testing the joint play. Correction of a restriction is the test plus an impulse.

Alternative Method of Manipulation (Fig. 5B.19)

Athlete: Same as above with the exception of the athlete being in a supine position.

Doctor: Standing and facing perpendicular to the involved arm. The knuckle of the doctor's index finger is placed deep in the antecubital fossa between the radial head and distal humerus to be used as a fulcrum. The other hand maintains pronation of the forearm.

Action: Apply a quick, sharp, impulse thrust with the distal forearm contact going toward the humerus, while at the same time applying a counterthrust with fulcrum contact going caudally and the radial head moving in a posterior direction.

Ulnohumeral Joint

The ulnohumeral hinge joint is the principal joint at the elbow that allows pure flexion and extension. A lack of full extension affects the throwing motion and also hinders a good follow-through in shooting a basketball.

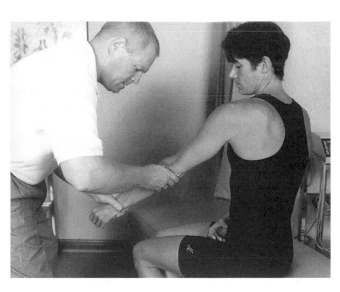

Figure 5B.18. Anterior glide of the radial head on the ulna.

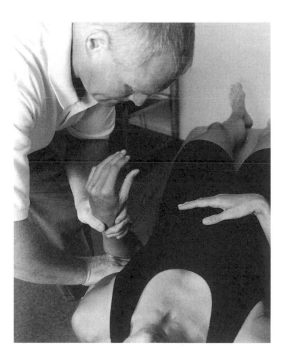

Figure 5B.19. Alternative method of manipulation.

EXAMINATION/MANIPULATION

Distraction in Flexion (Fig. 5B.20)

Athlete: Supine with the arm at the side, elbow bent, and forearm supinated.

Doctor: Standing and facing toward the involved elbow. The distal radius and ulna are grasped just above the wrist with the inferior hand while maintaining forearm supination. The thumb web is placed (palm down) on the most proximal portion of the forearm in the antecubital space, with the superior hand to be used as a fulcrum.

Action: Move the proximal forearm inferiorly with the superior hand while simultaneously applying flexion of the forearm with the inferior hand, affecting joint distraction. As movement increases, the elbow can be flexed progressively. Correction of restriction is the test plus an impulse.

Lateral Tilt of the Ulna on the Humerus (Fig. 5B.21)

Athlete: Supine with the arm at the side, slightly elevated and abducted, with the palm facing upward.

Doctor: Standing or sitting on the medial side of the involved arm. The distal radius and ulna are grasped just above the wrist with the inferior arm for stabilization. The superior hand grasps the proximal ulna, the doctor's palm upward. The elbow is a few degrees off complete extension and relaxed.

Action: Apply a lateral glide of the ulna on the humerus. There should be a springy endfeel. Correction of a restriction is the test plus an impulse. Only apply enough force for a correction; avoid excessive force.

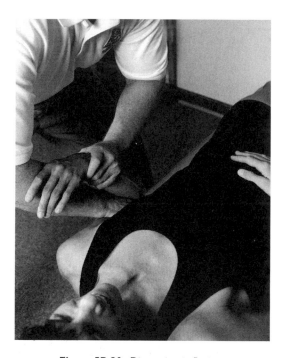

Figure 5B.20. Distraction in flexion.

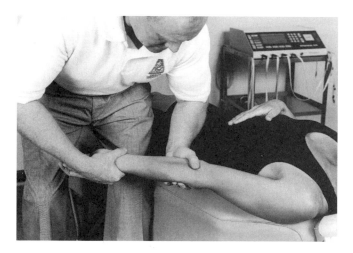

Figure 5B.21. Lateral tilt of the ulna on the humerus.

Medial Tilt of the Ulna on the Humerus (Fig. 5B.22)

Athlete: Same as above.

Doctor: Same as above with the exception of standing or sitting on the lateral side of the involved arm. The superior hand is reversed; the doctor grasps the lateral surface of the athlete's proximal ulna.

Action: Same as above with the exception of reversing the glide on the ulna by going lateral to medial. Correction of a restriction is the test plus an impulse.

Anterior (Extension) Glide of the Ulna on the Humerus (Fig. 5B.23)

Athlete: Standing or sitting with the involved arm flexed at 15°–20°, palm upward.

Doctor: Standing in front of the athlete and facing the involved elbow. The lateral hand grasps the distal radius and ulna just above the wrist for stabilization and to maintain the ath-

lete's palm facing upward in supination. The fingers of the active hand grasp the posterior proximal ulna. The thumb is relaxed in the fossa.

Action: Apply an extension glide of the elbow with the active hand testing joint play. There should be a springy endfeel. Correction of a restriction is the test plus an impulse. Note: The athlete must be totally relaxed. Do not apply an overcorrection thrust because this can cause a hyperextension insult.

Radiohumeral Joint

Complete mobility of the radiohumeral (ball and socket) joint in pronation and supination is necessary for full elbow extension. This can be achieved, to some extent, with the downward and upward glide of the radioulnar joint manipulation. It is further achieved with complete mobility of the distal radioulnar joint, as is seen in the next section.

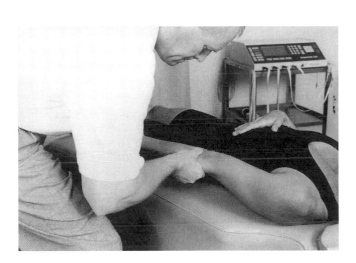

Figure 5B.22. Medial tilt of the ulna on the humerus.

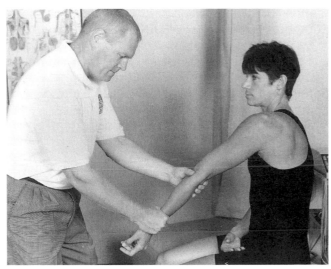

Figure 5B.23. Anterior (extension) glide of the ulna on the humerus.

THE WRIST

The wrist is composed of the distal radioulnar joint, radiocarpal joint, ulnomeniscotriquetral (ulnocarpal) joint, and midcarpal joint.

The wrist is the final link of joints that position the hand for its unique capabilities. It is multiarticular and allows for flexion, extension, radial deviation (abduction), ulnar deviation (adduction), rotation (supination and pronation), and circumduction.

Distal Radioulnar Joint

The distal radioulnar joint surfaces are enclosed in a capsule and held together by an articular disc.

This joint moves the proximal radioulnar joint as a functional unit for forearm and wrist pronation and supination.

EXAMINATION/MANIPULATION

Posterior and Anterior Glide (Fig. 5B.24)

Athlete: Supine or sitting with the elbow bent and palm facing away from the athlete.

Doctor: Facing toward the athlete with the athlete's elbow on the doctor's knee. The most distal ulna is grasped ventrally with the thumb pad and dorsally with the pads of the index and long fingers. The same pinch-grip is applied on the distal radius with the other hand.

Action: Stabilize with one hand and apply a push (posteriorly) and pull (anteriorly) with the other hand. Reverse this. Correction of a restriction is the test plus an impulse.

Rotation (Pronation and Supination) Glide (Fig. 5B.25)

Athlete: Same as above, except when testing the joint play for pronation the palm is facing toward the athlete.

Doctor: Same as above, except when testing the joint play for pronation the contact for the thumbs and fingers are in the exact opposite positions.

Action: Same as above, except to rotate, rather than push-pull. Apply a pronation rotation with the radius and a supination rotation with the ulna. There should be a springy endfeel at the end of the passive range of motion. Correction of a restriction is the test plus an impulse.

Radiocarpal Joint

The radiocarpal joint is the articulation between the distal end of the radius and the scaphoid and lunate carpal bones.

The proximal row of carpals slides in the direction opposite the physiologic motion of the hand. For example, in wrist flexion the proximal row moves dorsally, and in wrist radial deviation the proximal row slides in the ulnar direction.

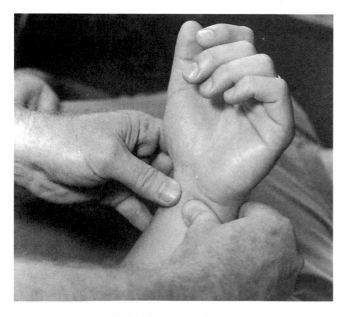

Figure 5B.24. Posterior and anterior glide.

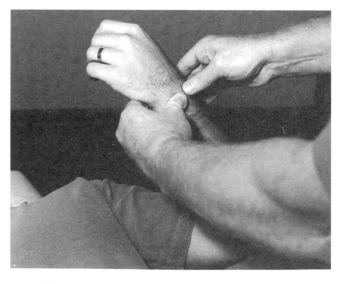

Figure 5B.25. Rotation (pronation and supination) glide.

EXAMINATION/MANIPULATION

Long-Axis Distraction (Fig. 5B.26)

Athlete: Standing with the elbow at 90° in the handshake.

Doctor: Standing directly in front of the athlete. The proximal row of carpals is grasped, just distal to the styloid processes, with the thumb on the radial side and the index finger on the ulna side. The stabilization hand is placed on the midproximal forearm as a counterpressure.

Action: Apply a distraction with the active hand on the carpals. The radius and ulna should seperate from the proximal carpal. Correction of a restriction is the test, plus a quick pull toward the doctor.

Anterior (Extension) and Posterior (Flexion) Glide (Fig. 5B.27)

Athlete: Sitting with the elbow flexed approximately 90°, palm downward.

Doctor: Standing on the lateral side of the involved wrist. The distal radius and ulna are grasped, with the thumb web on the dorsal aspect of the wrist just proximal to the styloid processes, with the stabilization hand. The other hand grasps the proximal row of carpals.

Action: The active hand applies a push downward (glide) and a pull upward to determine joint play of the radius and ulna on the proximal row of carpals. Correction of a restriction is with short, sharp impulses into the fixation. This is a general mobilization technique to increase joint play at the proximal row of carpals on the radius and ulna.

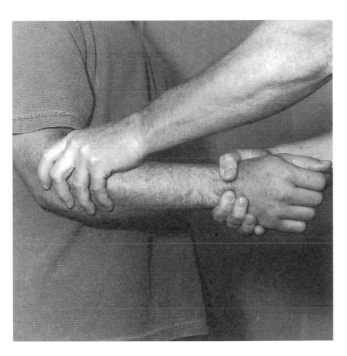

Figure 5B.26. Long-axis distraction.

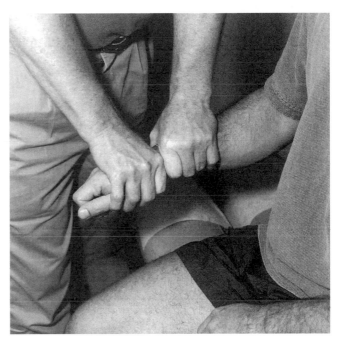

Figure 5B.27. Anterior (extension) and posterior (flexion) glide.

Extension and Flexion Glide of the Scaphoid and Lunate on the Radius (Fig. 5B.28)

Athlete: Sitting with the elbow flexed approximately 90°, palm downward.

Doctor: Standing or sitting on the lateral side of the involved wrist. The distal radius is grasped just proximal to the styloid process with the stabilization hand. The contact hand pinch-grips the scaphoid with the thumb on the dorsal surface and the index finger on the volar surface. The same pinch-grip is then applied to the lunate.

Action: The active hand applies a push downward (extension) and a pull upward (flexion) to determine joint play. Correction of a restriction is with a short, sharp impulse in the direction of the restriction.

Alternative Method of Manipulation (Fig. 5B.29)

Athlete: Same as above.

Doctor: Sitting or standing and facing toward the athlete. The fingers of both hands are placed in the palm of the athlete's hand with a double thumb contact on each carpal, one at a time.

Lateral Glide of the Scaphoid (Fig. 5B.30)

Athlete: Sitting or standing with the elbow at 90°, palm downward.

Doctor: Facing the athlete. The fingers of both hands are placed in the athlete's palm, and the thenar eminence of both hands is placed on the dorsal side of the hand. The index finger of the medial hand contacts the scaphoid.

Action: Apply a lateral (radial) deviation force to the scaphoid on the radius, feeling for a springy endfeel. Correction of a restriction is the test plus an impulse.

Ulnomeniscotriquetral (Ulnocarpal) Joint

The distal end of the ulna articulates with the triquetrum via an articular disc. A loss of joint play at this region generally restricts supination of the forearm and wrist.

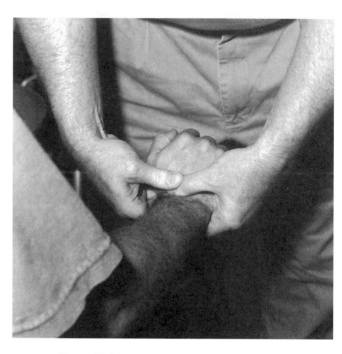

Figure 5B.29. Alternative method of manipulation.

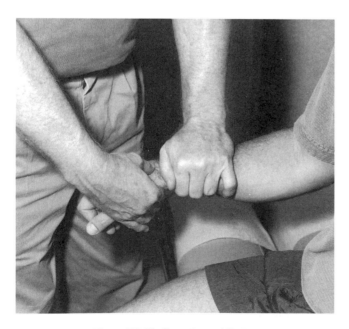

Figure 5B.28. Extension and flexion glide of the scaphoid and lunate on the radius.

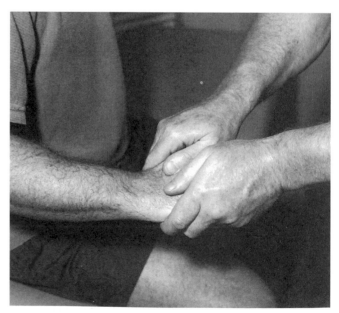

Figure 5B.30. Lateral glide of the scaphoid.

EXAMINATION/MANIPULATION

Long-Axis Distraction (Fig. 5B.31)

Athlete: Standing toward the elbow at 90°, palm inward.

Doctor: Facing toward the athlete. The athlete's hand is grasped in a hand-shaking position, with the doctor's index finger hooked over the triquetral bone. The other hand is placed over the radial side.

Action: Push downward on the radius while simultaneously pulling upward on the hand with the index-triquetral contact. There should be a separation at the ulnotriquetral joint. Correction of a restriction is the test plus an impulse.

Medial Glide of the Triquetrum (Fig. 5B.32)

Athlete: Sitting or standing with the elbow at 90°, palm downward.

Doctor: Facing the athlete. The fingers of both hands are placed in the palm of the athlete's hand, with the thenar eminence of the doctor's hands contacting the dorsal side of the athlete's hand. The index finger of the doctor's lateral hand contacts the triquetrum.

Action: Apply a medial (ulnar) deviation force to the triquetrum on the ulna, feeling for a springy endfeel. Correction of a restriction is the test plus an impulse.

ADDITIONAL JOINTS AND/OR SPECIFIC MOVEMENTS TO BE EVALUATED IN THE WRIST

The wrist joints in general, including the radiocarpal, ulnocarpal, midcarpal, intercarpal, and carpometacarpal joints, are to be evaluated and treated for restriction in the following directions: anterior (extension), posterior (flexion), medial, and lateral glide and long-axis distraction.

The distal row of carpals articulates with the proximal row of carpals. A loss of joint play at the midcarpal joint primarily restricts extension and secondarily restricts flexion of the wrist.

Long-Axis Distraction

The method of testing and manipulation is exactly the same way as that for the radiocarpal joint with the exception of hand placement. The active hand moves distally to grasp the distal row of carpals. This is a general mobilization technique to increase joint play at the midcarpal joint.

Anterior and Posterior Glide

The method of testing and manipulation is exactly the same as that for the radiocarpal joint with the exception of hand placement. The stabilization hand grasps the proximal row of carpals and the active hand grasps the distal row of carpals. This maneuver is a general mobilization technique to increase joint play at the midcarpal joint. It is an excellent maneuver to apply after a patient has a cast removed (healed fracture) or has any immobilization of the wrist.

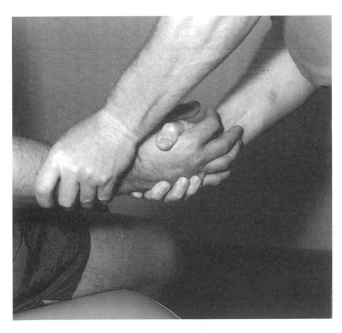

Figure 5B.31. Long-axis distraction.

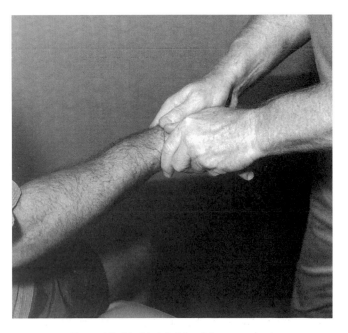

Figure 5B.32. Medial glide of the triquetrum.

Anterior and Posterior Glide of Each Distal Carpal on Each Proximal Carpal (Fig. 5B.33)

Athlete: Sitting or standing with the elbow flexed approximately 90°, palm downward.

Doctor: Standing or sitting on the medial or lateral side of the involved wrist. The proximal carpal bone is pinch-gripped, with the thumb on the dorsal surface and the index finger on the volar surface, with the stabilization hand. The contact hand pinch-grips the adjacent distal carpal bone in the same manner.

Action: The pinch-grip of the contact hand applies a push (anteriorly) and pull (posteriorly) with each carpal bone. The correction is the test plus an impulse.

Intercarpal Joints

EXAMINATION/MANIPULATION

Anterior and Posterior Glide of the Proximal and Distal Row of Intercarpals (Fig. 5B.34)

Athlete: Sitting or standing with the elbow flexed approximately 90°, palm downward.

Doctor: Sitting or standing and facing toward the athlete. One carpal in the proximal row is grasped with a pinch-grip from one hand, while the adjacent carpal from the same row is pinch-gripped with the other hand. One hand becomes the stabilization hand while the other hand becomes the active hand.

Action: Apply a push-pull on each carpal in the top row and then proceed with the same technique in the distal row of intercarpals. Correction of a restriction is the test plus an impulse.

Carpometacarpal Joints

The first carpometacarpal (thumb) or trapeziometacarpal joint is a unique joint cavity that is a separate articulation from the other four. The joint cavity of the four other carpometacarpal joints (fingers) articulate primarily with the large midcarpal joint and secondarily with the carpometacarpal joint cavity.

The trapeziometacarpal joint is a saddle-shaped joint that has a lax capsule with a wide range of motion, which allows the thumb to move away from the palm of the hand for opposition in prehension activities.

This joint is evaluated in long-axis distraction, posterior and anterior glide, and internal and external rotation. The other carpometacarpal joints are evaluated in long-axis distraction and posterior and anterior glide. This evaluation is performed by stabilizing the proximal bone with one hand while the contact hand grasps the adjacent distal bone and tests the joint play of each joint in each specific direction as specified above. The correction is the test plus an impulse.

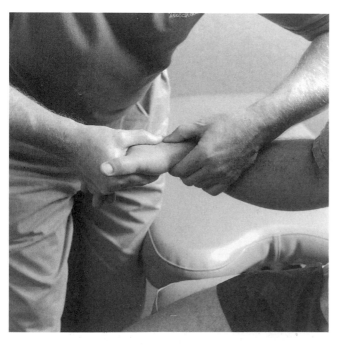

Figure 5B.33. Anterior and posterior glide of each distal carpal on each proximal carpal.

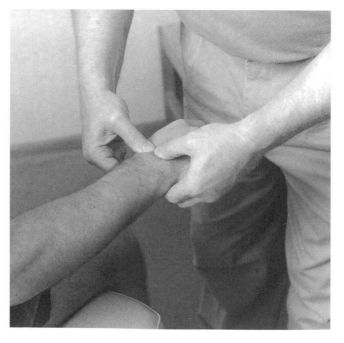

Figure 5B.34. Anterior and posterior glide of the proximal and distal row of intercarpals.

THE HAND

The hand is a unique body part, a balance of power, delicacy, and sensation. The understanding of this is personal for health-care professions such as chiropractic, in which manual skills are required for clinical practice.

The most common injuries in sports are to the hand. Although most are minor (e.g., jammed or sprained fingers), these injuries should not be taken lightly. Precise functioning of the hands is essential to almost every type of athletic activity.

Intermetacarpal Joints

EXAMINATION/MANIPULATION

Dorsal and Palmar Glide (Fig. 5B.35)

Athlete: Sitting or standing with the elbow flexed at approximately 90°, palm downward.

Doctor: Sitting or standing on either side of the involved wrist. The thumb is placed on the dorsal surface of one metacarpal with one hand (stabilization) and the thumb of the other hand (active) is placed on the adjacent metacarpal. The fingers of both hands are placed in the palm of the athlete's hand on the respective metacarpal.

Action: Apply a push-pull maneuver on each proximal metacarpal bone testing the intermetacarpal joint play. Correction of a restriction is the test plus an impulse. Now proceed onto the midintermetacarpal and distal intermetacarpal joints applying the same procedure.

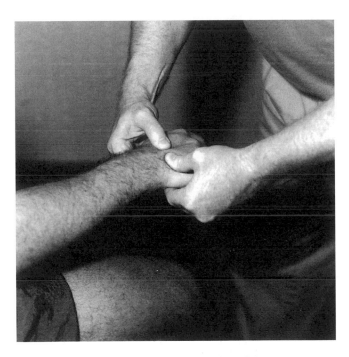

Figure 5B.35. Dorsal and palmar glide.

Metacarpophalangeal and Interphalangeal Joints

EXAMINATION/MANIPULATION

Long-Axis Distraction, Anterior (Extension), Posterior (Flexion), Lateral, Medial, Internal, and External Rotation Glides (Fig. 5B.36, A to G)

Athlete: Sitting or standing, palm downward and relaxed.

Doctor: Toward the medial or lateral side of the involved hand. The stabilization hand applies a pinch-grip on the distal shaft, near the joint line of the proximal bone. An example of this is the metacarpal bone of the metacarpophalangeal joint. The contact hand also applies a pinch-grip on the proximal shaft of the bone directly below the joint that is being tested and in this case would be the phalange.

Action: Move the distal phalanx with the contact hand in a gliding maneuver throughout the seven different directions (long-axis distraction, internal and external rotation, flexion, extension, and lateral and medial glide) within each joint, one direction at a time, testing for a springy endfeel. Correction of a restriction is the test plus an impulse.

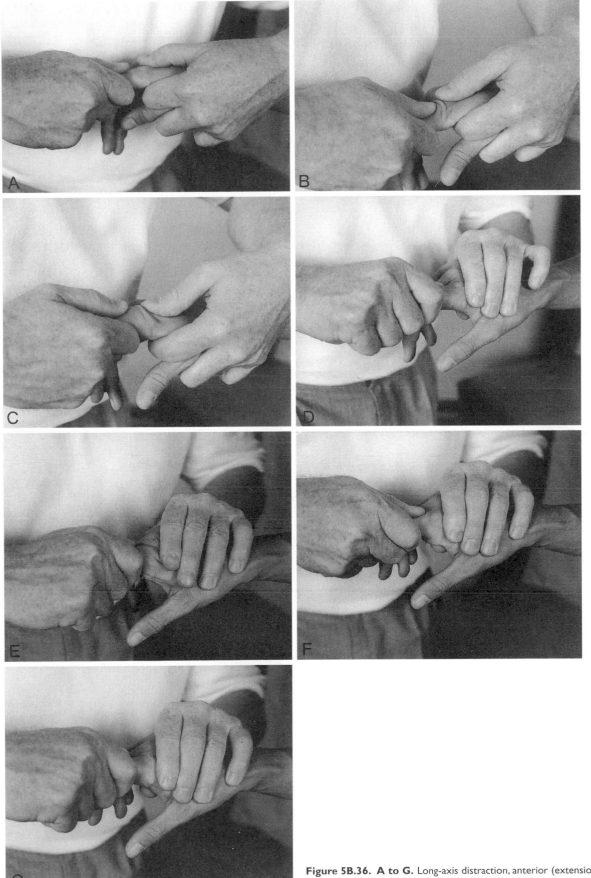

Figure 5B.36. A to G. Long-axis distraction, anterior (extension), posterior (flexion), lateral, medial, internal, and external rotation glides.

THE HIP

The hip is a ball-and-socket joint. It is formed by the articulation of the head of the femur into the acetabulum of the ilium. Unlike the shoulder, the hip is very stable and sturdy. It is practically impossible to dislocate the hip joint without first fracturing the socket. There is, however, a trade-off for high stability, which is low mobility.

Iliofemoral Joint

EXAMINATION/MANIPULATION

Long-Axis Distraction (Fig. 5B.37)

Athlete: Supine with the uninvolved leg at 90°, foot flat on the table. The involved leg is slightly abducted, externally rotated, and in a neutrally relaxed position.

Doctor: Caudal end of the table. The distal lower leg is grasped with both hands (avoiding the foot). The leg is elevated to approximately 15°–20° in the neutral position.

Action: Maintaining the neutral position, apply a long-axis traction by leaning backward. A separation (distraction) at the iliofemoral joint should occur. Correction of a restriction is the test plus an impulse. If the athlete has a knee disorder, both hands should be placed above the knee.

Anterior Glide (Fig. 5B.38)

Athlete: Prone with the involved leg near the side of the table. The knee should be flexed with or without slight abduction.

Doctor: Standing between the athlete's legs or on the opposite side of the table reaching across, and facing toward the involved hip. The athlete's knee is supported on the anterior aspect of the distal femur by the inferior hand, using slight elevation. The contact hand is placed on the posterior aspect of the greater trochanter.

Action: Apply pressure with the contact hand going in the anterior direction. The femur head should glide forward in the acetabular cavity. Correction of a restriction is the test plus an impulse.

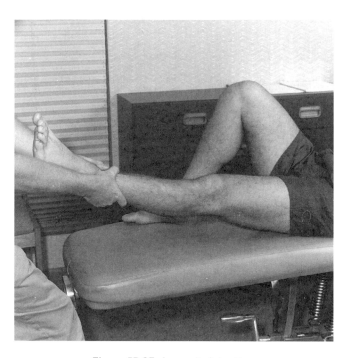

Figure 5B.37. Long-axis distraction.

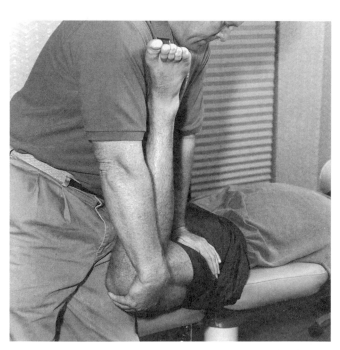

Figure 5B.38. Anterior glide.

Posterior Glide With Circumduction (Fig. 5B.39)

Athlete: Supine with the involved hip near the side of the table, or use a drop piece. Begin with the involved hip flexed to 90° and the knee relaxed.

Doctor: Standing on the involved side. The doctor's hands are interlocked over the knee and the doctor's chest is placed against the interlocked hands.

Action: First apply pressure down through the femur shaft posteriorly and then combine adduction with a circumduction mode going clockwise (9- to 12-o'clock range, left knee; 3- to 12-o'clock range, right knee) testing for a springy endfeel. Correction of any restriction within that range is the test plus an impulse. The impulse should be performed with a light body drop into the restriction (not toward the acetabular cavity).

Lateral Distraction (Fig. 5B.40)

Athlete: Supine with the involved leg flexed to approximately 40°–60°.

Doctor: Standing on the opposite side of involvement. The superior hand is placed on the table (grasping the edge) underneath the athlete's involved thigh. The forearm is slid as far up the thigh as possible to be used as a fulcrum. The contact (inferior) hand is placed on the lateral distal femur.

Action: Apply pressure with the contact hand on the distal femur going medially across the forearm. The femur is gently rocked over the forearm several times while testing the separation of the femur head from the acetabular cavity. The correction of a restriction is the test, plus several light to moderate impulses.

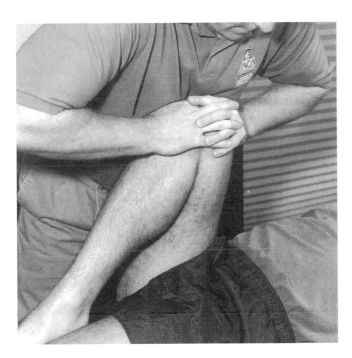

Figure 5B.39. Posterior glide with circumduction.

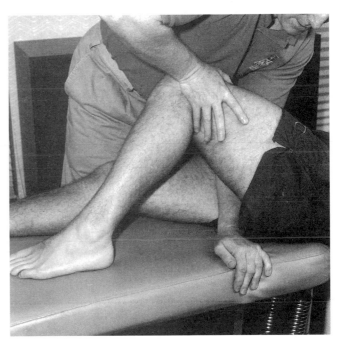

Figure 5B.40. Lateral distraction.

Internal Rotation (Fig. 5B.41)

Athlete. Supine with the involved hip flexed 90°.

Doctor: Standing on the involved side with the foot of the inferior leg on the table. The athlete's lower leg is placed over the doctor's thigh. The distal one third of the femur is grasped with both hands.

Action: Place the hands on the distal femur and the inferior forearm on the lower leg to guide the femur into internal rotation, testing for a springy endfeel. The correction of a restriction is the test plus an impulse.

External Rotation (Fig. 5B.42)

Athlete: Same as above.

Doctor: Standing on the involved side with the inferior knee resting on the table. The athlete's lower leg is placed over the doctor's upper arm and the distal one third of the femur is grasped with both hands.

Action: Place the hands on the distal femur and the upper arm on the lower leg to guide the femur into external rotation and test for a springy endfeel. The correction of a restriction is the test plus an impulse.

Figure 4 Glide (Fig. 5B.43)

Athlete: Prone with the involved leg near the side of the table in the figure 4 position by placing the hip and knee in flexion, abduction, and external rotation with the medial aspect of the foot resting on the table.

Doctor: Standing just below the involved lower leg on the same side facing cephalad. The involved medial aspect of the knee is grasped with the doctor's lateral hand. A pisiform contact with the active hand is placed directly over top of the posterolateral aspect of the head of the femur, just below the joint line.

Action: The stabilization (lateral) hand elevates the knee toward the ceiling while the active hand applies anterior pressure on the head of the femur testing for the springy endfeel. Correction of a restriction is the test plus an impulse. Many times this maneuver is used first to help loosen the hip joint when there is great difficulty with the long-axis distraction maneuver.

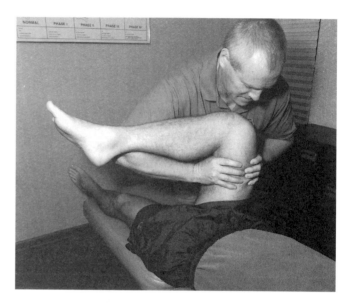

Figure 5B.42. External rotation.

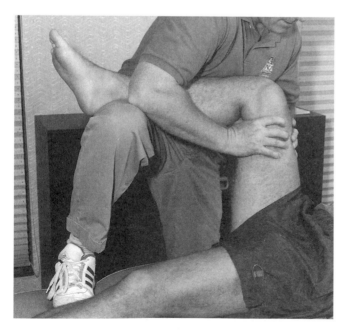

Figure 5B.41. Internal rotation.

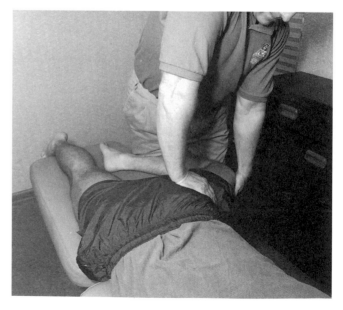

Figure 5B.43. Figure 4 glide.

THE KNEE

The knee is the most famous joint in sports and the largest joint in the body. The special attention it receives is due to its being the most frequent serious extremity injury in sports. Knee injury accounts for more time lost from competition by young athletes than any other type of injury. It also ends more athletic careers and disables more athletes in later years than any other sports injury. Its vulnerability is because of its basic structure, which is a hinge with long levers on either side. The combined functions of weight bearing and locomotion place considerable stress and strain on it. A strong and effective functioning knee joint is essential for most physical activities.

The knee is made up of three joints: the patellofemoral, tibiofemoral, and proximal tibiofibular.

Patellofemoral Joint

This joint consists of the largest sesamoid bone of the body, the patella, which is held in place laterally by the iliotibial band and retinaculum; these are opposed medially by the vastus medialis muscle. The patellar tendon anchors the patella inferiorly against the active pull of the quadriceps muscle superiorly. The patella glides inferiorly during knee flexion and superiorly during knee extension. Injury to the knee is generally followed quickly by atrophy of the quadriceps muscle group, primarily the vastus medialis muscle.

EXAMINATION/MANIPULATION

Inferior Glide (Fig. 5B.44)

Athlete: Supine with the involved knee in a slightly flexed (approximately 5°) and relaxed position. Place a pillow under the knee for support.

Doctor: Facing perpendicular on the side being tested. A thumb web contact is applied with the superior hand on the proximal, superior aspect of the patella. The thumb web of the stabilization hand is placed at the inferior aspect of the tibial tubercle.

Action: Apply pressure to the patella directly inferior (no downward pressure). The restriction is primarily soft tissue adhesions. Therefore corection is made with several impulse thrusts to break up and stretch the adhesive connective tissue.

Superior Glide (Fig. 5B.45)

Athlete: Same as above.

Doctor: Same as above with the exception of contacting the patella with the thumb web of the inferior hand on the distal, inferior aspect of the patella. The superior hand is placed on the lower one third of the femur for stabilization.

Action: Same as above with the exception of applying pressure to the patella going directly superior (no downward pressure).

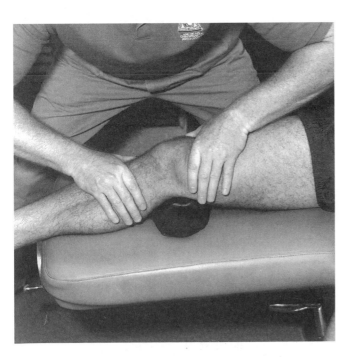

Figure 5B.44. Inferior glide.

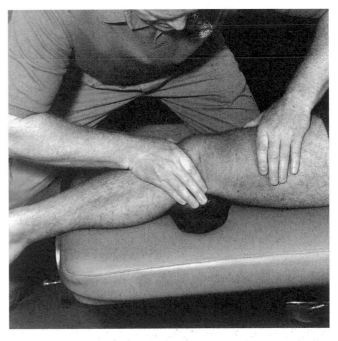

Figure 5B.45. Superior glide.

Medial Glide (Fig. 5B.46)

Athlete: Same as above.

Doctor: Same as above with the exception of placing the thumbs of both hands on the lateral border of the patella, then stabilizing with the fingers of both hands on the medial side of the knee.

Action: Same as above with the exception of applying a medial glide of the patella with both thumbs.

Lateral Glide (Fig. 5B.47)

Athlete: Same as above.

Doctor: Same as above with the exception of being on the opposite side of the involved knee. Place the thumbs on the medial border of the patella and stabilize with the fingers on the lateral side of the knee.

Action: Same as above with the exception of applying pressure with the thumbs in the lateral direction.

Tibiofemoral Joint

EXAMINATION/MANIPULATION

Posterior Glide (Fig. 5B.48)

Athlete: Supine with the involved knee flexed 90° and the foot flat on the table.

Doctor: Seated or kneeling on the distal aspect of the athlete's foot for stabilization. The doctor places the thenar eminence of both hands on each side of the anterior tibial tubercle. The fingers of each hand are placed on the posterior proximal aspect of the tibia for stabilization.

Action: Apply a posterior (push) glide of the tibia on the femur with the thenar testing for posterior joint play. Correction is made by adding a short, dynamic impulse into the restriction.

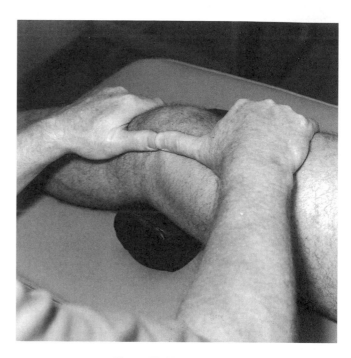

Figure 5B.47. Lateral glide.

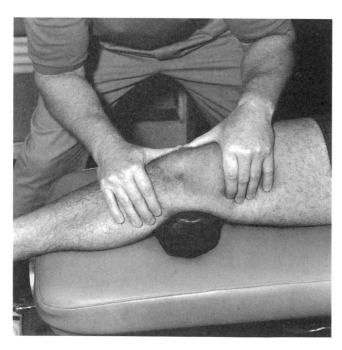

Figure 5B.46. Medial glide.

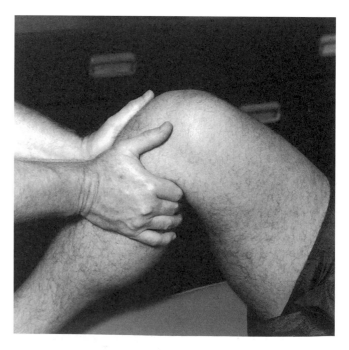

Figure 5B.48. Posterior glide.

Anterior Glide (Fig. 5B.49)

Athlete: Same as above.

Doctor: Same as above with the exception that the fingers of both hands on the most proximal aspect of the posterior tibia become the active part of the hands.

Action: Apply an anterior (pull) glide of the tibia on the femur with the fingers of both hands testing for anterior joint play. Correction is made by adding a short, dynamic impulse into the restriction.

Medial Glide (Fig. 5B.50)

Athlete: Supine with the involved leg in the extended but unlocked (5° flexion) position, and relaxed.

Doctor: Kneeling on the involved side. The superior hand is placed under the femur, palm facing laterally. The inferior hand is placed on the lateral aspect of the tibia, palm facing medially.

Action: Apply counterpressure with both hands, using primarily the inferior hand, testing medial glide of the tibia on the femur. Correction of a restriction is the test plus an impulse.

Alternative Method of Manipulation (Fig. 5B.51)

Athlete: Same as above with the exception of slightly more knee flexion.

Doctor: Standing on the involved side at the caudal end of the table. The distal lower leg is grasped with the medial hand. The thenar eminence of the contact hand is placed on the lateral epicondyle near the joint line.

Action: The contact hand drops the knee in the direction of extension and just before the knee is extended, a controlled short, sharp thrust is applied in the medial direction.

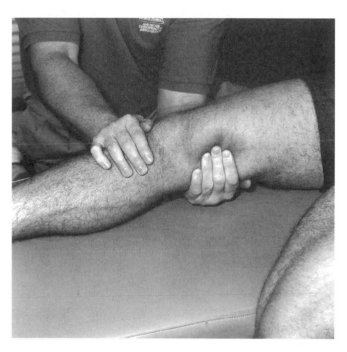

Figure 5B.50. Medial glide.

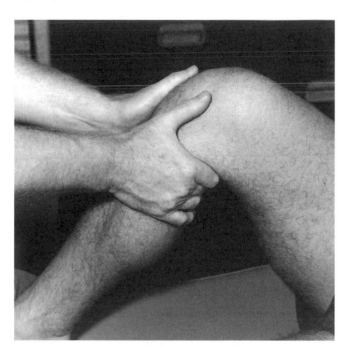

Figure 5B.49. Anterior glide.

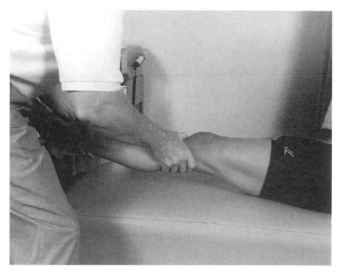

Figure 5B.51. Alternative method of manipulation.

Lateral Glide (Fig. 5B.52)

Athlete: Same as above.

Doctor: Same as above with the exception of reversing the hands. The superior hand is placed on the lateral femoral condyle, palm facing medially. The inferior hand is placed under the proximal tibia, palm facing laterally.

Action: Apply counterpressure with both hands, but primarily with the inferior hand, testing lateral glide of the tibia on the femur. Correction of a restriction is the test plus an impulse.

Alternative Method of Manipulation (Fig. 5B.53). This method is the same as the alternative method of manipulation for the medial glide of the tibia on the femur with the following exceptions.

Athlete: Same as above.

Doctor: Standing on the medial side of the involved knee. The medial hand is placed on the medial epicondyle near the joint line, and the other hand grasps the distal lower leg.

Action: Same as above, with the exception of applying a controlled short, sharp thrust in the lateral direction.

Internal Rotation (Fig. 5B.54)

Athlete: Supine with the hip and knee flexed at 90°.

Doctor: Facing perpendicular on the side being tested with the inferior foot on the table. The athlete's involved lower leg is placed over the doctor's distal thigh. The tibial epicondyle is grasped near the joint line with both hands. The superior hand is placed with the palm facing upward and the inferior hand facing downward.

Action: First remove the soft tissue slack, then apply internal rotation of the tibia on the femur with both hands testing for joint play. The correction of a restriction is the test plus an impulse.

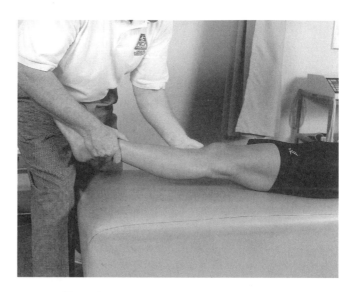

Figure 5B.53. Alternative method of manipulation.

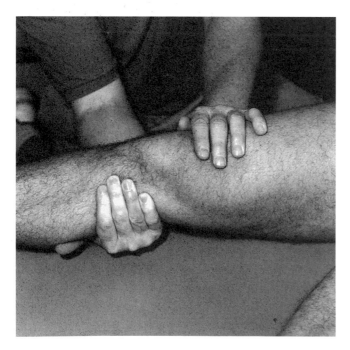

Figure 5B.52. Lateral glide.

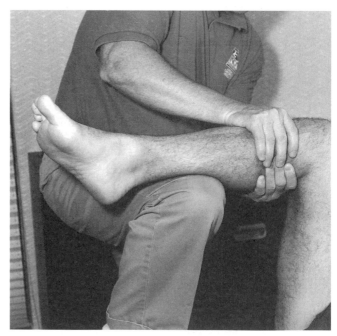

Figure 5B.54. Internal rotation.

External Rotation (Fig. 5B.55)

Athlete: Same as above.

Doctor: Same as above with the exception of taking a tissue pull toward external rotation as opposed to internal rotation.

Action: Apply an external rotation glide of the tibia on the femur with both hands testing for joint play. The correction of a restriction is the test plus an impulse.

Long-Axis Distraction (Fig. 5B.56)

Athlete: Supine with the uninvolved leg flexed at 90°, foot flat on the table. The leg being tested is extended on the table in the unlocked and relaxed position.

Doctor: Facing perpendicular with the involved ankle between the doctor's inner thighs. The tibiofemoral joint line is contacted with the index and thumb of both hands to palpate the joint separation.

Action: A separation at the joint is achieved by the doctor moving his or her body caudally. Correction of a restriction is achieved by the doctor moving his or her body caudally with a quick, short impulse.

Proximal Tibiofibular Joint

The proximal tibiofibular joint is not normally considered part of the knee joint; however, due to its location it is covered in this section.

Mobility at the head of the fibula occurs with knee and ankle movement. On knee flexion, the fibular head moves in the anterior direction; on knee extension, the fibular head moves in the posterior direction. Ankle dorsiflexion moves it in a superior direction, and ankle plantar flexion moves it in an inferior direction. Dysfunction at this joint causes knee pain.

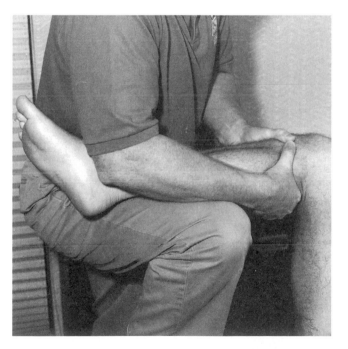

Figure 5B.55. External rotation.

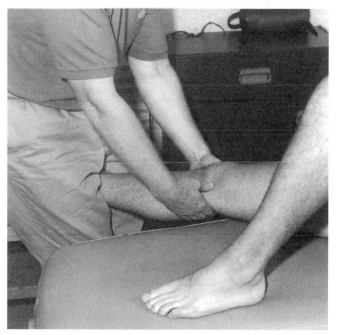

Figure 5B.56. Long-axis distraction.

EXAMINATION/MANIPULATION

Anterior and Posterior Glide (Fig. 5B.57)

Athlete: Supine with the involved knee flexed 90° and the foot flat on the table.

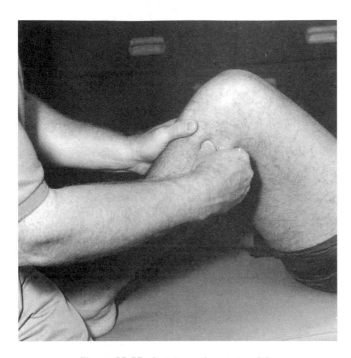

Figure 5B.57. Anterior and posterior glide.

Doctor: Seated or kneeling on the distal aspect of the athlete's foot for stabilization. The medial hand is placed just below the tibial tubercle of the tibia for stabilization. The head of the fibula is contacted with the lateral hand using a pinch-grip with the thumb on the anterior surface and the index and middle finger at the posterior surface.

Action: Apply a push in the posterior direction and pull in the anterior direction, testing for a springy endfeel. Correction of a restriction is the test plus an impulse.

Inferior Glide (Fig. 5B.58A and B)

Athlete: Supine with the leg being tested in a slightly flexed and unlocked position.

Doctor: Facing toward the medial side of the involved lower leg. The proximal tibiofibular joint is palpated with the index or middle finger of the superior hand while plantar flexing and inverting the foot with the inferior hand.

Action: The fibular head should glide in the inferior direction when the foot is moving in plantar flexion and inversion. Correction of a restriction is by placing the pisiform of the inferior hand on the proximal aspect of the lateral malleolus with the fingers stabilizing lightly on the Achilles tendon. The superior hand is placed over the contact hand for extra stabilization. Apply inferior pressure with the pisiform on the lateral malleolus followed by an added impulse.

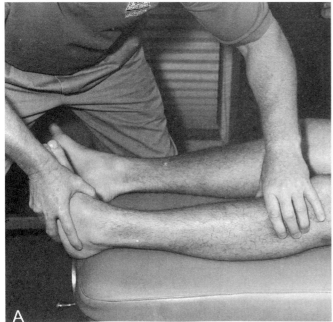

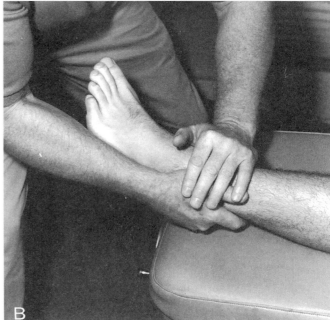

Figure 5B.58. Inferior glide.

Superior Glide (Fig. 5B.59A and B)

Athlete: Same as above.

Doctor: Palpate the proximal tibiofibular joint with the same hand as above. The inferior hand dorsiflexes and everts the foot, with the palm of the hand facing cephalad on the plantar surface of the foot.

Action: The fibular head should glide in the superior direction when the foot is moving in dorsiflexion and eversion. Correction of a restriction is achieved by placing the athlete on his or her side, opposite the involved leg, with the knee flexed and the medial lower leg on a soft table. The crease of the doctor's palm is placed at the inferior aspect of the lateral malleolus, and the other hand is used to grasp the wrist of the contact hand for stabilization. Apply pressure on the inferior malleolus going directly superior (not downward) in alignment with the lower leg, and add an impulse. To make a good impulse thrust on the malleolus, it is important that the lower leg does not slide. Therefore, place a skin contact of the lower leg on the table for better adherence.

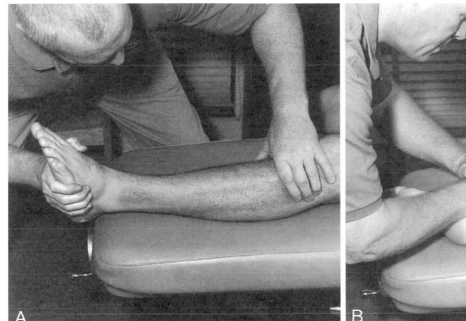
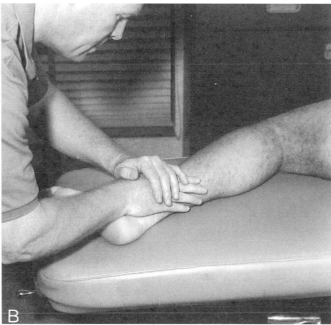

Figure 5B.59. Superior glide.

THE ANKLE AND FOOT

The many interconnecting bones of the ankle and foot result in the formation of numerous joints. The joints of the ankle and foot consist of the distal tibiofibular joint, mortise joint, tarsal joints, tarsometatarsal joints, intermetatarsal joints, metatarsophalangeal joints, and interphalangeal joints.

The joints of the foot and ankle must permit mobility in all planes to allow for minimal displacement of an athlete's center of gravity with respect to the base of support when walking over flat or uneven surfaces. Balance is dependent on proper functioning of the ankle-foot complex. Adequate mobility of the joints and proper structural alignment of the feet are also necessary for normal attenuation of forces transmitted from the ground to the weight-bearing extremities.

Distal Tibiofibular Joint

Due to the location of the distal tibiofibular joint and its involvement with the ankle, it is discussed in this section.

Mobility at the distal tibiofibular joint and the proximal tibiofibular joint can affect both the knee and ankle. Inferior or superior movement of the fibula directly influences ankle mechanics.

If the fibula is restricted from gliding in the superior direction, the ankle will compensate by remaining in a supinated position; if the fibula is not gliding in an inferior direction, the ankle will compensate by remaining in pronation.

EXAMINATION/MANIPULATION

Anterior and Posterior Glide (Fig. 5B.60)

Athlete: Supine with the knee flexed approximately 30°.

Doctor: Caudal end of the table. The doctor places one knee on the table, with the athlete's involved foot flat on the doctor's distal thigh for stabilization. The distal tibia is grasped with the medial (stabilization) hand and a pinch-grip is applied on the lateral malleolus with the active hand.

Action: Apply a push backward with the thumb (testing posterior glide) and a pull forward with the fingers (testing anterior glide) on the lateral malleolus. The correction is the test plus an impulse.

Talocrural (Mortise) Joint

The ankle is a hinge (ginglymus) joint, which is formed by the superior portion of the body of the talus fitting within the mortise, or cavity, formed by the combined distal ends of the tibia and fibula.

The mortise joint has two primary motions: dorsiflexion and plantar flexion with a slight amount of rotation. Perhaps the most common injury in all of sports is the sprained ankle. It is due to a combination of plantar flexion and inversion, and the structure damaged most often is the anterior talofibular ligament.

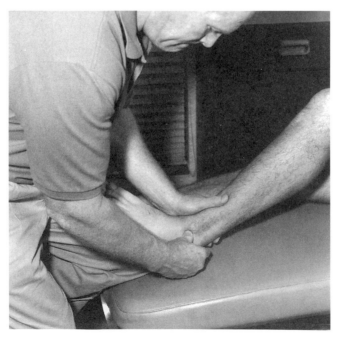

Figure 5B.60. Anterior and posterior glide.

EXAMINATION/MANIPULATION

Long-Axis Distraction (Fig. 5B.61)

Athlete: Supine with the lower leg hanging over the caudal end of the table at approximately 15° and relaxed.

Doctor: Standing in a crouched position at the caudal end of the table. The posterior tubercle of the talus is contacted with the pisiform or index and middle finger of the lateral hand, and the pisiform or distal forearm of the medial hand is placed over the dorsal aspect of the talus. The fingers of the medial hand grasp the wrist or lateral hand for stabilization.

Action: Apply a long-axis distraction with both contacts simultaneously in alignment with the lower leg, testing for a separation of the talus on the tibia. Correction of a restriction is the test plus an impulse.

Anterior and Posterior Glide (Fig. 5B.62)

Athlete: Supine, with the knee and ankle at 90°. The calcaneus is on the table.

Doctor: Standing at the caudal end of the table, the lateral hand grasps the midfoot for stabilization. The medial hand grasps the ankle just above the tibial malleolus.

Action: Apply a push (posterior) and pull (anterior) of the tibia on the talus with the tibial contact. Correction of a restriction is the test plus an impulse.

Talocalcaneal (Subtalar) Joint

The subtalar joint is the point of articulation between the talus and the calcaneus. The two motions allowed by the subtalar joint are pronation and supination. Normal pronation of the subtalar joint and foot is essential for normal adaptation to the terrain, shock absorption, and torque conversion, whereas supination is essential for propulsion with the foot and ankle as a rigid lever.

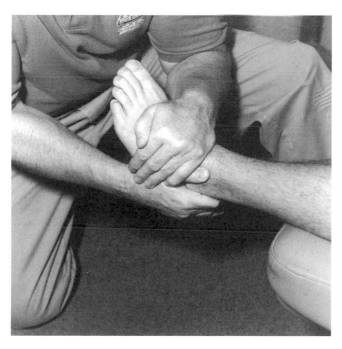

Figure 5B.61. Long-axis distraction.

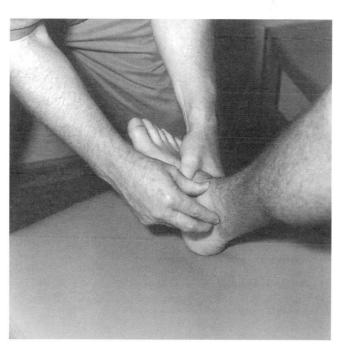

Figure 5B.62. Anterior and posterior glide.

EXAMINATION/MANIPULATION

Long-Axis Distraction (Fig. 5B.63)

Athlete: Supine with the lower leg hanging at approximately 15° and relaxed.

Doctor: Standing in a crouched position, the medial hand grasps the midfoot for stabilization. The lateral (active) hand grasps the calcaneus.

Action: Apply a long-axis distraction movement on the calcaneus with the lateral hand, testing for a separation of the calcaneus on the talus. If mobility is restricted, add a quick impulse thrust.

Medial (Eversion) Glide (Fig. 5B.64)

Athlete: Same as above.

Doctor: Standing in a crouched position at the caudal end of the table and toward the lateral side of the involved foot. The calcaneus is cupped with the lateral hand. The doctor's thenar eminence is placed on the superior, lateral aspect of the calcaneus, and the fingers of the same hand will grasp the medial, inferior aspect of the calcaneus. The medial hand (indifferent) will grasp the midfoot, palm downward (stabilization) with slight eversion of the foot.

Action: Apply the following movements simultaneously: medial push with the thenar and a pull laterally with the fingers testing the medial glide of the calcaneus on the talus. There should be a springy endfeel. Correction of a restriction is the test plus an impulse.

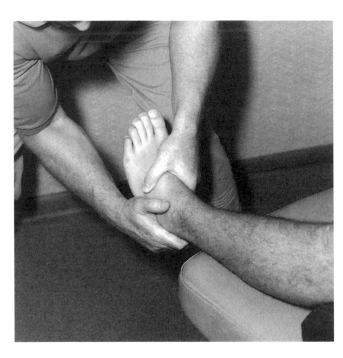

Figure 5B.63. Long-axis distraction.

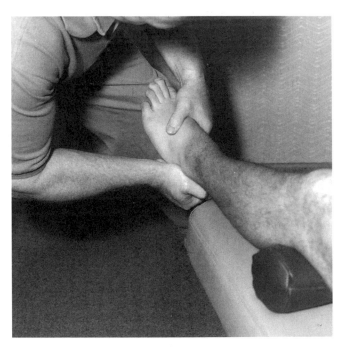

Figure 5B.64. Medial (eversion) glide.

Lateral (Inversion) Glide (Fig. 5B.65)

Athlete: Same as above.

Doctor: Standing in crouched position at the caudal end of the table and toward the medial side of the involved foot. Cup the calcaneus with the medial hand. The doctor's thenar eminence is placed on the superior, medial aspect of the calcaneus. The fingers of the same hand grasp the lateral, inferior aspect. The lateral hand (indifferent) grasps the midfoot, palm downward (for stabilization) with slight inversion of the foot.

Action: Apply the following movements simultaneously: lateral push with the thenar eminence and a pull medially with the fingers, testing the lateral glide of the calcaneus on the talus. Correction of a restriction is the test plus an impulse.

Talonavicular Joint

EXAMINATION/MANIPULATION

Navicular Dorsal and Plantar Glide (Fig. 5B.66)

Athlete: Supine with the involved knee flexed 90°, calcaneus on the table.

Doctor: Standing on the lateral side and facing the involved foot. The talus is stabilized with the thumb web of the superior hand (thumb on the lateral side of the foot). The contact hand is placed over the navicular in the same manner, except with the knuckle of the index finger on the superior aspect of the navicular and the finger on the inferior aspect of the navicular.

Action: The active hand applies a push downward and a pull upward, testing the joint play of the navicular on the talus. Correction of a restriction is the test plus an impulse.

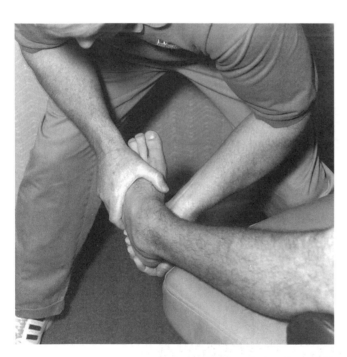

Figure 5B.65. Lateral (inversion) glide.

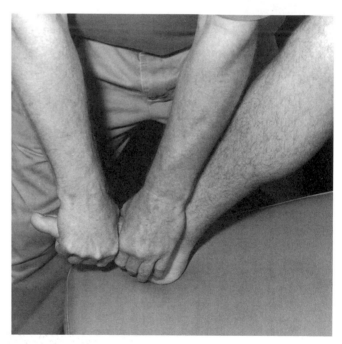

Figure 5B.66. Navicular dorsal and plantar glide.

Navicular Plantar Medial Glide (Fig. 5B.67)

Athlete: Supine or sitting with the lower leg over the end of the table at approximately 45°.

Doctor: Kneeling on the lateral side of the involved foot. The fingers of the superior hand grasp the calcaneus, and the thumb stabilizes the talus. The active hand grasps the forefoot, palm down, and hooks the superior aspect of the navicular with the distal phalanx of the index finger.

Action: Apply a plantar medial pressure on the navicular with the index finger and the forefoot, going in the direction of pronation. Correction of a restriction with the navicular is the test plus an impulse.

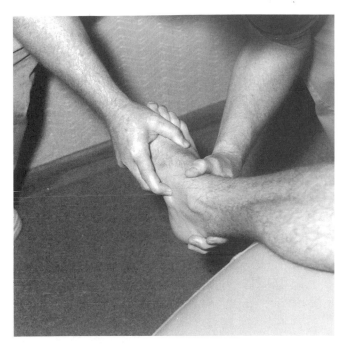

Figure 5B.67. Navicular plantar medial glide.

Navicular Dorsolateral Glide (Fig. 5B.68A and B)

Athlete: Same as above.

Doctor: Kneeling on the medial side of the involved foot. The fingers of the superior hand grasp the calcaneus with the thumb over the dorsal aspect of the talus. The inferior (active) hand grasps the forefoot, palm down, with the thumb placed on the medial, inferior aspect of the navicular.

Action: Apply a dorsolateral pressure on the navicular, with the foot going in the direction of supination. Correction of a restriction is the test plus an impulse. The thenar eminence of the stabilization hand can be used on the navicular in place of the thumb from the contact hand when performing the correction.

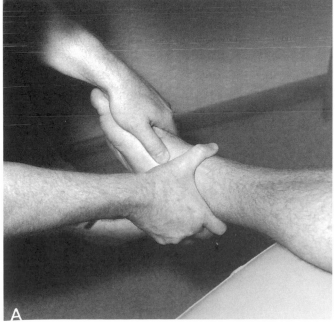
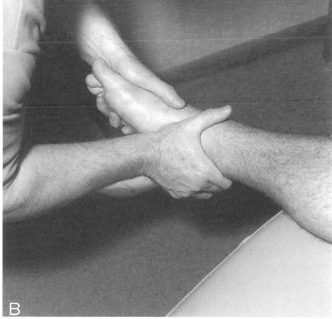

Figure 5B.68. Navicular dorsolateral glide.

Calcaneocuboid Joint

EXAMINATION/MANIPULATION

Cuboid Plantar and Dorsal Glide (Fig. 5B.69)

Athlete: Supine with the involved leg extended on the table and relaxed. The uninvolved knee is flexed at 90°, and the foot is flat on the table.

Doctor: At the caudal end of the table in a kneeling position and facing the plantar surface of the involved foot. The medial hand (stabilization) grasps the calcaneus with the fingers on the medial aspect and the thumb on the lateral aspect, palm facing upward. The lateral hand pinch-grips the cuboid with the index finger on the dorsal surface of the foot and the thumb on the plantar surface.

Action: The active hand applies a pulling downward on the cuboid in a plantar direction and a pushing upward on the cuboid in a dorsal direction. If mobility is restricted, the correction is the test plus an impulse.

Cuboid Plantar Lateral Glide (Fig. 5B.70)

Athlete: Same as above.

Doctor: Standing at the caudal end of the table and on the medial side of the involved foot. The calcaneus is grasped with the fingers of the superior hand, and the thumb is placed over the dorsal aspect of the talus for stabilization. The forefoot is then grasped with the contact hand, palm downward, with the thumb on the medial aspect of the arch and the superior aspect of the cuboid hooked by the distal phalanx of the index finger.

Action: The index finger of the contact hand applies a pulling downward on the cuboid, with the forefoot going in a supination direction. If mobility is restricted, an impulse is added.

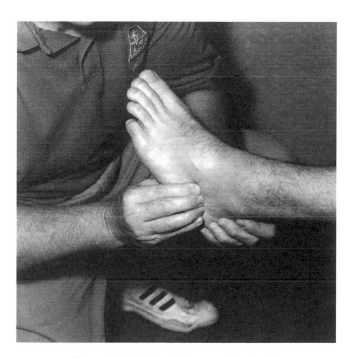

Figure 5B.69. Cuboid plantar and dorsal glide.

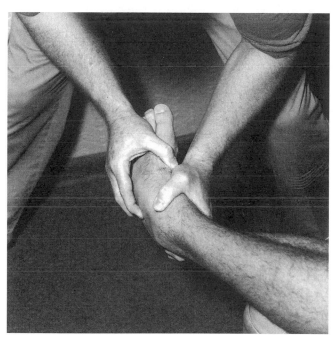

Figure 5B.70. Cuboid plantar lateral glide.

Cuboid Dorsomedial Glide (Fig. 5B.71A and B)

Athlete: Same as above.

Doctor: Facing the lateral side of the involved foot. The stabilization hand (inferior) grasps the forefoot, palm downward. The active hand grasps the calcaneus with the thumb placed on the lateral inferior aspect of the cuboid.

Action: The stabilization hand moves the forefoot in a plantar and everted direction. The thumb of the contact hand applies a pushing motion on the cuboid in the direction of pronation (dorsomedially). There should be a springy endfeel. Correction of a restriction is the test plus an impulse. The thenar eminence of the active hand can also be used in place of the thumb for the correction of the restriction.

Navicular Cuneiform Joint

EXAMINATION/MANIPULATION

Navicular-Cuboid Joint Play (Fig. 5B.72)

Athlete: Supine with the knee flexed 90°, heel on the table.

Doctor: Standing on the lateral side of the foot. The superior stabilization hand is placed over the navicular-cuboid region. The thumb is on the cuboid side of the foot, and the index finger is placed under the navicular bone along with the adjacent fingers. The inferior contact hand is placed in the same manner, except over the cuneiform.

Action: Apply a push downward and pull upward with the contact hand, testing the joint play of the cuneiform on the navicular. The correction is the test plus an impulse, in the direction of the restriction.

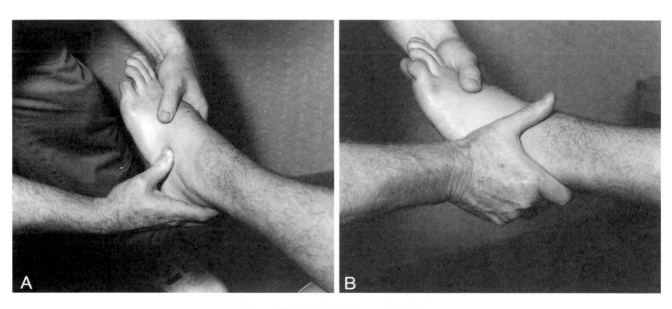

Figure 5B.71. Cuboid dorsomedial glide.

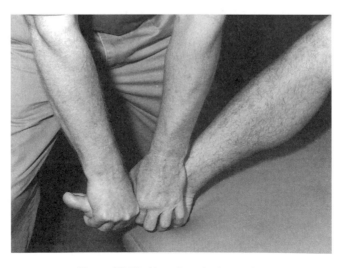

Figure 5B.72. Navicular-cuboid joint play.

Intercuneiform Joint Dorsal and Plantar Glide (Fig. 5B.73A and B)

Athlete: Supine with the involved leg extended and relaxed.

Doctor: Kneeling at the caudal end of the table and facing the medial plantar surface of the foot. The stabilization hand pinch-grips one cuneiform bone, with the thumb on the plantar surface of the foot and the index finger on the dorsal surface. The contact hand pinch-grips the adjacent cuneiform bone in the same manner.

Action: The contact hand applies a push upward with the thumb and a pull downward with the index finger, testing the joint play between each cuneiform. The correction of a restriction is the test plus an impulse.

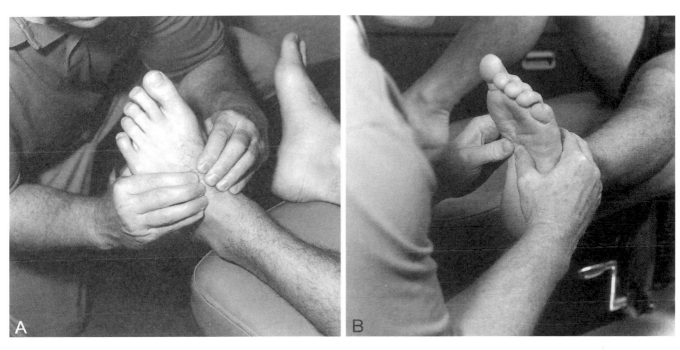

Figure 5B.73. Intercuneiform joint dorsal and plantar glide.

Tarsometatarsal Joints

EXAMINATION/MANIPULATION

Proximal Metatarsal Dorsal and Plantar Glide
(Fig. 5B.74A and B)

Athlete: Supine with the involved leg extended and relaxed.

Doctor: Kneeling at the caudal end of the table and facing the plantar surface of the foot. One hand stabilizes a cuneiform bone with a pinch-grip, and the other hand (contact) pinch-grips the proximal metatarsal directly below that cuneiform. The index fingers are on the dorsal surface, and the thumbs are on the plantar surface.

Action: The contact hand applies a pull downward with the index finger and a push upward with the thumb while testing joint play between each cuneiform and cuboid on the metatarsals. The correction is the test plus an impulse, in the direction of the restriction.

Alternative Method of Manipulation

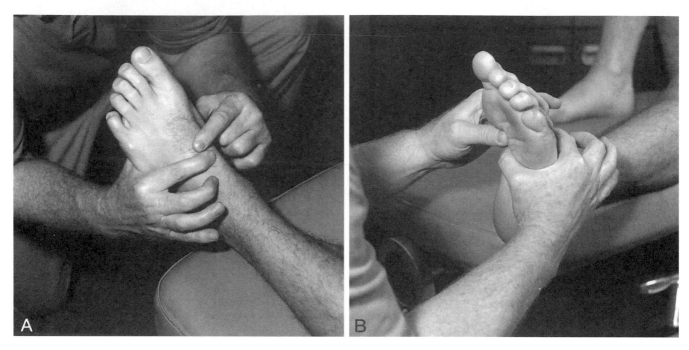

Figure 5B.74. Proximal metatarsal dorsal and plantar glide.

Plantar Glide (Fig. 5B.75A and B)

Athlete: Same as above.

Doctor: Same as above with the exception of applying a finger-over-finger (distal phalanx) contact on the proximal metatarsal while the thumbs are placed on the plantar surface of the foot in the same manner on the same distal metatarsal. The thumbs will stabilize the foot in a slightly dorsiflexed position.

Action: Apply an impulse thrust in a plantar direction with the index fingers while simultaneously applying pressure with the thumbs in a dorsal direction.

Alternative Method of Manipulation

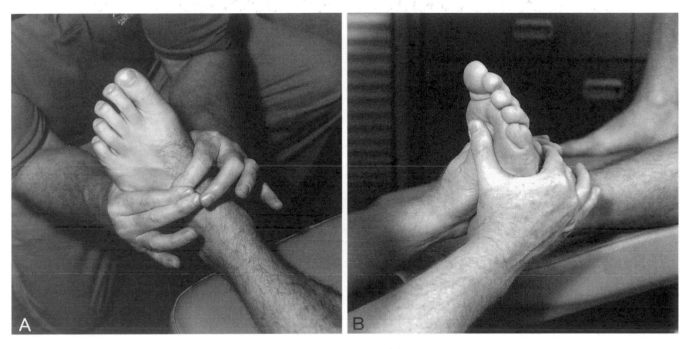

Figure 5B.75. Plantar glide.

Dorsal Glide (Fig. 5B.76)

Athlete: Standing with both hands on the wall for stabilization of balance, while lifting the involved foot off the floor. The involved foot will be directly alongside the other leg, with the toes pointing toward the floor.

Doctor: Kneeling directly behind the athlete and the involved foot. A thumb-over-thumb contact is applied on the plantar surface of the involved proximal metatarsal, with the index fingers on the dorsal surface of the distal phalanx of the same metatarsal.

Action: Elevate and lower the foot several times to ensure foot relaxation. Apply an impulse thrust with the thumbs going in a dorsal and downward (toward the floor) direction, taking care to avoid excessive plantar flexing of the foot.

Rotation of Tarsometatarsal Joints (Fig. 5B.77)

Athlete: Supine with the involved leg extended and relaxed.

Doctor: Kneeling or sitting and facing the plantar surface of the foot. The thumb web of the lateral hand is placed on the distal third of the fifth metatarsal shaft with the thumb hooking underneath the fifth metatarsal head. The medial hand is placed in the same manner on the first metatarsal. The fingers of both hands are placed lightly on the dorsal surface of the foot.

Action: Each hand will apply a clockwise and then a counterclockwise (combined eversion with pronation and inversion with supination) mobilizing maneuver of the metatarsals on the tarsals several times or until mobility is complete.

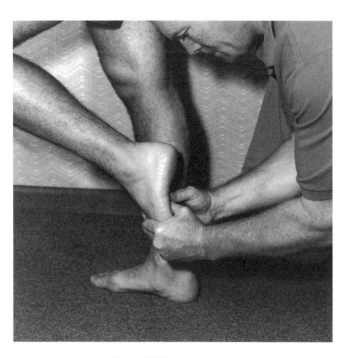

Figure 5B.76. Dorsal glide.

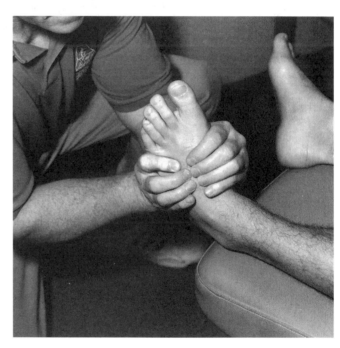

Figure 5B.77. Rotation of tarsometatarsal joints.

Intermetatarsal Articulation

EXAMINATION/MANIPULATION

Proximal and Distal Intermetatarsal Dorsal and Plantar Glide (Fig. 5B.78)

Athlete: Same as above.

Doctor: Kneeling or sitting and facing the plantar surface of the foot. The medial hand pinch-grips the proximal first metatarsal, and the lateral hand pinch-grips the proximal second metatarsal, with the index fingers on the dorsal surface and the thumbs on the plantar surface.

Action: One hand stabilizes while the other hand applies a push-and-pull maneuver on each proximal metatarsal progressively until mobility is complete between all the metatarsal bones. (Do the same maneuver with the distal metatarsals.)

Metatarsophalangeal and Interphalangeal Joints

EXAMINATION/MANIPULATION

Refer to the section on the hand. The testing procedure and manipulation of the metatarsophalangeal and interphalangeal joints are the same as that of the metacarpophalangeal and interphalangeal joints.

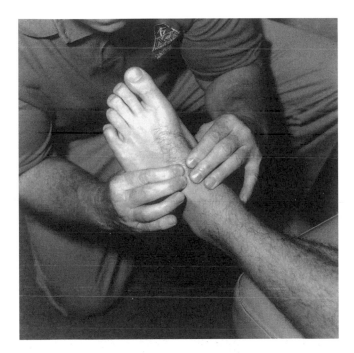

Figure 5B.78. Proximal and distal intermetatarsal dorsal and plantar glide.

THE RIBS

The ribs have multiple joint attachments, including the costovertebral joints, costotransverse joints, sternocostal joints, and costocostal (intercostal) joints. During respiration, these joints move in a superior-inferior and anterior-posterior expanding and compressing direction.

Trunk rotation allows the ribs to protrude posteriorly on the side to which the vertebral bodies rotate and to flatten on the contralateral side. Quite frequently, there are fixations in the thoracic spinal segment corresponding to the respective rib restriction. In this case, one should mobilize the thoracic spinal segments before mobilizing the rib.

Costosternal Joints

EXAMINATION/MANIPULATION

Posterior Glide (Fig. 5B.79)

Athlete: Supine with the head slightly elevated.
Doctor: Facing cephalad on the involved side. A pisiform or double thumb contact is placed on the rib, just lateral to the sternum.
Action: Apply an anterior-posterior glide with or without a superior or inferior angle depending on the direction of the restriction. There should be a springy endfeel of the rib on the sternum. Correction of a restriction is the test, plus a short, sharp impulse thrust into the restriction.

Costovertebral Joints

EXAMINATION/MANIPULATION

Anterior Glide (Fig. 5B.80)

Athlete: Prone.
Doctor: Same as above with the exception of using a pisiform or double thumb contact on the rib head, just lateral to the transverse process.
Action: Apply a light body drop with your contact hand in a posterior-anterior direction on the rib head just lateral to the transverse process testing the springy endfeel. Correction is the test plus an impulse. You may also combine superior or inferior glide with the posterior-anterior glide.

Alternative Method of Manipulation
Athlete: Prone.
Doctor: Standing on the opposite side to be tested and facing toward the rib cage. The doctor reaches over the athlete and grasps with the caudal hand the anterior iliac spine on the side to be tested. The fleshy pisiform of the other hand is placed on the respective rib head to be tested.
Action: The caudal hand lifts the anterior iliac spine off the table to introduce rotation on the lumbar spine.

The contact hand will follow the curve of the rib and test the springy endfeel while applying a light impulse thrust in the anterior-lateral (rotation) direction. The depth of the thrust is extremely shallow to avoid a rib injury.

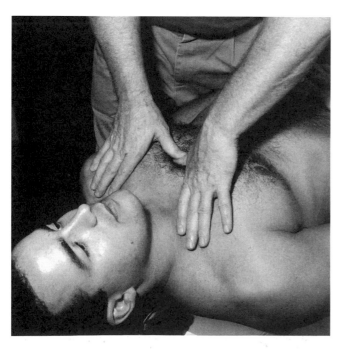

Figure 5B.79. Posterior glide.

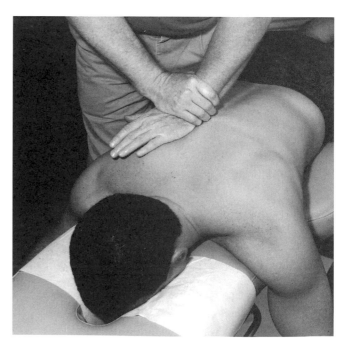

Figure 5B.80. Anterior glide.

First Rib Glide (Fig. 5B.81A and B)

Athlete: Sitting.

Doctor: Standing behind the athlete. One hand is placed on the top of the athlete's head (for stabilization), and the first rib head is palpated with the index finger of the other hand.

Action: Extend, laterally flex, and rotate the head with the stabilization hand. Rotate both away and toward the side of involvement to find the direction of greatest restriction. The palpating finger should feel the rib head move away, and the joint should have a springy endfeel. The correction of a restriction is as follows:

Athlete: Prone.

Doctor: On the involved side and inferior to the first rib. The stabilization hand is placed on the athlete's forehead. The head is extended, laterally flexed, and rotated in the direction of the greatest restriction. The index finger of the contact hand is placed on the rib head.

Action: Correction is applied with the contact hand in the direction of restriction.

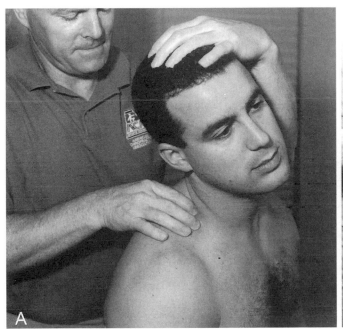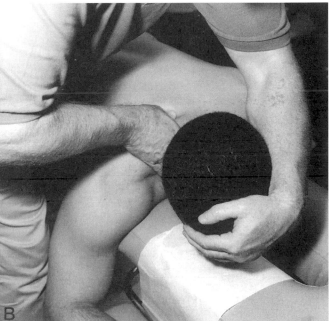

Figure 5B.81. First rib glide.

Intercostal Joints

EXAMINATION/MANIPULATION

Lateral Flexion Mobility (Fig. 5B.82A and B)

Athlete: Sitting with the head and neck in forward flexion.

Doctor: Sitting or standing toward the opposite side to be tested. The doctor's forearm and hand are draped across the athlete's shoulders. The inde finger of the palpating hand is placed between the ribs on the posterior, lateral rib cage near the rib angles.

Action: Side bend the athlete away from the side to be tested and the intercostal joint should open. Side bend the athlete toward the side to be tested and the intercostal joint should close. The correction is as follows:

Athlete: Prone.

Doctor: Standing on the involved side and inferior to the joint to be manipulated. The knife edge (little finger side) of the doctor's contact hand is placed on the involved fixated rib angle. The stabilization hand is placed on top of the contact hand for support.

Action: Correction is in accordance with the direction of the restriction with an impulse thrust. A flexion distraction table is very helpful. The table should be flexed in the opposite direction of the involved side to help facilitate the opening of the intercostal joints.

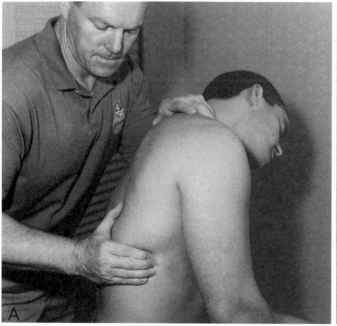
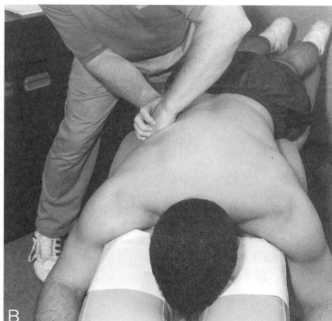

Figure 5B.82. Lateral flexion mobility.

THE JAW

Temporomandibular Joint

The paired temporomandibular joints (TMJs) are classified as condylar joints because one bone (the mandible) articulates with the other (skull) by two distinct articular surfaces or condyles. An articular disc of fibrocartilage divides the joint into two cavities, each lined with a synovial membrane.

The TMJ permits three types of motion: opening and closing of the jaw, protrusion and retrusion of the mandible (anterior and posterior motion), and medial or side-to-side motion.

EXAMINATION/MANIPULATION

Caudal Traction (Fig. 5B.83)

Athlete: Supine with the head slightly elevated.

Doctor: Standing on the side of the involved joint, facing the athlete. The cephalad hand stabilizes the athlete's forehead on the involved side. The thumb of the active hand (with surgical glove) is placed over the lower rear molars with the fingers wrapped around the lateral lower jaw on the involved side.

Action: Apply a slow traction downward several times, and then add a light to moderate impulse. Caudal traction may be combined with protrusion and retrusion. First apply the caudal traction; then add the protrusion or retrusion.

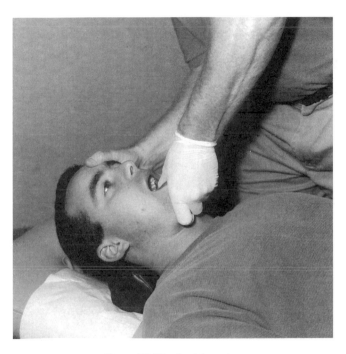

Figure 5B.83. Caudal traction.

Medial Glide (Fig. 5B.84A and B)

Athlete: Supine.

Doctor: Kneeling at the cephalad end of the table. The thenar eminence of each hand is placed on each side of the athlete's temporal region for stabilization. The pads of the fingers are then placed on each side of the ramus just below the TMJ.

Action: Apply a lateral (side-to-side) glide alternately with the fingers of each hand on the ramus to test joint play. The manipulation of the restricted joint is as follows:

Athlete: Supine with the head rotated so the involved joint is facing upward.

Doctor: Standing at the cephalad end of the table. The ear is cupped with the stabilization hand on the noninvolved side, with the thenar eminence contacting the temporal region just above the TMJ. The pisiform of the contact hand is placed on the mandible just below the TMJ, with the little finger extending along the ramus of the mandible.

Action: The athlete is asked to open his or her mouth slightly and relax, at which time a light to moderate short, sharp impulse thrust is given.

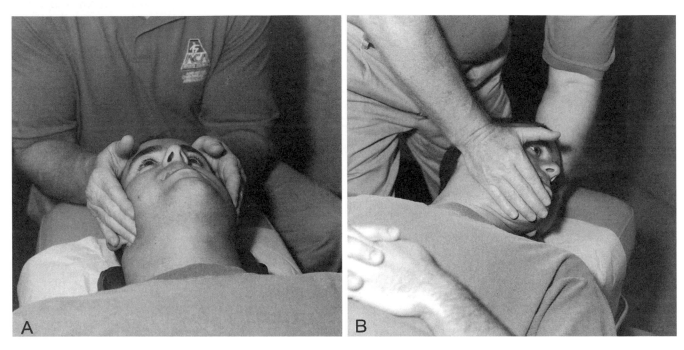

Figure 5B.84. Medial glide.

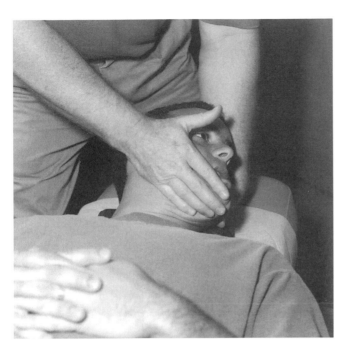

Figure 5B.85. Anterior-inferior glide.

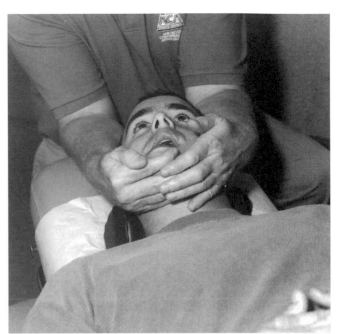

Figure 5B.86. Anterior-inferior malposition.

Anterior-Inferior Glide (Fig. 5B.85)

Athlete: Supine and facing toward the opposite side of the involved joint.

Doctor: Standing at the cephalad end of the table, on the side of involvement. The cephalad hand cups the ear with the stabilization hand on the noninvolved side and stabilizes the upper two or three cervical vertebrae with the last three fingers. The fleshy pisiform of the contact hand is placed on the angle of the mandible.

Action: Ask the athlete to open his or her mouth fairly wide several times. In the process of that movement, the doctor applies an inferior and anterior pressure on the mandible, testing the springy endfeel. The correction of a restriction is the test plus an impulse.

Anterior-Inferior Malposition (Fig. 5B.86)

Athlete: Supine with the head slightly elevated.

Doctor: Kneeling at the cephalad end of the table. The athlete's chin is cupped with the doctor's clasped fingers. The pisiform of the active hand is placed on the ramus of the involved side after removing the soft tissue slack.

Action: Ask the athlete to open his or her mouth as wide as possible, while you apply resistance in the opposite direction (superior-posterior) with both hands. Then have the athlete close the mouth, with resistance toward the involved side. Do this maneuver several times to normalize the joint structure. An alternative maneuver with manipulation is as follows: All the above remains the same with the exception that the athlete's jaw is in a relaxed, neutral position (slightly opened). Apply pressure with both hands going toward the involved side with a controlled impulse thrust. Do not hit the teeth together.

References

1. Mennell JM. Joint pain: diagnosis and treatment using manipulative techniques. Boston: Little, Brown & Co., 1964.
2. Hammer WI. Functional soft tissue examination and treatment: the extremities. Gaithersburg, MD: Aspen Publications, 1991;10:191–214.
3. Kapandji IA. The physiology of the joints. 2nd ed. New York: Churchill Livingstone, 1970;1–2.

Section II

SITE-SPECIFIC SPORTS INJURIES

Head Trauma in Sports

Dale K. Johns

EPIDEMIOLOGY

Participation in sports has increased significantly in recent years in the United States, with approximately 20% of the population engaged actively. Accordingly, the incidence of central nervous system trauma has also increased. However, a significant morbidity and mortality can be lowered by stricter adherence to established safety guidelines. The primary goal of medical personnel is to decrease the number and severity of athletic injuries (1–6).

The largest number of head injuries occurs in contact sports, particularly those in which the head is inclined forward or players collide with each other forcibly, receive blows, or are likely to fall. Football (1, 4, 7–10), rugby (11), boxing (11–18), hockey (15, 17), wrestling (19, 20), and the martial arts (21) are considered high-risk sports as are, to a lesser degree, soccer, vehicular racing, gymnastics (22), bicycling (23–26), horseback riding (27–29), diving (30–33), and parachuting (34). Considered to be low-risk sports are skiing (35, 36), roller skating (37), skateboarding, baseball (38), basketball (39), golf, and jogging (40). This classification is an arbitrary one, based primarily on the incidence of reported injuries.

Comprehensive statistics are kept by the National Football Head and Neck Registry (6). Their data report the mortality due to head injuries as slightly under 10 per year. The actual risk rate from 1980 to 1986 was 0.85 per 100,000 players, down from 1.5 per 100,000 players as reported by Schneider for 1959 to 1963 (10). The incidence of minor head injury per season has been estimated at 20% in high school players (41). The minor head injury rate was reported by Rimel et al. at the University of Virginia to be 8.2% in a group of 2350 collegiate football players over a 4-year period (42). Of the nearly 2.5 million participants in this sport annually, 66,000 are collegians. One fatality has been recorded for every 10 million athletic exposures at present. In 1964, it was one fatality for every 1.5 million exposures (43). The incidence of intracranial hemorrhage in football players is 1.2 per 100,000 players (44). Nonfatality injury rates varied from 20 to 81 injuries per 100 players per year, depending on the mode of reporting (1–5, 45–49).

Boxing has recently come under intense criticism from a number of authorities. Several deaths have been highlighted by television. Total boxing deaths numbered 353 in the years 1945 to 1983 (50), declining to 28 deaths from 1979 to 1985, for a 13.0 per 1000 participant risk rate (50). The result of repeated blows to the head is thought to produce not only acute focal injuries, such as contusion and intracranial hematoma, but also a chronic syndrome ranging from the "punch-drunk fighter" to "dementia pugilistica," a full-blown traumatic encephalopathy (51–53). Approximately 27,500 amateur boxers and 5000 licensed professionals are registered today (40). Advocates of the sport believe that progress has been made in decreasing the number of injuries by more careful monitoring of the boxers by the referee and ring physician and by rule changes, although others disagree. The minor head injury ("knockout") rate is approximately 5% in amateurs, rising to 6.3% in professionals.

Wrestling has also increased in popularity in recent years but has also come under criticism due to a relatively high incidence of serious injury to the participants (19, 20). One third of all wrestling injuries involve the head and neck (40). They are similar in nature to those that occur in boxing, including a chronic encephalopathy due to repeated injury.

Sports bicycling has also gained in popularity with an accompanying rise in the number of injuries. In 1980, there were nearly 1000 fatalities reported in bicyclists, of which 74% were head injuries (23, 24). Fife et al. reported 176 bicycling fatalities, all of which were due to injury to the head and neck; not one person was wearing a helmet (24).

Equestrian injuries have risen in number, with approximately 82 million Americans riding annually. Barber found two thirds of the injuries involved the head (27).

Those concerned with the medical supervision of athletes must be prepared to diagnose and treat acute head injuries and to recognize the sequelae of cerebral trauma.

ANATOMY

Understanding the pathophysiology of head injury requires a working knowledge of the anatomy of the skull and brain. The skull is essentially a closed, bony box with two apertures: the tentorium, which supports the cerebral hemispheres and gives hiatus to the midbrain, and the foramen magnum, through which the brain stem exits (Fig. 6.1).

The rough surface of the frontal floor, which also forms the orbital roof, is the major reason for the extensive injury to the frontal lobes in acceleration–deceleration trauma. The sharp edges of the sphenoid wings also produce bruising and laceration of the tips of the temporal lobes as they propel forward after an impact involving the skull.

The skull is compartmentalized by these unyielding structures into anterior, middle, and posterior fossae. Because of the surface irregularity and hardness of the bone, extensive damage can occur to the brain when it is set in motion, particularly when rotational forces are applied to the skull. The falx is a dense membranous structure that separates the cerebrum into right and left hemispheres. It contains the sagittal and straight sinuses. The meninges consist of three layers: the dura, a tough outer cover; the arachnoid, a filmy middle layer; and the pia mater, which is a thin, transparent layer closely adhered to the cortex.

The tentorium is a horizontal extension of the dura, which forms a membranous floor separating the anterior and middle fossae (supratentorial) from the posterior (infratentorial) fossa. It is attached anteriorly to the ridges of the petrous bone and posteriorly becomes contiguous with the investment of the dura forming the lateral sinuses. It is incomplete anteriorly, and it is through here that the midbrain exits. The third, fourth, and sixth cranial nerves are in close proximity to the tentorial edge on their way to the various foramina at the base of the skull, through which they exit to innervate the various organs of the face and neck.

The cerebral hemispheres are paired structures consisting of frontal, temporal, parietal, and occipital lobes separated by the falx, a vertical extension of the meninges dividing the cerebral hemispheres. Specific areas of specialized function exist within each lobe (Fig. 6.2). The frontal lobes contain the centers for intellectual function, eye movement, and motor speech. The posterior frontal lobe is concerned with motor and sensory function. The temporal lobe is primarily responsible for receptive speech and memory. The parietal lobes contain the association areas where information is processed. The occipital lobes deal primarily with vision.

The posterior fossa contains the cerebellum, the primary function of which is coordination and equilibrium, and the brain stem, which contains the nuclei for the cranial nerves and all tracts passing to and from the brain to the periphery.

The brain is suspended in the cerebrospinal fluid supported by the carotid arteries and brain stem and is separated from the dura by the fluid-filled subarachnoid space. Numerous veins connecting the dura and brain pass through here. The large venous sinuses within the dura drain the blood from the brain.

CEREBRAL BLOOD SUPPLY

The blood supply is primarily through the anterior circulation via the paired carotid arteries, which supply the majority of the blood flow to

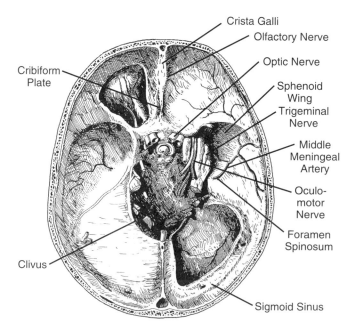

Figure 6.1. Anatomy of the skull. Note the rough surfaces of the frontal floor and sharpness of the sphenoid wings and crista galli. The middle meningeal artery enters the skull through the foramen spinosum at the base and courses across the floor as shown. The skull is essentially a closed box with a single opening—the foramen magnum.

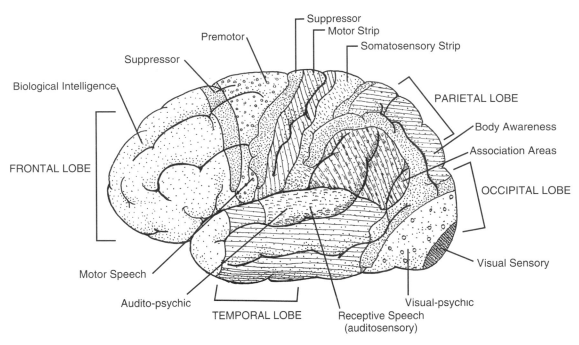

Figure 6.2. Neurophysiologic areas of the brain. The major neurophysiologic areas of the brain are portrayed across a gross lateral projection. The motor strip is considered the posterior boundary of the frontal lobe. Broca's area (motor speech) and the superior gyrus of the temporal lobe are vital in the dominant hemisphere. The parietal lobe contains the association areas, whereas the temporal lobe is important in memory. The temporal and occipital lobes contain visual radiations, with the primary area located at the occipital tip.

the brain. The remainder is carried by the vertebral arteries, with the left side commonly the larger. The carotid artery divides after passing through the base of the skull and cavernous sinus into the anterior and middle cerebral arteries, which supply the frontal, parietal, and temporal lobes. The occipital lobe, cerebellum, and brain stem are fed primarily by the posterior cerebral and vertebral arteries (Fig. 6.3).

The vertebral arteries enter the skull through the foramen magnum and join, shortly thereafter, on the ventral surface of the brain stem to form the basilar artery. This artery then bifurcates and joins the posterior communicating artery on either side at the circle of Willis, to form the paired posterior cerebral arteries. The middle meningeal artery arises from the external carotid artery and passes through the foramen spinosum at the base of the skull, where it enters the middle meningeal groove. It passes upward through the temporal and frontal bone, where it divides into frontal, middle, and posterior meningeal branches. It is vulnerable to laceration by fractures that traverse its path in the temporal bone.

PATHOPHYSIOLOGY

The majority of head injuries in sports are closed head injuries; i.e., the brain is damaged without penetration of the skull. They are due to direct impact with a ball, bat, other player's head, or a stationary object or they are due to a rapid acceleration-deceleration of the head. They encompass the entire spectrum, from simple loss of awareness without loss of consciousness to paralytic, irreversible coma and death. The severity of injury depends on a number of factors including velocity and direction of impact, position and motion of the head, and lines of force (54). The degree of injury depends, in general, on the amount of energy dissipated on impact. Fortunately, most of the injuries are minor.

The impact injuries are usually unidirectional (translational) applications of force without a significant rotary component (55). They produce movements of the brain within the skull due to rapid acceleration-deceleration of the head. Translational forces seldom produce loss of consciousness or neurologic deficit, but focal lesions, such as contusions and intracranial hematoma, may occur (54, 56).

Rotational forces are produced by a blow to the head, which causes it to twist and turn rapidly (57). Differential movement between the white and gray matter interfaces, causing stretching and tearing of neuronal tissue with resultant dysfunction (54, 57). This shaking of the brain produces diffuse brain injury, which is usually more severe than focal injuries and frequently re-

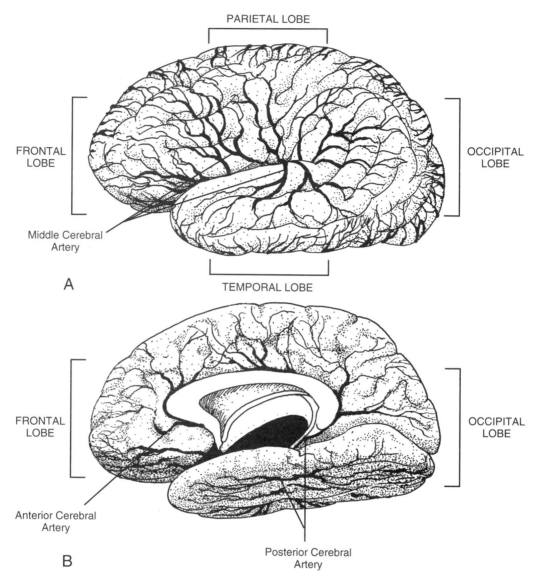

Figure 6.3. Blood supply to the brain. The major blood supply to the brain is via the carotid and vertebral arteries. The carotid branches into the anterior, middle, and posterior cerebral arteries, which supply the frontal, parietal, and occipital/temporal lobes, respectively.

sults in a loss of consciousness (57–59). A diffuse injury includes some degree of involvement of the entire brain, in contrast to a focal injury in which only a small area is involved, as in contusions and intracranial hematomas. They frequently occur as a result of rapid acceleration-deceleration of the head. Actual impact to the head is not required, as in the so-called whiplash injury, in which a rapid acceleration-deceleration occurs with inertial loading (55–57). Both translational and rotational forces can be produced.

Experiments have shown that if the head is immobile at the time of impact, a focal cerebral contusion or hematoma is likely to form under the site of impact (54). If, however, the head strikes an immobile object while moving, a simi-

lar lesion occurs on that portion of the brain opposite the area of impact. This situation explains the mechanism of coup-contra coup in-jury (54).

In acceleration-deceleration injuries, the head moving in space is stopped suddenly by a solid object, which causes the brain to strike the front of the skull (coup). The brain then rebounds with great force, striking the back of the skull, producing a contra coup injury.

In impact injuries, the skull deforms at the site of impact, striking the brain, producing a coup injury. The brain, which has been set in motion, then strikes the opposite side of the skull, producing a contra coup injury. Ommaya et al. found a direct relationship between the amount of inertial loading and rotation induced at the time of impact and the duration of loss of consciousness (54, 56, 60). Neuronal tissue is the most susceptible to trauma, particularly that located in the cerebral hemispheres.

Experiments performed on monkeys proved conclusively that the head must be allowed to rotate before loss of consciousness occurs (56, 60). When the forces were only in a straight line (translational), no loss of consciousness occurred but intracranial hemorrhage and contusions did (56, 60). Deceleration injuries produced cerebral and brainstem contusion as well as focal ischemia and intracranial hemorrhages in the frontal and temporal lobes, due to their close approximation to the rough bony surfaces that enclose them. Acceleration-deceleration injuries produced diffuse brain damage and were generally more severe than the impact injuries that produced focal lesions (54, 56).

The maximal tolerance of the brain to acceleration is between 188 and 230 gravitational forces (GF), with the time duration of 310 to 400 milliseconds (61). These levels are frequently exceeded in high-risk sports such as football, rugby, and boxing (8, 62).

Fortunately, most sports injuries are of low-velocity impact and inertial loading, so the majority are mild. The majority of athletes recover normalcy within 5 to 15 minutes after impact.

TYPES OF INJURIES

Scalp

The scalp consists of two layers: an outer one consisting of the epidermis and underlying subcutaneous tissue, which contains the hair follicles, and an inner dense fibrous layer, the galea. The latter structure allows the scalp to slide easily over the pericranium, which, along with the hair, protects the scalp from injury to some degree. The scalp is extremely vascular, being supplied by paired occipital arteries posteriorly, the superficial temporal arteries laterally, and the supraorbital arteries anteriorly; the supraorbital arteries exit the skull from the supraorbital foramen located just above the medial third of the eye.

An extensive laceration of the scalp can produce such profuse hemorrhage that hypovolemic shock occurs. Scalp bleeding, even from multiple arteries, can be controlled easily by placing a cord or even a large handkerchief around the

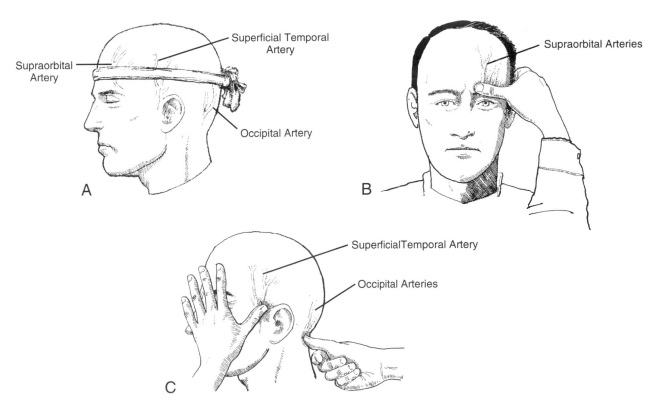

Figure 6.4. Blood supply to the scalp. The three major suppliers of blood to the scalp are shown (A) along with the appropriate locations for applying pressure to decrease scalp hemorrhage significantly (B,C). Twisting a handkerchief, rope, or belt tightly around the scalp can act as an effective tourniquet if more than one artery is torn, as seen in extensive laceration or avulsion injuries.

scalp in a band-like fashion, knotting it, and then twisting it to produce a tourniquet. It should be released for a short period every 20 minutes to prevent scalp necrosis (Fig. 6.4).

Hemorrhage from one or two arteries can be controlled by applying finger pressure just proximal to the laceration. The skull makes a good buttress against which to compress the artery.

The most common lesions seen are abrasions or contusions, which usually require no more than cleansing, followed by application of ice for several hours. Avulsion, or tearing of the scalp, is usually produced by a tangential blow and may be associated with profuse hemorrhage requiring referral to an emergency care facility. Scalp hemorrhage can often be controlled by packing the wound with sterile gauze, followed by tight application of an elastic bandage over the dressing to sustain pressure until the patient can be transported. If excessively tight, the dressing should be released for 1 or 2 minutes every 20 minutes. An effort should be made to leave the ears out of the dressing if possible. If not, gauze should be placed behind them to avoid pressure necrosis. Pressure can also be applied over the major arteries involved as an adjunct.

Skull Fractures

The skull is composed of a thick cortical inner and outer table, separated by a diploic layer. Blows to the calvarium distribute themselves radially, so the force on the impacted area is lessened. The act of the skull fracturing linearly dissipates much of the force rather than transmitting it to the brain. Fragments of bone driven into the dural covering, brain, or vessels can cause secondary injury, such as spinal fluid leaks, intracranial hematomas, infection, pneumocephalus, and other vascular complications. The primary significance of a skull fracture is that it is an index of the severity of the blow. However, it has no prognostic value.

A fracture significantly increases the likelihood of an intracranial hematoma. Approximately 25% of patients with skull fractures do not experience a loss of consciousness (63). It requires between

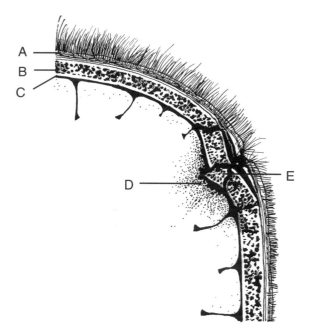

Figure 6.5. Open depressed skull fracture. Many depressed skull fractures produce underlying cerebral contusions and dural laceration. The fracture is often more extensive than seen on radiographs, and prompt surgical treatment is mandatory. Note the many anatomic elements affected: (A) scalp, (B) diploë, (C) dura, (D) cerebral contusion, (E) bone fragments.

900 and 1700 pounds of force over 0.001 second or less to fracture the frontal bone (61, 64). However, many patients with fractures do not sustain significant brain injury, and the converse is also true; that is, an individual may have no external signs of head injury but have irreversible brain damage. Table 6.1 presents a simple classification of skull fractures.

Linear fractures comprise 80% of the total, of which half are in the midportion of the skull (65). Fractures are classified as either open or closed, depending on whether there is an overlying scalp laceration communicating with the outside. This ragged wound could expose the brain to infection if the dura is lacerated. In more severe injuries, multiple linear fractures may coalesce to produce a "cracked eggshell" appearance on radiographic study, referred to as a comminuted fracture. Linear or comminuted fractures seldom, if ever, have surgical indications.

Depressed fractures are usually the result of a large force exerted over a small area of the skull. They often require elevation, particularly if the outer table of the depressed fragment is below the inner table of the skull. Open depressed fractures should always be elevated to inspect the dura for laceration. Forty percent of patients with closed depressed fractures have a neurologic deficit. This percentage is even higher in open depressed fractures (Fig. 6.5).

Table 6.1. Skull Fractures

Classification	
Linear fractures	Diastatic fractures
Open	Basilar fractures
Closed	Perforating
Depressed fractures	fractures
Open	
Closed	

Diastatic fractures are those that travel along a suture line. Because of the large venous sinuses in close approximation, special attention should be given to monitoring these patients.

Basilar fractures are difficult to diagnose by radiograph. Even on special basilar views, the yield is less than 40%. Located here are foramina through which the cranial nerves and major arteries pass, making them subject to injury by displaced bone. External indications of basilar fractures are otorrhea, otorrhagia, hemotympanum, rhinorrhea, and panda bear and Battle's signs. The panda bear or raccoon sign is produced by a fracture across the floor of the frontal fossa, which allows blood to extravasate down into the eyelids. Initially, it may be unilateral but often it becomes bilateral in several hours. The bilateral periorbital ecchymoses that result give the victim a panda bear or raccoon appearance (Fig. 6.6).

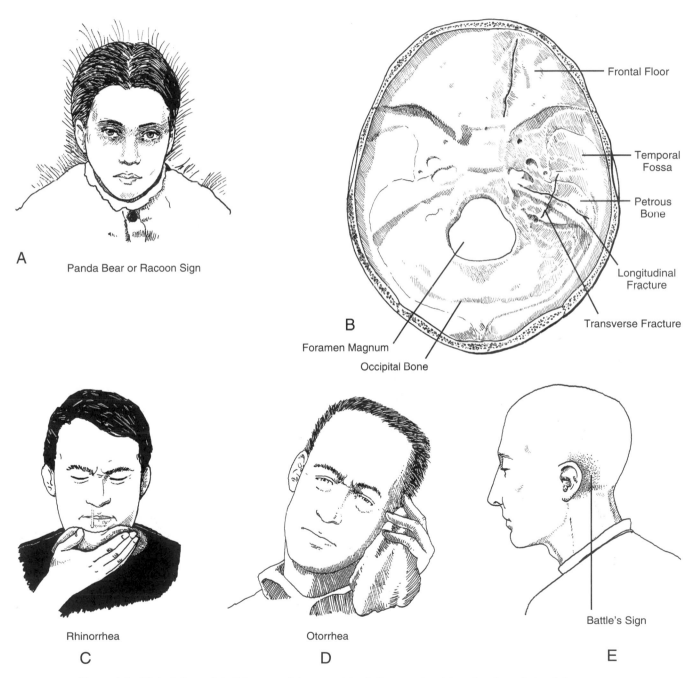

Figure 6.6. Clinical signs of skull fracture. A fracture of the skull may result in bilateral ecchymosis (panda bear or raccoon sign) (A) or rhinorrhea (C). Fractures through the petrous bone (B) can cause otorrhea (D). Basilar fractures may result in spinal fluid leaks from either the ear or nose. Basilar fractures may also cause the development of Battle's sign: ecchymosis behind the ear (E).

An area of discoloration behind the ear or over the mastoid process, due to extravasation of blood from a fracture across the transverse sinus, is known as a Battle's sign. Delayed cranial nerve palsies can occur, especially facial nerve dysfunction that produces a unilateral facial weakness with drooping of the angle of the mouth and inability to close the eye. Rhinorrhagia or otorrhagia, which is much more rare, can easily be diagnosed by the observation of blood-tinged fluid dripping from the nose or ear, particularly if that structure is dependent. By catching some of the fluid on a clean white cloth, one can easily discern a red ring in the center surrounded by a halo, which becomes progressively lighter as it goes peripherally. This halo appearance is diagnostic of bloody cerebrospinal fluid. If clear fluid is present, it can be tested for glucose using urosticks, which confirm the diagnosis. (No other nasal secretion shows a positive test for glucose.)

Blood oozing from the ear without a laceration of the pinna or external injury to the canal is diagnostic of petrous bone fracture. Blood behind the tympanic membrane or clear spinal fluid exiting the ear indicates the same. If any of the above signs are observed, the athlete should be referred to a facility with neurosurgical coverage.

Perforating fractures are usually due to gunshot or knife wounds but may result from accidents involving spear guns or archery. The object striking the skull is often metallic and small, traveling with sufficient velocity to penetrate the skull, driving bony fragments ahead of it into the brain. The degree of brain damage is usually in direct correlation with the mass and velocity of the object.

CONCUSSION

Concussion is an ambiguous term, which covers a wide range of conditions, from a brief loss of awareness without amnesia to prolonged loss of consciousness (42, 54, 66–68). Physiologically, it is a disruption of the neural activity of the brain stem, secondary to trauma. Clinically, it represents a reversible loss of consciousness due to temporary dysfunction of the mesencephalic reticular activating formation (69), a result of diffuse bilateral hemispheric injury, with midbrain injury also present in the more severe cases.

The parameters determining the severity of injury are the duration of unconsciousness and the length of post-traumatic amnesia (PTA). PTA can occur even in patients appearing only slightly dazed (54, 70). An injury must be diffuse and severe enough to produce a physiologic disconnection between the cortex and the brain stem. Following loss of consciousness, recovery of awareness precedes motor and sensory recovery. After a head injury, the victim should improve. If not, it is important to look for secondary complications, such as an intracranial hematoma, hypoxia, or signs of brain swelling. In the past, it was a common belief that no structural damage occurred as a result of concussion, but Oppenheimer found neuronal loss on postmortem examinations of patients who suffered concussion as the only known head injury (71). Many neuropathic and clinical studies, including a retrospective one at the University of Virginia, have left little doubt that many people with minor head injuries do suffer organic brain damage manifested clinically by difficulty with cognitive functions and inability to process information at a normal rate (42, 61, 67, 72–76). Evidence of neuronal cell damage in the reticular formation, even in cases of mild concussion, has been demonstrated conclusively.

To produce a loss of consciousness, the degree of force exerted must be sufficient to physiologically disconnect the cerebral hemispheres from the brain stem reticular activating system. If it is less, it does not produce a "classic concussion" but only a brief loss of awareness. It also adversely affects memory, which is a function of the temporal lobes, suggesting that the hemispheres are more sensitive to mild trauma than is the brain stem, which appears to be the least vulnerable portion of the central nervous system. It is unlikely that damage occurs to the brain stem without severe diffuse hemispheric injury.

FOCAL BRAIN INJURIES

Contusion

Contusion is a bruising of the brain, resulting in subpial hemorrhage accompanied by neuronal injury and death, which heals only by scarring. The ventral surfaces of the frontal lobes and the tips of the temporal lobes are commonly involved because these areas impact the irregular bony surfaces of the orbital roof and sharp edges of the sphenoid wings (16, 18, 77, 78). Contusion can also result from a direct blow to the skull (coup injury) that sets the skull rapidly into motion, striking the brain, which is not moving as rapidly due to inertia. The contra coup injury occurs when the skull, having stopped, is struck by the brain, which is now in motion. Later hemorrhage into the necrotic area is not unusual and may produce sudden neurologic deterioration (62).

Frequently, some degree of subarachnoid hemorrhage is present as evidenced by subhyoid hemorrhages seen on ophthalmoscopic examination. Nuchal rigidity, severe headache, photophobia, and frequent alterations in the level of consciousness are suggestive of subarachnoid hemorrhage, which frequently produces severe vasospasm and decreased cerebral blood flow resulting in ischemia, hypoxia, and cerebral edema.

INTRACRANIAL HEMATOMAS

Intracranial hematomas are of three basic types, based on their location: epidural, subdural, and intracerebral. They are present in approximately 10% of all head injuries (79).

Epidural Hematomas

Nearly 2% of head injuries have concomitant epidural hematomas (79). Eighty-five percent occur as a result of fractures across the middle meningeal groove of the temporal bone, lacerating of one of the branches of the middle meningeal artery (Fig.6.7) (61, 80, 81). The mechanism of injury is usually a direct blow to the head, as is often seen in athletic injuries. These head injuries are true neurosurgical emergencies; death can occur rapidly from cerebral herniation due to the rapidly expanding mass within the skull. Venous epidural hematomas are produced by leakage of blood from one of the large dural sinuses lacerated by fragments of bone resulting from skull fracture. The symptoms are of slower onset and the neurologic deterioration is not nearly as rapid. Eighty percent of hematomas are located within the temporal fossa (79). They are rarely bilateral. In approximately 40% of cases, they are associated with other traumatic intracranial lesions. The morbidity and mortality rate in older series was nearly 70%, but with better diagnostic methods and prompt neurosurgical treatment, it has decreased to approximately 20% (82).

Approximately one third of patients does not gain consciousness after impact, whereas another one third does not lose consciousness, perhaps for days. The classic syndrome occurs in the remaining one third, which everyone responsible for the medical care of athletes should familiarize themselves with (55). The initial impact is usually a blunt, low-velocity blow, which results in a brief period of loss of consciousness, followed by a variable period of wakefulness,

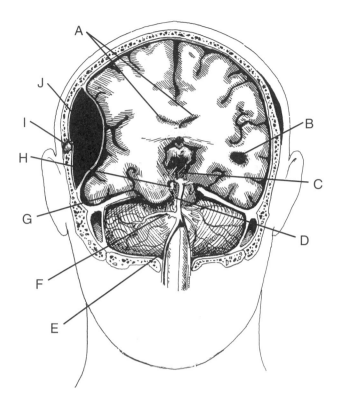

Figure 6.7. Intracranial injuries. Intracranial injuries most often result in hematoma formation with associated secondary signs. (A) Hematomas can result in the mass effect that produces compression of the brain and ventricles. (B) Parenchymal hematoma. (C) Compression of the posterior cerebral artery by swelling and hematoma can produce contralateral blindness. (D) Brain stem shift and compression result in hemiparesis and positive Babinski sign, loss of consciousness, and respiratory and vasomotor paralysis. (E) Herniation of cerebellar tonsils causes brain-stem signs. (F) Pressure on the oculomotor nerve (III) causes ipsilateral pupillary dilation and loss of the light reflex. (G) Location of tentorium. (H) Uncal herniation can produce cranial nerve palsies and midbrain signs. (I) Skull fracture lacerating the middle meningeal artery. (J) Epidural hematoma.

ranging from 15 minutes to as long as 1 month, depending on whether the source of the hematoma is arterial or venous. If arterial, the lucid interval is much shorter. Once the mass has reached sufficient size, rapid neurologic deterioration occurs, characterized by progressive loss of alertness, severe headache, nausea, vomiting, contralateral hemiparesis, and ipsilateral pupillary dilatation in 30 to 50% of cases (65). Cushing's triad, i.e., bradycardia, hypertension, and respiratory depression, are terminal events produced by uncal herniation. The pathophysiology is that of a rapidly expanding mass compressing the brain that, in turn, causes impairment of circulatory function with resultant hypoxia, venous stasis, and brain swelling, with resultant cerebral edema. This swelling results in an increase in brain volume, producing a rise in intracranial pressure.

After the compliance of the brain becomes exhausted, the temporal lobes are driven downward and medially through the tentorial notch (uncal herniation) that, in turn, compresses the midbrain and oculomotor nerve. If the hematoma is in the posterior fossa, the cerebellum is forced into the foramen magnum, causing irreversible brain-stem damage. The onset of symptoms can be either acute or chronic. Headaches, ataxia, vomiting, incoordination, paresis, and cranial nerve palsies are clinical indications of an expanding posterior fossa mass with Cushing's triad developing in the terminal stages (Fig. 6.8). Nearly 30% of patients that recover have residual neurologic deficit. Frequently, swelling of the scalp can be seen over the hematoma site.

Subdural Hematomas

Subdural hematomas are associated with 5% of all head injuries, roughly three times that of epidural hematomas (55). The precipitating injury is one of a high-velocity impact, producing sudden jarring of the brain, with stretching and tearing of the bridging veins. Gennarelli et al. produced predictable subdural hematomas in animals by rotational head acceleration; no impact was required to produce these lesions (72). Approximately 50% are associated with skull fractures, and between 15% and 20% are bilateral. Most occur over the convexities, and 84% have associated hemorrhagic contusions or in-

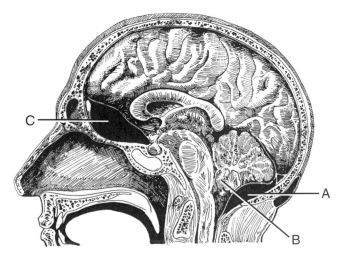

Figure 6.8. Other hematomas. (A) Posterior fossa hematomas are often difficult to diagnose. They may result in sudden death, ataxia, dysmetria, and dysarthria due to brain-stem and cerebellar compression. (B) Cerebellar compression may obstruct spinal fluid pathways, causing hydrocephalus. (C) Subfrontal hematomas are often associated with frontal contusions, with loss of intellect, affect, inhibition, and cognitive functions.

tracerebral hematomas with resultant brain swelling (55).

Acute subdural hematomas are often associated with massive injuries to the brain. The morbidity and mortality rate usually depend on the latter rather than the blood clot and run between 50% and 80% (44, 55). The symptoms are those seen with all rapidly expanding intracranial lesions and are not so much due to the blood clots themselves, as to the concomitant brain contusion and resultant swelling. The earliest and most sensitive sign is a change in mental status, followed by hemiparesis and pupillary changes. One should be suspicious if the loss of consciousness is prolonged or if a rapid deterioration occurs in the neurologic status. The onset of symptoms usually occurs within the first week of injury, most within 24 hours.

Subacute and Chronic Hematomas

These hematomas develop much more slowly and are seldom associated with diffuse brain contusion. Symptoms do not appear for more than 20 days after injury. The mechanism is essentially the same as that seen in acute hematomas but of lesser force. The head injury may even be trivial. The onset of symptoms is much more insidious and manifested initially by headache and personality changes, followed by a gradually deteriorating sensorium. The onset of hemiparesis is more gradual, and the prognosis is significantly better. Mortality in simple hematomas without associated brain injuries is approximately 20%.

Intracerebral Hematomas

Free blood within the brain substance itself (intracranial hematoma) is frequently associated with other brain lesions. The incidence is approximately 2% of head injuries (83). Severe neurologic deficits are common, such as loss of consciousness, hemiparesis, aphasia, and visual disturbances, depending on the area of the brain involved. Many of the injured have only partial neurologic recovery. The mortality rate is nearly 50% (84). Symptoms and signs depend on the location and size of the hemorrhage. Some individuals do not lose consciousness or demonstrate any focal neurologic signs, but an intracerebral hematoma is seen as an incidental finding on magnetic resonance imaging (MRI) or computed tomography (CT) scan. They are usually produced by translational rather than rotational forces. Hemorrhage can occur into a contusion, even weeks later, which may produce a sudden deterioration of the clinical picture.

MANAGEMENT

The management of athletes with head injuries is a dynamic and constantly evolving science, requiring ordered thinking and adherence to established protocols that are familiar to everyone involved. A fundamental knowledge of anatomy, pathophysiology, and neurology, accompanied by sound clinical judgment, is essential. An accurate diagnosis must be made quickly, followed by institution of appropriate treatment. There is no place for panic on the part of the medical team, whose primary goal is the prevention of further injury (85). There must be quick, efficient handling of each injury, without fumbling or confusion that might cause harm to the athlete.

A team member should be appointed and should direct the other members and be responsible for all decisions. Essential qualities should include resourcefulness, ordered thinking, calmness, and the ability to perform a rapid and concise general physical and neurologic examination. The leader must be proficient in cardiopulmonary resuscitation (CPR) and in Advanced Cardiac Life Support (ACLS) as well (86). It is advisable that this team member be readily available for any on-site emergency. A physician, if present, usually assumes this position and supervises the on-field management of the athlete. A physician or paramedical team should be present at all high-risk sporting events. Prior training and mock drills are necessary to allow the individuals to function as a unit and to understand their responsibilities fully.

All team members should be trained in advanced first aid and trauma management, including the removal of protective equipment and transport of the injured, and should be proficient in CPR as well. All members should have preassigned specific tasks for which they have been trained (87–89). Emergency equipment must be readily available and include, at the minimum, a spine board or rigid stretcher, sandbags, cervical collars, oxygen, and the equipment for CPR. Occasionally, bolt cutters may be required to remove certain types of football face masks. The location of all emergency equipment should remain unchanged, and all team members should be proficient in its use. An ambulance should be present at high-risk sporting events for transport to a facility located in the immediate vicinity. Even in low-risk sports, an ambulance should be on stand by availability.

An ideal trauma team would consist of a medical professional as leader and four assistants, all trained in CPR and familiar with the techniques of immobilization, handling, and transport of injured players. Prearrangement with a nearby hospital should be made before high-risk sporting events take place.

MILD HEAD INJURY

Mild head injuries represent the lower end of the spectrum of mechanically induced, diffuse injuries. They can be the result of either direct impact or impulse-producing sudden movement of the head due to impact elsewhere (54). It is possible to produce them without actual impact to the head, as is seen in the so-called whiplash injury, in which a rapid flexion extension of the neck imparts kinetic energy to the brain as a result of inertial loading. Focal lesions can be produced as well as diffuse injury, particularly if a rotary component is present as well as a transitional one (90). Under extreme circumstances, the pure force of acceleration alone can cause brain damage, as proven by neuropathic studies.

A number of researchers (20, 44, 59, 73, 89, 91–94) have used a wide variety of criteria to define cerebral concussion. Russell et al. defined minor head injury as a loss of consciousness of less than 20 minutes, a Glasgow coma scale of 13 to 15, and hospitalization of less than 48 hours (92). Other authors describe mild concussion as a loss of awareness with a short-term memory loss of up to 60 minutes after impact (PTA) (38, 42, 83). Jennett classified head injuries according to the duration of PTA, as listed in Table 6.2 (95).

The exact criteria for defining concussion have varied widely in the literature, but those of Ommaya and Gennarelli (Table 6.3) appear most suited to use in athletes (59).

Careful observation of all athletes, particularly those engaged in high-risk sports, is mandatory during practice and training sessions and during games. Anyone who appears dazed or confused or is staggering or stumbling around should be removed from play and examined. Dave Megesy, a former football player, defined the "ding" as, "getting hit on the head so hard that memory is affected but you are able to walk around and even

Table 6.2. Jennett Classification of Head Injuries

Less than 5 minutes	Very mild
Less than 1 hour	Mild
1 hour to 24 hours	Moderate
1 to 7 days	Severe
Longer than 7 days	Very severe

Table 6.3.   Classification of Concussion

Grade I—Transient confusion with rapid return to normal without amnesia. This is the mildest from of head injury and is completely reversible, usually within 15 minutes, without post-traumatic amnesia (PTA). These are the football players who have been "dinged" or "had my bell rung," or the boxer who is "out on his feet." They are often dazed or confused and may suffer headache, nausea, and vertigo.

Grade II—Greater and more prolonged confusion accompanied by a short period of PTA, which begins approximately 10 minutes after injury. The symptoms usually resolve quickly but can persist several weeks or more in rare instances.

Grade III—A still greater degree of initial confusion with both retrograde amnesia and PTA, which is present from the time of impact. The athlete may continue to play without recall of prior events. Retrograde amnesia is a loss of memory for events before the accident. Ataxia may also be seen in these individuals to the point of their being nonambulatory. Visual and auditory hallucinations occur in approximately 3%. Headache, nausea, vomiting, and incoordination are not infrequent symptoms.

Grade IV (classic concussion)—A brief period of loss of consciousness, followed by a period of confusion and some degree of retrograde amnesia and PTA. A gradual recovery then begins, with a return first of lucidity and mental function, followed by recovery thereafter of the motor and sensory functions, and lastly a return of memory and other cognitive functions.

Coma—The individual is unresponsive to external stimulation. If unconsciousness persists for longer than 1 hour, the patient is defined as being comatose. Cardiorespiratory collapse may be present.

continue playing without any pain, and the only way that other players or coaches realize what happened is that you cannot remember the plays" (96). Zeliska et al. and Yarnell and Lynch describe several types of short-term amnestic syndromes for football players with head injuries (39, 70). Recall of recent events is primarily affected; therefore, questions regarding recent events such as, "What's the score?" "What's your assignment?" "What's the game plan?" can confirm concussion as having occurred. Do not ask questions requiring immediate memory or cognitive function, such as digital recall and reverse spelling (70). The initial examination should also include an assessment of the player's mental status. Is he confused, disoriented, or dazed? Is he steady on his feet and is his gait normal? Is there any degree of PTA or retrograde amnesia? Is there any neurologic deficit? These questions must be answered before a decision can be made as to whether the player should be allowed to return to play, be observed on the sidelines, or be sent to the hospital.

Table 6.4 is an algorithm that provides guidelines for the evaluation and disposition of athletes with head injuries.

The secondary complications of head injury are usually responsible for any deterioration in the neurologic status. The most common of these are brain swelling, cerebral edema, intracranial hematoma or hemorrhage, ischemia, and hypoxia

(69, 97, 98). Hypoxia appears to be related to a brief hypotensive episode that commonly occurs after even mild head injuries (99). Respiratory and cardiac function, as well as motor activity, often fail temporarily. The integrity of the cerebrovascular system becomes compromised. This process can be self-perpetuating, with an increase in cerebral edema, a decrease in brain compliance, and subsequent uncal herniation (97, 98).

Moderate and Severe Head Injuries

Moderate concussion has been defined arbitrarily as a loss of consciousness of less than 5 minutes, and severe concussion as one greater than 5 minutes (100). Another criterion is based on the duration of PTA. If it exceeds 1 hour after impact, the injury is considered to be of moderate severity (101). Coma represents a period of unconsciousness lasting more than 1 hour and is simply a prolonged state characterized by no speech or purposeful response to painful stimulation or other external stimuli. The eyes are usually closed and the body tone flaccid. Severe head injuries can occur as a

Table 6.4.   On-Site Assessment of Head Injury

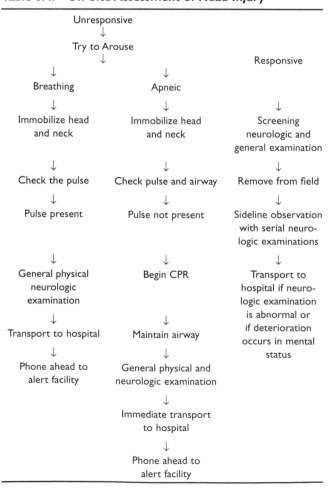

result of the initial impact or can be due to the consequences of the secondary factors of brain injury.

Those who suffer severe head injuries with a prolonged loss of consciousness are likely to demonstrate focal neurologic findings including decorticate and decerebrate rigidity. A decorticate response consists of flexion of the arms on the chest and extension of the legs to external stimulation. This response reflects a physiologic level of injury between the cortex and the red nuclei (midbrain). A decerebrate response consists of extension of all four limbs, with pronation of the arms and plantar extension of the feet. This response reflects injury to the brain stem between the red nuclei and the vestibular nuclei. Approximately 40% of patients with severe head injuries need a neurosurgical operative procedure (84).

ON-SITE EVALUATION

As one approaches an unconscious player on the field, an assessment should be made of the relationship between the head and neck to the rest of the body (Fig. 6.9). The player should be assumed to have a cervical spine injury until proven otherwise; approximately 15% of severe head injuries have associated cervical fractures (102).

If lying face down, carefully logroll to a supine position (Fig. 6.10). This move is best accomplished by the leader controlling the head while commanding the other members of the team to roll the individual over back in unison. The leader should use the crossed arm technique, which makes controlling the head much easier while performing this maneuver. From this position, slight traction should be applied to the head, which is maintained in a neutral position. The other members of the team should station themselves at the shoulders, hips, and knees. With one simultaneous movement, the player should be rolled toward them onto the spine board, keeping the head, neck, and spine in line. The leader should control the head at all times and instruct the others about their duties and plan of action. Everyone should remain calm; the goal is prevention of further injury.

At this time, a rapid assessment should be made to ensure that the player is breathing and that a pulse is present. Apnea may normally occur for up to 60 seconds after a head injury. If pulse or respirations are absent, any obstructing equipment, such as the face mask, is removed and CPR is begun. Hyperventilation can be accomplished, if necessary, by using manual resuscitation methods and supplemental oxygen. Normally, an athlete with a head injury hyperventilates spontaneously.

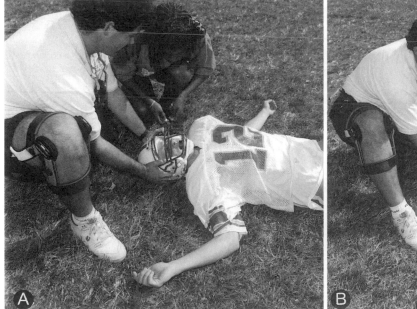
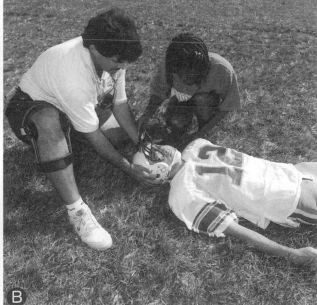

Figure 6.9. Initial assessment of athletes with head or cervical injury. The athlete should be approached from the head and urged to keep the head still if conscious. Consciousness and breathing should be assessed. The leader should immobilize the athlete's head with fingers spread as shown. Mouth guards should be removed, if present. If the athlete is unconscious, airway, character of breathing, and pulse should be checked. If pulse is absent, appropriate measures including cardiopulmonary resuscitation should be initiated. If the athlete is conscious, simple questions should be used to assess mental status. Appropriate responses indicate intact cerebral function.

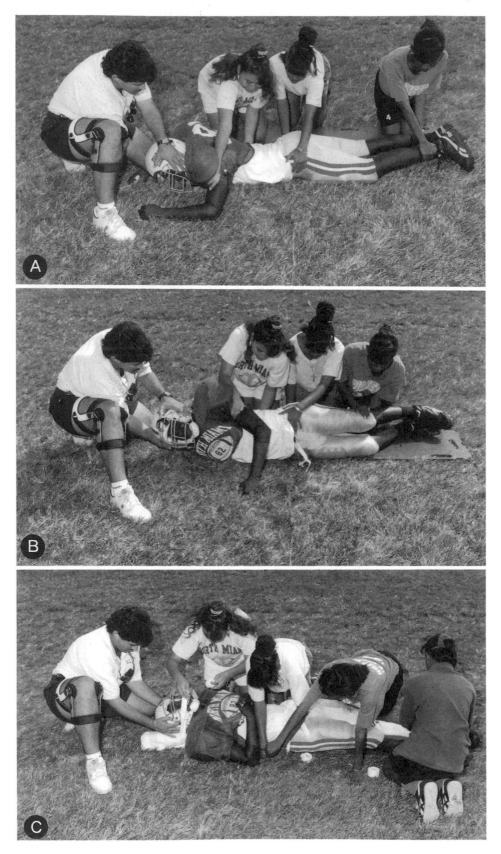

Figure 6.10. Control and transport of athletes with head or cervical injury. The team leader is responsible for immobilization of the head. Others should position themselves at the shoulders, hips, and knees of the athlete. Note the crossed-arm techniques of the leader. The athlete should be logrolled by a simultaneous movement of the assistants at the leader's command, keeping the spine in alignment.

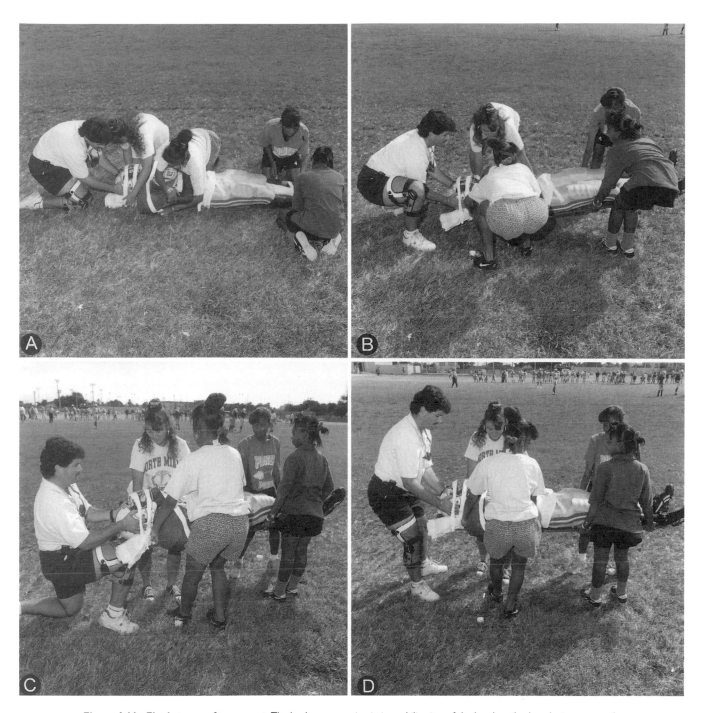

Figure 6.11. Final stages of transport. The leader must maintain immobilization of the head until other devices are available, such as sandbags or total immobilization devices. This restraint can be difficult if the injured person is confused, combative, or both. Four team members are required for transport. If the athlete also suffers from cardiac arrest or hemorrhaging, additional personnel are required.

If pulse and respirations are present, the spine board can be lifted by four members of the medical team, with the leader stationed at the head to keep it immobile and in slight traction (Fig. 6.11). An alternative method is to place large sandbags on either side of the head, but not if the player is restless or agitated. The final step is transporting the player off the field to the waiting ambulance.

A rapid evaluation of the individual should include mental status, facial appearance, ability to speak, weakness, pupillary response, and presence of abnormal posturing. A brief physical examination of all major systems should follow. Restlessness is often present after head injury, particularly in the young, but it may be secondary to a full bladder or a dressing that is too tight.

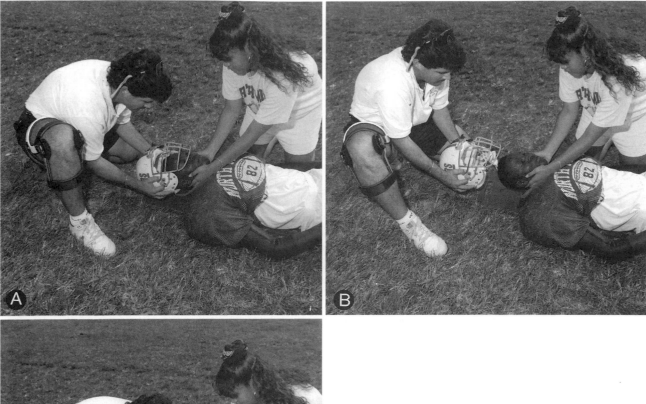

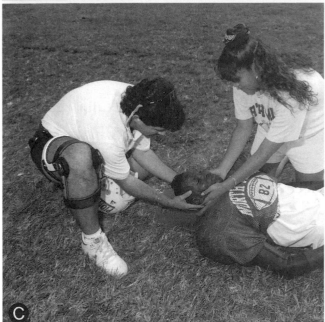

Figure 6.12. Helmet removal. Unless the patient's condition (e.g., respiratory or cardiac arrest or extreme hemorrhage from under the helmet) makes it mandatory, the helmet should be left in place until arrival at a medical facility. Should the helmet require removal, the head should be supported by a team member while the leader spreads the flaps and removes it, after first removing the chin strap.

Close monitoring of the respiratory rhythm and rate is imperative. Abnormal respiratory patterns may be indicative of the area of injury; e.g., a Cheyne-Stokes pattern of periodic hyperpnea followed by apnea suggests bilateral hemisphere damage, and apneustic breathing (prolonged inspiration) favors a pontine lesion. An ataxic or totally irregular pattern indicates a medullary lesion. Attention should also be given to changes in skin color, such as paleness or cyanosis, which may indicate hypovolemic shock or respiratory insufficiency. Check carefully for airway obstruction by food, secretions, or foreign objects. Airway maintenance is of prime impor-

tance in an unconscious individual. Cervical collars, helmets, or other protective gear should be left in place, unless the patient's condition requires removal, until the cervical spine is proven intact (Fig. 6.12). If the helmet must be removed, the face mask should come off first, followed by the helmet. The athlete's head and neck should be stabilized by one team member, while the other spreads the flaps and pulls it straight backward. On-site airway maintenance can be performed by several methods recommended by the American Heart Association (87). The most common and easiest to use are the jaw thrust and head tilt techniques. The jaw thrust maneuver is performed by grasping the angles of the lower jaw and lifting gently with one hand on either side; this action allows the mandible to swing forward as the head is tilted backward (Fig. 6.13). This position can be more easily maintained by placing one's elbows on the board on which the injured player is lying. This technique is the safest to use if a cervical spine injury is suspected.

If the above maneuver is unsuccessful, the head tilt, jaw lift maneuver can be instituted (Fig. 6.14). One hand tilts the head back, taking care not to overextend it whereas the other is placed under the mandible and lifted, which moves the chin upward and anteriorly. The fingers must not compress the soft tissue between the rami of the mandible because of possible airway obstruction.

DISPOSITION OF HEAD INJURIES

Before the athlete is allowed to return to play, certain criteria should be met.

A. Players suffering Grade I concussion, as described by Ommaya, can return to play if they are completely lucid and asymptomatic, and if they can move at their usual speed and dexterity and are neurologically negative. Serial examinations should be performed on the sidelines. If the symptoms (headache, nausea, dizziness) do not clear, referral to a physician is necessary (41, 102).

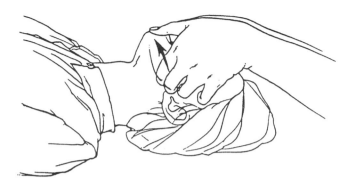

Figure 6.14. Head tilt-chin lift maneuver for opening of the airway. (Reproduced with permission. Instructor's manual for basic life support, 1990. Copyright American Heart Association.)

B. Those with Grade II concussions should be treated essentially the same as those with Grade I injuries. If retrograde amnesia exists or disorientation persists, however, return to play is not indicated. Before the athlete resumes play, all symptoms must have cleared and the results of the neurologic examination must be normal.

C. Those with Grade III concussions should not return to the game. If the period of disorientation lasts longer than 1 hour, or if symptoms such as headache, confusion, fatigue, nausea, ataxia, and vomiting persist, physician referral is indicated (85). Visual or auditory hallucinations are infrequently seen. If focal neurologic symptoms become manifest, the athlete requires immediate neurosurgical attention. Return to practice should not be allowed until the player is perfectly lucid and devoid of all symptoms and the results of a neurologic examination are normal (54, 85).

D. In Grade IV (classic concussion), the athlete is initially unresponsive and usually flaccid. This state usually passes in a few minutes, followed by a period of semistupor, improving to disorientation and diminishing confusion, and finally returning to lucidity. Later, motor skills and sensory function begin to improve, followed by a gradual return of memory, usually with some degree of post-trauma (PTA) or retrograde amnesia. Cognitive thinking is the last function to return and may be impaired for several months or more (73).

A true loss of consciousness is a contraindication to further participation (31, 54, 76, 103). The same guidelines as those for Grade III concussions should be followed. A loss of consciousness lasting longer than several minutes mandates

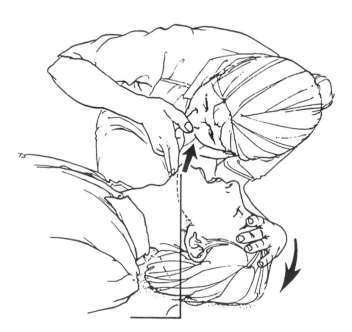

Figure 6.13. Jaw-thrust maneuver for opening of the airway. (Reproduced with permission. Instructor's manual for basic life support, 1990. Copyright American Heart Association.)

prompt transport to a hospital for observation (31, 85, 104). Anyone who has had more than one concussion during the season should undergo a complete neurologic examination by a specialist, including diagnostic studies because of the potential for progressive neurologic injury (69, 105, 106). An athlete who has a concussion with loss of consciousness is four times more likely to have a second one than the player who has not (106, 107). The receiving medical facility should be alerted before arrival of the victim, so that proper preparations can be made and the appropriate specialist contacted (108). The examiner should not be misled by what appears to be a relatively insignificant head injury, as severe brain damage can occur without evidence of significant external trauma. With the advent of CT and MRI scans, many athletes who have only "mild head injury" without neurologic deficit have been shown to have impressive intracranial hemorrhages or contusions, primarily in silent areas of the brain.

E. In Grade V, those in a coma with cardiorespiratory collapse require CPR and immediate transport. Jennett observes that the degree of trauma is not as important as the consequences of it (109). In mild head injury, no correlation exists between the length of unconsciousness and the severity of the symptoms. In severe head injury, however, a rough correlation exists. The athlete's neurologic status immediately after the injury does not reliably indicate the degree of pathology produced, the severity of the injury, or the prognosis.

NEUROLOGIC ASSESSMENT

After the player has been stabilized from a cardiorespiratory standpoint, a neurologic examination should be performed. A classic neurologic examination on the field is not practical; therefore, a quick assessment of the player's neurologic status can be obtained by using the Glasgow coma scale (Table 6.5). In the past a strong need existed for a standardized method of describing patients with head injuries. Teasdale and Jennett developed such a system—the Glasgow coma scale—which relies on eye opening and motor and verbal responses to "score" each victim on a scale from 1 to 15 (94). By reducing the patient's injury to a numeric figure, communication between medical personnel is facilitated, the severity of the injury established, and neurologic changes easily identified. It also has predictive value as to outcome.

Table 6.5. Glasgow Coma Scale

Eye Opening	
Score	
4	Opens eyes spontaneously without stimulation
3	Opens eyes to command
2	Opens eyes to pain (pinch or press on nailbeds)
1	No response
Best verbal response	
Score	
5	Oriented to time, place, and person; carries on conversation
4	Confused
3	Inappropriate words—verbalizes but makes no sense
2	Incomprehensible, garbled words; moaning
1	None—no sound of pain
Best motor response	
Score	
6	Obeys commands
5	Localizes noxious stimuli, tries to remove stimulus with hand
4	Withdrawal, does not localize pain but withdraws in flexion
3	Abnormal flexion, adducts shoulder, flexes and pronates arm, flexes wrist, and makes a fist in response to pain
2	Abnormal extension, adduction, internally rotates shoulder, extends forearm, flexes wrist, and makes a fist in response to pain
1	No motor response to command or pain
_____	Total score

Patients with a Glasgow coma scale less than 7 have a 40% mortality rate, with one half of the survivors remaining in a vegetative state (102). The Glasgow coma scale is not meant to replace the comprehensive neurologic examination; however, it has become an integral part of the diagnosis and treatment of head injuries.

The score of each category is totaled. A Glasgow coma scale score between 13 and 15 indicates a mild head injury; scores from 9 to 12 are considered moderate. If less than 7, the individual is considered to be in a coma; if less than 3, the individual is considered to be in a deep coma (42, 94, 110, 111).

The most important indicator of cerebral function is mental status, which always changes before more severe indicators of increased intracranial pressure are seen, such as pupillary inequality and hemiparesis. Alterations in vital signs, e.g., hypertension, bradycardia, and respiratory abnormalities, occur late and often signal an irreversible pathologic process (uncal herniation). The likelihood of survival is negligible, and in those who do survive, severe neurologic impairment is invariably present.

Neurologic Examination

A complete neurologic examination should follow at the earliest opportunity after removal of the athlete from the field. This exam consists of a mental status evaluation, which should include level of awareness, orientation, and speech. Cranial nerve examination should emphasize examination of the pupils, including size, equality, and briskness of reaction. A familiarity with the various pupillary aberrations is necessary for proper evaluation.

A Marcus-Gunn pupillary reaction may be the result of direct trauma to the eye, injuring the retina or optic nerve. The consensual pupillary response is stronger than the response to direct light in the damaged eye because of the afferent pupillary defect. One check is to shine a light first in the damaged eye and observe the response to light, then swing the light to the other eye and observe the reaction in the damaged eye. It should be more brisk than when the light shines directly into it.

Anisocoria, or unequal pupils, can also be an important diagnostic sign. A unilateral, dilated, and fixed pupil can indicate uncal herniation but may also be due to local injury to the eye or be present in certain metabolic states such as diabetes mellitus. Significant alterations in the mental status and probably other neurologic signs accompany the blown pupil, if mental state reflects uncal herniation. Anisocoria can also indicate injury to the cervical sympathetic ganglion in the neck. Sympathetic denervation to the ipsilateral eye produces the classic triad of miosis, ptosis, and anhidrosis, known as Horner's syndrome.

In pontine injuries, the pupils are miotic, frequently anisocoric, and poorly reactive to light. This sign would not be present without severe neurologic deficit and accompanying alterations in mentation. The ciliospinal reflex elicited by pinching the neck and causing pupillary dilation is likely to be absent if a brain-stem lesion is present.

Extraocular movements can be tested only in an individual who is able to cooperate. The player should follow an object (such as one's finger) with the eyes, first in a horizontal and then in a vertical direction. Impairment of extraocular movement can be due to direct trauma to the eye; injury to the third, fourth, or sixth cranial nerves; brain-stem injury; or damage to Brodmann's area 8 in the frontal lobes.

Injury to the pontine gaze center causes conjugate deviation of the eyes to the opposite side, whereas in frontal lobe injuries, the individual "looks to the side of the lesion."

Abducens (VI) nerve palsy can be an early sign of increased intracranial pressure. Its long length and small size make it susceptible to trauma. Dysfunction is seen as an inability to move the affected eye past the midline on a horizontal plane. An inability to direct the eye down and inward suggests trochlear (IV) nerve paresis, and inability to move the eye inward and upward indicates oculomotor (III) nerve dysfunction. The integrity of the trigeminal (V) nerve can be tested by checking sensation over the face with a pin, or by stimulating the cornea with a wisp of cotton. Injury to the facial (VII) nerve produces an ipsilateral flaccid paralysis of the face, characterized by drooping of the angle of the mouth and inability to close the eye. Those affected cannot purse their lips, smile, or whistle because of facial weakness. Drooling from the affected side is common. Peripheral seventh nerve injuries produce the above picture, whereas a central lesion, that is, one above the facial (VII) nerve nucleus in the pons, produces a lower facial paralysis but spares the periocular motor function, thus allowing the individual to blink because of bilateral supranuclear innervation.

The doll's head maneuver (oculocephalic) should not be performed until a concomitant cervical spine injury has been ruled out.

The gag reflex (glossopharyngeal nerve, IX) can be elicited by stimulating the uvula with a tongue blade. Hypoglossal (XII) nerve function is affirmed by asking the individual to stick out the tongue. Injury to the peripheral nerve makes the tongue deviate to the side of the injury, whereas injury to the brain stem above the hypoglossal nuclei results in the tongue protruding toward the side opposite the injury, due to decussation of the fibers in the lower brain stem.

Motor movement and strength testing are performed by testing each extremity independently and comparing it with the extremity on the opposite side. Asking the patient to elevate each extremity independently, squeeze the fingers, and push the foot against the hand gives an accurate assessment of motor function. For symmetry and strength, one side can be compared with the other. Table 6.6 presents grades commonly used to describe the degree of weakness. Reduction in a numeric score establishes a baseline for future

Table 6.6. Rating Motor Strength

Grade 5/5	Normal strength
Grade 4/5	Mild to moderate weakness
Grade 3/5	Can move the extremity against gravity, but it is weak
Grade 2/5	Minimal movement possible but unable to move against gravity
Grade 1/5	Twitching of the muscles but no perceptible movement of the extremity
Grade 0/5	No movement

comparison and facilitates communication with other medical personnel.

Sensory examination can be performed by running a safety pin or pinwheel over the body and comparing one side to the other. Then run it vertically to look for a sensory level. A hemihypesthesia would suggest injury to the contralateral postcentral gyrus, if on the basis of head injury. One side of the body can be compared with the other for symmetry. Position sensation can be determined by moving the great toe up or down and asking the individual to give its location with eyes closed.

The deep tendon reflexes should be normoreflexic and symmetrical. The presence of pathologic reflexes, such as sustained clonus or a positive Babinski sign, is an important indicator of upper motor neuron dysfunction. The latter can be elicited by stroking a blunt object upward along the lateral aspect of the sole of the foot and then across the ball in a medial direction. A positive response would be extension of the great toe and fanning of the remaining ones. Pressing forcefully against the sole of the foot to sustain it in dorsiflexion may elicit clonus, which is a repetitive beating of the foot in a rhythmic manner until the pressure is released. Clonus must be sustained to be considered indicative of upper motor neuron injury.

Cerebellar function can be assessed easily by using the Rhomberg maneuver, finger-to-nose test, tandem walking, or heel-to-shin maneuver. For the Rhomberg maneuver, the individual stands erect, places both feet together, and closes the eyes. If the patient tends to fall consistently to one side, the test result is considered positive and usually indicates a cerebellar lesion on the side toward which the patient falls. This maneuver checks the integrity of the vermis or midline portion of the cerebellum. Incoordination of the extremities indicates injury to the cerebellar hemispheres. Impaired coordination may well predispose the athlete to further injury and should be a contraindication to further participation.

Serial examinations may be more important than the initial one, especially in diagnosing focal lesions such as hematomas and secondary complications, which may arise from the prime injury.

Conclusion

Theoretically, no athlete who regains consciousness after a head injury should die or suffer major disability. With accurate diagnosis and swift, effective management of athletes with head injuries, the morbidity and mortality can be lowered.

Mild head injuries without loss of consciousness and no focal neurologic signs may be observed on the sidelines with repeated examinations. Athletes should not be allowed to participate in further play unless they become perfectly lucid and have no further symptoms or neurologic deficit.

Patients with moderate head injuries plus a short loss of consciousness and some degree of amnesia, if improved, after several shortly spaced neurologic examinations, should be transported to the hospital for further neurologic testing. They should not be allowed to return to play that day and must be completely free of symptoms before they are allowed to practice (31, 55, 85).

Patients with severe head injuries and prolonged loss of consciousness or focal neurologic deficit should undergo immediate transport to a facility with neurosurgical coverage.

SEQUELAE OF HEAD INJURIES

Postconcussion Syndrome

After recovery from a head injury, the individual may regain motor function and coordination fully but continue to have severe headaches, fatigue, recent memory loss, problems with cognitive thinking, periods of confusion and disorientation, personality changes, irritability, or dizziness (42, 47, 111–114). This mélange of symptoms is commonly known as postconcussive syndrome. Its incidence yearly is approximately 20% in football players and 6% in boxers. The symptoms may persist from a few days after the injury to many months or more (8, 68, 73, 115, 116). Hugenholtz and Stuss found gradual improvement occurred over 3 months, suggesting a recovery process (100). Repeated episodes of trauma are likely to increase the risk of further injury, even if the initial trauma produces neurologic damage so minor as to be unobservable clinically (67). Gronwall et al. reported that recovery of cognitive function is slower after a second injury than it was after the first, as demonstrated by slowness in processing information (68, 73). Repeated episodes of trauma have shown an accumulative impairment (67). Return to sports activity should not be permitted until all symptoms have resolved. Postconcussive syndrome is more frequent in mild head injuries than in severe ones and appears to combine organic and functional disorders (117).

Impaired attention and information processing are more affected, whereas intellectual function and reaction times are less affected with this syndrome (73, 115, 116, 118–120). Stretching and tearing of brain substance producing diffuse neuronal injury are known to occur during commotio cerebri. Even a mild concussion may be followed by incapacitating symptoms lasting more than 1 month after the injury (42, 67, 121). A study of high school football players at Allegheny Hospital in Pittsburgh, Pennsylvania, revealed that 25% of them continued to have abnormal psychiatric tests 6 months after having three separate incidents of minor head trauma (41). Furthermore, of those with five head injuries, 40% were affected 6 months after injury. The preponderance of evidence, therefore, supports Sir Charles Symonds' statement, "It is questionable whether the effects of concussion, however slight, are ever completely reversible" (76).

Post-traumatic Encephalopathy

A single massive head injury or repeated episodes of minor trauma have proved detrimental to cerebral function and intellect and may accumulate to produce the syndrome of post-traumatic encephalopathy (13, 51, 52, 67, 122, 123). This condition is characterized by the punch-drunk fighter, as described by Martland (63). The number of bouts in which a boxer competes correlates with the severity of the symptoms that he later experiences, which include diminished motor performance, spasticity, rig-idity, ataxia, tremor, impaired cognitive func-tion, Parkinson-like symptoms, and personality changes (3, 11, 13, 14, 32, 124, 125). This syndrome has been reported in 17% to 55% of professional boxers (52, 124, 126). The medical personnel supervising athletes must recognize the symptoms of brain injury, even if subtle, and protect the individual from further insult, even if it calls for recommending retirement from the sport. Elimination or restriction of sports activities, particularly in young athletes, should be discussed in detail, not only with the individual but also with his parents and the involved coaching staff. Coaches, trainers, and parents should be made aware of the possible consequences of repeated minor head injury. They must be particularly concerned about sports such as football, rugby, horse riding, and boxing, in which repetitive injury is common (29, 47, 52, 127). Structural brain damage and severe functional impairment have been described in boxers so often that numerous authors are calling for the sport to be banned (52, 53, 77, 78, 123, 128).

Post-traumatic Seizures

Seizures are rare complications of closed head injury, particularly in sports. Frequently, it is directly related to the severity of the injury. The incidence is approximately 5% in severe closed head injuries, increasing to nearly 40% in those with dural penetration (129, 130). In mild head injuries, such as those commonly seen in sports, the incidence is only 0.4%. Onset is usually within 24 hours of the injury but can occur for up to 2 years afterward (129).

If a player has a seizure, no attempt should be made to restrain him. A padded tongue blade should be readily available in the emergency gear, and inserted between the teeth to prevent laceration of the tongue. Fingers should never be used for this purpose because severe laceration is likely. Immediate evacuation to an emergency facility is necessary. The airway must be scrupulously maintained during transport. A single grand mal seizure should be a sufficient criterion to preclude the individual from further contact sports. Oxygen, if available, can be administered by nasal cannula or mask, if the seizure is prolonged.

Vomiting

Vomiting can be extremely dangerous in a comatose individual because of the dangers of airway obstruction and aspiration pneumonia. It occurs in approximately 20% of head injuries, being more common in milder cases (83). If unconscious, the victim should be logrolled to the side, so that the mouth is dependent. Before returning the victim to an upright position, one should check for food particles lodged in the throat. All personnel should be proficient in performing the Heimlich maneuver. Vomiting may also be a sign of increased intracranial pressure, mandating serial neurologic examinations. If a cervical spine injury is suspected, care must be taken to keep the spine in alignment with the head at all times.

Cranial Nerve Palsies

Anosmia occurs in 3 to 10% of head injuries (103). Once lost, the sense of smell returns in only one half of the patients (103). Its loss is often unrecognized because of a failure to test for it. Partial or complete blindness can also occur as a rare complication of head trauma (1–2%), usually from bruising the optic nerve as it enters the orbit through the optic foramen or from orbital fracture (103). Approximately half recover some degree of vision. Basilar skull fractures may involve the fourth or sixth cranial nerves, resulting in extraocular nerve palsies. Abducens nerve injury is present in 2 to 10% of all head injuries, resulting in horizontal diplopia (17). Trochlear nerve paresis causes vertical diplopia, with the injured player frequently tilting the head to correct it.

Shock

Essentially, two types of shock—hypovolemic and neurogenic—are associated with head trauma. Hypovolemic shock is produced by a rapid decrease in circulating blood volume and is almost never seen in isolated head injury unless extensive scalp lacerations have occurred. Associated long bone or viscus injuries should be sought if it is present. Hypovolemic shock is characterized by a rapid thready pulse and hypotension, with the victim appearing pale, apprehensive, and cool to the touch. Neurogenic shock is produced by activation of the vasomotor center of the brain stem with peripheral vasoconstriction. The patient appears to be in shock, but blood pressure and pulse are normal. These features help differentiate between these two types of shock.

Vascular Lesions

Carotid cavernous sinus fistula is a rare complication that usually occurs from injury to the face or front of the skull. It is the result of laceration of the carotid artery within the cavernous sinus from a penetrating object, most commonly bone. Traumatic aneurysms resulting from injury to the arterial wall are even more rare and are the result of indriven bone or missiles.

Hydrocephalus

Post-traumatic hydrocephalus is usually the result of disruption of the normal subarachnoid pathways for absorption of cerebrospinal fluid. The mechanism is thought to be fibrin deposits from free blood within the cerebrospinal fluid occluding the pacchionian granulations. Headache, lethargy, and other symptoms of increased intracranial pressure occurring weeks after head injury should alert the physician to this possibility.

Miscellaneous

Other rare conditions include diabetes insipidus and respiratory distress syndrome. Neurologic sequelae can also occur as a result of fat embolism from long-bone fractures. The sudden onset of confusion, disorientation, high fever, and possible focal neurologic deficit in an alert individual after an injury should point to this diagnosis.

DIFFERENTIAL DIAGNOSIS

The conditions listed in Table 6.7 produce sudden alterations in the level of consciousness and, in certain instances, mimic the symptoms and signs of head injury.

PREVENTION

Although the number of participants engaged in sports has increased, the number of injuries has decreased, primarily because of new equipment, rule changes, better coaching, supervision, and education. A number of factors should receive consideration, and the major factors are listed in Table 6.8.

A comprehensive preseason examination provides a baseline for future comparisons and screening of future participants. A detailed history, including in-depth inquiry into the presence of earlier injuries, other medical conditions, and offseason participation in other sports should be obtained. The examination should include a general physical examination, including the individual's vital signs, height, and weight; detailed neu-

Table 6.7.   Differential Diagnosis of Head Trauma

I. Structural lesions
  A. Tumors
    1. Intraparenchymal hemorrhage within the mass, producing a rapid increase in size
    2. Obstruction of cerebrospinal fluid pathways, producing acute hydrocephalus
II. Cerebrovascular accidents
  A. Ruptured aneurysms or arteriovenous malformations
  B. Thrombosis or infarction
    1. Intracranial
    2. Extracranial
  C. Spontaneous intracranial hemorrhage
    1. Telangiectasia
    2. Hypertension
III. Cardiac abnormalities
  A. Arrhythmias
  B. Mural thrombi with embolization to the brain
  C. Myocardial pathology
  D. Myocardial infarction
IV. Metabolic
  A. Drugs
  B. Diabetes mellitus (diabetic coma)
  C. Hypoglycemic shock
V. Syncope (vasovagal)
VI. Associated injuries
  A. Visceral rupture (hypovolemic shock)
  B. Long bone fractures (fat embolism)
VII. Infections, acute
  A. Viral
  B. Bacterial

Table 6.8. Factors That May Decrease Injury

Preseason screening examinations	Proper conditioning and training
Education of participants	Education and supervision
Interval physical examinations	Rule changes
Properly designed equipment	Good sportsmanship

rologic examination; and any laboratory studies that are indicated. Special attention should be paid to examination of the visual, auditory, cardiovascular, and musculoskeletal systems. Careful evaluation of the individual's gait, balance, and coordination is also important.

Interval physical examinations during the season should be performed routinely to detect any abnormal variation from the initial examination. Examination is also mandatory after a head injury, no matter how minor, because of the accumulative effects of repeated trauma. Neuropsychologic testing should be considered if postconcussive symptoms persist. Education of coaches, trainers, athletes, and officials concerning the hazards of improper and dangerous techniques should be continuous.

Dangerous maneuvers, such as high-sticking, (6, 86, 131), head-butting, and spearing should be condemned. Rule changes outlawing the use of the helmeted head as the initial point of contact significantly reduced the number of head injuries (132). The mandatory use of helmets has decreased the incidence of head injury in a number of sports (15, 26, 38, 45, 133). Failure to use or poorly fitting head gear is associated with a high incidence of skull fracture, intracranial hematomas, and head injuries (26, 130, 132, 134). In sports for which sufficient data exist, i.e., football, gymnastics, and wrestling, the principal factors resulting in injury are improper technique and conditioning (132). Alley reported violation of fundamental skills in blocking or tackling in 34% of injuries to high school football players in his series (1). Good sportsmanship should be encouraged at all times. A thorough explanation of the sport, along with the possibility of injury, should be rendered to players and their parents before the athlete begins play.

In adolescence, two episodes of minor concussion or a single one producing a loss of consciousness longer than 5 minutes suggests that the individual should stop playing the sport. Supervision by the coaching staff and trainers should be required at all times. The staff must be proficient not only in teaching physical education, but also in giving first aid and CPR. A concern for the safety of the athlete must assume top priority.

Properly designed, well-fitting equipment with safety devices is essential, as are proper conditioning and training under skilled supervision. The most important factor in preventing injury is evaluation of the potential athlete before allowing participation in a particular sport (130, 135). Some individuals are not physically capable of competing in certain sports. The responsibility of the team physician is to guide them toward activities that they are capable of performing. Periodic discussions with team personnel concerning injury prevention could be rewarding. The use of anabolic steroids or other drugs, including alcohol, should receive blanket condemnation. Biochemical assays have been performed on athletes with head injuries who were involved in football, rugby, and boxing; these assays have demonstrated an elevated creatine kinose-BB (BB designates the isozyme). These elevated levels may reflect early injury to the central nervous system and may help to prevent chronic encephalopathy (12, 136).

In conclusion, the team physician should provide the safest medical environment possible for those engaged in sports activities. By doing so, the goals of decreasing injury, providing an accurate diagnosis, giving appropriate treatment, and providing maximum safety for the participants can be met.

References

1. Alley RH. Head and neck injuries in high school football. JAMA 1964;188:418–422.
2. Allman FL Jr. Problems in treatment of athletic injuries. JAMA 1964;53:381–383.
3. Henry NH. A study of football injuries in fifty North Carolina high schools in 1948 (thesis). Eugene: University of Oregon, 1949.
4. Krause MA. The nature and frequency of injuries occurring in Oregon high school football (thesis). Eugene: University of Oregon, 1959.
5. Minnesota State High School League. Major injuries and fatalities: 1971–1980. Anoka, MN: Minnesota State High School League, 1980.
6. Torg JS, Truex R Jr, Quedenfeld TC, et al. The national football head and neck injury registry: reports and conclusion. JAMA 1979;241:1477–1479.
7. Murphy RJ, Tarner H, Spence O, et al. Five-year football injury survey. Phys Sports Med 1978;6:94–102.
8. Reid SE, Ried SE Jr. Football, neck muscles and head impact. Surg Gynecol Obstet 1978;147:513–517.
9. Schneider RC, Antine BE. Visual-field impairment related to football head gear and face guards. JAMA 1965;192:616–618.
10. Schneider RC. Head and neck injuries in football. Baltimore: Williams & Wilkins, 1973.
11. Walker AE, Caveness WF, Critchley M, eds. The late effects of head injury. Springfield, IL: Charles C. Thomas, 1969:408.
12. Brayne CEG, Calloway SP, Dow L, et al. Blood creatinine kinase isoenzyme BB in boxers. Lancet 1982;2:1308–1309.
13. Casson IR, Sham R, Campbell EA, et al. Neurologic and CT evaluation of knocked-out boxers. J Neurol Neurosurg Psychiatry 1982;45:170–174.

14. Cohen L. Should the sport of boxing be banned? Can Med Assoc J 1984;130:767–768.
15. Fekete JF. Severe brain injury and death following rigid body accidents: the effectiveness of the safety helmet of amateur hockey players. Can Med Assoc J 1968; 99:1234–1239.
16. Hillman H. Boxing. Resuscitation 1980;8:211–215.
17. Hughes B. Acute injuries of the head. 4th ed. Baltimore: Williams & Wilkins, 1964.
18. Lampert PW, Hardman JM. Morphological changes in brains of boxers. JAMA 1984;251:2676–2679.
19. Kersey RD, Rowan L. Injury accounting during the 1980 NCAA wrestling championships. Am J Sports Med 1983; 11:147–151.
20. Strauss RH, Lanese RR. Injuries among wrestlers in school and college tournaments. JAMA 1982;248:2016–2019.
21. McLatchie GR, Davies JE, Caulley JH. Injuries in karate, a case for medical control. J Trauma 1980;2: 956–958.
22. Goldberg MJ. Gymnastics injury. Orthop Clin North Am 1980;11:717–726.
23. Ballhom A, Absoud EM, Kotecha MB, et al. A study of bicycle accidents. Injury 1985;16:405–408.
24. Fife D, Davis J, Tate L, et al. Fatal injuries to bicyclists: the experience of Dade County, Florida. J Trauma 1983;23:745–755.
25. Lehman LB. Neurological trauma resulting from cycling accidents. Emerg Med 1987;19:2–16.
26. Lehman LB. The sorrows of cycling. Emerg Med 1987; 19:2–3, 16.
27. Barber HM. Horse play: survey of accidents with horses. Br Med J 1973;3:532–534.
28. Barclay WR. Equestrian sports. JAMA 1978;240: 1892–1893.
29. Foster JB, Leiguarda R, Tiley PJB. Brain damage in national hunt jockeys. Lancet 1976;1:981–983.
30. Davis JC. Medical examination of sport scuba divers. In: Strauss RH, ed. Sports medicine. Philadelphia: WB Saunders, 1984:513–523.
31. Dempsey RJ, Schneider RC. The management of head injuries in sports. In: Schneider RC, Kennedy JC, Plant ML, et al., eds. Sports injuries: mechanisms, prevention, and treatment. Baltimore: Williams & Wilkins, 1984: 652–675.
32. Lanphier EH. Diving medicine. N Engl J Med 1957;256: 120–131.
33. Robey JM, Blyth CS, Mueller FD. Athletic injuries: application of epidemiologic methods. JAMA 1971;217: 184–189.
34. Krel FW. Parachuting for sport: study of 100 deaths. JAMA 1965;194:264–268.
35. Dowling PA. Prospective study of injuries in United States Ski Association freestyle skiing 1976-1977 to 1979-1980. Am J Sports Med 1982;10:268–275.
36. Ellison AE. Skiing injuries. JAMA 1973;223:917–919.
37. Ferkel RD, Mai LL, Ullis KC, et al. An analysis of roller skating injuries. Am J Sports Med 1981;10:24–30.
38. Goldsmith W, Kabo JM. Performance of baseball head gear. Am J Sports Med 1982;10:31–37.
39. Zeliska JA, Noble HB, Porter MA. A comparison of nerves and movements: professional basketball injuries. Am J Sports Med 1982;101:297–299.
40. Lehman LB. Nervous system sports-related injuries. Am J Sports Med 1987;15:494–499.
41. Gerberich SG, Priest JO. Concussion incidence and severity in secondary school varsity football players. Am J Public Health 1983;73:1370–1375.
42. Rimel RW, Giordani B, Barth JT, et al. Disability caused by minor head injury. Neurosurgery 1981;9:221–228.
43. Clarke AJ, Sibert JR. Why child cyclists should wear helmets. Practitioner (London) 1986;230:513–514.
44. Jennett B, Teasdale G. Management of head injuries. Philadelphia: FA Davis, 1981.
45. Clark DM. Neglect blamed for injuries in sports program. JAMA 1964;190:36.
46. Gennarelli TA. Head injury mechanisms. In: Torg JS, ed. Athletic injuries to the head, neck, and face. Philadelphia: Lea & Febiger, 1982.
47. Lidvall HF, Linderoth B, Norlin B. Causes of the post-concussional syndrome. Acta Neurol Scand 1974; (suppl 156):144.
48. Moretz A, Raskin A, Grana W. Oklahoma high school football injury study: a preliminary report. Oklahoma State Med Assoc J 1978;71:85–88.
49. National Athletic Injury/Illness Reporting System. NAIRS sport-related incidence charts. University Park: Pennsylvania State University, 1976–1979.
50. Moore M. The challenge of boxing: bringing safety into the ring. Phys Sports Med 1980;8:101–105.
51. Corsellis JAN, Brutan CJ, Freeman-Browne D. The aftermath of boxing. Psychol Med 1973;3:270–303.
52. Jedlinski J, Gatarski J, Szymusik A. Encephalopathia pugilistica (punch drunkenness). Acta Med Pol 1971; 12:443.
53. Neuberger KT, Sintar DW, Denst J. Cerebral atrophy associated with boxing. Arch Neurol Psychiatry 1959;81: 403–408.
54. Ommaya AK, Gennarelli TA. A physiopathologic basis for noninvasive diagnosis and prognosis of head injury severity. In: McLaurin RL, ed. Head injuries: proceedings of the second Chicago symposium on neurologic trauma. New York: Grune & Stratton, 1975:229–237.
55. Bruno LA, Gennarelli TA. Management guidelines for head injuries in athletes. Clin Sports Med 1987;6:17–29.
56. Ommaya AK, Hirsch AE. Tolerance of cerebral concussion from head impact and whiplash in primates. J Biomech 1971;4:13–22.
57. Holbourn AHS. Mechanics of head injury. Lancet 1943; 2:438.
58. Bruno LA. Focal intracranial hematomas. Head Injuries 105–121.
59. Ommaya AK, Gennarelli TA. Cerebral concussion and traumatic unconsciousness. Brain 1974;97:633–654.
60. Ommaya AK, Hirsch AE, Flamin ES, et al. Cerebral concussion in the monkey: an experimental model. Science 1966;153:211–212.
61. Bakay L, Glasover FE. Head injury. Boston: Little, Brown, & Co., 1980.
62. Reid SE, Tarkington JA, Epstein HM, et al. Brain tolerance to impact in football. Surg Gynecol Obstet 1971;133:929–936.
63. Martland HS. Punch drunk. JAMA 1928;91:1103–1107.
64. Thomas LM. Skull fractures. In: Wilkens RH, Rengachary SS, eds. Neurological surgery. New York: McGraw-Hill, 1985:1623–1626.
65. Bakay L, Lee JC, Lee GC, et al. Experimental cerebral concussion: part I. an electron microscope study. J Neurosurg 1977;47:525–531.
66. Gennarelli TA. Cerebral concussion and diffuse brain injuries. In: Cooper PR, ed. Head injuries. Baltimore: Williams & Wilkins, 1982.
67. Gronwall D, Wrightson P. Cumulative effect of concussion. Lancet 1975;2:995–997.
68. Gronwall D, Sampson H. The psychological effects of concussion. Auckland: Auckland University Press, 1974.
69. Bruce DA, Gennarelli TA. Resuscitation from coma to head injury. Crit Care Med 1978;6:254–268.
70. Yarnell PR, Lynch S. Retrograde memory immediately after concussion. Lancet 1970;1:836.
71. Oppenheimer DR. Microscopic lesions in the brain following head injury. J Neurol Neurosurg Psychiatry 1968; 31:299–306.
72. Gennarelli TA, Thibault LE, Adams JH, et al. Diffuse anodal injury and traumatic coma in the primate. Ann Neurol 1982;12:564–574.
73. Gronwall D, Wrightson P. Delayed recovery of intellectual function after minor head injury. Lancet 1974; 2:605–609.

74. Jennett B. Early complications after mild head injuries. NZ Med J 1976;144–147.

75. MacFlynn G, Montgomery EA, Fenton GW, et al. Measurement of reaction time following minor head injury. J Neurol Neurosurg Psychiatry 1984;47:1326–1331.

76. Strich SJ. Diffuse degeneration of the cerebral white matter in several dementia. J Neurol Neurosurg Psychiatry 1956;19:163–185.

77. Lehman LB. Pros and cons of boxing. The New York Times 1985;62.

78. Lundberg GC. Boxing should be banned in civilized countries. JAMA 1983;62:249–250.

79. Thomas LM, Gurdjian ES. Intracranial hematomas of traumatic origin. In: Youmans JR, ed. Neurological surgery. Philadelphia: WB Saunders, 1973:960–967.

80. Friedman WA. Head injuries. Clin Symposia Ciba 1983; 35(4):2–32.

81. Galbraith S. Age distribution of extradural hemorrhage without skull fracture. Lancet 1973;1:1217.

82. Jamieson KG, Yelland JDN. Extradural hematoma: report of 167 cases. J Neurosurg 1968;29:13.

83. Gurdjian ES, Webster JE. Head injuries. Boston: Little, Brown, & Co., 1958:169.

84. Becker DP, Grossman RG, McLaurin RL, et al. Head injuries: panel 3. Arch Neurol 1979;36:750–758.

85. Wilton P, Fulco J, O'Leary J, et al. Body slam is no sham. N Engl J Med 1985;313:188–189.

86. Lehman LB. Preventing nervous system sports injuries. Nurse Practitioner 1989;14(3):42–46.

87. American Heart Association. Standards and guidelines for cardiopulmonary resuscitation (CPR) and emergency cardiac care. JAMA 1988;244:453.

88. McIntyre KM, Lewis AJ, eds. Textbook of advanced cardiac life support. Dallas: American Heart Association, 1981.

89. Stang JM. Cardiopulmonary resuscitation. In: Schneider RC, Kennedy JC, Plant ML, et al., eds. Sports injuries: mechanisms, prevention, and treatment AEMD-NMAF. Baltimore: Williams & Wilkins, 1985:797–808.

90. Ommaya AK, Faas F, Yarnell P. Whiplash injury and brain damage. JAMA 1968;204:285–289.

91. Committee on Head Injury Nomenclature of the Congress of Neurological Surgeons. Glossary of head injury including some definitions of injury to the cervical spine. Clin Neurosurg 1966;12:386–394.

92. Russell WR. The traumatic amnesias. New York: Oxford Press, 1971.

93. Schacter DL, Crowitz HF. Memory function after closed head injury: a review of the quantitative research. Cortex 1977;13:150–176.

94. Teasdale G, Jennett B. Assessment of coma and impaired consciousness: a practical scale. Lancet 1974; 2:81–84.

95. Jennett B. Severity of brain damage, altered consciousness and other indicators. In: Odom GL, ed. Central nervous system trauma research status report. Bethesda: NIH Public Health Service, 1979:204–219.

96. Meggyesy D. Out of their league. Berkeley: Ramparts Press, 1970:125.

97. Adams JH. The neuropathology of head injuries. In: Vinken PJ, Bruyn GW, eds. The handbook of clinical neurology. Injuries of the brain and skull, part I. Amsterdam: North-Holland Publishing, 1975:23:35–65.

98. Adams JH, Graham DI. The pathology of blunt head injuries. In: Critchley M, O'Leary J, Jennett B, eds. The scientific foundations of neurology. London: William Heinemann Medical Books, 1972:478–491.

99. Dila C, Bouchard L, Meyer E, et al. Microvascular response to minimal brain trauma. In: McLaurin RL, ed. Head injuries. New York: Grune & Stratton, 1976: 213–215.

100. Hugenholtz H, Stuss DT. How long does it take to recover from mild concussion? Neurosurgery 1988;22: 853–858.

101. Lehman LB. Scuba and other sports diving: nervous system complications. Postgrad Med 1986;80:68–70.

102. Dacey RG Jr, Jane J. Craniocerebral trauma. Clin Neurol 1984;30:1–61.

103. Symonds C. Concussion and its sequelae. Lancet 1962; 2:81–84.

104. Baker EP Jr. Diagnosis and treatment of head injuries. In: Cave EF, Burke JF, Boyd RJ, eds. Trauma management. Chicago: Yearbook Medical Publishers, 1974.

105. Gerberich SG, Priest JD, Grafft J, et al. Injuries to the brain and spinal cord: assessment, emergency care, and prevention. Minnesota Med 1982;65:691–696.

106. Gerberich SG. Analysis of high school football injuries and concomitant health care provision (thesis). Minneapolis: University of Minnesota, 1980.

107. Gerberich SG. Evaluation of injury/illness incidence and health care provision for football participants in the secondary schools of Minnesota (thesis). Minneapolis: University of Minnesota, 1977.

108. Schneider RC, Kriss FC. Head and neck injuries in football: mechanisms, treatment and preventions. Baltimore: Williams & Wilkins, 1972.

109. Jennett B. Assessment of the severity of head injury. J Neurol Neurosurg Psychiatry 1976;39:647–655.

110. Bowers SA, Marshall LF. Outcome in 200 consecutive cases of several head injuries treated in San Diego County: a prospective analysis. Neurosurgery 1980;6: 237–242.

111. Rimel RW. Moderate head injury: completing the clinical spectrum of brain trauma. Neurosurgery 1982;11:344–351.

112. Cartlidge NEF, Shaw DA. Head injury. London: WB Saunders, 1981.

113. Caveness WF. Post traumatic sequelae. In: Walker AE, Caveness WF, Critchley M, eds. The late effects of head injury. Springfield: Charles C. Thomas, 1969:209–219.

114. McKinlay WW, Brooks DV, Bond MR. Post-concussional symptoms, financial compensation and outcome of severe blunt head injury. J Neurol Neurosurg Psychiatry 1983;46:1084–1091.

115. Alexander MP. Traumatic brain injury. In: Benson DF, Blumer D, eds. Psychiatric aspects of neurologic disease. New York: Grune & Stratton, 1982;2:219–249.

116. McLaurin RL, Titchener JL. Post-traumatic syndrome. In: Youmans JR, ed. Neurological surgery. 2nd ed. Philadelphia: WB Saunders, 1982;4:2175–2187.

117. Alves WM. Mild brain damage and outcome. In: Becker DD, ed. Purlichock

118. Benton A. Behavioral consequences of closed head injury. In: Odom GL, ed. Central nervous system trauma research status report. Bethesda: NIH Public Health Service, 1979:220–231.

119. Binder LM. Persisting symptoms after mild head injury: a review of the postconcussive syndrome. J Clin Exp Neuropsychol 1986;8:323–346.

120. Reitan RN. Psychological testing after craniocerebral injury. In: Youmans JR, ed. Neurological surgery. 2nd ed. Philadelphia: WB Saunders, 1982;4:2195–2204.

121. Merskey H, Woodforde JM. Psychiatric sequelae of minor head injury. Brain 1972;95:521–528.

122. Casson I, Siegal O, Sham R, et al. Brain damage in modern boxers. JAMA 1984;251:2663–2667.

123. Maudsley C, Ferguson FR. Neurological disease in boxers. Lancet 1983;2:795–801.

124. Roberts AH. Brain damage in boxers. London: Pitman, 1969.

125. Schneider RC. Serious and fatal neurosurgical football injuries. Clin Neurosurg 1965;12:226.

126. Lacava G. Boxers encephalopathy. J Sports Med Phys Fitness 1963;3:87–92.

127. Yarnell PR, Lynch S. The ding amnestic states in football trauma. Neurology 1973;23:186.

128. Vegso JJ, Lehman RC. Field evaluation and management of head and neck injuries. Clin Sports Med 1987;6:1–6.

129. Jennett B. Epilepsy after non-musculoskeletal head injuries. ed. 2. London: William Heinemann Medical Books, 1975.
130. Miller JD, Jennett WB. Complications of depressed skull fracture. Lancet 1968;2:991.
131. Lehman LB. Reducing neurologic trauma in sports. NY SJ Med 1988;88:15–17.
132. Clarke KS. An epidemiological view. In: Torg JS, ed. Athletic injuries to the head, neck and face. Philadelphia: Lea & Febiger, 1982:15–25.
133. Krantz KP. Head and neck injuries to motorcycle and moped riders with special regard to the effect of protective helmets. Injury 1985;16:253–258.
134. Lehman LB. Skull fractures: dispelling some misconceptions affecting management. Postgrad Med 1988;83:53–63.
135. Lehman LB. The preseason athletic screening examination. Med Times 1988;116:29–31.
136. Brayne CEG, Dow L, Calloway SP. Creatine kinase-BB isoenzyme in rugby football players. J Neurol Neurosurg Psychiatry 1984;47:568–569.

7

Cervical Spine

Rick S. Saluga

There are now more individuals participating in athletic activities than ever before in history. It has been estimated that approximately 100 million men and women of all ages are engaged in some type of sport (1). Subsequently, there are more opportunities for injuries to occur. Contact and team sports are played more regularly through the early teens and twenties and are the most responsible for cervical injury. It is these contact sports, such as American football, hockey, wrestling, and soccer, that lend themselves to the injury of the cervical spine. It must be remembered, however, that any activity or sport that places the cervical spine in a compromising position and overloads the spinal structures can result in injury.

FUNCTIONAL ANATOMY

To comprehend all the various mechanisms of injury in the neck, one must first thoroughly understand the functional anatomy of the normal upper and lower cervical spine. The occipito-atlanto-axial complex is the most cephalad region of the cervical spine that begins articulation with an egg-resting-in-a-saucer description. The C1 vertebra articulates around the odontoid of C2 (a trochlear joint) and is responsible for approximately 50% of the rotation of the entire cervical spine. These bony and cartilaginous articulations are held together by the active (muscular) and passive (ligamentous) tissues. All the ligamentous structures in the upper cervical spine—including the alar ligaments and tectorial membrane, which anchor the odontoid process directly to the base of the skull—are probably the strongest and most important of the cervical spine (2).

The function of the alar ligaments is to help prevent excessive rotation and lateral flexion of C1 on C2. Rotation takes place through approximately 45° in each direction around the eccentrically placed odontoid process (3). In times of significant trauma, the spaces formed by these tissues, which are seen on plain film radiography,

help demonstrate the injury. In the case of an alar ligament tear, there can be asymmetry of the paraodontal space on an anterior-posterior (AP) open mouth radiograph. The alar ligaments limit axial rotation of the atlantoaxial complex (to the right by left alar ligament and vice versa) and lateral flexion. The right alar ligament should prevent right slippage of the atlas and occiput during right lateral flexion and vice versa (Fig. 7.1). The alar ligament is maximally stretched and subsequently most vulnerable to injury when the head is rotated and flexed (4). This is a common mechanism of athletic injury.

The transverse ligament (atlantodental ligament) is also capable of being injured in athletic competition. This ligament arises from the anteromedial aspect of the C1 vertebra and runs posterior to the odontoid process (Fig. 7.2). Radiographically, it is responsible for the maintenance of the atlantodental interval visualized on the lateral cervical radiograph. The transverse ligament prevents atlantoaxial subluxation with its subsequent potential for spinal cord compression. Atlantoaxial subluxation has been recognized to occur in 10–20% of Down's syndrome patients (5). The reasons postulated for this occurrence include agenesis, congenital ligamentous weakness, and intrinsic connective tissue defects. Thus, all participants in the Special Olympics that have Down's syndrome are required to undergo radiographic procedures to rule out atlantoaxial instability, which precludes contact sports if present.

Radiographic measurements of the distance between the anterior aspect of the odontoid and the posterior aspect of the anterior arch of the atlas range from 3 mm in adults to 5 mm in adolescents. This measurement should not only be taken in the neutral position but also in flexion and extension. Measurements greater than the established normals are significant of a "loose joint" complex from trauma, congenital variations, or metabolic processes.

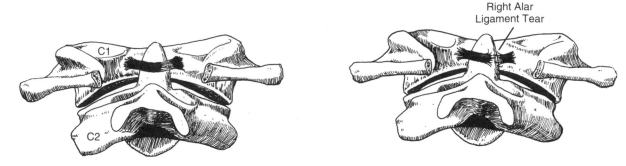

Figure 7.1. Right alar ligament tear. The right alar ligament normally prevents the right slippage of the atlas and occiput during right lateral bending.

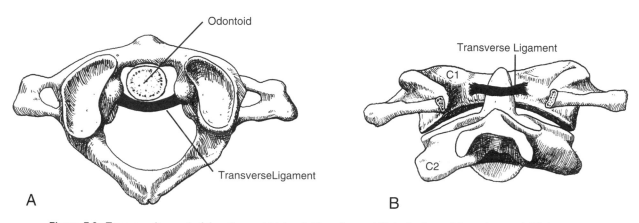

A   B

Figure 7.2. Transverse ligament of the atlantoaxial joint. **A.** The atlantoaxial joint is pictured from above and **(B)** from the front. The transverse ligament secures the odontoid against the anterior arch of the atlas.

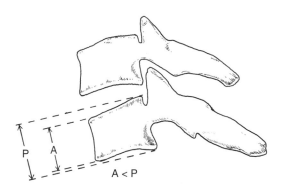

Figure 7.3. Comparison of anterior to posterior height in cervical vertebrae. The cervical discs are approximately 40% higher anteriorly than posteriorly. Combined with the differences in anterior and posterior vertebral height of the vertebrae, this accounts for cervical lordosis.

The cervical lordosis is formed by the cervical discs, which are approximately 40% higher anteriorly than posteriorly (6). The vertebral bodies are neutral to mildly kyphotic (7) (Fig. 7.3). In a study of 200 asymptomatic men and women, the mean cervical lordosis was found to be 23° (Fig. 7.4) with only 9% of the study group demonstrating hyperlordosis (9). The paired cervical facets are almost horizontal in the upper cervical spine (Fig. 7.5) and gradually become more vertical progressing to the lower cervical spine; they are oriented approximately 45° to the

longitudinal and anterior to posterior axes of the vertebra (3). The lateral inner body joints or joints of Luschka contribute to the lateral stability of the cervical spine and are found from C3 gradually disappearing at or around C5-C6, with anatomic remnants to C7. Agenesis or hypoplasia of these joints can yield a destabilizing element to the spinal motor unit with accelerated degeneration.

The cervical facets are innervated by the dorsal ramus, which is composed of three branches: the medial, lateral, and intermediate. The medial branch is a mixed sensory and motor nerve that is sensory to the joint capsule, ligamentum flava, and interspinous and supraspinous ligament (nuchal ligament), and 100% motor to the multifidus (10). The lateral branch is also a mixed sensory and motor nerve and is sensory to the fascial structures of the cervical musculature and motor to the long regional muscles, such as the splenius capitis and cervicis.

Specifically, the C1 dorsal ramus innervates the suboccipital muscles (obliques capitus superior and inferior, and rectus major and minor) but has no cutaneous branch. The medial branch of the C2 dorsal ramus becomes the greater occipital nerve, which innervates the cranium to the coronal suture and communicates with the supraorbital

nerve. The C3 dorsal ramus becomes the lesser occipital nerve and innervates the posterior cervical
region and cranium below the external occipital
protuberance. The remaining cervical multifidi are
innervated by the medial branch, numbered one
segment more than the spinous attachment. For
example, the C3 multifidus is innervated by the C4
medial branch of the dorsal ramus (10). The facet
joints of C2-C3 are innervated by the medial
branch of the dorsal ramus of C3. Below this level,
each facet joint receives innervation from its own
medial branch and from the segment above and
below. For example, the C5 facet joint is innervated by C4-C5-C6 (11). Consequently, any injury
that involves the cervical facet joints could refer
pain to the head, shoulder, and chest (12) (Fig.
7.6). Specific disorders of C1-C3 are associated
with pain referral to the head, whereas disorders
of C4-C7 can refer pain to the shoulders, scapula,
and chest wall.

The cervical discs are innervated by the sinuvertebral nerve and the vertebral nerve, which
penetrate the outer one third of the disc annulus
and have both somatic and autonomic connections (13). The pattern of innervation is similar in
the lumbar spine. Recently, Jinkins (14) demonstrated a vertebrogenic (discogenic) cause of autonomic dysfunction in the lumbar spine. Because the innervation patterns are similar in
both the cervical and lumbar spine, it would
stand to reason that involvement of a cervical
disc could cause pain and autonomic dysfunc-

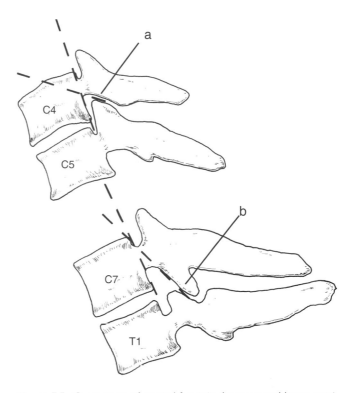

Figure 7.5. Comparison of cervical facets in the upper and lower cervical spine. The paired cervical facets are almost horizontal in **(A)** the upper
cervical spine and become more vertical in **(B)** the lower cervical spine.

tion in much the same way as it does in the lumbar spine. This vertebrogenic (discogenic) symptom complex could include local and referred
pain as well as autonomic reflex dysfunction. The
cervical discogenic syndromes can consist of pain
radiating to the head, shoulder, and upper arm
and are often associated with paresthesias without neurologic deficit (15). Any involvement of a
cervical disc that could cause mechanical or
chemical nocioreaction could subsequently be responsible for pain production. Very often, this
has been referred to as internal derangement of
the disc and is an explanation for the pain associated with provocation discography (16).

Considering the fact that both the cervical
facets and cervical discs have been shown to be
potent sources of pain, it would be wise to consider their possible role in any athletic injury.
The clinical relevance in discussing the articular and discal neuroanatomy provides an
anatomic substrata for the question of pain
origination. For example, in the case of a cervical sprain, which usually involves the posterior
ligamentous complex, there would be a pain
stimulus from the medial branch of the dorsal
ramus. The mixed motor and sensory nature of
this nerve could evoke a motor response of the
multifidus and a scleratogenous type of pain
distribution (Fig. 7.7). Considering the spino-
transverse orientation of the multifidus, which

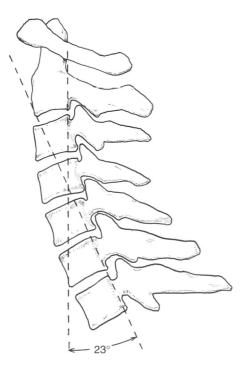

Figure 7.4. Measurement of cervical lordosis. The mean cervical lordosis
in asymptomatic men and women has been found to be 23° (8).

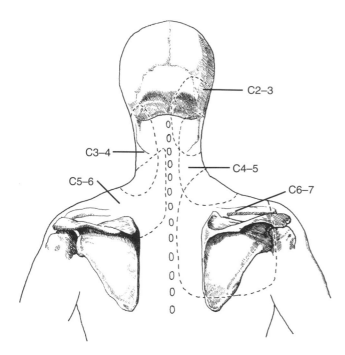

Figure 7.6. Pain referral patterns for cervical facet joint injury. Injuries to the cervical facet joints can refer pain to the head, shoulder, chest, and scapula.

is able to cause a mild degree of extension, rotation, and axial compression, ensuing somatic dysfunction could occur (C. April, personal lecture, 1989). The idea of the multifidus functioning as a component of somatic or articular dysfunction (chiropractic subluxation complex) can be demonstrated electromyographically by the presence of continuous spontaneous activity. Thabe demonstrated this in his evaluation of patients with somatic dysfunction in either the upper cervical or sacroiliac regions (17). He also found manipulation (thrust technique) to result in the immediate disappearance of the spontaneous activity. In another study, Vorro determined that asymmetric motion of the cervical spine, as determined by manual diagnosis, demonstrated significant EMG findings (increased activity) compared with a normal symmetric motion group (18). Furthermore, the muscles in the asymmetric group were slower to initiate action with a reduction in both time and strength of contraction. This is probably one of the factors responsible for the anecdotal reports of increased athletic performance after undergoing manipulative procedures.

One of the goals of manipulation is the restoration of symmetry to and normalization of the internal joint environment. Both quicker muscular reaction and increased strength could follow the procedure. The involvement of the multifidus and dorsal ramus has been termed the dorsal ramus

loop syndrome and can be a perpetuating factor of any injury or disorder (19).

The models of spinal dysfunction such as disc protrusion, sprain injury, deconditioning of the cervical muscles, or abnormal facet geometry could all distort facet load transmission and cause this self-perpetuating lesion (19) (Fig. 7.7). For instance, disc injury to the lumbar spine has been shown to alter the mechanical properties of the spinal motor unit, with secondary facet joint motion asymmetry (8). In Panjabi's study (8), flexion and extension and coupled motions were all disturbed whenever facet joint motion asymmetry was documented. In their case of a simulated lumbar posterior lateral disc protrusion, the contralateral facet impacted the pars interarticularis, which would stimulate the dorsal ramus. In the cervical spine, it could be postulated that abnormal coupling would also occur in disc injury with ipsilateral versus contralateral pars impaction occurring.

It has been shown in the lumbar spine that weakness or imbalance of the prime movers activates the intersegmental muscles (multifidi and intraversari), which are primarily kinesiologic monitors, and loads the spine in a more injury-prone posture (20). This same scenario probably occurs in the cervical spine.

Abnormal facet geometry of developmental, degenerative, or injury etiology could all cause abnormal load displacement characteristics causing facet capsule stress. The various models of dysfunction such as sprain, disc injury, weakness, or altered posture could conceivably exist singularly or in any combination of involvement (19). Unfortunately, definitive research to substantiate most of these concepts has only been performed in the lumbar spine. It is believed, however, that the cervical spine would behave similarly with only minor differences.

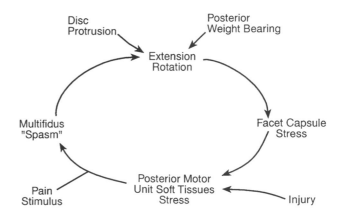

Figure 7.7. Cyclical development of pain syndromes in cervical sprains. The mixed motor and sensory nature of the dorsal ramus could evoke a motor response of the multifidus and a scleratogenous pain distribution.

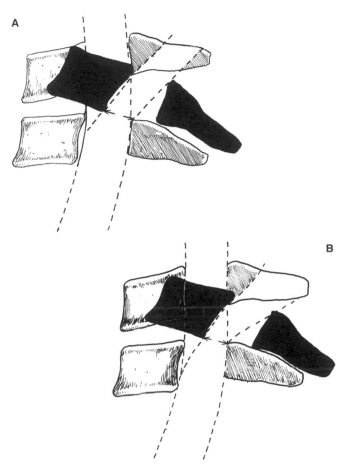

Figure 7.8. Pincer mechanism of spinal stenosis. With the pincer mechanism, the spinal cord is compressed by opposing vertebral bodies during **(A)** extension and **(B)** hyperextension.

STENOSIS

Congenital spinal stenosis has received much attention as a predisposition to serious cervical spine injury (21). In a study of athletes who presented with transient quadriparesis after injury, congenital cervical spinal stenosis was implicated as a primary factor (22). Penning studied the relationship of stenosis dynamically in flexion and extension (23). To accomplish this, he measured the sagittal diameter of the spinal canal from the inferior portion of the superior vertebral body to the nearest point on the spinolaminar line of the inferior vertebra. He described what could occur as the pincer mechanism (Fig. 7.8). With a pincer mechanism, the spinal cord is compressed by the opposing vertebral bodies.

Torg also described a methodology of assessing cervical spinal stenosis. He proposed a ratio method of mensuration to eliminate the radiographic magnification error. Essentially, measurements were taken from a neutral lateral radiograph (72 film focal distance [FFD]) of the distance between the posterior vertebral body and spinolaminar line (which becomes the numerator) and the mid anterior-posterior width of the vertebral bodies (which becomes the denominator) (Fig. 7.9). He considered any ratio below 0.8 as significant for spinal stenosis.

In two separate studies, Odor (24) and Hertzog (25) found the ratio method to be highly unreliable as a predictive value of cervical spine stenosis (only 12%). A newer approach to this very real clinical entity is the assessment of "functional" spinal stenosis (26). Functional ascertainment involves the standards of the magnetic resonance imaging (MRI), computed tomography (CT) scan, or contrast-enhanced studies. Functional spinal stenosis is defined as a loss of the cerebrospinal fluid around the cord, with a possibility of cord deformation in the most severe cases. It is now becoming increasingly apparent that the spinal cord and neural canal shape are unique in each individual. Subsequently, a diagnosis of spinal stenosis should not be made from plain film radiography alone. It has been concluded that, "patients who have stenosis should be advised to discontinue participation in contact sports" (26). Furthermore, the Torg ratio should not be relied on as a definitive answer to the question of stenosis. Instead, it would appear from the literature, if a positive Torg ratio is present, either an MRI or postcontrast CT should be performed to define significant spinal stenosis.

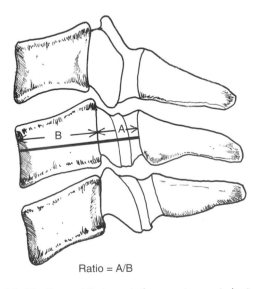

Ratio = A/B

Figure 7.9. The Torg and Pavlov ratio for assessing cervical spine stenosis. The ratio is composed of **(A)** the distance between the posterior vertebral body and spinolaminar line and **(B)** the midanteroposterior width of the vertebral body. A ratio below 0.8 is considered significant for spinal stenosis.

NEURAPRAXIAS

The only prototypical cervical spine sports injury, is "the burner," also known as "the stinger." Technically, this type of injury is a neurapraxia of the brachial plexus, which is a contusion or stretching of the nerve resulting in transient disruption of nerve function, less severe than axonotmesis (nerve plasma disruption) or neurotmesis (complete transection). This injury occurs with cervical rotation coupled with lateral flexion and contralateral shoulder depression or cervical rotation with extension and ipsilateral shoulder depression (Fig. 7.10).

Neurapraxias are the most common cervical spine injuries, often associated with spinal canal stenosis. The salient diagnostic point is their short duration and pain-free cervical range of motion. Neurapraxias include burning and paresthesias with a possible complete loss of sensation in the upper extremities. Motor changes range from mild weakness to complete paralysis, all with a pain-free cervical range of motion. To completely dismiss disc or facet involvement may, however, be an erroneous assumption. Pointdexter and Johnson (27) examined 20 football players with the diagnosis of stinger and found a C6 radiculopathy rather than a stretch or nerve contusion disorder in all 20 subjects. However, the athletes were receiving care directed at the brachial plexus versus that of the spinal structures.

Spinal Cord Neurapraxias

In a survey of athletes at 503 colleges, a history suggesting neurapraxia of the spinal cord was found to exist in approximately 1.3 in 10,000 athletes. A stenotic neural canal was found in most cases (28). Just as in neurapraxias of the brachial

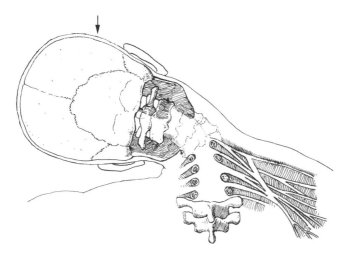

Figure 7.10. Mechanism of injury in the cervical burner or stinger. Arrow indicates a force propelling the head to the shoulder, thus stretching the brachial plexus nerves.

plexus and nerve roots, spinal cord neurapraxia is associated with sensory changes that include burning, pain, numbness, and tingling, whereas the motor changes range from weakness to complete paralysis or transient quadriplegia (21). Spinal cord neurapraxias, like stingers and burners, generally only last from 10 to 15 minutes, although in some patients they may gradually resolve in 36 to 48 hours. Again, neck pain is absent. It is the author's opinion that if any presentation or history of either brachial plexus or spinal cord neurapraxia exists, further evaluation is warranted.

Evaluation should include cervical functional radiography consisting of neutral lateral, flexion, and extension views, with orthopedic and neurologic assessment. The radiographs would be used for the preliminary evaluation of spinal stenosis, degenerative disc disease, instability, congenital malformations, and for help with the diagnosis of hypomobility or hypermobility of the cervical spinal joints (29). If the examiner is trained in manual diagnosis or has access to a manual diagnostician (D.C. and D.O.), this part of the examination could also be used to ascertain somatic dysfunction (chiropractic subluxation complex). Treatment would consist of addressing all functional loss or pain with spinal manipulation, cervical spine strengthening exercises, and physical therapy modalities. Specifically, manipulation is directed at the hypomobile joints demonstrated through functional radiography and/or manual diagnosis (palpation). Physical therapy would consist of ice and the electrotherapies, such as high-volt galvanism or interferential current for pain control and antiinflammatory effects. Cervical spine strengthening exercises range from the simple self-administered isometric program to the sophisticated computer-assisted exercise machine. Obviously, some of these techniques are more effective and safer than others.

One of the most difficult decisions that a team physician encounters is the determination of who stays and who plays after a cervical spine injury. Unfortunately, there is no definitive answer to this question because "a normal neurologic on-field screening does not rule out serious underlying neck injury if the patient has severe neck pain or persistent apprehension" (30). To help with this decision-making process, Watkins (31) designed a relative risk return-to-play score card (Fig. 7.11). To complete this score card assessment, however, radiographic evaluation for cervical stenosis is required, making it unsuitable for on-site decision-making. Subsequently, any athlete who sustains an injury should not return to his or her sport until a thorough evaluation, including radiographs, can be performed. It is important to remember that the

Rating	Extent of deficit
1	Unilateral arm pain or dysesthesia, loss of strength
2	Bilateral upper extremity loss of sensory or motor function
3	Any loss of sensory or motor function
4	Transient quadriparesis
5	Transient quadriplegia
Rating	Time
1	Less than 5 min
2	Less than 1 hr
3	Less than 24 hr
4	Less than 1 wk
5	More than 1 wk
Rating	Central canal diameter
1	Greater than 12 mm
2	10–12 mm
3	10 mm
4	10–8 mm
5	Less than 8 mm

Risk course to assess total return to play risk

Points	Risk
Less than 6	Minimal
6–10	Moderate
11–15	Severe

Figure 7.11. Score card for making return-to-play decisions. (Courtesy of R.G. Watkins, M.D.)

symptoms of neurapraxias are short lived and possibly associated with stenosis and radiculopathy.

CERVICAL SPRAIN/STRAIN

Acute cervical sprain/strains are frequently seen in the field of athletic endeavor and are sometimes associated with thoracic outlet syndromes (32). The soft tissue structures, including muscles, ligaments, discs, and joint capsules, are all capable of being injured. Most cervical sprains sustained in athletic competition involve a hyperflexion axial compression mechanism of injury, compared with the hyperextension axial distraction seen in motor vehicle accidents (33). Subsequently, it could be expected that different anatomic tissues would be involved. Generally, a hyperflexion type of injury will involve the posterior ligamentous and soft tissue complex, whereas hyperextension injury will injure the anterior ligamentous and soft tissue structures (and possibly posterior bony elements). If the traumatic stresses are significant enough in either hyperflexion or hyperextension, fracture/dislocation or injury to the anterior and posterior tissues can occur. Two of the most notorious and preventable causes of cervical injury in contact sports are the "high tackle" in rugby football and "spearing" in American football. In both situations, hyperflexion and rotation are implicated.

In the evaluation of a suspected cervical sprain, two main types of assessment tools are used. The first is that of manual diagnosis, which is the skilled palpation of both the static and dynamic components of the spinal structures. This type of examination is used by chiropractic physicians, osteopathic physicians, physical therapists, and manual medicine practitioners and is shown to be highly accurate (34). Functional radiography is the second primary examination tool for cervical spine trauma and is considered the most important means of cervical spine injury evaluation in Europe (23). To perform functional radiography, passive maximum end range of motion is templated on a clear acetate with degrees of excursion measured between flexion and extension (Fig. 7.12). In a

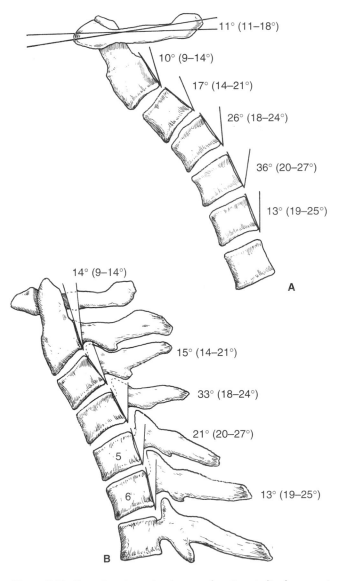

Figure 7.12. Examples of templated range of motion studies from cervical spine plain film radiography. **A.** The results of flexion extension templating after vehicular trauma, revealing hypermobility of C5 (36°) with reactive hypomobility of C6. This signifies a grade 2 sprain injury of C5 ligaments. **B.** Hypermobility of C4 (33°) with reactive hypomobility of C6 (13°) and possibly C3 (15°). Expected normal ranges at each level are shown in parentheses.

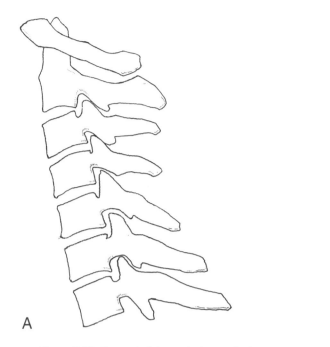
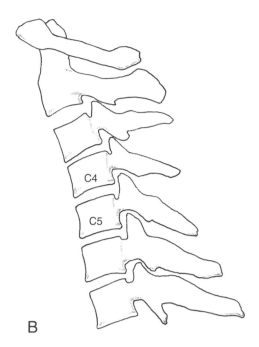

Figure 7.13. Reversal of the cervical curve. **A.** A nonangular reversal of the cervical lordosis. This form may suggest a lesser grade of traumatic reversal or a postural aberration. It is difficult to select one or two segments at which the lordosis is reversed. **B.** Clear angular reversal of the cervical lordosis. This form is almost always the result of a more significant sprain injury or from disc degeneration. It is relatively easy to isolate the segment of reversal, in this case C4 on C5.

sprain type of injury, the demonstrable findings are hypermobility at one or two segments with reactive hypomobility, either above or below the level of excessive motion. In a study by Dvorak, the normal intersegmental mobility ranged from 11–18° at C1 to 17–25° at C7 (29).

- C1: 11–18°
- C2: 9–14°
- C3: 14–21°
- C4: 18–24°
- C5: 20–27°
- C6: 17–25°

Another critical point in the radiographic evaluation is the careful scrutiny of the neutral lateral cervical radiograph. Consideration is made regarding the smooth uninterrupted lordotic character or the presence of a sharp angular reversal either segmentally or, in some instances, bisegmentally of the lordosis. Angular loss is a significant indicator of soft tissue trauma (Fig. 7.13).

In another study, Amevo described a more sophisticated type of functional radiography that used a computer-assisted digitized methodology (35). These findings of radiographic plain film abnormalities in patients with traumatically induced neck pain were described as an abnormal instantaneous axis of rotation. An analogy could be made between a functional spinal unit—which consists of two vertebrae, disc, and the supporting soft tissue elements—and a speed-balanced

tire. If the tire happens to be out of balance, it wobbles slightly when spun at high speed, much like a traumatized spine does with active motion. Amevo's study, however, lacked specific information for treatment application but instead functioned as a marker for medical-legal cases.

Diagnosis of cervical sprain is made by the lack of positive neurologic findings, i.e., hyporeflexia with true upper extremity motor weakness, limited range of motion, and positive manual diagnosis correlated with functional radiography. There is, however, the possibility of dermatomal paresthesias in a grade 2 or 3 cervical sprain or of upper extremity dysesthesia from thoracic outlet syndrome. The author's criteria for grading cervical sprains are as follows.

1. Grade 1—loss or angular loss of the cervical lordosis (unisegmental or bisegmental) with intermittent referred pain pattern, trigger points, and segmental hypomobility.
2. Grade 2— angular loss of the cervical lordosis (unisegmental or bisegmental), frequent or constant referred pain pattern or sensory radicular symptom pattern, and segmental hypermobility.
3. Grade 3—angular loss of the cervical lordosis (unisegmental or bisegmental), 3.5 mm of horizontal vertebral displacement on the lateral cervical radiograph or an angular difference of 11° or greater than an adjacent

cervical segment with soft tissue swelling of the retropharyngeal or retrotracheal air space (Fig. 7.14).

Unfortunately, allopathic treatment of this disorder has relied on a dependence of passive modalities such as pain medication, antiinflammatory medications, soft cervical collars, rest, and physical therapy. For example, Mealy compared a group of patients with cervical sprain/strain injuries arising from cervical acceleration/deceleration trauma who received early active mobilization with a group who received conventional therapy such as rest, cervical collar, and muscle relaxants. The group that received the early active mobilization had increased range of motion and decreased pain at the end of 8 weeks compared with the passive treatment control group (36).

In another study, Amesis stated that rest is not benign and can become pathologic. Soft tissue shortens if not regularly stretched (37). Ultimately, rest and immobility may cause symptomatic spinal degeneration (38). Medication in the form of nonsteroidal antiinflammatory drugs has been shown to suppress proteoglycan synthesis in the herniated nucleus pulposus of canines (39). This suppression could interfere with healing by decreasing the building blocks used in tissue repair and damaging the uninvolved healthy tissue, to say the least.

In a recent literature search, Florian distinguished useful from useless treatment of neck pain (40). The scientific literature delineated only two types of beneficial therapy: manipulation and mobilization. With this consideration of manipulation and mobilization being the only viable treatments with proven efficacy, they should be the primary modes of conservative management of athletic cervical spine injury. Manipulation addresses the hypomobility found through manual diagnosis and functional radiography, whereas mobilization is a more generalized method of restoring range of motion.

Research has demonstrated an increase in cervical strength and flexibility through rehabilitative exercise (41, 42). It has been postulated that appropriate rehabilitation can aid in recovery and decrease noncatastrophic injury. Subsequently, a manipulative rehabilitative approach would be well suited to the treatment of cervical sprain injury. Rehabilitation, in the form of progressive resistive exercise, starts approximately 8 weeks after injury, sometimes earlier in less severe cases. Generally, some type of quantitative assessment tool is used to ascertain muscular strength in the various planes of motion. A normal hierarchy of strength exists that shows extensors being approximately 20% stronger than flexors, with decreasing strength in the order of extensors, flexors, rotators, and lateral flexors (43). A normative strength data base is starting to emerge that will allow for comparisons among different groups of individuals. Unfortunately, each of the various manufacturers of the testing equipment has different normative data, making the strength hierarchy values the most usable information for a return to normal. Return to play is allowed after rehabilitation is complete. The normal strength ratios should be documented or the injury adequately healed, with the patient demonstrating a pain-free range of motion and negative neurologic examination.

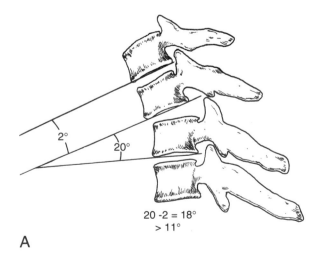

A

20 -2 = 18°
> 11°

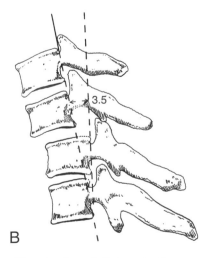

B

Figure 7.14. Grade 3 cervical spine sprain injury. Signs of a grade 3 sprain on a neutral lateral radiograph. **A.** A greater than 11° difference in angulation between two adjacent segments. **B.** A greater than 3.5 mm forward translation of one segment on another. Grade 3 injuries are unstable and require immediate orthopedic care.

Acute Cervical Instability

The purpose of this section is to alert the practicing clinician to this diagnostic entity. Subacute cervical instability is defined as the radiographic evidence of cervical instability within 3 weeks of cervical spine injury after the results of adequate initial radiographic examination were negative (44). It must be emphasized emphatically that negative is not really negative in this case, but is instead a misdiagnosis in the initial radiographic impression. A closer review of the radiographic findings would have allowed the diagnosis of a grade 3 cervical sprain and possible subacute cervical instability. Those findings are as follows:

1. Interspinous widening,
2. Anterior subluxation,
3. Vertebral compression fracture, and
4. Loss of the cervical lordosis.

These findings may present singly or in combination. The criteria of radiographic instability are 3.5 mm of horizontal displacement or an angular difference of greater than 11° on an adjacent level segment. An enlargement of the retrotracheal or retropharyngeal space can also be a warning sign of possible cervical instability. The mechanism of the subacute instability is thought to occur from the elastic and plastic deformation of the ligaments and disc in the cervical spine. The clinical bottom line of conservative management of grade 3 cervical sprains would be the immediate referral for neurosurgical consultation and comanagement of the patient with this practitioner. The therapeutic goal would be to prevent a fixed deformity such as unilateral facet dislocation.

Cervical Disc Syndrome

Cervical disc herniations with neurologic symptoms are reported to be relatively uncommon in athletes but are known to occur (45). The presentation of a limited cervical range of motion, neck and referred pain into the upper extremity or hand, hyporeflexia, and weakness or paresthesias corresponding to a segmental level all suggest a herniated nucleus pulposus. Specifically, neurologic examination would include reflex, sensory, and motor evaluations. Reflex examination would include the biceps (C5), triceps (C7), brachioradialis (C6), and ulnar (C8-T1). Sensory examination would include pinwheel sensitivity testing of the various dermatomes of the cervical spine. Motor examination would include manual muscle testing procedures of the cervical spine's segmental innervation. Orthopedic testing would include any physiologic or physical stress that replicates or reduces the patient's symptoms, e.g., Spurling's test, Valsalva's maneuver, Brakody's sign, axial traction, or nerve traction hyperabduction stresses. Unfortunately, the sensitivity and specificity have never been proven either for or against the use of these tests, yet they are commonly relied on in the initial clinical assessment. All these procedures could be correlated to the more sensitive radiographic analysis (MRI and CT) or electrodiagnostic test (EMG, NCV, and SSEPS).

Conservative treatment would consist of specific spinal manipulation (46) and rehabilitative strengthening exercises (47) coupled with pain control and antiinflammatory modalities. Conservative care is not continued with any signs of spinal cord compression or radiculopathy that do not show improvement after a short therapeutic trial. Long tract signs, such as ataxia, hyperreflexia, or urinary incontinence, suggest a neurosurgical emergency. Return to play is permissible when the results of the patient's physical and rehabilitative examinations are normal.

CERVICAL FRACTURES AND DISLOCATIONS

Fortunately, fractures and/or dislocations do not occur frequently. These types of injuries, when they do occur, may be stable or unstable and with or without neurologic deficit. The danger, of course, with these types of injuries is the possibility of spinal cord damage with paralysis. Diagnosis of these types of injuries is made from the physical examination and plain film radiographs or CT scan. Treatment ranges from the closed reduction of a dislocation with surgical tongs to decompressive surgery. These types of severe injuries do not warrant conservative care in the initial phase. This is not to say that these types of athletic injuries would not benefit from postemergency manipulative and rehabilitative care on a case-by-case basis. In fact, it is the author's opinion that this type of functional treatment would be most beneficial.

ON-SITE EVALUATION

On-site evaluation could involve some of the most important decisions regarding an athlete's health that he or she will ever receive. For example, suppose that you are the team physician at a local high school football game and witness one of your team's players "really getting hit." From your perspective, it appears that he may have hyperflexed his neck. The player is down on the field and is not moving. You rush to the player's side and your first concern is to guard the spine from further damage if damage has occurred (Fig. 7.15). It

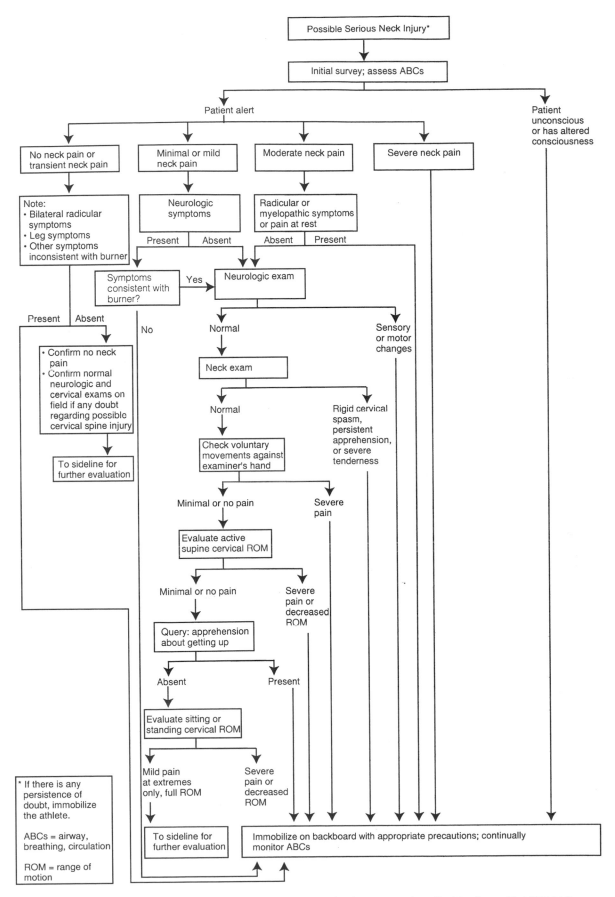

Figure 7.15. On-field process of assessing neck injuries. (Reprinted with permission from Physician Sports Med 1993;21:8).

has been estimated that 50% of neurologic deficits are created after the initial trauma (30). It is always assumed that a cervical injury has occurred until proven otherwise. Your initial assessment reveals a conscious athlete in a supine position. You check for signs and symptoms of serious neck injury, such as severe neck pain, tenderness, or muscular spasm. The lack of these findings, however, does not preclude serious, unstable neck injury.

The ABCs (airways, breathing, and circulation) of cardiopulmonary function should be followed. If the patient is unconscious and the airway is blocked, it must be opened immediately with immobilization being secondary (45). In the case of a football player with a helmet and face mask, the face mask can be removed with bolt cutters (Fig. 7.16) and the possibility of such should be planned for ahead of time. A forward jaw thrust technique is used that may be sufficient to open the airway. Make sure to double check for foreign objects, such as the player's mouthpiece or possibly vomitus. If this is not sufficient to obtain a clear airway, cervical malalignment may be present. This can be corrected by using gentle, two-handed traction of approximately 10 pounds of force, while slowly turning the head into alignment with the trunk. It is important to avoid either flexion or extension because these positions are likely to exacerbate spinal cord compression.

After the airway has been reestablished, the head should be immobilized in this new position. If the patient is unconscious or has altered consciousness, he will be immobilized on a backboard (Fig. 7.17). Loss of consciousness, posttraumatic amnesia, headache, dizziness, impaired orientation, or any central nervous system signs all suggest cerebral concussion (Table 7.1).

In the absence of any cervical spine injury, the greatest risk to an athlete who has sustained a concussion and wishes to return to play is the second impact syndrome (see return to play in Table 7.1) (48). The second impact syndrome can be described as a second head injury that is superimposed on an unresolved preexisting concussion. This second impact syndrome can cause cerebral edema and possible death. A classification system for the rating of cerebral concussions and return to play is provided in Table 7.2.

If the patient needs to be turned over from a prone to a supine position, a "log-rolling" technique is used. This procedure involves a minimum team of four persons. The one person supporting and controlling the head is referred to as the chief and is not responsible for any lifting or positioning other than controlling the head. The other individuals should be positioned on each side of the shoulders, waist, and feet. The person supporting the head will grasp the clavicle and trapezius while cradling the injured athlete's head with his or her forearms, while the others turn the patient over with the chief's arms rotating into a neutral position. If the injured athlete

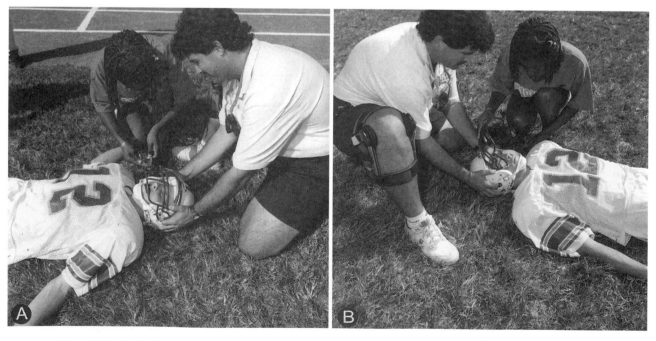

Figure 7.16. Football mask removal. **A.** Remove single and double bar masks with bolt cutters. Remove cage-type masks by cutting the plastic loops with a utility knife. Make the cut on the side of the loop away from the face. **B.** Remove the entire mask from the helmet so it does not interfere with further resuscitation efforts.

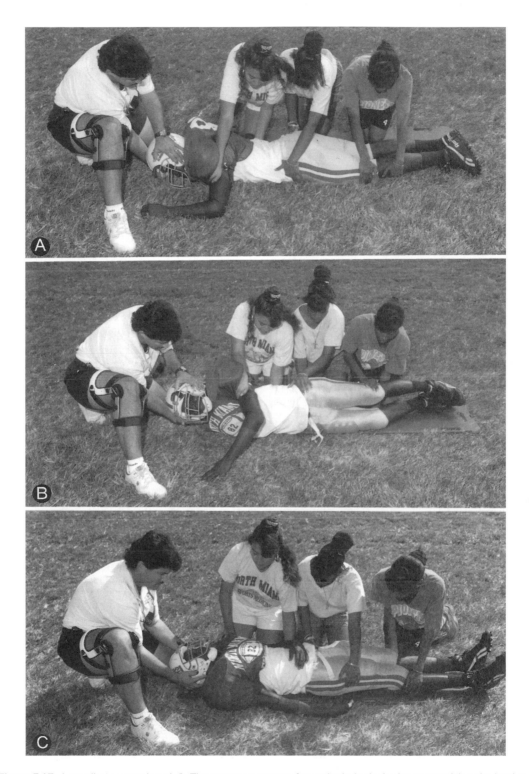

Figure 7.17. Log-roll to a spine board. **A.** This maneuver requires four individuals, the leader to immobilize the head and neck and to command the support team and three individuals who are positioned at the shoulders, hips, and lower legs. **B.** The leader uses the cross-arm technique to immobilize the head. This technique allows the leader's arms to unwind as the three assistants roll the athlete onto the spine board. **C.** The three must maintain body alignment during the roll.

Table 7.1. Classification of Concussion

Colorado Classification	
Grade 1	Confusion without amnesia
	No loss of consciousness
Grade 2	Confusion with amnesia
	No loss of consciousness
Grade 3	Loss of consciousness
Cantu's Classification	
Grade 1	No LOC, PTA <30 min
Grade 2	LOC <5 min or PTA >30 min
Grade 3	LOC >5 min or PTA >24 h

From Chiropractic Sports Medicine 1994;8(2):720
LOC, loss of consciousness; PTA, posttraumatic amnesia.

Table 7.2. Recommended Timetable[a] for Return to Play and Practice After Successive Concussions

Concussion Severity	First Concussion	Second Concussion	Third Concussion
Bell ringer	Return to game if asymptomatic after 10–30 min[b]	Return in 1 wk if asymptomatic	Return in 1 wk if asymptomatic
Grade 1	Return in 1 wk if asymptomatic	Return in 2 wk if asymptomatic after 1 wk	Terminate season (no play for 3–6 mo)
Grade 2	Return in 1 wk if asymptomatic	Return in 1 mo if asymptomatic for final 1 wk	Terminate season (no play for 3–6 mo)
Grade 3	Return in 1 mo if asymptomatic for final 1 wk	Terminate season (no play for 3–6 mo)	

Adapted from Cantu RC. Guidelines to return to contact sport after a cerebral concussion. Phys Sports Med 1986: 14:75–83.
[a]Recommendations are for return within a contact or collision sport season (3 months).
[b]No headache; dizziness; or impaired orientation, concentration, or memory at rest or with exertion.

is already in the supine position, the individual supporting the head directs the others to reach underneath and to clasp their hands and lift while a backboard is placed under the player. This maneuver should be practiced in a drill before a real emergency situation arises, necessitating perfection (see Chapter 6).

The injured athlete will then be taken to the sidelines or the locker room on the spine board for further evaluation, and a decision will be made regarding the therapeutic plan. Players are not allowed to return to play with any symptoms, motor weakness, or paresthesias of the arms or legs. If this is a football injury and neurologic symptoms are present, the helmet should remain in place until adequate radiography can be performed to rule out fracture and/or dislocation. Essentially, evaluation at this point would proceed in the usual fashion. Return to play is based on clinical evaluation. Any athlete who sustains a cervical spine injury should undergo a thorough examination that includes orthopedic, neurologic, and radiographic procedures (31).

References

1. Nicholas JA. Orthopedic problems in athletes. Compr Ther 1985;11:48–56.
2. Rauschning W. In: Haldeman S. Modern developments in the principles and practice of chiropractic. East Norwalk, CT: Appleton-Lange 1992:64–65.
3. Moroney SP. Load displacement properties of lower cervical spine motion segments. J Biomech 1988;21:769–779.
4. Dvorak J. Functional anatomy of the alar ligament. Spine 1987;12:183–189.
5. Cope R. Abnormalities of the cervical spine in Down's syndrome. South Med J 1987;80:33–36.
6. Pooni JS. Comparison of the structure of the human intervertebral disc in the the cervical, thoracic and lumbar regions of the spine. Surg Radiol Anat 1986;8:175–182.
7. Gilad I, Nissan M. A study of vertebra and disc geometric relations of the human cervical and lumbar spine. Spine 1986;11:154–157.
8. Panjabi MM. The effects of disc injury on the mechanical behavior of the spine. Spine 1984;9:707–713.
9. Gore DR. Radiographic findings of the cervical spine in asymptomatic people. Spine 1986;11:52.
10. Bogduk N. The clinical anatomy of the cervical dorsal rami. Spine 1982;7:319–329.
11. Bogduk N. The cervical zygapophyseal joints as a source of pain. Spine 1988;13:610.
12. Dwyer A. Cervical zygapophyseal joint pain patterns: part 1. a study of normal volunteers. Spine 1990;15:453–457.
13. Bogduk N. The innervation of the cervical intervertebral disc. Spine 1988;13:2–8.
14. Jinkins JR. The anatomic basis of vertebrogenic pain and the autonomic syndrome associated with lumbar disc extrusion. Am J Neuroradiol 1989;10:219–231.
15. Bogduk N. Neck pain: an update. Aust Fam Physician 1988;17:75.
16. April C. Cervical zygapophyseal joint pain patterns: part 2. a clinical evaluation. Spine 1990;15:458–461.
17. Thabe H. Electromyography as a tool to document diagnostic findings and therapeutic results associated with somatic dysfunctions in the upper spinal joints and sacroiliac joints. Manual Med 1986;2:53–58.
18. Vorro J. Clinical biomechanical correlates for cervical function, part 2: a myoelectric study. J Am Osteopathic Assoc 1987;87:353–367.
19. Banks. SD. Biomechanical/spinal disorders lecture series. 1:13.
20. Paniapour M. The triaxial coupling of torque generation of trunk muscles during isometric exertions and the effect of fatiguing isoinertial movements on the motor output and movement patterns. Spine 1988;13:982–992.
21. Torg J. Neurapraxia of the cervical spinal cord with transient quadriplegia. J Bone Joint Surg Am 1986;68:1354–1370.
22. Ladd AL. Congenital cervical stenosis presenting as transient quadriplegia in athletes: a report of two cases. J Bone Joint Surg Am 1986;68:1371–1374.
23. Penning L. Some aspects of plain radiography of the cervical spine in chronic myelopathy. Neurology 1962;12:513–519.
24. Odor JM. Incidence of spinal stenosis in professional and rookie football players. Am J Sports Med 1990;18:507–510.
25. Hertzog RJ. Normal cervical spine morphometry and cervical spinal stenosis in asymptomatic professional football players. Spine 1991;166(Suppl):178–186.
26. Cantu R. Functional cervical spinal stenosis: a contraindication to participation in contact sports. Med Sci Sports Exerc 1993;25:316–317.
27. Pointdexter DP, Johnson EW. Football shoulder-neck injury: a study of the stinger. Arch Phys Med Rehabil 1984;65:601–602.
28. Christensen KD. Chiropractic rehabilitation: cervical spine. Ridgefield, WA: C.R.A. publisher, 1991.
29. Dvorak J. Functional radiographic diagnosis of the cervical spine: flexion-extension. Spine 1986;13:148.

30. Anderson C. Neck injuries. Phys Sports Med 1993;21: 21–34.
31. Watkins RG. Neck injuries in football players. Clin Sports Med 1986;5:215–246.
32. Capistrant T.D. Thoracic outlet syndrome and cervical strain injury. Minn Med 1986;69:13–17.
33. Roy S, Irvin R. Sports medicine: prevention, evaluation, management, and rehabilitation. Englewood Cliffs, NJ: Prentice-Hall, 1983:250.
34. Jull G. The accuracy of manual diagnosis for cervical zygapophyseal joint pain. Med J Aust 1988;148:233.
35. Amevo B. Abnormal instantaneous axis of rotation in patients with neck pain. Spine 1992;17:748–756.
36. Mealy K. Early mobilization of acute whiplash injuries. Br Med J 1986;292:656–657.
37. Amesis A. Cervical whiplash: considerations in the rehabilitation of cervical myofascial injury. Can Fam Physician 1986;32:1871–1876.
38. Kahanovitz N. The effects of internal fixation on articular cartilage of unfused canine facet joint cartilage. Spine 1984;9:268–272.
39. Yoo JU. Suppression of proteoglycan synthesis in chondrocyte cultures derived from canine intervertebral disc. Spine 1992;172:221–224.
40. Florian T. Conservative treatment for neck pain distinguishing useful from useless therapy. J Back Musculoskeletal Rehabil 1991;15:55–66.
41. Stump JA. Comparison of two modes of cervical exercise in adolescent male athletes. J Manipulative Physiol Ther 1993;16:155–160.
42. Leggett SH. Quantitative assessment and training of isometric cervical extension strength. Am J Sports Med 1991;19:653–659.
43. Beimborn DC, Morrisseu MC. Review of the literature related to trunk muscle performance. Spine 1988;13: 655–660.
44. Herkowitz HN. Subacute instability of the cervical spine. Spine 1984;9:348–357.
45. Jackson DW. Cervical spine injuries. Clin Sports Med 1986;5:373–383.
46. Siciliano M. Reduction of a confirmed C5-C6 disc herniation following specific chiropractic spinal manipulation: a case study. J Chiro Res Clin Invest 1992;8:17–23.
47. Highland T. Changes in isometric strength and range of motion of the isolated cervical spine after 8 weeks of clinical rehabilitation. Spine 1992;17(Suppl):77–82.
48. Roberts WO. Who plays, who sits?. Physician Sports Med 1992;20:66–72.

Thoracic Spine Injuries

Steven M. Skurow

Conservative management of thoracic spine injuries presents a challenge to the sports physician to diagnose the condition properly and to administer treatment so that the athlete can resume activity as quickly as possible. Fortunately, most thoracic spine injuries can be treated conservatively.

The thoracic spine is not often a site of sports-related injuries, as are the cervical and lumbar spines or extremities. This is because of two kinematic differences in the thoracic spine: decreased intervertebral motion and the protective shell and immobilizing presence of the rib cage (1).

Although there is a debate in the literature about the actual amount of movement in the thoracic spine (2), rotation and lateral flexion allow the predominant amount of movement as the vertical alignment of the facets limits flexion and extension. Furthermore, the attachments of the ribs between the vertebral bodies limit the amount of lateral flexion (1).

Thoracic disc spaces are narrow. The spinous processes extend downward in the thoracic spine overlapping each other, often resting on another spinous process. This in turn increases the leverage of the interspinous ligaments because the spinous processes have to separate as the spine flexes forward (Fig. 8.1).

This rigidity in the thoracic spine helps protect it against some of the common injuries that can occur in the much more mobile cervical and lumbar spines. Thoracic spine injuries become more likely with prolonged static loading, vibratory stress, and repetitive bumps and shocks (3). These aspects are further influenced by the muscle strength and skill of the athlete and the presence or absence of degenerative changes.

It is the stability of the thoracic spine that makes it an infrequent site of fractures, dislocations, sprained ligaments, or herniated discs. Contusions and muscle strains, however, are common in this region. Fractures, when they occur, usually are compression fractures of the vertebral body or of the spinous or transverse processes (Fig. 8.2) (1, 4). Dislocations—although rare—can occur, and when present often cause spinal cord damage (5). Costovertebral joint dysfunction and intrathoracic injuries also occur in certain sports. Understanding the biomechanics of the thoracic spine and the causative mechanism of injury will help the treating physician diagnose the condition and begin treatment.

DEVELOPMENTAL ANATOMY

It is important to understand the time frame for the appearance and fusion of thoracic ossification centers. Knowledge of this sequence will help reduce the risk of erroneously identifying unfused ossification centers as fractures. These centers are also potential sites of injury during growth.

The arches, in the thoracic spine, usually become fused to the vertebral body around the ages of 4 to 5. Secondary centers of ossification begin to develop around the ages of 11 to 16 in the tips of the spinous processes, in the tips of the transverse processes, and in the growth cartilage between the discs and the bony vertebra (Fig. 8.3). Ossification normally is completed by the age of 25.

Secondary centers of ossification appear around the age of 15 or 16 in the head and in the tubercle of the rib. There may be one or two centers in the tubercle, but usually just one in the head. These centers begin to fuse somewhere between the ages of 22 and 25.

Thoracic vertebrae are distinguished by articulations with the ribs. Vertebral foramina are circular and small. Transverse processes point laterally backward and upward and possess facets for articulation with the tubercles of the ribs. Spinous processes are typically long and thin. The articular processes are flat facet-type joints. The superior articular facets lie behind the pediculi and face upward, backward, and slightly laterally. The inferior facets are found in front of the lamellae and face exactly opposite the superior facets.

Only the middle four thoracic vertebrae—levels 5, 6, 7, and 8—are considered typical. The upper four share some features in common with the cervical spine, and the lower four share features in common with the lumbar vertebrae and are thus considered atypical.

Articulations for the heads of the ribs span between two vertebrae. Accommodating facets on the upper posterolateral angles of the inferior vertebrae and the lower posterolateral angles of the superior vertebrae occur, except for T1, T11, and T12, which have single facets. On T1 there is a full facet at its superolateral posterior angle and a hemifacet on the posterolateral inferior angle. On T11 and T12 there are single facets for the head of the ribs on their pedicles.

The spinous processes of the middle four thoracic vertebrae are long and overlapping and are almost vertical. The 1st and 2nd and the 11th and 12th have nearly horizontal spinous processes. T3, T4, T9, and T10 have spinous processes between these two extremes.

The intervertebral disc in the thoracic region is thin and nearly uniform in thickness. The tho-racic region receives its kyphotic curve predominantly from the wedge shape of the vertebral bodies and not from the shape of the discs. The joint formed by the intervertebral disc and intervertebral bodies is a stiff, slightly movable joint that allows for bending and rotation as well as gliding movements in small degrees.

Facet joints, whose orientation has been described previously, are synovial joints with supporting capsules. They allow for flexion, extension, rotation, and lateral bending. Their movements are

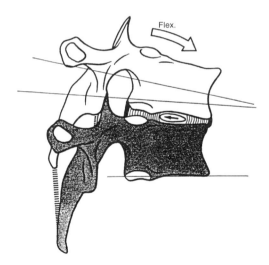

Figure 8.1. Thoracic spinous processes are long, providing increased leverage. From Kapandji IA: The Physiology of the Joints, 2nd ed, volume 3: the trunk and the vertebral column. New York, Churchill Livingstone, 1974.

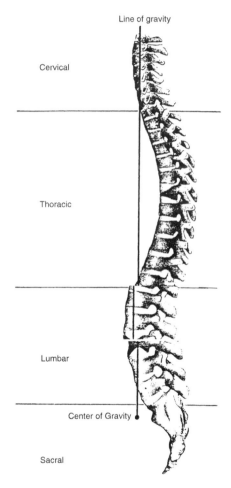

Figure 8.2. Anterior wedge shaped fractures (compression fractures are common in the thoracic region. From Bullough PG, Boachie-Adjei O: Atlas of Spinal Diseases. Philadelphia, JB Lippincott.

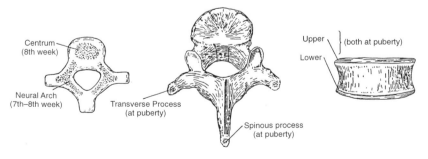

Figure 8.3. Ossification of the vertebral column: Left, typical vertebra, center, typical vertebra at puberty, right, vertebral body at puberty. From Clements CD: Gray's anatomy. Philadelphia, Lea & Febiger, 1985.

abdominal quadrants. This tests the integrity of nerve fibers from segmental levels T7–T12 (12). Barkman's reflex specifically centers on the upper abdominal quadrant of T7–T9 and is performed with cutaneous stimulation just below the nipple, resulting in homolateral contraction of the rectus abdominis (12). The obliquus reflex confirms the response of the lower abdominal reflex (T8–T12). Stimulation of the skin below the inguinal ligament contracts a part of the ipsilateral external oblique muscle (14). For Beevor's sign, the athlete is supine and flexes the neck or sits up. The abdominal muscles are palpated and the umbilicus is observed, which should stay centered. If there is functional weakness or paralysis, the umbilicus will move to the side opposite the weakness (12).

LABORATORY TESTING

Athletic injuries involving the thoracic spine are usually straightforward musculoskeletal problems not requiring extensive laboratory workups. There are circumstances, however, which may require an intelligent use of laboratory tests (Table 8.3). These circumstances would include the following.

1. Suspected metabolic, nutritional, or absorption problems that would adversely affect musculoskeletal strength, particularly disorders affecting calcium, vitamin D, parathormone, magnesium, phosphate, and creatinine.
2. Suspected spondyloarthropathy.
3. A history of malignancy.
4. Signs or symptoms suggesting that the spinal complaints are referred from a visceral source.
5. Suspected infections.

Table 8.3. Abnormal Findings That May Indicate Further Testing

	Multiple Myeloma	Visceral	Infection	Inflammation
CBC			X	
ESR				X
SGOT		X		
SGPT		X		
LDH		X		
Lipase		X		
Amylase		X		
Bilirubin		X		
Plasma protein electrophoreses	X			
Urine Bence Jones protein	X			
HLA-B27				X

CBC, complete blood count; ESR, erythrocyte sedimentation rate; SGOT, serum glutamic-oxaloacetic transaminase; SGPT, serum glutamate pyruvate transaminase; LDH, lactate dehydrogenase; HLA-B27, human leukocyte antigen B27.

Specific Recommendations

Because the marrow of the vertebrae is one of the primary locations for hematopoiesis, disorders affecting the blood-forming elements may adversely affect the strength of the vertebrae. Most of these disorders, when severe enough to affect vertebral strength, have other more severe and obvious systemic manifestations that bring the disorder to the attention of the physician. A complete blood count with differential can uncover a large number of these disorders including anemias and leukemias. Some disorders, such as multiple myeloma, may be more difficult to uncover and require more sophisticated testing such as plasma protein electrophoresis and urine Bence Jones proteins.

Visceral causes of thoracic pain again usually have more severe primary symptoms and signs; thus, they are not typically difficult to differentiate from musculoskeletal injuries. Myocardial infarction, pancreatitis, and cholecystitis are three of the more common visceral disorders to refer pain to the thoracic region; cardiac enzymes (serum glutamic-oxaloacetic transaminase, lactate dehydrogenase, creatine phosphokinase), serum lipase and amylase, and serum bilirubin, respectively, are routine laboratory tests that can be used to help establish the presence of these conditions.

Nonspecific tests for inflammation such as C-reactive protein and erythrocyte sedimentation rate are inexpensive and sensitive tests for the detection of inflammatory disorders. They are, however, nonspecific and susceptible to laboratory error.

Antinuclear antibody, rheumatoid factor checked by RA-latex, and human leukocyte antigen B27 are helpful when considering conditions such as lupus erythematosus, rheumatoid arthritis, Reiter's syndrome, or ankylosing spondylitis. These tests are expensive when compared with nonspecific tests for inflammation, and although more specific, they are far from pathognomonic. They are most useful when there is a strong clinical suspicion of these disorders.

Infections causing osteomyelitis and discitis or infections in the soft tissues in the areas contiguous to the dorsal spine when well contained may show no positive laboratory findings. Tests that are done are usually directed at detecting the antibody response to these infections. The fault with this type of test is that its result can remain positive long after the disease has been eradicated.

The scope of this chapter does not permit a more detailed discussion of laboratory medicine. The interested reader is referred to standard laboratory medicine texts.

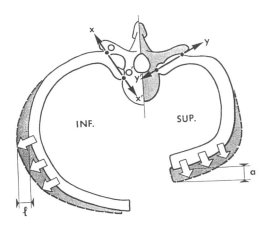

Figure 8.4. Difference in movement of superior (SUP) and inferior (INF) ribs. From Kapandji IA: The Physiology of the Joints, 2nd ed, volume 3: the trunk and the vertebral column. New York, Churchill Livingstone, 1974.

significantly curtailed by the intimate connection of the thoracic spine to the thoracic cage, the intervertebral disc, and by strong check ligaments.

The costovertebral joints and costotransverse joints are both synovial joints with surrounding capsules. A line drawn between the costotransverse and costovertebral joints defines the axis of rotation of the ribs. Superiorly this axis is more in the frontal plane and inferiorly more in the sagittal plane. Consequently, upper ribs move in an anterior-posterior (AP) fashion and lower ribs move medial to lateral, with the middle region being a mixture of the two motions (Fig. 8.4).

HISTORY OF THE INJURY

Contusions and muscle strains occur most commonly in the thoracic spine, whereas fractures, dislocations, sprained ligaments, and herniated discs occur much less commonly (6). The physician must be alert for other disorders, such as neoplastic diseases of the thoracic spine, that also must be considered in the differential diagnosis of the athlete, just as one would with a nonathletic patient (7).

It is of paramount importance that the physician obtain a thorough history. The information gleaned from this history, combined with an understanding of the physical actions common to the sport in which the injured athlete participates, greatly aid in the formulation of a differential diagnosis, prognosis, and treatment plan (Table 8.1).

In obtaining a thorough history, the first questions should be directed at determining what hurts and how the injury occurred (8). It is often helpful to question a witness to the injury as the athlete may not know how it occurred or may have the wrong idea about its occurrence. An injury caused by a single event is often easier for the athlete to describe than one caused by repet-

itive trauma or overuse. In this latter case, the athlete may not be aware of an event that initiated the pain but can describe what movement causes the pain (8).

The injured athlete should be questioned about the chief complaint and its frequency, the severity of pain (graded 1 to 10), and the mode of onset (gradual versus sudden). Other questions should include any functional limitations, related symptoms, type of pain, previous injuries, and relapses to the area (8, 9).

Specific questions should be asked after obtaining the answers to the above initial questions that will help the physician in planning the examination of the injured athlete. The athlete should be asked whether the thoracic pain goes up and down between the spine and the medial border of the scapula. If so, the neck may be the source. Respiration also should be checked to note any correlation with the symptoms. Increased pain with inspiration, when the patient is seated in a trunk flexed forward position, implies a nonmusculoskeletal cause (1). The athlete should also be questioned whether the pain is radicular or nonradicular. Nonradicular pain is often caused by muscle spasm, but could also be due to bony deformities (7). Any tingling and numbness warrants careful consideration because these symptoms in the extremities of an athlete with a thoracic spine injury may suggest spinal cord trauma (5).

Because the varying types of injuries that occur to the thoracic spine of the athlete are limited, it is important to ascertain the mechanism of the injury (4). This mechanism is determined by the important question, "How did it happen?" Certain history suggests a common thoracic injury site. These mechanics and their corresponding injuries will be discussed later in this chapter.

PHYSICAL EXAMINATION OF THE THORACIC SPINE

Inspection

After obtaining a thorough history from the injured athlete, a visual inspection of the thoracic spine should be made. The examiner should note the athlete's motion, the nature of his or her stride,

Table 8.1. Information Gained from Standard History Questions

Onset (and course)
Palliative and provocative (aggravating and alleviating)
Quality
Radiation or referral
Site
Timing

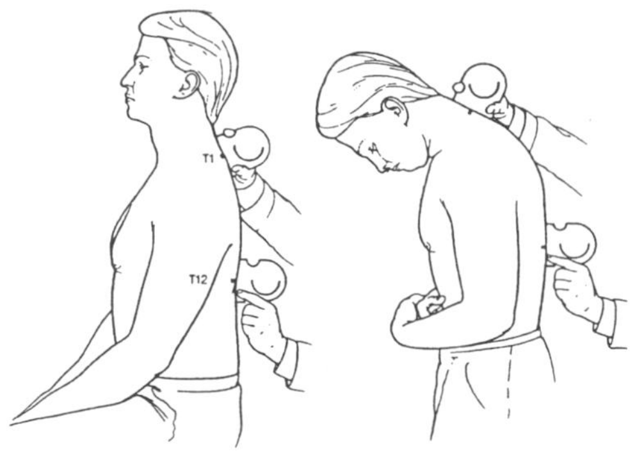

Figure 8.5. Good method of measuring active range of motion is the use of dual inclinometers or computer assisted inclinometers. AMA: Guides to the Evaluation of Permanent Impairment, 4th ed.

and any antalgic posture. (Examination of motion of activities of daily living and motions associated with the sport, e.g., the tennis stroke or throwing motion, can provide important clues.) The examiner should also check for swelling, atrophy, effusion, hypertrophy, and deformation. The epidermis and subcutaneous tissues should be inspected for wounds, swelling, edema, color, depressions, and scars (9). Observe the athlete from all sides, checking for excessive thoracic kyphosis. A long and smooth kyphosis is indicative of an adolescent postural roundback, whereas a sharply angled and rigid kyphosis presents in Scheuermann's disease (Fig. 8.5) (7).

Palpation and Percussion

Very gently palpate the area of pain first. This helps to assure the athlete that the examiner knows where the pain is located. Being gentle at this stage of the examination prevents the athlete from becoming anxious and tense. The injured area can be examined in greater detail later.

Palpate and percuss the uninjured side or the area above or below the injured site. Vary the pressure to palpate sequentially from superficial to deep structures. Palpating and percussing similar but uninjured areas lets the athlete know what to expect; this also offers both examiner and athlete a chance to contrast and compare the injured to the uninjured structures.

Because the athlete may experience pain at a point distant from the actual site of injury, it is wise to palpate potentially associated regions. For example, the source of interscapular pain frequently is found in the cervical region.

Next palpate the area of pain again using the technique described above for the uninjured side. Make sure to include the spinous processes, costovertebral joints (effusions, form, pain), muscles (tone, swelling, mobility, and crepitation), myofascial trigger points, skin (temperature, adhe-

sions, swelling, edema), and fasciae (thickening, swelling, mobility) (5, 9).

If the history indicates a potential fracture, point tenderness will often be revealed over the involved vertebrae. Percussion of the thoracic spinous processes while the patient is flexed can help elicit painful areas (5).

Ranges of Motion

Active and passive ranges of motion of the thoracic spine should be evaluated. Execute active range of motion including flexion, extension, lateral bending, and rotation, then passive range of motion in the same direction, comparing and contrasting the active and passive movements (10). Note the athlete's willingness or hesitancy to do motions. Consider the extent of motion (also evasive movements), execution of motion, noise, and pain (9). The examiner should watch how the athlete returns to the upright position. Whereas active ranges of motion are determined by the athlete, passive ranges of motion are determined by the examining physician. Information from the active and passive ranges of motion will help identify the injured area. If active and passive movements are limited and/or painful in the same direction, the injured area is most likely in noncontractile structures. Conversely, if active and passive movements are limited and/or painful in opposing direction, the injured area is probably in contractile structures. Passive movements limited in various directions suggest an injury of the joint capsule (9).

Contractile structures (muscle fibers, connective tissue components, muscle-tendon transitions, tendon insertions) can be further tested by resistance, noting amounts of pain and strength. Resistance testing can help identify the injury site (9) (Table 8.2).

Joint Testing

Joints and the intraarticular structures are tested by accessory movements such as traction and gliding (9). If fractures have been ruled out, joint dysfunction can be diagnosed accurately. Findings of localized tenderness over the dysfunctional joint or spinous process and palpation for joint play and skinfold rolling help to determine joint involvement (5). Segmental joint play can be

Table 8.2.   Resistance Testing for Contractile Structures

Pain + good strength = small muscle-tendon injury
Pain + poor strength = large muscle-tendon injury
No pain + good strength = normal condition
No pain + poor strength = neurologic defect

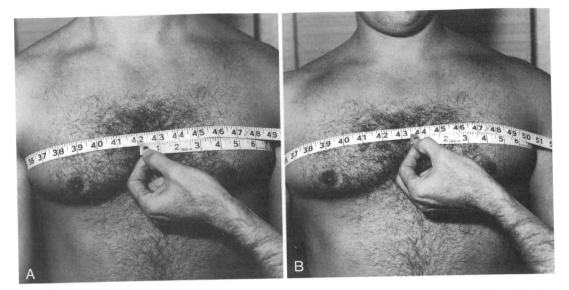

Figure 8.6. A and **B.** Chest expansion as measured at the fourth intercostal space should be greater than 2.5 cm (1 inch).

evaluated by a springing test of the transverse process with the examining doctor's thumbs (11).

Soft Tissue Testing

Soft tissue testing is also important in the evaluation; studies have shown that more than 75% of all athletic injuries are in soft tissues (9). Superficial skin palpation can evaluate temperature and skin moisture. Palpation of the musculature can evaluate tone and consistency (also painful regions). While the doctor is examining the osseous structures such as the spinous processes, transverse processes, and costovertebral angles, tenderness arising from irritation of the juxtaposed soft tissues should also be sought (11).

Orthopedic Signs and Tests

Other tests for thoracic lesions include chest expansion test, Forestier's bowstring sign, Lewin supine test, and Kernig's sign (12, 13).

The chest expansion test measures the thoracic cage during inspiration and expiration. Subnormal expansion (less than 2.5 cm) suggests thoracic fixation and is an important sign in ankylosing conditions such as ankylosing spondylitis (Fig. 8.6).

Forestier's bowstring sign consists of having the athlete stand and bend to the side. If positive, as in ankylosing spondylitis, ipsilateral tightening and contracture of the paraspinal musculature will occur (12).

For Lewin's supine test, the examining doctor stabilizes the lower trunk and the patient attempts to sit up. If the patient cannot do this, the test is positive for possible ankylosing dorsolumbar spinal lesion (12).

Kernig's sign is performed by the examining doctor passively flexing the patient's thigh to a

right angle and then attempting to extend the leg completely. If the patient is unable to do so, with the pain on the side of involvement, the sign is positive and is an indicator of meningeal irritation or possible spinal cord lesion (12, 13).

For suspected fractures of the thoracic spine, the Soto Hall test should also be done. The athlete is placed supine and his or her head is bent forward toward the chest. If local pain is produced (usually it is severe), a fracture should be suspected (12, 13).

Although the preceding tests and signs may be of some benefit, they are rarely very specific for any one disorder. However, they can be helpful in localizing injuries and in leading to new lines of diagnostic thought when they are unexpectedly present or absent. They should always be considered in light of the history and physical findings such as reflexes, sensations, muscle strength, and selective testing of passive, active, and resisted movements.

Neurologic Examination

A neurologic examination should be performed to identify possible cord injuries (14). Both deep and superficial reflexes should be tested (5). When testing sensations, it may be helpful to remember the following landmarks and their related neurologic levels: the medial forearm (T1), medial side of the upper arm (T2), medial aspect of the upper arm and the axilla to the nipple line (T3), and the umbilicus area (T10) (15).

Significant neurologic signs and tests for the thoracic spine include the abdominal reflex, Barkman's reflex, Beevor's sign, and Obliquus reflex. The abdominal reflex is tested by running a blunt-ended object along the upper and lower

COMMON THORACIC SPINE INJURIES

Contusions

Contusions to the thoracic spine occur often but are not usually serious (14). Contusions are common after blows to the back because of the many muscles that attach to the thoracic spine and the subcutaneous position of the spinous processes of the thoracic vertebrae (6). In contact sports, athletes commonly suffer from painful contusions of the lower rib cage (costochondral contusions) (16). Contusions are also common in baseball (infielders hit by errant balls) (3) and soccer (blows from another player). The most common contusion is of the muscles lateral to the spinous processes. Contusions over the bone are more common with a severe blow or a hard kick, as in soccer or martial arts (3, 10). Contusions may also cause hematomas within the muscles, but unlike muscles of the thigh, the thoracic muscles are not a common site of myositis ossificans (4).

For contusion over a spinous process, observation and gentle palpation expediently identify the area. A radiographic examination of AP and lateral views should be made to rule out a fracture (10).

For minor contusions of the thoracic spine, conservative treatment may simply consist of rest from the athletic activity until pain subsides while still participating in the athlete's conditioning program (16). If the contusion is over a spinous process, physiologic therapeutics such as cryotherapy and electrotherapy are the recommended course of treatment. It is also recommended to use a protective pad over the area when resuming athletic participation (4–10). Contusions that have caused hematomas within the muscle should be treated with cold packs for the first 24–48 hours followed by contrast therapy.

Some common complications of contusions are residual stiffness, aching, and restricted motion. These complications are best treated by heat, massage, manipulation, and exercise (7). If latent trigger points develop, vapocoolant stretch and spray therapy can be effective in eliminating them.

Deep massage and aggressive mobilization or manipulation should be delayed until acute symptoms have subsided. Inordinately aggressive early treatment will impede the healing process and may lead to excessive scar tissue formation with a poor long-term result. However, immobilization is usually not needed and is usually detrimental.

Intrathoracic Injuries

Because of the protection offered by the rib cage, intrathoracic injuries are uncommon, except for athletes participating in such sports as motocross, auto racing, and horse racing—these participants may suffer great forces in an accident (16). Contact sports such as karate can produce injuries of the thoracic viscera such as internal bleeding (from blows to the right subcostal region), splenic rupture (from heavy round house kicks to the left posterior and lower thoracic region), and lung collapse (3, 10). Treatment of these injuries is out of the conservative scope of this text.

The most common intrathoracic injury is pneumothorax, which is usually caused by rib fractures. Pneumothorax may resolve itself, but usually produces significant dyspnea; therefore, it is best treated with a referral for placement of a chest tube. Pneumothorax can be visualized on chest radiographs (16).

Rib fractures without pneumothorax occur with greater frequency in males involved in contact sports such as soccer, martial arts, and football. Symptoms are pain and difficulty with breathing. Chest examination may find splinting with a noticeable difference in respiratory excursion between the right and left sides (16). Chest radiographs (AP and lateral) should be obtained to rule out pneumothorax. Upper and lower rib views, or spot films of the involved area, may also be necessary to demonstrate the fracture. Radiographs taken shortly after the injury unfortunately show only half to two thirds of the actual number of fractures (17). The diagnosis may have to be made on clinical evidence alone, but if deemed necessary a bone scan taken 3 days or more after the time of injury will usually demonstrate increased uptake if a fracture is present.

Recommended treatment for rib fractures is withdrawal from the sport until chest pain subsides. Recovery is usually rapid. Taping is not usually recommended because it further inhibits respiration without offering protection or pain relief. Local anesthetics have been suggested by some (18) as a means of controlling pain, but they are not without risk. Injections may cause a pneumothorax. Using anesthetic injections to return an injured player to competition is extremely dangerous and shows a disregard for the athlete's safety.

Costovertebral Joint Dysfunction

Costovertebral joint injuries are usually due to compression traumas to the thorax. For example, wrestlers may suffer side-to-side compressions in takedowns, and football players may suffer chest compression falling on a ball with a player on their back. A similar injury can occur in a rugby pileup (15). Landing hard on the feet can produce flexion injuries, as in gymnastic dismounts, which also can cause joint dysfunction. Swimmers specializing in butterfly are prone to this injury when they encounter rough water during the recovery phase between strokes.

The complaints are of pain and intercostal spasms referred along the associated rib. Coughing, sneezing, and deep inspiration may be painful. Costovertebral dysfunction is easily overlooked when pain radiates along the rib because it can be mistaken for an intercostal muscle spasm (5).

Diagnosis can be accomplished by palpation from the injured joint that will elicit pain. Radiographs should be obtained to preclude more serious causes of pain (15). Treatment consists of manipulation of the costovertebral articulations. Modalities to control initial inflammation and muscle spasm such as cryotherapy, pulsed ultrasound, and interferential currents may also be helpful. Recovery is usually immediate or within 48 hours if manipulation can be performed (5).

MUSCLE SPASM (SOFT TISSUE INJURY)

Nonradicular pain in the thoracic region may be caused by muscle spasms. It is more common in the general populace than in the athlete. Diagnosis is accomplished by palpation of the soft tissue and discovery of a firm tender area (the spastic muscle) (7). Radiographs are of no use in this diagnosis. Treatment consists of limiting rotation of the trunk, heat, massage, and gentle mobilization of the spine.

For persistent symptoms over several weeks, radiographs (AP and lateral) and laboratory testing (complete blood count, urinalysis, SMA, and sedimentation rate or C-reactive protein) should be obtained to rule out occult fracture and other disease processes (7).

Strains

Thoracic strains are common in athletes. Racket sports with the sudden changes from spinal extension to flexion, exacerbated with high torque of the upper body with an attempt to return a shot, overload the attachments of the thoracic spinal muscles, resulting in strains. Martial arts athletes also frequently suffer strains. The most common strain they suffer is of the large muscles supporting the spine. These are often injured in warm-up exercises by overstretching or when an assisting athlete pushes the stretching athlete's back and chest down onto his or her legs and toward the floor (10).

Diagnosis of a strain is begun with the history of no direct trauma. Active range of motion and then passive range of motion with a search for trigger points should be performed. If pain is

Table 8.4. Classification of Strains

Grade 1	Minimal damage
Grade 2	Moderate damage—intact muscle fibers
Grade 3	Moderately severe damage—muscle fibers partially torn
Grade 4	Complete rupture

present, in the active examination particularly, a strain is most likely the cause (10).

Strains are usually classified into four grades (Table 8.4). In a grade 1 strain, there is injury to a few fibers and the muscle sheath is intact. This is usually treated with vapocoolant or ice, compression, and ultrasound. A grade 2 strain is one in which the sheath is intact but there is more bleeding in the tissues. Ice, pressure bandage, rest, and isometric contractions are recommended. In a grade 3 strain, a large area of muscle is involved and the sheath is partially torn. This is treated the same as a grade 2 strain. A grade 4 strain consists of a complete rupture. Immediate splint immobilization, ice, and elevation are recommended; emergency transport to a hospital is necessary (3).

Chronic strains are difficult to manage in sports-related cases because the athlete is usually not willing to allow sufficient time for the injury to heal before resuming athletic participation. The diagnosis of a chronic strain is also difficult unless there is a previous history of an acute strain in the area. Idiopathic fibrositis syndrome and ankylosing spondylitis should be ruled out in reaching the diagnosis (10).

To help return the athlete to participation, strapping may be used. The upper thoracic spine is difficult to protect, but the lower thoracic spine can be well protected with elastic adhesive cross-stretch tape. The strapping should be applied to limit forward and lateral flexion. As the strain improves, long-stretch tape (not as supportive) or a corset can be used (Fig. 8.7) (4).

Sprains

Sprains infrequently occur in the thoracic spine (6). Sprains do occur in power events such as shot put, where the athlete has used heavy weights in training and then uses sudden violent contraction of the back muscles in throwing. This can cause tears of the thoracic muscles from their attachment or through the muscle belly, as well as tearing of spinal ligaments (3).

The only ligament easily palpated in the thoracic spine is the supraspinous. When injured, tenderness can be elicited when this ligament is palpated along its course or at its bony attachment. If the supraspinous, interspinous, or interlaminal ligaments are sprained, extension will be pain-free but flexion of the thoracic spine will cause pain (3).

Radiographs, though to be of little help in the diagnosis of a sprain, should be obtained to rule out bone damage. A minimum of AP and lateral views should be obtained, and bending views are helpful in diagnosis of a rupture of the suprainterspinous ligaments. If the tear is complete, there will be greater separation of the affected spinous process than of the ones above and below in forward flexion. This is a rare thoracic spinal injury (3).

Sprains of recent onset should be treated with relative rest. Depending on the severity of the sprain, relative rest may vary from simple adhesive tape strapping, without lost time from sports participation, to complete immobilization.

Immobilization for prolonged periods causes scar tissue that is not well organized to withstand high degrees of stress. However, unguarded movements may cause repeated reinjuries and lead to excessive scar tissue formation or complete rupture of the damaged ligament. As a general rule, aim to keep the athlete's movements within the pain-free or almost pain-free range and increase the degree of motion as soon as pain permits.

During the acute phase, apply cryotherapy for 20 minutes (depending on how much subcutaneous fat there is) followed by a 1-hour "defrost." Continue to repeat this cycle throughout the first

48 hours. Electrical stimulation therapy such as high-volt galvanic, interferential, or microcurrent may be applied during this phase as well, but muscle contraction should be avoided.

After the first 48 to 72 hours, thermal therapies such as hot packs, short-wave diathermy, ultrasound, infrared, and whirlpool baths may be added. Gentle massage of the surrounding soft tissues can usually be added at this time also. This phase of treatment may last from a few days to a number of months. As the pain decreases, gradually add more aggressive forms of treatment such as mobilization, manipulation, and exercise.

During all phases of care, the athlete should continue to maintain his or her conditioning by exercising their noninjured parts. This is beneficial to the healing of the injury and allows for a quicker and safer return to sports participation.

A total dislocation would be very unusual in the thoracic spine (4). Emergency treatment would be to splint the area, apply ice, and prevent the athlete from moving until he or she can be transported safely to a hospital (3).

Apophyseal Joint Problems

The capsule of the apophyseal joint can tear or stretch during extreme rotation or prolonged partial rotation of the thoracic spine. The joint surfaces then move out of opposition, causing pain and spasm; there is an inability for them to glide back.

Palpation may find tenderness over the injured joint and pain increased by rotation. The athlete usually complains of pain over the injured joint and may have radiation around the corresponding dermatome (19).

Treatment by manipulation is very successful and gives rapid results. Once "set" by manipulation, the remainder of the treatment is the same as that for sprains. The athlete should allow several days of rest for the capsule to heal. Recurrence is common because of some residual laxity of the capsule (19).

Fractures

Most fractures are stable fractures such as a compression or wedge fracture of the vertebral body. Approximately 1 in 10 fractures is unstable (15), such as the fracture dislocation. This unstable fracture typically occurs at the T12/L1 junction and is caused by a flexion-rotation injury. Cord involvement is also common as the cord is larger at the T12/L1 junction because of the origin of the great nerves for the lower limbs. Because dislocation fractures are wholly unstable, they are

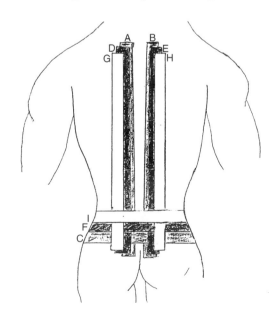

Figure 8.7. Strapping form stabilization of the lower thoracic spine. Six or more crossing strips of elastic tape should be used. Pelvic straps should extend around to the front. Elastic cross-stretch tape should be utilized, and the athlete may want to shave the area to be taped. Letters A to I indicate order of taping.

out of the scope of this conservative management text. Fractures should be suspected in falls from horseback (e.g., polo), motocross, skiing, and snowmobiling accidents. Avulsion fractures of the spinous and transverse processes have also been found to occur in the thoracic spine in power throwing events such as the shot put.

Thoracolumbar fractures can occur in various sports including snowmobiling; Nordic, Alpine, and freestyle skiing; tobogganing; and ultralight aircraft flying (20, 21). In these sports, wedge compression and burst fractures occur more often. There is one additional question to pursue with the patient with a thoracolumbar fracture: genitourinary dysfunction. This deficit is not detectable with the physical examination but can occur in patients with a thoracolumbar fracture. A careful history of genitourinary function should be obtained for a possible referral for urologic workup.

Athletes who have sustained thoracolumbar fractures also may suffer from chronic vertebral instability and complain of persistent midline back pain. To test for stability, have the athlete lie prone and apply pressure to the injured site. The pressure should reproduce the pain. Then have the athlete contract the paraspinous musculature and apply pressure again. If the pain is diminished or relieved, the test is positive and indicates instability.

The most common fracture in the thoracic spine is the compression fracture (6). The athlete will usually give a history of sharp forward flexion with a forceful fall on the buttocks. The anterior aspect of the vertebrae is compressed, and the anterosuperior corner of the vertebrae may be broken off (4, 5). If the force is directed axially up the thoracic spine, a fracture of the hyaline cartilaginous endplate of the intervertebral disc may occur. Nuclear material extruding into the body of the vertebrae may result in a Schmorl's nodule (5). Compression injuries can occur in missed falls such as in judo (8) or horseback falls. Roughly 17% of parachute jumping injuries have been found to be compression fractures of the thoracic spine (22). Snowmobiling injuries also frequently cause compression fractures (23).

Signs and symptoms of the compression fracture will include local pain, tenderness, decreased range of motion, and paravertebral muscle spasm (23).

Examination of the athlete with a suspected compression fracture should include palpation of the area of tenderness and paravertebral muscles. With the athlete supine, his or her head should be flexed forward to force the chin against the chest; this will usually elicit pain at the fracture area. Range of motion studies will usually find forward flexion to cause pain at the area of fracture (4). A neurologic examination should be done to rule out any spinal cord injury from displaced fragments (14).

Radiographs should be obtained consisting of AP, lateral, and oblique views (10). The compression fracture can be overlooked easily or missed on the initial radiograph, only becoming apparent at a later stage when the bony callus becomes visible (3, 4). Some compression fractures are relatively asymptomatic and go clinically unrecognized but can cause much pain and disability later in the athlete's life (15). Close examination of the radiographs is therefore important. Inspection of the bone appearance may reveal a fracture line or increased density due to compaction (14). The vertebrae should be measured anteriorly to determine whether a single vertebra is narrower than the others (4). Sequential radiographs may be necessary. A bone scan may be obtained 3 to 5 days after the injury. A positive technetium pyrophosphate bone scan will confirm the diagnosis (24). A magnetic resonance imaging (MRI) scan will also demonstrate the injury and is preferable to computed tomography (CT) because CT does not adequately demonstrate fractures parallel to the axial plane. An MRI will also demonstrate any ligamentous injury that CT or regular radiographs cannot (25).

Recommended treatment usually consists of some type of bracing such as the Jewett or Griswald brace and the Taylor thoracolumbar brace. Both braces use a biomechanical principle to relieve the weight on the anterior vertebral bodies and place more of the load on the posterior elements of the thoracic vertebrae (Fig. 8.8) (1).

Hyperextension exercises can be added after a period of complete rest followed in a few weeks by flexion exercises (14). Ankylosis usually develops at the injury site after healing (26).

Prolapsed Disc Lesions

Prolapsed disc lesions are not common in the thoracic spine, but when they occur they usually do so in the lower thoracic region (24) or at the apex of a scoliosis or kyphosis (19).

Examination may find pain over the spine and related dermatome. There will be hypoalgesia if the nerve root is compressed. MRI will confirm the diagnosis; MRI is superior to CT in clarifying multiple levels of abnormality (27).

Treatment may include rest and later exercise to build the paraspinal muscles. Because of the potential for serious neurologic damage (spinal cord), a neurosurgical consultation is recommended.

A complete herniation with spinal cord compression may cause symptoms ranging from in-

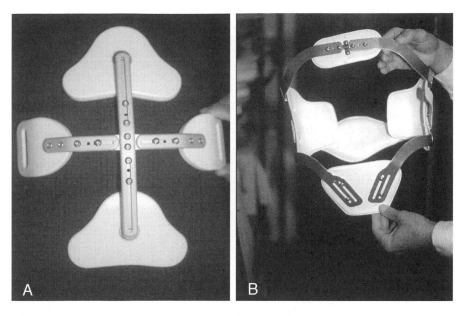

Figure 8.8. Two examples of hyperextension braces that can be used in the treatment of thoracic compression fractures. **(A)** Cruciform brace, **(B)** Jewett brace.

tercostal pain to severe spastic paraparesis. Diagnostic procedures should include CT scan, myclography, and nuclear resonance. Referral should be made for possible surgical intervention (28).

SCOLIOSIS

Although scoliosis is not traumatically induced by a sports-related injury, scoliosis can affect an athlete's performance and his or her ability to participate in a sport (24). Certain sports, such as power canoeing, can promote a scoliotic condition. Paddling on one side of the canoe exclusively can cause the thoracic musculature to develop asymmetrically, shortening on the paddling side and becoming lax on the opposite side (3). If scoliosis is caught early and treated, it will not restrict the athlete's participation. Seventy percent of cases are idiopathic and occur 8 times more often in female athletes than in male athletes (14, 24).

Evaluation of the patient should include questions of the age at onset, family history, developmental history (rapid growth etc.), and symptoms such as fatigue and pain. Examination visually should include a check of shoulder level, elbow height, and waist symmetry (15). Assessment of the curve should include range of motion, degree of flexibility or rigidity, and radiographic evaluation (14). Radiographic evaluation should include AP and lateral views of the thoracic spine and a left hand and wrist in the adolescent for determination of boneage appropriate to chronologic age (15). The curve is then measured and graded us-

ing the Cobb method (14, 15). Regular reexaminations approximately every 3 months are necessary to follow the evolving scoliosis.

There are general suggested guidelines for athletic participation with scoliosis. Athletes with scoliosis of 20° or more should avoid contact sports. Adolescents with up to 30° of curvature should participate in noncontact sports. Weight training should be restricted to lifting 10–15% of body weight or bench pressing no more than 50% of body weight (15).

Treatment should include manipulation and physiologic therapeutics, exercise, and stretching. Referral for surgical consultation is necessary for rapidly progressing cases, curves greater than 45° in adolescents, and decreased cardiopulmonary function (14).

SCHEUERMANN'S DISEASE

Scheuermann's disease (juvenile epiphysitis or spinal osteochondrosis) strikes roughly 30% of the general adult population. There is a disruption of the vertebral growth plate causing irregular transition of cartilage to bone. This results in wedging of a number of the thoracic vertebrae (5). It is most common in young males aged 10 to 25 years (15). Studies have found a much higher incidence of Scheuermann's disease in trampolinists, rowers, and gymnasts. The growing tissues of the adolescent are sensitive to mechanical stress such as those that occur in gymnastics, trampoline, high diving, wrestling, and canoeing (9, 29). Weight training and long distance running also impose excessive stress or

there may be a postural precipitant such as riding a racing bike with low-set handlebars (19).

The young athlete may present with a round back deformity (24). The athlete usually complains of localized interscapular or lower thoracic pain, aggravated by sitting, standing, or bending (7). In the acute stage, pain is not relieved by lying down (19). Palpation usually finds tenderness over the thoracic spine and interspinous ligaments with marked muscle spasm.

Radiographic evaluation will show thoracic vertebral wedging (a minimum of three is needed for diagnosis of Scheuermann's (24)) anteriorly greater than 5°; sometimes the vertebral endplates are irregular (7). Radiographs may be negative initially but after several weeks, changes can be seen with fragmentation of the epiphyseal ring or wedging. A technetium scan will reveal a hot patch over the involved vertebrae (19).

Minor laboratory testing should include a complete blood count to exclude other conditions, such as infection or tumor, in reaching the Scheuermann's diagnosis (19).

Treatment should consist of manipulation and mobilization and rest. As pain subsides, strengthening exercises should be begun; exacerbating movements that accentuate rounding of the back should be avoided (15). Flexibility exercises for the thoracic spine are also helpful (30). Usually, the pain takes several weeks to subside but often recurs. Generally, the young athlete should avoid participation in his or her sport (except swimming) for approximately 6 months (19). If a severe deformity has developed, a hyperextension brace may be necessary during the adolescent's remaining growth years.

FEMALE ATHLETES

Unusually large breasts can put a strain on the spine, leading to thoracic discomfort or pain. It is recommended that female athletes with this situation use supportive sports bras. If breast size interferes with the athlete's ability to compete comfortably, she may want to consider breast-reduction surgery.

For a more complete discussion of problems specifically affecting the female athlete, the reader is referred to Chapter 17.

References

1. Gould JA, Davies GJ. Orthopedic and sports physical therapy. St. Louis: C.V. Mosby, 1986:32–33.
2. White A. Analysis of the mechanics of the thoracic spine in man. Acta Orthop Scand 1969: 11–93.
3. Reilly T. Sports fitness and sports injuries. London: Faber and Faber, 1981:107–108.
4. O'Donahue DH. Treatment of injuries to athletes. Philadelphia: WB Saunders, 1984:89–92.
5. Roy S, Irvin R. Sports medicine: prevention evaluation, management and rehabilitation. Englewood Cliffs, NJ: Prentice-Hall, 1983:264–266.
6. Haycock CE. Sports medicine for the athletic female. Med Econ 1980:303–4.
7. Mellon MB. Office management of sports injuries and athletic problems. Philadelphia: Hanley and Belfus, 1988: 205–206.
8. Bernhardt D. Sports physical therapy. New York: Churchill, Livingstone, 1986:107–108, 138–140.
9. Kuprian W. Physical therapy for sports. Philadelphia: WB Saunders, 1982:12.
10. Birrer RB. Medical injuries in the martial arts. Springfield, IL: Charles C. Thomas, 1981:89–92.
11. Dvorak J, Dvorak V, Schneider W. Manual medicine. Berlin: Springer Verlag, 1984:127–170.
12. Mazion J. Illustrated manual of neurological reflexes, signs & tests: orthopedic signs, tests, & maneuvers for office procedure. Arizona: JM Mazion, 1984:30–31, 94–95, 276, 308–309, 359.
13. Schafer R. Motion palpation and chiropractic technic principles of dynamic chiropractic. Huntington Beach, CA: Motion Palpation Institute, IV:150–154.
14. Birrer RB. Sports injuries for the primary care physician. East Norwalk, CT: Appleton-Century-Crofts, 1984:15.
15. Birrer R. Common sports injuries in youngsters. Oradell, NJ: Medical Economics, 1987:6.
16. Appenzeller O, Atkinson R. Sports medicine, fitness, training & injuries, 3rd ed. Baltimore: Urban and Schwarzenberg, 1988:267–268.
17. Fam AG. Chest wall pain: if not cardiac disease, then what? part 1: pain arising from the ribs and sternum. J Musculoskeletal Med 1987;2:65–74.
18. Powell HD. Local anesthetics for the broken rib. Lancet 1980;1:1032–1033.
19. Lachmann S. Soft tissue injuries in sports. Oxford: Blackwell Scientific Publications, 1988:96–98.
20. Keene J. Thoracolumbar fractures in winter sports. Clinical orthopaedics and related research 1987;216: 39–49.
21. Zwimpfer T, Gertzbein S. Ultralight aircraft crashes: their increasing incidence and associated fractures of the thoracolumbar spine. Trauma 1987;27:431–436.
22. Petras A, Hoffman E. Roentgenographic skeletal injury patterns in parachute jumping. Am J Sports Med 1983; 11:325–328.
23. Roberts V, Noyes F, Hubbard R, et al. Biomechanics of snowmobile spine injuries. J Biomech 1971;4: 569–577.
24. Micheli L. Pediatric and adolescent sports medicine. Boston: Little, Brown & Co., 1984:110–113.
25. Goldberg AL, Rothfus WE, Deeb ZL. The impact of magnetic resonance of the diagnostic evaluation of acute cervicothoracic spinal trauma. Skeletal Radiol 1988;17:89–95.
26. Hanley E, Eskay M. Thoracic spine fractures. Orthopedics 1989;12:689–696.
27. Goldberg AL, Rothfus WE, Deeb ZL, et al. Thoracic disc herniation versus spinal metastases: optimizing diagnosis with magnetic resonance imaging. Skeletal Radiol 1988;17:423–426.
28. Greco P, Ruosi C, Mariconda M, et al. Intervertebral disc herniation at D3-4. The Italian journal of orthopedics and traumatology 1989;15;3:377–381.
29. Lehman L. Preventing and anticipating neurological injuries in sports. Am Fam Pract 1988;38:181–184.
30. Smith N. Sports medicine: a practical guide. Philadelphia: WB Saunders, 1987:111.

9

Lumbar Spine Injuries

Scott D. Banks

Sports place the spine at significant risk of injury similar to what is seen in the knee and ankle. Up to 20% of all athletic injuries involve the neck and lower back (1). A 5-year prospective study of a women's NCAA Division I gymnastics team reported that lower back injuries were the most common type of existing injury at the beginning of the study and the most common new injury during the study (2). Lower back injuries accounted for more than 15% of all new injuries during the study period. Damage to the structural components of the lumbar spine is very common in sports that involve repetitive impact or end range-of-motion loading. Examples of this observation include the 3- to 10-fold increase in the incidence of spondylolysis in athletes in several sports (3); a 2.5-fold increase in the incidence of magnetic resonance imaging (MRI) established disc degeneration in elite level gymnasts compared with age-matched control subjects (4) and an increased incidence of Schmorl's nodes and vertebral body abnormalities in gymnasts (3).

It is not yet known if these structural abnormalities associated with sports relate to a significantly increased incidence of functional impairment either during the actual time of athletic participation or in the years after retirement from a particular sport. In the evaluation of the incidence of back pain in athletes, some studies have suggested that it is no greater than in nonathletic control subjects (3, 5), whereas others have found an increased incidence (4, 6). Very little data exist on the incidence of back pain in former athletes with participation-acquired structural abnormalities of the spine. Whether structural injury to the spine affects future spinal morbidity is unknown, and there is little basis by which to counsel young athletes with back pain about returning to the associated sports activity.

The relationship between spinal biomechanical function and injury predisposition is now better understood than in the past. The future would seem to hold promise for our ability to intervene at the level of predisposing pathomechanical function to prevent some athletic injury. Any comprehensive evaluation of the injured lumbar spine should encompass traditional orthopedic and neurologic testing as well as biomechanical testing. Injury to tissue will often elicit secondary pathomechanical adaptations that may persist after the initial tissue injury has resolved, causing persistent pain and limitation of function. Reflex joint dysfunction is perhaps as common as other secondary disorders that occur as the result of trauma such as muscle weakness. Failure to identify secondary joint dysfunction may prevent resolution of lumbar spine pain or make the individual susceptible to reinjury.

LUMBAR BIOMECHANICS

The cervical and lumbar lordoses are significantly different in origin. The cervical lordosis is solely the result of lordotic wedging of the discs. The anterior disc height in the cervical spine is approximately 40% greater than the posterior (7). The vertebral bodies, however, are slightly kyphotic and thus do not contribute to lordosis (8).

The lumbar lordosis, in contrast, is due to a combination of wedging of the discs and vertebral bodies in the lower lumbar spine (7, 8). It is the lordotic shape of the lumbar vertebrae that make them at risk of bony injury to the neural arch during extension loading. The lordotic attitude of the lower lumbar spine is thought to counteract the high anterior shear forces inherent to this region because of the tilt of the lumbosacral junction. However, this same anatomical relationship that helps to counteract load in flexed postures may actually be a detriment in extension postures. In the transition area from the lower to upper lumbar spine, the vertebral bodies lose this wedging and are actually kyphotic in the upper lumbar spine (8–10). Any lordosis in this area is then the result of persistent lordotic wedging of the discs.

A large amount of variation in this pattern exists, and certain patterns of variation seem to predispose to specific low back dysfunction. Although most discussion of lumbar posture and back pain emphasizes the assumed relationship between increased lumbar lordosis and pain, this relationship is not well established and may be relatively rare. More recent data suggest that decreased lumbar lordosis may be a more common cause of pain/injury predisposition (11–14).

Although low back pain is common in athletes, there are only a few areas in which its diagnosis or treatment is unique to athletics. With the exception of only a few sports, back pain is probably as common in nonathletes. Athletes may be afforded more protection from low back pain than nonathletes by their general physical conditioning. The epidemic of low back pain in society has been linked to poor trunk muscle strength (15–17) and poor general cardiovascular health (18), two factors that are not prevalent in athletes.

As with other lordotic areas, flexion injury to the lumbar spine usually results in soft tissue injury (disc and/or ligaments), whereas extension injury more often results in injury to bone. The general rule is that in significant or repetitive extension trauma, presume fracture until proven otherwise. The addition of axial loading to either flexion or extension is usually far more injurious than single-plane forces.

Mechanical or functional low back pain is the most common category of back pain, accounting for perhaps 80–90% of all cases. Even when specific tissue injuries or pathologies have been found, they are often not the source of ongoing pain and dysfunction (19). Many injuries or tissue deficits cause secondary pathomechanics or "secondary lesions" that may be the ongoing source of pain (19). Correcting the secondary coexisting functional lesion may return the patient to a symptom-free state despite the persistence of a demonstrable tissue lesion such as disc degeneration (19).

It is important to use a comprehensive evaluation format of the athletic lumbar spine, assessing for both tissue injury or pathology and for pathomechanical dysfunction. Although in many cases it may be possible to assign the cause or effect role to either tissue injury or pathomechanical function, evaluation and treatment should be aimed equally at both areas.

CLINICAL EVALUATION

Clinical evaluation of the lumbar spine should comprehensively evaluate tissue integrity and functional capacity. Functional capacity testing may provide information regarding the extent of the injury, such as loss of range of motion, and information regarding injury predisposition, such as muscle weakness or imbalance. In many cases, it is impossible to distinguish predisposing factors from the result of trauma. However, evaluation of functional factors serves as a good guide for the appropriate return to athletic activity.

History

History is of prime importance in the diagnosis of injury to the lumbar spine, as it is in almost all other anatomical areas. The mechanism of injury will often be the most efficient guide to an orderly progression of diagnostic testing. An in-depth understanding of the mechanics of stresses to the lumbar spine in various sports is important in establishing mechanism of injury, particularly in "overuse" or repetitive stress injuries in which a single inciting event is not known.

Because the center of sagittal plane rotation of the lumbar spine is in the posterior portion of the disc, flexion trauma must be looked at much differently than extension trauma. Flexion of the lumbar spinal segments causes significant distractive force on the soft tissues of the posterior motor unit or neural arch, or of the posterior disc anulus before bone apposition of the vertebral bodies can occur anteriorly. Significant flexion trauma should elicit suspicion of posterior soft tissue or disc anulus injury. Suspicion of vertebral body bony injury should increase if flexion is combined with axial compression.

During spinal extension, there is early bone apposition in the neural arch, and this mechanism of trauma should begin an orderly process of investigation of bone injury to the neural arch, particularly the pars interarticularis. In approximately one third of individuals, maximum physiologic extension causes direct contact to the superior surface of the pars interarticularis by the inferior facet tip of the cephalad vertebra (20). Because this contact occurs within maximum physiologic extension, sports involving repetitive maximum extension cause repeated bony stress to the pars. Stress fractures of the neural arch in sports involving repetitive extension loading of the lumbar spine are well documented (21–24). In the other two thirds of individuals, physiologic lumbar extension is limited by imbrication of the spinous processes on the interspinous ligament (20) and can be a source of back pain of soft tissue origin.

Examination

Examination of the lumbar spine, pelvis, and lower extremities should encompass an orderly progression of challenging the structure and function of all components. The pelvis is included in the examination of the lumbar spine because the two areas are functionally dependent and capable of causing secondary dysfunction in each other. Associations have been drawn between the coexistence of primary lumbar spine lesions and secondary sacroiliac joint dysfunction (19) and between hip joint mobility and back pain (25). At times it is difficult to distinguish primary lesions from secondary lesions such as reflex joint dysfunction. All lesions should be assessed; a therapeutic program to return an athlete to full functional capacity will require the correction of primary and secondary functional lesions.

Examination of the lumbar spine should encompass orthopedic, neurologic, and biomechanical/functional testing. The considerable overlap between these areas in the lumbar spine makes it impractical to discuss them as unique entities. Failing to look at the total structural and functional entity of the lumbar spine concurrently has perhaps been a significant factor in the lack of practical diagnostic and therapeutic programs for disorders involving this area. Failing to integrate orthopedic, neurologic, and biomechanical factors in examination may lead to inadequate diagnosis or to an incomplete assessment of secondary factors, which may limit the restoration of full functional capacity or greatly increase reinjury risk.

Examination of the lumbopelvic complex begins with the observation of stance and gait. Lumbar spine pain may alter gait, or gait abnormalities (such as those seen in leg length inequality [LLI]) may predispose to the development of a repetitive stress back injury. Mechanical dysfunction of the sacroiliac joint has been shown to alter temporal and kinetic parameters of gait as measured on a force platform (26–28), although the ability to detect these asymmetries by observation is unproven. The author's experience with videotaped gait analysis of several thousand distance runners has been that valuable information regarding sacroiliac dysfunction can be obtained by observation of gait.

The observation of a static list or antalgia is suggestive of a lumbar disc lesion (29, 30) and should orient examination and imaging decisions in that direction. In more subtle cases, antalgia in the coronal plane may only be observed under stress (Fig. 9.1). Flexion of the spine causes increased posterior disc bulging or protrusion (31, 32) and may make small amounts of antalgia or lateral list obvious.

Observation of the static alignment of the lower extremities should also be done in the standing position. Both unilateral and bilateral abnormalities of lower extremity alignment can cause functional stress to the lumbar spine. Unilateral factors such as knee valgus or subtalar pronation may simulate the pathomechanics of LLI. Excessive bilateral subtalar pronation may

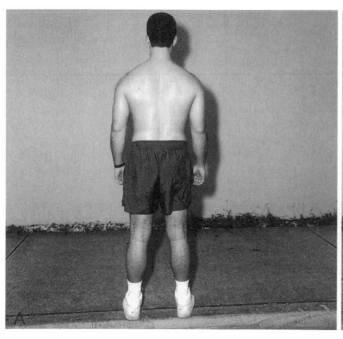 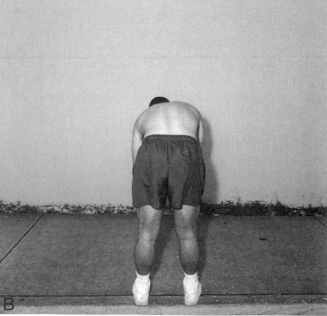

Figure 9.1. Flexion stress antalgia. **A.** Statically, antalgia is not apparent. **B.** With flexion stress, antalgia becomes more apparent.

cause insufficient shock attenuation during running sports and may be a contributing factor to lumbar spine pain.

Examination should next progress to the sitting posture. Although this is a convenient posture to examine the lower extremities neurologically, it also serves as a "stress test" to the lumbar disc. Intranuclear pressure in the lumbar discs is greatest in the sitting and flexed sitting postures (33). Small disc protrusions may only produce symptoms and objective signs while internal disc pressure is increased in this fashion. For example, the sitting straight leg raise (SLR) test for radicular pain from disc compression may be positive, whereas the more typical supine SLR test can be negative because of internal disc pressure reduction in the supine posture (Fig. 9.2). This differentiation may be particularly helpful in the common patient who only has symptoms suggestive of radiculitis with prolonged sitting.

In the sitting posture, sensory, motor, and reflex testing of the lower extremities can be performed. Neurologic innervation patterns to the lower extremities from the lumbar spine are well established and allow for an orderly assessment of impairment of sensory or motor function. Both reflex and manual muscle testing should be done to isolate motor involvement completely. For example, slight motor weakness of the L4 nerve root from a third lumbar disc protrusion may be imperceivable when testing the patellar reflex because this reflex is governed by mixed L4 and L3

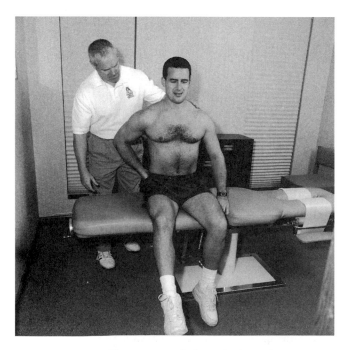

Figure 9.2. The sitting straight-leg or Bechterew's test.

innervation. However, manual testing of eversion of the foot may demonstrate this slight impairment because the peroneus muscle is entirely L4 innervated.

Sensory testing in athletes is best performed with a pinwheel. Although this has the disadvantage of being more subjective than testing contrasting sharp and dull sensation, it has the advantage of being able to elicit more subtle amounts of sensory alteration. Athletes are usually well motivated to return to activity, and the concern about malingering or exaggeration that is required in examining nonathletes in third-party claims is usually unimportant. Pinwheel testing should be done by comparing the degree of sensation between different dermatomes on the involved leg and between the same dermatome on the uninvolved leg. This allows for the detection of mild sensory impairment and yet is fairly objective if responses correlate. A comprehensive understanding of the innervation of the lower extremity is of great clinical utility in assessment of lumbar spine disorders.

Examination should proceed to the supine posture. The SLR test is performed both on the uninvolved leg and involved leg if radicular complaints exist. The position at which the test is positive should be recorded because it may reflect the extent of nerve root compression and serve as a reference point for monitoring clinical improvement, since the degree of limitation of SLR has been shown to correlate directly to the size of the protrusion (34). The exact site of pain should be recorded, as the distribution of pain with SLR has been shown to correlate with the surgical location of the disc approximately 88% of the time (34). Central protrusions usually cause back pain only during SLR, whereas lateral protrusions tend to cause only radicular pain. Intermediate protrusions tend to cause radicular and back pain (34). The prognosis of the conservative treatment of disc protrusion has been shown to vary with the relative position of the disc to the nerve root (35). A positive well leg raise test or contralateral SLR test is highly suggestive of significant disc protrusion or prolapse (Fig. 9.3) (30, 36).

Because the SLR test is basically a root traction test for the lower lumbar nerve roots that become distal in the sciatic nerve, the test can be reinforced by other maneuvers that increase root tension, such as flexion of the cervical spine and dorsiflexion of the foot during SLR (Fig. 9.4). These reinforcements may be most helpful in cases in which the SLR test produces back pain only and doubt of its radicular sig-

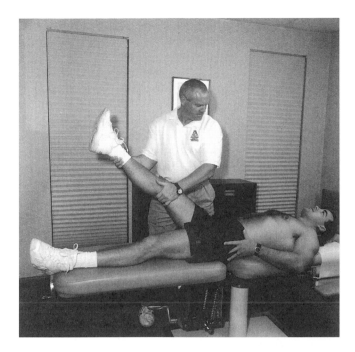

Figure 9.3. The well leg raise test. Raising the uninvolved leg reproduces radicular pain in the involved leg.

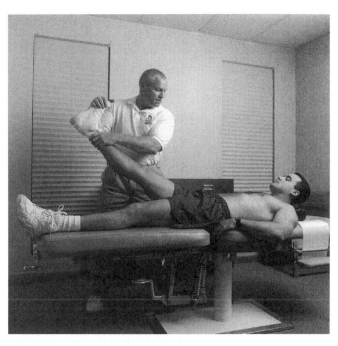

Figure 9.4. Reinforcement of the straight-leg raise test. Straight leg raise reinforced with flexion of the cervical spine and with dorsiflexion of the foot.

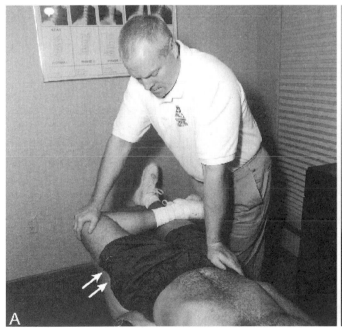
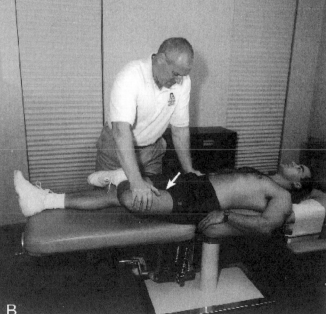

Figure 9.5. Pain referral patterns during the Fabère test. **A.** Pattern from sacroiliac joint pain. **B.** Pattern from hip joint pain.

nificance exists. If SLR produces back pain only, its increase by reinforcing maneuvers suggests root tension.

The Fabère test—which includes abduction, external rotation, and extension of the hip joint—is an important part of the lumbar spine examination because of the overlapping pain referral patterns of the hip joint and lumbopelvic complex. Perhaps the greatest difficulty is in dif-

ferentiating between sacroiliac pain and hip joint pain. Although both areas are stressed by the Fabère test, the area of pain referral is often different. The hip usually refers pain to the groin and medial thigh; sacroiliac pain is most often perceived as in the buttock (Fig. 9.5). If there is any question after the Fabère test, the hip joint can be stressed by maximal internal rotation of the leg. This produces very little stress to the sacroiliac joint but stresses the hip joint capsule early because of the orientation of the capsular ligaments (Fig. 9.6).

The anterior spine can also be palpated in the supine position, although the ability to produce information with this procedure varies with the size and muscle mass of the patient. Approximately one in three peripheral disc herniations of the spine has been found to be anterior (37), and palpation for segmental tenderness may be most appropriate through the abdomen.

The prone position is the most appropriate position to palpate the spine for segmental tenderness. The entire posterior motor unit is seg-mentally innervated by the dorsal ramus (38). Referred tenderness is usually present throughout the posterior motor unit when any of the bony or soft tissues are injured. There is probably an overlap in dorsal ramus innervation to atleast one caudal and cephalad level (38), but maximal tenderness to palpation is usually felt at the level of injury. Although palpation of the lumbar spine may be segmentally specific, it is not tissue-specific because of shared innervation throughout the posterior motor unit. Deep palpation of the spine may produce only local tenderness or may reproduce referred pain patterns.

The palpation of intersegmental motion and motion palpation may be performed standing or seated, but is discussed here for continuity. Although motion palpation of the lumbopelvic com-

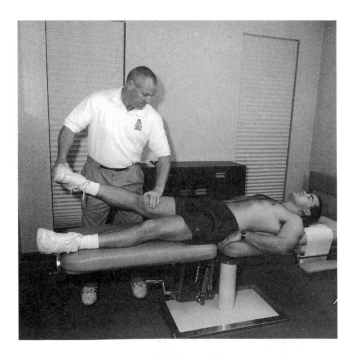

Figure 9.6. Internal rotation of the hip to differentiate true hip joint pain from sacroiliac joint pain.

plex has not been proven to have high interexaminer reliability in research trials, this procedure seems to be valuable in assessing joint dysfunction. The use of motion palpation of the lumbar spine to assess primary or secondary joint dysfunction is being advocated by many researchers and clinicians (19, 39–41). The increased emphasis on the functional nature of a large percentage of back pain, and the understanding that the common dysfunction is that of a painful restriction of motion (42), suggest that intersegmental motion analysis should be a routine part of examination of the lumbar spine. Motion palpation is a clinical procedure requiring a considerable amount of study and practice, and those aware of the importance of this type of analysis to a comprehensive evaluation of the lumbar spine and pelvis will want to read a comprehensive text or participate in an instructional course on this subject.

The presence of muscle spasm is also evaluated in the prone position. The concept of generalized spasm of the back muscles is questioned by electromyography (EMG) (43–46) and newer understanding of the muscle innervation of the back. The primary back extensors are the more superficial muscles and are multisegmentally innervated (47, 48). The ability of segmental pain stimulus to cause "spasm" of this multisegmentally innervated muscle group is questioned. The multifidus muscle, in contrast, is unisegmentally innervated and probably has the clinical ability to react to segmental injury by "spasm" (47–49). Limited study with insertional EMG has shown multifidus to be overactive in response to segmental joint dysfunction, and normalization of this activity has occurred with treatment (49). The ability to palpate spasm accurately in the segmental multifidus muscle has not been tested. Diffuse lumbar muscle spasm probably does not occur, and the failure to observe or palpate such spasm may reflect the selection of the muscle group examined rather than the presence of "spasm." Innovations in the area of detecting "spasm" may come in the area of EMG monitoring of posture and movement. Evaluation of EMG monitoring in various postures and during movement has demonstrated that increased and asymmetric EMG activity does occur in back pain subjects versus control subjects (44, 45, 50). The concept of palpation of segmental spasm during motion palpation seems logical, although this procedure is untested in research trials.

The heel to buttock test is also performed prone. The lower leg is flexed on the thigh. At the end of knee flexion, the sacroiliac joint and lower

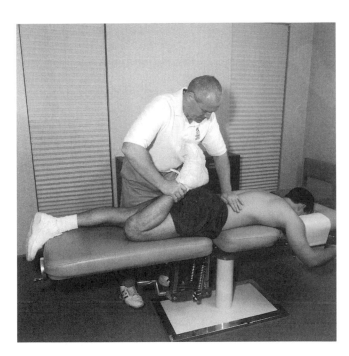

Figure 9.7. Heel to buttock test.

spine are extended (Fig. 9.7). Any lesion such as a facet or bony pars injury may be stressed by this maneuver. Although the test is not site specific, the exact location of the pain during the test may help localize the lesion.

Standing functional examination should assess lumbar range of motion for symmetry, amounts of each motion compared with normal reference ranges, and pain reproduction with reference to direction of trunk motion. Comparison of individual motions to expected normals is probably least productive of useful clinical information, whereas pain reproduction during loading in a specific plane is probably the most helpful in diagnosis. Normal range of motion of the lumbar spine has been shown to vary widely based on factors such as age, sex, and weight, making it difficult to perceive individual differences attributed to spine dysfunction (51). Generally, posterior motor unit pain such as that with facet disorders, is increased with lumbar extension as this motion loads the involved structures (12, 52). The facet joint structures appear to be oriented to restrict primarily the high anterior shear and rotational loads inherent to the lumbar spine and less adapted to resist extension loading (53). Extension of the spine causes significant loading of the bony and soft tissue structures of the posterior motor unit (54). The physiologic range of lumbar extension is 30° but may be normally more in flexible athletes. Restriction by pain is indicative of pain within the posterior motor unit.

The anterior motor unit, especially the intervertebral disc, is loaded in flexion. Flexion produces a posterior shift in the disc nucleus (27) and increased nerve root compression in disc protrusion (31), which is consistent with the clinical finding of increased symptoms during this loading. Lateral bending and rotation have the advantage over flexion and extension of being able to compare side-to-side symmetry. Restriction of lateral bending and rotation has been shown to correlate more closely with the presence of low back pain than do other lumbar spine movements (55). The combination of these movements with extension, or the Kemp's test, can be used to assess symmetry of side-to-side movement and thus the presence of joint dysfunction. A similar assessment of this motion can be done with lateral bending radiographs and has been correlated to the correction of joint dysfunction in those with back pain (56). The Kemp's test may also be useful in reproducing the radicular pain in disc protrusion and has been suggested as able to determine the medial or lateral position of the protrusion relative to the nerve root (57). Reproduction of radicular pain with the Kemp's test to the side of pain is thought to indicate that the disc is lateral to the nerve root. Reproduction with the test to the side away from the radicular pain is thought to indicate a protrusion medial to the nerve root (Fig. 9.8) (57).

Standing trunk flexion will also allow for the observation or palpation of the flexion relaxation response in the paraspinal musculature. During normal flexion of the trunk, the spine flexes to its physiologic limit during the first two thirds of total trunk flexion. It is believed that as the spine "senses" this limit, at which point it is "hanging" from the posterior spine ligaments, eccentric contraction of the back extensor muscles to control the rate of spinal flexion is no longer necessary. At this point, the paraspinal muscles relax and trunk flexion from approximately 60–80° to that of full trunk flexion at approximately 100° occurs by flexion of the pelvis under eccentric control of the hamstring muscles (58). Back pain is known to abort or negate this flexion relaxation response (58, 59). Although clinical trials have not examined the ability of palpation to detect this muscular relaxation, it is the author's experience that this is a clinically useful procedure.

In the standing position, the relative motion of the sacroiliac joints may be assessed. Sacroiliac syndrome, or a painful mechanical restriction of the sacroiliac joint, may be one of the most overlooked primary causes or secondary perpetuating causes of back pain (19, 60–62). In a large case observation study of almost 1300 patients, Bernard and Kirkaldy-Willis found that sacroiliac syndrome occurred as a primary or secondary diagnosis in approximately 1 in 4 patients, being the most common condition found of the 23 causes of back pain examined (19).

Motion palpation of the sacroiliac joint is performed by palpating points on the sacrum and pelvis, usually the posterior superior iliac spine (PSIS) and the second sacral tubercle, while the patient flexes the thigh and thus hemipelvis on the trunk (Fig. 9.9). Although most of this motion occurs through flexion of the hip joint, a small but significant amount of motion occurs through extension rotation of the hemipelvis at the sacroiliac joint (63). As the ilium extends, the PSIS should move inferiorly in relation to the sacral tubercle. Side-to-side asymmetry of this motion is readily visible during this maneuver.

This basic examination will provide the examiner with a good understanding of the location, tissue source, and nature of back and referred pain in the athletic patient. The examiner should be familiar with several additional reinforcing examination procedures for each phase of the examination. Areas of positive findings should be examined in more depth to formulate an orderly progression of diagnostic testing such as imaging or the appropriate initiation of treatment.

DIAGNOSTIC IMAGING

Diagnostic imaging of the lumbopelvic complex should be an orderly process guided by the results of a comprehensive history and examination. Imaging is often used as a more preliminary tool; this is probably a very inefficient mode of operation regarding the lumbar spine. Back pain has been found to be the most common symptom in general clinical practice for which radiographs are ordered (64), yet their yield of useful diagnostic information that will have a significant impact on treatment is questioned (64–67). This is not to say that radiographs or diagnostic imaging as a whole are not valuable in the evaluation of the lumbar spine and pelvis, but rather that an appropriate and logical

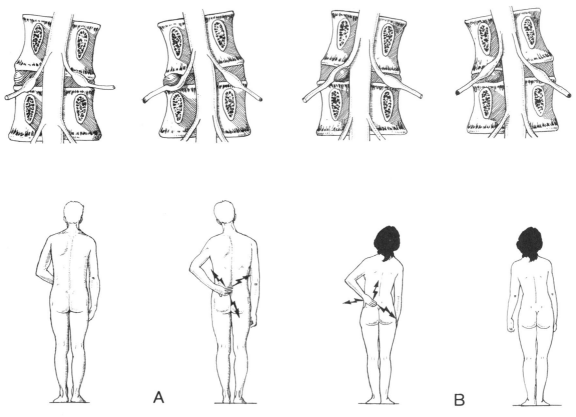

Figure 9.8. Kemp's test. **Left Two Figures.** Rotation and lateral bending to the side of leg pain may reproduce radicular pain if the disc protrusion is lateral to the nerve root. **Right Two Figures.** Rotation and lateral bending away from the side of leg pain may reproduce radicular pain if the disc protrusion is medial to the nerve root. (Adapted from White AA, Panjabl MM. Clinical biomechanics of the spine. Philadelphia: JB Lippincott, 1972.)

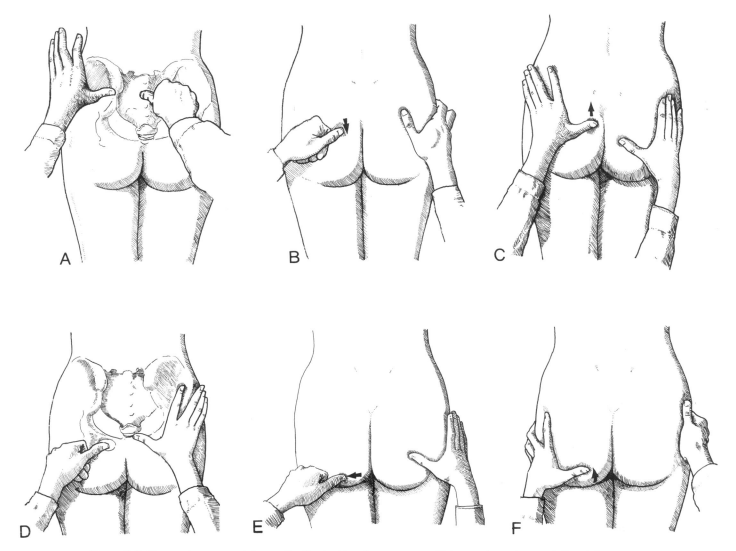

Figure 9.9. Tests to demonstrate left sacroiliac fixation. Tests for upper part of joint are shown in parts A, B, and C; tests for lower part of joint are shown in parts D, E, and F. **A.** The examiner places the left thumb on the posterior superior iliac spine and right thumb over one of the sacral spinous processes. **B.** When movement is normal, the examiner's left thumb moves downward as the patient raises the left leg. **C.** When the joint is fixed, the examiner's left thumb moves upward as the patient raises the left leg. **D.** The examiner places the left thumb over the ischial tuberosity and the right thumb over the apex of the sacrum. **E.** When movement is normal, the examiner's left thumb moves laterally as the patient raises the left leg. **F.** When the joint is fixed, the examiner's left thumb moves slightly upward as the patient raises the left leg.

decision-making process regarding this type of testing is important.

Several imaging tools, such as radiology, scintigraphy, computed tomography (CT), and MRI scanning, are useful in evaluating the injured lumbar spine. Each test is more suited to studying particular tissues and pathologic processes. It is important that the use of diagnostic imaging be guided by history and clinical evaluation, and the limitations of each procedure be weighed in making a final diagnosis. The high incidence of structural abnormalities such as disc degeneration or spondylolysis in asymptomatic persons requires that careful correlation between imaging and clinical evaluation be used to prevent inappropriate treatment.

SPINAL INJURIES

Spinal injury in sports may occur from a single supramaximal stress or from repeated submaximal stress. Both types of injuries are common and usually associated with a specific mechanism of injury. Understanding the mechanism of injury is important in diagnosis because of the limitations in actually "viewing" injured tissue or function. Distinguishing the mechanism of injury from the biomechanics or pathomechanics of a particular sport is often one of the most helpful diagnostic tools.

For the purpose of understanding and categorization, it is useful to study sports injuries to the lumbar spine in terms of their mechanism of causation. This will usually correlate with the mechanism of stress that must be placed on the tissue involved to reproduce symptoms during clinical testing. Generally, pain stimulus can be broken down into two general categories: that arising from the posterior motor unit and that arising from the anterior motor unit (Fig. 9.10). The bone and soft tissue structures of the anterior motor unit are innervated by the sinuvertebral nerve and its branches that originate from both the ventral ramus of the spinal nerve root and the sympathetic trunk (64). They have the ability to cause local segmental pain, to refer pain through segmental neural connections or through the lumbar sympathetic nerve distribution, and to cause secondary dysfunction in the posterior motor unit that may refer pain through the dorsal ramus neural system.

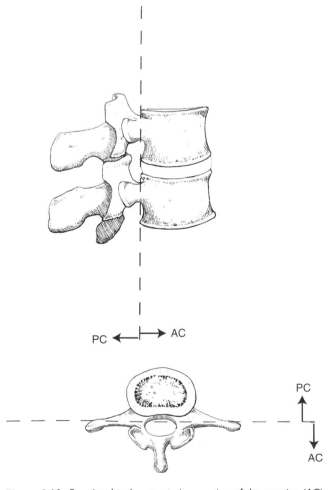

Figure 9.10. Functional and anatomical separation of the anterior (AC) and posterior (PC) compartments of the vertebral motor unit. The division occurs just posterior to the posterior longitudinal ligament. Structures in the anterior compartment are innervated by the sinuvertebral nerve and projections from the sympathetic trunk. Structures in the posterior compartment are innervated by the dorsal ramus.

Anterior Compartment Injuries

The major functional structure in the anterior motor unit is the intervertebral disc. The disc is responsible for the combination of high–load-bearing characteristics of the lumbar spine along with the high mobility inherent to this area. The disc, when injured, is perhaps the most common source of anterior motor unit pain. The complexity of diagnosis of the vertebral motor unit comes from the functional codependence of the anterior and posterior motor units. Tissue injury in one may cause pathomechanics in the other, which then becomes the site of pain perpetuation. An example of this is disc protrusion. Studies imaging the anatomical lesion in disc protrusion found that the tissue injury or the protrusion persists after symptomatic resolution of pain with treatment (65–67). This suggests that other factors, such as secondary mechanical joint dysfunction, must often occur concurrently with disc protrusion to produce the acute symptomatic state (19). It has been further suggested that the persistence of the secondary mechanical joint dysfunction following disc injury causes eccentric motion of the vertebral motor unit as a whole and will lead to subsequent reinjury (68).

INTERVERTEBRAL DISC INJURY

It is difficult to estimate the frequency of injury to the intervertebral disc in sports because of the atypical presentation of disc injuries in some athletes (69) and because of the coexistence of disc injuries with other lesions that, when treated, may lead to symptomatic resolution and an end to the diagnostic evaluation. Day et al. confirmed 12 cases of disc protrusion in one college football team in 4 years (69). This suggests a relatively high incidence given the small numbers of players studied.

Disc injuries may be peripheral or central, involving the peripheral disc margin or the adjacent vertebral endplate, respectively. In peripheral disc anulus injuries, protrusion may be either posterior or anterior with the intervertebral foramen (IVF) as the boundary (Fig. 9.11). Disc protrusion classically is diagnosed by the presence and location of involvement of the adjacent nerve root. It should be remembered, however, that peripheral protrusions anterior to the intervertebral foramen and central protrusions into the vertebral endplate will not involve the nerve root. These types cause a clinical picture similar to several other types of mechanical back pain, with local pain and referred rather than radicular pain to the lower extremity. The referred pain patterns

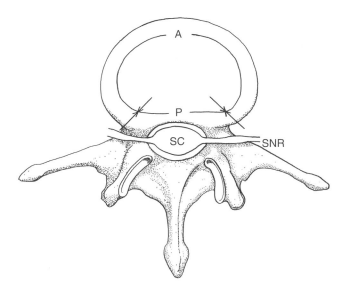

Figure 9.11. Anterior (A) versus posterior (P) disc herniation. SC: spinal cord; SNR: spinal nerve root.

The signs and symptoms of disc injury are broken into two categories: mechanical and neurologic. The presence of signs and symptoms in both categories makes the diagnosis more obvious when nerve root involvement is not present. Neurologic symptoms typically include pain, paresthesia, and burning confined to the neurologic level of involvement. Sensory dermatomes are well known and specific. Because the nerve root that passes over the posterolateral portion of the disc exits through the next caudal intervertebral foramen, specific nerve root symptoms usually indicate protrusion of the next cephalad numbered disc (Table 9.1). For example, an L4 disc protrusion will usually involve the L5 nerve root. Symptoms may be intermittent and present only with flexion stress such as bending or sitting. In their study of college football players, Day et al. found clear dermatomal pain patterns to be rare (69). Most players had proximal leg pain pat-

not corresponding to a particular nerve root are thought to originate from the afferent fibers in the disc anulus that enter the spinal cord through the sinuvertebral nerve and sympathetic trunk connections (37). The disc afferents that enter the cord through the sinuvertebral/sympathetic connections do so at only two levels: S2 and L2 (37). The upper lumbar disc afferents travel in the sympathetic trunk to the L2 level before entering the cord, and the lower lumbar disc afferents descend the sympathetic trunk to enter the cauda equina at the S2 level (37). Pain referred from the disc anulus at a lower lumbar level will tend to have sympathetic characteristics such as vasomotor, sudomotor, and pilomotor characteristics, and will refer into the S2 distribution (Fig. 9.12). Another unique component of disc pain referred through these neural mechanisms is that it is often bilateral (37). A large number of the afferents from the disc anulus entering the cauda equina decussate before synapsing. The synapses to both sides of the cord give the disc anulus the ability to refer pain to both lower extremities.

High suspicion of a protruded disc not involving the spinal nerve root should be elicited by an athlete with mechanical examination signs suggestive of a disc injury and a referred pain pattern of burning pain, paresthesia, and autonomic signs confined to the back of the buttocks and thigh corresponding to the S2 dermatome either unilaterally or bilaterally. Similarly, these symptoms referred to the lateral and anterior thigh above the knee should raise suspicion of an upper lumbar disc anulus lesion.

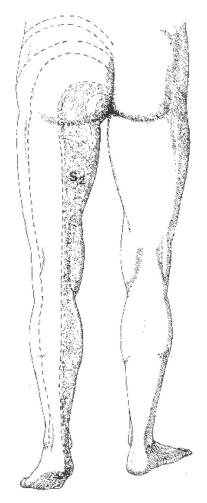

Figure 9.12. The S2 dermatome. Anterior disc herniation at all lower lumbar levels may refer pain into this distribution as the sympathetic disc anulus afferents from L3 down all enter the spinal nerve root at S2.

Table 9.1. Disk Protrusion Level Versus Nerve Root Involvement

Root	Disc	Muscles	Reflex	Sensation	EMG	Myelogram
L4	L3–L4	Tibialis anterior	Patellar	Medial leg	Fibrillation or sharp waves in tibialis anterior	Bulge in spinal cord adjacent to L3–L4
L5	L4–L5	Extensor hallucis longus	None (tibialis posterior)	Lateral leg and dorsum of foot	Fibrillation or sharp waves in extensor hallucis longus[a]	Bulge in spinal cord adjacent to disc L4–L5
S1	L5–S1[b]	Peroneus longus and brevis	Achilles tendon	Lateral foot	Fibrillation or sharp waves in peroneus longus and brevis[c]	Bulge in spinal cord adjacent to disc L5–S1

EMG, electromyography.
[a]Extensor digitorum longus and brevis, medial hamstring, gluteus medius muscles.
[b]Most common level of herniation.
[c]Flexor hallucis longus, gastrocnemius, lateral hamstring, gluteus maximus muscles.

terns typically not associated with nerve root patterns (69). However, clinical signs such as root tension signs were present, as is more typical of radicular pain.

Neurologic signs should be elicited by sensory, reflex, and muscle testing of the lower extremities. Equivocal neurologic signs can be evaluated with electrodiagnostic testing. Although this testing is specific, demonstrating the nerve structure involved, it is not sensitive as significant impairment of the nerve root is necessary before abnormalities can be demonstrated. The SLR test will usually reproduce nerve root pain, and its improvement corresponds to the recovery of nerve root compression. In Day et al.'s study, SLR was invariably positive in confirmed cases of disc protrusion even when patient symptoms were nonspecific (69). Another significant neurologic sign is the Valsalva maneuver. Reproduction of leg pain while increasing intraabdominal and thus intrathecal pressure is highly suggestive of nerve root compression.

The most typical mechanical sign of disc injury is reproduction of pain in limitation of trunk flexion, although the entire range of motion may be impaired. Flexion has been shown to increase typical posterior disc protrusion (31). Antalgia or list may be present statically or occur only when the disc is stressed during flexion. Kemp's test may reproduce radicular pain or may produce back pain only. Segmental tenderness and spasm may help localize the level of involvement when nerve root signs are nonspecific. An athlete with strong mechanical indicators of disc injury should progress into imaging for the investigation of disc protrusion even in the absence of a classic radicular pattern of symptoms. This is especially true of the athlete with an absence of classic radicular symptoms but with mechanical signs of disc injury and a positive SLR test. Adhering to the older philosophy that disc injury is only suspect when classic radicular symptoms and signs are present may lead to the oversight of many disc injuries in athletes, particularly in those that participate in contact sports.

Postural radiographs may be helpful in the diagnosis of disc injury and in differentiating bony injuries. However, a high incidence of old bony injury has been found to occur in football players with established disc injuries, clouding the diagnosis (69). Postural radiographic signs of disc protrusion include a decrease in the disc angle or relative flexion of the joint (12, 13, 70), decreased sacral base angle (11–13), and decreased lumbar lordosis (Fig. 9.13) (11–13, 71). The altered intersegmental and regional postural relationships seen in disc protrusion are thought to be the result of altered segmental mechanics from displacement of the disc nucleus center and due to adaptive neurologic mechanisms such as antalgesia.

It has been suggested that a decreased or flattened sacral base angle is also predictive of an increased risk of disc injury (11). In a study of nonathletes, DeCyper (11) found that those with a decreased sacral base angle, which would decrease lordosis, had a sixfold increase in disc protrusion over the 5-year observation period. This seems logical because the lumbar lordosis compensates the forward shear and flexion stress on the disc in the neutral posture. A decreased sacral base angle and the resulting decrease in lordosis would increase the flexion stress on the posterior disc anulus.

More advanced imaging of the disc injury itself can be accomplished with CT and MRI. CT scanning has the advantage over plain radiographs and myelography of actually imaging the disc itself because of the soft tissue contrast available. Radiographs the secondarily by showing the relative postural position of the vertebral adjacent to it, and myelography only by imaging the neural deficit that results from disc protrusion.

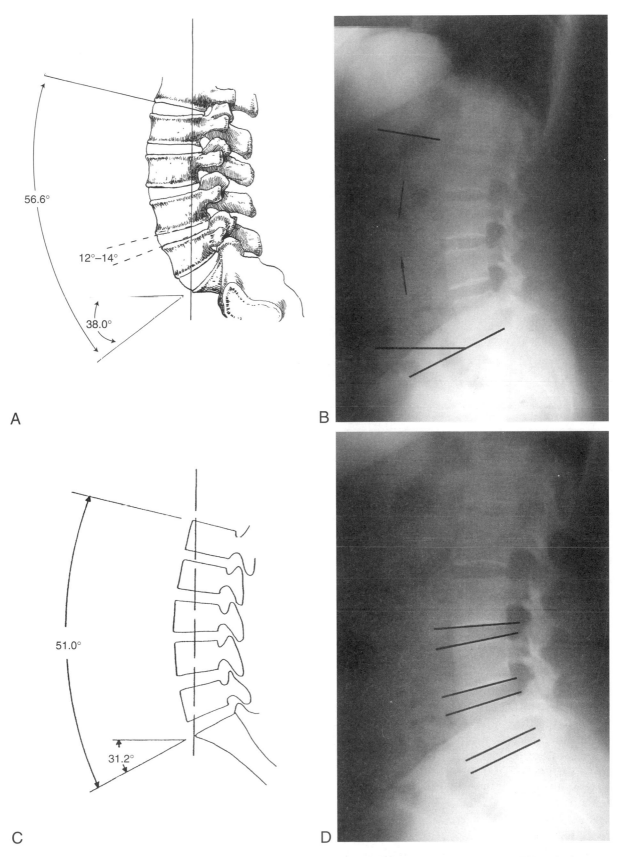

Figure 9.13. Alteration of postural parameters in disc protrusion. **A.** Normal sacral base angle, lordosis, and lower lumbar disc angles. **B** and **C.** Acute disc protrusion. Lordosis and sacral base angle reduction. **D.** Acute disc protrusion at L4. Reduction of the L4 and L5 disc angles. (C: Reprinted with permission from Banks SD. Lumbar facet syndrome. J Manipulative Physiol Ther 1983;6:179.)

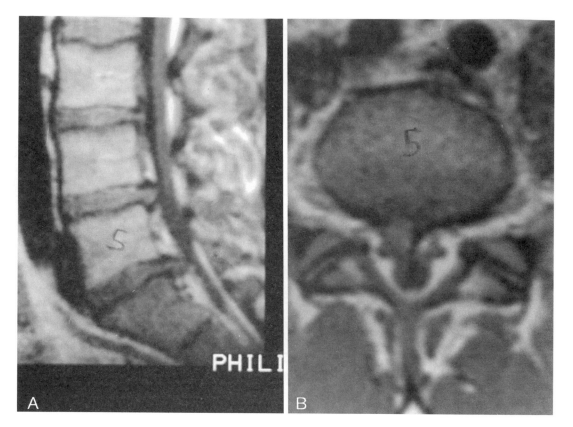

Figure 9.14. Lumbar sagittal cut MRI. **A.** Protruded disc at L4. Dark outer rim is disc anulus and posterior longitudinal ligament. Lighter area is protruded nucleus. Annular disruption at L5. Disc nucleus is degenerative—loss of water gives darker signal. **B.** Axial cut of L5 disc.

Although CT scanning is superior to plain radiographs in diagnosing disc injury, it is less sensitive and less specific than MRI (72). In a correlation of imaging with surgical findings, CT scanning was found to be 83.3% sensitive and 71.4% specific compared with 91.7% and 100% for MRI. Because CT scanning also involves significant exposure to ionizing radiation, MRI is the preferred imaging modality. MRI has the additional advantages of contrasting different water densities within the disc, making it possible to detect early disc degeneration and to differentiate nuclear from anular material (Fig. 9.14).

The treatment of lumbar disc injury varies with the initial clinical presentation. The presence of significant early motor weakness or signs of cauda equina pressure are an indication for immediate surgical decompression, and appropriate referral should be made. Conservative therapy in the absence of these signs is indicated and usually effective. Rest from the inciting activity and from movements and postures that stress the disc or increase root pain should be avoided. The use of complete rest, as in bed rest, should be avoided whenever possible. Bed rest has been shown to be of little value in most back

pain (73, 74) and has been shown to increase the time lost from activity when used for more than 2 days (75).

In a study of patients with disc prolapse, those who had resolution of the injury and those who had emergence of a chronic back and sciatic pain syndrome correlated with the respective lack of or development of a fibrinolytic defect within the disc (76). The authors of this study suggest that the possibility of the development of this fibrinolytic defect, and thus the emergence of a chronic disc syndrome, may be associated at least partially with the use of prolonged bed rest. Animal study has found that inactivity interferes with the normal metabolic pathways of the disc and increases the degenerative enzyme activity (77). The presence of significant radicular pain may be an indication for the use of bed rest, but early mobility should be encouraged in those without pronounced neurologic deficits.

The use of spinal manipulation is being advocated increasingly for lumbar disc protrusion (35, 66, 67, 78–86). The exact mechanism by which manipulation improves the acute symptomatic state associated with lumbar disc protrusion is unknown. Cox and Aspergren have suggested that manipulation actually reduces the size of the protrusion and this mechanism seems to be at least contributory (67). However, post-treatment imaging in those with symptomatic resolution of lumbar disc protrusion suggests that conservative treatment does not significantly correct the imaged tissue defect (65, 66). The reduction of secondary mechanical restriction of the facet joints, which when combined with the disc protrusion cause the symptomatic state, seems like a more feasible mechanism for the positive effects of manipulation on patients with disc protrusion. In those without signs of cauda equina compression or with significant acute neurologic deficits, manipulation is perhaps the preferred conservative treatment alternative.

Other conservative treatment modalities, such as physical therapy, can be used to augment manipulation, although the value of many of those commonly used is questioned. Trials supporting the use of electrical stimulation, back supports, conventional traction, and other common modalities are lacking (74). There is evidence, however, that the coupling of multiple physical modalities in the patient with back pain enhances the results compared with any single treatment (83).

Cauda equina compression, pronounced neurologic deficit, and progressive neurologic deficit are indications for referral for surgical consultation in lumbar disc protrusion or prolapse. Lumbar disc surgeries appear to yield no better long-term results than conservative therapy (87), result in persistent loss of physical performance, and yield a low return to athletic participation (69). Day et al. found that only two of six college football players who had undergone surgical procedures were able to return to the sport despite a good surgical result (69). They suggest that the definition of a good result typical in studies of surgical intervention in a nonathlete is insufficient in an athlete, and that only a "perfect" result will allow return to contact sports.

Full rehabilitation is important before return to sport activity following a lumbar disc injury. Dysfunctional factors such as muscle imbalance, muscle weakness, poor range of motion, and regional incoordination may occur secondary to lumbar disc injury or they can exist as a predisposing factor. Rehabilitation should emphasize flexibility, return of trunk muscle strength, and correct strength ratios. The most consistent strength abnormality found in back pain patients is weakness of the trunk extensors or a reduction in the trunk extensor/flexor ratio (16). The guidance of lumbar spine rehabilitation by trunk strength testing may prove to be one of the most significant factors regarding return to athletic competition after injury.

The other significant injury classification in the anterior motor unit is that of bony injury to the vertebral body. Injuries may involve compression fracture to the vertebral body or fracture of the end plate by herniation of the disc nucleus. Both injuries can result from a single significant flexion injury and should be part of the differential diagnosis if this mechanism of injury is known.

Posterior Compartment Injuries

The posterior compartment or motor unit begins just posterior to the posterior longitudinal ligament (Fig. 9.15). Functionally, this anatomical

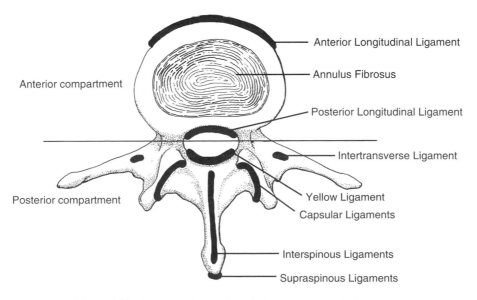

Figure 9.15. Anterior and posterior spinal compartment soft tissues.

boundary approximately separates the vertebral motor unit into anterior and posterior sections, with the center of rotation in the sagittal plane as the dividing point. Structures posterior to the center of rotation are distracted during spinal flexion, while those anterior to the center of rotation are compressed during the same movement. A single spinal movement, such as flexion, would be expected to exert different types of loads on the two functional spinal compartments.

Structurally, the posterior compartment is designed to help resist axial rotation and the high anterior shear loads on the lower lumbar spine; such stresses are inherent to an area with a significant amount of lordosis. Whereas the lower lumbar facet joints are adapted to help resist the high anterior shear stresses inherent to this area, it would appear that they are less oriented to resist extension loading. Sports that repetitively load this area in extension are known to cause a high incidence of injury to these structures.

BONY INJURIES TO THE NEURAL ARCHES

A considerable amount of study is appearing on the high incidence of injury to the bony neural arches in athletes (21–24, 88–91). The mechanism of injury appears to be direct loading of the pars interarticularis by the tip of the inferior facet of the cephalad vertebra. Yang and King have demonstrated that segmental extension is limited by this mechanism (54). Adams et al. (92) found that bony imbrication of the facet joint was the limiting mechanism in segmental extension in approximately one third of the specimens tested. The remaining specimens were limited in extension motion by imbrication of the spinous processes. Individual differences in segmental anatomy and regional posture may account for the different mechanism of extension limitation in different spines. The identification of these factors may provide the ability to predict which spine may be at risk of neural arch injury in sports involving extension loading.

At least two studies suggested that increased lumbar lordosis may be a predisposing factor to back pain in athletes in sports in which neural arch injuries are common. This suggests that increased lumbar lordosis may be a factor in neural arch injuries. Ohlen et al. (93), studying female gymnasts, found the mean lumbar lordosis to be 40.6° in female gymnasts with back pain versus 35.4° in those without back pain. Because these were surface measurements that do not account for most of the lordosis contributed by the L5 disc and vertebral body, they probably represent 15–20° less lordosis than radiographic measurement would yield. Addition of a 20° correction for L5 would suggest a lordosis of 60° in those with back pain versus 55° in those without back pain.

Ohlen et al. also found that those with greater lordosis had less lumbar extension motion (93). This suggests that the lordotic posture causes relative segmental extension in the resting posture, allowing less dynamic extension before segmental imbrication occurs.

Mahlamaki et al. also found increased lumbar lordosis in an athletic population with low back pain (94). In a group of 39 young cross-country skiers with low back pain, they found a mean radiographic lordosis of 69°. This is well in excess of studies of healthy populations. In another study of nonathletes, increased lordosis has been correlated with a high incidence of spondylolysis (95). Comparing 18 adolescents with a mean lordosis of 53° to 18 adolescents with Scheuermann's kyphosis resulting in a mean lumbar lordosis of 72°, the incidence of spondylolysis was found to be 6% versus 50%, respectively (95). Further data on this relationship may give doctors the ability to screen young athletes posturally, to steer those with a biomechanical predisposition for bony neural arch injuries away from sports known to cause considerable extension loading of the lower lumbar spine.

The diagnosis of bony neural arch injuries is made by the combined use of physical examination, radiography and scintigraphy, or bone scanning. Suspicion of neural arch injury should be high in an athlete in whom pain reproduction occurs predominantly in extension. Flexion of the spine may produce the complaint of stiffness from secondary muscle grading but is generally painless. The unilateral extension test as described by Micheli (24) can be used to locate the symptomatic side in unilateral lesions. The patient flexes one knee and then extends the spine (Fig. 9.16). This maneuver causes greater intersegmental extension on the weight-bearing leg and should be compared side to side. Approximately 50% of young athletes with positive radiographs and bone scans prove to have a unilateral lesion (88). The remainder of the physical examination findings in these patients is unremarkable, and the results of neurologic examination of the lower extremities are typically normal.

The persistence of back pain with conservative treatment in an athlete in a sport involving extension loading, and an examination that reproduces pain primarily in extension, are indications for imaging. Postural radiographs, includ-

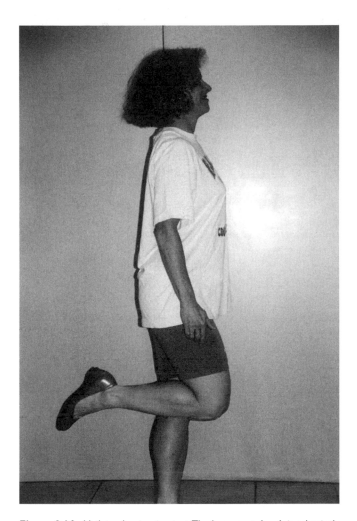

Figure 9.16. Unilateral extension test. The bony neural arch is selectively loaded to the side of the leg with increased weight bearing.

cent injury that has a chance of healing if treated properly. A positive bone scan in a patient with negative radiographs indicates a stress reaction in bone suggesting an impending stress fracture (Table 9.2) (88).

It may be found that a stress reaction to bone is occurring on the side opposite from a radiographic pars defect. This suggests that the pars defect is old and that the opposite stress reaction is the symptomatic injury (88). Once unilateral pars injury occurs, the opposite pars becomes the limiting factor in segmental extension. It is probable that bilateral pars defects in a patient with a recurrent history of back pain were actually unilateral lesions that developed at different times.

Active bone lesions including stress reactions and bony defects with an active bone scan should be treated as acute stress fractures. As with any fracture, treatment involves reduction of the defect or the stress area and immobilization. Neural arch injuries are reduced by flexion of the lower lumbar segments. This can be accomplished by the fitting of a semirigid orthosis in the zero lordosis position. The patient is flexed forward until the lumbar lordosis straightens and is fitted in this position (Fig. 9.17). Using a modified Boston brace, Micheli found that 32% of full spondylolytic injuries obtained full bony healing (24). Although exact statistics are unavailable, the rate of prevention of pars defects by appropriate treatment of stress reactions to bone should be very high.

With an active pars injury, the orthosis is worn throughout the day for 6 months or until an initially active bone scan becomes negative. Even if union of the pars defect is not obtained, symptomatic resolution allows almost 90% of patients to return to full athletic activity (24). Spondylolisthesis or anterior slippage rarely occurs from recent acquired spondylolysis because the disc affords the vertebral motor unit considerable stability.

Micheli emphasizes that spondylolysis is a stable injury that does not contraindicate vigorous sports activity (24). Spondylolisthesis usually is

ing oblique views, give both an evaluation of the neural arch and postural information, such as the magnitude of lordosis, that may be contributory to diagnosis. Initial negative radiographs and poor segmental mobility as detected by segmental motion palpation suggest mechanical facet pain, and appropriate treatment such as manipulation and physiotherapy is indicated. Examining a young athletic population referred for imaging for suspected neural arch injury because of chronic back pain, Papanicolaou et al. still found that more than one third of this selective group proved to have mechanical back pain and negative imaging (88). This suggests that the majority of the general athletic population with acute back pain will prove to have mechanical back pain rather than bony neural arch injury.

If initial radiographs demonstrate a neural arch defect or if there is sclerosis of the pars interarticularis, bone scanning is indicated. A positive bone scan in a patient with a bony defect seen radiographically would indicate a more re-

Table 9.2.   Classification of Neural Arch Injuries in Athletes

	Symptoms	Bone scan	Radiographs
Mechanical back pain	Variable	−	−
Early stress reaction of bone	5–8 wk	+	−
Stress reaction of bone	1–5 mo	+	Sclerosis
Stress fracture	2–6 mo	+	Sclerosis
Spondylolysis (old injury)	Variable	−	Lytic defect

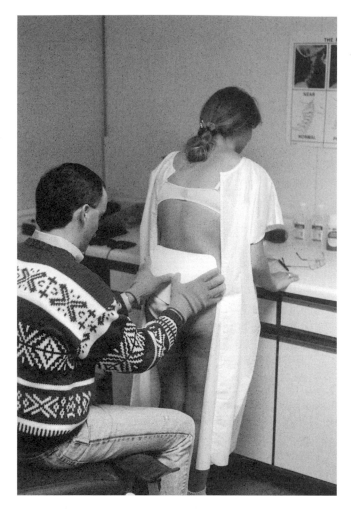

Figure 9.17. Fitting of a thermoplastic orthosis. The patient is fitted in the zero lordosis position.

equally stable, and sports participation with lower grades is acceptable. The tendency for spondylolisthesis to produce symptoms seems to originate more from segmental instability than from the degree of slippage (96). The ability to assess true instability, however, has not been well established. It has been suggested that greater than 3 mm of sagittal plane segmental translation between flexion and extension lateral radiographs is diagnostic of instability (97). More recently, Friberg has used traction and compression radiographs to evaluate instability of spondylolisthesis (98). She found that 5 mm of sagittal plane translation between axial traction and compression correlated with the presence of symptoms, whereas those with less translation were typically without symptoms.

Cox correlated the response to treatment with spinal manipulation to test the clinical value of determining stability (99). Using a variation of Friberg's criteria, Cox classified patients as stable or unstable based on a limit of 3 mm or more of translation between a neutral lateral radiograph and one taken in axial traction. In this limited case study, 100% of patients classified as stable had at least 75% subjective improvement with manipulation. Of those classified as unstable, only 20% obtained this level of improvement. Although this somewhat confirms this type of analysis, further verification of these techniques of evaluating instability is necessary. At this point, the determination of instability in spondylolisthesis suggests a poorer prognosis with treatment and return to sports activity but it is not a fail-safe prognostic sign. Virta compared surgical and conservative treatment outcomes in patients with spondylolisthesis and found that assessment of instability did not predict either (100).

One of the standards by which the necessity of fusion is judged is the response to extensive conservative treatment and rehabilitation (101). Although less-favorable prognosis is indicated by radiographic instability, response to treatment including exercise rehabilitation should be the ultimate test. Return to sport should be a comprehensive decision based on radiographic assessment, response to treatment and rehabilitation, and load-bearing demands placed on the lower lumbar spine in the sport involved.

FACET SYNDROME—MECHANICAL BACK PAIN

It should be stressed that the majority of patients presenting with examination findings consistent with posterior compartment pain will prove not to have bone injury but rather mechanical back pain or facet syndrome. The common facet syndrome is a painful restriction of motion in a lower lumbar facet joint. However, because of the use of this term for several disorders of the facet joints, the research literature is confusing.

Facet syndrome can present as localized back pain or back pain with radiation to one or both lower extremities. The lower extremity pain is referred, not radicular pain, and is not confined to a specific dermatomal location. The referred pain patterns that originate from the facet joints have been termed scleratogenous pain or lumbar dorsal ramus syndrome (102). The dorsal ramus of the spinal nerve root innervates the soft tissue structures of the posterior compartment, including the facet joint capsules (38). The lateral branches of the lumbar dorsal rami become cutaneous over the buttock and lateral thigh area as well as innervating the lumbodorsal fascia (33). This innervation area is in the proximal leg only and would not be expected to cause distal radiation. This neural pattern is the probable neurologic pathway for pain referred from the lumbar facet joints to the proximal leg such as in lumbar myofascial pain syndrome. Although dissection study has not identified these same sensory fibers to the lower extremity from the fifth lumbar level, indirect evidence would suggest that they exist and are the source of referred proximal leg pain associated with facet syndrome at this level (103–105). Scleratogenous or referred pain patterns to the proximal lower extremity can be induced by infiltration of the lower lumbar facet joints to produce capsular irritation (103, 105), and scleratogenous pain patterns can be abolished by anesthetic injection into the facet joints (104, 106, 107).

The common mechanical facet impingement syndrome needs to be separated from other causes of facet pain in the nonspecific category called facet syndrome. The more pathomechanically descriptive term of dorsal ramus loop syndrome (DRLS) is suggested by the author (Fig. 9.18). The lesion appears to involve a pain reflex originating from soft tissue impingement by extension rotation of the facet joint. This pain reflex causes a "spasm" of the multifidus muscle, which receives 100% of its innervation from the medial branch of the dorsal ramus of the level of the spinous process at which the muscle attaches. Whereas the larger erector spinae muscles receive multisegmental innervation for the lateral and intermediate branches of the dorsal ramus, this is not the case with the multifidus muscle (38). The

multifidus muscle is more susceptible to "spasm" than are the muscles of the erector spinae group because of this innervation difference. With its spinous process attachment, the multifidus is capable of causing extension rotation fixation of the facet joint and thus further capsular soft tissue impingement pain, continuing the reflex. Primary posterior compartment soft tissue sprain may begin this loop syndrome, or repeated mechanical impingement from sports involving hyperextension positioning of the lumbar spine may account for its initiation.

This reflex intersegmental hypomobility involving the multifidus muscle mediated through the dorsal ramus has been tested clinically. Thabe examined 20 patients with restriction of a sacroiliac joint by insertional electromyography of the S1 portion of the multifidus muscle (49). Increased spontaneous activity or "spasm" was demonstrated in the multifidus muscle when joint restriction was present. Additionally, spontaneous multifidus activity could be resolved immediately with manipulation of the joint. Comparative treatments of mobilization, joint injection, and intramuscular injection were all less effective than manipulation in resolving abnormal multifidus activity. Although this was an uncontrolled study, it should serve as a model for similar controlled trials of this concept.

The clinical diagnosis of mechanical facet syndrome or DRLS includes well-localized joint tenderness, a referred rather than true radicular pain pattern, exacerbation of pain with a sustained posture and temporary relief with movement, exacerbation of pain with hyperextension, and a negative result of a neurologic examination of the lower extremities (12, 108).

Pathologic evaluation of radiographs is usually unremarkable in DRLS, but spinographic or postural analysis may be helpful both in the diagnosis and in determining postural predisposition (12, 13). The relative segmental extension position, as determined by measurement of the "disc angle," has been demonstrated to be significantly greater in those with clinical DRLS and to normalize with resolution of the acute state with manipulative treatment (Fig. 9.19) (12, 13). Taylor has demonstrated a similar increase in the disc angle at the symptomatic level in those with back pain and spondylolisthesis (109).

In a comparative study of patients with DRLS and lumbar disc syndrome, the author found that the overall shape of the lumbar posture was different in both patient groups compared with asymptomatic control subjects with no back pain

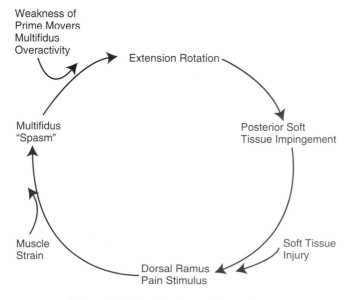

Figure 9.18. The dorsal ramus loop syndrome.

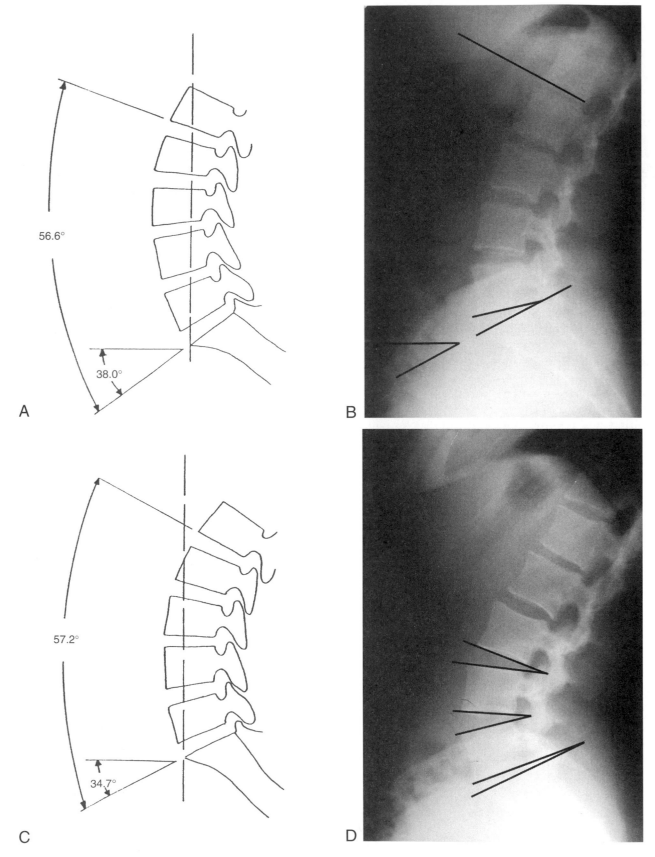

Figure 9.19. Postural parameters in dorsal ramus loop syndrome. **A.** Normal postural parameters. **B** and **C.** In dorsal ramus loop syndrome. **D.** Increased disc angle at L4 in acute dorsal ramus loop syndrome. (A and C: Reprinted with permission from Banks SD. Lumbar facet syndrome. J Manipulative Physiol Ther 1983;6:179.)

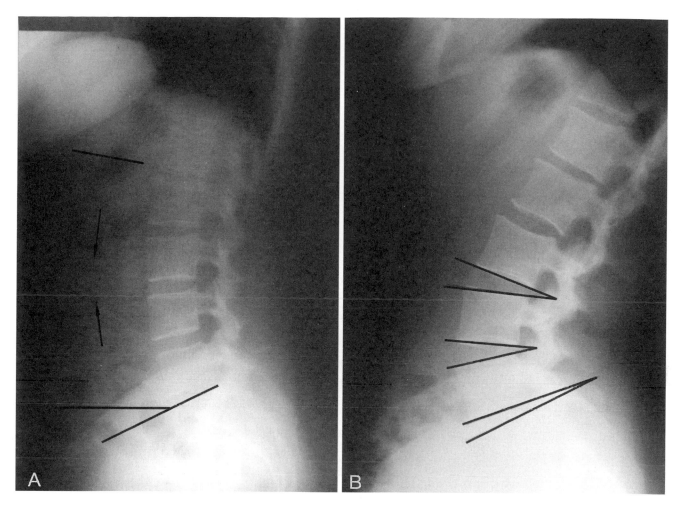

Figure 9.20. Lumbar spine postural parameters. **A.** Disc protrusion. Reduced sacral base angle and reduced lordosis. **B.** Dorsal ramus loop syndrome. Reduced sacral base angle but with a normal lordosis.

history (Fig. 9.20) (12). After resolution of acute DRLS with manipulation, the intersegmental extension rotation was found to correct significantly, but the overall postural configuration changed little (3). This suggests that the extended posture with a relatively normal amount of lordosis and yet a shallow sacral base angle is predisposing to mechanical facet pain, just as a large lordosis with an increased sacral base angle predisposes to bony pars injury.

DRLS may be one of the most responsive disorders to manipulative treatment. In a large case study of 1300 patients with low back pain, Bernard and Kirkaldy-Willis reported good or excellent results in 88% of patients receiving manipulation for facet syndrome (19). Several other studies have suggested that manipulation is an effective treatment for back pain, although they have not been condition specific in selection of a patient population other than usually to select those with "mechanical" back pain (39, 41, 42, 110–113). It is logical that the majority of these

patients had DRLS given its predominance in mechanical back pain populations. Facet joint or medial branch nerve blocks and, rarely, facet denervation by radiofrequency or surgical lysis of the medial branch have been used in those refractory to resolution with manipulation (19). The need for these procedures in a young athletic population should be rare. Exercise may play an important role in the control of recurrent DRLS, but for reasons in contrast to those often hypothesized. Most back exercises are given to correct postural relationships such as anterior or posterior pelvic tilt. However, their success is probably more dependent on dynamic changes rather than postural correction. It is the author's experience that the postural predisposition of DRLS is not altered by postural exercise, although the recurrent nature of this syndrome is improved.

An emerging theory suggests that the longer, more superficial muscles of the erector spinae group are the prime movers of the back, and that some of the deeper, shorter muscles of the back form a distinct group with a separate function (47, 48). Looking at macroscopic and microscopic data on the multifidus muscle, it is now thought to be separate from the erector spinae group and to serve as a secondary mover rather than as a prime mover. The multifidus has been demonstrated to have a greater concentration of muscle spindle cells than the erector spinae, suggesting that it is as much a sensory monitor as a prime mover (114). Its attachment to the spinous process, and therefore its mechanical ability to cause extension rotation of the joint of origin (115), further suggests that the multifidus is not an active prime mover of the lumbar region. The attachment of the erector spinae group to the transverse process area, which is close to the center of rotation of the motor unit in the sagittal plane, makes it more suited for controlling regional movement without adversely affecting intersegmental position.

Both fatigue of the prime movers (116) and activation of the secondary movers after soft tissue injury (117) have been suggested to cause excessive use of the secondary muscles such as the multifidus. Overactivity of this muscle causes extension loading of the facet joints and is perhaps a significant causative mechanism of DRLS or facet syndrome. Most back exercise programs designed to change posture may actually be effective more because they reestablish dominance of the prime movers of the lower back, breaking the dorsal ramus loop activity, than because they alter postural weight bearing. Exercise should include complete strength training of the back extensor mechanism, concentrating on strength through a full range of concentric and eccentric motion.

Sprain/Strain

Sprain/strain of soft tissue injury to the ligament or muscle units themselves is probably more common in athletes than in other patient populations. In nonathletes, this is probably a much overworked diagnosis whose use reflects the nonspecific nature of most conservative treatment in the early stages of back pain. An absolute necessity for the diagnosis of sprain and strain is significant tissue stress. Insidious back "injuries" should elicit a diagnostic evaluation more oriented toward mechanical or reflex back pain.

One of the great difficulties in establishing the relative frequencies of mechanical/repetitive stress injuries and sprain/strain injuries is the fact that they often coexist. Soft tissue sprain/strain may be one of the most common causes of repetitive mechanical back pain in athletes because of the reflex induction of secondary joint dysfunction in response to the associated neural stimulus from tissue injury.

Sprain or ligament injury usually occurs when the posterior soft tissues are loaded by flexion of the spine. Acute back pain associated with a sudden flexion stress is suggestive of ligament injury. Because the back muscles are active either concentrically or eccentrically in most non-neutral postures and during all movement, the mechanism of strain or injury to the muscular structures is less associated with a specific motion. The fact that sprain and strain commonly occur together further clouds the distinction of the two injuries and perhaps accounts for the common use of the combined terminology.

Once a history consistent with a mechanism sufficient to cause sprain/strain has been established, clinical examination will usually help delineate the nature of the injury. The most difficult differentiation is among sprain/strain, disc injury without radicular pain, and facet syndrome. Sprain/strain causes localized back pain that can refer into the dorsal ramus distribution. This is similar to facet syndrome but is easily differentiated from disc injury that has accompanying radicular or nerve root pain. Whereas facet syndrome causes pain almost exclusively with lumbar extension, posterior soft tissue injury limits extension by compression of the inflamed soft tissues, but also limits flexion by distraction of the same tissues. Disc injury tends to cause pain with flexion but with accompanying antalgia, and extension pain is infrequent and milder. If radicular pain is present, disc injury is much more likely.

The ability to differentiate sprain from strain in the spine by pain or passive versus active motion is questionable. This procedure is difficult to impossible to perform and has never been shown to be of practical clinical value. As the treatment of the two types of tissue injuries is similar, the differentiation is probably not important clinically.

Treatment should involve aggressive management of the acute inflammatory response and protection of the injured tissues from load stress. Immediate and repetitive ice applications are perhaps the best early therapy for control of inflammatory response. Hourly ice applications from 20 to 30 minutes should be begun immediately and continued until significant pain reduction occurs. The injured tissue should be protected but not immobilized in most cases. Immobilization with bed rest has never been shown to be beneficial and may prolong associated disability or return to activity (74, 75). Recent research on the use of passive motion in the healing of soft tissue suggests that nonstressful movement is important in healing (118). Early active motion has also been shown to enhance the ultimate strength and quality of tendon repair (119).

The balance between avoiding stress-inducing motion and maintaining controlled motion is usually obtained by limitation of sports and trunk flexion until pain-free range of motion is obtained. An elastic support may be used in the early stages of return to sports activity but should be discontinued as full muscle strength and coordination return.

Soft tissue injury creates secondary joint dysfunction, and treatment/rehabilitation is not complete until factors such as joint and muscle dysfunction are resolved. Reflex joint activity has been found to inhibit normal muscular training with exercise and can prevent adequate rehabilitation (120). Sprain/strain injury cannot be considered resolved until assessment of intersegmental joint motion has occurred and any dysfunction such as secondary DRLS has been resolved with manipulation. Manipulation is a more controlled procedure than is typically thought by those not actively involved in this clinical specialty. Only one study has been done to date on the use of spinal manipulation in the early stages of soft tissue injury (121). In a study of 61 patients with acute cervical spine soft tissue injuries, Mealy et al. demonstrated significantly better return of motion and pain reduction in those receiving controlled manipulation after 24 hours of ice applications versus those patients receiving rest and immobilization. Although there are no similar trials on the lumbar spine, early manipulation of clinically demonstrated intersegmental joint dysfunction would seem to be appropriate and preferred.

THE LUMBOPELVIC COMPLEX

Sacroiliac Joint Dysfunction

The sacroiliac joint can be involved in athletic back pain as a primary and secondary source of pain because of its shared function with the lumbar joints during static and dynamic tasks. The lumbopelvic complex should be viewed as a kinetic chain rather than two distinct functional areas. During gait, a single stride is a complex integrated motion involving hip flexion, hemi-pelvic posterior rotation occurring through the sacroiliac joint, and coupled rotation/lateral bending of the spine. Although the amount of normal motion inherent to the sacroiliac joint has been found to be only 2–3° (63), this movement plays an important role both in performing overall movement and in keeping the sacrum level to spare the lumbosacral area from excessive torsion during gait.

There is only a small amount of literature available on the sacroiliac joint, and it is even less specific about the role of this joint in sports injuries. What is available, however, makes it seem logical that sacroiliac joint dysfunction is a significant factor in athletic back pain syndromes. In a nonathletic population, sacroiliac joint dysfunction has been suggested as a major overlooked source of back pain, accounting for as many as one in four cases of mechanical-type back pain (19). Furthermore, sacroiliac joint dysfunction or sacroiliac syndrome was found to be the most common secondary perpetuating factor in other types of mechanical back pain (19).

Sacroiliac joint dysfunction or syndrome is a painful restriction of motion usually occurring unilaterally. Thabe has suggested that the mechanism of restriction may be reflex activity in the lower lumbar multifidus muscles, which attach across the joint and receive innervation from the S1 dorsal ramus (the sensory innervation of the joint) (49). This reflex activity can be initiated either by impingement or sprain of the joint, or secondarily from multifidus activity that can be the result of other lower lumbar posterior compartment pain stimulus. A common source of secondary sacroiliac joint dysfunction is facet syndrome (19).

Sacroiliac joint dysfunction is suggested by a history of mechanical-type back pain that localizes to the joint/buttock area. Pain may refer to the posterior and lateral thigh, similar to other scleratogenous patterns. Pain may occur consistently during the same phase of the gait cycle. Examination for root tension signs is negative as is neurologic evaluation of the lower extremities. Tenderness may localize to the posterior, superior iliac spine and adjacent area. Testing that stresses the joint, such as the Fabère test or Gaenslen's maneuver, may produce pain over the sacroiliac area rather than the hip joint proper. Patients may complain of pain on the SLR test, but it is localized to the joint area rather than radiating to the leg. The mainstay of sacroiliac diagnosis is demonstration of side-to-side movement asymmetry with motion palpation. The procedure involves comparing side-to-side joint movement during flexion of the hemipelvis simulating gait (Fig. 9.9). The procedure has been shown to be reproducible by experienced examiners (122–124).

Manipulation is the initial treatment of choice in sacroiliac joint dysfunction. Manipulation improves subjective and objective pain assessments, static lumbopelvic posture, joint mobility, hamstring muscle peak torque, abnormal spontaneous activity in the multifidus muscle, and ground reaction forces through the lower extremities during gait as measured by force plate analysis (19, 49, 125–128). Rarely, manipulation does not resolve sacroiliac syndrome and injection of a local anesthetic with cortisone may be helpful (19). Other pathomechanics that may contribute to the development of sacroiliac joint dysfunction, such as LLI, should be corrected to prevent recurrence.

LLI—Functional Scoliosis

Perhaps the greatest difficulty when discussing LLI is how to place the disorder under the most appropriate heading. The effects of LLI have been shown to be diverse, but are perhaps most pronounced on the lumbopelvic complex and on the coordination of function of this area with that of the lower extremities. Whereas LLI by itself is not a clinical disorder but rather a pathomechanical predisposition, it is a contributing factor in many sports injuries. Failure to evaluate LLI in an athlete with a repetitive stress injury such as muscle tendon strain of the pelvis may preclude resolution with otherwise appropriate treatment.

LLI has been shown to disturb many parameters associated with static posture and kinetic function. LLI has been shown to affect spinal posture and balance (129); paraspinal EMG symmetry (130, 131); position of the center of pressure (132); extent of postural sway (132); weight stress distribution through the hip joint (133); kinematic symmetry throughout the lower extremity and foot (134, 135); risk of developing back (133, 136, 137), hip (133, 138), and knee pain (139–141); and maximum oxygen uptake (142). This diverse impact on the musculoskeletal system and on the kinetics of gait suggests a significant role for LLI in the predisposition for a wide variety of sports injuries.

Clinical evaluation of LLI should include physical and radiographic measurements. Obvious imbalance on physical examination or repetitive injuries to the kinetic chain without apparent causation are indications for radiographic examination. Physical examination involves direct and indirect measurements. There is a considerable amount of disagreement about the accuracy of different physical examination techniques to assess LLI. Direct physical measurements involve measuring from a point on the pelvis to a bony prominence on the lower leg. Gogia and Braatz found that measures using the anterior superior iliac spine and the medial malleolus correlated accurately with radiographic measurements (143). Woerman and Binder-MacLeod, however, found this method to be less accurate than indirect measurement by placing blocks of known thickness under the short leg until the pelvis was visibly leveled (144). Friberg et al. compared direct and indirect physical measurements to radiographic measurements and found that none of the physical methods correlated highly with radiographic findings if 5 mm was used as the standard of clinical importance (145).

The author's experience suggests that the indirect method of observation of height symmetry of the iliac crests is the best physical screen for the need for radiographic examination. However, the more methods of physical examination that yield the same result, the higher correlation between suspected findings and true radiographic measurements.

The radiographic assessment of LLI should include standing anterior-posterior and lateral films. Care must be taken during positioning to minimize patient rotation, which will give projectional error in measurement of the femur head heights because these structures are not at the height of the central ray of the radiographic tube. Errors of several millimeters can be introduced to this measurement by rotation. The Winterstein method of rotational determination will allow the calculation of rotational error (146). This method has been demonstrated to be accurate when compared with leg length measurements from radiographs with the central ray at femur head height, where rotation cannot cause distortion (146).

To be confident that correction of the LLI will have a positive biomechanical impact, the lumbopelvic compensation or pathomechanics should match that expected from LLI. The side of the short leg would be expected to cause an ipsilateral pelvic and sacral tilt and ipsilateral spinal curvature beginning with the lowest mobile spinal segment. Compensatory spinal curves are typically gradual and less than 10° in magnitude (Fig. 9.21). Contralateral curves or atypical curves suggest other pathomechanics and may not correct with correction of the LLI.

For discrepancies greater than 0.5 inch, a modified orthoroentgenogram or scanogram should be taken. The classic scanogram involves sectional

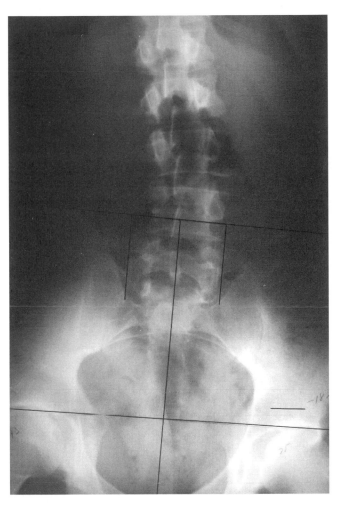

Figure 9.21. Lumbopelvic postural radiograph of significant leg length inequality.

radiographs of the ankle, knee, and hip joints taken on the same film. The modified scanogram is a sectional view of the hip and knee joints on the same weight-bearing film (Fig. 9.22). Because the feet are in a fixed position, the relative lengths of the tibias are determined by direct comparison of the tibial plateau heights; the relative femoral lengths are determined by direct comparison of the femur head heights plus or minus any contralateral or ipsilateral tibial difference. Although this method does not allow for the measurement of discrepancy resulting from structures below the distal tibia, these are rare and can be first screened for by physical examination. If, for example, there is pronounced pronation on one side with a supinated or cavus foot on the opposite side, an approximate 0.25-inch shortening on the pronated side is assumed. This foot pattern, however, is rare.

For discrepancies greater than 0.5 inch, complete correction of the LLI may not always be ideal. If the discrepancy is entirely in the femur, complete correction will cause unleveling of the knee joints (Fig. 9.23). With the known pathomechanical effect of LLI on the knee, complete correction of the femoral shortening may level the pelvis and spine, but increase the stress on the knee. In those cases, a 50% correction usually is a good compromise. When LLI is solely the result of tibial shortening, complete correction levels the knees, pelvis, and spine and is preferred.

Correction of LLI should be gradual and accompanied by ongoing correction of lumbopelvic

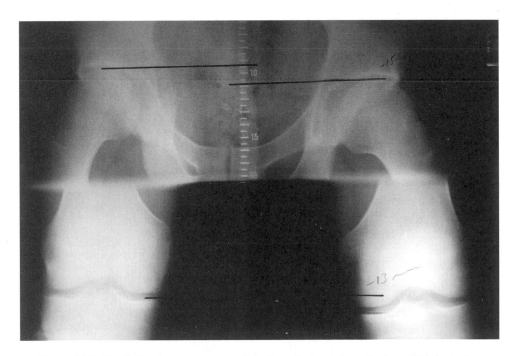

Figure 9.22. Modified orthoroentgenogram of significant leg length inequality from tibial shortening.

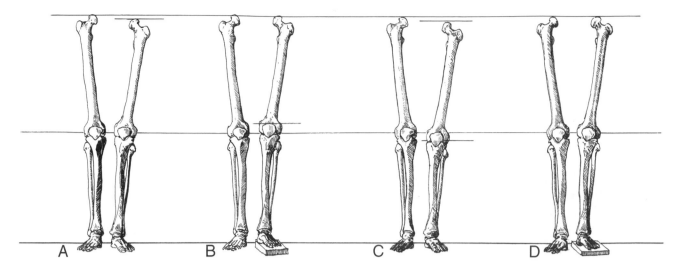

Figure 9.23. Leg length inequality. **A.** Femoral shortening. **B.** Corrected femoral shortening with a shoe lift causing asymmetry of height of the knee joints. **C.** Tibial shortening. **D.** Correction of tibial shortening with a shoe lift.

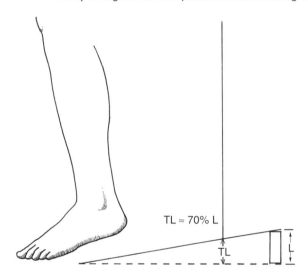

$$TL \approx 70\% \; L$$

Figure 9.24. Relationship between the ankle joint and the heel. Heel lifts result in only an approximate 60–70% correction of leg length as the ankle joint is approximately 30% of the foot length away from the heel.

adaptation pathomechanics by manipulation. Papaiounnou et al. found that scoliosis persisted or even occurred contralateral to shoe lifts in several patients (129). This probably reflects adaptive pathomechanics that should be corrected with manipulation and exercise. Heel lifts can be used in smaller discrepancies but are uncomfortable and alter foot mechanics if greater than approximately 10 mm or 0.25 inch. Beyond this amount, full sole lifts are required. Heel lifts will only correct approximately 60–70% of their thickness because of the position of the ankle mortise relative to the heel (Fig. 9.24). Actual correction with heel lifts is usually limited to only approximately 7 mm with a 10-mm heel lift. Corrections of greater than 7 mm (heel lift greater than 10 mm) require a sole lift.

References

1. Haldeman S. Spinal manipulative therapy in sports medicine. Clin Sports Med 1986;5:277–293.
2. Sands WA, Shultz BB, Newman AP. Women's gymnastics injuries: a 5 year study. Am J Sports Med 1993;21: 271–276.
3. Sward L. The thoracolumbar spine in young elite athletes. Sports Med 1992;13:357–364.
4. Sward L. Disc degeneration and associated abnormalities of the spine in elite gymnasts: a magnetic resonance imaging study. Spine 1991;16:437–443.
5. Kujala UM, Salminen JJ, Taimela S, et al. Subject characteristics and low back pain in young athletes and nonathletes. Med Sci Sports Exerc 1992;24:627–632.
6. Locke S, Allen GD. Etiology of low back pain in elite board sailors. Med Sci Sports Exerc 1992;24:964–966.
7. Ponni JS, Hukins DWL, Harris PF, et al. Comparison of the structure of human intervertebral discs in the cervical, thoracic and lumbar regions of the spine. Surg Radiol Anat 1986;8:175–182.
8. Gilad I, Nissan M. A study of vertebra and disc geometric relations of the human cervical and lumbar spine. Spine 1986;11:154–157.
9. Berry JL, Moran JM, Berg WS, et al. A morphometric study of human lumbar and selected thoracic vertebrae. Spine 1987;12:362–367.
10. Busche-McGregor M, Naiman J, Grice AS. Analysis of the lumbar lordosis in an asymptomatic population of young adults. JCCA 1991;25:58–64.
11. DeCyper H, Heijnen B. The lordotic angle as a predictor of low back pain. Medica Physica 1988;11:21.
12. Banks SD. The use of spinographic parameters in the differential diagnosis of facet and disc syndromes. J Manipulative Physiol Ther 1983;6:113–116.
13. Banks SD. Lumbar facet syndrome: spinographic assessment of treatment by spinal manipulative therapy. J Manipulative Physiol Ther 1983;6:175–180.
14. Sward L, Eriksson B, Peterson L. Anthropometric characteristics, passive hip flexion, and spinal mobility in relation to back pain in athletes. Spine 1990;15:376–382.
15. Smidt G, Herring T, Amundsen L, et al. Assessment of abdominal and back extensor function: a quantitative approach and results for chronic low back pain patients. Spine 1983;8:211–219.
16. Mayer TG, Smith SS, Keeley J, et al. Quantification of lumbar function. part 2: sagittal plane trunk strength in chronic low back pain patients. Spine 1985;10:765–771.
17. Kishino ND, Mayer TG, Gatchel RJ, et al. Quantification of lumbar function. part 4: isometric and isokinetic lift-

ing simulation in normal subjects and low back dysfunction patients. Spine 1985;10:921–927.

18. Svensson HO, Vedin A, Wilhelmsson C, et al. Low back pain in relation to other diseases and cardiovascular risk factors. Spine 1983;8:277–285.

19. Bernard TN, Kirkaldy-Willis WH. Recognizing specific characteristics of nonspecific low back pain. Clin Orthop 1987;217:266–280.

20. Adams MA, Dolan P, Hutton WC. The lumbar spine in backward bending. Spine 1988;13:1019–1026.

21. Ireland LM, Micheli LJ. Bilateral stress fracture of the lumbar pedicles in a ballet dancer. J Bone Joint Surg 1987;69:140–142. Abstract.

22. McCarrol JR, Miller JM, Ritter MA. Lumbar spondylolysis and spondylolisthesis in college football players. Am J Sports Med 1986;5:404–406.

23. Letts M, Smallman T, Afanasiev R, et al. Fracture of the pars interarticularis in adolescent athletes: a clinical-biomechanical analysis. J Pediatr Orthop 1986;6:40–46.

24. Micheli LJ. Back injuries in gymnastics. Clin Sports Med 1985;4:85–93.

25. Mellin G. Correlations of hip mobility with degree of back pain and lumbar spine mobility in chronic low back pain patients. Spine 1988;13:668–670.

26. Robinson RO, Herzog W, Nigg BM. Use of force platform variables to quantify the effects of chiropractic manipulation of gait symmetry. J Manipulative Physiol Ther 1987;10:172–176.

27. Herzog W, Nigg BM, Robinson RO, et al. Quantifying the effects of spinal manipulation on gait using the patients with low back pain: a pilot study. J Manipulative Physiol Ther 1987;10:295–299.

28. Herzog W, Nigg BM, Read LJ. Quantifying the effects of spinal manipulation on gait using patients with low back pain. J Manipulative Physiol Ther 1988;11:151–157.

29. Porter RW, Miller CG. Back pain and trunk list. Spine 1986;11:596–600.

30. Khuffash B, Porter RW. Cross leg pain and trunk list. Spine 1989;14:602–603.

31. Schnebel BE, Watkins RG, Dillin W. The role of spinal flexion and extension in changing nerve root compression in disc herniations. Spine 1989;8:835–837.

32. Krag MH, Seroussi RE, Wilder DG, et al. Internal displacement distribution from in vitro loading of human lumbar and thoracic spinal motion segments: experimental results and theoretical predictions. Spine 1987;12:1001–1007.

33. White AA, Panjbi MM. The clinical biomechanics of spine pain. In: Clinical biomechanics of the spine. Philadelphia: JB Lippincott, 1978:334.

34. Shiqing X, Quanzhi Z, Dehao F. Significance of the straight-leg raising test in the diagnosis and clinical evaluation of lower lumbar intervertebral-disc protrusion. J Bone Joint Surg 1987;69:517–522. Abstract.

35. Cox JM. Care of the intervertebral disc. In: Low back pain: mechanism, diagnosis and treatment. Baltimore: Williams & Wilkins, 1985:203–217.

36. Kosteljanetz M, Bang F, Schmidt-Olsen S. The clinical significance of straight-leg raising (Lasegue's sign) in the diagnosis of prolapsed lumbar disc: interobserver variation and correlation with surgical finding. Spine 1988;13:393–395.

37. Jinkins JR, Whittemore AR, Bradley WG. The anatomic basis of vertebrogenic pain and the autonomic syndrome associated with lumbar disc extrusion. AJR 1989;152:1277–1289.

38. Bugduk N. The innervation of the lumbar spine. Spine 1983;8:286–293.

39. Arkuszewski Z. The efficacy of manual treatment of low back pain: a clinical trial. Man Med 1986;2:68–71.

40. Stevens A. Manual medicine: a description of some strategies. Medica Physica 1988;11:151–163.

41. Kirkaldy-Willis WH, Cassidy JD. Spinal manipulation in the treatment of low back pain. Can Fam Physician 1985;31:535–540.

42. Cassidy JD. An overview of the problem of low back pain. DC Tracts 1989;1:345–356.

43. Roland MO. A critical review of the evidence for a pain-spasm-pain cycle in spinal disorders. Clin Biomech 1986;1:102–109.

44. Arena JG, Sherman RA, Bruno GM, et al. Electromyographic recordings of 5 types of low back pain subjects and non-pain controls in different positions. Pain 1989;37:57–65.

45. Ahern DK, Follick MJ, Council JR, et al. Comparison of lumbar paravertebral EMG patterns in chronic low back pain patients and non-patient controls. Pain 1988;34:153,160.

46. Miller DJ. Comparison of electromyographic activity in the lumbar paraspinal muscles of subjects with and without chronic low back pain. Phys Ther 1985;65:1347–1357.

47. MacIntosh JE, Valencia F, Bogduk N, et al. The morphology of the human lumbar multifidus. Clin Biomech 1986;1:196–204.

48. Kalimo H, Rantanen J, Viljanen T, et al. Lumbar muscles: structure and function. Ann Med 1989;21:353–359.

49. Thabe H. Electromyography as tool to document diagnostic findings and therapeutic results associated with somatic dysfunctions in the upper cervical spinal joints and sacroiliac joints. Man Med 1986;2:53–58.

50. Triano JJ, Luttges M. Myoelectric paraspinal response to spinal loads: potential for monitoring low back pain. J Manipulative Physiol Ther 1985;3:137–145.

51. Batti'e MC, Bigos SJ, Sheehy A, et al. Spinal flexibility and individual factors that influence it. JAPTA 1987;5:653–657.

52. Helbing T, Lee CK. The lumbar facet syndrome. Spine 1988;13:61.

53. Stokes IAF. Mechanical function of facet joints in the lumbar spine. Clin Biomech 1988;3:101–105.

54. Yang KH, King AI. Mechanism of facet load transmission as a hypothesis for low back pain. Spine 1984;9:557–565.

55. Mellin G. Correlations of spinal mobility with degree of chronic low back pain after correction for age and anthropometric factors. Spine 1987;5:464–468.

56. Carrick FR. Treatment of pathomechanics of the lumbar spine by manipulation. J Manipulative Physiol Ther 1981;4:173–178.

57. Cox JM. Diagnosis. In: Low back pain: mechanism, diagnosis and treatment. Baltimore: Williams & Wilkins, 1985:86–88.

58. Kippers V, Parker AW. Posture related to myoelectric silence of erectors spinae during trunk flexion. Spine 1984;9:740–745.

59. Triano JJ, Schultz AB. Correlation of objective measure of trunk motion and muscle function with low back disability ratings. Spine 1987;12:561–565.

60. McGill SM. A biomechanical perspective of sacroiliac pain. Clin Biomech 1987;2:145–151.

61. Kidd R. Pain localization with the innominate upslip dysfunction. Man Med 1988;3:103–105.

62. Greenman PE, Tait B. Structural diagnosis in chronic low back pain. Man Med 1988;4:114–117.

63. Sturesson B, Selvik G, Uden A. Movements of the sacroiliac joints: a roentgen sterophotogrammetric analysis. Spine 1989;2:162–165.

64. Bogduk N. The anatomy of the intervertebral disc syndrome. Med J Aust 1976;1:878–881.

65. Boumphrey FRS, Bell GR, Modic M, et al. Computed tomography scanning after chymopapain injection for herniated nucleus pulposus. Clin Orthop 1987;219:120–123.

66. Cox JM. Pre and post CT scans on chiropractic-treated disc protrusion patients. Digest Chiro Economics Jan/Feb1985:38–41.

67. Cox JM, Aspergren DD. A hypothesis introducing a new calculation for discal reduction: emphasis on stenotic factors and manipulative treatment. J Manipulative Physiol Ther 1987;10:287–295.

68. Panjabi MM, Krag MH, Chung TQ. Effects of disc injury on mechanical behavior of the human spine. Spine 1984;9:707–713.

69. Day AL, Friedman WA, Indelicato PA. Observations on the treatment of lumbar disc disease in college football players. Am J Sports Med 1987;15:72–75.

70. Chung H, Fang S, Hsueh T. A correlative study of 108 cases of lumbar disc herniation. Chih 1989;23:101–103.

71. Nzeh DA, Komolafe F. Radiographic patterns of lumbar spinal degenerative changes in symptomatic patients. Rays 1987;12:35–38.

72. Forristall RM, Marsh HO, Pay NT. Magnetic resonance imaging and contrast CT of the lumbar spine. comparison of diagnostic methods and correlation with surgical findings. Spine 1988;13:1049–1054.

73. Gilbert JR, Taylor DW, Hildenbrand A, et al. Clinical trial of common treatments for low back pain in family practice. Br Med J 1985;291:791–794.

74. Deyo RA. Conservative therapy for low back pain: distinguishing useful from useless therapy. JAMA 1983;250:1057–1062.

75. Deyo RA, Diehl AK, Rosenthal M. How many days of bed rest for acute low back pain? a randomized clinical trial. N Engl J Med 1986;315:1064–1070.

76. Klimiuk PS, Pountain GD, Keegan AL, et al. Serial measurements of fibrinolytic activity in acute low back pain and sciatica. Spine 1987;12:925–928.

77. Holm S, Nachemson A. Variations in the nutrition of the canine intervertebral disc induced by motion. Spine 1983;8:866.

78. Raftis KL, Warfield CA. Spinal manipulation for back pain. Hosp Pract 1989;24:89–90.

79. Quon JA, Cassidy JD, O'Connor SM, et al. Lumbar intervertebral disc herniation: treatment by rotational manipulation. J Manipulative Physiol Ther 1989;12:220–227.

80. Cailliet R. The conservative management of disc disease. a common denominator. Disc Disease May/June 1990:173–175.

81. Nwuga VCB. Relative therapeutic efficacy of vertebral manipulation and conventional treatment in back pain management. Am J Phys Med 1982;61:273–278.

82. Kinalski R, Kuwik W, Pietrzak D. The comparison of the results of manual therapy versus physiotherapy methods used in treatment of patients with low back pain syndromes. Manual Med 1989;4:44–46.

83. Coxhead CE, Meade TW, Inskip H, et al. Multicenter trial of physiotherapy in the management of sciatic symptoms. Lancet 1981;1:1065–1068.

84. Ouellette J. Low back pain: an orthopedic medicine approach. Can Fam Phys 1987;33:689–694.

85. Hollingworth GR, Wood WE. Spinal manipulation for low back pain: an office procedure. Can Fam Phys 1987;33:2051–2055.

86. Kuo PP, Loh Z. Treatment of lumbar intervertebral disc protrusions by manipulation. Clin Orthop 1987;215:47–55.

87. Weber H. Lumbar disc herniation: a controlled prospective study with ten years of observation. Spine 1983;8:131–140.

88. Papanicolaou N, Wilkinson RH, Emans JB, et al. Bone scintigraphy and radiography in young athletes with low back pain. AJR 1985;145:1039–1044.

89. Abel MS. Jogger's fracture and other stress fractures of the lumbosacral spine. Skeletal Radiol 1985;13:221–227.

90. Matheson GO, Clement DB, McKenzie DC, et al. Stress fractures in athletes: a study of 320 cases. Am J Sports Med 1987;15:46–57.

91. Ciullo JV, Jackson DW. Pars interarticularis stress reaction, spondylolysis, and spondylolisthesis in gymnasts. Clin Sports Med 1985;4:95–110.

92. Adams MA, Dolan P, Hutton WC. The lumbar spine in backward bending. Spine 1988;13:1019–1026.

93. Ohlen G, Wredmark T, Spangfort E. Spinal sagittal configuration and mobility related to low back pain in the female gymnast. Spine 1989;14:847–850.

94. Mahlamaki S, Soimakallio S, Michelsson J-E. Radiological findings in the lumbar spine of 39 young cross country skiers with low back pain. Int J Sports Med 1988;9:196–197.

95. Ogilvie JW, Sherman J. Spondylolysis in Scheuermann's disease. Spine 1987;12:251–253.

96. Amundson GM, Wenger DR. Spondylolisthesis: natural history and treatment. state of the art reviews. Spine 1987;1:323–338.

97. Dupuis P, Yong Hing K, Cassidy JD, et al. Radiographic diagnosis of degenerative lumbar instability. Spine 1987;10:262–276.

98. Friberg O. Lumbar instability: dynamic approach by traction-compression radiography. Spine 1987;12:119–128.

99. Cox JM, Trier K. Chiropractic adjustment results correlated with spondylolisthesis instability. Manual Med 1991;6:67–72.

100. Virta L, Osterman K. Radiographic correlations in adult symptomatic spondylolisthesis: a long-term follow-up study. J Spinal Dis 1994;7:41–48.

101. Frennered AK, Danielson BI, Nachemson AL, et al. Midterm follow-up of young patients fused in situ for spondylolisthesis. Spine 1991;16:409–416.

102. Bogduk N. Lumbar dorsal ramus syndrome. Med J Aust 1980;2:537–541.

103. McCall IW, Park WM, O'Brien JP. Induced pain referral from posterior lumbar elements in normal subjects. Spine 1979;4:441–446.

104. Fairbank JCT, Park WM, McCall IW, et al. Apophyseal injection of local anesthetic as a diagnostic aid in primary low back pain syndromes. Spine 1991;16:598–605.

105. Marks R. Distribution of pain provoked from lumbar facet joints and related structures during diagnostic spinal infiltration. Pain 1989;39:37–40.

106. Lau LSW, Littlejohn GO, Miller MH. Clinical evaluation of intraarticular injections for lumbar facet joint pain. Med J Aust 1985;143:563–565.

107. Murtagh FR. Computed tomography and fluoroscopy guided anesthesia and steroid injection in facet syndrome. Spine 1988;13:686–689.

108. Warfield CA. Facet syndrome and the relief of low back pain. Hosp Pract 1988;30:41–48.

109. Taylor DB. Foraminal encroachment syndrome in true lumbosacral spondylolisthesis: a preliminary report. J Manipulative Physiol Ther 1987;10:253–256.

110. Waagen GN, Haldeman S, Cook G, et al. Short term trial of chiropractic adjustments for the relief of chronic low back pain. Man Med 1986;2:63–67.

111. Tobis JS, Buerger AA. Rotational manipulation of the lumbosacral paravertebral area: effect of straight leg raising tests. Arch Phys Med Rehabil 1976;57:565.

112. Halder NM, Curtis P, Gillings DB, et al. A benefit of spinal manipulation as adjunctive therapy for acute low back pain: a stratified controlled trial. Spine 1987;12:703–706.

113. Bonfort G. Chiropractic treatment of low back pain: a prospective survey. J Manipulative Physiol Ther 1986;9:99–112.

114. Nitz AJ, Peck D. Comparison of muscle spindle concentrations in large and small human epaxial muscles acting in parallel combinations. Am Surg 1986;52:273–277.

115. Macintosh JE, Bogduk N. The biomechanics of the lumbar multifidus. Clin Biomech 1986;1:205–214.

116. Parnianpour M, Nordin M, Kahanovitz N, et al. The triaxial coupling of torque generation of trunk muscles during isometric exertions and the effect of fatiguing isoinertial movements on the motor output and movement patterns. Spine 1988;13:982–992.

117. Panjabi M, Abumi K, Duranceau J, et al. Spinal stability and intersegmental muscle forces: a biomechanical model. Spine 1989;14:194–200.

118. O'Driscoll SW, Salter RB. The repair of major osteochondral defects in joint surfaces by neochondrogenesis with autogenous osteoperiosteal grafts stimulated by continuous passive motion: an experimental investigation in the rabbit. Clin Orthop 1986;208:131–140.

119. Mabit CH, Bellaubre JM, Charissoux JL, et al. Study of the experimental biomechanics of tendon repair with immediate active mobilization. SRA 1986;8:29–35.

120. Beimborn DS, Morrissey MC. A review of the literature related to trunk muscle performance. Spine 1988;13:655–660.

121. Mealy K, Brennan H, Fenelon GCC. Early mobilization of acute whiplash injuries. Br Med J 1986;292:656–657.

122. Wiles MR. Reproducibility and intraexaminer correlation of motion palpation findings of the sacroiliac joints. JCCA 1980;24:59–69.

123. Carmichael JP. Inter and intraexaminer reliability of palpation for sacroiliac joint dysfunction. J Manipulative Physiol Ther 1987;10:164–171.

124. Brunarski DJ. Chiropractic biomechanical evaluations: validity of myofascial low back pain. J Manipulative Physiol Ther 1982;5:155–161.

125. Atha J, Yeadon MR, Quinell R. Low back configuration changes following osteopathic therapy: a pilot study. Clin Biomech 1988;3:197–203.

126. Cibulka MT, Delitto A, Koldehoff RM. Changes in innominate tilt after manipulation of the sacroiliac joint in patients with low back pain. Phys Ther 1988;68:1359 1363.

127. Herzog W, Nigg BM, Read LJ. Quantifying the effects of spinal manipulations on gait using patients with low back pain. J Manipulative Physiol Ther 1998;11:151–157.

128. Cibulka MT, Rose SJ, Delitto A, et al. Hamstring muscle strain treated by mobilizing the sacroiliac joint. Phys Ther 1986;66:1220–1223.

129. Papaiounnou T, Stokes I, Kenwright J. Scoliosis associated with limb length inequality. J Bone Joint Surg 1982;64:59–62. Abstract.

130. Triano JJ. Objective electromyographic evidence for use and effects of lift therapy. J Manipulative Physiol Ther 1983;6:13.

131. Vink P, Kamphuisen HAC. Leg length inequality, pelvic tilt and lumbar back muscle activity during standing. Clin Biomech 1989;4:115–117.

132. Mahar RK, Kirby RL, MacLeod DA. Simulated leg length discrepancy: its effect on mean center-of-pressure position and postural sway. Arch Phys Med Rehabil 1985;66:822–824.

133. Friberg O. Clinical symptoms and biomechanics of lumbar spine and hip joint in leg length inequality. Spine 1983;8:643.

134. Bandy WD, Sinning WE. Kinematic effects of heel lift use to correct lower limb length differences. J Orthop Sports Phys Ther 1986;7:173–178.

135. D'Amico JC, Dinowitz HD, Polchaninoff M. Limb length discrepancy. Am Podiat Med Assoc 1985;75:639–643.

136. Helliwell M. Leg length inequality and low back pain. The Practitioner 1985;229:483–485.

137. Friberg O. Biomechanical significance of the correct length of lower limb prostheses. a clinical and radiological study. Prosthet Orthot Int 1984;8:124–129.

138. Friberg O. Hip-spine syndrome. Man Med 1988;3:144–147.

139. Dixon AS, Campbell-Smith S. Long leg arthropathy. Ann Rheum Dis 1969;28:359–365.

140. Kujala UM, Kvist M, Osterman K, et al. Factors predisposing army conscripts to knee exertion injuries incurred in a physical training program. Clin Orthop 1986;210:203–212.

141. Kujala UM, Osterman K, Kvist M, et al. Factors predisposing to patellar chondropathy and patellar apicitis in athletes. Int Ortho 1986;10:195–200.

142. Delacerda FG, McCrory ML. A case study: effect of leg length differential on oxygen consumption. J Orthop Sports Phys Ther 1981;3:17–20.

143. Gogia PP, Braatz JH. Validity and reliability of leg length measurements. J Orthop Sports Phys Ther 1986;8:185–186.

144. Woerman AL, Binder-MacLeod SA. Leg length discrepancy assessment: accuracy and precision in 5 clinical methods of evaluation. J Orthop Sports Phys Ther 1984;5:230.

145. Friberg O, Nurminen M, Korhonen K, et al. Accuracy and precision of clinical estimation of leg length inequality and lumbar scoliosis: comparison of clinical and radiological measurements. Int Disabil Studies 1988;10:49–53.

146. Winterstein JF. Determining the accuracy of leg length measurement. Chiropractic Spinography, 1970; February: Chapter V.

The Trunk and Viscera

Donald D. Aspegren

Injuries to the trunk represent a much different area of didactic study compared with other topics discussed in this text. Minor injuries, such as contusions or costochondral separations, are frequently found in sports. Almost any team physician, athletic trainer, or coach can readily identify and treat these maladies. However, the challenge that confronts anyone who works as a team physician is the serious injury that may be masked as a minor abrasion. This is always the concern of any team physician because it is easy to become complacent and relaxed after seeing mostly sprains and strains. While working in the game situation and being confronted with many of the cases described herein, the team physician must work with the most fundamental tools and equipment to rule out some of the most potentially life-threatening disorders that may confront him or her in clinical practice. Three fundamental elements that should be used in a field situation are as follows.

1. Clinical knowledge. There is no substitute for staying abreast of current information and literature so that we are capable of recognizing the small subtleties that can lead to a proper diagnosis.
2. Knowledge of the game. The author sincerely believes that a physician serving a particular sport should be very familiar with all aspects of that activity. The physician should be able to empathize with the athlete—and thus better understand the athlete's reaction—to help differentiate between behaviors that suggest frustration and behavioral instances that suggest a more serious illness.
3. Common sense. This quality cannot be taught; it comes with time and experience. However, if the author were to offer one bit of advice to young team physicians, it would be to take the safest approach in all cases, especially if there are any doubts in the mind of the physician. This may mean pulling the star receiver from a league contending football squad during a tight game. However, as is described in the splenic rupture section of this chapter, such an action may be necessary.

Contusions

Contusions are extremely common, particularly in high-velocity contact sports such as football. Although not terribly serious in themselves, a deep contusion many times mimics rib fractures or other related rib pathology. The athlete will commonly present with similar findings to those of a rib fracture, i.e., difficulty breathing, pain on palpation, and discomfort on distal compression of the ribs. If pain persists after a short period, radiographs would be indicated to help rule out a rib fracture or, perhaps, an underlying pneumothorax.

Ice therapy should be initiated as soon as possible over the injured area to help control swelling and offer some pain relief. Once rib fractures or other underlying disorders have been ruled out, and the athlete is to be returned to a contact sport, various forms of protection may be implemented. For example, various forms of rib pads are available that offer minimal restriction to football players (Fig. 10.1). If rib pads are unavailable, or the athlete prefers not to wear them, taping in conjunction with high-density foam is also useful. One of the foam suppliers whose products the author has found useful is Cramer Products (Gardner, KS); several degrees of foam concentration and thickness are offered (Fig. 10.2).

While the athlete is not competing, e.g., during leisure time, a rib belt may be useful. This would help offer the athlete comfort and assist in the healing process.

Rib Fractures

As mentioned previously, one of the greatest concerns a team physician has when an athlete

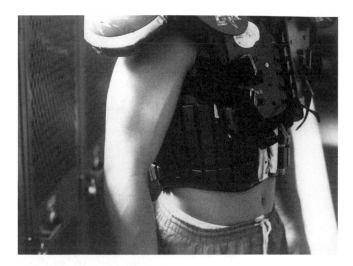

Figure 10.1. Rib pads offer protection for ribs and upper quadrant visceral organs.

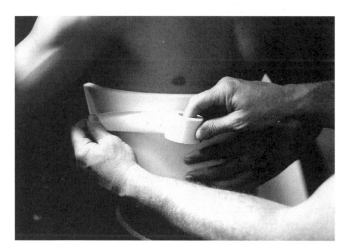

Figure 10.2. High-density foam used to protect ribs.

complaining of rib pain is that he or she may have sustained a rib fracture. These disorders are commonly downplayed by athletes because they would seem to represent little concern other than tolerating a fair amount of pain. However, the physician should always remain aware of the secondary problems, which may manifest in the athletes playing with broken ribs. Such disorders as pneumothorax or lacerated spleen have been reported to occur in concurrence with rib fractures (1, 2).

While the team physician evaluates for possible rib fractures, it is best to keep in mind the underlying structures in case the rib did penetrate deeper organs at the time of contact. To evaluate for possible rib fracture while in the field setting, compress the rib cage away from the side of injury (Fig. 10.3). Although a contusion may also exhibit a positive response from the athlete, a rib fracture is commonly far more symptom

producing. Immediate therapy would consist of ice and compression. A rib belt should be used in these cases to help allow for proper union between the two rib segments (Fig. 10.4). The athlete should be restrained from competition until the rib is healed. Healing of this condition commonly takes 3 to 4 weeks, and the athlete may be returned to the sport with proper padding and taping.

Traumatic and Spontaneous Pneumothorax

Pneumothorax occurs in athletes via two principal methods. The first, traumatic pneumothorax, is a result of a rib fracture that lacerates the pleura. The second, spontaneous pneumothorax, may occur in an athlete participating in a non-contact sport, such as running, who experiences a sudden onset of shortness of breath and sharp pains within the chest. Spontaneous pneumothorax occurs most commonly in young, otherwise

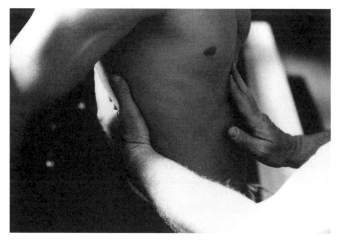

Figure 10.3. Distal compression used to evaluate for possible rib fractures.

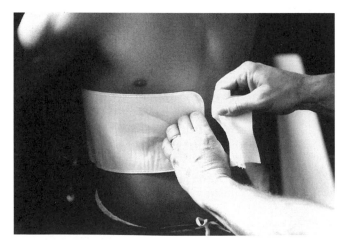

Figure 10.4. Rib belt used to stabilize ribs during healing.

healthy adults between the ages of 20 and 40, with recurrence experienced by approximately 50% of individuals (3). In situations in which the pneumothorax is quite large, the patient may become cyanotic, experience shortness of breath, and present in acute distress.

In both pneumothorax types, signs will be similar, such as shallow, rapid breathing due to air being unable to inflate the damaged lung. Percussion will be hyperresonant over the region of involvement. However, in situations of traumatic pneumothorax, percussion will be difficult due to the overlying rib fracture or contusion. An athlete suspected of having a pneumothorax should be transported immediately to an emergency facility for further observation and evaluation. Chest films will need to be performed, and vital signs will need to be monitored.

The diagnosis of pneumothorax is commonly confirmed by the standing posterior-anterior (PA) chest radiograph. Pulmonary vessels are usually observed extending up to a thin, smooth line representing the visceral pleura, bordered by air that has entered the pleural space. The pneumothorax is most frequently observed in the lung apex; however, subpulmonic and medial collections of air may also be seen. The lateral standing chest radiograph is useful to confirm the suspected pneumothorax and help rule out other pathology. Although not as sensitive or specific as the PA view, the lateral view offers a confirmatory degree of information for the diagnosis.

Glazer et al. (4) recently evaluated 122 separate cases of pneumothorax, appraising the usefulness of the standing PA view compared with the lateral projection. They were able to identify the pneumothorax from the PA projection in 97% of examinations (118 of 122). The pneumothorax was observed in a lateral projection in 89% of patients (109 of 122). The authors went on to conclude that in 14% of examinations, the lateral view was helpful in arriving at a diagnosis of a pneumothorax; in 11% of cases, the lateral projection demonstrated the condition far better. Further, 3% of patients presenting with a pneumothorax revealed that only the lateral projection was able to confirm the diagnosis; the PA projection was not conclusive.

Some of the problems encountered in relying solely on the lateral projection would be that more structures overlap compared with PA views. For example, skinfolds are capable of mimicking a pleural visceral line, offering a false-positive reading. One of the more common types of patients in whom this might be observed would be those who had undergone a previous mastectomy and now have a fold of skin that might simulate a lung edge. Another potential pitfall in relying heavily on the lateral projection would be that the scapular spine overlying the lung apex could also be mistaken for a pneumothorax.

The diagnosis of pulmonary embolism should be included in the differential diagnosis of pneumothorax. Although this condition is rare in young, athletic adults, the pattern of signs and symptoms would be very similar to that of pneumothorax. Cough or dyspnea may occur suddenly in an otherwise healthy athlete. The development of thromboembolic events is more common in women who are taking oral contraceptives and smoke cigarettes. Otherwise, pulmonary embolisms are commonly associated with trauma, strenuous and repetitive exercise, or underlying illnesses.

Seasonal Allergies

The athlete with hypersensitivity to differing environmental antigens poses a common problem for the team physician. Symptoms may range from a seasonal rhinitis, asthma, or urticaria and advance to anaphylaxis. One of the first steps the physician should take toward better understanding which antigens may be affecting the athlete is to obtain information regarding seasonal variations in the major pollens in the region. In moderate to severe cases, workouts may need to be tailored to help circumvent some of the daily and seasonal fluctuations in the pollens. Many athletes with known allergies will carry prescription drugs or over-the-counter antihistamines to control their symptoms. Unfortunately, these medications may tend to make the athlete drowsy or lethargic. The author has used several homeopathic formulas which contain Ephedra extract, as well as manipulation and diathermy over the sinuses and chest region.

Exercise-Induced Bronchospasm

A common problem confronting the asthmatic athlete is the experience of exercised-induced bronchospasm characterized by airway obstruction following hyperpnea or physical exertion. Adelman and Spector (3) report that approximately 75% of asthmatic individuals would experience a postexercise fall in forced expiratory volume in 1 second (FEV_1) of greater than 10%. The mechanism by which exercise induces bronchial constriction remains unclear. However, it is widely believed that the cause is a respiratory heat loss and airway cooling (5). Cold air is inhaled through the mouth, and ultimately contacting the alveoli with heat and water added continuously. During episodes of strenuous exercise, large volumes of air travel through the upper and lower respiratory tract, further promoting a falling temperature at any point in the airway. In certain asthmatic patients, it is believed that they have thermally sensitive neural receptors in the airway that mediate obstructive responses to cooling (6). The body responds by rewarming the airways through the dilation of local bronchial vessels. As a result, the mucosa becomes hyperemic edematous and ultimately the small airways become obstructed.

Antihistamines and vitamin C may be used to help control the reactions. Certain prescription medications may also be useful in severe cases. Manipulation and percussion should be used to help clear the congestion.

Some patients may require a respiratory inhalant or other medication. If these are prescription drugs and a referral is indicated, be aware that some athletes will need to pass a drug test. General practitioners or internists may not be aware of which drugs are allowed by the various governing bodies. Be certain to contact the governing body before use. This list of medications does change, so be sure to update your records.

Costochondral Separations

Costochondral separations are a relatively common occurrence in such sports as wrestling, football, and weight lifting. In many of these activities, the rib cage is put under a high level of compression, allowing for the separation to occur. The separation might not be limited only to the costochondral region, but to the region where the rib cartilage attaches to the sternum and posteriorly at the costovertebral junction. In many situations in which there is a separation to one of these three different areas, the other area may become symptomatic and need to be treated as well. In situations in which a costochondral or chondralosternal separation occurs, pinpoint tenderness will be experienced by the athlete and typically is able to be reproduced by the physician. If the activity is repeated habitually, as in performing a bench or leg press during weight lifting, separation may become chronic as the supportive ligaments become lax. The athlete may feel the rib pop out of its normal articulating position.

Therapy would commonly consist of gentle manipulation to the region, a rib belt, taping, and a reevaluation of the technique being performed, as in weight lifting. The author finds acupuncture to be useful in these disorders because this circumvents the use of an electrical modality, which may interfere with the normal conductivity of the heart.

Differential diagnosis should include heart disorders and epigastric reflux. It is important to rule out these potentially life-threatening disorders, especially in middle-aged patients. However, costochondral separations are extremely common and relatively easy to treat.

Keating (7) recently reported an unusual case involving a high school wrestler who was originally believed to have a costochondral separation injury. The young male athlete originally experienced acute anterior chest pain while performing a hyperextension trunk stretching exercise. Closer examination revealed extreme tenderness and a slightly palpable prominence over the anterior sternum approximately 2 cm distal to the sternal angle. Plain film studies of the sternum revealed an unusual formation believed to be a stress fracture. A bone scan was used to confirm the stress fracture diagnosis, noting the increase and uptake at the suspected region. Modification of athletic activities followed, allowing for proper healing and leaving the patient asymptomatic 2 months after the initial diagnosis. Obviously, a stress fracture of the sternum is exceptionally rare in a non–weight-bearing osseous structure. However, noting the high degree of competitiveness currently found within sports, certain elite athletes will definitely stress the upper body through weight lifting and related activities; thus, other more common conditions are mimicked.

INJURY TO DEEP TRUNCAL STRUCTURES

Injuries to the torsal contents are most commonly associated with contact sports, particularly the abdominal viscera. The spleen is the most commonly injured visceral organ. However, other areas such as the bowel, liver, kidneys, and bladder must also be considered in the differential diagnosis when there is acute trauma.

The history of the onset of symptoms is of extreme importance in this situation; abdominal complaints can vary from such minor disorders as a "stitch" in the side to nausea from a peptic ulcer to a lacerated spleen or kidney. The history should offer a detailed description of the events before the injury, answering such questions as the following. "Was the athlete kicked in the abdominal region or posterior flank area?" "Did the athlete receive a blow from a blunt end of a helmet?" "Was the athlete stepped on by another player's cleats?" "How long ago did the injury occur?" "Is this something from the previous play in which the player had to be helped off the field, or was this one or two quarters prior in the game and only now has the player become acute with distress, suggesting that a fulminating disorder may be occurring?"

Splenic Trauma

The spleen is typically protected by the left lower ribs. However, in certain situations the athlete may extend himself or herself outward, i.e., when catching a pass, or the athlete may have an enlarged spleen (i.e., from mononucleosis), which predisposes the spleen to a greater risk of injury. As Kulund's report (8) states, mononucleosis will make the spleen large and weak from hyperplasia of white pulp, an extensive lymphocytic infiltration into the red pulp. If the disease is allowed to progress, the enlargement and weakening process will take approximately 14–28 days to advance. Thus, the spleen is usually not susceptible to rupture before 2 weeks into the disease. At this 14-day stage, it is possible for the spleen to rupture from the slightest blow to the left upper quadrant of the abdomen or lower left set of ribs.

Cardinal signs of mononucleosis are lymphadenopathy, sore throat, fever, and fatigue. An athlete who has these symptoms, along with lethargic play in performance, should prompt one to perform a monospot test. The spleen should be palpated for possible enlargement if mononucleosis is suspected. However, in the case of an acute injury, palpation may be difficult.

Treatment of this disease in athletes should be supportive care, fluids, lots of rest, monitoring of fever, and laboratory studies. When the fever subsides, the patient may be allowed to return to normal daily activities. However, restrictions from physical activity, particularly contact sports, should continue for 3 to 6 months. The author is aware of many athletes allowed to return to a contact sport much sooner than 3 to 6 months. However, the team physician should keep the following statistics in mind. DeShazo (9) reported a much higher incidence of splenic rupture in those football players who had mononucleosis before the diagnosis of the rupture. Specifically, of the 17 of 22 ruptures involving football athletes, 8 of these individuals had mononucleosis before splenic rupture.

Splenic rupture may also occur in athletes not afflicted by mononucleosis. These cases will usually present in one of three modes. First, the acutely injured athlete who just received a sharp blow to the left upper quadrant or left lower ribs. This athlete is unable to return to activity on the playing field and needs to be helped to the sidelines. Second, an athlete may experience trauma to the abdominal region, be able to regain apparently normal ambulation, and then later in the game present with increasing symptoms and develop left shoulder pain, due to intraperitoneal irritation against the diaphragm by blood coming from the spleen. Third, the delayed splenic rupture, which may occur up to 1 month after the abdominal trauma has been experienced. This may have weakened the spleen, making it susceptible to minor trauma, and a ruptured spleen results.

Aspegren et al. (2) recently reported on a case of acute splenic rupture in a high school football player whose team physician was a chiropractor. Midway through the second quarter of a high school football game, one of the players was preparing to make a tackle while covering a punt. At that time, the player making the tackle was legally blocked by an opponent, striking the left anterior axillary region. The injured player remained on his back, offering an initial impression of "having the wind knocked out of him." After approximately 1 minute, he began breathing better but still with effort. It was at that point that the player asked the field physician to lift the sternal section of his shoulder pads off his chest. This was the first clue suggesting that a more severe injury may have occurred than was initially suspected. On lifting the sternal section of the pads, tenderness was elicited off the left fifth through seventh ribs on palpation, suggesting a possible fracture and at least contusions.

Abdominal examination was difficult because the patient had difficulty relaxing sufficiently to allow for palpation. At that time, it was decided to transport the player to the local emergency department for evaluation of a possible rib fracture and splenic rupture. While waiting for transportation to be brought to the locker room, the patient's condition began to worsen and initial signs of shock developed. Later, the emergency department physician agreed with the initial impression of the field physician and ordered chest and rib plain film studies as well as a computed tomography (CT) study of the spleen.

Plain films revealed a nondisplaced fracture of the left seventh rib (Fig. 10.5). The radiologist believed this rib fracture was the culprit in lacerating the spleen. The CT scan with contrast material performed the night of the injury demonstrated findings consistent with a lacerated spleen (Fig. 10.6). Specifically, the radiologist commented on the observation of an enlarged spleen with an abnormal contour and a large amount of fluid in and around the organ.

The patient was monitored closely during the

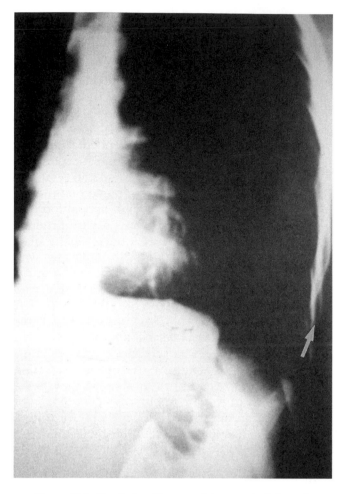

Figure 10.5. Nondisplaced fracture of the seventh rib (arrow).

next 10 days. Of prime importance were the heart rate, hemoglobin level, and temperature. The patient had a low-grade fever of 100°F over the next 3 days, and his hemoglobin count gradually decreased from 13.0 to 10.4 mg/mL. At that point, the patient received two units of whole blood from a parent. The hemoglobin level stabilized over the next day and then gradually increased to 14.2 mg/mL 6 days later.

A follow-up CT scan with contrast material performed 3 weeks later showed the lacerated spleen more clearly, due to the change in attenuation values of the blood during the interval. The laceration to the spleen was evident, as was the consolidating hematoma in and around the spleen (Fig. 10.7).

A third CT scan was performed, now 60 days past the injury, demonstrating improvement in many of the previously described areas. The hematoma in and around the spleen had diminished, and there was evidence of viability and healing of all areas of the spleen since the prior CT scan study (Fig. 10.8). From that point on, recovery was uneventful. However, in further discussion with the player's coach, it seemed to take almost 1 year before the athlete regained the full levels of energy that he had before the incident.

At one time, it was believed to be beneficial to remove the traumatized spleen because it was considered to serve a relatively minor role in the function of the reticuloendothelial system. How-

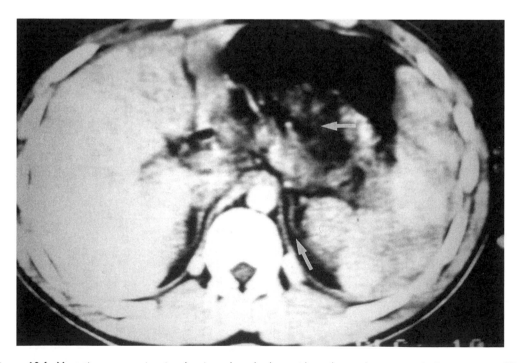

Figure 10.6. Magnetic resonance imaging showing enlarged spleen with an abnormal contour and a large amount of fluid (white arrows) in and around the spleen.

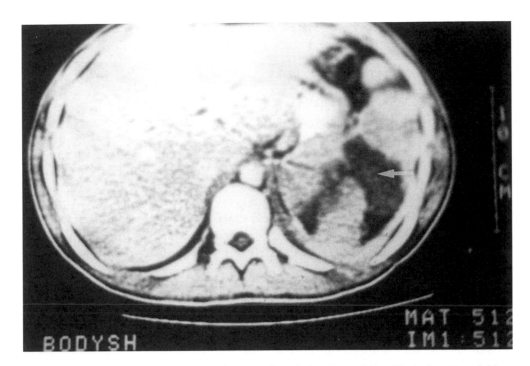

Figure 10.7. Magnetic resonance imaging showing laceration through the spleen and consolidating hematoma (white arrow) in and around the spleen.

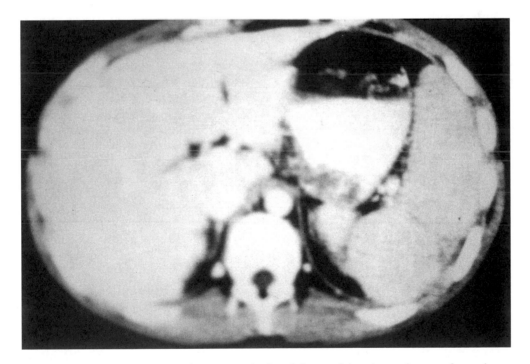

Figure 10.8. Magnetic resonance imaging demonstrating healing of all areas of the spleen and return of normal contour.

ever, this trend has changed in more recent years for several reasons (10). First, there have been many reported problems for patients as a result of splenectomy. These include such problems as sepsis, long-term suppressed immune function, and death. Now all attempts are made to salvage the spleen. The second reason for being able to save more spleens has been brought about by a more widespread use of CT (11–19) or ultrasound (19–22) to evaluate and monitor the spleen. CT is probably the most frequently used instrument to monitor and to assess prognosis of the spleen.

The decision of when to remove the spleen and when it is best to attempt splenic salvage through a nonoperative conservative approach is very controversial. Buntain et al. (13) have attempted to develop a spleen grading system for the use of CT for these particular situations. In their recent study, 46 patients with blunt splenic trauma were evaluated and graded I–IV with CT findings. The grading score depended on capsular or subcapsular disruption, parenchymal injury, vessel involvement, and fragmentation/devascularization. Of the patients who underwent surgery, their grading system appeared accurate for tissue assessment and seemed useful in identifying spleens that would best be treated via splenectomy.

Other elements used to monitor patient progression or regression while in the hospital after splenic rupture had been identified are the hemodynamic findings (23, 24). These would include hemoglobin levels and heart rate as the two principal telltale indicators as to whether the patient required a transfusion and also whether the patient was losing blood into the peritoneum. As was mentioned in the case of the football player with the splenic injury, the subsequent hemoglobin levels were of major concern. In his situation, if his hemoglobin had continued to fall below the 10.4 mg/mL level and the two units of blood had not stabilized the hemodynamics of his system, the spleen would have been removed.

The field physician should always remain aware and sensitive to the possibility of a delayed rupture of a traumatized spleen (16, 25–27). Even in players with mild abdominal trauma, stomach rupture can occur at a later time, and these individuals should be questioned days and even weeks after a blow to the abdomen to avoid the oversight of such a malady. Schultz and Froelich (26) recently presented a case of delayed splenic rupture 23 days after abdominal trauma. Results of the initial scintigram of the spleen were normal. However, the second scintigram performed before splenectomy showed a persistent defect.

Sziklos et al. (27) reported delayed splenic ruptures occurring in two of their patients. One rupture was on day 31 after the injury, and the other was on day 26. To help identify these spleens, which are likely to undergo a delayed rupture, they suggest an initial study to identify splenic damage soon after the accident. A follow-up study is mandatory to demonstrate proper healing. Lack of such healing is a sign of possible impending delayed splenic rupture.

Rib pads would be considered useful in helping to avoid such injuries to the spleen, liver, and proximal small bowel. At this time, rib pads are considered an optional piece of equipment; however, it may be considered in the best interest of players who are rendered susceptible to such blows, i.e., receivers, halfbacks, and quarterbacks, that this equipment be used routinely.

Hepatic Rupture

The liver may become predisposed to rupture in several different ways, such as direct trauma or episodes of contagious hepatitis. In the situation of acute trauma, the liver may be damaged in a similar mode as the spleen, but now involving the right upper quadrant of the abdomen or right lower ribs. If the spleen is traumatized, the capsule will help control the amount of bleeding if the capsule remains intact. If, however, the capsule is lacerated (e.g., from a fractured rib), bleeding will occur into the intraperitoneal cavity, leading to irritation of the right diaphragmatic region with possible right shoulder pain. As in the situation of a ruptured spleen, the person with hepatic rupture should also be followed by immediate transport to an emergency department facility for observation and further testing.

In the situation of hepatitis, a commonly reported form that may affect an entire team would be hepatitis A. Hepatitis B is most commonly transferred in athletes through open cuts allowing for exposure to the infected individual's blood.

Hepatitis A is transported most frequently through a fecal-oral route. In situations where entire teams are involved, a common water supply has become contaminated, leading to widespread infection. In 1969, members of the Holy Cross football team became infected after drinking contaminated water. Of 97 players, coaches, and trainers, 32 individuals (34%) tested positive for hepatitis A disease (28). It was later determined that contaminated surface water had entered the team's drinking water as the result of a freak back-siphonage. Approximately 1 month later, team members became symptomatic over 15 days.

It is far more common to have one or two members of a team afflicted by the disease rather than the entire team. In such situations, supportive care should be instituted for those individuals involved. Observing for more serious complications of hepatitis (such as hepatic failure, which may necessitate hospital admission), and precautions to protect the other members of the team should be instituted. There should be close observation of those individuals who have had close personal contact with the afflicted patient, and these individuals should be monitored for early signs and symptoms. If questionable contact may have occurred with another individual on the team, passive immunization with immunoglobulins may be used to help the severity of the illness. All water supplies should be cleaned thoroughly to control the spread of the disease. As is commonly known in hepatitis A, most of the cases are subclinical, meaning that other individuals on the team may be afflicted by the disease. These other individuals, however, may not be expressing enough of the symptoms to suggest the presence of infection. Thus, it may be necessary to perform liver function studies on the entire team to help find these subclinical cases. In those individuals with abnormal liver function, Decker and Overby (29) state that the presence of the immunoglobulin M antibody to hepatitis A confirms an acute infection. This was the test used to confirm and rule out a true infection in serum samples of the Holy Cross football squad (28).

Hepatitis B will be transferred via blood and blood products between individuals. Although transmission between athletes is quite rare, it can occur via open wounds between an infected and susceptible host. Cuts and abrasions are the most concerning lesions lending to potential spread.

Hepatitis B infection may be documented by the presence of hepatitis B surface antigen (Hbs Ag) in serologic studies. Once a case is identified, care is supportive. The patient should be monitored for advancing liver pathology such as cirrhosis. Furthermore, infected athletes should be monitored for the potential of becoming carriers of the disease. If this is the case, the athlete may need to terminate participation because of the risk of infecting others (30).

Rupture of the Bowel

During instances of acute abdominal trauma, the previously described structures (such as the kidney, spleen, and liver) are more commonly involved than the gastrointestinal tract. Although it may be rare for the small and large bowel to be involved, ruptures can occur and should certainly be included in the differential diagnosis after an acute trauma to the abdominal sections.

Murphy and Drez (31) recently reported on a case of jejunal rupture in a high school football player. The athlete was struck in the abdomen with a helmet. He experienced sharp, midepigastric pain and appeared to "have the wind knocked out of him." The athlete regained his feet and was able to continue with the game after a short rest. However, shortly after the game was over, the athlete experienced generalized abdominal pain. It would be common for athletes to experience pregame nervousness in the stomach; however, observing this in a postgame setting should alert the team physician to a possible underlying abdominal injury. In this case, the athlete was transported to an emergency department and demonstrated the vital signs of pulse rate of 120 beats/min, normal blood pressure, increased rate of respiration at 30/min, and a slightly increased temperature of 99.8°F. Diffused abdominal tenderness was noted with extreme rigidity and rebound tenderness. Bowel sounds were decreased. Laparotomy revealed a 1.5-cm jejunal perforation. The damaged bowel was surgically closed, and the patient recovered uneventfully.

The most common segments of the small bowel to be injured are the duodenum, proximal jejunum, and terminal ilium. These areas are the most susceptible because they are attached to the peritoneal wall; consequently, they are unable to escape episodes of trauma. Other regions of the small bowel are freely movable, unattached, and far less likely to be injured. The bowel is most commonly to be injured by a crushing blow to the abdominal region, pinning the bowel against the spine. Those signs and symptoms may vary considerably among athletes who have experienced trauma to the bowel. There does seem to be a consistent finding of sharp midepigastric pain followed by signs of chemical peritonitis within a few hours.

In addition to the midepigastric pain and abdominal guarding commonly observed, the patient will have a notable decrease or loss in bowel sounds, abdominal rigidity, cold and clammy skin, and further signs of initial stages of shock. Blood may enter the peritoneum and irritate the diaphragm, resulting in consequential irritation of the phrenic nerve and ultimately shoulder pain. It is common for hours or even days to elapse before symptoms of abdominal damage begin to appear.

Trauma to the Solar Plexus

As has been described in several of the previous sections, athletes will commonly experience the situation of "having the wind knocked out of them." The greatest concern for the team physician is to be aware of other possible injuries, such as to the bowel or spleen. However, these situations are rare; most commonly, the athlete has simply lost the ability to breathe due to a traumatic blow to the abdomen. The athlete will present in a state of anxiousness, unable to catch his or her breath and unable to speak. In these situations, the team physician should take steps to calm the athlete while making certain that the airway is not blocked by a mouthpiece or foreign object, such as a piece of equipment or tongue.

Athletes will regain their breath sooner if you can calm them, loosen their belt, and bend their knees to help relax the abdominal region. The athlete should be taken from playing field and quickly examined. If all systems initially check out, the athlete should be allowed to return to the game without restriction. However, the athlete should be watched closely from this time on for several days to even weeks for signs of abdominal involvement and early stages of shock, further identifying greater involvement beyond that of solar plexus trauma.

"Stitch in the Side"

A common occurrence in untrained runners who are beginning to increase their training is the expression of sharp pains under the right lower ribs. The common name given to this is a "stitch in the side" or "side ache." The list of causes includes gas in the large bowel, anoxia in this region of the diaphragm, diaphragmatic spasm, or possible liver congestion with stretching of the liver capsule. Pain is usually alleviated by having the athlete take deep breaths. If the athlete is currently involved in an event in which he or she cannot stop, the athlete may try breathing out with the lips pursed. Once the pain has subsided, the athlete may typically resume the workout without a recurrence of symptoms. As the individual becomes better conditioned, the frequency of this condition decreases.

Renal Injury

Kidney damage caused by a blow to the flank region is always a concern to the team physician while supervising contact sports. Athletes may complain of back pain and may demonstrate blood in the urine on micturition. An athlete who sustained a blow to the flank region and who complains of persistent pain in this area should have a urinalysis performed for microscopic hematuria.

Obviously, the patient with the above-described symptoms and a positive urinalysis offers a suggestion of a possible renal rupture or laceration and requires further investigation by a urologist. However, difficulty in diagnosis arises from the report by several studies that hematuria and other elements of urinary sediment are found to be abnormal after episodes of strenuous exercise.

Alvarez et al. (32) recently investigated hematuria and microalbuminuria induced by prolonged exercise in 26 runners who participated in a 100-km race. The authors collected urine samples before and after the race and 24 hours later.

Microscopic hematuria was observed in two runners before the race and in nine runners (34.6%) after the race. In addition, five runners (19.2%) demonstrated macroscopic hematuria after the race. No red blood cell casts were observed. Albuminuria was observed in 18 of 26 athletes immediately after the event. Additional studies were performed 24 hours later, and all the results returned to a normal level, except for five runners who had demonstrated macroscopic hematuria and one with microalbuminuria without hematuria.

Gardner (33) reported his urinary sediment observations of a college football team for which he observed results over 2 weeks during the midseason. He noted that the severity of proteinuria and cylindruria was found to correlate with the degree of individual physical exertion. The study went on to demonstrate not only an abnormal degree of proteinuria and increased number of granular and hyaline casts, but also red blood cell casts in some of the specimens. The phenomenon of abnormal findings after exertion, without known clinical consequences, has been described as pseudonephritis of athletes (Table 10.1).

Kulund (8) reported how boxers must have a normal urinalysis before entering the ring. However, most boxers will have an abnormal urinalysis after a boxing match. The most common findings observed in these athletes are hematuria and albuminuria, and the urine may also contain granular and hyaline casts. As Kulund goes on to explain, some of this may be explained by the boxer's position taken while competing. This is known as a crouched position. The position apparently increases the intraabdominal pressure and thus compresses the boxer's renal vessels. In addition, the "grunt reflex" may adversely affect kidney function. The grunt reflex is said to affect the kidneys by causing the diaphragm and ab-

---

Table 10.1.   Features of Athletic Pseudonephritis

Proteinuria
  Albuminuria
  Globulinuria
  Myoglobinuria (usually mild and transient)
  Hemoglobinuria (mild; presence parallels hematuria)
Formed elements
  Hyaline casts
  Granular casts
  Red blood cells
  White blood cells
  Red blood cell casts
Clinical setting
  Occurs within 7 days of last exertion
  Abnormalities clear with rest
  Abnormalities do not occur immediately postexercise *with*, but later (more than 1 day) *without*, depression of glomerular filtration rate

dominal muscles to contract during a boxer's attack. This may further increase abdominal pressure, partially displace the kidneys, and perhaps cause ptosis.

In runners, the mechanism initiating abnormal urinary studies is believed to be attributed to the shunting of blood to active muscles away from the renal system. As a result, the renal blood flow decreases by approximately 50%, leading to a relative renal ischemia and hematuria. Other related causes may include direct kidney damage, trauma to the kidney tubules, renal vein kinking, and bladder contusions.

CARDIOVASCULAR DISEASES IN ATHLETES

Every year, the media carries tragic reports of young, well-trained athletes suddenly dying of cardiac disease. When we envision someone dying of a cardiomyopathy, the scene of an elderly man who perhaps had a heart attack once, was attempting to regain a heightened level of physical activity, and suddenly dies due to overexertion usually comes to mind. However, several studies have described the incidence, occurrence, and pathophysiology leading to sudden cardiac death in younger athletes. The reported rate of death during such activities as jogging or cross-country skiing is 4 to 7 times greater than that experienced during sedentary pursuits (34, 35). In addition, during vigorous activities, the incidence of sudden death has been observed to raise from 5 to 56 times that of rest (35, 36). However, we should keep in mind the rate of cardiac arrest is lower among physically active individuals while they are at rest. The above figures do suggest that various levels of exercise can provoke sudden cardiac death in susceptible individuals.

Waller (37) reported on 15 individuals, ages 13 through 29, who suddenly died shortly after strenuous exercise. All individuals had been exercising several times a week before the incident. Cardiovascular abnormalities were observed in 14 of 15 individuals, suggesting an etiology for the premature deaths. Structural abnormalities observed included congenital coronary artery anomalies, hypertrophic cardiomyopathy, mitral valve prolapse, and tricuspid valve incompetency (one patient).

Maron et al. (38) reported mortality findings on 29 well-conditioned competitive athletes ages 13 through 30. Their findings demonstrated that 22 died during or shortly after high levels of physical exertion, 2 died during or soon after mild exertion, and 5 died during sedentary activities. Structural cardiovascular abnormalities were observed in 28 of 29 subjects. Twenty-two of 28 had abnormalities that were considered significant enough to have been the likely cause of death. Six of 28 had autopsy findings that were suggestive of likely cardiac involvement leading toward death. One individual of the 29 listed in the study had no cardiomyopathy observed. Common findings observed during autopsy were as follows: 14 athletes were found to have hypertrophic cardiomyopathy, 5 had a concentric left ventricular hypertrophy, and 3 had significant coronary artery disease with a decrease in lumen diameter up to 75%. A dissecting aortic aneurysm and rupture were observed in two individuals. The remaining individuals had combinations of disorders such as coronary artery malformation, valvular abnormalities, and unusual myocardial cell formation.

The death of mature athletes, those older than 30 years of age, seems to be well epitomized by the premature death of author Jim Fixx. Fixx was previously observed to be a healthy, well-conditioned athlete who would seem least likely to die of cardiac disease. However, autopsy findings demonstrated advanced coronary artery disease in several of the vessels with associated myocardial necrosis of the left ventricular wall. Predisposing factors leading to Fixx's death were a history of cigarette smoking, elevated cholesterol level observed in a postmortem finding of 254 mg/100 mL, and a family history of premature coronary artery disease (39).

Thompson et al. (34) have estimated the incidence of death during jogging for men, ages 30 through 64, to be 1 death per year for every 7620 joggers. This rate is a seven-fold increase over the normal death rate expected during sedentary activities for the general population in the same age group. Of the studies demonstrating autopsy findings in athletes who have experienced sudden death due to cardiac factors, one trend has been found consistently over the years. This is that atherosclerotic coronary arteries appear to be the major contributing factor to sudden cardiac death in older athletes; as discussed previously, a wide array of disorders are believed to be involved in younger individuals who experience cardiac involvement. Virmani et al. (40) reported their work on 23 joggers older than 30 years of age. Their autopsy findings demonstrated severe coronary artery disease in 22 of 23 individuals. Of the same 23 deceased athletes, 13 were found to have healed or acute myocardial infarction. All these individuals were believed to be in excellent physical condition, compiling high numbers of miles in weekly workouts, and generally determined to be experienced runners.

Rogota et al. (41) reported on 75 athletes older than 30 years of age who died during recreational activities. Causes of death were listed as follows: 71 from atherosclerotic coronary heart disease, 2 from hypertensive cardiovascular disease determined by clinical diagnosis, 1 from cerebrovascular accident, and 1 by aortic aneurysm dissection.

The Detection of Cardiac Risk in Athletes

Described above is an overview of how both younger and older athletes are affected by cardiac dysfunction. These situations are certainly tragic; however, they represent a small fraction of individuals currently active in some form of athletic participation. Consequently, it becomes virtually cost-prohibitive to perform an extensive cardiac evaluation on every individual seeking to increase their level of physical activity.

As a result, one should seek to identify factors elicited from the patient that might help identify the need for further, more extensive tests. A great deal of emphasis should be placed on taking a thorough history and thus eliciting possibly previously diagnosed cardiac disorders within the patient or his or her relatives. For example, the patient may describe how a parent or sibling may have experienced a cardiovascular disease prematurely compared with the general population. Perhaps someone in the athlete's family carries an elevated serum lipid level, possibly suggesting a need for evaluation in this area. The patient might also describe some previous illnesses of their own that may include conditions affecting the heart, such as rheumatic fever; hypertension; diabetes mellitus; history of smoking; various arrhythmias; unusual heart sounds or murmurs; or perhaps chest symptoms on previous exertion. All these would tend to suggest the possibility of underlying cardiac disease.

A large number of cardiac conditions have been associated with exercise-related sudden death. Sadaniantz and Thompson (35) outline the most common etiologic factors (Table 10.2). As Waller (37) has observed, the most frequent cause of death in individuals older than 40 years of age is atherosclerotic coronary artery disease. For those athletes younger than 40 years of age, congenital conditions such as hypertrophic cardiomyopathy and anomalous origin of the coronary arteries are the most frequent causes.

Those patients with the above-described disorders should undergo further evaluation in such preliminary areas as laboratory tests to measure serum lipid levels; an exercise electrocardiogram would be ordered in individuals with arrhythmias or confirmed, elevated cholesterol levels.

If the patient does not have a history of elevated blood fats and is younger than 40, serum lipids levels are not commonly evaluated. However, if the individual is older than 40, even without a history suggesting serum fat elevation, it is generally considered a good idea to evaluate this area to help assess for possible premature coronary artery disease.

Van Camp (38) offers the following suggestions for performing an electrocardiogram. Exercise electrocardiograms should be performed before beginning vigorous exercise in those individuals identified as the following:

1. Men 45 years of age or older;
2. Women 55 years of age or older;
3. Adults who have described chest discomfort on exertion, irregular heart rate, or syncope;
4. Men younger than 45 years of age or women younger than 55 years of age identified as having a significant risk of coronary artery disease.

These individuals might also have a serum cholesterol level greater than 250 mg/100 mL, high-density lipoprotein rating less than 35 mg/ 100 mL, blood pressure with a systolic level of 170 mm Hg and a diastolic level of 90 mm Hg, cigarette smoking, diabetes mellitus, family history of sudden cardiac death, or coronary artery disease in relatives younger than 60 years of age.

Ambulatory electrocardiograms should be performed in those individuals with arrhythmias

Table 10.2. Causes of Exersise-Related Sudden Death in Athletes

Factors that cause myocardial ischemia
  Atherosclerotic coronary artery disease
  Coronary artery spasm
  De novo coronary artery thrombus
  Intramyocardial bridging
  Hypoplastic coronary artery
  Anomalous coronary arteries
Structural abnormalities
  Hypertrophic cardiomyopathy
  Mitral valve prolapse
  Valvular heart disease
  Lipomatous infiltration of the right ventricle
  Marfan's syndrome
Arrhythmias
  Wolff-Parkinson-White syndrome
  Lown-Ganong-Levine syndrome
  Ventricular arrhythmias
  Medial hyperplasia and intimal proliferation of the main sinus node artery
Miscellaneous
  Subarachnoid hemorrhage
  Gastrointestinal hemorrhage
  Myocarditis

and/or syncope. If the individual intends to begin any degree of physical activity and has a noticeable arrhythmia, it is best to have this condition stabilized before beginning such events. Resting electrocardiograms may be performed on individuals between the ages of 30 and 45 years for men and 30 and 55 years for women, who are now believed to have a significant risk of coronary artery disease. However, the resting electrocardiogram is of limited value when attempting to identify those levels of dysfunction that may be related to physical activity.

Chest radiographs may be useful in identifying aortic enlargement or congestive heart failure and related disorders. However, the chest radiograph is of limited value and typically not performed unless clinical findings or history is suggestive.

Echocardiography is an extremely useful test to identify various heart chamber and related pathologic anatomical development. However, this test is expensive and should be ordered on a selective basis only for those patients with identified indications.

Prevention of a Cardiac Disaster

One of the primary goals in preventing an athlete from experiencing a sudden cardiac death would be to identify those conditions before the expression of a cardiac condition. The physician should be aware of conditions such as murmurs, arrhythmias, and a history of connective tissue disease (e.g., Marfan's syndrome). Some of these athletes may have been previously instructed to limit their athletic participation due to a possible cardiac disorder. However, other athletes may not have had their cardiomyopathy previously discovered.

Sadaniantz and Thompson (35) recently reported on a 57-year-old runner who collapsed and died approximately 1 minute after setting a US eastern regional indoor masters record in the 3000 meter run. This man had never complained of any symptoms that were suggestive of cardiovascular disease and had completed a normal exercise stress test 22 months before his run. Autopsy failed to reveal thrombi or hemorrhage of the coronary arteries, and there was no evidence of an acute myocardial infarction. However, further evaluation of the left anterior interventricular coronary artery, left circumflex artery, and right coronary arteries revealed extensive atherosclerotic plaquing occupying 75–80% of the cross-sectional area. Evaluation of the left ventricular wall demonstrated patchy fibrotic foci suggestive of prior infarctions.

This is an example of a patient dying of atherosclerotic coronary artery disease and a case that offers a challenge to all physicians confronted with individuals attempting to either increase athletic activity or maintain a high level of strenuous exercise. Not only does this case demonstrate how difficult it may be to identify those individuals with advancing coronary artery disease, but further brings to light limitations and concerns regarding the effectiveness of a stress electrocardiogram.

For young athletes, the most common cause of sudden cardiac death is that of anomalous origin of the coronary arteries. The most common congenital coronary deformity is the origin of the left anterior interventricular coronary artery off the right coronary artery. The right coronary artery does not receive nearly the blood supply of the left. It is also believed that a precipitating factor behind the myocardial ischemia in these individuals is that during heightened exertion, there is an increase in stroke volume, which may compress the coronary artery's origin and thereby reduce its flow.

Signs and symptoms suggesting that a young patient may have anomalous coronary artery system would be an exercise-induced syncope, angina pectoralis, or acute cardiac distress. Those individuals demonstrating a definite exercise-induced syncope should have a full cardiovascular evaluation, including coronary angiogram to evaluate for these disorders.

In many sports, height offers a tremendous advantage to some individuals. However, for those players who are exceptionally tall, the team physician should maintain an awareness of the possibility of Marfan's syndrome. Interest in this disease as a possible etiologic factor resulting in sudden cardiac death was greatly heightened after the death of a 31-year-old female Olympian during a volleyball game. It is reported that during the third game of the match, she left the playing floor during a routine substitution, sat down, and silently slid to the floor. Autopsy revealed a rupture of the aorta, with microscopic histologic studies consistent with Marfan's syndrome. Elements that should suggest possible Marfan's syndrome in the athlete are excessive height when compared with family members, unusually long limbs, an increase in lower extremity length, and very long slender fingers. A high-arched palate, sternal deformities, and lens dislocations are also commonly observed. In addition to the aortic dilation, the mitral valve has a tendency to prolapse more frequently than in those nonafflicted individuals.

The therapeutic and/or preventative measures to be taken with the cardiac case will be determined by the degree of involvement of disease the athlete may have experienced. For instance, measures to control lipid levels with diet regulation and perhaps use of such products as niacin may be all that is required. In other individuals, the level of competition may need to be regulated so as not to potentiate a cardiovascular accident. The use of aspirin in athletes and nonathletes has become commonplace in everyday practice. Aspirin will inhibit the enzyme cyclooxygenase, thereby attenuating platelet aggregation and interfering with atherosclerotic processes. Several well-controlled clinical studies (42, 43) have demonstrated the positive effects of using aspirin in those individuals who are at risk of recurrent myocardial infarction. Aspirin has even reduced the incidence of myocardial infarction in healthy individuals.

De Meersman (43) recently addressed a concern many athletes and team physicians have regarding the consumption of aspirin and its effects on the body's ability to regulate temperature, body fluids, respiratory functions, and hormonal responses during exercise. During his studies and rather impressive review, he concluded that 325 mg/day would not have adverse effects on the above-stated functions, as this dose has been shown to be effective in reducing heart attacks and, further, has been found to be safe when combined with exercise.

References

1. Roy S, Irvin R. Sports medicine: prevention, evaluation, management, and rehabilitation. Englewood Cliffs, NJ: Prentice-Hall, 1983.
2. Aspegren D, Phillip S, Benak D. Acute splenic rupture in a high school football player. Chiro Sports Med 1989;3: 120–123.
3. Adelman D, Spector S. Acute respiratory emergencies in emergency treatment of the injured athlete. Clin Sports Med 1989;8:71–79.
4. Glazer H, Anderson D, Wilson B, et al. Pneumothorax: appearance on lateral chest radiographs. Radiology 1989; 173:707–711.
5. Strauss RH, McFadden ER, Ingram RH, et al. Enhancement of exercise-induced asthma by cold air. N Engl J Med 1977;297:743–747.
6. McNally JF, Enright P, Hirsch JE, et al. The attenuation of exercise-induced bronchoconstriction by oropharyngeal anesthesia. Am Rev Respir Dis 1979;119:247–252.
7. Keating T. Stress fracture of the sternum in a wrestler. Am J Sports Med 1987;15:92–93.
8. Kulund, D. The injured athlete. 2nd ed. Philadelphia: JB Lippincott, 1988.
9. DeShazo WF III. Returning athletes to athletic activity after infectious mononucleosis. Phys Sportsmed 1980;8: 71–72.
10. O'Connor G, Geelhoed G. Splenic trauma and salvage. Am Surg 1986;52:456–462.
11. Resciniti A, Fink M, Raptopoulos V, et al. Non-operative treatment of adult splenic trauma: development of a computed tomographic scoring system that detects appropriate candidates for expectant management. J Trauma 1988;28:828–831.
12. Meredith J, Trunkey D. CT scanning in acute abdominal injuries. Surg Clin North Am 1988;68:255–268.
13. Buntain W, Gould H, Maull K. Predictability of splenic salvage by computed tomography. J Trauma 1988;28: 24–34.
14. Brick S, Taylor G, Potter B, et al. Hepatic and splenic injury in children: role of CT in the decision for laparotomy. Radiology 1986;165:643–646.
15. Mahboubi S. Abdominal trauma in children: role of computed tomography. Pediatr Emerg Care 1985;1:37–39.
16. Sutton C, Hoaga J. CT evaluation of limited splenic trauma. J Comput Assist Tomogr 1987;11:167–169.
17. Federle M, Griffiths B, Minagi H, et al. Splenic trauma: evaluation with a CT. Radiology 1987;162:69–71.
18. Sortland O, Nerdrum H, Solheim K. Computed tomography and scintigraphy in the diagnosis of splenic injury. Acta Chir Scand 1986;152:453–461.
19. Adler D, Blane C, Coran A, et al. Splenic trauma in the pediatric patient: the integrated roles of ultrasound and computed tomography. Pediatrics 1986;78:576–580.
20. Weill F, Rohmer P, Didier D, et al. Ultrasound of the traumatized spleen: left butterfly sign in lesions marked by echogenic blood clots. Gastrointest Radiol 1988;13: 169–172.
21. Filialrault D, Longpre D, Patriquin H. Investigation of childhood blunt abdominal trauma: a practical approach using ultrasound as the initial diagnostic modality. Pediatr Radiol 1987;17:373–379.
22. Booth A, Bruce D, Steiner G. Ultrasound diagnosis of splenic injuries in children: the importance of the peritoneal fluid. Clin Radiol 1987;38:395–398.
23. Mucha P Jr, Daly R, Farnell M. Selective management of blunt splenic trauma. J Trauma 1986;26:970–979.
24. Johnson H Jr, Shatney C. Splenic injuries in adults: selective nonoperative management. South Med J 1986;79:5–8.
25. Mahon P, Sutton J Jr. Nonoperative management of adult splenic injury due to blunt trauma: a warning. Am J Surg 1985;149:716–721.
26. Schultz D, Froelich J. Delayed rupture of the spleen: a case report. Clin Nucl Med 1985;10:642–645.
27. Sziklos J, Spencer R, Rosenberg R. Delayed splenic rupture: a suggestion for "predictive monitoring." J Nucl Med 1985;26:609–611.
28. Friedman L, O'Brien T, Morse L, et al. Revisiting the Holy Cross football team hepatitis outbreak (1969) by serological analysis. JAMA 1985;254:774–776.
29. Decker R, Overby L. Serologic studies of transmission of hepatitis A in humans. J Infect Dis 1979;139:74–82.
30. Volpicelli N, Spector M. In: Appenzeller O, ed. Sports medicine: fitness, training, injuries. 3rd ed. Baltimore: Urban & Schwarzenberg, 1988.
31. Murphy C, Drez D. Jejunal rupture in a football player. Am J Sports Med 1987;15:184–185.
32. Alvarez C, Mir J, Obaya S, et al. Hematuria and microalbuminuria after a 100 kilometer race. Am J Sports Med 1987;15:609–611.
33. Gardner K Jr. In: Appenzeller O, ed. Sports medicine: fitness, training, injuries. 3rd ed. Baltimore: Urban & Schwarzenberg, 1988.
34. Thompson P, Funk E, Carleton R, et al. Incidence of death during jogging in Rhode Island from 1975 through 1980. JAMA 1982;247:2535–2538.
35. Sadaniantz A, Thompson P. The problem of sudden death in athletes as illustrated by case studies. Sports Med 1990;9:199–204.
36. Siscovick D, Weiss N, Fletcher R, et al. The incidence of primary cardiac arrest during vigorous exercise. N Engl J Med 1984;311:874–877.
37. Waller B. Exercise-related sudden death in young (age <30 years) and old (age >30 years) conditioned subjects. Cardiovasc Clin 1985;15:9–73.

38. Maron B, Roberts W, McAllister H, et al. Sudden death in young athletes. Circulation 1980;62:218–229.
39. Van Camp S. Advances in sports medicine and fitness. Chicago: Year Book, 1988;1.
40. Virmani R, Rominowitz M, McAllister H Jr. Nontraumatic death in joggers: a series of 30 patients at autopsy. Am J Med 1982;72:874–882.
41. Rogota M, Crabtree J, Sturner W. Death during recreational exercise in the state of Rhode Island. Med Sci Sports 1968;16:339–342.
42. Hennekens C, Eberlein K. A randomized trial of aspirin and B carotene among U.S. physicians. Prev Med 1985;14:165–168.
43. DeMeersman R. Aspirin and exercise as a prophylaxis for heart disease. is it safe? Sports Med 1990;9:71–75.

The Shoulder

Margaret E. Karg and John J. Danchik

To describe the anatomy of the shoulder, it is more accurate to use the term "shoulder joint complex" because of its many joints and relationships. The shoulder joint complex is unique in that it connects the axial skeleton and the remainder of the upper extremity. Built more for flexibility and gliding motions, the shoulder joint complex provides the ability to use the upper extremity in a multitude of positions and motions.

A thorough understanding of the anatomy and biomechanics of the shoulder and its examination are paramount in ensuring an accurate diagnosis and appropriate treatment. Pain in the shoulder region may be due to intrinsic disease of the shoulder joints and/or surrounding soft tissue. Pain may also be referred from other structures, such as the spine or viscera. The possibility of referred pain or of more than one lesion occurring at a time can make examination and diagnosis complex. It is for this reason that the authors recommend a complete physical examination to determine general health before a regional examination of the shoulder.

ANATOMY

There are three true articular anatomical joints and two physiologic "joints" in the shoulder (1).

True Anatomical Joints of the Shoulder

The glenohumeral joint can be compared to a golf ball sitting on a tee. It is classified as a multiaxial ball-and-socket synovial joint that depends on muscle rather than bones or ligaments for its support and integrity. The joint capsule and ligaments provide static stability. The surrounding muscles, particularly the rotator cuff, provide dynamic stability. The glenohumeral joint, by virtue of its three axes of rotation and three degrees of freedom, is also capable of circumduction.

The glenoid itself articulates with only 30% of the humeral head; however, the surface contact between the glenoid and the humerus increases to 75% because of the presence of the glenoid labrum. The labrum is thought to be a fibrocartilaginous structure surrounding the glenoid and is considered a redundant fold of capsular tissue continuous with the articular cartilage of the glenoid (2).

The glenoid cavity is pear shaped. The relaxed humerus rests in the upper narrower half of the glenoid cavity. Contraction of the rotator cuff muscles pulls the humerus down into the lower, wider part of the glenoid cavity. If this dropping down or depression does not occur, full abduction is not possible (3).

The close-packed position of the glenohumeral joint is combined full abduction and external rotation. The loose-packed position/resting position is at 30° horizontal abduction/55° abduction. The capsular pattern for the glenohumeral joint is external rotation and abduction (80–120°) (4).

The acromioclavicular joint is composed of the acromion process of the scapula and the distal end of the clavicle. This plane synovial joint augments the range of motion of the humerus. A fibrous capsule surrounds the joint that contains an articular disc. This joint depends on its ligaments for its strength: the acromioclavicular and coracoclavicular, with the medial conoid and lateral trapezoid.

The S shape of the clavicle exhibits varied angles of articulation at the acromioclavicular joint. These variations have been categorized as types I, II, and III, with type I being relatively more vertical and type III being relatively more horizontal. It is thought that type I acromioclavicular joints are more prone to degenerative processes because of the increased shear forces in this type of joint (5).

The close-packed position of the acromioclavicular joint is at 90° arm abduction. The resting position/loose-packed position is at the anatomical position of the arm at the side. The capsular pattern is at endrange, 180° arm abduction and flexion (4).

The sternoclavicular joint is the only connection between the shoulder and the spine. Medially, the clavicle articulates with the manubrium sternum and the cartilage of the first rib, forming a saddle-shaped synovial articulation containing a substantial disc. Only 50% of the clavicle articulates with the manubrium and first rib, the remainder being prominent superiorly. Like the acromioclavicular joint, it depends on ligaments for strength.

The close-packed position of the sternoclavicular joint is at maximal rotation of the clavicle with the arm at full elevation and flexion. The resting position/loose-packed position is at the anatomical resting position. The capsular pattern is at endrange, 180° abduction and full flexion, like that of the acromioclavicular joint (4).

Two Physiologic "Joints" or Relationships

The scapulothoracic "joint" consists of the body of the scapula and the muscles and bursae covering the posterior chest wall; therefore, it is not a true joint. Because of this, it does not have a close-packed position or capsular pattern. The superohumeral relationship refers to the relationship of the humeral head to the overlying coracoacromial arch or ligament. This is also known as the subdeltoid "joint" or supraspinatus "outlet" (6). This is where impingement can happen if:

1. Normal depression by the rotator cuff does not occur.
2. There is compression of subacromial bursa and/or its subdeltoid and subcoracoid extensions, the supraspinatus tendon, or long head of the biceps tendon due to overuse or congenital anomalies (7).

The intraarticular biceps tendon is the only sheathed tendon of the shoulder. The synovial lining of the long head of the biceps is also an extension of the synovium of the glenohumeral joint and rotator cuff. It runs along the anterior surface of the humerus in the intertubercular groove between the lateral greater tuberosity and the medial lesser tuberosity (8).

Shoulder Bursae

There are many bursae around the shoulder. Of greatest interest is the subacromial bursa with its varied extensions, the subcoracoid and subdeltoid bursa, and the scapulothoracic bursa, which plays a role in the "snapping scapula syndrome" when it becomes inflamed. Bursitis may occur at the inferior angle of the scapula owing to poor trunk and lower body mechanics. For example, during the serve in tennis, inadequate pelvic rotation and back movement may lead to excessive shoulder movement in the cocking position, creating excessive friction at the bursa.

BIOMECHANICS

Mobility

An important aspect of the shoulder in terms of its mobility is the scapulohumeral rhythm. For the arm to be abducted from the side to overhead, there must also be simultaneous synchronous motion of the scapula. Clinically, patients with restricted humeral movement will commonly demonstrate abnormal scapular movement. Thus, clinical rehabilitation of restricted humeral movement may also necessitate scapular manipulation and rehabilitation (Table 11.1).

Along with the scapulohumeral movement, the clavicle must also move. From 0–30° of scapular rotation, the clavicle also elevates 30°. From 30–60° scapular rotation, the clavicle—because of its S shape—does not elevate further, but rather rotates around its long axis so that the distal portion moves upward and forward. The crank shape thus elevates the distal end via rotation with no change in angle of elevation at the proximal sternoclavicular joint (1).

Shoulder abduction is thus a complex process. We often only think of the large muscles involved with abduction, i.e., the deltoid, supraspinatus, and contralateral upper trapezius. However, there must be combined contraction of the supraspinatus, infraspinatus, and subscapularis, which adduct the humeral head into the glenoid, to even begin the movement of abduction. The infraspinatus, subscapularis, and latissimus dorsi also have a downward pull on the humeral head. Therefore, the supraspinatus, infraspinatus, and subscapularis together tighten the joint, lowering the center of rotation of the humeral head with a downward/inward gliding motion. If the humeral head were not lowered during abduction, the greater tuberosity would impinge on the coracoacromial ligament. Therefore, weakness of the rotator cuff will result in lack of clearance and cause superohumeral or "supraspinatus outlet" impingement.

Table 11.1.   Scapulohumeral Rhythm

Arm Abduction	90°	180°
Glenohumeral rotation	60°	120°
Scapular rotation	30°	60°
Clavicle elevation/ rotation	30°	Rotates upward and forward at its distal end, about its long axis

Stability

The biomechanical features of the shoulder, regarding stability, also need to be evaluated. The glenoid fossa itself is a very shallow depression in the scapula. The glenoid labrum forms a rim that encircles the fossa and provides a greater surface area of contact for the humerus. This is similar to the knee in which menisci on the tibia deepen the contact area for the femur. As with the menisci of the knee, the labrum is wider at its periphery and narrows at its center (2). In addressing the capsular action during glenohumeral movement in the 90° abducted arm, the superior portion of the capsule is relaxed and the lower portion becomes taut. In the 45° abducted arm, both superior and inferior capsules are relaxed; thus, this position is one of instability of the glenohumeral joint.

There are also numerous ligaments in the shoulder. The glenohumeral ligaments reinforce the anterior capsule. Internal rotation of the humerus relaxes these three ligaments; external rotation tenses them. During shoulder abduction, the middle and inferior glenohumeral ligaments become taut; the upper ligament relaxes.

The coracohumeral ligament, connecting the coracoid process of the scapula to the humerus, is a broad band that strengthens the upper part of the capsule. It consists of two bands: the anterior inserting into the greater tuberosity, and the posterior merging with the remainder of the capsule. During extension, tension develops mainly in the anterior band. During flexion, tension develops mainly in the posterior band (9).

The coracoclavicular ligament serves to connect the coracoid process of the scapula with the clavicle. It consists of two ligaments: the trapezoid ligament (anterior and lateral) and the conoid ligament (posterior and medial). The trapezoid ligament is stretched when the clavicle moves posteriorly, limiting posterior motion. The conoid ligament is seen to limit the clavicle from moving anterior from the scapula. Together these two ligaments maintain the proper relationship between the distal clavicle and acromion. Thus, in acromioclavicular separations, these two ligaments become involved in the injury (10).

EXAMINATION OF THE SHOULDER

When possible, the mechanism of injury to the athlete's shoulder should be ascertained. The shoulder may be injured in its role as a prime mover, such as in repetitive activity during the golf swing or tennis stroke; it may be injured in its role as a stabilizer, such as in supporting a weight during weight lifting or vaulting in gym-

nastics; or it may be injured as a result of direct trauma such as a fall or blow to the shoulder. Therefore, a thorough history is an essential guide to physical examination.

After the history of the injury has been obtained, other specific questions may be useful.

1. What is the character, duration, frequency, and/or intensity of the symptomatology?
2. Is there audible painful/nonpainful clicking or crepitus?
3. What is provocative?
   A. Positions at rest, i.e., night pain, versus positions during movement, occupational component.
   B. Previous treatment.
4. What is palliative?
   A. Rest versus movement.
   B. Heat versus ice.
   C. Nonsteroidal anti-inflammatory drugs (NSAIDs).
   D. Previous treatment.
5. Has there been recent injury to the cervical spine?
6. Is there previous history of fractures, i.e., stress fractures?
7. Is there previous personal or family history of organic disease?
   A. Rheumatoid arthritis.
   B. Gouty arthritis.
   C. Diabetes.
   D. Alcoholism.
   E. Cancer.

Observation Checklist

1. Ascertain side of dominance.
2. Observe contour, symmetry, muscular development.
3. Signs of atrophy, subluxation, dislocation.
4. Color, edema, temperature.
5. General posture to include carrying angle of the elbow.
6. Conscious/unconscious guarding.

Active Range of Motion (Table 11.2)

In the event that the patient exhibits a painful arc of 80°–120° abduction, one should immedi-

Table 11.2. Active Range of Motion

Flexion	180°	Extension	50°
Abduction	180°	Adduction	50°
Internal rotation	90°	External rotation	90°
Horizontal flexion (Adduction)	120°	Horizontal extension (Abduction)	50°

ately consider the possibilities of instability and/or impingement.

Resisted Range of Motion (Using Gross Range of Motion or Specific Muscle Testing)

Examination for strength should include the following.

1. Upper trapezius.
2. Deltoid.
3. Biceps.
4. Supraspinatus.
5. Infraspinatus.
6. Teres minor.
7. Subscapularis.
8. Latissimus dorsi.
9. Pectoralis—major and minor.
10. Rhomboid—major and minor.

Passive Range of Motion and Examination for Joint Integrity

Gross ranges of motion are to be examined for stability (as listed for active range of motion).

Examination of Joint Play in the Following Directions (Listed in the Order of Most Common to Least Common Instabilities)

1. Anterior/inferior.
2. Anterior.
3. Inferior.
4. Superior.
5. Posterior.
6. Multidirectional.

The integrity of the anterior/inferior capsule is tested with the elbow flexed 90° and the arm abducted 90°. The glenohumeral joint is externally rotated as a simultaneous posterior-to-anterior force is applied. In an unstable capsule there will be pain, apprehension, and/or subluxation.

Other stability tests are best performed with the athlete supine at the edge of a table. Stress is applied into the joint in each of the anterior, posterior, superior, and inferior directions, while the arm is moved in varying degrees of rotation to provoke the instability.

A common finding of inferior and multidirectional instabilities is the presence of a "sulcus sign," a prominent depression below the acromion when inferior traction is applied to the arm of the upright patient.

Impingement Syndrome Tests

PAINFUL ARC SIGN

Between 60° and 130° abduction (11).

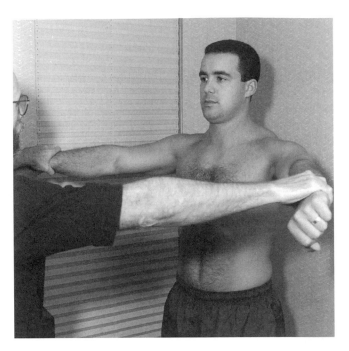

Figure 11.1. Supraspinatus test. Note the position of the arms, which are 45° to the body with the thumbs pointed down. The patient attempts to push up as the examiner provides resistance. An inability to resist the examiner, resulting in weakness and/or pain, is indicative of a tear of the supraspinatus muscle, tendon, or neuropathy of the suprascapular nerve.

MUSCLE TESTING OF SUPRASPINATUS

Arm at 90° abduction, 30° anterior circumduction, and internal rotation with thumb downward. Resistance to abduction is applied by the examiner, testing for pain and weakness (Fig. 11.1).

LOCKING POSITION TEST

Performed to evaluate for an impingement syndrome of the supraspinatus and/or bicipital tendon. The arm is extended and internally rotated, while watching for pain at the inferior aspect of the acromion.

The examiner passively flexes the arm slightly, with the elbow flexed and the forearm pronated. Upward pressure is applied along the axis of the humerus to produce pressure at the inferior surface of the acromion (12).

The examiner blocks scapular motion along the lateral border with one hand, while the other hand forces forward elevation of the patient's affected shoulder, anywhere between flexion and abduction. This forces the greater tuberosity against the acromion, compressing the soft tissues that lie between (12).

The examiner blocks the acromial arch, preventing scapular motion superiorly with one hand while flexing and abducting the patient's affected shoulder at varying degrees with the other hand (12).

The examiner flexes the patient's elbow and shoulder 90° with slight shoulder adduction and then internally rotates the forearm and shoulder. Gerber et al. believe that this method is most useful in determining subcoracoid impingement owing to an enlarged coracoid process (13, 14).

Biceps Tendon Tests

SPEED'S TEST (FIG. 11.2)

The patient's shoulder is flexed forward with the elbow fully extended and the forearm supinated against the examiner's resistance (3).

LUDINGTON'S TEST (FIG. 11.3)

The patient clasps both hands behind his or her head in an effort to relax the biceps bilaterally. The examiner palpates the bicipital tendon as the patient alternately contracts the biceps. Lack of movement of the biceps tendon is indicative of rupture (3).

ABBOT-SAUNDER'S TEST

The patient's arm is passively abducted to 150° and externally rotated, after which the arm is passively lowered to the patient's side. If pain is experienced in the bicipital groove and/or there is a

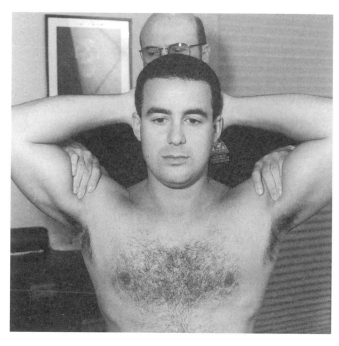

Figure 11.3. Ludington's test. Both arms are clasped behind the patient's head with the biceps relaxed bilaterally. The examiner then palpates the bicipital tendon as the patient alternately contracts the biceps. Lack of the ability to palpate the biceps tendon on the involved side is indicative of rupture of the long head of the biceps.

palpable click around this groove, tenosynovitis of the long head of the biceps and/or subluxation of the bicipital tendon is suggested.

GILCREST SIGN

Identical to the Abbot-Saunder's test, except the patient performs procedure while holding a 5-lb weight. The significance of the findings is identical to that of the Abbot-Saunder's test.

LIPPMAN TEST

The biceps are relaxed by passively bending the elbow to 90°. Pressure is applied to the tendon of the long head approximately 3 inches distal to the glenohumeral joint. The examiner attempts to displace the tendon from side to side in the groove. Pain and/or a palpable subluxation will indicate tenosynovitis of the long head of the biceps and/or subluxation of the tendon out of the groove.

YERGASON'S TEST (FIG. 11.4)

The patient flexes the elbow and pronates the forearm. The examiner applies resistance as the patient then tries to flex the elbow actively and supinate the forearm simultaneously. Pain at the bicipital groove indicates tenosynovitis and/or subluxation of the biceps tendon.

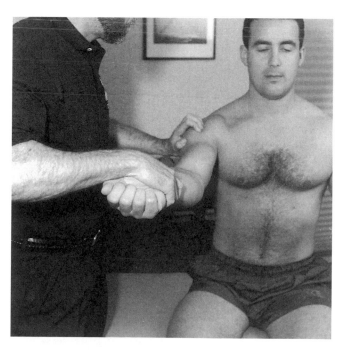

Figure 11.2. Speed's test. The patient's shoulder is flexed forward with the elbow fully extended and the forearm supinated against the examiner's resistance. Pain reproduced in the bicipital groove or tenderness indicates biceps tendinitis.

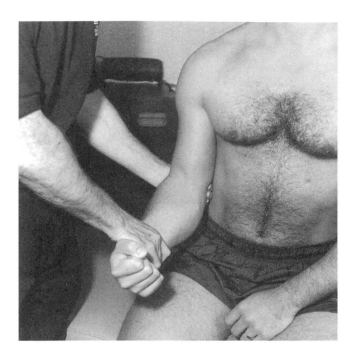

Figure 11.4. Yergason's test. The patient flexes the elbow and pronates the forearm. The examiner applies resistance as the patient then tries to actively flex the elbow and supinate the forearm simultaneously. Pain at the bicipital groove would indicate tenosynovitis and/or subluxation of the biceps tendon.

BICEPS TENDON STABILITY TEST

Identical to Yergason's test, except that as the patient attempts to supinate the forearm actively and flex the elbow, he or she also tries to rotate externally the upper arm simultaneously. Pain over the bicipital groove or a palpable click will indicate tenosynovitis of the long head of the biceps and/or subluxation of the tendon.

BOOTH AND MARVEL TRANSVERSE HUMERAL LIGAMENT TEST

Performed by passively abducting the arm to 90° and flexing the elbow to 90°. The examiner palpates the bicipital groove as he or she passively rotates the arm internally and externally. A palpable snap with attendant pain indicates loss of integrity of the transverse humeral ligament (12).

Rotator Cuff Tests

DROP ARM TEST (FIGS. 11.5 AND 11.6)

This test can be performed by passively abducting the patient's arm to 150°. The patient is then instructed to slowly drop the arm toward the side of the body. If the arm drops quickly due to pain, it suggests a rotator cuff tear of the supraspinatus tendon. If the patient is able to

perform this test adequately, the examiner proceeds with Codman's drop arm test (15).

CODMAN'S DROP ARM TEST

The patient's arm is passively abducted to 150°. The patient then is asked to slowly lower

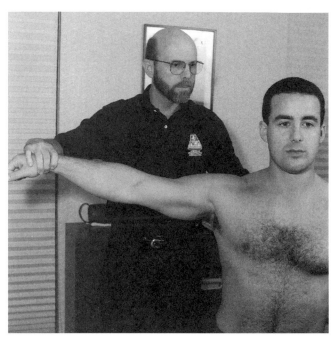

Figure 11.5. Arm drop no. 1. The patient's arm is passively abducted to 90° by the examiner.

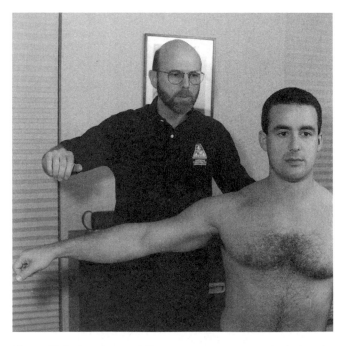

Figure 11.6. Arm drop no. 2. The patient is instructed to slowly drop the arm toward the side of the body. If the arm drops quickly due to pain, with the patient unable to return the involved arm slowly to the side, a rotator cuff tear is suggested.

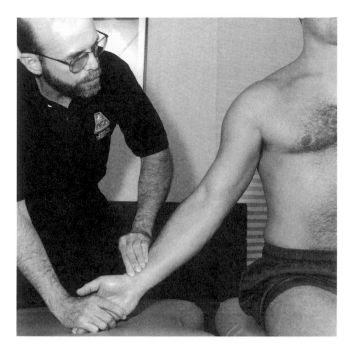

Figure 11.7. Costoclavicular maneuver. While taking a deep breath, the patient draws the shoulders backward and down. The examiner palpates the radial pulse as the patient performs the maneuver. An absence of the radial pulse indicates thoracic outlet syndrome.

the arm to the side. As the patient does so, the examiner applies a gentle downward force to the arm. If the arm drops quickly due to pain, one should suspect a rotator cuff tear of the supraspinatus tendon.

Thoracic Outlet Tests (16)

1. Inspection of posture:
   A. Shoulder asymmetry.
   B. Poorly developed musculature/drooping shoulders.
   C. Unusually large breasts.
2. Palpation: Reveals tenderness over supraclavicular fossa, check for increased tone of the scalene muscles.
3. Listen for bruits: Over supraclavicular fossa while arm is in a provocative position.
4. Provocative maneuvers: Examiner looks for obliteration of radial pulse and/or exacerbation of symptoms.
   A. Costoclavicular maneuver (Fig. 11.7). Patient shrugs shoulders with deep inhalation while drawing the shoulders backward in an exaggerated military position.
   B. Scalenus anticus maneuver. Patient turns the head away from the involved side and opens and closes the involved hand 5 times and is then examined for blanch-

ing of the hand. This may also be done by turning the head toward the involved side.
   C. Adson's maneuver (Fig. 11.8). Patient extends and turns head toward involved side with deep inhalation, and the examiner laterally rotates and extends the shoulder.
   D. Wright's hyperabduction. Patient turns head away from involved side, and with deep inhalation the arm is abducted and externally rotated. The pectoralis minor muscle forces compression against the fulcrum of the coracoid process.
   E. Arm elevation stress test (AEST). With arms overhead, patient rapidly flexes and extends fingers. Reproduction of symptoms or fatigue is a positive sign.

Radiographic Examination

A trauma series is the recommended radiographic examination of the shoulder. This includes anterior-posterior, lateral (also known as the Y view or the supraspinatus tunnel view), and axillary views of the scapula. Other suggested views include the anterior-posterior thorax view in neutral, medial, and lateral rotation and the West Point view (17).

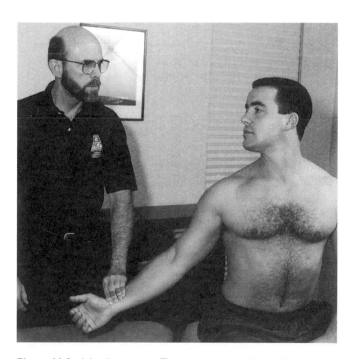

Figure 11.8. Adson's maneuver. The patient extends the head toward the side of involvement while taking a deep breath. The examiner takes the patient's pulse. Diminution or obliteration of the radial pulse is indicative of thoracic outlet syndrome.

ANTERIOR DISLOCATIONS OF THE SHOULDER

Traumatic injuries to the shoulder may create dislocation of the glenohumeral joint. The resultant resting position of the humeral head, in relation to its adjacent anatomy, will classify an anterior dislocation into one of four categories discussed below (18).

The subcoracoid dislocation is the most common type of injury of the anterior shoulder and is the most common type of dislocation of a major joint in the body. The humeral head is displaced anteriorly with respect to the glenoid and inferior to the coracoid process.

The subglenoid dislocation is the second most common type of acute anterior shoulder dislocation, with the posttraumatic resting position of the humeral head located anterior to and below the inferior glenoid fossa. Together, the subcoracoid and subglenoid dislocations account for approximately 99% of anterior dislocations of the humeral joint (18).

The subclavicular dislocation is a rare type of acute anterior shoulder dislocation, with the posttraumatic resting position of the humeral head being displaced medial to the coracoid process just inferior to the lower border of the clavicle.

The intrathoracic dislocation is also a rare type of acute shoulder dislocation in which a lateral force has driven the head of the humerus medially between the ribs and the thoracic cavity. The latter two dislocations are usually associated with severe trauma and may be accompanied by fracture of the greater tuberosity of the humerus and/or rotator cuff avulsion.

Mechanism of Injury

A direct force, such as a traumatic impact to the lateral or posterior/lateral aspect of the shoulder, can produce an injury to the anterior stabilizers of the joint, with resultant sprain, subluxation, or dislocation. However, the most common injury occurs from indirect forces. The injury is secondary to forces applied to the arm that indirectly injure the supporting structures of the joint. An outstretched arm that is forced into extension, abduction, and external rotation will cause a stretching and/or tearing of the anterior capsule and ligaments. When the humerus is in abduction and internal rotation, or in forward flexion and external rotation, the acromial arch limits complete elevation of the arm. Further forceful elevation uses the arch as a fulcrum and dislocates the proximal head by causing it to descend and move forward.

Visual Examination and Diagnosis

Diagnosis is usually not difficult if one is present when the athlete sustains the injury. There is an immediate disability with severe pain, and the athlete is unable to move the arm without significant discomfort. The corresponding muscles are in spasm, attempting to stabilize the joint, and the humeral head may be palpable anteriorly. The posterior shoulder shows a depression beneath the acromion, and the arm is held in slight abduction and external rotation. Any attempt to adduct and rotate internally the arm will be met with immediate resistance by the athlete. Because of the frequent association of nerve injury (particularly the axillary nerve and to a lesser extent radial injuries), an essential part of examination is the assessment of the neurovascular status of the upper extremity. The examination should include sensory changes to the lateral arm (axillary nerve), the lateral aspect of the forearm (musculocutaneous nerve), and the forearm and hand (brachial plexus nerves). Strength of the forearm, wrist, and fingers should be evaluated. Palpation of the radial pulse and a check of peripheral circulation to the fingernails of the affected limb should be performed.

Complications of Reduction of an Anterior Dislocation

There are several potential complications that a physician must be aware of before the reduction of an anterior dislocation. This includes the possibility of damage to the nerves around the glenohumeral joint, in particular the axillary, musculocutaneous, and ulnar nerves. A rotator cuff tear may occur, especially in conjunction with an inferior type of anterior dislocation, regardless of the patient's age. Fractures of the humeral head, glenoid, and greater tuberosity are all complications that can occur while spontaneously reducing the dislocation.

The ideal time to reduce a shoulder dislocation is immediately after it has occurred. If there is a delay, pain and involuntary muscle spasm can make reduction difficult and necessitate a general anesthetic. Unless there are extreme circumstances, it is imperative that radiographs be taken before any attempt at reduction is made. It is important for the physician to know the direction of the dislocation (subcoracoid dislocations are more difficult to reduce than subglenoid) (19), the possible existence of associated fractures, and any possible barriers to relocation. Postreduction films should be obtained immediately after reduction. Also, regardless of the method used, postreduction tests are performed including the sensory and motor function of all five major nerves in the upper extremity. The strength of the pulse is verified and compared with the noninjured side.

Common Techniques of Reduction

MODIFIED HIPPOCRATIC METHOD

The athlete lies supine with the affected arm held between 30° and 40° of abduction. Countertraction is performed by means of a swathe around the patient's upper thorax, the direction of force being opposite to the traction applied on the affected arm. The affected arm is very gently pulled in its longitudinal axis, while the patient is reassured and encouraged to relax. The traction should be very gentle, with a slow increase in the amount of force exerted. It should be steady and held for approximately 60 seconds. In most cases, the arm will be felt to slip back into the glenoid fossa as the athlete relaxes. The arm should then be placed into internal rotation and held in place across the chest.

THE HIPPOCRATIC METHOD

The stockinged foot of the physician is used as countertraction. The heel should not go into the axilla but should extend across the chest wall. Traction should be slow and gentle. As with all traction techniques, the arm may be rotated gently internally and externally to disengage the humeral head. This is the method of reduction that is least recommended and should only be used in an emergency situation, i.e., when the physician is alone.

STIMSON'S TECHNIQUE

The patient lies prone on the edge of the examining table, while downward traction is gently applied to the upper arm. This is usually accomplished through the use of weights, which are attached to the wrist of the dislocated shoulder, permitting the arm to hang freely off the edge of the table. Five pounds is usually sufficient, but more or less weight may be used depending on the size of the patient. When using this technique, one should be patient because it may take 15 to 20 minutes for the reduction to occur.

KOCHER MANEUVER

The modified Kocher maneuver can be performed when the preceding three methods have failed to relocate the dislocation. There have been complications when the Kocher maneuver has been used in a forceful manner by an unskilled person.

The arm of the patient is gently externally rotated, while traction is being applied through the longitudinal axis of the humerus. This usually results in the humeral head slipping back into the glenoid. As this is felt to occur, the arm is then brought into a slightly adducted and internally rotated position, which should complete the reduction.

Postreduction Care

The rotator cuff is evaluated by observing the isometric strength of external rotation and abduction. Because recurring glenohumeral instability is the most common complication of a glenohumeral dislocation, postreduction treatment focuses on optimizing shoulder stability and/or strength. Thus, two potentially important elements of postreduction treatment are protection and muscle rehabilitation. It is important that the shoulder be immobilized until it is asymptomatic, usually 10 days to 3 weeks, and then be treated with a vigorous but controlled rehabilitation program. The role of an extensive rehabilitation program is paramount in returning the athlete to participation.

The risk of recurring dislocation will depend on the patient's age at the time of initial dislocation. Recurrent dislocation of the shoulder is a problem of youth, with peak incidence occurring at age 20. After age 70, the incidence of recurrence is extremely low (20). In Rowe and Sakellarides' classic study of 324 anterior dislocations, the redislocation rate in patients younger than 20 was greater than 90%, whereas after the age of 40, the rate fell below 25% (21). Although uncommon in patients older than 50, recurrences do happen. This has been associated with excessive generalized ligamentous laxity.

Recurrent Anterior Dislocation/Instability

Recurrent anterior shoulder instability can be the result of either traumatic or atraumatic forces placed on a stretched glenohumeral joint. In those patients who present with a definite history of trauma, the direction of shoulder instability is related to the structural damage of the joint. When the direction of the trauma is anterior, the shoulder commonly has ruptures of the glenohumeral ligaments at its inferior/anterior glenoid attachments, referred to as Bankart lesions. Frequently, surgery is required to achieve shoulder stability. Patients that have no history of significant trauma may have multidirectional and, in some instances, bilateral instability. Rehabilitation is often limited to extensive rotator cuff strengthening and coordination exercises. If surgery is performed, laxity of the inferior capsule must be the area that is reinforced.

ANTERIOR SHOULDER SUBLUXATION

Shoulder subluxation may be defined as humeral head translation greater than one half the width of the glenoid but less than the sum of one half of the glenoid and one half of the humeral head (22). Certain athletes, such as swimmers and baseball players, are predisposed (because of the nature of the activity) to excessive glenohumeral motion/instability. However, they will remain asymptomatic unless the capsule and/or the labrum begins to deteriorate and tear. Frequently, this will result in an anterior subluxation of the humeral head.

Once again, the goals of conservative management should include restoration of strength and range of motion. It is important to realize that there needs to be an initial period of complete rest with patients who have had an acute anterior shoulder subluxation. In these cases it is common for the patient's shoulder to be immobilized, with the arm internally rotated at the side, for 3 to 5 weeks, or until there is a decrease in pain or inflammation. Both internal and external rotator cuff strength contribute to anterior and posterior stability. Coordinated actions of the rotator cuff muscles help hold the humeral head within the glenoid. Therefore, rotator cuff strengthening exercises should be performed. This is accomplished most safely and effectively by keeping the humerus close to the body with the elbow flexed 90°.

SURGICAL PROCEDURES

Stabilization of the glenohumeral joint by means of surgery should only be considered after a reasonable time has passed in an attempt to strengthen the internal and external rotators.

Before selection of the surgical procedure to be used, recognition of the existence of a Bankart lesion or a Hill-Sachs defect of the humeral head must be identified through proper radiologic diagnostic examination. If a Bankart lesion is present, the lesion should be anatomically reattached to the glenoid with surgery. Arthroscopic

findings indicate that the incidence of Hill-Sachs lesions after one anterior dislocation can be as high as 47% (23). These lesions are present in more than 80% of recurrent dislocations and in only 25% of patients with subluxation (24). The size of the lesion should not be of concern if the anterior soft tissue repair is performed adequately.

Surgical techniques for recurrent anterior shoulder dislocations and subluxations should include the Bankart, Putti-Platt, Magnuson-Stack, and Bristow operations (25–28). In the Bankart operation, the surgeon reattaches the torn labrum to the inferior glenoid rim and reinforces the inferior capsule and lax glenohumeral ligaments by means of an "inferior capsular shift" (29). In the Putti-Platt operation, the capsule and distal part of the subscapularis tendon are attached to the soft tissue around the glenoid rim. This operation limits external rotation of the shoulder. The Magnuson-Stack operation entails transferring the subscapularis tendon from its insertion into the lesser tuberosity of the humerus laterally across the bicipital groove to the greater tuberosity. The Bristow operation is a transfer of the coracoid tip and its conjoined tendon to the glenoid rim that will block and sharply reduce the dislocation but will result in limited external rotation.

Postoperatively, the arm is immobilized in adduction and internal rotation. Some authors recommend postoperative immobilization for 4 to 6 weeks, after which a rehabilitation program is begun. However, Rowe and associates (28) recommend immobilization for just 2 to 3 days, after which the arm is completely free. Then the patient is instructed to increase gradually the motion and function of the extremity.

POSTERIOR SHOULDER INSTABILITY/DISLOCATION

A posterior dislocation is rare in an athlete, accounting for less than 2% of shoulder dislocations (30). The exact incidence is hard to determine because the literature on posterior dislocation and subluxation is relatively sparse. Symptomatic posterior subluxation is increasingly recognized in the athlete, whereas posterior dislocation is uncommon.

Mechanism of Injury

The mechanism of injury for posterior dislocation is usually from either a direct blow to the anterior shoulder or, more commonly, indirect forces applied to the shoulder that combine flexion, ad-

duction, and internal rotation. These forces will drive the humeral head posteriorly, while the arm is in flexion, usually below 90° and internal rotation, finally resting under the acromion process. This most common mechanism of injury accounts for the statement that 98% of all posterior dislocations are in the subacromial position. Only rarely do subglenoid and subspinous dislocations occur (18).

Clinical Findings

Clinical signs or symptoms of posterior dislocations are often overlooked. Repeated instances of misdiagnosis on the first examination have been documented, with an incidence estimated at 60–80% (18). Symptoms consist of generalized shoulder pain and an inability to externally rotate or adduct the arm. In contrast to the anterior dislocation, the athlete with posterior dislocation may not realize that the shoulder is actually dislocated. The arm is held across the front of the chest wall, and any attempt to elevate it results in an inability to supinate the hand. When viewed from above, there is a bulge posteriorly with a prominent coracoid process. The standard trauma radiograph series for the shoulder should be obtained, in which a classic roentgenographic finding of a vacant glenoid sign will be observed. The vacant glenoid sign refers to the void seen in the anterior half of the glenoid fossa in posterior dislocations on a standard anterior-posterior film of the shoulder (31).

Reduction

Reduction is achieved with the patient in the supine position. Lateral traction is applied with internal rotation to remove the notch from the glenoid, followed by external rotation to relax the posterior capsule. Posterior pressure is then placed on the humeral head to facilitate reduction. As reduction is achieved, the arm is then gently adducted into external rotating and placed at the side. Immobilization is from 4 to 6 weeks in slight abduction and external rotation.

Recurrent Posterior
Dislocation and Subluxation

This is an unusual condition that is more commonly seen in those with loose ligaments and may occasionally be combined with anterior instability. If recurrent subluxation occurs posteriorly, the posterior glenoid lip may erode the humeral head. Recurrent posterior subluxation and dislocation by flexing the arm below 90°, with internal rotation, with repetitive forceful

movements (e.g., archer's shoulder) can also create posterior shoulder instability (32).

CONSERVATIVE CARE

Conservative management begins with the avoidance of any voluntary episodes of instability or positions that are likely to result in subluxation. Early restoration of normal shoulder motion must be achieved before beginning to strengthen the internal and external rotators. Rehabilitative emphasis should be on the external rotation in positions that will not aggravate any preexisting tendinitis.

SURGERY

Athletes who have symptoms that are severely disabling, or who have had no success with nonoperative treatment, should be treated surgically with a posterior capsulorrhaphy (33). When the posterior aspect of the glenoid is severely damaged or flattened, and the posterior portion of the capsule of the infraspinatus tendon is attenuated, a bone block should augment the reconstruction (34).

MULTIDIRECTIONAL AND INFERIOR INSTABILITY

Multidirectional and inferior instability are seen in athletic, active patients with or without generalized joint laxity. The mechanism of injury can include various combinations of (1) repetitive microtraumas, (2) inherent joint laxity, and (3) one or more major injuries to the glenohumeral joint (35). Proper detection depends on suspecting its possibility in all types of patients regardless of age.

Examination should include recognition of the sulcus sign (36), positive apprehension test in multiple directions, stress radiographs, and fluoroscopy. Arthroscopy may be helpful in doubtful cases, but the findings require clinical interpretation. Initial treatment for multidirectional instability is nonsurgical. Patients with joint laxity are more likely to respond to rehabilitation than patients with a major traumatic injury.

The rehabilitation program consists of three phases: (1) range of motion exercises performed with the shoulder in the scapular plane avoiding stress on the capsule, (2) eccentric and isotonic strengthening exercises started with the arm at the side, and (3) isokinetic internal and external rotation performed at varying degrees of shoulder abduction. Sports-specific exercises are added when strength and endurance are 80% of function compared with the uninvolved side.

Selection of surgical candidates in patients with multidirectional instability can lead to indecision because of the difficulty in recognizing all the directions of instability, determining the motivation of the patient, and excluding the other possibilities for joint laxity. The surgical procedure most often performed to reduce capsular laxity on all three sides of the glenohumeral joint is the inferior capsular shift.

ACROMIOCLAVICULAR DISLOCATIONS

The acromioclavicular joint is relatively weak and inflexible for the constant burden and repeated stress it bears. Those who expose the joint to excessive and repetitive trauma (e.g., heavy laborers, weight lifters, contact sport participants) risk injury by contusion, sprain, or separation. The mechanism of acromioclavicular disruption is primarily of two types. In the first type of injury, when a force is applied to the acromion or glenohumeral joint from above, it causes the scapula to rotate around the coracoid, which then becomes a fulcrum. The acromioclavicular ligament, being intrinsically weak, gives way and the joint dislocates. The second type of injury occurs when a downward force of great intensity forces the clavicle on the first rib. The rib becomes the fulcrum, tearing the coracoclavicular and acromioclavicular ligaments, which causes a complete acromioclavicular separation (Fig. 11.9).

The two most common injuries that result in acromioclavicular separation are falling on the point of the shoulder and falling on the hand of an outstretched arm. Two rare mechanisms of injury include a direct lateral blow on the shoulder, such as being crushed (i.e., in a pileup), or a posterior blow to the scapula.

Classification of Acromioclavicular Dislocations

Rockwood's classification of injuries to the acromioclavicular and coracoclavicular complex allows the effective grouping of injuries for diagnosis, treatment, and prognosis (37).

In a Type 1 sprain, only the acromioclavicular ligament is sprained, with minimal swelling, tenderness, and limitation of motion.

With a Type 2 sprain, the acromioclavicular ligament is damaged along with a partial sprain or stretching of the coracoclavicular ligaments. There is an increase in swelling and tenderness as well as a greater limitation of motion. There is also a slight elevation of the clavicle.

In Type 3 sprain, there is a complete tear of the acromioclavicular and coracoclavicular ligaments with damage often to the deltoid and trapezius. The arm will be found to be supported; the symptoms increase significantly when it hangs freely. There is significant swelling, tenderness, and elevation of the clavicle.

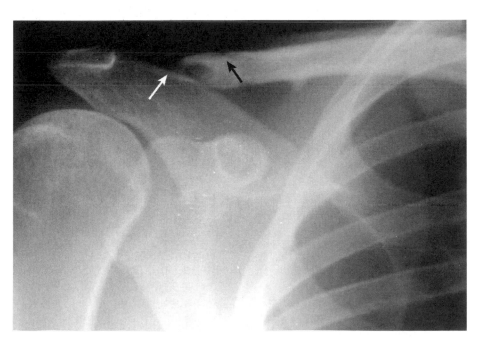

Figure 11.9. Acromioclavicular separation. Note the widened gap between the acromion process and the distal clavicle (white arrow). A fracture of the distal clavicle is also seen (dark arrow).

A Type 4 sprain is a posterior dislocation of the clavicle on the acromion, with complete disruption of the acromioclavicular joint and ligaments, although the coracoclavicular ligaments may remain intact.

A Type 5 sprain represents a complete loss of the acromioclavicular joint, ligaments, and coracoclavicular ligaments as well as the trapezius and deltoid muscle attachment to the clavicle and acromion. Often the acromion buttonholes through the muscle.

A Type 6 sprain represents the clavicle being displaced inferior to the coracoid. This is a rare injury in athletes and usually only occurs with massive trauma.

Examination

A helpful test in evaluating the acromioclavicular joint is to interlock the fingers over it and then squeeze. The examiner should feel for any abnormal motion. This is only helpful in Type 1 sprains; in the Type 2 and 3 sprains, the clavicle is visually elevated and can be confirmed by radiographs.

In a Type 1 sprain, there is no separation and the radiograph will be of no assistance. In a Type 2 sprain, the initial radiograph will usually show the separation. An anterior-posterior radiograph of the entire upper thorax allows the vertical distance between the coracoid and the clavicle on both the involved and uninvolved side to be compared. A second radiograph, with 10-lb weights attached to both wrists rather than having the patient hold them, makes the separation more dramatic. (When the weight is held in the hand, the increased muscular effort required to hold it may mask the degree of separation.) In the case of a Type 3 sprain, the radiograph shows the complete separation and a weighted view is unnecessary.

Treatment

Treatment of an acute Type 1 injury is symptomatic and should include antiinflammatory modalities, ice, and padding of the shoulder to prevent direct pressure over the joint. The athlete is often able to return to competition immediately and certainly within 2 days to 2 weeks, depending on the sport.

In treatment of a Type 2 separation, immobilization of the acromioclavicular joint is of utmost importance. The use of a modified Kenny Howard sling, which approximates the joint by depressing the clavicle and elevating the arm simultaneously, will often effectively accomplish this goal. The length of treatment depends on the symptoms, the healing time of the athlete, and the sport involved. The return to athletic competition will be from 1 to 4 weeks. It is common for the initial deformity, associated with a Type 2 separation, to be permanent.

Treatment of a Type 3 acromioclavicular separation will fall into two categories: a conservative closed symptomatic treatment or surgical intervention (38, 39).

The two most commonly used forms of conservative care are a sling and harness immobilization device, such as the above-mentioned Kenny Howard sling, and what is known as "skillful neglect" (17). The sling and harness device must be continuously worn for 6 weeks to maintain the reduction. During this time, isometric exercises are instituted and periodic checks of the position of the sling are made. This is an uncomfortable experience for the athlete, and patient compliance drops off dramatically as time proceeds. Skillful neglect consists of nothing more than a standard sling that is discontinued when the symptoms allow, usually after 7 to 10 days.

While the patient is wearing the sling, isometric exercises are begun. The sling is loosened for range of motion exercises, and the exercises are performed with the athlete supporting the acromioclavicular joint. Progressive resistance exercises are begun as soon as they can be tolerated.

Currently, there are three basic surgical procedures that are commonly performed to reduce a Type 3 acromioclavicular joint separation. These are (1) acromioclavicular joint fixation with wires, (2) circumferential Dacron or wire immobilization of the coracoid and clavicle, and (3) screw fixation of the clavicle to the coracoid (37, 40). Recently, surgical intervention of a Type 3 separation has fallen out of favor with orthopedists, who have elected conservative treatment of this condition. A report by Walsh et al. showed that there was no decrease in strength compared with the normal shoulder in the third-degree acromioclavicular separations treated by nonoperative means, as opposed to a 9.8% deficit of those shoulders treated surgically (41). A similar study by Galpin et al. concluded that nonoperative care of this injury returned the athlete to physical activities, sports, and work earlier than surgical repair (42). These reports tends to give support to nonsurgical treatment of this problem, especially in an athlete who requires optimum strength in his or her shoulder.

There are problems and complications that should be considered in both conservative and surgical methods of Type 3 reductions. These include posttraumatic arthritis, deformity, calcification of soft tissues (especially the coracoclavicular ligaments), pain, and disability in sports activity.

Treatment of Type 4-5-6 Dislocations

These acromioclavicular joint separations/injuries will be difficult, if not impossible, to treat without surgical reduction because of the anatomical disrelationship of the involved structures as a result of severe trauma.

STERNOCLAVICULAR DISLOCATIONS

The sternoclavicular joint is involved in practically every motion of the upper extremity, because of its anatomical configuration and strong supporting ligamentous structure. It is one of the least commonly dislocated joints in the body. It may be dislocated in an anterior or posterior direction by significant traumatic forces applied to the shoulder. These forces may be direct or indirect and commonly occur in sports injuries (43, 44). A force applied directly to the front aspect of the medial clavicle will cause it to move posterior, directly landing behind the sternum and into the mediastinum. This can occur from a head butt, from a kick, or by being fallen on. Because of the anatomy, it is uncommon for a direct force to produce an anterior sternoclavicular dislocation.

If a force is applied laterally, with the shoulder rolled forward and the hand in front of the athlete, this force is directed down the clavicle producing a posterior dislocation of the sternoclavicular joint (9). The most common mechanism of injury to the sternoclavicular joint is from indirect forces that are applied from the anterior-lateral or posterior-lateral direction.

Anterior Dislocations of the Sternoclavicular Joint

The anterior dislocation is the most common type of sternoclavicular dislocation, with accompanying rupture of the capsular and intraarticular ligaments. The medial end of the clavicle can be seen and palpated anterior to the sternum. It may be either fixed or mobile. If the shoulder is traumatized laterally and rolled backward with the hand behind the athlete, the force is directed down the clavicle producing an anterior dislocation of the sternoclavicular joint (9). This may occur when an outfielder is running to chase a fly ball and runs directly into a wall, producing a lateral to medial force. It may also occur in racquetball or handball when the athlete attempts to get a low drive, cannot stop, and hits the side wall, once again transmitting a force from lateral to medial. Another type of indirect force that may cause anterior dislocation occurs when an athlete falls on an outstretched abducted arm, driving the shoulder medially in the same manner as described for a lateral trauma to the shoulder.

Posterior Dislocations

Posterior dislocations of the sternoclavicular joint are rare. Clinically, they can be palpated as a depression between the sternal end of the clavicle and the manubrium. The patient with a posterior dislocation will have much more pain than one with an anterior dislocation. The patient may complain of tightness of the throat, difficulty in breathing, shortness of breath, or even choking sensation. In acute injury, vascular circulation to the affected arm may be decreased. This can be a life-threatening situation.

Reduction

An anterior dislocation may be reduced with the athlete supine, by administering combined 90° humeral flexion and long axis traction while simultaneously manipulating the clavicle with the opposite hand. Many acute anterior dislocations are unstable after reduction, and in some instances surgical intervention may be required to repair or reconstruct the injured joint (9). After reduction, an attempt should be made to hold the athlete's shoulders backward, trying to maintain stability in the sternoclavicular joint. In some instances, this can be accomplished by the use of a soft figure-eight support using a soft foam pad that applies direct pressure over the anterior dislocation. Immobilization should be maintained for at least 4 to 6 weeks, after which the arm is taken out of the support for an additional 2 weeks before any strenuous activity is undertaken.

Posterior dislocations of the sternoclavicular joint should be reduced immediately. The preferred reduction procedure has the athlete lying supine with a sandbag between the shoulders, while the shoulders are extended over the edge of the table. Traction is then applied to the arm with the shoulder abducted and extended. The clavicle may have to be manipulated in a superior/inferior manner until it can maneuver into position (9). Unlike the anterior dislocation, the posterior reduction leaves the sternoclavicular joint with a very stable end result. After reductions, the shoulder should be held back in a figure-eight support for 4 to 6 weeks, followed by 1 week of rest before strenuous exercise begins.

IMPINGEMENT SYNDROME

Impingement syndrome is the most common shoulder problem seen in athletes (45). The lesion consists of an irritation to the rotator cuff tendons and/or the long head of the biceps tendon. During combined shoulder movements of flexion, abduction, and rotation, these tendons may become compressed by structures of the supra-spinatus outlet (6). These structures include the anterior-inferior one third of the acromion process of the scapula; the bursa, with its subacromial-subdeltoid and sometimes subcoracoid extensions forming a 3- to 7-mm diameter cap over the rotator cuff (44); the coracoacromial ligament, thought to be an unnecessary vestigial structure (46); the acromioclavicular joint; the coracoid process; the head of the humerus; and the glenoid (47).

As previously mentioned, the shoulder is designed more for mobility than stability. The shoulder capsule and ligamentous structures statically stabilize the shoulder, exerting a restraining effect on glenohumeral motion. The rotator cuff and scapular rotator muscles dynamically stabilize the shoulder, centering the humeral head in the glenoid while simultaneously creating maximal leverage and movement. It is imperative that these structures function in perfect concert with one another. When stability is compromised for the sake of function, injury will occur. Therefore, it is important to recognize that impingement may be a direct result of instability, and that instability must be taken into account before attempting to correct for impingement. A continuum of instability, subluxation, and impingement will finally result in rotator cuff tear (48).

Much controversy surrounds the exact etiology of impingement syndrome. The lesions of the rotator cuff are produced by the interaction of four elements: vascular, degenerative, traumatic, and mechanical anatomic factors (49).

Vascular Factors

An area of vascular insufficiency, termed the critical zone by Codman (50), exists approximately 1 cm medially to the insertion of the supraspinatus tendon (49). Avascularity has been noted in the upper part of the infraspinatus and biceps tendon as well. There is an intimate relationship between the rotator cuff and biceps: as the biceps tendon passes through the bicipital groove and crosses the glenohumeral joint, it also passes directly under the critical zone of the supraspinatus. Therefore, both structures are subject to compression on arm elevation in a site of relatively poor vascularity (51). According to Rathbun and McNab, there is also a "wringing out effect" to the vessels as they stretch over the humeral head with the arm at rest. An apparent relationship exists between these areas of avascularity and where degeneration and eventual tendon ruptures occur (52).

Degenerative Factors

Many investigators have noted degenerative changes in the rotator cuff tendons associated with aging. Rotator cuff rupture is a common finding in older patients and often occurs bilaterally. There is also evidence of enthesopathy, i.e., tendinopathy at the insertion at the joint related to degenerative changes. This may be associated with spur formation (49).

Traumatic Factors

When ruptures of the rotator cuff occur, they are usually seen in athletes between 20 and 30 years of age and are associated with specific violent injury, such as shoulder dislocations and fractures of the greater tuberosity. Researchers contend that repeated overuse, particularly in the overhead position of external rotation and abduction, may also be categorized as trauma and may be the result of subtle instability (49).

Mechanical/Anatomic Factors

Neer (7) was the first to postulate mechanical impingement of the supraspinatus and long head of the biceps against the antero-inferior third of the acromion process of the scapula when the arm is elevated and forward flexed. Neer thought it to be the primary etiologic basis for 95% of rotator cuff tears. Acromion morphology has since been studied and three types of acromion processes have been identified: Type 1, flat; Type 2, curved; and Type 3, hooked.

A study by Morrison showed 80% of rotator cuff tears to be associated with Type 3 acromions, 19.5% associated with Type 2 acromions, and none with Type 1 acromions (53). Furthermore, two studies showed the occurrence of Type 3 acromions to be approximately 40%, Type 2 approximately 40%, and Type 1 approximately 18%. Findings also support the hypothesis that acromial morphology can be identified with a modified lateral scapula radiograph (53). Generally, an acromion with less slope and an undersurface with a prominent anterior edge will predispose to the problem of impingement (47).

CLASSIFICATION OF IMPINGEMENT LESIONS (ADAPTED FROM NEER, 1987)

1. Outlet impingement—narrowing supraspinatus outlet.
    A. Shape of acromion (overhanging curve or spur).
    B. Slope of acromion (flat).
    C. Prominent acromioclavicular joint (shape or excrescences).
2. Less frequent—outlet is normal.
    A. Prominent greater tuberosity (malunion, faulty prosthesis).
    B. Loss of humeral depressors (cuff, biceps).
    C. Loss of glenohumeral fulcrum (laxity or bone loss).
    D. Loss of suspensory mechanism (trapezius palsy or acromioclavicular separation may impair scapular rotation).
    E. Unfused acromial epiphysis.
    F. Nonunion or malunion of acromion (6).

Another mechanical consideration is impingement between the head of the humerus and the coracoid process of the scapula. The space between the humeral head and the coracoid process must accommodate the articular cartilage, joint capsule, and subacromial bursae and must allow for the movement of the rotator cuff muscles as well as the long head of the biceps. This space may be compromised due to an altered enlarged coracoid process, from trauma, or iatrogenic changes and may be the culprit in cases of chronic "idiopathic impingement syndrome." It is thought that this can be detected during examination combining shoulder movements of abduction, flexion, and internal rotation, as opposed to external rotation (32).

Three Progressive Stages of Impingement Lesions (47)

STAGE I: EDEMA AND HEMORRHAGE OF THE ROTATOR CUFF

This stage is characteristically observed in athletes younger than 25 years old, but may occur at any age. It is the result of repetitive overhead use with the shoulder in combined abduction and external rotation. Differential diagnosis must include that of shoulder instability, subluxation, and acromioclavicular arthritis. The signs and symptoms of Stage I may be the same as those of Stage III; therefore, a rotator cuff tear may easily be missed. The treatment at this stage is conservative, and the condition is considered reversible.

STAGE II: FIBROSIS AND TENDINITIS OF THE ROTATOR CUFF

This lesion characteristically occurs in athletes 25 to 40 years of age. In this stage, the bursa may become fibrotic and tendinitis may ensue. The shoulder may function asymptomatically with light activity but will become painful with more vigorous overhead use. Calcium deposits and frozen shoulder must be ruled out. The likelihood of recurrent pain with activity is high. Treatment should be conservative.

STAGE III: TEARS OF THE ROTATOR CUFF, RUPTURE OF THE BICEPS, AND BONY CHANGES

These lesions are common and occur almost exclusively in athletes older than 40 years of age. Considered to be chronic or attritional, tears constitute 90% of all injuries to the rotator cuff (54). Unrelenting impingement will ultimately result in partial or complete tears of the rotator cuff, lesions in the biceps, and/or various bony alterations around the shoulder joint. Cervical radiculitis and neoplasm must be ruled out. There may be progressive disability, and surgery may be necessary. It has been shown that most torn rotator cuff tendons show evidence of degeneration, and many patients describe having had shoulder pain before the injury. It is apparent that trauma may enlarge a tear, but is rarely the principal factor (47) (Fig. 11.10).

Impingement and the Long Head of the Biceps Tendon

Tears of the supraspinatus will usually accompany tears of other tendons and occur before ruptures of the biceps in a ratio of approximately 7 to 1. The biceps may rupture first if subjected to excessive impingement wear owing to shallowness or laterality of the bicipital groove (55). The synovial lining of the long head of the biceps is an extension of the synovium of the shoulder joint and the rotator cuff. Therefore, any inflammation of the cuff muscles or in the joint itself will inherently extend down along the biceps sheath. A narrow bicipital groove and restrictive transverse humeral ligament will further provoke the tenosynovitis, usually beneath or just distal to the transverse ligament, and the situation will become chronic (8).

Most biceps tenosynovitis and ruptures are thought to be caused by subacromial impingement. Also, because the biceps function to depress the humeral head, injury as in rupture or dislocation of the long head may escalate im-

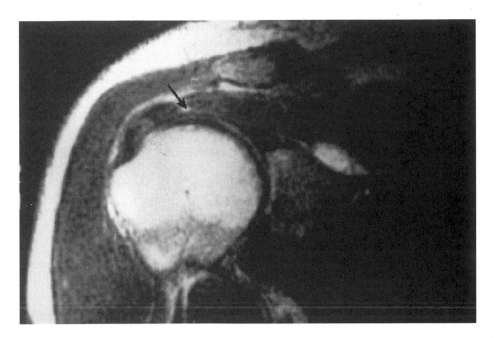

Figure 11.10. Tear of the supraspinatus (white arrow). Edema is visible in this tear of the supraspinatus tendon in a 64-year-old male tennis player. The supraspinatus muscle and its tendon are easily seen as they pass under the acromion process.

pingement as its restraining action is lost. Rupture of the biceps tendon is rare, even in the young adult sustaining severe trauma (47). Such injury occurs in young weight lifters, in whom acute rupture is provoked by a single violent effort. Usually, however, the tendon will become worn by repetitive stress, and the tear will occur in the weakened area. Steroid injections into such a weakened area can expedite the development of a complete tear of the biceps tendon (55).

The biceps tendon may become worn due to a narrow tunnel-shaped intertubular groove or it may dislocate medially. Acute fixed medial displacement or subluxation is rare but can occur due to a tear in the coracohumeral ligament. In cases of trauma, it is important to rule out osteochondral fracture involving the bicipital groove, or damage to the lesser tuberosity or subscapular tendon. A bicipital groove radiograph is necessary in diagnosis of any bony irregularities. The dimensions of the intertubercular groove can be measured radiographically and may help to assess the state of the bicipital tendon. An arthrogram may also be necessary to detect the position of the tendon.

Presentation

The clinical presentation of impingement syndrome and ensuing pathology can be nonspecific. In the initial stage of impingement syndrome, the

athlete may complain of a poorly localized deep ache in the shoulder, particularly following overhead activity. The shoulder may be painful and uncomfortable to lie on at night. The shoulder range of motion is usually unimpaired and pain will decrease with rest. As the condition progresses, the athlete may complain of shoulder stiffness and pain during and after activity involving combined movements of shoulder elevation, abduction, and rotation. Eventually, during later stages, pain and weakness will prohibit athletic activity, most likely because of resultant partial or complete tears in the rotator cuff, rendering arm elevation difficult or impossible (7).

In instances of rotator cuff tear, one of the most classic symptoms is night pain. The pain will frequently radiate down the arm, rarely extending below the elbow. It can also extend toward the clavicle and up the side of the neck. The classic case is the middle-aged patient who tears his or her rotator cuff, sometimes feels a snap sensation in the shoulder in the course of heavy lifting, and is unable to lift the arm. The signs and symptoms seen during clinical examination may indicate overt weakness but could possibly be nonspecific and even absent, causing a missed diagnosis (56).

Examination for Impingement Syndrome

Proper examination when considering impingement must include a thorough visual examination of the back and front of the patient. Scapular elevation and rotation, as well as muscular development and possible atrophy, should be noted. Examination of the cervical spine including bilateral neurologic examination of the upper extremity is mandatory; cervical radiculopathies at the fifth, sixth, and seventh nerve root level and peripheral neuropathies commonly refer pain to the shoulder. The examiner must then check for palpable tenderness at the point of impingement. Points of tenderness include the supraspinatus and biceps tendons and the anterior edge of the acromion, greater tuberosity, and acromioclavicular joint (7, 35, 48, 57, 58). Next, active range of motion is observed. Range of motion may be normal, but there will be a painful arc at approximately 60–130° abduction. Passive range of motion is examined with the patient supine, avoiding accessory movement of the spine. Resisted range of motion in all directions should be attempted, with particular attention to the rotator cuff and especially the supraspinatus. The supraspinatus is best tested by specific tests previously described.

In the absence of frank dislocation, impingement may be difficult to differentiate from instability. An athlete with instability will usually report that he or she feels the shoulder is coming out of joint. The tests for shoulder instability should be performed routinely.

Impingement tests cause pain in impingement lesions of all stages and can be elicited in different ways, as described in the examination section of this chapter. Note that these tests are relatively nonspecific. Therefore, it is important to understand the progression of impingement syndrome to differentiate the stage of the condition. Patients with tendinitis may also exhibit a positive impingement sign (59). Individual muscle strength testing should also be performed but will be difficult if the shoulder is very painful.

In the event of partial-thickness rotator cuff tears, active range of motion may be normal. Unless associated with impingement, passive range of motion may not be painful. Resisted muscle testing should be both painful and weak. A positive drop arm test may be elicited. Full-thickness tears will likely prevent active abduction. Passive range of motion may again be unremarkable. Muscle testing should reveal significant pain and weakness, and a positive drop arm test will be elicited (12).

In cases of large rotator cuff tears, partial or complete rupture of the long head of the biceps tendon is not unusual. Although thought by Lippman (60) to be an unimportant vestigial structure, the long head of the biceps serves as an eccentric decelerator of the forearm in throwing (12). In examination of the bicipital tendon, first test for pain or weakness with a resisted biceps' test. It is important to rule out arthrosis, calcific changes in the tendons or bursa, or bone lesions such as cystic changes of the greater tuberosity or subcortex of the acromion and localized osteopenia (56). Pain, at greater that 120° abduction to end range of shoulder flexion and abduction, may be indicative of acromioclavicular or glenohumeral joint pathology (11, 58). For this reason, plain films can be very useful. The majority of patients with rotator cuff disease will have abnormal plain films.

Radiographic signs compatible with a complete tear of the rotator cuff include (1) decrease in height of the acromiohumeral compartment, (2) osteoporosis of the greater tuberosity, (3) acromiohumeral nearthrosis, (4) lack of alignment of the humeral head, (5) spurs at the acromial insertion of the coracoacromial ligament, and (6) osteoarthritis of the acromioclavicular and glenohumeral joints (61). Many conditions are incorrectly diagnosed as bursitis. This diagnosis is usually used inappropriately, and physical and roentgenographic signs are not always reliable. An arthrogram may be necessary in distinguishing the various impingement lesions (47).

Treatment of Impingement Syndrome

Effective treatment of impingement syndrome depends largely on the specificity of the diagnosis. The physician must not only identify which structure has been irritated, but more importantly must identify the underlying cause. Patients must be questioned thoroughly. In the event of a trauma, such as in a fall or blow to the shoulder, the physician must ask the following questions. Was a snap or pop heard? How did the arm feel immediately after the injury? Were there signs of numbness or tingling? How has the condition progressed since the injury? Is there pain at night? The answers to these questions, along with radiographic and examination findings, will help to discern an underlying instability or rotator cuff tear that may disguise itself as impingement, particularly in the early stages.

In the event of insidious onset of pain due to repetitive activity, it is useful to observe the patient performing the activity. Then one can determine what aspect of that activity is provocative and can educate the patient more effectively about what is more biomechanically correct. Commonly, an athlete may be contacting the ball late, as in a racket sport, or may be lacking appropriate external rotation before abduction, as in throwing. Both mechanisms force the humeral head against the acromion, inflaming the underlying structures.

Initial, in-office treatment should include electrical stimulation modalities that decrease inflammation in conjunction with ice. Cross-friction massage, to the supraspinatus and/or biceps tendon as appropriate, may also help to decrease pain. This should be done discriminately, so as not to create further irritation. Pathomechanics of the joints and of the spine, thorax, and extremities should be addressed.

Home instructions are imperative and serve not only for rehabilitation of the injury, but also encourage patient participation and responsibility. On the first day of treatment, at-home icing is encouraged for 10 to 20 minutes every hour. The next day, the affected shoulder should be treated with moist heat and pendulum exercises with a dumbbell of appropriate weight strapped to the wrist, followed by ice. This routine can be followed 2 to 3 times a day the first week. The patient should be instructed to avoid overhead activity. As the inflammation and pain decrease, moist heat followed by gentle stretching can be started. Stretching should include the supraspinatus, biceps, pectoralis, upper trapezius, and levator scapula, avoiding provocative positions of arm abduction. Stretching should be followed by ice. As the condition improves, strengthening of the external rotators can be introduced, followed by nonpainful wall-walk exercises. When the painful arc sign can no longer be elicited, and muscle grading of the shoulder and cervical spine musculature is 5/5, a comprehensive stretching and strengthening program (including scapular stabilization and core strengthening exercises) is recommended. Sport-specific skills and instruction regarding biomechanics can be introduced in the final phases of rehabilitation.

The physician must remember that in the older patient, degenerative changes may have already set in. This increases the likelihood of a tear masquerading as impingement. Patients unresponsive to conservative measures must be examined with a computed tomography (CT) arthrogram to further assess the injury.

Conclusions/Considerations

It is Neer's belief that 95% of rotator cuff tears are caused by impingement wear, as opposed to circulatory deficiency or trauma. He postulates this because 50% of those patients with rotator cuff tears are unable to recall any injury and 40% cannot be attributed to physical work; the tears must develop because of compromising anatomical variances (i.e., genetic makeup creating a space problem). This naturally supports the necessity for surgical intervention involving removal of the anterior acromion, affording decompression of the rotator cuff, bicipital tendon, and subacromial bursa (6, 47).

This theory, however, is not supported by all surgeons; many are not satisfied with the results of the acromioplasty procedures and claim surgical results have been poor (62). According to James E. Timbon, M.D., Associate Clinical Professor of Sports Medicine at USS School of Medicine, "Surgical decompression of the subacromial arch is good for pain relief but is highly unpredictable for allowing a high level athlete to return to his or her competitive status" (62). Today the concept of overuse as an etiology is gaining wider acceptance. Symptoms of impingement and eventual rotator cuff pathology may simply be a matter of mileage (48). Thus, impingement may be the end result of a breakdown or stretching of the static stabilizers due to overuse, allowing for anterior subluxation and impingement of the humeral head, particularly during abduction and external rotation. Nirschl (63, 64) emphasizes the muscular component of overuse: if a weakened and inflamed rotator cuff is unable to counter the forces of the deltoid pulling the humeral head superiorly, the impingement is then secondary, rather than primary to an inherited defect. A thorough history and examination that take all possibilities into account are most important.

OTHER MISCELLANEOUS SHOULDER CONDITIONS

Osteolysis of the Distal Clavicle

Osteolysis of the distal clavicle is a relatively rare condition that may occur after an acute injury or may be the result of repetitive microtraumas placed on the acromioclavicular joint. The diagnosis is usually made by radiographic evaluation, with the distal clavicle visualized showing all or any of the following changes: osteoporosis, osteolysis, tapering, or osteophyte formation. These changes are unilateral and do not involve the acromion (65, 66).

CLINICAL SIGNS AND SYMPTOMS

Pain in the region of the acromioclavicular joint with limitation of extreme shoulder motion in flexion and abduction appears to be the predominant symptom. Hypertrophy of the surrounding soft tissues may be visualized with point tenderness to palpation.

TREATMENT

These symptoms have been proven to be self-limiting and may take anywhere from 6 to 12 months of complete rest and elimination of the symptomatic activities to resolve. In rare cases that are resistant to conservative treatment, surgical removal of the distal clavicle may be necessary.

Biceps Tendon Subluxation

Another shoulder injury that produces anterior pain in the form of popping or snapping is subluxation of the biceps tendon. Normally the tendon on the long head of the biceps rests in the intratubercular groove, which is formed by the greater and lesser tuberosities of the humerus. On elevation of the arm, the intraarticular portion of the tendon is only a few centimeters long, but on extension this length increases to approximately 4 cm (9). Because the tendon is fixed at the superior glenoid rim, the head of the humerus must move against the tendon on elevation and extension, creating a gliding mechanism that is controlled by the coracohumeral ligament (67). The tendon does not actually slide into the groove, but rather the groove slides over the tendon. This occurs primarily when the arm is moved from internal to external rotation and from external to internal rotation (68).

MECHANISM OF INJURY

Subluxation may occur by an initial forceful injury, such as arm resisting abduction and external rotation. This action causes the transverse humeral ligament to become stretched, which permits the subluxation. The anatomical shape of the intratubercular groove regarding its shallowness and flatness of the lesser tuberosity may predispose the athlete to recurrent subluxation.

SYMPTOMS

Most symptoms are associated with pain, snapping, dull ache, and crepitation in the anterior aspect of the shoulder. Point tenderness is located over the bicipital groove, and this area of tenderness may move laterally when the arm is externally rotated and medially when the arm is internally rotated.

TREATMENT

Conservative treatment should be initiated in the acute subluxation by means of antiinflammatory modalities and resting the arm for 4 to 7 days in internal rotation. As swelling and tenderness subside and functional capacity returns,

a progressive rehabilitation program should be prescribed. Surgical intervention is rare but has proven to be successful; it consists of the removal of the long head of the biceps from the superior glenoid rim and suturing it into the bicipital groove (9).

Rupture of the Long Head of the Biceps Tendon

In younger active patients involved in overhead sports such as weight lifting, a sudden overload can result in an isolated biceps rupture. This may be within the muscle tendon junction, rather than the long head tendon itself.

In older athletes, the long biceps tendon becomes degenerative by persistent rubbing in a tight, steep-walled intratubercular groove. Extraarticular tears of the long biceps tendon almost always occur in or near the bicipital groove between the tuberosities of the humeral head. The rupture results in a very characteristic prominence of the muscle belly owing to contracture of the biceps. In the majority of elderly patients, little disability will result from this injury. However, there will be some measurable loss of flexion and supination power. In young active athletes, persistent weakness and pain may result. In these patients with high athletic expectations, an early surgical intervention is the best alternative.

The long head of the biceps spans two joints, and repairs usually restore only the part nearest the elbow. If the tendon is left unrepaired, the athletes will lose approximately 20% of supination strength and 8% of elbow flexion strength: however, they will have no weakness in grip, pronation, or elbow extension (61). Similar to the subluxating biceps tendon surgery, the tendon is removed from the superior glenoid and sutured into the floor of the bicipital groove. The arm is then immobilized for 3 weeks. Passive flexion exercise should begin on the second postoperative day. Patients usually can return to activity with some lifting at approximately 6 months.

Anterior Lateral Humeral Exostosis

Repetitive traumatic compressive forces to the anterior lateral aspect of the humerus can result in a painful bony prominence. This exostosis is a result of damage at the insertion of the deltoid or at the brachialis origin with tearing due to periosteal trauma. Immediately after the injury, the athlete's upper arm will swell acutely, become tender, and a hematoma may develop. This contusion should not be massaged soon after injury because this may cause further bleeding and irritation resulting in myositis ossificans. A true exostosis usually occurs in older athletes, whereas myositis ossificans occurs more frequently in younger athletes. The connective tissue associated with the bruised brachialis muscle becomes ossified in myositis ossificans.

The area should be iced immediately after the injury. The arm should be rested and further protected with the use of a fiberglass soft cast during competition. Rarely will radiographs reveal any abnormality other than soft tissue swelling. However, if pain persists, radiographs taken 2 or 3 weeks after the injury may confirm the beginnings of callus formation, which in time evolves into a mature exostosis. If mature bone forms, the area will continue to be sore despite any extra padding. If the region continues to be painful, the exostosis may need to be removed surgically.

THROWING INJURIES

The mechanism of throwing involves hundreds of coordinated body movements synchronized for the purpose of covering a specific measurable distance in the shortest time. Unfortunately, when this repetitive act is overused or biomechanically abused, specific injuries to the shoulder joint occur. Understanding the four biomechanical phases of throwing, and the actions of the primary muscles involved in each movement, may help the physician to recognize more easily selected shoulder injuries when they are correlated with the throwing motion. For example, acute and chronic overuse injuries to the shoulder are common in baseball pitchers, who are repetitively attempting to accelerate a 5-oz, 9-in. (circumference) baseball a distance of 60 ft, 6 in. at speeds approaching or greater than 90 miles/hr in $\frac{1}{10}$ second. To understand the various injuries that occur, it is necessary to be familiar with the dynamic phases of the throwing motion and the associated osseous and muscular stresses that are placed on the shoulder and upper arm.

The action of throwing is an extremely complex motion that involves parts of the entire body to varying degrees in a coordinated manner. In pitching, velocity is directly related to the magnitude of the force used by the athlete to throw the baseball and to the speed of the hand at the moment of release. The speed that the hand is able to achieve depends on the distance through which it moves in the preparatory part of the act of throwing and the summed angular velocities of the contributing body segments. Hence, the longer the

preparatory backswing and the greater the distance that can be added by means of rotating the body, shifting the weight, and perhaps even taking a step, the greater the opportunity for accelerating. Approximately 50% of the ball speed is obtained from the forward step and body rotation (69). The remaining speed is contributed by the joint actions in the shoulder, elbow, wrist, and fingers as well as through the coordination of the lower extremity, in particular, the ipsilateral and contralateral leg motion while pivoting. This is why the technique of a baseball pitcher is designed to allow maximum time and distance over which to accelerate the ball before its release.

The Four Phases of Throwing

Regardless of the sporting activity, the throwing action can be divided into four phases: (1) windup (cocking phase), (2) early acceleration (stage I), (3) acceleration (stage II), and (4) follow-through (70).

During the windup or cocking phase, the shoulder is abducted to 90° in hyperextension and extreme external rotation. The scapula is compressed against the chest wall, slightly elevated, and the wrist is extended. This is achieved by the synchronized contractions of the posterior deltoid, infraspinatus, teres minor, trapezius, and serratus anterior muscles. This prestretching phase prepares the anterior shoulder structures for violent muscular contraction.

In early acceleration (stage I), as the athlete strides forward or "opens up," the body and shoulder are brought forward while the arm and forearm are left behind. Muscular movements of the pectoralis major and the deltoid will bring the humerus forward to perform this action.

Acceleration (stage II) begins as the shoulder violently moves from external to internal rotation and longitudinal flexion. The wrist is simultaneously snapped from an extended to a flexed position to give added speed to the throw. This short phase of less than $\frac{1}{10}$ second can generate a ball velocity of 90 miles/hr (71). The pectoralis major, latissimus dorsi, and subscapularis are the main internal rotators that perform this motion.

With follow-through, the body's weight is firmly transferred onto the front foot. The speed of movement continually increases from the trunk to the hand, putting a considerable pull on the glenohumeral joint and causing the humeral head to leave the glenoid by more than 2.5 cm (69). The triceps decelerates the arm as the elbow extends and the forearm pronates. Once again the internal rotators are responsible for this action.

SELECTED THROWING INJURIES OF THE SHOULDER

Injuries to the shoulder may be classified into groups ranging from acute (consisting largely of soft tissue injuries) to subacute to chronic. In the chronic type, acute flare-ups or recurrences due to abuse or overuse can occur. For the purpose of discussion, throwing injuries of the shoulder can be simplified by grouping them according to anatomic region and relating them to specific phases of throwing when possible.

Anterior Shoulder Injuries

Bicipital tenosynovitis was named by many as the most common of the anterior shoulder injuries in throwers and involves pain over the long head of the biceps in the bicipital groove (72). This injury is most commonly seen in the windup phase, as the upper arm initially goes into extreme external rotation. However, it also occurs in the acceleration stage II phase, as the humerus is violently moved from external to internal rotation. It moves from the anterior part of the shoulder medially when the arm is internally rotated and laterally when the arm is externally rotated.

The pectoralis major, anterior deltoid, and latissimus dorsi muscles and other internal rotators can be injured in the early acceleration phase. When the subscapularis muscle is injured, symptoms include localized pain and tenderness over its insertion at the lesser tuberosity. The force of strong internal rotation in the acceleration stage II phase may rupture the pectoralis major or latissimus dorsi, or create an avulsion fracture of the humerus.

Subluxation of the tendon of the long head of the biceps is a rare injury. It usually causes a snapping or popping symptom in front of the shoulder joint when the arm is drawn back into external rotation at the end of the windup phase and in the beginning of the acceleration phase.

Repeatedly throwing too hard and too often may produce inflammatory reactions to the subacromial bursa. This occurs in pitchers who have poor pitching mechanics or continue to pitch with pain. Adhesions develop within the bursa that keep the rotator cuff from gliding smoothly under the acromion process and the coracoacromial ligament.

The tenderness is felt over the long head of the biceps but remains persistently anterior despite internal or external rotation of the humerus. The pain occurs mainly during the acceleration and early follow-through phases.

An excessively forceful pitch and accompanying follow-through can create an anterior subluxation of the glenohumeral joint, resulting in shoulder instability.

Impingement syndrome usually consists of inflammation and/or thickening of the structures (subacromial bursa, supraspinatus tendon, tendon of the long head of the biceps) lying under the coracoacromial arch (anterior edge of the acromion, coracoid process, coracoacromial ligament) and is aggravated during shoulder abduction and external rotation during the acceleration phases (73).

Through arthroscopy, tears of the anterosuperior portion of the labrum, near the origin of the tendon of the long head of the biceps muscle, have been visualized. These injuries occur during the high-velocity deceleration of elbow extension by the biceps brachii during the follow-through phase of throwing (72).

Posterior Shoulder Injuries

Because the teres minor and infraspinatus form the posterior portion of the rotator cuff, small tears might occur in these muscles due to their repeated "wringing" during the extremes of external rotation in the follow-through phase. Other terms used to describe this injury are posterior cuff strain, posterior capsulitis, teres minor capsular strain, and infraspinatus syndrome (74).

Ossification at the posteroinferior part of the glenoid, Bennett's lesion, is often associated with tears of the glenoid labrum and posterior capsule. The ossification is, in part, an inflammatory response to microtrauma and is also caused by posterior subluxation of the humeral head during windup or posterior "cuffitis" in the region of the teres minor during follow-through (69).

Conclusion

Although one is able to define the phases of throwing and to identify specifically the interaction of muscle groups at different stages of action, one can only hypothesize that a specific injury will occur during a particular phase of the throwing motion. Variables such as the presence of weakness, fatigue, incoordination of motion, degree of chronic degenerative changes, and scarring from previous injury are responsible for the difficulty in qualifying these injuries.

NEUROVASCULAR INJURIES TO THE SHOULDER

Neurovascular injuries in athletes are common in the world of sports. In discussing neurovascular injuries of the shoulder, one must have thorough knowledge of the neurologic innervation and vascular supply in relation to the soft tissue and bony anatomy. The C4-T1 spinal nerve roots or ventral rami supply innervation to the upper extremity; thus, their junctions comprise the brachial plexus. The five ventral rami unite to form three trunks. The upper trunk is formed by the fifth and sixth cervical nerve, the middle trunk by the seventh cervical nerve, and the lower trunk by the eighth cervical and first dorsal nerves. Passing underneath the clavicle, these trunks divide into anterior and posterior branches (75).

The anterior branches of the upper and middle trunk form the outer or lateral cord that gives rise to the musculocutaneous nerve, upper fibers of the median nerve, and external anterior thoracic nerves. Posterior branches of all three trunks unite to form the posterior cord that gives rise to the subscapular, circumflex, and musculospinal nerves and ultimately the radial and axillary nerves. The anterior branch of the lower trunk gives rise to the ulnar nerve, lower fibers of the median nerve, and internal anterior thoracic nerve (75).

The neurovascular bundle refers to the subclavian and axillary arteries and veins and the brachial plexus. These structures pass through several narrow spaces from the cervical spine and the lower border of the pectoralis major muscle in which compression may occur. These spaces, according to Poitevin (76), may be static or dynamic, depending on the nature of the boundaries. Static spaces are described as independent of upper limb position, whereas dynamic spaces are dependent on upper limb position.

Anatomical Entities Involved in Neurovascular Injuries of the Shoulder

PLEURAL SUSPENSORY APPARATUS

The pleural suspensory apparatus is composed of the suprapleural membrane and three ligaments from the lower cervical spine and first ribs.

INTERSCALENE SPACE

The interscalene space is made up of the three scalene muscles: anterior, middle, and posterior. These muscles constitute a singular muscular mass and are subject to congenital variation. The subclavian artery and brachial plexus pass through the interscalene space with the subclavian vein passing anterior to the scalenus anterior muscle. The scalenus posterior divides the interscalene space into an anterior vascular passage, containing the subclavian artery, and a posterior neural passage, containing the inferior trunk of the brachial plexus.

PRESCALENE SPACE

This is bounded by the clavicle and sternoclavicular joint, scalenus anterior, and first rib. It is crossed by the subclavian vein.

CLAVIPECTORAL REGION

This extends from the clavicle to the medial border of the pectoralis minor muscle. There are two bundles of the coracocostoclavicular ligament linked to and reinforcing the subclavian muscle sheath, joining the coracoid process to the medial first ribs.

COSTOCLAVICULAR SPACE

This is bounded by the clavicle, subclavian muscle, and first rib at the apex of the axilla. Its size is dependent on upper limb position.

RETROPECTORALIS MINOR SPACE

The retropectoralis minor space is located between the pectoralis minor muscle and the posterior wall of the axilla. Its size is dependent on upper limb position.

PREHUMERAL HEAD PASSAGE

This is a confined space created due to traction of the head of the humerus with combined 90° humeral abduction and retraction, possibly compressing the axillary artery and/or brachial plexus.

Median Nerve Compass

This compass is located where the axillary artery passes through a Y-shaped passage formed between the median nerve roots. The axillary artery may be compressed with extreme movements of humeral abduction and retraction.

The presence of a cervical rib may also cause neurovascular compression. Cervical ribs are present in less than 1% of the population, with less than 10% of those causing thoracic outlet syndrome. Cervical ribs can be short or long and can sometimes form a true joint with the sternum or first rib. The anterior aspect of shorter ribs can have a fibrous attachment to the first rib and may produce compression of the subclavian artery or the brachial plexus lower trunk.

Compromise of the brachial plexus and subclavian vessels may occur because of elongation, bending, and/or compression within any of the aforementioned spaces. Static compressions may be due to anatomical variations or downward migration of the shoulder girdle or to hypotonicity of the shoulder elevators. Dynamic compressions are created by sustained forced positions of the upper limb with exaggerated structural narrowness, thereby creating entrapment. This is particularly significant for the throwing athlete (Table 11.3) (76).

Thoracic Outlet Syndrome

This condition is also referred to as the thoracic inlet syndrome (77). It may be neurologic, usually involving the lower trunk of the brachial plexus, and/or vascular, involving the subclavian artery and vein (16).

Compromise of these structures depends on the varying architecture of the anatomy, i.e., congenital anomalies, and dynamic stresses placed on them. Compression of these structures may result in neck pain, pain radiating into the arm and forearm, paresthesia, weakness, fatigability, swelling, discoloration, ulceration, and possible Raynaud's phenomenon (78, 79).

There are basically three symptom patterns in thoracic outlet syndrome. The most common pattern is the result of lower trunk compression invoking paresthesia, weakness, and pain along the medial aspect of the arm, forearm, hand, and ulnar half of the ring and little fingers. Less common is upper trunk compression, which results in more proximal symptomatology often mimicking C5-C6 disc herniation. The third symptom pattern involves vascular components of the subclavian artery and vein. Venous compression often results in swelling and cyanosis. The possibility of venous thrombosis must also be considered, whereas arterial compression results in coolness, paresthesia, blanching, and fatigability. Compressions may affect neurologic and vascular structures simultaneously (78, 79).

Costoclavicular Syndrome

This is defined as compression of the neurovascular structures in the space between the clavicle and the first rib and is usually dynamic. Elevation of the arm with combined retraction of the shoulder entails backward movement of the clavicle. Both movements narrow the costoclavicular space. The healed callus of a clavicular fracture may also compromise this space. Symptoms of costoclavicular syndrome can best be reproduced by asking the patient to shrug the shoulders while elevating the chest with deep inhalation (16).

Scalenus Anticus Syndrome

This syndrome is the result of compression within the interscalene space that may be due to hypertrophy, spasm, or swelling of the scalenus musculature. Symptoms usually occur over the ulnar and median nerve distribution. Pressure over the interscalene space will reproduce symptoms, as will scalenus anticus maneuvers such as turning the head away from the involved side and opening and closing the involved hand 5 times and then examining for blanching of the hand. This may also be done by turning the hand toward the involved side (16).

Hyperabduction Syndrome

This condition is caused by compression just proximal to the axilla and anterior to the pectoralis minor muscle insertions into the coracoid process that acts as a fulcrum under the neurovascular structures when the arm is elevated. Repeated hyperabduction or hypertrophy of the pectoralis minor may both cause compression (80).

Postural abnormalities of low shoulder carriage and poor shoulder mechanics can also result in compression of these neurovascular structures.

Cervical Burner

Cervical burner and "stinger" are terms used to describe a traction injury that creates a burning sensation, usually along the upper trunk distribution of the brachial plexus. This injury is most commonly seen in athletes who participate

Table 11.3. Compressions of the Brachial Plexus and Subclavian Vessels

Static Compressions	Dynamic Compressions
Downward pull of the arm	Elongation of C8 and to a greater extent T1 nerve roots, as well as the subclavian artery around the first rib
90° Abduction and retraction of the arm	Humeral head compression and retraction of the axillary artery and brachial plexus terminal branches
180° Hyperabduction	Compression of C5/C6/C7 nerve roots against the posterior border of the clavicle; possible medial nerve or axillary artery compression by humerus; compression of the neurovascular bundle as it bends around the pectoralis minor muscle

Adapted from Poitevin LA. Thoraco-cervico-brachial confined spaces: an anatomic study. Annales de Chirurgie de la Main 1988;7:5–13.

in contact sports such as football, rugby, and wrestling (81). The mechanism of injury is combined contralateral cervical lateral flexion and ipsilateral shoulder depression. The athlete will present with a limp arm, describing initially a sharp burning pain and weakness and thereafter numbness and radiating pain in specific or generalized areas from the supraclavicular region down the arm and forearm into the hand and fingers. Sensory loss and paralysis are usually transient, lasting only minutes, although players often experience repeated episodes. Examination will reveal tenderness in the supraclavicular fossa over the brachial plexus and upper trapezius on the affected side (82). Shoulder depression along with contralateral cervical flexion away from the side of injury will be provocative.

These burner syndromes have been classified by Clancy (81). Grade 1 is defined as a neurapraxia without axonal injury and with complete recovery occurring within 2 weeks. Grade 2 is defined as axonotmesis with symptoms lasting 2 to 3 weeks, with EMG testing indicating axonal injury. Grade 3 is defined as neurotmesis with symptoms lasting more than 1 year (83).

It is necessary to differentiate this injury from cervical nerve root lesions, for which the symptomatology may be more confined. Cervical radiculopathy is more likely to present with tenderness along the cervical spine. Cervical compression, forward flexion, extension, and/or lateral flexion ipsilaterally are likely to reproduce the symptomatology (70).

TREATMENT

Rest is imperative. The athlete should not return to play until all symptoms have abated and full preinjury strength has been restored. Modalities that reduce inflammation, such as ice, NSAIDs, and ultimately neck strengthening exercises may also be useful. Christman et al. (84) found a high incidence of lateral flexion injury in players of average build, rather than in those with shorter, thicker, or long necks. Protective gear such as neck rolls and heightened shoulder pads can be used to limit cervical movement, although their efficacy is unknown. EMG studies may remain abnormal long after the symptoms have been resolved; therefore, return to play should be based on clinical examination findings. Cervical burner and cervical radiculopathy may be difficult to distinguish. There is some controversy over the exact mechanism of injury, in that the possibility of concomitant involvement of cervical nerve root damage and whether this is causative in cases of prolonged recovery. The study by Speer and Bassett demonstrated a questionable relationship between weakness and electrical evidence of axonal loss (82).

Acute Brachial Neuropathy

Another similar entity to the cervical burner, although relatively uncommon, is brachial neuropathy or brachial plexopathy. As opposed to the cervical burner, it has no known etiology. It will usually affect the dominant shoulder and proximal arm. It may present with an acute onset of shoulder pain without trauma, muscular weakness, and sometimes winging of the scapula and sensory loss, all continuing despite cessation of activity. The muscles commonly involved include the serratus anterior, deltoid, supraspinatus, infraspinatus, biceps, and triceps. It is necessary to diagnosis this differentially from other more common shoulder disorders such as impingement syndrome, instability, or nerve entrapment. Although this entity is termed brachial neuropathy, there is often involvement of muscles that are not innervated by the brachial plexus, i.e., serratus anterior and trapezius, and may involve muscles innervated by a peripheral nerve. Therefore, this entity would be more accurately termed single or multiple axon loss mononeuropathy or proximal upper extremity mononeuropathy multiplex. Electromyography and nerve conduction studies are necessary to confirm the diagnosis (85).

TREATMENT

Treatment should include rest, NSAIDs, initial support of the extremity with gentle range of motion exercises, spinal manipulation if indicated, and eventually a complete strengthening program. Full recovery of strength may not be possible; therefore, return to play must be dealt with on an individual basis.

In the likely event of dynamic neurovascular compression in which surgical decompression is unnecessary, a conservative approach is best. It is important that the diagnosis be accurate. Initially plain films should be taken. Postural mechanics and observation of activities that may be provocative (i.e., overhead hyperabduction movements such as those involved in throwing) must be addressed. The necessity of chiropractic manipulation must be examined to ascertain proper rib, shoulder, and spinal biomechanics. Rest, ultrasound, electrical stimulation or transcutaneous electrical nerve stimulation (TENS), and appropriate stretching (anterior neck and shoulder muscles) and strengthening (trapezius, levator, scapular, and rhomboid muscles) programs to improve shoulder posture and spinal biomechanics should be prescribed. Electrodiagnostic studies, Doppler imaging, arteriogram, venogram, or magnetic resonance imaging (MRI) may be necessary for the unresponsive patient.

Peripheral Neuropathies

SUPRASCAPULAR NERVE

Suprascapular nerve palsy without scapular fracture is rare. Branches from C5-C6 give rise to the suprascapular nerve that passes underneath the trapezius muscle along the supraspinatus fossa into the infraspinatus fossa, innervating the supraspinatus, infraspinatus, shoulder joint, and scapula. This nerve is vulnerable to injury at two sites: the suprascapular notch and the lateral border of the spine of the scapula, where the nerve enters the infraspinatus muscle. Blunt trauma or movements of anterior circumduction, or combined forward flexion and external rotation, may result in lesions to the suprascapular nerve (86, 87). Backpack palsy is another term used to describe this entity. The pressure of the straps and postural strain can irritate the suprascapular nerve. It has also been documented in weight lifters and volleyball players (88, 89). Denervation of this nerve will result in weakness and atrophy of the supraspinatus and infraspinatus muscle, limiting initial abduction and external rotation (90). Suprascapular nerve palsy with isolated denervations of the infraspinatus muscle has also been documented (87). One case study revealed infraspinatus atrophy, with weakness of external rotation and a positive impingement sign. Atrophy and weakness are cardinal signs of suprascapular nerve lesions; electromyography will confirm the diagnosis.

QUADRILATERAL SPACE SYNDROME

Compression of the posterior humeral circumflex artery and axillary nerve can occur in the quadrilateral space that is bordered superiorly by the teres minor, inferiorly by the teres major, medially by the long head of the triceps, and laterally by the humerus. Shoulder abduction and external rotation will exacerbate symptoms of paresthesia and vague shoulder pain of the arm, forearm, and hand and has been documented in baseball pitchers. A subclavian arteriogram is necessary to confirm the diagnosis. Approximately 75% of patients showing evidence of occlusion do not have symptomatology to warrant surgery (91).

AXILLARY NERVE

The axillary nerve arises as the last branch of the posterior cord of the brachial plexus C5 and C6 nerve roots and, accompanied by the posterior circumflex humeral artery, passes between the subscapularis and teres major. It then travels lateral to the long head of the triceps into the quadrilateral space innervating the deltoid and teres minor muscles and glenohumeral joint. Axillary nerve lesions unrelated to anterior dislocations are rare, but may occur from a traumatic infraclavicular brachial plexus stretch injury (92, 93). When the shoulder is internally rotated, the axillary nerve is taut as it winds around the surgical neck humerus. Cases of axillary nerve injury due to heavy blows to the shoulder while tackling in rugby have been documented in the literature. Symptoms include immediate numbness over the lateral aspect of the shoulder, which persists over several weeks with the inability to elevate the shoulder. Examination will reveal obvious wasting of the deltoid. EMG testing is necessary to determine the presence/absence of electrical activity (93).

LONG THORACIC NERVE

The long thoracic nerve arises from C5, C6, and C7 nerve roots that unite within the mass of the middle scalene muscle and extend down beneath the brachial plexus, along the lateral chest wall, and into the serratus anterior muscle. Because of its superficial location, it is vulnerable to injury from direct blows; it can also be injured through excessive traction and overuse (94). Symptoms include limited shoulder movement, owing to weakness or paralysis of the serratus anterior with or without pain, along with classic winging of the scapula. EMG studies will confirm this diagnosis, and treatment is conservative. Rest and eventual strengthening of the serratus anterior will help return the athlete to play, although the scapular winging may never completely resolve (89).

Referred Pain

Other conditions that cause shoulder pain range from benign and cancerous tumors and aseptic necrosis to pain referred from other systems. These systems may include the cervical spine, central nervous system, thorax and gallbladder, as well as distal upper extremity pain such as in carpal tunnel syndrome (95). A complete physical examination is imperative in serving the best interests of the patient. Diagnostic procedures such as CT, MRI, arthrography, arteriography, and EMG may be useful in confirming a diagnosis. These tools, however, should not be abused in an effort to rule out various conditions, but rather to confirm and clarify one's findings.

References

1. Kapandji IA. The physiology of the joints. In: Annotated diagrams of the mechanics of the human joints. upper limb. 5th ed. Honore LH, trans. New York, NY: Churchill Livingstone, Longman Group Limited, 1982;1:2–70.
2. Moskowitz E, Rashdokff ES. Suprascapular nerve palsy. Connecticut Med 1989;53:639–640.
3. Magee DJ. Orthopedic physical assessment. Philadelphia: WB Saunders, 1987:62–91.
4. Cyriax J. Textbook of orthopaedic medicine: diagnosis of soft tissue lesions. 8th ed. East Sussex, England: Bailliere-Tindall, 1982;1:127–167.
5. DePalma AF. Surgery of the shoulder. 2nd ed. Philadelphia: JB Lippincott, 1973.
6. Neer CS, Poppen NK. Supraspinatus outlet. Orthopaedic transcripts of the meeting of The American Shoulder and Elbow Surgeons. New York, NY. 1987;11:234.
7. Neer CS II. Anterior acromioplasty for the chronic impingement syndrome in the shoulder. J Bone Joint Surg Am 1972;54:41–50. Abstract.
8. Neviaser TJ. The role of the biceps tendon in the impingement syndrome. Orthop Clin North Am 1987;18: 383–386.
9. Rockwood CA, Matsen FA, eds. The shoulder. Philadelphia: WB Saunders, 1990;1.
10. Urist MR. Complete dislocation of the acromioclavicular joint; the nature of the traumatic lesion and effective methods of treatment with an analysis of 41 cases. J Bone Joint Surg 1946;28:813–837.
11. Kessel L, Watson M. The painful arc syndrome. clinical classification as a guide to management. J Bone Joint Surg Br 1977;59:166–172.
12. Hammer WI. Functional soft tissue examination and treatment by manual methods: the extremities. Gaithersburg, MD: Aspen Publishers, 1991:27–62.
13. Gerber C, Terrier F, Ganz R. The role of the coracoid process in the chronic impingement syndrome. J Bone Joint Surg Br 1985;67:703–708.
14. Hawkins RJ, Hobeika P. Physical examination of the shoulder. Orthopedics 1983;6:1270–1278.
15. Wilson CL. Lesions of the supraspinatus tendon. Arch Surg 1943;46:307–325.
16. Karas SE. Thoracic outlet syndrome. In: Hershman EB, ed. Clinics in sports medicine: neurovascular injuries. Philadelphia: WB Saunders, 1990;2:297–310.
17. Bergfeld JA. Acromioclavicular complex. In: Nicholas JA, Hershman EB, eds. The upper extremity in sports medicine. St. Louis: CV Mosby, 1990:169–180.
18. Rockwood CA. Subluxations and dislocations about the shoulder. In: Rockwood CA, Green DP, eds. Fractures in adults. Philadelphia: JB Lippincott, 1984:722–860.
19. Canales-Cortes V, Garcia-Dihinx-Checa L, Rodriguez-Vela J. Reduction of acute anterior dislocations of the shoulder without anaesthesia in the position of maximum muscular relaxation. Int Orthop 1989;13:259–262.
20. Ganel A, Chechick A, Heim M. Approaches to senior care: recurrent dislocation of the shoulder in an elderly patient. Orthop Rev 1990;19:633–635.
21. Rowe CR, Sakellarides HT. Factors related to recurrences of anterior dislocation of the shoulder. Clin Orthop 1961;20:40.
22. Schwartz RE, O'Brien SJ, Warren RF, et al. Capsular restraint to anterior posterior motion of the shoulder. Orthop Trans 1988;12:727.
23. Calandra JJ, Baker CL, Uribe J. The incidence of Hill-Sachs' lesions in initial anterior shoulder dislocations. Arthroscopy 1989;5:254–257.
24. Pavlov H, Warren RF, Weiss CB Jr, et al. The roentgenographic evaluation of anterior shoulder instability. Clin Orthop 1985;184:153.
25. Hill JA, Lombardo SJ, Kerlan RK. The modified Bristow-Helfet procedure for recurrent anterior shoulder subluxations and dislocations. Am J Sports Med 1981;9: 283–287.
26. Lombardo SJ, Kerlan RK, Jobe FW, et al. The modified Bristow procedure for recurrent dislocation of the shoulder. J Bone Joint Surg Am 1976;58:256–261.
27. Osmond-Clarke H. Habitual dislocations of the shoulder. the Putti-Platt operation. J Bone Joint Surg Br 1948;30:19.
28. Rowe CR, Patel D, Southmayd WW. The Bankart procedure: a long term end result study. J Bone Joint Surg Am 1978;60:1–16.
29. Neer CS, Foster CR. Inferior capsular shift for involuntary inferior and multidirectional instability of the shoulder. J Bone Joint Surg Am 1980;62:897.
30. Boyd HB, Sisk TD. Recurrent posterior dislocation of the shoulder. J Bone Joint Surg Am 1972;54:799.
31. Skyhar MJ, Warren RF, Altchek DW. Instability of the shoulder. In: Nicholas JA, Hershman EB, eds. The upper extremity in sports medicine. St. Louis: CV Mosby, 1990:181–212.
32. Fukuda H, Neer CS II. Archer's shoulder. recurrent posterior subluxation and dislocation of the shoulder in two archers. Orthopedics 1988;11:171–174.
33. Lipscomb AB. Treatment of recurrent anterior dislocation and subluxation of the glenohumeral joint in athletics. Clin Orthop 1975;109:122–125.
34. Fronek J, Warren RF, Bowen M. Posterior subluxation of the gleno-humeral joint. J Bone Joint Surg Am 1989; 7:205–216.
35. Neer CS II. Involuntary inferior and multidirectional instability of the shoulder: etiology, recognition and treatment. Instr Course Lect 1985;34:232–238.
36. Warren RF. Subluxation of the shoulder in athletes. Clin Sports Med 1983;2:339.
37. Neer CS, Rockwood CA. Fractures and dislocations of the shoulder. In: Rockwood CA, Green DP, eds. Fractures in adults. Philadelphia: JB Lippincott, 1984:1.
38. Bjerneld H, Hovelius L, Thorling J, et al. Acromioclavicular separations treated conservatively. Acta Orthop Scand 1983;54:743.
39. Smith MJ, Stewart MJ. Acute acromioclavicular separation. Am J Sports Med 1979;7:65.
40. Bosworth BM. Acromioclavicular separation: a new method of repair. Surg Gynecol Obstet 1941;73:866.
41. Walsh WM, Peterson DA, Shelton G, et al. Shoulder strength following acromioclavicular injury. Am J Sports Med 1985;13:153–158.
42. Galpin RD, Hawkins RJ, Grainger RW. A comparative analysis of operative versus non-operative treatment of Grade III acromioclavicular separations. Clin Orthop 1985;193:150–155.
43. Nettles JL, Linscheid R. Sternoclavicular dislocations. J Trauma 1968;8:158–164.
44. Waskowitz WJ. Disruption of the sternoclavicular joint: an analysis and review. Am J Orthop 1961;3:176–179.
45. Jobe FW. Painful athletic injuries of the shoulder. Clin Orthop 1983;173:117–124.
46. Richardson A. Overview of soft tissue injuries of the shoulder. In: The upper extremity in sports medicine. St. Louis: CV Mosby, 1990:221–236.
47. Neer CS II. Impingement lesions. Clin Orthop 1983;173: 70–77.
48. Jobe FW, Frank W. Impingement problems in the athlete. Instr Course Lect 1989;38:205–209.
49. Neviaser RJ, Neviaser TJ. Observations on impingement. Clin Orthop 1990;254:60–63.
50. Codman EA. The shoulder. 2nd ed. Boston: Thomas Todd, 1934.
51. Warren RF. Lesions of the long head of the biceps tendon. Instr Course Lect 1985;34:204–209.
52. Rathbun JB, MacNab I. Microvascular pattern of the rotator cuff. J Bone Joint Surg Br 1970;52:540–553.

53. Morrison DS. Clinical significance of acromial morphology. Orthopaedic transcripts of the meeting of The American Shoulder and Elbow Surgeons Long Beach, CA. 1987;11:234–235.

54. Neviaser RJ. Ruptures of the rotator cuff. Orthop Clin Am 1987;18:387–394.

55. Ellman H. Shoulder arthroscopy: current indications and techniques. Orthopedics 1988;11:45–51.

56. Crass JR. Current concepts in the radiographic evaluation of the rotator cuff. Diagn Imaging 1988;28:23–73. Critical reviews.

57. Brems J. Rotator cuff tear: evaluation and treatment. Orthopedics 1988;11:69–81.

58. Cone RO III, Resnick D, Danzig L. Shoulder impingement syndrome: radiographic evaluation. Radiology 1984;150: 29–33.

59. Bonutti PM, Hawkins RJ. Rotator cuff disorders. Bailliere Clin Rheumatol 1989;3:535–550.

60. Lippman RK. Frozen shoulder; periarthritis; bicipital tenosynovitis. Arch Surg 1943;47:283–296.

61. Bernageau J. Roentgenographic assessment of the rotator cuff. Clin Orthop 1990;254:87–91.

62. Nash HL. Rotator cuff damage: reexamining the causes and treatments. Phys Sports Med 1988;16:129–135.

63. Nirschl RP. Shoulder tendinitis. In: Petrone P, ed. American Association of Orthopaedic Surgeons symposium on the upper extremity in sports. St. Louis: CV Mosby, 1986:322–337.

64. Nirchl RP. Prevention and treatment of elbow and shoulder injuries in the tennis player. Clin Sports Med 1988;7:289–308.

65. Cahill BR. Osteolysis of the distal part of the clavicle in male athletes. J Bone Joint Surg Am 1982;64:1053.

66. Jacobs P. Post-traumatic osteolysis of the outer end of the clavicle. J Bone Joint Surg Br 1964;46:705.

67. Paavolainen P, Bjorkenheim JM, Slatis P, et al. Operative treatment of severe proximal humeral fractures. Acta Orthop Scand 1983;54:374–379.

68. DePalma AF, Callery GE. Bicipital tenosynovitis. Clin Orthop 1954;3:69.

69. Kulund DN. The injured athlete. Philadelphia: JB Lippincott, 1982: 267–270.

70. Roy S, Irvin R. Sports medicine prevention, evaluation, management, and rehabilitation. Englewood Cliffs, NJ: Prentice-Hall, 1983:211–216.

71. Pettrone FA. The pitching motion. In: Pettrone FA, ed. American Academy of Orthopaedic Surgeons symposium on upper extremity injuries in athletes. St. Louis: CV Mosby, 1986:59–63.

72. Andrew JR, Carson WG Jr, McLeod WD. Glenoid labrum tears related to the long head of the biceps. Am J Sports Med 1985;13:337–341.

73. Atwater AE. Biomechanics of overarm throwing movements and of throwing injuries. Exerc Sport Sci Rev 1979;7:43–85.

74. Lombardo SJ, Jobe FW, Kerlan RK, et al. Posterior shoulder lesions in throwing athletes. Am J Sports Med 1977;5:106–110.

75. Gray H. Gray's anatomy, descriptive and surgical. New York: Crown Publishers, 1977:768–776.

76. Poitevin LA. Thoraco-cervico-brachial confined spaces: an anatomic study. Annales de Chirurgie de la Main 1988; 7:5–13.

77. Howell JW. Evaluation management of thoracic outlet syndrome. In: Donatelli RA, ed. Clinics in physical therapy: physical therapy of the shoulder. New York: Churchill Livingstone, 1991:151–160.

78. Roos DB. The place for scalenectomy and first-rib resection in thoracic outlet syndrome. Surgery 1982;92: 1077–1085.

79. Sellke FW, Kelly TR. Thoracic outlet syndrome. Am J Surg 1988;1556:54–57.

80. Nichols HM. Anatomic structures of the thoracic outlet. Clin Orthop 1986;207:13–20.

81. Clancy WG, Brand RL, Bergfield JA. Upper trunk brachial plexus injuries in contact sports. Am J Sports Med 1977;5:209–216.

82. Speer KP, Bassett FH III. The prolonged burner syndrome. Am J Sports Med 1990;18:591–594.

83. Hershman EB. Brachial plexus injuries. In: Hershman EB, ed. Clinics in sports medicine: neurovascular injuries. Philadelphia: WB Saunders, 1990;2:311–330.

84. Christman OD, Snook GA, Stanitis JM, et al. Lateral-flexion neck injuries in athletic competition. JAMA 1965; 192:117–119.

85. Hershman EB, Wilbourn AJ, Bergfeld JA. Acute brachial neuropathy in athletes. Am J Sports Med 1989;17; 655–659.

86. Bateman JE. Nerve injuries about the shoulder in sports. J Bone Joint Surg Am 1967;49:785–792.

87. Black KP, Lombardo JA. Suprascapular nerve injuries with isolated paralysis of the infraspinatus. Am J Sports Med 1990;18:225–228.

88. Ferretti A, Gugielmo D, Russo G. Suprascapular neuropathy in volleyball players. J Bone Joint Surg Br 1987; 69:260–263.

89. Pianka G, Hershman EB. Neurovascular injuries. In: Nicholas JA, Hershman EB, eds. The upper extremity in sports medicine. St. Louis: CV Mosby, 1990:691–710.

90. Moseley HF, Overgaard B. Anterior capsular mechanism in recurrent anterior dislocation of the shoulder. morphological and clinical studies with special reference to the glenoid labrum and the gleno-humeral ligaments. J Bone Joint Surg Br 1962;44:913–927.

91. Cormier PJ, Matalon TAS, Wolin PM. Quadrilateral space syndrome: a rare cause of shoulder pain. Radiology 1988;167:797–798.

92. Friedman AH, Nunley II, JA, Urbaniak JR, et al. Repair of isolated axillary nerve lesions after infraclavicular brachial plexus injuries: case reports. Neurosurgery 1990;27:403–407.

93. Hopkins GO, Ward AB, Garnett RAF. Lone axillary nerve lesion due to closed non-dislocation injury of the shoulder. Injury 1985;16:305–306.

94. Foo CL, Swann M. Isolated paralysis of the serratus anterior. J Bone Joint Surg Br 1983;65:552–556.

95. Spiegel MPH, Crues JV III. The painful shoulder: diagnosis and treatment. In: Liang MH. ed. Primary care: clinics in office practice. musculoskeletal pain syndromes. Philadelphia: WB Saunders, 1988;4:709–724.

The Elbow, Wrist, and Hand

Joel P. Carmichael

The purview of this text is conservative management. Conservative sports medicine practice allows a wide variety of therapeutic options for most elbow, wrist, and hand injuries. The usefulness of splints, braces, and supports is perhaps greatest for injuries to this area of the body. Due to the relatively low ratio of muscle to bone, fractures and dislocations to the upper extremity distal to the elbow are common. Hence, the best treatment of some injuries discussed in this section will involve surgical intervention. This is especially true in the context of high-level athletic competition. The necessity of operative treatment has been discussed when appropriate. The level of diagnostic or therapeutic invasiveness depends on the present and future needs of the athlete, type of sport in question, age of the athlete, and level of athletic competition encountered. As in every area of conservative practice, decisions regarding treatment of a specific athlete must always be made on the basis of the best available evidence.

THE ELBOW

Most sports require controlled use of the hand. The ability to orient the hand in space is vital. This ability, whether in throwing a baseball, shooting a free throw, or performing a handstand, depends on functional, painless motion at the elbow. Because forces at the wrist and hand are multiplied at the elbow in some sporting activities, ligamentous stability and healthy articular cartilage are very important.

The movements of the elbow and forearm are complex. The forces placed on the elbow during sports are often disproportionately large, and failure of soft tissues is common. To address elbow injuries effectively, it is essential to have a thorough working knowledge of the anatomy and biomechanics of this region.

Clinically Relevant Anatomy of the Elbow

The elbow, also known as the cubital joint, is composed of three parts: the ulnohumeral, radio-capitellar, and proximal radioulnar articulations (Fig. 12.1). The ulnohumeral joint joins the trochlea of the humerus and the trochlear notch and coronoid process of the ulna. The trochlea has articular cartilage covering its anterior, posterior, and inferior surfaces. Posteriorly, the trochlea is oriented obliquely; with full extension of the elbow in the anatomical position, the forearm creates a valgus angle with the humerus. This is known as the carrying angle, and its average measure is 10°–15°. There is a lack of continuous cartilage coursing from the articular surface of the coronoid process anteriorly to the articular surface of the olecranon posteriorly. This is a finding often misinterpreted as pathologic at the time of arthroscopy (1). The radio-capitellar joint is formed by articular surfaces of the humeral capitellum (or capitulum) and the head of the radius. The capitellum is spheroidal and covered with articular cartilage at its anterior and inferior surfaces. The head of the radius has a slightly concave articular end for the corresponding convex surface of the capitellum.

The radial head is also composed of a convex, circumferential expansion of bone above the more narrow radial neck. This area is smooth and covered with hyaline cartilage for articulation with the radial notch at the proximal ulna. This forms the proximal radioulnar joint. The head of the radius is held in place by the strong annular (orbicular) ligament of the radius. This ligament is funnel-shaped, particularly in adults, being of a smaller circumference below than above.

Medial and lateral stability are conferred in full elbow extension by locking of the olecranon process of the ulna into the olecranon fossa of the humerus. When the olecranon apparatus is unlocked, stability is provided by the ulnar and radial collateral ligaments. The ulnar (medial) collateral ligament is composed of three bands: a strong anterior oblique band, a thin fan-like posterior band, and a transverse ligament spanning the distal insertions of the anterior oblique and

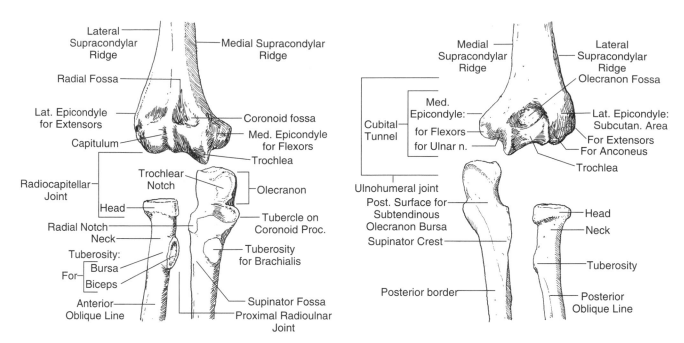

Figure 12.1. The elbow, also referred to as the cubital joint, is composed of three parts: the ulnohumeral, radiocapitellar, and proximal radioulnar articulations.

posterior bands on the proximal ulna. Knowing the points of attachment of this ligament complex is important in understanding medial ligament injuries. The humeral attachment is at the distal tip of the medial epicondyle, somewhat medially placed on the "underside" of the condyle. The bulk of the ligament, and the cord-like anterior oblique band in its entirety, attaches to the medial edge of the coronoid process of the ulna. The weak posterior band is attached to the medial edge of the olecranon. The anterior oblique band becomes taut in extension of the elbow, whereas the posterior band becomes taut in flexion. The transverse ligament merely deepens the socket for the trochlea of the humerus (Fig. 12.2).

Laterally, the elbow is stabilized by the radial (lateral) collateral ligament. Its apex attaches proximally to the lateral epicondyle of the humerus, and its base blends with the annular ligament of the radius. The annular ligament loops around the radial head and its ends attach to the margins of the radial notch.

The thin joint capsule completely encloses the cubital joint's three articulations. The joint cavity is continuous between the proximal radioulnar, ulnohumeral, and radiocapitellar joints. The joint capsule is bounded anteriorly by the biceps and brachialis muscles and posteriorly by the triceps muscle and tendon. This relationship is important in posterior dislocations and supracondylar fractures at the elbow. These serious injuries may contuse or lacerate the brachialis and/or biceps muscle, giving rise to heterotopic ossification (myositis ossificans) (Fig. 12.3). The synovial lining of the joint capsule extends slightly distal to the annular ligament of the radius. Its distal extension underneath the annular ligament is known as the saccular recess. The fibrous capsule completely encloses the elbow joint. Its anterior and posterior aspects are thin and weak. Laterally, the fibrous capsule is strengthened by the collateral ligaments, described above. The fibrous capsule is attached to the proximal margins of the coronoid and radial fossae anteriorly, but not to the upper limit of the olecranon fossa posteriorly. The fibrous capsule's distal attachments include the margins of the trochlear notch, anterior border of the coronoid process, and annular ligament.

The brachial artery courses anterior to the capsule just medial to the biceps tendon in the antecubital space. The elbow joint derives an abundant collateral circulation from this artery. However, Haraldsson (2) has shown that the blood supply to the humeral capitellum is limited past age 10 in adolescents. Deficient blood supply, superimposed by repeated trauma in the young pitcher or gymnast, can cause enough disruption to disturb the circulation. This is believed to give rise to capitellar osteochondrosis (also known as Panner's disease) in the younger athlete and osteochondritis dissecans in the older adolescent athlete. Osteochondritis dissecans is an ischemic necrosis of the capitellum.

There is an intimate relationship between the joint capsule and the neurovascular structures of the arm. The median nerve courses anterior to the joint capsule, medially adjacent to the brachial artery. This nerve also lies medial to the biceps tendon. The musculocutaneous nerve innervates the biceps and brachialis above the level of the elbow. It terminates as the lateral antebrachial cutaneous nerve. The radial nerve descends anterior to the lateral epicondyle beneath the brachialis and brachioradialis muscles. The ulnar nerve traverses the elbow in the cubital tunnel beneath the medial epicondyle. The course of nerves around the elbow are described in greater detail as lesions to each are discussed later in this chapter.

The flexor-pronator muscles arise from the medial epicondyle. The extensor muscles of the wrist and hand originate from the lateral epicondyle. The extensor carpi radialis longus arises above the common extensor origin at the lateral supracondylar ridge. The extensor carpi radialis brevis (ECRB) arises from the lateral epicondyle at the common extensor origin (Fig. 12.4). Its origin is clinically important because the tendon of the ECRB, according to many, is the most commonly involved site of inflammation in tennis elbow (3–7). The bony origin of the ECRB tendon is small in comparison with the vast bony origin of the extensor carpi ulnaris and the extensor carpi radialis longus muscles (8). The lateral epicondyle lacks a periosteal lining and contains a matrix of fibrocartilage, hyaline cartilage, calcified cartilage, and bone where the tendon inserts.

The ECRB tendon is superficially continuous with the antebrachial fascia and distally with the intermuscular septum, which separates the ECRB and the extensor digitorum muscle. The tendon is thin and narrow superficially, whereas the deep portion more distally widens into a broad base. Parts of the extensor carpi radialis longus and extensor digitorum muscles are also attached to the septum and tendon from which the ECRB arises. Hence, additional forces act on

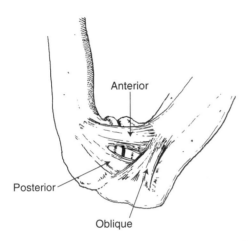

Anterior

Posterior

Oblique

Figure 12.2. The three divisions of the ulnar (medial) collateral ligament. 1: Anterior; 2: posterior; 3: oblique.

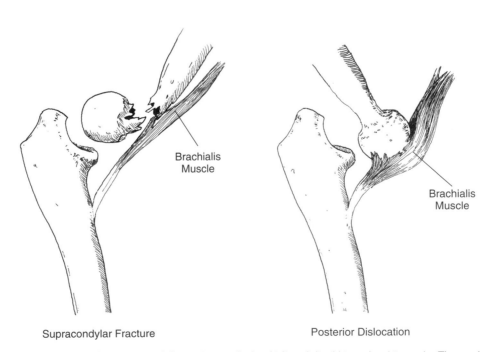

Brachialis Muscle

Brachialis Muscle

Supracondylar Fracture

Posterior Dislocation

Figure 12.3. Myositis ossificans can result from injury to the brachialis and distal biceps brachii muscles. The usual mechanism is supracondylar fracture or posterior dislocation. Intermuscular bleeding leads to heterotopic bone formation.

the ECRB tendon each time the extensor carpi radialis longus and extensor digitorum contract or lengthen. When the forearm is fully pronated, the head of the radius rotates anteriorly against the ECRB tendon, producing a fulcrum of mechanical irritation. This irritation is maximized when combined with elbow extension and palmar flexion at the wrist. These anatomical concepts will be particularly important as we consider the pathomechanics of tennis elbow.

Only two of the many bursae about the elbow are clinically important—the two olecranon bursae (9). The subcutaneous olecranon bursa is located in the subcutaneous connective tissue over the olecranon process. The subtendinous olecranon bursa lies between the tendon of the triceps and the olecranon, just proximal to its insertion into the olecranon.

The supracondylar process is an anomalous structure that has no known function in humans. In climbing animals, such as lemurs and members of the cat family, it protects the neurovascular bundle as it passes the elbow joint and provides a large area for attachment of the pronator teres muscle (10). Its occurrence in humans is esti-

mated to be between 1% and 3%, and it is often bilateral. With direct trauma to the area, as in contact sports, the symptoms of pronator syndrome may develop.

BIOMECHANICAL RELATIONSHIPS AMONG THE HUMERUS, ULNA, AND RADIUS

The elbow contains two independent axes of motion. The axis for forearm rotation lies within the radiocapitellar joint, and the axis for flexion and extension lies within the ulnohumeral joint. Any injury or condition that constrains either axis of motion will limit function and performance. Although most daily activities can be performed between 30° and 130° of elbow flexion/extension, 50° of forearm supination, and 50° of forearm pronation, these standards are inapplicable to athletes. Participation in sports places great biomechanical demands on the elbow and related soft tissues.

Ulnohumeral and Radiocapitellar Joints

The ulnohumeral joint is classified as a diarthrodial hinge, permitting flexion and extension. The instantaneous axes of rotation of this joint are clustered at the center of the arc formed by the trochlear sulcus of the humerus. The radiocapitellar joint is classified as a diarthrodial hinge in its movements with the ulnohumeral articulation, and as a diarthrodial pivot joint as it acts in conjunction with the proximal radioulnar joint. The axis of hinge motion (Fig. 12.5) can be approximated by a line that connects the center of the arc of the trochlear sulcus with the center of the arc of the capitellum. This axis creates a 94°–98° angle with the long axis of the humeral shaft, and it lies perfectly within the coronal plane of the forearm.

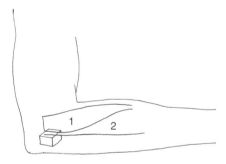

Figure 12.4. The extensor carpi radialis brevis tendon is the most common site of soft tissue inflammation in tennis elbow. Here, the cube of the lateral epicondyle is depicted in relation to (1) the extensor carpi radialis longus and (2) the extensor carpi radialis brevis muscles.

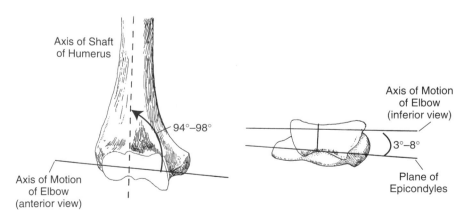

Figure 12.5. The axis of hinge motion at the ulnohumeral joint.

Proximal Radioulnar Joint

The proximal (superior) radioulnar joint is classified as a diarthrodial pivot joint. It is a true synovial joint between the convex circumferential surface of the radial head and the concave radial notch of the ulna. Proximally, the center of rotation at the radial head must always be the center of the fibroosseous annular ligament. On cursory analysis it would appear that forearm supination and pronation consist of simple pivot-type rotations of the radius around a stationary ulna. However, pronatory and supinatory movements of the forearm are far more complex than this. The axis of rotation of pivotal movements around the proximal radioulnar joint is a moving axis. This axis shifts to either the radial or ulnar side of the forearm depending on the functional activity of the arm. Movement of the axis is possible because the ulna does not remain stationary during the supination or pronation accompanying most functional activities. The distal end of the ulna moves laterally during pronation and medially during supination. This movement of the ulna in the frontal plane carries the distal end of the forearm axis with it. Ulnar movement in the frontal plane (with the elbow flexed) is made possible at the ulnohumeral joint because frontal plane translations occur along the saddle-like surfaces of this joint. Ulnar translations in the frontal plane are minimized by full elbow extension with the olecranon process locked in the olecranon fossa. This can be readily confirmed by the reader by observing the ulna in full supination/pronation while the elbow is locked in extension.

Carrying Angle

The anatomical valgus angulation (carrying angle) at the elbow creates asymmetrical valgus loading both in static positional activities, such as a handstands, and in more dynamic settings, such as throwing a javelin or baseball. The valgus angulation is especially important in gymnasts who frequently bear weight through their upper extremities. As they perform handstands or handsprings on a variety of gymnastic paraphernalia, the weight-bearing axis falls medial to the elbow joint, creating high valgus loads. To attenuate these loads, gymnasts usually hyperextend to lock the olecranon posteriorly and reduce the stress on the flexor muscles. A minimal loss of extension can be a profound detriment to the gymnast—as functionally disabling as a flexion contracture. Without this capacity for slight hyperextension, the strength required to sustain a motionless handstand position is much greater, exceeding the abilities of most athletes. Attempts to compensate will compromise safe, proper technique and predispose to additional injury.

Bony Alignment

When the elbow is flexed to 90°, three major bony landmarks should occupy the apices of an equilateral triangle. These landmarks are:

1. The tip of the medial epicondyle,
2. The tip of the lateral epicondyle, and
3. The tip of the olecranon process.

In addition, radiographically these three points should occupy points along a straight line. Variations from these spacial relationships on palpation and radiographic examination represent the presence of some clinical abnormality of the elbow.

Clinical Evaluation of the Elbow

INSPECTION/OBSERVATION

A complete history should be obtained before an examination begins. A detailed description of the mechanism of injury, including direction and magnitude of trauma, will be of great benefit in ascertaining the nature and extent of the problem. The location of pain should be defined as precisely as possible by clinical history.

Physical examination of the injured elbow begins with inspection for any variations from normal. Acute or subacute injuries to the elbow are observed for swelling, redness, abrasions, lacerations, and bone and joint alignment, including carrying angle. This angle normally measures 10°–15°. Measurement may be important in cases of medial elbow pain produced by valgus overload. The athlete's spontaneous use or guarded disuse of the upper extremity is noted. At this time observation of the cervical spine, shoulder, wrist, and hand should also be performed. In throwing athletes who have elbow pain, there may be flexion contracture of the dominant arm. Documentation of differences between dominant and nondominant arms is important for later comparison. Circumferential measurements may be appropriate in cases of prolonged disuse or immobilization. Surgical scars will be noted with previous open reduction of fracture/dislocations or from arthroscopic procedures at the elbow. A complete surgical history should be obtained.

PALPATION

Palpation can often precisely localize the injured structure(s). Begin with gentle palpation for localized tenderness and signs of inflammation. The medial and lateral epicondyles and the tip of the olecranon process are easily palpated in their subcutaneous positions. Bony alignment of these structures should be confirmed with simultaneous three-finger palpation. With the elbow flexed to 90°, these landmarks form an equilateral triangle. This configuration may be disrupted in the presence of fracture, particularly among pediatric patients.

The position of the ulnar nerve is located with palpation medially. The position of the nerve should be checked with the elbow in both flexion and extension, as this is the easiest way to assess ulnar nerve subluxation. Tenderness at the ulnar collateral ligament should be checked. Sensitive fingertips are essential to this procedure. Palpation of the subtleties of the ulnar collateral ligament insertion requires repeated practice (1).

Palpation of the bony origin of the ECRB is indicated in the presence of lateral elbow pain. With the patient's elbow flexed to 90°, this origin is a small site at the lateral epicondyle of the humerus in the direct vicinity of the muscle fibers of the extensor carpi radialis longus muscle (8). This site can be located precisely (with elbow flexed to 90°) by envisioning the intersection between the line described by the anterolateral margin of the triceps tendon and the proximal extension of a line described by the lateral aspect of the radius. The bony origin of the ECRB is localized along the horizontal line as it approaches the vertical line (Fig. 12.6). Distal to the lateral epicondyle, the superficial part of the ECRB tendon can be palpated. It lies between the belly of the extensor carpi radialis longus muscle and the origin of the extensor digitorum muscle (Fig. 12.4). Tenderness of any part of the ECRB tendon indicates the presence of tendinitis (also referred to as lateral epicondylitis and tennis elbow.)

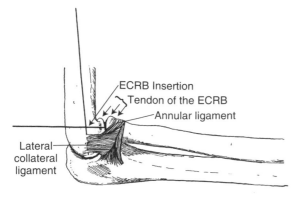

Figure 12.6. Locating the origin of the extensor carpi radialis brevis. The point of bony insertion is located along a horizontal line as it approaches the vertical line depicted here.

Light pressure is used for palpation of the radial head over the radiocapitellar joint while the forearm is gently supinated and pronated. Intraarticular effusion may be noted by superficial palpation just posterior and lateral to the head of the radius. Detecting effusion is more difficult and less reliable at the medial elbow.

Flexion of the elbow to 15° allows for palpation of the olecranon fossa posteriorly. Both medial and lateral aspects may be palpated using this method, allowing the examiner to distinguish between posteromedial and posterolateral problems.

RANGE OF MOTION

Active and Passive Ranges

Normal active elbow range of motion measures 0° extension and 145° flexion. The elbow can be moved passively to 160° of flexion. The ability to hyperextend the elbow by as much as 5° or 10° is normal in some people.

Pronation and supination are measured from the neutral position in which the hand is held in a plane perpendicular to the transverse plane of the elbow joint. From neutral, supination and pronation both measure between 85° and 90°. All ranges of motion pertinent to a particular injury should be compared with the uninjured side because this is the best barometer of normal for any particular patient.

Joint Play Examination

Accessory (joint play) movements of the elbow include long axis distraction of the ulna on the humerus, varus/valgus movement of the ulna on the humerus (with elbow flexed), superior/inferior glide of the radius on the ulna, and dorsal/ventral glide of the head of the radius on the ulna and capitellum in elbow extension. Rotation of the head of the radius at the proximal radioulnar joint is limited in supination primarily by the pronating muscles of the forearm, and in pronation by the compression of soft tissues covering the shafts of the radius and ulna as the two bones are crossed. Therefore, reliable joint play assessment of the head of the radius in rotation is not possible. Joint play movements at the elbow may be influenced by loss of joint play at the distal radioulnar joint, and assessment here must be included when examining the elbow's accessory mobility.

Long axis distraction of the ulna on the radius is assessed with the patient lying supine, elbow flexed to 90°, with the forearm supinated. The examiner grasps the proximal forearm in the antecubital space using his or her own web space for

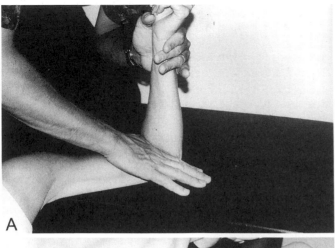

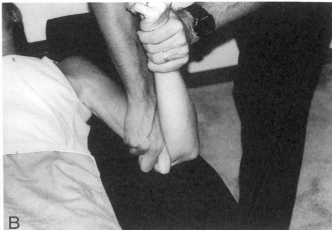

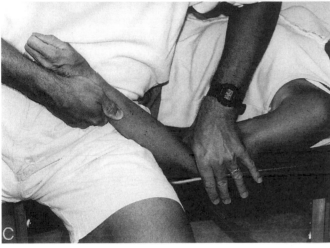

Figure 12.7. A, B, and C depict three methods for assessing long axis distraction of the ulnohumeral joint. There are specific advantages to each.

contact. The opposite hand is used to stabilize the patient's wrist in forearm supination. The proximal ulna is moved inferiorly by exerting distal pressure with the web space of the examiner's hand along a line described by the long axis of the humerus (Fig. 12.7A).

A second technique involves stabilization of the antecubital space against the examining table with the web space of the examiner's hand while exerting a distractive force at the wrist (Fig. 12.7B). With this technique, the elbow can be mobilized into greater flexion should joint play be found to be deficient.

A third technique involves anchoring the distal humerus with the elbow in 20° to 30° flexion. The distal ulna is grasped between thumb and fingers, and a distractive force is exerted by pulling at the distal ulna in combination with outward rotation of the examiner's body (Fig. 12.7C). Therapeutically, this technique has the advantage of allowing mobilization of the elbow into extension during inferior ulnar glide. All these techniques stretch the fibrous capsule of the elbow joint.

Medial and lateral translation of the trochlea (humerus) on the sellar surface of the coronoid (ulna) is assessed by positioning the patient supine on the examining table with the elbow unlocked in a slight degree of flexion, forearm supinated. The distal end of the ulna is anchored between the examiner's hand and body. The posterior aspect of the elbow is cupped by the examiner's other hand as he or she exerts gentle medial and lateral pressures at the joint to assess for normal, springy joint play movements (Fig. 12.8). Loss of joint play in these movements will prevent important contributions of motion by the ulna in pronatory and supinatory movements of the forearm.

Superior and inferior glide of the radius on the ulna is examined by anchoring the distal humerus against the table with the patient supine. The forearm is held in neutral position as the radius is grasped by the examiner's free hand. A long axis distraction is produced by pulling the radius away from the elbow joint along its long axis. One or two fingers of the anchoring hand may be used to monitor movement of the head of the radius (Fig. 12.9).

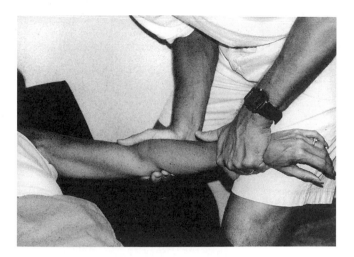

Figure 12.8. Assessment of medial and lateral glide of the ulna with respect to the humerus.

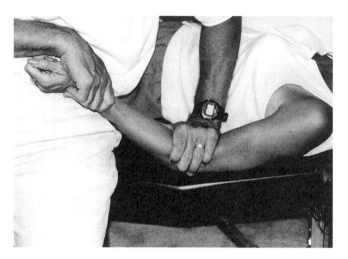

Figure 12.9. Distal glide of the radius on the ulna at the proximal radioulnar joint.

Dorsal and ventral glide of the radial head is performed by grasping the inner aspect of the patient's distal brachium while the patient grasps the examiner's arm in similar fashion. The patient's arm is thus stabilized while the free examining hand grasps the head of the radius between the thumb and medial aspect of the flexed first finger at the proximal interphalangeal (PIP) joint. The radial head is then moved dorsally and ventrally. This technique can also be considered a joint play assessment of the radiocapitellar joint. Restriction of this accessory movement will, however, primarily affect pronation and supination of the forearm.

A second method for assessing joint play at the head of the radius in ventral glide places the patient's forearm into a degree of pronation with the elbow fully extended. The distal end of the

radius is stabilized in pronation and elbow extension while the free examining hand gently springs the radiocapitellar joint into extension, using the thumb as a monitoring point of contact (Fig. 12.10). This accessory joint play movement is often absent after immobilization or casting of the elbow in flexion, in throwing athletes with flexion contractures of the elbow, and in tennis players. Dysfunction here is most often associated with lateral elbow pain.

NEUROLOGIC EXAMINATION

A relatively small but significant number of sports injuries involve the peripheral nervous system (11). At times these lesions are difficult to differentiate clinically from the more commonly encountered abnormalities of bone or soft tissue (12). Occasionally neurologic deficit will accompany severe injuries such as fractures or dislocations.

Neurologic evaluation at the elbow and forearm begins with inspection. Trophic skin changes, including a red, shiny appearance, loss of arm hair, and thin skin, are associated with reflex sympathetic dystrophy after fracture to the elbow or wrist. The arm is held in guarded fashion. Muscle wasting may also be evident in peripheral neuropathy involving the ulnar or radial nerves at the elbow. The median nerve may be compressed near the elbow via the pronator syndrome or the anterior interosseous syndrome.

The nature of neurologic examination precludes an evaluation that would be restricted to the elbow and forearm. Deep tendon reflexes, cutaneous sensation, and motor strength must be assessed for both upper limbs. Sensory examination should determine the precise distribution of

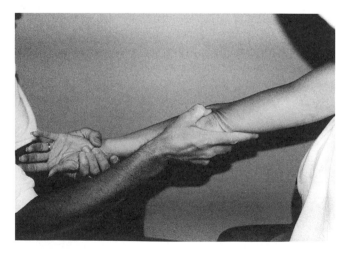

Figure 12.10. Examination of joint play in extension at the radioulnar joint.

any paresthesias. Although peripheral nerve lesions associated with elbow injury usually involve the ulnar nerve, they may occasionally involve portions of the median and radial nerves. A thorough knowledge of muscle testing is essential for the differential diagnosis of these syndromes. Figure 12.11 lists abnormal findings from muscle testing of the elbow, forearm, and hand in a diagnostic, correlative fashion. Other details of neurologic examination are discussed where nerve lesions are discussed later in this chapter.

ORTHOPEDIC EXAMINATION

Flexion of the elbow to 15° unlocks the olecranon process from the olecranon fossa, allowing for examination of the medial and lateral ligaments. The radial collateral ligaments are best stressed with the humerus internally rotated. The ulnar collateral ligament is best evaluated with the humerus externally rotated. As the examiner grasps the sides of the elbow with both hands, the distal end of the forearm can be stabilized between examiner's own arm and body (Fig. 12.12). Stabilization of the humerus is essential but often difficult to achieve. Evidence of ligamentous instability is often subtle, requiring attention to detail, not unlike cruciate insufficiency at the knee. Complete compromise of the ulnar collateral ligament can be masked as a stable joint, even under anesthesia.

Even when no weakness is produced with muscle testing, resisted muscle contractions may reproduce the pain or paresthesia of chief complaint. This may be associated with peripheral nerve entrapment, as noted earlier, or with soft tissue injuries. Resisted wrist extension performed with the elbow extended (Cozen's test) produces loading of the extensor carpi radialis longus and brevis tendons. When tendinitis/epicondylitis is suspect by history and location of pain, resisted eccentric contraction may be necessary to reproduce the pain; isometric contraction may fail to produce pain in mild cases. Resisted eccentric contraction forces the extended wrist into flexion against resistance. It places a greater stress on contractile tissues. This method of tissue tension testing should be used whenever the clinical scenario gives rise to a suspicion of injury to tendon or muscle when initial isometric testing is unproductive.

Alternatively, it is sometimes useful to place the suspected muscle and tendon at full tension (fully lengthened position) and ask the patient to contract (shorten) the muscle against resistance. This has been effective is eliciting the pain of chief complaint in subtle cases. Passive tensile loading of the contractile structure is often all that is necessary to reproduce the pain of chief complaint. For example, maximal passive stretch of the wrist extensors with elbow extended, forearm pronated, and wrist flexed often reproduces the discomfort associated with lateral epicondylitis. In this context, the diagnostic maneuver is known as "Mills' test." It is worth emphasizing that a thorough understanding of the principles of tissue tension testing will lead naturally to the formulation of an appropriate test. It is the author's opinion that the recall of eponymic designations (13, 14) for these maneuvers is tertiary.

These muscle testing principles apply to all resisted orthopedic muscle tests of the elbow, forearm, wrist, and hand. Medial elbow pain may result from injury and inflammation to the flexor/pronator group of muscles. Resisted testing or passive maximal stretch will usually reproduce the pain of chief complaint in such instances. Local palpation will correlate with the anatomical site of inflammation. Resisted supination is often important in distinguishing entrapment sites in pronator and radial tunnel syndromes. In these instances paresthesias, not pain, may be the major symptom reproduced. Lateral elbow pain and/or paresthesia, produced by resisted extension of the middle finger with the elbow extended (e.g., Maudsley's test (14)), is suggestive of radial tunnel syndrome.

DIAGNOSTIC IMAGING

A routine radiographic examination consists of an anterior-posterior view in full extension and a lateral projection with the elbow flexed to 90°. Oblique views, with the elbow fully extended, and a radial head–capitellum view are also obtained when additional information is desired. The radial head–capitellum view is performed by positioning the patient as for routine lateral elbow projection but tilting the tube 45° toward the joint (15). This enables better visualization of the capitellum and coronoid process, freeing the radiocapitellar joint from overlap by the ulna. This view is especially useful for detecting subtle fractures of the radial head, capitellum, and coronoid process. It is generally used when a fracture is not identified by standard views but is strongly suspected.

Anterior and posterior fat pads are intracapsular structures that provide valuable information about intraarticular injuries. On a normal lateral view the anterior fat pad sign is present, but the posterior fat pad is absent or seen as a linear, paper-thin lucency. Hemarthrosis from intraar-

Chief Complaint	Neurological Exam Findings	Diagnosis
Pain in the volar aspect of the forearm with numbness and paresthesias in all or part of median nerve distribution of the hand	Dysesthesias in the cutaneous distribution of median nerve & local discomfort over compression site, AND: a) Pain with resisted elbow flexion with elbow positioned at 120°–135° b) Pain with resisted elbow flexion & forearm supination. c) Pain with resisted forearm pronation with the elbow flexed and the fingers and wrist relaxed in flexion. d) Pain with resisted contraction of the flexor digitorum superficialis muscle to the middle finger.	**Pronator Syndrome** (Median neuropathy) a) Trauma to supracondylar process with median nerve compression. b) Median nerve compression at the bicipital aponeurosis. c) Median nerve compression at the pronator teres muscle *(Most frequent site of compression.)* d) Compression of the median nerve at the proximal margin of the flexor digitorum superficialis. *(Second most frequent site of compression.)*
Vague feeling of discomfort in the proximal forearm	No sensory deficits. Weakness with resisted testing of the: 1) Flexor pollicis longus 2) Flexor digitorum profundus 3) Pronator quadratus ± loss of ability to pinch between thumb and 1st finger Positive EMG of deep forearm muscles (but false negative EMG if electromyographer fails to achieve proper needle placement)	**Anterior Interosseous Syndrome** (Compression of the motor branch of the median nerve.)
Wrist drop or weakness of wrist extensors	± Sensory deficit of the dorsomedial aspect of the hand. Weakness of wrist extensors. Positive EMG for motor deficit involving radial nerve.	**Radial Nerve Palsy**
Paralysis or paresis of wrist extension with ulnar deviation ± paralysis	No sensory deficits. Weakness on resisted testing of extensor carpi ulnaris and occasionally the extensor digitorum (1 or more) at the MCPs. Usually EMG is positive for compressive neuropathy.	**Posterior Interosseous Nerve Syndrome**
Chronic lateral elbow pain and paresthesias ± weakness	Deep, dull tenderness at the radial tunnel. Pain always reproduced by resisted forearm supination with the elbow flexed and the forearm positioned in full pronation. EMG usually normal, but occasionally nerve conduction velocity is slowed across the elbow. Maudsley's test (resisted extension of the 3rd ray with the elbow fully extended) reproduces the pain of chief complaint.	**Radial Tunnel Syndrome**
Paresthesias of the 4th and 5th digits. Pain along medial joint line of the ulna Clumsiness or heaviness of the hand and fingers with use	Decreased sensation in the 4th and 5th digits. Sustained elbow flexion ("elbow flexion test") × 3 min. increases pain, numbness and tingling. ± Tinel's sign at the cubital tunnel. ± EMG. When positive, correlates with a more severe case. ± Motor weakness of the flexor carpi ulnaris (often masked by hypertrophy in athletes.) ± Atrophy of hypothenar eminence (often masked by hypertrophy in athletes.)	**Ulnar Neuritis/Cubital Tunnel Syndrome**
Painful "snapping" or "popping" at the elbow during flexion and extension	Palpable snap or shift of tissue crossing medial elbow with flexion and extension repetitively.	**Ulnar Nerve Subluxation**

Figure 12.11. Areas of focal muscle weakness in the diagnosis of compressive neuropathies about the elbow and forearm.

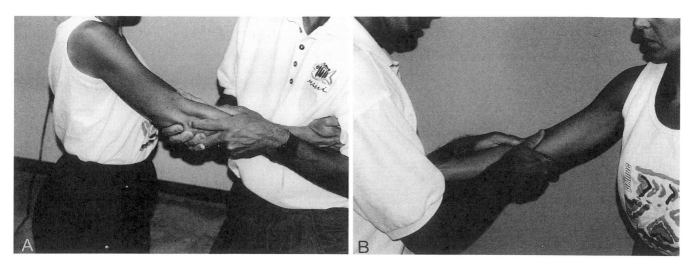

Figure 12.12. A. Varus. **B.** Valgus stress tests for the ligaments of the medial and lateral elbow.

ticular fracture causes the anterior fat pad to bulge further anteriorly, and the posterior fat pad will be displaced posteriorly and proximally, rendering it visible on the standard lateral projection. Fat pad displacement can also be caused by synovial hypertrophy and pyarthrosis. Therefore, clinical correlation of fat pad displacement is always required. The supinator fat stripe lies anterior to the radial head and neck. This fat stripe may be displaced or obliterated in the presence of a fracture involving the elbow. In all cases in which fat pad displacement or blurring of the supinator line is detected on plain radiography, further views of the elbow are mandated.

Fractures

In the pediatric elbow (patients younger than age 16), minimally displaced or incomplete supracondylar fractures are difficult to diagnose. Fracture is confirmed when, on the lateral projection, a line drawn tangent to the anterior humeral cortex is ventral to or intersects the anterior third of the capitellum. In patients with a Monteggia fracture-dislocation, the radiocapitellar line draws attention to the proximal radius where dislocation is often overlooked.

Medial epicondylar avulsion only occurs in the pediatric population (16). It results from a fall on an outstretched hand or violent contraction of the flexor-pronator group during throwing. In some cases, comparative views with the normal elbow will be required to visualize subtle displacements of the medial epicondyle. If a positive fat pad sign or small metaphyseal flake fracture is present, extension of the fracture to the unossified trochlear ossification center must be suspected because the medial epicondyle is largely

excluded from the joint space. The elbow may be examined under anesthesia to detect instability, or arthrography may be used to outline the articular surfaces and demonstrate an intraarticular fracture (17). Magnetic resonance imaging (MRI) may also be used to assess the cartilaginous humeral ossification center.

The most common elbow injury in adults is fracture of the radial head or neck (16). This includes injuries from all causes, not just athletic injuries. The absence of fat pad displacement does not conclusively rule out the presence of fracture in an adult. A radial head fracture appears as a linear lucency along the joint surface. The site of fracture is often depressed. Impaction fractures of the radial neck often cause mild discontinuity of cortical bone best appreciated with the radial head–capitellum view.

A capitellar fracture is typically displaced proximally above the radial head and coronoid process. This is distinguished from radial head fractures, which are often nondisplaced. The capitellar fracture fragment may be rotated 90° so that the articular surface faces ventrally. The fracture is not often seen on the anterior-posterior view. In some cases the displacement of fat pads is the only clue to the presence of fracture.

Osteochondral fractures and intraarticular fracture fragments are best evaluated by computed tomography scan (CT) or CT arthrography (18). Double-contrast arthrography, using injection of 0.5 to 1.0 mL of iodinated contrast followed by injection of 6 to 10 mL of air, allows for clear visualization of the articular surfaces and clearly outlines the joint space and the nature, number, and position of intraarticular bodies. The indications for arthrography, using either conventional tomography or CT, are seven-fold: (1) detection of the presence, size, and number of intraarticular loose bodies; (2) determination of whether juxtaarticular calcifications are intraarticular; (3) evaluation of articular cartilage surfaces; (4) delineation of juxtaarticular soft tissue masses; (5) demonstration of joint capacity; (6) evaluation of synovial abnormalities; and (7) documentation of needle position during arthrocentesis (19). Of these, only (1), (2), and (3) are often applicable to injuries directly related to sports.

Dislocations

Elbow dislocations are easily detected by standard radiographs. The radius and ulna are displaced posteriorly or posterolaterally in approximately 90% of patients with elbow dislocation. There is a high frequency of associated fractures, most commonly involving the medial condyle or epicondyle, radial head, and coronoid process. Fractures are more easily seen radiographically once the dislocation has been reduced. If the joint is incongruous after reduction, an entrapped intraarticular fragment should be suspected. This usually represents an avulsed medial epicondyle in children and a fragment from the tip of the coronoid process in adults (20).

Franklin et al. identified six conditions under which the addition of CT scanning was useful in evaluating adult elbow injuries (21). These conditions include (1) severe or complex injury; (2) presence of foreign bodies; (3) dislocations; (4) when radiographic positioning is difficult for interpretable films; (5) when conventional radiography is insufficient, as in casted fractures; and (6) when no fracture was discerned by plain radiography in the presence of joint effusion. These investigators found that the additional information gleaned from CT scans ordered under these conditions changed the diagnosis in 45% and changed management in 31% of adult patients. These criteria for adults were subsequently applied to a pediatric population (22). Ten cases of pediatric elbow trauma were evaluated, and in no case did the CT evaluation change therapy. The authors concluded that although CT imaging may infrequently be helpful to confirm or delineate suspicions raised by clinical examination or conventional radiography, it should be relegated to the status of an occasional adjunct in the management of pediatric elbow trauma.

Radionuclide Imaging

Radionuclide imaging of the joints has proven useful for documenting the presence and severity of inflammatory arthritis, differentiating septic arthritis from osteomyelitis, and detecting early evidence of avascular necrosis (23). This modality has limited usefulness in the context of sports injuries of the elbow. Other, less expensive modalities are generally sufficient for the purposes of appropriate management. One notable exception to this is bone scanning to determine the presence or absence of active heterotopic bone formation.

MRI

The superior soft tissue resolution of MRI makes it useful in the evaluation of musculoskeletal injuries. MRI can aid in the diagnosis of osteonecrosis (osteochondritis dissecans), neoplasms, trauma, and infection. MRI for elbow disorders has not been studied as aggressively as MRI for the shoulder and knee.

Elbow examinations are best performed at a facility where off-center zooming with surface coils is available. The T1-weighted spin-echo thin section technique with four averages provides good definition of the joint, soft tissues, and bone. If off-center zooming is not available, the patient's arm must be raised overhead to place the elbow as close to the center of the bore as possible. The elbow may then be flexed or extended, depending on the area of interest. The raised-arm position is much more difficult for the patient to maintain. Planes of imaging and sequences should be modified to expedite completion of an MRI study of the elbow performed in this fashion.

A wide variety of diagnostic imaging modalities may be required for complete evaluation of elbow and forearm injuries. Diagnostic imaging for specific disorders is discussed in later sections of this chapter.

Common Athletic Injuries Related to the Elbow and Forearm

FRACTURES

Recognition of distinctive fracture injuries is important to the conservative sports physician. Although many of these injuries can be treated nonoperatively, some cannot. It is important for the sports medicine specialist to differentiate between the two to ensure proper management from the very beginning. In some cases, special diagnostic procedures are necessary to clarify further the best treatment approach. Fractures to the elbow and forearm can result in permanent deformity or compromised athletic capacity if incorrectly managed.

Due to the varied nature and complexity of fractures of the elbow and forearm, certain axioms must be adhered to in conservative management. Anatomical reduction is essential to preserve optimal function. Before any reduction, however, a careful evaluation of neurovascular status must be performed. Any deficit or compromise must be treated before reduction. Furthermore, the neurovascular status of the arm may change over time; thus, close observation is essential after reduction during the early immobilization phase.

General conservative treatment measures will be provided for every fracture injury at some point during rehabilitation, even after open reduction. No more than 3 to 4 weeks of immobilization are appropriate in most cases, with even shorter periods in some fractures. After the cast is removed, a custom-molded fracture orthosis may be used, extending from the axilla to wrist and spanning the elbow with adjustable hinges. This brace can be extended with hinges across the wrist as necessary. Early, controlled mobilization of the injured elbow can then begin. The brace provides adjustable restriction of movement in flexion, extension, supination, and pronation. Torsional movements of the forearm are best avoided early on, especially in severely comminuted fractures.

Using the functional brace, range of motion is increased by 15° per week at the elbow and wrist, depending on the fracture pattern. Usually by 8 weeks the brace can be modified to allow full range of motion and activity. Radiographic and clinical evidence should be monitored for evidence of healing at intervals. If radiographs at 8 weeks still demonstrate a significant gap or significant radiolucency across the fracture site, an additional 4 to 6 weeks of bracing is indicated before full activation.

Once full, unbraced, pain-free range of motion is possible, restrengthening exercise should be aggressive. Return to upper limb weight-bearing activities (e.g., handstands in gymnastics) depends on the type of fracture, type of fixation used, quality of anatomical reduction, level of pain (if any), and freedom of movement of the elbow. These factors will vary from patient to patient and will require careful consideration before return to full sporting activity can be recommended. A description of fracture patterns and currently accepted treatment regimens follows to provide the reader with a reference for the most common types of elbow and forearm fractures sustained by athletes.

Galeazzi's Fracture

A fracture of the distal to middle one third of the radius coupled with subluxation or dislocation of the distal radioulnar joint is known as the Galeazzi's fracture. Other eponyms by which this fracture is known include the Piedmont fracture, the fracture of necessity, and the reverse Monteggia fracture.

Galeazzi's fractures usually result from a direct blow over the dorsal aspect of the distal forearm. In some cases this type of injury is produced by a fall on an outstretched hand with forced pronation of the forearm.

Moore et al. (24) have described the following four radiographic criteria to aid in the recognition of the Galeazzi's fracture.

1. Widening of the distal radioulnar joint space.
2. Dislocation of the ulna relative to the radius on the lateral view.
3. Greater than 5 mm of shortening of the radius with the anterior-posterior radiograph.
4. Fracture at the base of the styloid process of the ulna.

It is important for the conservative physician to recognize this fracture; while the rather "simple-looking" radius fracture is easily identified, the radioulnar joint injury may initially be overlooked. The conservative sports physician who fails to recognize the distal joint injury and opts for closed reduction of the radial fracture can expect unsatisfactory results. Hughston (25) cites the following four adverse mechanical factors that contraindicate closed reduction of Galeazzi's fractures.

1. The effect of gravity acting on the distal radioulnar joint may cause subluxation with subsequent angulation of the radial fracture, even within a cast.
2. The pronator quadratus can rotate the distal radius in an ulnar and volarward direction.
3. The brachioradialis can exert adverse rotational forces on the fracture site, shortening the radius.
4. The outcropping forearm muscles can rotate the fracture and also cause shortening.

For these reasons, most authors advocate open reduction and rigid internal fixation.

The most salient point for the conservative physician regarding Galeazzi's fractures is early recognition and appropriate referral.

Reverse Galeazzi's Fracture

Dolan and Dell (26) have described a reverse Galeazzi's fracture in which the distal ulna is fractured rather than the radius. The distal radioulnar joint is again subluxated or dislocated. Hypersupination of the forearm results in a spiral fracture of the ulna. As with the Galeazzi's fracture, the reverse Galeazzi's fracture may be misdiagnosed as a simple "nightstick" fracture of the ulna. The distal radioulnar joint injury may be overlooked. This again underscores the need to examine the joints at either end of a fractured bone.

Watson (27) indicates that open reduction and internal fixation (ORIF) are required in reverse Galeazzi's fracture if there is an associated fracture of the dorsoulnar aspect of the distal radius.

Both Bone Fractures (Radius and Ulna)

As noted in the discussion of the biomechanics of supination and pronation, forearm function is complex. Particularly great demands for forearm function are made by athletes. For this reason, fractures of the forearm demand near-anatomical reduction. When both radius and ulna are fractured, good reduction for the preservation of optimal function requires ORIF. The ulna is easily approached along its subcutaneous border, whereas approaches to the radius vary depending on the location of the fracture.

Monteggia Fractures

Monteggia fractures consist of radial head dislocation and fracture within the proximal one third of the ulna. Bado (28) has expanded the classic definition of Monteggia fractures based on the direction of radial head dislocation. In athletes, Monteggia fractures typically involve anterior radial head dislocation (Bado Type 1) with ventrally angulated ulnar fracture.

The Monteggia fracture is produced either by a direct blow to the ulna or axial loading of the forearm with forced pronation. As with Galeazzi's fractures, it is important to identify the dislocation in addition to the obvious fracture. Radial head dislocations are often missed due to lack of appropriate imaging of the elbow. Radiographic examination of forearm fractures must always include at least two views of the elbow.

Closed reduction of Monteggia fracture is acceptable in children, owing to easy reduction of radial head dislocations. However, the more skeletally mature patient requires operative treatment (27) to ensure anatomical alignment of the ulna. In adults, the radial head can be blocked from easy reduction by enfolding of the annular ligament or when the radial head "buttonholes" completely through the joint capsule and annular ligament proximally.

Isolated Ulna (Nightstick) Fractures

The nightstick ulnar fracture is relatively common among football and hockey players. It is most often caused by a direct blow to the forearm. Careful examination of the radial head and distal radioulnar joints must be performed to exclude the presence of Monteggia or reverse Galeazzi's fracture. Only then can the diagnosis of nightstick fracture be made with confidence.

After the diagnosis of isolated ulnar fracture is confirmed, the severity of displacement and degree of angulation are used to determine whether treatment will be conservative or operative. A majority of these fractures can be treated conservatively because they are less than 50% displaced and have angulation of less than 10°. In such cases, these fractures are not likely to displace because the radius and its proximal and distal articulations are intact and there is minimal soft tissue disruption.

High-energy impact can produce displaced ulnar fractures of greater than 50%, with more than 10° angulation. Extensive comminution often accompanies these injuries, and operative reduction with compression plating is needed.

When the criteria for conservative management are met (as is most often the case), splinting or casting should be provided for 7 to 10 days. This should allow the initial discomfort and swelling to subside. The arm is then transferred to a functional fracture brace, and the patient is given permission to use the arm within the limits of comfort. This treatment protocol has been described by Sarmiento et al. (29). Pollock et al. (30) report that isolated ulnar fractures treated with this simple method can heal in as little as 6 weeks.

Olecranon Fractures

A history of avulsion force without direct impact trauma suggests olecranon stress fracture (31–33), triceps avulsion, or traction apophysitis (34, 35) in the adolescent with posterior elbow pain. Forceful contraction of the triceps against a fixed forearm (as in gymnastics) or repetitive throwing with extensor overload (especially during follow-through) can provide sufficient avulsive force to give rise to any of these injuries. In cases in which repetitive overload has produced an avulsive injury to the posterior elbow in the adolescent athlete, avoidance of the aggravating activity will allow symptoms to resolve. Continued overload of the extensor mechanism can lead to microfractures of the olecranon physis and delayed closure of the plate.

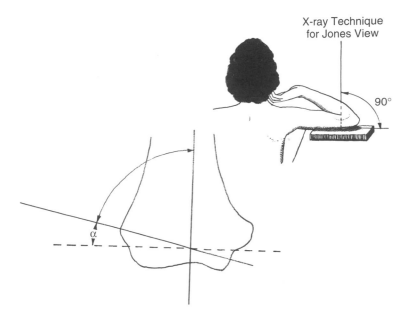

Figure 12.13. Baumann's angle on the Jones view of the elbow. Any discrepancy of greater than 5° compared with the injured side signifies unsatisfactory reduction in supracondylar fractures.

er flexion or extension trauma. In extension trauma, the supracondylar fracture is generally an oblique fracture passing from the posterior aspect of the humerus. The humeral shaft is displaced anteriorly, presenting the possibility of injury to the soft tissue and neurovascular structures in the cubital fossa.

Flexion trauma is a less common cause of supracondylar fracture. In these cases, the shaft of the humerus is displaced posteriorly and the distal fracture fragment displaces anteriorly. Examination will reveal moderate to significant soft tissue swelling and some degree of malalignment. Posterior displacing supracondylar fractures can be differentiated clinically from posterior dislocations by examining the relationship between the epicondyles and the tip of the olecranon process. In supracondylar fractures, the anatomical relationships between the epicondyles and the tip of the olecranon (equilateral triangle in flexion, straight line in extension) are maintained, whereas in posterior dislocation, these relationships will be distorted. The diagnosis is confirmed by radiographic examination.

Neurovascular examination is extremely important in children with supracondylar fractures. Any neurovascular deficits are immediate indications for open reduction. In lieu of such deficits, closed reduction should be attempted. This is best performed under anesthesia and muscle relaxation (47, 48). In an extension-type injury with anterior displacement of the humerus, longitudinal traction is applied first to overcome the compressive force of the biceps and triceps at the fracture site. The forearm is placed in extension for this maneuver. Next, the distal fragment is manipulated medially or laterally to realign any displacements in the frontal plane. Finally, the proximal humeral shaft is stabilized while the distal fragment is pulled anteriorly as the elbow is flexed.

In flexion-type injury with posterior displacement of the proximal fragment, longitudinal traction is applied as before. Then the proximal shaft is stabilized and the distal condylar region is pushed posteriorly while maintaining the arm in an extended position.

The most frequent complication in the conservative treatment of supracondylar fractures is malreduction. External fixation for extension injuries should avoid immobilizing in extremes of flexion because of the possibility that the neurovascular structures have been traumatized (48). After reduction has been achieved, maintaining reduction becomes the primary concern; malreduction leads to a change in carrying angle and cubitus varus deformity. Good reduction requires evaluation of Baumann's angle on the Jones view of the elbow (48). This angle is formed by a line perpendicular to the shaft of the humerus and a line passing through the physis of the lateral condyle (Fig. 12.13). Any discrepancy of greater than 5° compared with the injured side signifies unsatisfactory reduction.

A recent study of 108 patients correlated quality of reduction with the angle of elbow flexion used in external fixation (47). The authors found that in those patients who could achieve and

Clinical history will differentiate fracture separation of the olecranon from avulsion injuries. Fracture separation is usually the result of a direct blow over the proximal aspect of the olecranon (36) or is due to tremendous tensile loads through the triceps associated with javelin throwing (37–39). Smooth bony surfaces on either side of the acute separation are characteristic of a delayed union or chronic separation. With sufficient impact the fracture may be comminuted, often with articular depression. However, comminution is rare in athletes and is most often encountered with polytraumatized patients.

Fractures of the olecranon must be differentiated into displaced versus nondisplaced types by radiography. If the fracture fragment is separated less than 2 mm from the ulna, it is considered a nondisplaced olecranon fracture. This assessment is made only after inspection of lateral radiographs with the elbow flexed. If greater than 2-mm fragment separation is noted, the patient has a displaced olecranon fracture. The current consensus is that displaced olecranon fractures require ORIF to reconstitute the extensor mechanism of the elbow. Also, delayed closure in fracture separation of the olecranon epiphysis is heralded by sclerotic margins at the edges of the lesion. Curettage and bone grafting are then advocated to bring about closure.

Nondisplaced olecranon fractures may be treated with closed methods, using 2 to 3 weeks of external fixation with the elbow in a semiflexed position (40). However, Watson (27) contends that most olecranon fractures are intraarticular, requiring open, anatomical reduction. Watson believes that closed methods rarely achieve satisfactory reduction of the intraarticular component of the fracture. Clinical trials are needed to resolve this controversy.

Radial Head Fractures

Fractures of the radial head are common in athletes. Mason (41, 42) proposed a classification system for radial head fractures as follows: Type I, nondisplaced fracture; Type II, marginal fractures with displacement including impaction, depression, and angulation; and Type III, comminuted fractures involving the entire radial head.

Type I fractures are initially treated with 3 to 5 days of immobilization. After the pain has subsided, gentle, active range of motion at the elbow should begin. The immobilizing elbow splint should be replaced by a sling as range of motion exercises begin. In undisplaced (Type I) or minimally displaced (Type II) fractures, a sling is frequently the only form of therapy used, without

splinting. F
10 and 21 c
no further di
tient may retu
to 4 weeks in m
return to activit
criterion used fo
comfort reported

When Type II fra
ture line with displa
when the articular
ment diverges more
screws is recommende
tive results occur in tho
ture line is noncomminu
the articular surface of tl

In most Mason Type II
with numerous fracture lir
ment and/or comminution
ographs, the elbow joint sho
injected with local anestheti
careful passive range of moti
determine the presence or abse
blockage due to displaced fragm
articular surface. If no mechan
identified, and if the fracture is n
angulated extensively, conservativ
appropriate.

Conservative treatment of Type II
fractures of the radial head consists
lization for 7 to 10 days in a poste
Splinting the elbow in flexion versus
does not affect outcome (44). The elbow
be splinted at the angle of greatest comf
Again, repeat radiographs should be per
at appropriate intervals to ensure that f
displacements or loose body formation ha
occurred. At 7 to 10 days (if comfort levels are
equate and displacement is unchanged or
proved), the patient is placed in a functional fra
ture brace with controlled hinges across th
elbow. Graduated mobilization is achieved using
this brace with gentle, active range of motion exercises. The brace also avoids the late complication of radial head dislocation. Several reports show excellent results using conservative treatment measures for even the most extensive comminuted radial head fractures (45, 46). The keys to success are exclusion of cases in which mechanical blockage is present and the institution of early, controlled active range of motion.

Supracondylar Fractures

Supracondylar fractures are sustained in young athletes before the physes at the elbow have closed. Fracture mechanics can include ei-

maintain external fixation at 120° elbow flexion, closed reduction was stable. However, reduction was lost in 19 of 22 patients in whom an angle of less than 120° was used. In light of the fact that loss of reduction is not uncommon, many methods of stabilization have been proposed, including olecranon traction, percutaneous pinning with K-wires, and ORIF. Current opinion indicates the best results with percutaneous K-wire pinning (48).

For the conservative physician treating supracondylar fractures, it is most important to distinguish flexion-type versus extension-type injuries and then to choose the most appropriate method of fixation. Operative stabilization will be necessary in some cases.

High-energy intraarticular comminutions are very rare and will not be addressed in this chapter.

Medial and Lateral Condylar Fracture

Fractures of the distal humerus are uncommon in athletes but do occur. Such injuries include supracondylar fracture, condylar fractures (e.g., medial and lateral), and epicondylar fractures (medial and lateral). Condylar fractures are more prevalent in athletes because this injury is sustained by a direct blow or by the repetitive axial loading forces placed on the elbow. Milch (49) devised a classification system for distinguishing stable and intrinsically unstable fractures. The lateral trochlear ridge (Fig. 12.14) is the key to analyzing condylar fractures on radiographs. Milch Type I fractures are those in which the lateral trochlear region remains with the intact condyle (Fig. 12.15). In such cases the lateral trochlear ridge, anchored to intact bone, will prevent dislocation of the radius and ulna. Provided

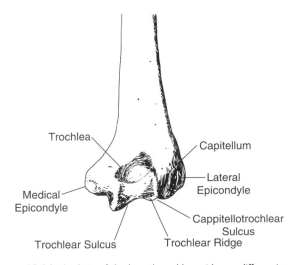

Figure 12.14. Analysis of the lateral trochlear ridge to differentiate stable from unstable fractures at the elbow.

there is no intraarticular step-off or incongruency, Type I fractures can be managed nonoperatively. These fractures must be followed closely for evidence of loss of reduction. If the slightest displacement occurs, ORIF must be performed.

Milch Type II fractures involve the lateral trochlear ridge as part of the fractured condyle (Fig. 12.15). These injuries usually involve fracture-dislocation and are therefore unstable. When the lateral trochlear ridge is lost, the radius and ulna may dislocate medially or laterally. Type II fractures must undergo open reduction because, even in the presence of congruent joint surfaces after reduction, conservative management can result in malalignment of one condyle with another and cause a loss of range of motion and intrinsic instability. This is an unacceptable outcome for the competitive athlete.

Lateral condylar fractures occur more commonly than medial ones and may be associated with rupture of the medial collateral ligament. After reduction has been obtained in Type II fractures, stress radiographs should be obtained. If gross instability remains, medial collateral ligament repair is indicated.

Intercondylar Fractures

Figure 12.16 illustrates the four types of intercondylar fracture as classified by Riseborough and Radin (50). Type I fractures are nondisplaced. Type II fractures exhibit some displacement between trochlea and capitellum, but no rotation of either fracture fragment. Type III intercondylar fractures show evidence of rotation with separation of fragments. Type IV fractures show significant comminution and displacement.

Intercondylar fractures occur when forces acting through the proximal ulna force the end of the ulna in wedge-like fashion between the articular surfaces of the distal humerus. The ulna acts as a cleaver, separating medial from lateral fracture fragments.

Current opinion reflects the following treatment guidelines.

1. Type I intercondylar fractures—plaster immobilization using a posterior mold for 3 weeks, followed by active range of motion.
2. Type II intercondylar fractures—internal fixation is recommended because of fragment displacement and joint incongruity. Early range of motion is encouraged.
3. Types III and IV—internal fixation with interfragmentary screws and various types of plating. With severe comminution, fixation may not be possible. In such cases, olecra-

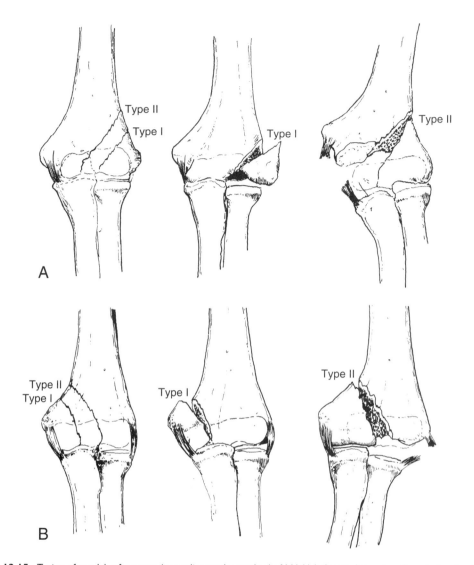

Figure 12.15. Typing of condylar fractures (according to the method of Milch) helps to determine if surgical reduction and internal fixation are required. Type II fractures require surgical reduction. **A.** Lateral condylar fractures. **B.** Medial condylar fractures. In Milch Type I fractures, note how the fracture line does not cross the trochlear ridge; therefore, the trochlear ridge is not part of the distal fracture fragment. In Milch Type II fractures, the lateral trochlear ridge (and the condyle) are part of the distal fracture fragment. The fracture line crosses the trochlear ridge.

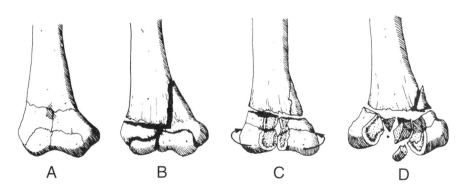

Figure 12.16. Milch classification of the four types of intercondylar fractures. **A.** Type I, undisplaced intercondylar fracture. **B.** Type II, displaced but not rotated T-shaped intercondylar fracture. **C.** Type III, displaced and rotated T-shaped intercondylar fracture. **D.** Type IV, displaced, rotated, and comminuted T-shaped intercondylar fracture.

non traction is used for 3 or 4 weeks, followed by placement of a collar cuff and early range of motion.

In a study of 29 patients with fractures of the distal humerus, the 22 who were able to begin range of motion therapy within 6 weeks of injury obtained acceptable results from treatment. More than half of those patients starting therapy after 6 weeks had unsatisfactory outcomes. Early range of motion and rigid fixation (when applicable) are essential to satisfactory end results (40).

Epicondylar Fractures

Fractures of the epicondyles are common in children, especially in throwing athletes. Chronic, repetitive valgus stress may give rise to injury not only to muscle, tendon, ligament, or articular cartilage, but also to the physeal plate of the medial epicondyle. This spectrum of injuries at the medial elbow is known as Little League elbow and includes the consideration of fracture separation of the medial epicondylar epiphysis. The diagnosis of epicondylar fracture is confirmed when comparative radiographs of left and right elbows demonstrate increased density of the bony apophysis with widening and irregularity of the physeal line on the symptomatic side. Clinical history ranges from that of painful limitation of motion during throwing to the report of an acute injury from avulsion of the medial epicondyle or direct trauma to the elbow. When direct trauma to the elbow is sustained, elbow subluxation or dislocation must be ruled out. Grana and Rashkin (51) studied 80 Little League pitchers age 9 to 14 and found that 45% had experienced elbow pain. Eighty percent of these athletes showed radiographic abnormalities on the involved side. Symptoms are more often associated with sidearm pitching when the athlete uses a whipping motion to increase velocity.

When fractures of the medial epicondyle are identified, the degree of displacement and instability determines the most appropriate course of therapy. Nondisplaced, stable fractures can be treated with simple immobilization followed by early range of motion. When the epicondyle is displaced more than 3 mm, ORIF will prevent the possibility of nonunion (52). However, successful outcomes with conservative management have been reported with up to 1 cm of displacement (53).

Radiographic assessment of medial collateral instability (with epicondylar fracture) has been described elsewhere in the literature and will not be detailed here (54). Significant instability necessitates early anatomical reduction and internal fixation, followed by early protected range of motion. Other indications for operative treatment in epicondylar fractures include ulnar nerve symptoms postinjury or mechanical blockage of motion indicating incarceration of fracture fragments within the joint. Lateral epicondylar fractures are usually produced by a direct blow and can usually be treated by simple immobilization. If significant displacement, comminution, or incarceration of fragments is present, surgical reduction is recommended (48).

Capitellar Fractures

Fractures of the capitellum are caused by a direct fall on the outstretched hand. Patients present with significant soft tissue swelling, limited range of motion, and effusion. Radiographs will reveal a large displaced capitellar fragment (Type I), a fracture fragment containing mostly articular cartilage with very little attached bone (Type II), or comminution (Type III). Current recommendations are operative for all three types of capitellar fractures (47). As with most fractures of the elbow, instituting early range of motion exercise is essential to good outcome.

OTHER BONE INJURIES

Osteochondrosis and Osteochondritis Dissecans of the Capitellum

Vague lateral elbow pain in the athlete older than 12 years of age may herald the presence of osteochondritis dissecans of the capitellum. This is thought to occur secondary to repetitive valgus stress applied to the elbow during throwing. This injury has also been reported in gymnastics and racket sports (40). Discomfort and swelling are usually present over the lateral aspect of the elbow. Examination will reveal effusion, tenderness at the radiocapitellar joint, possible crepitus, and decreased range of motion. Plain radiographs may not show abnormality. Conventional tomography or CT scanning of the capitellum can be helpful in delineating the lesion. Thin-section CT scanning or tomography (with or without contrast) should always be performed on athletes with elbow pain when radiographs are negative in the presence of joint effusion.

Range of motion examination is especially important. Locking or catching with flexion/extension of the elbow, when radiographs do not demonstrate fracture or loose bodies, is a hallmark of osteochondritis dissecans. This clinical finding also differentiates osteochondritis dissecans from osteochondrosis of the capitellum, in which no locking or catching is produced. Osteochondrosis of the capitellum (also known as Panner's disease (55)) usually occurs in athletes younger than the age of 12. Radiographs exhibit characteristic fragmentation of the capitellar ossification center due to sclerosis and resorption of this structure.

Treatment of osteochondrosis consists of resting the affected limb. This may be difficult to enforce in the active population younger than 12 years of age. Treatment of the older osteochondritis dissecans population is dictated by the status of the necrotic intraarticular fragment. If the fragment gives rise to frequent or irreversible locking or blockage, arthroscopy or arthrotomy is necessary because bony changes resulting from this disorder can produce lifelong functional deficits. Osteochondritis dissecans can be difficult to manage by relative rest. It is important for parents, coaches, and the athlete to understand that there is a significant potential for lifelong consequences when the lesion is not allowed to heal properly. The best treatment of this disorder is prevention because the radiocapitellar joint has a propensity for arthritic change once the capsule has been surgically disrupted. Prevention consists mainly of maintaining athletic activity within reasonable limits (e.g., limiting the number of innings pitched.) Throwing athletes should also be advised about restricting the amount of practice throwing at home and on the playground.

DISLOCATIONS

Dislocations of the elbow are most common in athletes who participate in a contact sport, such as gymnastics, football, or wrestling. Injury usually involves axial loading of the arm coupled with an extension force to the elbow. Dislocations can, however, occur with the elbow in the flexed position (34).

Dislocations can produce an extensive amount of soft tissue damage with disruption of both anterior and posterior capsules, collateral ligaments, brachialis muscle, and common wrist flexor muscle mass. Neurovascular insult may also occur. When neurologic deficits are present, intraarticular loose bodies are the cause.

Best results occur with early reduction of the dislocation. Posterior dislocations are most common. Even when ligaments have been disrupted, good results with conservative treatment have generally been reported. A recent study reported that there was no statistically significant difference between those elbow dislocations treated surgically versus nonsurgically (56).

Reduction of the dislocation begins with gently positioning the forearm in supination to unlock the coronoid process and radial head. Then gentle, nontraumatic traction is exerted through the forearm while stabilizing the distal humerus. The physician can push distally on the olecranon if necessary. Some authors report that even when using gentle traction, neurologic compromise can occur (57). Postreduction examination must reassess neurologic status. The elbow should be immobilized to allow soft tissue swelling and pain to stabilize. A protected active range of motion program should begin within 2 or 3 days after reduction unless the elbow demonstrates a propensity to redislocate. Excessive pain during rehabilitation should be avoided because this seems to aggravate swelling and inflammation. Return to activity is generally within 3 to 6 weeks of injury and should be guided by an assessment of the return of muscle strength and range of motion. Protective bracing is recommended on return to contact sports.

The most common long-term complaint of patients who have suffered an elbow dislocation is loss of extension mobility. Acute valgus instability does not appear to present a long-term problem after the elbow has healed fully.

LIGAMENT INJURIES/MEDIAL INSTABILITY/THROWING INJURIES

In most athletic endeavors, the medial aspect of the elbow is subjected to repetitive tensile stresses, whereas the lateral aspect is exposed to compressive forces. Ligaments fail under tensile loads; therefore, ligamentous elbow injuries usually affect the medial elbow. The ulnar collateral ligament is the ligament most commonly injured, especially its anterior oblique band. Skill in palpating this structure requires much practice.

Throwing Injuries

Ulnar collateral ligament injury is the most common cause of medial instability at the elbow. It is caused by repetitive valgus extension overload. This is most often encountered in baseball pitching. Other throwing sports, such as javelin and shot put, involve more transference of torsional energy from the legs and trunk, whereas pitching a baseball involves an independent whip-like action of the arm designed to impart great velocity to the ball. During the acceleration phase, the trunk and pelvis have already rotated forward and the arm is "catching up" to the motion of the rest of the body (58). During this phase, the elbow rapidly extends and a large valgus force is produced. This force results in a variety of injuries to the medial elbow, depending on the age of the child. We have already discussed fractures of the medial epicondyle as a cause of pain and swelling in the younger throwing athlete. The curve ball has been cited as the primary cause of Little League elbow, and this pitch has been banned in many places. However, studies have shown that a properly thrown curve ball is no more injurious than a traditional fastball (59). Properly thrown curve balls are produced by an increase in the rate of elbow extension while throwing a curve, not by increased supination during release. Improper supination during release increases the likelihood of injury.

Ulnar collateral ligament sprains present with pain and possibly swelling at the medial aspect of the elbow. Symptoms are better with rest and worse with use. Stiffness may also be present. Examination reveals pain on palpation, well localized to the anterior oblique portion of the ulnar collateral ligament. Valgus stress increases familial pain at the medial elbow and will demonstrate instability in more advanced cases. Severe cases will also reveal the presence of flexion contracture at the elbow. Bony changes can be seen radiographically, ranging from medial spur formation at the proximal ulna to actual avulsion fractures including heterotopic calcification of the degenerated ligament. Resisted wrist flexion will not produce pain unless the flexor pronator group is also strained.

Conservative treatment includes rest from pitching, ice, and electrical stimulation for pain control. Ice is also applied to the elbow (and shoulder if necessary) after throwing to decrease the inflammatory response. Ice should not be used injudiciously over the cubital tunnel because this may give rise to ulnar nerve dysfunction. Contrast fomentation with ice and heat can be useful. Gentle stretching and range of motion exercises are performed early for the elbow flexor and extensor musculature. Light transverse friction massage may be applied to realign collagen fiber and mobilize scar tissue within the ligament. The patient can be taught how to perform this procedure at home. As with other ligamentous injuries, ulnar collateral ligament sprains take a long time to heal (1).

The best treatment of collateral ligament sprains in throwing athletes is prevention (58). The following principles are used.

1. Proper conditioning. Maintain flexibility and endurance in the off-season by tossing the ball without maximal effort. The athlete should avoid beginning the season with pitching at maximum velocity without a good base of endurance and conditioning exercise.
2. Avoid pain and inflammation.
   A. Strictly avoid pitching when fatigued. An accurate pitch count should be kept during the game, with the pitcher's limit known in advance. If the pitcher begins to show loss of control, this can mean fatigue. Fatigue can cause improper pitching mechanics leading to injury. Also, although Little League games are usually well supervised and pitching limits enforced, some parents may have their child throwing hard on off days as part of practice. The parents, coaches, and athlete must be counseled against excessive practice.
   B. Ice the elbow after pitching in practice and in competition. On off days, continue stretching and light tossing, again without maximal effort.

Overuse injuries before skeletal maturity can lead to permanent dysfunction of the elbow. Although the child's successful performance in athletics is often the focus of attention, the parents must know the importance of rest and rehabilitation for the child pitcher with a painful medial elbow. A defined schedule of rehabilitation should be established; this gives the athlete (and parents, if necessary) a timetable. Ill-defined treatment plans may cause the athlete to lose confidence and abandon rehabilitation. Rehabilitation plans have been outlined elsewhere in detail (60).

Although lateral elbow pain is the most common disorder encountered in tennis, the elite tennis player is more likely to develop medial elbow pain due to the high overhand serve. The mechanics of this serve are similar to pitching in that both involve high valgus loads to the medial elbow in an effort to impart high velocity to the object of play. Treatment principles remain the same for the elite tennis player with tension overload injuries to the medial elbow.

Chronic instability of the ulnar collateral ligament that persists after all rehabilitative efforts may require surgery. This most often involves the professional baseball pitcher. The operative procedure, described by Jobe et al. (61), is technically demanding, but has been met with good results. Outcome depends on a carefully monitored postoperative rehabilitation program.

Hyperextension Injuries

Hotchkiss (58) notes that hyperextension injuries of the elbow have not been described in the literature. However, he states that these injuries do occur. Unfortunately, such injuries are more difficult to treat than extension injuries involving fracture or posterior dislocation.

Hyperextension produces a traumatic stretch to the anterior joint capsule and flexor musculature. Collateral ligaments and the biceps tendon remain intact. Heterotopic ossification of the brachialis can occur if it is torn.

Early active range of motion is encouraged to regain extension mobility. Immobilization for more than a few days should be avoided. Pain and swelling may persist for weeks, precluding a full range of motion. Full recovery may be protracted, and it is best to inform the patient, parents, and coach of this early in the course of management. This injury can severely restrict the athlete's participation in sports, despite the best efforts at conservative rehabilitation. There is a potential for long-term disability. If participation in sports is continued, the elbow must be taped to prevent further hyperextension (58).

Rodeo cowboys are at increased risk for hyperextension injuries to the elbow during bull riding and bronco riding. The elbow should be taped protectively at slightly less than the angle of elbow flexion used during riding to prevent hyperextension injury before it occurs.

RADIAL HEAD SUBLUXATION

In children younger than age 7 (62), the head of the radius is relatively smaller than in adults so the grip of the annular ligament is not as firm as in later life. In addition, the capsule is lax and its distal attachment to the radius is thin and weak. A sudden longitudinal traction force on the child's extended, pronated forearm can subluxate the head of the radius at the proximal radioulnar joint. The annular ligament tears from its attachment to the radius during traction force. When traction is released, the ligament becomes incarcerated between the capitellum and the proximal tip of the radius, preventing reduction. Supination of the forearm with the elbow slightly flexed restores the annular ligament to its normal position. This fact is used in therapeutic reduction.

History typically reveals a sudden pull on the extended forearm, as in pulling a child from the monkey bars or pulling the child quickly from the ground to avoid danger. There is an immediate onset of pain, and the child will refuse to use the affected limb. Physical examination reveals an arm limply held close to the body and slight tenderness over the radial head. Full elbow flexion, extension, and forearm pronation are possible,

but the child screams at the slightest attempts at active supination (62).

Traumatic radial head subluxation must be differentiated from radial head dislocation. In patients with radial head dislocation, all movements may be guarded, but pronation and supination are equally painful. Radial head dislocation is rare. The two disorders can also be differentiated radiographically, with disruption of normal roentgenometric relationships in the case of dislocation. A line drawn through the center of the long axis of the radius will pass through the center of the the capitellar epiphysis in a normal elbow and in radial head subluxation, but not in radial head dislocation (62).

Reduction of traumatic radial head subluxation is made by first cooling the elbow with ice for 5 minutes. Next, the child's elbow is gently flexed and extended to ensure relaxation. With the elbow partially flexed, the child's attention is then diverted. Gentle but firm thumb pressure is applied over the radial head, and the forearm is gently but quickly supinated. This maneuver is accompanied by a palpable and sometimes audible reduction click. Postreduction immobilization is unnecessary. Traction to the child's forearm should be avoided, and the inciting mechanism of trauma fully explained to the parents.

JOINT DYSFUNCTION AT THE PROXIMAL RADIUS

Proximal radioulnar or radiocapitellar joint dysfunction, characterized by loss of joint play, is common (especially in conjunction with tennis elbow or throwing-related flexion contractures of the elbow). This condition is also seen frequently after immobilization. Immobilization after trauma or surgery may lead to progressive contracture of capsular and pericapsular structures, intraarticular fibrofatty connective tissue encroachment, adhesions with collagen fiber cross-linking, articular cartilage fibrillation, and primitive mesenchymal tissue invasion of the subchondral plate. McVay notes that there are pads of fat filling the coronoid, radial, and olecranon fossae that may become fibrocartilaginous, project into the joint space, and cause locking (63).

Loss of joint play can be restored by direct, high-velocity, low-amplitude manipulation. A short impulse in a posteroanterior direction is applied to the radius with the elbow extended and forearm pronated (64, 65). Articular release is often attended by an audible click. Reassessment after successful manipulation will demonstrate restoration of joint play. Several manipulations may be necessary to restore joint play fully. When successfully regained, normal accessory movements of the radiocapitellar and radioulnar joints will contribute to smooth, synchronous, pain-free elbow function during athletic activities.

High-velocity, low-amplitude manipulative therapy is a highly specialized skill and should not be attempted by an untrained physician. This procedure usually requires referral to a knowledgeable chiropractor. Elbow manipulation under general anesthesia has been reported in the literature (66). Ten of 11 patients studied had undergone at least one form of surgical procedure before manipulative intervention. These patients not only lost joint play, they were also unable to achieve a full passive range of motion up to the zone of accessory joint movement. A single elbow manipulation under anesthesia was found to improve motion in more than 50% of patients in whom well-supervised rehabilitation with analgesics, intraarticular anesthesia, ice, continuous passive motion, active assisted range of motion, muscle strengthening, and static and dynamic splint therapy had failed.

TENDON AND MUSCLE INJURY

Tennis Elbow

The nomenclature for soft tissue injuries at the lateral elbow is extensive. Synonyms for tennis elbow include carpenter's elbow, dentist's elbow, tiller's elbow in yachtsmen, potato pickers' plight, and politician's paw. Diagnostically this entity has been referred to as an epicondylitis and a tendinitis. The most common pathologic finding from operative material has been macroscopic and microscopic tears in the musculotendinous structures, especially at the tendinous insertions into bone over and around the lateral epicondyle at the humerus (67). In this respect, the lesion represents both a tendinitis and an epicondylitis.

Tennis elbow tends to be a self-limiting disorder. Lateral epicondylitis is between 3 and 10 times more common than medial epicondylitis. Fifty percent of all tennis players can expect to experience tennis elbow at some time during their playing lifetime. One third of these cases will be severe enough to limit tasks of daily living. The peak incidence is between the ages of 40 and 50. Ninety percent of players who have had tennis elbow never have recurrence of symptoms. This may be due to increased extensibility of the ECRB once a first tear has occurred. The majority of cases resolve well with conservative therapy.

In general, tennis elbow is thought to be the result of overuse of the wrist extensors at the lateral epicondyle. The most commonly involved tendon is the ECRB. (3–8, 67–69) According to a recent review of literature (70), most authors consider the primary cause of tennis elbow to be mechanical. Microscopically, most tears occur where the ECRB tendon inserts, via Sharpey's fibers, into the junction of hyaline cartilage and calcified cartilage at the lateral epicondyle. There is least elasticity at this junction. A secondary, chronic, inflammatory response is brought about by continued overuse of the extensor tendon complex, with granulomatous tissue formation, ingrowth of free nerve endings, neovascularization, and continued bleeding. This can be noted deep to the ECRB tendon at surgery in what is known as the subaponeurotic space. In severe injuries there can also be a microavulsion fracture at the tendinous insertion of the ECRB (69). The end result is nonresolving, painful scar tissue tending toward mucinoid degeneration rather than repair. These advanced lesions have been termed enthesopathies, meaning a pathologic entity of the specialized insertion of tendons and ligaments into bone.

Clinical history will reveal lateral elbow pain with athletic activity, especially with the backhand in novice tennis players. In approximately one third of cases, symptoms are severe enough to limit normal activities. Some patients may have associated numbness or dysesthesia from elbow to hand. Examination demonstrates well-localized tenderness at the lateral epicondyle and along the tendon of the ECRB. When sensory changes are present, these are often reproduced or intensified by myofascial trigger points in one or more of the wrist extensor muscles. Neurologic examination is normal. Orthopedic examination reproduces the familiar pain with three tests. Mills' test is a passive stretch of the extensor tendons produced by full elbow extension, forearm pronation, wrist flexion, and ulnar deviation of the hand (13). This test will stretch the injured tissue, provoking pain. Resisted contraction of the ECRB and related tendons (Cozen's test) is performed with the elbow and wrist fully extended. Pain may not be provoked until the patient's strength is overcome and the wrist is forced into flexion by the examiner. This produces eccentric loading of the extensor tendons. With Maudsley's test, there is pain on resisted extension of the middle finger at the metacarpophalangeal joint (MPJ) when the elbow is in full extension (14).

Rest, ice, and compression will curb inflammatory response in acute injuries, although compression is less important than in foot and ankle injuries. Ice massage, refreezeable ice packs, or crushed ice works best for cryotherapy. Application for 10 to 20 minutes several times per day is indicated during the first 72 hours of acute injury. Pulsed ultrasound and transcutaneous electrical nerve stimulation (TENS) or interferential electrical stimulation may also be helpful in limiting inflammation and pain.

Postacute care for tennis elbow includes continuous ultrasound and/or phonophoresis and transverse friction massage to the ECRB. Transverse friction should be performed gently, transverse to the ECRB tendon, with lightly progressive increase in pressure as tolerated by the patient over 2 to 4 minutes. This procedure realigns collagen fiber to the direction of tensile stress, mobilizes scar tissue, and produces a temporary pressure paresthesia. Ice should always follow this type of massage. Myofascial trigger point therapy to flexor and extensor muscles is indicated by the presence of referred pain from the elbow to hand. Digital ischemic compression or spray and stretch therapy works very well. Postisometric relaxation techniques to stretch the wrist extensors are also effective.

A loss of joint play at the radiocapitellar or proximal radioulnar joint are common. However, other areas of joint play restriction may be noted in any direction in the elbow, between radius and ulna along the forearm, or at the wrist or shoulder. Gentle, high-velocity, low-amplitude manipulative therapy is essential in such cases and may require several applications to restore full accessory mobility. Soft tissue adhesions may also respond well to appropriate high-velocity manipulative procedures in an effort to break down resistance to the normal gliding movements between myofascial tissues.

Resistant and chronic cases may require a more aggressive manipulation, classically described by Mills (13). Mills reported that the primary indication for manipulation was loss of full elbow extension. He reported immediate cure rates of approximately 65% using this manipulation, with a 17% delayed cure rate. The procedure is performed with the forearm fully pronated and the elbow fully flexed. The elbow is then forced from flexion into full extension. A successful manipulation is accompanied by an easily audible crack. Wadsworth (69) reports that in more than 100 patients treated with Mills' manipulation for resistant cases of tennis elbow, most cases were resolved. Several patients had reduced pain for several months before resolution. Six patients required remanipulation. One required subsequent surgical release. Wadsworth performs this maneuver with the patient fully re-

laxed under general anesthesia. After manipulation, the patient is told to avoid strain on the area for 3 months.

The cracking sound accompanying Mills' manipulation is attributed to either the completion of a partial tear of the common extensor tendon (in effect, a closed lateral release) or the breakdown of adhesions that have formed at the common extensor origin. The latter explanation is favored, although simple articular cavitation may explain this phenomenon.

If aggressive manipulation fails in patients who have fully complied with instructions for appropriate cessation of athletic activity for 3 months, nerve conduction studies should be performed to confirm possible compression of the posterior interosseous nerve at the supinator muscle. The nerve is compressed where it delves distally into the supinator. Thirty percent of the population will have a well-defined arcade of Frohse (Fig. 12.17), which enhances the likelihood of compression neuropathy at this site. Surgery is rarely necessary.

Other conservative measures sometimes offered include corticosteroid injection and laser therapy. In a retrospective study, patients injected with a corticosteroid preparation showed higher short-term relief but also higher incidence of recurrence than patients treated conservatively without injection (71). Gallium-arsenide (Ga-As) and helium-neon (He-Ne) laser radiation were studied in a randomized controlled trial for the treatment of tennis elbow (72). The investigators concluded that laser treatment is no better than placebo in reducing tennis elbow pain. Furthermore, laser radiation designed for conserva-

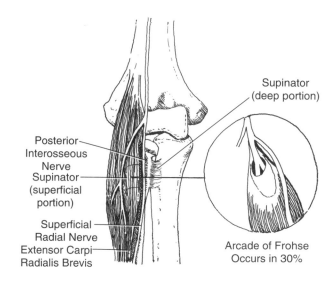

Figure 12.17. The arcade of Frohse at the supinator muscle.

tive clinical use had no effect on conduction velocity of sensory nerves, nor did it have a thermal effect on subcutaneous tissue. These modalities currently have no compelling supportive evidence for use in tennis elbow.

Clinical progress can be monitored by gently performing Cozen's test. Changes in strength and threshold to pain are noted. Early return to sports activity should be accompanied by a constrictive band placed several centimeters distal to the origin of the ECRB. This will prevent reinjury by reducing the magnitude of tensile loads at the site of initial injury. Strengthening exercises for the wrist extensors should be performed during the early stages of return to sports activity. Wrist rolling resistance exercises can be performed, elbows extended, using wrist or ankle weights suspended from 1-inch PVC pipe. The author has found this to be an inexpensive, effective means of forearm restrengthening. As strength increases, the patient should be weaned from the constrictive band.

Because tennis elbow is more common among those who have poor backhand technique, patients should be encouraged to receive instruction in this regard. Although epidemiologic studies have not shown a significant relationship between grip size and incidence of tennis elbow, it would still seem appropriate to have all patients with tennis elbow measured for grip size. The length of a line drawn along the radial border of the fourth finger from its tip to the proximal palmar crease should closely approximate the circumference of the grip. When the tennis racket is gripped properly, there should be approximately 0.5 inch between the tip of the longest finger and the thenar eminence. The common mistake is that grip sizes are too small. Overgrip can easily be added to remedy this. Racket head size does not correlate with the incidence of tennis elbow. Whereas rackets with larger heads absorb vibrations better than standard-size rackets, the oversize rackets offer a greater potential for producing torque injury from off-center hits. There seems to be no significant advantage or disadvantage in using larger rackets with respect to injury prevention. Excessive racket vibration has not been shown to cause tennis elbow (70).

Higher racket string tension requires that a greater amount of shock be absorbed by the arm. Players recuperating from tennis elbow should be advised to use low string tensions (28 to 32 lb) as they return to the courts.

The differential diagnosis of tennis elbow at the lateral epicondyle includes biceps tendinitis, periarthritis of the shoulder, carpal tunnel syndrome, cubital tunnel syndrome, medial epicondylitis, cervical radiculopathy, and other soft tissue lesions (69). Arthritis at the elbow is usually obvious and is associated with prior trauma or history of rheumatoid disease. Radiographs will define whether lateral elbow pain is related to arthritic or ectopic calcifications in the elbow.

Golfer's Elbow and Other Lesions

Medial epicondylitis has been termed golfer's elbow but is also one of the group of conditions referred to as pitcher's elbow and Little League elbow. We have discussed throwing injuries in detail earlier in this chapter. We now consider soft tissue injury of the common flexor tendon at the medial epicondyle, flexor-pronator tendons, and triceps insertion.

Medial epicondylitis, flexor-pronator tendinitis, and triceps tendinitis involve strain from overuse of the common flexor tendon, pronator teres tendon, and triceps tendon, respectively. The pathology involves microtearing of musculotendinous tissue with subsequent inflammatory response. As with lateral epicondylitis, pain is activity related, as revealed by clinical history.

In medial epicondylitis and flexor-pronator tendinitis, examination will reveal painful resisted wrist flexion and/or forearm pronation. Tenderness is localized to the medial epicondyle and proximal flexor-pronator tendons. In triceps tendinitis, pain is provoked by resisted elbow extension and is localized at the insertion of the triceps into the olecranon process.

Treatment of these conditions is generally the same as for lateral epicondylitis in the acute, postacute, and chronic stages. However, manipulative therapy has not been reported in the literature and would not appear to be appropriate other than for restoration of joint play, if lost. Mills' manipulation is not indicated for these conditions. Conservative modalities for pain control and inflammation (ice, pulsed ultrasound, electrical stimulation/TENS) are followed by soft tissue rehabilitation procedures (transverse friction massage, stretching, restrengthening) as the lesion progresses.

For medial epicondylitis and flexor-pronator tendinitis, wrist flexion and forearm pronation exercises are used in conjunction with a constrictive elbow cuff as the patient resumes participation in sports. As the patient gains strength, the cuff is set aside. Recurrence is prevented by continued stretching and restrengthening exercise on a periodic basis.

BURSAL INJURY

Olecranon Bursitis

Subcutaneous olecranon bursitis at the elbow can occur any time this area is subjected to repeated impact trauma or friction. Falls on the artificial turf in football, soccer, or baseball lead to a higher incidence because of the low pliability on the underlying surface of older turf. Bursitis may also result from repeated blows to the elbow in unpadded football linemen or, paradoxically, from repeated hyperextension at the elbow joint (i.e., in basketball) in older athletes. Application of ice with compression to the swollen area is usually all that is indicated in early stages. Ultrasound may accelerate resolution of the problem in subacute cases. If a distended bursa interferes with motion, aspiration may be considered. Excision of this bursa is seldom necessary (58), although this should be considered in chronic, nonresolving cases. Bursitis of the subtendinous olecranon bursa is rare in sports.

NERVE INJURIES

The ulnar, median, radial, and musculocutaneous nerves are vulnerable to direct and indirect trauma in athletic competition. Nerve injuries at the elbow are most often seen in throwing and racket sports, weight lifting, gymnastics, and contact sports.

Ulnar Nerve Disorders at the Elbow

The most common neurologic problem in the elbow region in athletes is compression of the ulnar nerve at the cubital tunnel (1). The ulnar nerve passes from the anterior compartment of the brachium into the posterior compartment by penetrating a thick fibrous raphe of the medial intermuscular septum (73). The ulnar nerve then passes through the arcade of Struthers, formed by a thickening of the deep investing fascia of the distal brachium, by the superficial muscular fibers of the medial head of the triceps, by the attachment of the internal brachial ligament, and by the medial intermuscular septum. This arcade is located 8 cm above the medial epicondyle and is present in 70% of anatomical specimens. The arcade of Struthers may be a source of ulnar nerve entrapment, especially as a result of tethering after ulnar nerve transposition anteriorly. Distally the ulnar nerve lies medial to the intermuscular septum, then passes posterior to the medial epicondyle into the cubital tunnel where it rests against the posterior portion of the ulnar collateral ligament.

The boundaries of the cubital tunnel are the ulnar collateral ligament anteriorly, the medial edge of the trochlea, and the medial epicondylar groove (74). The roof of the tunnel is formed by the triangular arcuate ligament that extends from the medial epicondyle to the medial border of the olecranon.

With elbow flexion, the arcuate ligament stretches approximately 5 mm for each 45° of flexion, thus narrowing the volume of the cubital tunnel with elbow flexion (Fig. 12.18) Furthermore, the ulnar nerve elongates an average of 4.7 mm during elbow flexion, and it has been noted that the medial head of the triceps can push the nerve 7 mm medially as the elbow flexes (75). Ulnar neuropathy at the elbow has four etiologies. First, traction injuries to the nerve can result from dynamic valgus forces at the elbow, as in pitching, or in static valgus deformity secondary to previous fracture or injury at the growth plate. Second, anatomical irregularities within the ulnar groove, such as arthritic spurs, can result in friction irritation and impingement of the nerve. Third, the ulnar nerve may subluxate due to trauma or a lax triangular arcuate ligament. Fourth, progressive compression of the ulnar nerve within the cubital tunnel may occur spontaneously, due to space-occupying lesions (e.g., granulomas, ganglions, neoplasms), after traumatic injuries (e.g., fracture, tethering lesions, epiphyseal injuries), or in metabolic conditions such as diabetes, alcoholism, or advancing malignancy. Spontaneous

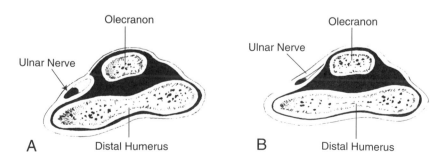

Figure 12.18. Cross-section through the elbow at the cubital tunnel. **A.** Elbow extension. **B.** Elbow flexion. Note compression of the tunnel with flexion.

compression within the cubital tunnel is known as cubital tunnel syndrome.

The athlete involved in overhand activities (e.g., pitching, tennis, and javelin) is particularly prone to ulnar nerve traction and compression lesions. Normally the ulnar nerve is free to move in its groove longitudinally and medially. Repeated stress or injury may lead to inflammation, adhesions, and restriction of ulnar nerve mobility within the cubital tunnel. Subsequent fibrosis can compromise the vasa nervosum—the vascular supply to the nerve.

The symptoms of ulnar neuritis at the elbow initially consist of intermittent dysesthesias in the fourth and fifth digits. Often the first symptom in the throwing athlete will be medial joint line pain at the elbow, with pain and paresthesias along the ulnar aspect of the forearm to the hand as inflammation progresses. Clumsiness or heaviness of the hand and fingers, especially during throwing, may also be reported. When ulnar nerve subluxation is present, there may be a sensation of painful snapping behind the medial epicondyle during flexion and extension of the elbow.

Clinical examination reveals tenderness along the course of the ulnar nerve in the cubital tunnel, in its passage into the flexor carpi ulnaris, and sometimes at the arcade of Struthers. The elbow flexion test (75) is performed by having the patient sit for 3 minutes with both elbows fully flexed with full extension of the wrist and supination of the forearms. This provides both traction and compression to the ulnar nerve. When ulnar neuritis is present for any reason (including cubital tunnel syndrome), the test will reproduce pain, numbness, and tingling. Tinel's sign will often be present at the cubital tunnel or more distally where the nerve enters the flexor muscle mass. Neurologic examination usually does not reveal sensory deficits, and motor weakness and intrinsic atrophy are hard to detect in well-developed athletes.

"Double crush" syndrome occurs when a nerve is compressed or compromised at two or more separable points along its course (76–78). The most common upper extremity double crush association is seen with cervical spondylosis and carpal tunnel syndrome. However, double crush phenomena involving the ulnar nerve would include cervical disc protrusion or thoracic outlet compression in combination with compression at the cubital tunnel, or compression at the cubital tunnel in conjunction with compression of the distal portion of the ulnar nerve at the level of Guyon's canal. Poor treatment outcome in ulnar neuropathy may be the result of failure to consider the possibility of additional sites of entrapment in a double crush syndrome.

Many transient episodes of ulnar neuritis in the athlete can be treated conservatively. Accurate electrodiagnostic studies are essential in outlining a treatment plan. Radiographs or CT scans may show degenerative changes that compromise the cubital tunnel. The goal of treatment is to decrease pressure and irritation around the nerve. Rest, immobilization, ultrasound, and concomitant myofascial release therapy can be used. Ultrasound at the cubital tunnel can be performed with the elbow immersed in water to optimize penetration and avoid the bony prominences in the area. Activities that require repetitive elbow flexion should be avoided. Some patients sleep with elbows at acutely flexed angles. Elbow braces that prevent flexion from occurring may be effective for patients who report nocturnal aggravation of symptoms.

Muscle fibrillation or conduction slowing on electrodiagnostic examination indicates that a prolonged course of conservative therapy should not be undertaken in the absence of significant clinical progress. Surgical transfer of the ulnar nerve is recommended if conservative therapy fails or when electromyographic (EMG) changes are profoundly positive (1). A comprehensive review of the literature (79) used a staging system to evaluate operative and nonoperative treatment results for ulnar nerve entrapment in more than 2000 patients reported in 50 papers from 1898 through 1988. This staging system appears in Figure 12.19. This re-

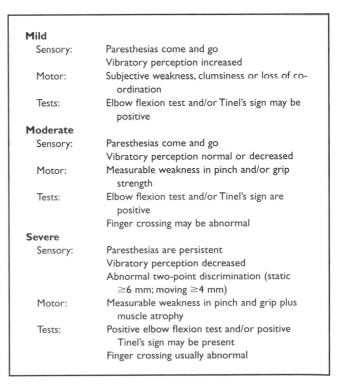

Mild
Sensory:	Paresthesias come and go
	Vibratory perception increased
Motor:	Subjective weakness, clumsiness or loss of coordination
Tests:	Elbow flexion test and/or Tinel's sign may be positive

Moderate
Sensory:	Paresthesias come and go
	Vibratory perception normal or decreased
Motor:	Measurable weakness in pinch and/or grip strength
Tests:	Elbow flexion test and/or Tinel's sign are positive
	Finger crossing may be abnormal

Severe
Sensory:	Paresthesias are persistent
	Vibratory perception decreased
	Abnormal two-point discrimination (static ≥6 mm; moving ≥4 mm)
Motor:	Measurable weakness in pinch and grip plus muscle atrophy
Tests:	Positive elbow flexion test and/or positive Tinel's sign may be present
	Finger crossing usually abnormal

Figure 12.19. Staging of ulnar nerve compression at the elbow.

view indicated that 50% of patients in the mild category of compression did well with nonoperative treatment. The remainder of these, and all moderate and severe cases, required surgical intervention. This staging system may be useful to the conservative practitioner in determining those athletes who would best benefit from conservative versus operative management.

Children usually suffer ulnar neuropathy in conjunction with posterior dislocation and with medial epicondylar fracture. The onset of neurologic symptoms after fracture may range from 7 days to 40 years; hence (with delayed onset over years) the diagnostic term "tardy ulnar nerve palsy" (80). Surgical outcomes are best with early intervention.

Median Nerve Compression

Median nerve compression at the elbow is rare in athletes (1). Two compressive neuropathies near the elbow involve the median nerve: the pronator syndrome and the anterior interosseous syndrome.

Pronator syndrome involves pain in the volar aspect of the forearms with numbness and paresthesias in all or part of the median nerve distribution of the hand. Symptoms are aggravated by exertion and are relieved by rest. Sensory disturbances are seldom nocturnal, and patients rarely report awakening with paresthesias of the hands. This differentiates pronator syndrome from median nerve compression more distally, at the carpal tunnel. In all cases of pronator syndrome, Phalen's test at the wrist will be negative unless there is concomitant entrapment at the carpal tunnel.

The most frequent site of compression of the median nerve in pronator syndrome is at the pronator teres muscle. In such instances, resisted forearm pronation with the elbow in flexion will reproduce the chief complaint. During resisted testing, the wrist and fingers must be relaxed in the flexed position so that the flexor digitorum superficialis (FDS) is relaxed. This muscle must be relaxed to differentiate compression at the FDS versus the pronator teres muscle. The second most frequent site of median nerve compression is at the FDS.

When compression occurs at the FDS, resisted flexion of this tendon to the middle finger will increase the familiar pain of chief complaint. The site of compression is the proximal margin of the muscle where the nerve sometimes passes deep to a fibrous arch.

A third site of median nerve compression in pronator syndrome is beneath the bicipital apo-

neurosis. In this case, resisted elbow flexion and forearm supination will increase symptoms.

Finally, median nerve compression can result from trauma and compression at a structure known as the supracondylar process. This structure is present in an estimated 1% to 3% of humans. With trauma to this area with resultant swelling, pressure to the median nerve can result. The symptoms and signs of high median nerve compression will develop. The key to examination is the palpation of a bone mass located 5 to 7 cm proximal to the medial epicondyle on the medial border of the brachialis muscle. The mass will be tender, and percussion over it may produce distal paresthesias. Resisted flexion, with the elbow positioned in acute flexion at between 120° and 135°, will reproduce pain. Compression of the median nerve is least common at the supracondylar process. However, when present, this lesion can be treated conservatively with rest, elevation, and immobilization of the elbow. Symptoms should resolve as swelling subsides. If symptoms persist, operative excision of the supracondylar process is indicated.

Resisted muscle tests in the diagnosis of pronator syndrome are summarized in Figure 12.20. Conservative measures such as pulsed ultrasound and heat may be attempted. However, in more severe cases, operative release at the site of compression has been recommended (81).

Anterior interosseous syndrome has traditionally been thought to represent compression of the anterior interosseous nerve, usually due to fibrous bands located deep to the ulnar head of the pronator teres muscle or due to a tendinous origin of the flexor superficialis. As a pure motor branch of the median nerve, anterior interosseous nerve compression is not typically associated with sensory deficits, although a vague feeling of discomfort may be reported in the proximal forearm. Weakness is confined to three muscles: the flexor pollicis longus, flexor digitorum profundus to the index (and sometimes the long) finger, and the pronator quadratus.

Miller-Breslow et al. (82) reported eight cases of anterior interosseous syndrome treated by observation alone. All patients showed signs of recovery in 6 months, with full recovery in 1 year. The authors believed that anterior interosseous syndrome represented a neuritis rather than a compression neuropathy because several of the cases involved additional sensory losses in other nerves, and four cases presented with shoulder pain initially.

The diagnostic hallmark on clinical examination is a loss of the ability to pinch the thumb and index fingers together due to thumb and first finger weakness. However, this finding is not always present. Careful examination will, however, reveal weakness of the three muscles noted above. Testing the pronator quadratus involves resisted forearm pronation with the elbow in complete flexion.

EMG of the forearm muscles should be carried out in all suspected cases of neuropathy and often confirms the diagnosis. However, due to the difficulties of needle placement, a negative EMG

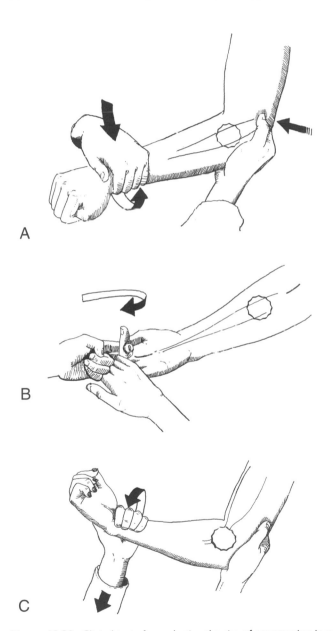

A

B

C

Figure 12.20. Clinical tests for evaluating the site of compression in a pronator syndrome. **Top.** Compression at the pronator teres muscle. Pain will be reproduced by resisted forearm pronation and extension of the elbow. **Middle.** Compression at the flexor superficialis arch. Pain will be reproduced by resisted flexion of the flexor superficialis tendon to the middle finger. **Bottom.** Compression at the bicipital aponeurosis. Pain will be reproduced by resisted flexion at the elbow and supination of the forearm.

does not exclude the diagnosis of anterior interosseous syndrome. Differential diagnosis includes tendon rupture or stenosing tenosynovitis of one of the flexor tendon sheaths.

Initial treatment should be conservative, consisting of 6 to 8 weeks of rest. The treatment goal is to reduce nerve compression and/or inflammation. Decongestion of the area may be facilitated by ultrasound. Gentle massage and electrical stimulation may help to maintain muscle condition and facilitate healing. If conservative therapy fails to restore motor strength, operative decompression may be necessary. However, at least one group of investigators advises that the disorder be followed for at least 6 months before a decision regarding surgery is made (82).

Radial Nerve Compression

Acute radial nerve compression follows displaced fractures of the shaft of the humerus, improper use of axillary crutches, and deep intramuscular injections into the posterior or lateral aspects of the brachium. Acute radial nerve compression is secondary to tourniquet compression, either after surgery or in drug addicts. Also, strenuous activities that require repeated elbow extension against resistance may lead to an acute compressive neuropathy of the radial nerve.

In acute compression, weakness or even total paralysis (wristdrop) of the wrist and digital extensors occurs. Dorsal sensory loss at the hand may also be present. In exercise-related cases, the site of compression is in the region of the lateral intermuscular septum, which the nerve pierces as it enters the anterior arm 10 cm proximal to the lateral epicondyle. Direct palpation or percussion of this area will increase symptoms. Treatment of acute compression is rest and cessation of all strenuous activities. Most cases resolve within several weeks. Surgical decompression is recommended for recurrent episodes of weakness after strenuous exercise.

Posterior interosseous syndrome develops in the following manner. After the radial nerve pierces the lateral intermuscular septum, it enters the anterior aspect of the arm where it innervates the brachioradialis and extensor carpi radialis longus muscles. At or a few centimeters below the elbow, the nerve bifurcates into its sensory and motor components. The motor component is the posterior interosseous nerve, which passes between the two heads of the supinator muscle. At the superficial head of the supinator, a fibrous semicircular arch provides passage for the nerve. In 30% of anatomical specimens, the arch remains fibrous throughout its length medially and is referred to as the arcade of Frohse (Fig. 12.17) (83). The arcade is absent in fetuses and develops as a response to rotational movements of the forearm. Due to its fibrous nature, the arcade of Frohse serves as an unyielding restraint, limiting the space occupied by the posterior interosseous nerve when injury produces swelling in the area.

The posterior interosseous nerve is purely motor, producing a typical attitude of the hand at the time of clinical presentation. Ulnar deviation of the wrist is compromised or impossible due to weakness or paralysis of the extensor carpi ulnaris muscle. The extensor carpi radialis longus is never affected, and the brevis is often spared due to its more proximal innervation. Paralysis of the digital extensors prevents the ability to extend the fingers or thumb. However, paralysis may be incomplete, involving only one or two digits. Electrodiagnostic studies will usually confirm the diagnosis of compressive neuropathy.

Treatment depends on the length of time paresis and paralysis have been present. If there is no improvement after 6 to 8 weeks of conservative therapy, surgery is necessary to prevent advancing nerve degeneration and muscle atrophy. Conservative therapy, as with anterior interosseous syndrome, is directed toward reducing nerve irritation. If swelling is present, ice and pulsed ultrasound are appropriate. Continuous ultrasound, gentle massage, and electrical stimulation may be beneficial, and the patient must curtail all activities that aggravate the symptoms. Posterior interosseous syndrome must be considered in the differential diagnosis of tennis players whose lateral elbow pain is unresponsive to conservative therapy.

Radial tunnel syndrome is characterized by chronic lateral elbow pain with paresthesias and, in some cases, weakness. Roles and Maudsley (14) first coined the term radial tunnel syndrome in their report of a study of patients with chronic tennis elbow. The syndrome differs from posterior interosseous syndrome, which produces purely motor deficits without pain. In radial tunnel syndrome there are several different complaints, including pain, paresthesias, and muscular weakness (in some cases).

The radial tunnel is bounded medially by the brachialis muscle, anterolaterally by the brachioradialis, and more distally by the extensor carpi radialis longus (14, 81). The tunnel is approximately 5 cm long. It begins at the level of the capitellum, which forms its posterior wall, and proceeds distally to the end of the supinator muscle. The radial tunnel includes the ar-

---

1. At fibrous bands at the proximal end of the radial tunnel
2. At a sharp tendinous margin along the ECRB muscle
3. At a "fan" of radial recurrent vessels, which become dilated during exercise
4. At the arcade of Frohse
5. At a fibrous band at the distal edge of the supinator muscle.

Figure 12.21. Sites of radial nerve compression in radial tunnel syndrome.

cade of Frohse. There are five sites of potential compression in radial tunnel syndrome, listed in Figure 12.21.

Examination must carefully localize the site and quality of pain. Pain overlying the lateral epicondyle or radial head that is described as dull or deep (rather than sharp or knife-like) is more likely to represent pain from radial tunnel syndrome. To differentiate radial tunnel syndrome from lateral epicondylitis, the most useful test is resisted forearm supination. With the patient's elbow fully flexed and the forearm fully pronated, the patient is asked to supinate against resistance. If the supinator muscle is responsible for abnormal pressure on the nerve, this test will worsen neurogenic symptoms. Extension of the middle finger against resistance (Maudsley's test) may also reproduce familiar symptoms but is positive less often. Electrodiagnostic tests should be ordered, with particular attention to nerve conduction studies. In lieu of definitive electrodiagnostic test results, the diagnosis must be based on the patient's history and clinical findings.

Conservative treatments are most often ineffective in treating radial tunnel syndrome. In fact, it is the failure of response to conservative therapy (for a presumptive diagnosis of tennis elbow) that often alerts the clinician to the possibility of radial tunnel syndrome. Surgical decompression of the radial tunnel and arcade of Frohse successfully alleviates symptoms. The elbow is splinted for 1 week after surgery. Postsurgical rehabilitation usually lasts several months before normal muscle tone and endurance are restored for the resumption of full activities.

MYOFASCIAL/REFERRED PAIN SYNDROMES

Myofascial syndromes may coexist with or mimic radiculopathy and peripheral neuropathy (84). As an example, myofascial trigger points in the infraspinatus, subscapularis, or teres major may masquerade as—and be misdiagnosed as—ulnar neuropathy or C8 radiculopathy. Scalene and pectoralis trigger points can mimic C7 radiculopathy or radial tunnel syndrome. Even when neurologic compromise is present, active myofascial trigger points must not be left untreated. If effective conservative or surgical intervention is provided when active trigger points are left untreated, a less than optimal clinical outcome may be realized. This is because myofascial trigger points can remain even after elimination of the primary, inciting irritation (84). Therefore, the conservative sports physician must always include palpation for myofascial trigger points in the clinical examination.

Treatment of trigger points that affect the elbow and forearm should consist of digital ischemic compression and/or spray and stretch techniques. Moist hot packs are applied in conjunction with stretching techniques. Home stretching exercises are essential and should be performed at least 3 to 5 times daily. Self-application of ischemic compression may also be taught, if appropriate.

CUTS AND SCRAPES TO THE ELBOW

Although most cuts and scrapes to the elbow may appear minor, a significant disruption of deeper structures is occasionally present. This can happen as a result of falling on an asphalt track, running into a fence in the outfield, or being swiped by a cleat in almost any field sport.

Abrasions confined to the skin and subcutaneous tissue should be cleansed with mild soap and/or antibiotic solution, then inspected for foreign bodies. Gravel, asphalt, or other debris can be visible after healing and can result in skin discoloration ("traumatic tattoo") at the wound site. Debridement of abrasions is best accomplished with a brush. Accordingly, local anesthesia may be necessary in severe cases to minimize pain with cleansing. Devitalized tissue is simultaneously removed with this process.

Lacerations are first debrided using forceps, and devitalized tissue is removed with a scalpel or scissors. Delayed closure of lacerations over 8 hours increases the risk of infection (85). High-pressure irrigation of the laceration removes minute foreign bodies and minimizes the chance of infection. A rubber-bulb syringe can be used for this purpose. Normal saline is an adequate lavage solution. Closure of the laceration should be performed carefully, sparing dermal insult if possible. Lacerations into the dermis will require the use of absorbable intradermal suture to minimize the deposition of collagen in the scar during the healing phase.

Injury to underlying tendon, muscle, and nerve as well as vascular damage must be considered in cases of deeper lacerations. Tetanus

prophylaxis is important to consider with any wound. Follow-up wound care is directed at maintaining a clean environment for healing. Prolonged splinting of the elbow is rarely necessary, although temporary immobilization may be needed to prevent dehiscence early in recovery.

THE WRIST AND HAND

Hand and wrist injuries comprise approximately one fourth of all general athletic injuries (86). The high prevalence of hand and wrist injuries relates to the requirement of hand or wrist involvement in almost all sports. Figure 12.22 lists the prevalence of hand injuries in various sporting events.

Patterns of hand and wrist injury are usually characteristic to specific types of sports. As an example, hamate fractures are particular risks in racket or stick sports such as golf, tennis, and baseball (63). Metacarpal fractures are seen in sports in which the hand is used to strike, such as boxing and karate. Vascular injuries are most common in ball sports in which the hand is used to decelerate the ball from high velocity, e.g., baseball and handball. Compression neuropathy is usually encountered in athletes who are required to contact other hard surfaces continuously or repetitively (e.g., compression of the digital nerve in bowler's thumb and ulnar nerve compression in cyclists.)

In many cases injury is unavoidable due to the nature of hand involvement in various sports. However, in some cases injury might be prevented by the development and use of more protective gear, better training techniques, or a more efficient interface between athlete and sporting devices.

Clinically Relevant Anatomy of the Wrist and Hand

Due to its complexity, the relevant anatomy of the wrist and hand is discussed briefly in this chapter. The carpus, or wrist, is the most complex joint in the body owing to its unique arrangement

Sport	Percentage	Sport	Percentage
Handball	30	Boxing	31
Volleyball	23	Judo	10
Basketball	19	Skiing	16
Soccer	10	Ice Hockey	5
Gymnastics	17		

Figure 12.22. Relative frequency of hand injuries compared to total injuries. (Reprinted with permission from Amadio PC. Epidemiology of hand and wrist injuries in sports. Hand Clin 1990;6:379–381.)

and functions. It is formed by the articulations between the distal end of the radius and two rows of carpal bones, proximal and distal. The proximal row of carpals, from lateral to medial, consists of the scaphoid (or carpal navicular), lunate, triquetrum (triangular), and pea-shaped pisiform. The pisiform is a sesamoid bone within the tendon of the flexor carpi ulnaris and is easily palpable as an anatomical landmark. The distal row of carpals contains the trapezium and trapezoid laterally, the capitate, and the hamate medially. The hook of the hamate, or hamulus, can be palpated distolaterally to the pisiform near the base of the fourth and fifth metacarpals. The capitate, largest of the carpals, articulates with seven other bones and serves as a central attachment from which most of the intercarpal ligaments radiate. With the exception of the pisiform, there are no insertions of forearm muscles into the carpus. As a result, wrist movements are the product of muscle contractions whose tendons cross the joint completely.

The distal radius and the articular disc of the distal radioulnar joint form a concavity for articulation with the convex surfaces of the scaphoid, lunate, and triquetrum. This is known as the radiocarpal joint. The large convex articular surface formed by the unified proximal row of carpals allows for significant movements in flexion, extension, adduction, abduction, and circumduction. The fibrous joint capsule enclosing the radiocarpal joint attaches proximally to the radius and ulna and distally to the proximal row of carpals. The synovial capsule within presents numerous folds, especially at the dorsal aspect. The radiocarpal joint cavity does not communicate with the midcarpal joint.

Much of the apparent movement at the radiocarpal joint actually occurs at the midcarpal joint, the articulation between the proximal and distal rows. Each row acts as a unit in producing flexion, extension, adduction, and abduction of the wrist. The articulations of the midcarpal joint share a common joint space and synovial lining.

The ulnomeniscotriquetral joint is the articulation joining the ulna, articular disc, and triquetrum. This joint has no capsule and no separate synovial cavity, but is considered a joint due to its contribution to joint gliding in supination and pronation of the forearm. This region contains the triangular fibrocartilage complex (TFCC). The TFCC is a cartilaginous, ligamentous structure interposed between the ulna and the ulnar carpus that arises from the lunate fossa of the radius and inserts into the distal ulnar styloid base, ulnar carpal bones (triquetrum and hamate), and base of the fifth metacarpal. It incorporates the

dorsal and volar radioulnar ligaments and the ulnar collateral ligament. These are anatomically poorly defined structures. The TFCC also incorporates the well-defined articular disc and extensor carpi ulnaris sheath (Fig. 12.23). The peripheral ligamentous portion of this structure is highly vascularized, whereas the triangular fibrocartilage itself is relatively avascular. The TFCC functions as a cushion for the ulnar carpus, carrying approximately 20% of the axial load of the forearm in cadavers (87). If excised, the load borne by the ulnar carpus during axial loading is reduced to 6%. The TFCC contributes significantly to proximal wrist stability as an extension of the radiocarpal articulation and also stabilizes the ulnar carpus. When it is injured, radioulnar and radiocarpal stability are often compromised.

The carpometacarpal joint is a combination of articulations between the medial four metacarpals and the distal row of carpals. This distal row, together with the second and third metacarpal rays, can be regarded as a central fixed unit in the hand, around which the thumb rotates in a large arc on the radial side and the ring and little finger metacarpals rotate to a lesser degree on the ulnar side (88). These bones establish the functional transverse and longitudinal arches of the gently cupped hand. The joint capsule defines a separate joint cavity from the rest of the carpus.

The trapeziometacarpal joint is a true saddle joint. Its surfaces allow a wide range of motion for the thumb, including flexion, extension, abduction, adduction, and combinations of these that allow for thumb opposition and circumduction.

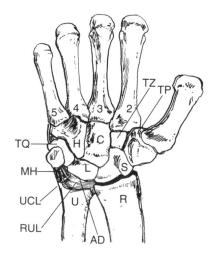

Figure 12.23. The component parts of the triangular fibrocartilage complex are fourfold: (1) articular disc (AD); (2) meniscus homolog (MH); (3) ulnar collateral ligament (UCL); and (4) dorsal and palmar radioulnar ligaments (RUL). H: hamate; C: capitate; TZ: trapezoid; TP: trapezium; S: scaphoid; L: lunate; TQ: triquetrum; R: radius,; U: ulna. (Reprinted with permission from Palmer AK, Werner FW. J Hand Surg 1981;6:153.)

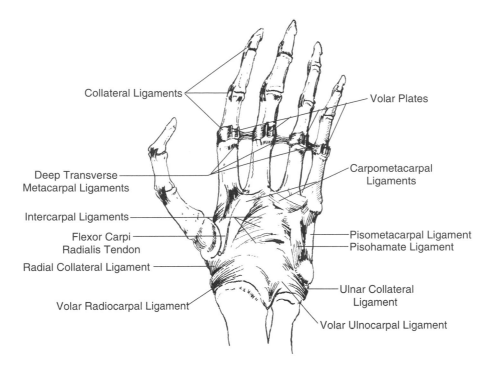

Figure 12.24. Volar anatomy of the wrist and hand. Note the volar plates.

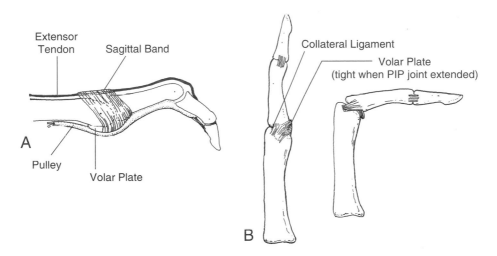

Figure 12.25. A. Proximally, the volar plate is loosely attached to the metacarpal head to allow for hyperextension at the metacarpophalangeal joint. **B.** The volar plate extends over the metacarpal head in a visor-like fashion. If injured and subsequently immobilized in flexion, adhesions can form between the volar plate and the distal volar surface of the metacarpal, restricting extension at the metacarpophalangeal joint.

The five metacarpals in articulation with the proximal phalanges form the MPJ. MPJ 2 through 5 have joint capsules that are reinforced dorsally by the dorsal hood apparatus and volarly by the volar plates. The volar plates, or palmar ligaments (Fig. 12.24), are fibrocartilaginous structures whose distal, cartilaginous portions are firmly fixed to the proximal phalanges. The proximal portions of these structures are membranous and loosely attached to the metacarpal heads via the joint capsule, permitting hyperextension at the MPJ (Fig. 12.25A). They provide an additional confining structure for synovial fluid and stabilization against dorsal dislocation during MPJ hyperextension. The volar plates may be injured by trauma during sports. Because each plate extends proximally in a visor-like fashion over the metacarpal head during flexion (Fig. 12.25B), adhesions may form between the membranous surfaces if the joint is immobilized in flexion. Similar plates are noted at the proximal and distal interphalangeal (DIP) joints, although at the PIP joint there is a bony attachment that provides resistance against hyperextension. The thumb MPJ is similar to the other MPJ arthrokinematically, but it does not contain a volar plate.

The PIP joints, DIP joints, and thumb interphalangeal joint are bicondylar, uniplanar joints. The collateral ligaments of these joints are concentrically placed and are of equal length. They are maximally taut throughout the range of motion (89).

Movements of the hand are accomplished by a combination of intrinsic and extrinsic musculature. These muscles are innervated by the radial, median, and ulnar nerves. It is helpful to consider the muscles acting on the wrist and hand as distinct layers. Three volar and two dorsal layers are presented in Figure 12.26 (89).

All extrinsic volar tendons pass through the carpal tunnel with the exception of two: the flexor carpi ulnaris, whose tendon attaches to the pisiform, and the palmaris longus tendon, which passes superficial to the flexor retinaculum. The flexor retinaculum is often described as the volar carpal ligament and transverse carpal (or transverse retinacular) ligament. The palmaris longus tendon is an important anatomical landmark. Although absent on one or both sides in 13% of individuals, when present this tendon can easily be seen as it bisects the distal skin crease, exactly at the middle of the wrist. Just deep and lateral to this tendon lies the median nerve, beneath the flexor retinaculum.

The extrinsic dorsal tendons pass through six synovial sheaths at the wrist, shown in Figure 12.27. Figure 12.27 also shows how Lister's tubercle is used to mechanical advantage by the extensor pollicis longus tendon, which takes a 45° turn at this tubercle to enter the dorsal aspect of the thumb. The lateral-most compartment contains

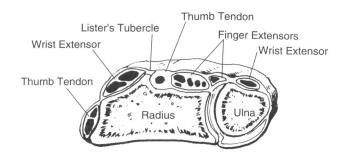

Figure 12.27. The six extensor tendon sheaths at the dorsum of the wrist.

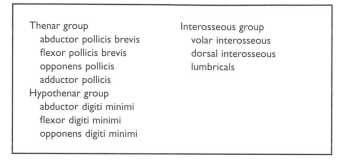

Thenar group	Interosseous group
abductor pollicis brevis	volar interosseous
flexor pollicis brevis	dorsal interosseous
opponens pollicis	lumbricals
adductor pollicis	
Hypothenar group	
abductor digiti minimi	
flexor digiti minimi	
opponens digiti minimi	

Figure 12.28. The intrinsic muscles of the hand.

the abductor pollicis longus and extensor pollicis brevis tendons. Inflammation and tenosynovitis involving this synovial sheath from overuse or disease is termed deQuervain's syndrome. A similar overuse syndrome is sometimes noted in the sheath containing the extensor pollicis longus tendon. The extensors are innervated by the posterior interosseous nerve, a terminal branch of the radial nerve.

The intrinsic hand muscles consist of the thenar muscle group, hypothenar muscle group, and interosseous muscles (Fig. 12.28). In general, the medial intrinsic musculature derives its innervation from the ulnar nerve, and the lateral intrinsic musculature derives its innervation from the median nerve.

Blood is carried to the wrist and hand by the radial and ulnar arteries and their branches. The radial artery can be palpated dorsolaterally at the floor of the anatomical snuffbox formed by the scaphoid and trapezium. The ulnar artery enters the hand as part of the "ulnar trio." This trio consists of the ulnar artery, ulnar nerve, and flexor carpi ulnaris. The artery and nerve pass through the canal of Guyon under the pisohamate ligament.

The blood supply to the hand consists of two vascular arches: the superficial volar arch born primarily by the ulnar artery (with frequent attachment on the radial aspect to the superficial branch of the radial artery) and the deep volar

Volar musculature	Dorsal musculature
Superficial Layer	*Superficial Layer*
Pronator teres	Brachioradialis
Flexor carpi radialis	Extensor carpi radialis
Palmaris longus	longus
Flexor carpi ulnaris	Extensor carpi radialis
Middle Layer	brevis
Flexor digitorum	Extensor digitorum
superficialis	communis
Deep Layer	Extensor digiti minimi
Flexor digitorum	Extensor carpi ulnaris
profundus	*Deep*
Flexor pollicis longus	Supinator
Pronator quadratus	Abductor pollicis longus
	Extensor pollicis brevis
	Extensor pollicis longus
	Extensor indicis

Figure 12.26. Muscle layers of the wrist and hand.

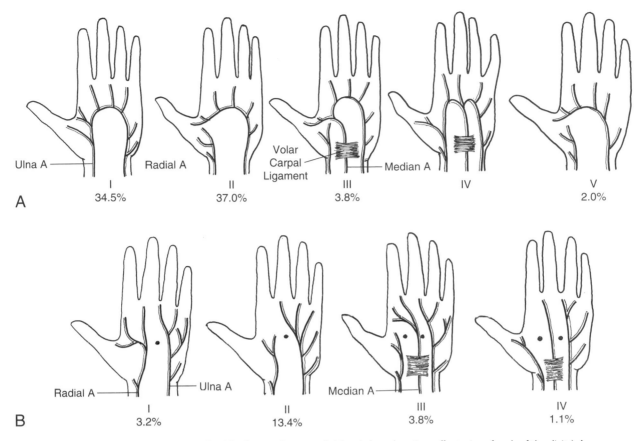

Figure 12.29. **A.** Five variations (I to V) of a complete superficial arch (one that gives off arteries of each of the digits). Approximately 80% of hands have a complete arch. **B.** (I to IV) Areas of circulatory discontinuity. Approximately 20% of hands have incomplete superficial arches. (Reprinted with permission from Rettig AC. Neurovascular injuries in the wrists and hands of athletes. Clin Sports Med 1990;9:389–417.)

arch supplied mainly by the primary branch of the radial artery. The ulnar artery forms the main source of the superficial volar arch and is usually the most important contributor to digital circulation. Approximately 80% of hands have a complete superficial volar arch, the remainder having one of four variations of arterial supply involving terminal branching of the radial, ulnar, and sometimes median arteries (Fig. 12.29A and B).

Biomechanics of the Wrist and Hand

The reader is encouraged to study the following biomechanical concepts carefully. They are difficult to grasp in just one reading. However, a good understanding will contribute significantly to the clinical evaluation of wrist motion and to an understanding of intercalated segmental instabilities discussed later in this chapter.

RADIOCARPAL AND MIDCARPAL JOINTS

Clinically relevant ligaments of the wrist are illustrated in Figures 12.30, 12.31, and 12.32. The volar radiocarpal ligamentous complex is com-

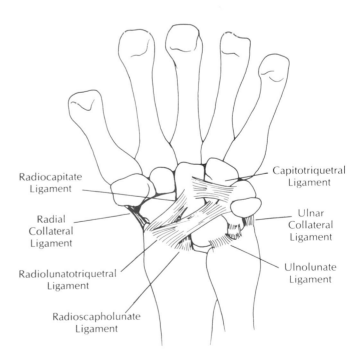

Figure 12.30. Volar intracapsular ligaments of the wrist. (From Barry MS, Kettner NW, Pierre-Jerome C. Carpal instability: pathomechanics and contemporary imaging. Chiro Sports Med 1991;5:38–44.)

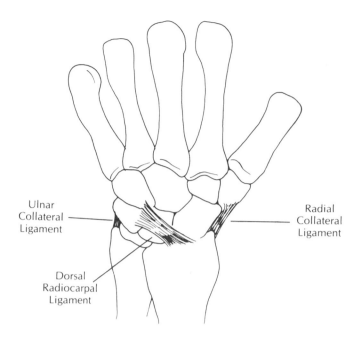

Figure 12.31. Dorsal extrinsic ligaments of the wrist. (From Barry MS, Kettner NW, Pierre-Jerome C. Carpal instability: pathomechanics and contemporary imaging. Chiro Sports Med 1991;5:38–44.)

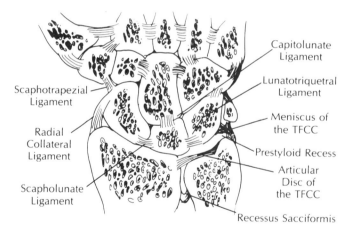

Figure 12.32. Intrinsic ligaments of the wrist. (From Barry MS, Kettner NW, Pierre-Jerome C. Carpal instability: pathomechanics and contemporary imaging. Chiro Sports Med 1991;5:38–44.)

posed of three strong intracapsular ligaments: radiocapitate, radiotriquetral (radiolunatotriquetral), and radioscaphoid (radioscapholunate). The radiocapitate ligament is at maximal tension on wrist extension with ulnar deviation. The radiotriquetral ligament is the largest ligament of the wrist and is placed in tension with wrist extension. These two ligaments separate on wrist extension, creating what is known as the space of Poirier. This interligamentous space is an area of potential volar weakness with axial loads imposed on the extended wrist, as in gymnastic handsprings. The radiotriquetral ligament extends

from the volar aspect of the radius across the lunate, where it sends slips of tissue to insert on the triquetrum—hence its alternative designation, the radiolunatotriquetral ligament. The third volar radiocarpal ligament, the radioscaphoid ligament, is a large, distinct ligament arising from the volar tip of the distal radius to insert into the proximal volar aspect of the scapholunate joint.

The scapholunate ligament is an interosseous structure that is triangular in cross section. The thickest ligamentous attachments are proximal and dorsal, so that more motion occurs between the scaphoid and the lunate at the volar side of the joint. According to Mayfield (90), most intercarpal injuries begin at the scapholunate joint. The scapholunate ligament is more often overstretched than torn. In a study of wrist ligament failure, the scapholunate ligament was found to sustain the largest degree of strain or elongation before failure under tension (91). This finding suggests that partial ligament failure (e.g., tensile strength loss and elongation or overstretching) in association with a grossly intact ligament can be associated with carpal instability. Hence, the scapholunate interosseous ligament must be considered an important structure whose (sometimes insidious) injury is the first step in a progression of perilunar instability.

The dorsal radiocarpal ligament extends from the dorsal radius to the triquetrum, serving to maintain apposition of the lunate to the distal radius (92).

Flexion/Extension Movement

The proximal carpal row is stabilized to the distal forearm by five ligaments; the distal carpal row is stabilized by only one, the radiocapitate ligament. Dorsiflexion (e.g., wrist extension) is initiated at the midcarpal articulation owing to the insertion of wrist extensors to the base of the metacarpals dorsally. However, although initiated at the midcarpal joint, most wrist extension appears to take place at the radiocarpal joint due to the locking of proximal and distal carpal rows by the taut radiocapitate ligament (93). As the volar radiocarpal ligaments become taut with wrist extension, a sling is created across the scaphoid waist, dorsiflexing the scaph-oid and capitate as a unit. The scapholunate interosseous ligament transfers movement to the lunate, which dorsiflexes as well. Hence, in the normal, uninjured wrist, the lunate and the capitate share the same longitudinal axis (e.g., they are coaxial) from the neutral position through extension of the wrist due to the integrity of the scapholunate interosseous ligament (Fig. 12.25A). The volar radiocapitate ligament acts as a sling to provide further resistance preventing palmar flexion of the lunate during wrist extension.

As palmar flexion occurs from the neutral position, the dorsal carpal ligament becomes taut, initiating migration of the triquetrum along the slope of the hamate, toward the radius. This movement can be appreciated by anterior-posterior radiographs of the wrist in neutral and in full flexion. Most wrist flexion takes place at the midcarpal articulation (e.g., between proximal and distal rows) because flexion of the proximal row is limited by a taut dorsal ligament (93).

Ulnar/Radial Deviation

The biomechanics of the carpus in the frontal plane are perhaps the most complex set of arthrokinematic movements anywhere in the body, even when compared with the foot. From a biomechanical standpoint, the wrist can be divided into radial and ulnar longitudinal carpal columns. The ulnar column is the "control column": the architecture of the ulnar column is such that movement here initiates all subsequent carpal movements. The majority of force transmission occurs through the radial column.

The ulnar column contains what Weber (93) describes as a "control surface," that is, the articulation whose movement dictates all subsequent carpal kinematics. This surface is the triquetrohamate articulation. Movement between the triquetrum and hamate give rise, through articular facet orientation and ligamentous tensions, to the primary movements in all other carpals except the trapezium and trapezoid (Fig. 12.33). These latter two bones remain fairly well in place as the scaphoid glides along their stationary articulating surfaces. Because the trapezium and trapezoid articulate with the base of the thumb and because they are relatively stationary, the thumb is able to maintain mechanical advantage for movement in both radial and ulnar deviation of the wrist.

The configuration of the dorsal to volar, oblique, sloping articular surface of the hamate gives rise to biplanar motion of the triquetrum. As the wrist moves from neutral into ulnar deviation, the triquetrum translates laterally along the hamate as the hamate moves proximally toward the ulna. Simultaneously, due to the sloping surface of the hamate, the triquetrum moves volarly. Also simultaneously, the hamate glides proximally with respect to both triquetrum and capitate, interposing itself between these two bones like a keystone (Fig 12.33A). Figure 12.33A illustrates that in the ulnar-deviated wrist, the proximal pole of the hamate is closer to the radius (and lunate) than in any other position. As a result of hamate move-

ment, the proximal end of the capitate moves proximally and radially. This exerts a compressive force on the lunate. Coupled with triquetral translation volarly, compressive forces acting on the lunate rotate it into a dorsally facing attitude. Viewed from a lateral vantage point, the lunate thus rotated no longer shares the same long axis as the capitate (Fig. 33B). This movement can be appreciated radiographically. The dorsiflexion of the lunate exerts a similar dorsiflexory force on the scaphoid via the scapholunate interosseous ligament, and the pole of the scaphoid moves dorsally. This movement can be appreciated clinically. The scaphoid tubercle (palpable volarly when in the neutral wrist position) moves dorsally during ulnar deviation, disappearing under the palpating finger.

As the wrist moves from neutral into radial deviation, the triquetrum translates medially and

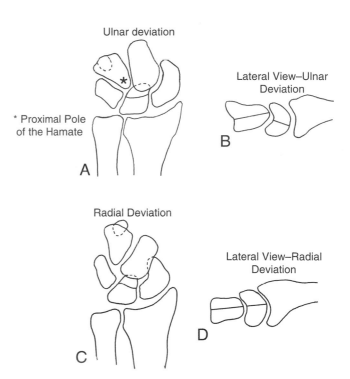

Figure 12.33. The orientation of the lateral articular surface of the hamate dictates the complex biplanar movements of the triquetrum. **A.** Dorsal view of left carpus in ulnar deviation. Note that proximal pole of hamate is closer to radius and ulna than in any other position of the wrist. Note also that the hamate is wedged between the capitate and triquetrum like a keystone. **B.** Lateral view of capitate, lunate, and radius with longitudinal axes of capitate and lunate drawn in. The lunate dorsiflexes during ulnar deviation of the wrist. **C.** Dorsal view of left carpus in radial deviation. Note how much of the lateral articulating surface of the hamate is exposed compared with 12.33A. **D.** Lateral view of capitate, lunate, and radius with longitudinal axes of capitate and lunate drawn in. Note that the capitate and lunate are coaxial during radial deviation of the wrist. (Adapted from Weber ER. Concepts governing the rotational shift of the intercalated segment of the carpus. Orthop Clin North Am 1984;15:193–207.)

dorsally along the slope of the hamate as the hamate moves away from the radius and ulna (Fig. 12.33C). As this occurs, the lunate and capitate become coaxial (Fig. 12.33D), and the scaphoid simultaneously flexes to its neutral position. In the last 10° of radial deviation, the radiolunotriquetral ligament's attachment to the lunate forces the lunate dorsal to the axis of the capitate, and compressive forces acting through the capitate cause the lunate to palmar flex slightly. The scapholunate interosseous ligament transmits this palmar flexion to the scaphoid, bringing the scaphoid tubercle volarward, where it may be palpated clinically. Again, the trapezoid and trapezium remain relatively stationary, accommodating scaphoid movement at the scaphotrapeziotrapezoid joint.

In summary, the hamate acts as an inclined plane on which the triquetrum slides up or down to produce volar or dorsiflexion movement to the lunate relative to the more stable capitate. The lunate and scaphoid remain associated throughout radial and ulnar deviation owing to the strong scapholunate interosseous ligament. Palpation of the scaphoid tubercle in radial and ulnar deviation can provide clues about the biomechanical integrity of the scapholunate articulation. This joint is considered the first area of ligamentous breakdown and dissociation, frequently progressing to significant wrist instability.

CARPOMETACARPAL JOINTS AND FINGER JOINTS

The four distal carpals and the second and third metacarpals function as a central fixed unit around which the thumb, and to a lesser degree the fourth and fifth rays, rotate. This unit is stabilized by closely interlocking bony architecture and strong interosseous ligaments. All gripping, hand-cupping, and pinching movements involve rotations at the carpometacarpal joints, especially those of the first, fourth, and fifth rays.

The fourth and fifth metacarpals articulate with the slightly saddle-shaped distal surface of the hamate. Eight degrees of motion are available at the fourth ray, whereas approximately 15° of motion can be produced at the fifth ray (88). These movements facilitate opposition of the fourth and fifth fingers with the thumb.

The carpometacarpal joint of the thumb is far more mobile and less stable than the other carpometacarpal joints. This joint is biconcave, allowing for motion in all directions, including rotation. It is supported by the ulnar-volar ligament and is dynamically stabilized by the abductor pollicis longus tendon.

The DIP and PIP joints are bicondylar with great congruency between joint surfaces. These joints have 1° of freedom, allowing for flexion and extension.

Clinical Evaluation of the Wrist and Hand: Examination of the Wrist

Specific orthopedic and neurologic tests for the injured wrist are discussed in the following section in conjunction with the conditions in which an abnormal finding may be encountered.

HISTORY

Too often history is abandoned after the patient states, "I fell and hurt my wrist." The diagnosis of sprained wrist is inadequate in establishing a proper treatment regimen. There are several common conditions of the wrist that are frequently misdiagnosed, owing to cursory history and examination. Clues to the nature of the injury are provided by knowing the exact position of the hand and wrist, point of impact, and activity performed at the time of trauma. Although the patient will not recall each detail, some gentle probing may yield valuable diagnostic information. For example, the scaphoid is fractured with wrist extension and with falls impacting the thenar side of the hand. The scaphoid is rarely injured when the wrist is in flexion. The diagnosis of fracture of the hook of the hamate might be overlooked if the patient with dorsoulnar wrist pain were not to describe the injury as occurring during a "fat swing" with a golf club. Occult wrist ganglions are common but often misdiagnosed because the pattern of pain can only be obtained by a good clinical history. Characteristically, a patient presenting with an occult ganglion will complain of a vague, intermittent wrist pain aggravated by use (e.g., waxing and waning pattern). The central, dorsal pain is maximum when bending the wrist back and pushing to get out of a chair (stressed dorsiflexion). Occult wrist ganglia represent entities that are diagnosed by exclusion. The diagnosis of dorsal occult scapholunate ganglion will be confirmed by negative wrist radiographs together with the clinical finding of well-localized tenderness at the dorsal scapholunate junction.

INSPECTION

Inspection before specific palpation and testing procedures can be useful in the evaluation of the traumatized wrist. Swelling may assist in localization. Excessive hemorrhage may indicate the presence of fracture rather than merely ligamentous injury.

PALPATION

Palpatory examination of the wrist must be methodical, like a "search pattern" when reading radiographs. Emphasis is placed on completeness. Gentle but firm pressure should always be used and will always cause some discomfort. Therefore, positive findings should always be compared with the opposite wrist. Beckenbaugh (94) describes a method of wrist palpation that uses the dorsal pole of the lunate as a key topographic point. Tenderness is pinpointed by palpating firmly with the pad of the thumb or first finger. The suspected site of injury is palpated last. Figure 12.34 lists the specific sites of palpation, together with the diagnostic implications of tenderness noted in that location.

Dorsal Wrist Palpation

When tenderness is noted while palpating the radial styloid, pressure applied to the distal radius may uncover a nondisplaced Colles' fracture. Palpation should then proceed to the anatomical snuffbox, where tenderness has traditionally been used as an indicator of scaphoid fracture.

Palpation of the lunate and scapholunate ligament uses the dorsal pole of the lunate as a landmark. Volar pressure is applied to the dorsal pole of the lunate. By slightly flexing and extending the wrist while sliding the thumb radially from the dorsal pole of the lunate, a distinct sulcus can be felt when scapholunate dissociation is present.

Gently passing the thumb ulnarly and distally provides opportunity for assessing the triquetrum and triquetrolunate junction. In severe injuries of the triquetrolunate ligament, the triquetrum will be ballottable, associated with a sharply painful click. Avulsion fractures of the triquetrum will result in exquisite point tenderness.

To palpate the ulna, distal radioulnar joint, and extensor carpi ulnaris tendon, the thumb is gently passed proximally to the distal dorsal radioulnar ligaments. If tenderness is present at the radial border of the ulnar head, gently supinate and pronate the forearm to detect abnormal motion. The dorsal ulna is ballotted for abnormal motion as well. Then palpation progresses to the extensor carpi ulnaris sheath. Again, if locally tender, flex the wrist. A distinct snap of the extensor carpi ulnaris tendon when the wrist is supinated indicates rupture of the extensor retinaculum. Injuries of the TFCC may reproduce pain in this area; any snap or click felt in this region during pronation, supination, or flexion must raise the index of suspicion of injury to the TFCC.

The ulnar snuffbox (94) is bounded by the flexor carpi ulnaris and extensor carpi ulnaris. This is a palpable sulcus on the ulnar border of

Site	Diagnostic Implication(s)	Comments
Radial styloid	Direct contusion and/or fracture of styloid.	Degenerative changes are not pain-producing to palpation here
Snuffbox	Tenderness is hallmark of scaphoid fracture and/or scapholunate ligament injury.	Arthritis at the scaphotrapezial joint will result in more distal snuffbox pain.
Trapezium and carpometacarpal joint of the thumb	Trapezial tenderness indicates radial collateral ligament injury.	Compression of the first metacarpal reproduces pain in carpometacarpal arthrosis.
Index and long	Tender metacarpal bases imply carpometacarpal sprain with or without fracture.	
Capitate	Rarely tender here. Painful in both scapholunate and triquetrolunate instability patterns.	Palpate proximal to 3rd metacarpal for sulcus of the neck of the capitate.
Lunate and scapholunate ligament	Tender in lunate fracture and scapholunate dissociation.	
Triquetrum and triquetrolunate junction	Local pain in triquetrolunate sprains.	
Ulna, distal radioulnar joint and extensor carpi ulnaris	Tender in radioulnar instability. Ballottement may be possible at the ulna with instability. Extensor retinacular rupture.	
Ulnar snuffbox	Lunatotriquetral sprain	Important and commonly missed diagnosis.

Figure 12.34. Site of dorsal wrist tenderness correlated with diagnostic implications.

the wrist. Radial deviation of the wrist brings a rounded bony prominence to this sulcus. This prominence is the triquetrum. Firm pressure applied here may reveal a click or snap, strongly suggestive of lunotriquetral ligament injury. The triquetrum may be ballottable. This is an important and commonly missed injury of the wrist. Exquisite tenderness without a click or snap indicates triquetral fracture, which is rare.

It must be remembered that fractures of the hook of the hamate produce dorsal wrist pain and tenderness along the carpometacarpal joints dorsally. Care must be taken to evaluate volar tenderness when tenderness is elicited dorsally in this area.

Volar Wrist Palpation

Palpation then moves to the volar surface. The volar aspect of the radial styloid should be palpated with firm, direct pressure. The radial artery is accessible as the palpating finger or thumb moves ulnarly from the styloid. The flexor carpi radialis sheath, tuberosity of the trape-zium, hook of the hamate, and pisiform should be included in palpatory examination of the volar wrist. Recall that the hamate is located distally and radially to the pisiform.

RANGE OF MOTION

Range of motion of the wrist, both active and passive, should be noted. Limited motion in specific directions gives clues to areas of injury. Passive motion, as noted previously, is used to elicit clicks or snaps evidencing ligamentous disruptions within the wrist.

Clinical Evaluation of the Wrist and Hand: Examination of the Hand

Specific orthopedic and neurologic tests for the injured hand are discussed in the following section in conjunction with the conditions in which an abnormal finding may be encountered.

INSPECTION/OBSERVATION

Inspection is the key to diagnosis in those athletic injuries that result in a characteristic deformity (e.g., boutonnière deformity, mallet finger, and trigger finger). The degree of pain and swelling provides clues as to the location and severity of injury.

PALPATION

Screening palpation of the hand begins with the carpometacarpal joints to localize areas of tenderness along the metacarpals and phalanges. A tuning fork may be used with palpation to screen for fractures. Every attempt should be made to localize the precise area of pain so that correlation with an anatomical structure can be made. As with wrist injuries, the mechanism of trauma is important and if known can guide the examiner in palpatory examination.

ORTHOPEDIC/NEUROLOGIC EXAMINATION

Active and passive range of motion of the metacarpophalangeal, interphalangeal, and carpometacarpal joints is carried out in all planes of movement, including opposition and reposition of the thumb and the fourth and fifth digits. Hand-cupping movements and clenching the fist can reveal subtle motor deficits or aid in localization of pain.

Careful neurologic evaluation is important in those syndromes presenting with loss of sensation and/or motor strength. Detailed motor testing may be necessary to localize involvement to a specific peripheral nerve or tendon. The examiner must never forget that injuries proximal to the hand and wrist can manifest themselves predominantly within the hand. History will usually provide the necessary information in this regard. Handgrip strength can be evaluated using a dynamometer; interrater and test-retest reliability are reported at 0.98 and 0.88, respectively. The most consistent measure of strength over time is the average of three separate recordings (95). Hand dynamometry is suitable for assessing clinical progress over the treatment period when weakness has been detected.

Diagnostic Imaging in Evaluation of the Wrist

Static bony pathologic states can often be demonstrated with plain film radiographs. In addition, several dynamic pathologic conditions have been defined, fostering an array of dynamic x-ray imaging techniques. Conventional tomography, CT, MRI, arthrography, and scintigraphy all play important roles in evaluation of various disorders producing a painful wrist.

A routine radiographic study of the wrist consists of the posteroanterior (PA), lateral, and PA (or external) oblique views. One well-recognized imaging center, the Mallinckrodt Institute of Radiology, St. Louis, Missouri, adds a PA ulnar deviation view to the standard series (96). This view is valuable in detecting dynamic instability of the scapholunate interosseous ligament not always visible with the other three views. A gap of more than 3 mm present between scaphoid and lunate is indicative of significant ligamentous disruption. Furthermore, in ulnar deviation the scaphoid normally dorsiflexes, bringing it more parallel to the plane of the carpus. This expands its length and will demonstrate fractures of the scaphoid that might otherwise be missed (94).

Care should be taken to position the dorsum of the radius with the metacarpals to obtain a "true" neutral lateral projection; this will be important in biomechanical evaluation. Other supplemental views may include oblique views at variable increments of tube angulation of pronation/supination (e.g., the Gilula series), the carpal tunnel view to evaluate the bony tubercles (trapezial tuberosity and hamulus) and soft tissue structures of the carpal tunnel, and coned-down spot films of specific areas obtained fluoroscopically. Radiographs are studied for cortical disruptions, erosions, bony proliferations and periosteal reaction, and degree and pattern of mineralization. Soft tissue abnormalities, including calcifications, swelling, and abnormal articular cartilage, are also sought.

CARPAL INSTABILITY AND PLAIN RADIOGRAPHY

The integrity of bony and ligamentous architecture of the wrist is assessed by determining whether the three arcs of the wrist and the parallelism of the joints are maintained (Fig 12.35) on the neutral PA view. Disruption of any of these arcs signifies dislocation or subluxation and ligament injury.

A true neutral lateral radiograph can be used to perform biomechanical assessments of the wrist.

Roentgenometric angles between the individual carpals can be drawn on the lateral view, including the scapholunate, radiolunate, radioscaphoid, and capitolunate angles. The scapholunate angle is formed by the long axes of the scaphoid and lunate. It normally measures 30°–60°. The capitolunate angle is formed by the long axes of the lunate and capitate. These two angles are most commonly used to identify abnormal carpal alignment and ligamentous instability patterns, such as dorsal intercalated segment instability (DISI) and volar intercalated segment instability (VISI). These and other angles appear, together with their normal values, in Figure 12.36A. McMurtry's index, used to assess ulnar translocation (e.g., with dorsal dislocations of the distal ulna), is drawn on the PA view (Fig. 12.36B).

Finally, aside from the PA ulnar deviation view, other dynamic studies can be revealing. Motion radiographs taken laterally in palmar flexion and extension, in PA radial deviation, and in PA forced-grasp (fist) position will cause compression forces that may reveal dynamic instability. For example, consider the patient with dynamic scapholunate instability who has a click in the wrist with forceful grip but no dissociation on the PA ulnar deviation view. The clenched-fist position forces the capitate into the scapholunate interval, separating it during forceful grasp. This separation will be appreciated on the clenched-fist PA view. A good working knowledge of the biomechanics discussed earlier in this chapter will aid greatly in the interpretation of dorsiflexion and volarflexion motion radiographs. In mid-

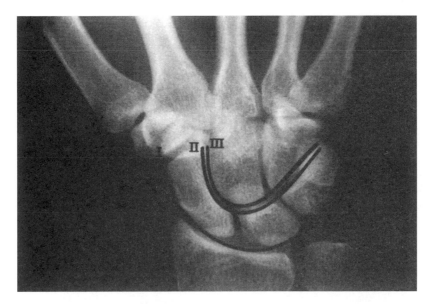

Figure 12.35. The parallelism of the three arcs of the wrist, seen on the neutral posterior-anterior view, indicates normal anatomical integrity. (From Barry MS, Kettner NW, Pierre-Jerome C. Carpal instability: pathomechanics and contemporary imaging. Chiro Sports Med 1991;5:38–44.)

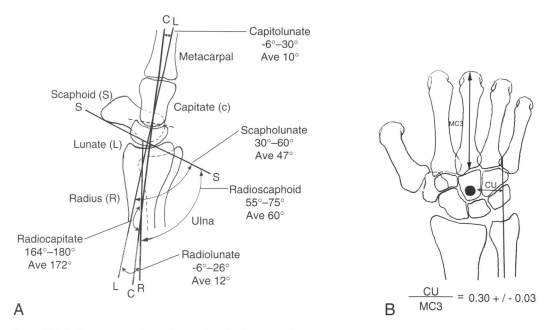

Figure 12.36. Roentgenographic angles used in the diagnosis of volar intercalated segment instability and dorsal interca-lated segment instability. The scapholunate and capitolunate angles are the most commonly used angles. **A.** The carpal angles as measured on the lateral view and their normal ranges. **B.** McMurtry's index for ulnar translocation. (Reprinted with per-mission from Linn MR, Mann FA, Gilula LA. Imaging the symptomatic wrist. Orthop Clin North Am 1990;21:515–543.)

carpal VISI instability, the lunate may increase its palmar-flexed position with motion studies. In scapholunate DISI instability, the lunate fails to move with the scaphoid in normal palmar (volar) flexion and appears abnormally dorsiflexed.

SELECTION OF WRIST IMAGING MODALITIES IN ATHLETIC TRAUMA

Radiographic evaluation should begin with a standard three-view (or preferably four-view) (in-cluding PA ulnar deviation) wrist series. If nega-tive, supplementary views should be selected based on the location of pain. If again negative or equivocal, scintigraphy, CT, or MRI should be chosen to evaluate the painful joint.

Wrist fractures are most completely evaluated with CT. CT is also of reported value in imaging carpal ganglion cysts (97) and carpal osteonecro-sis (96). Scintigraphy is most useful when all other radiographic studies are normal. A charac-teristic hot spot on bone scan indicates the pres-ence of fracture undetected radiographically. Oc-casionally an increased technetium 99 uptake will be noted with ligamentous injury, but the re-sponse will not be as vigorous as with fracture. Furthermore, a negative bone scan is significant because it clearly excludes fracture as the cause of wrist pain.

Wrist arthrography is valuable in assessing ligamentous and soft tissue disruptions in the

wrist. A triple injection technique (87), including injections into the radiocarpal, distal radioulnar, and midcarpal joints, allows for superior visual-ization of complex abnormalities of the TFCC and lunotriquetral ligament.

MRI is sensitive for fracture at many sites (e.g., knee, long bones) owing to its ability to demon-strate marrow hemorrhage and edema. However, as yet only anecdotal instances of MRI demon-stration of carpal fractures have been identified (96). MRI is useful in evaluating tears of the TFCC. MRI can demonstrate subradiographic ab-normalities such as tenosynovitis, subtle fluid collections, and the effect of a wrist lesion on the surrounding neurovascular structures.

Algorithms for acute wrist trauma and for the chronically symptomatic wrist summarize this discussion and appear in Figures 12.37A and B.

Diagnostic Imaging in Evaluation of the Hand

Routine radiographic evaluation of the hand includes the PA, lateral, and oblique views. Ra-diographs of individual digits are used to evalu-ate a particular area of complaint. Stress views are usually obtained to rule out ligamentous injury.

Collateral ligament injuries of the thumbs are often misdiagnosed as a simple sprain, leading to chronic instability and pain (16). The routine ra-diographs are often negative because almost half of all ligament tears occur without fracture. Stress views of both thumbs should be obtained for comparison. Localized widening or subluxation indicates ligament disruption.

As with other occult bone injuries, nuclear scintigraphy may be useful for demonstrating fractures of the metacarpals and phalanges not visible on routine radiographs. MRI and CT scanning are not used routinely in the evaluation of athletic injuries of the hand, although these modalities may be useful for demonstrating secondary inflammatory changes and vascular injuries of the palm.

Goals of Recovery	Technique
Stability	Splinting
Decrease pain	TENS, oral supplements or medications
Decrease inflammation	Ice, oral supplements or medications
Increase strength	Stress loading, isometric exercise, splinting
Mobility	
Increase functional range	Active/passive ROM, continuous passive motion, diathermy, ultrasound, massage
Endurance	
Increase strength	Work hardening
Work performance	Isokinetic conditioning, isotonic conditioning, variable resistance training

Figure 12.38. Goal-oriented rehabilitation of wrist injuries. (Adapted from Koman LA, Mooney JF, Poehling GG. Fractures and ligamentous injuries of the wrist. Hand Clin 1990;6(3):477–491.)

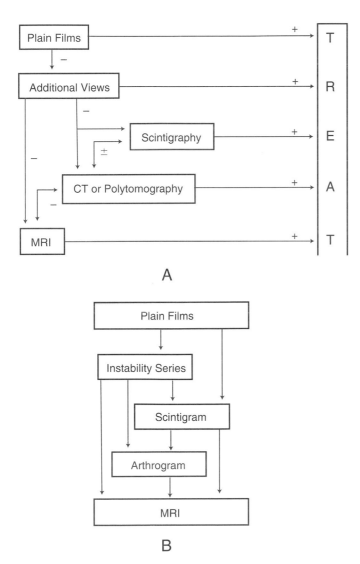

A

B

Figure 12.37. Algorithms for the radiographic assessment of wrist pain. **A.** Algorithm for acute trauma. "+": definitive diagnosis; "−": normal; "±": indeterminate or equivocal. **B.** Algorithm for the chronically symptomatic wrist. The decision to treat can be made at any algorithm level, depending on the clinical problem and information obtained. Many cases will not reach the end of the algorithm. (Reprinted with permission from Linn MR, Mann FA, Gilula LA. Imaging the symptomatic wrist. Orthop Clin North Am 1990;21:515–543.)

Common Athletic Injuries of the Wrist and Hand

Although treatment must be based on the pathology involved, the level of participation in sports (e.g., professional or national/international amateur versus local/state level) is an important factor in managing injuries. The most pressing concerns are often when or whether the patient will be able to resume competition. In some injuries several treatment options are available, and the appropriate choice depends on the immediate and long-term needs of the athlete. These needs may determine conservative versus nonconservative management. For many ligamentous injuries and more complex injuries such as TFCC lesions, definitive treatment may be postponed until the end of the season without compromising long-term treatment outcome.

Although osseous injuries may be healed and structurally sound at 6 to 8 weeks, collagen maturation in ligamentous injuries may require 6 to 9 months for full recovery (98). Flexibility, mobility, and strength must be maintained or restored during the rehabilitation period. These goals are reflected in Figure 12.38. Reentry into sports practice and competition depends on the type of injury and the speed of recovery.

FRACTURES OF THE WRIST AND HAND

Too often hand and wrist injuries are ignored—by athlete and trainer alike—in the heat of battle. Unfortunately, a seemingly trivial hand or wrist pain can lead to significant disability without timely and proper treatment. Prompt attention on the playing field can even improve final outcome of recovery in some cases. If good judgment allows for the continuation of play, protection with the use of padding and tape will provide safety to the injured area while definitive diagnosis and treatment are postponed until after competition.

Immediate field treatment of fractures of the wrist and hand involve the local application of ice, elevation, analgesics, and splinting. Neurovascular status should always be determined as soon as possible. Appropriate radiographs must be taken—and the nature and extent of trauma must be ascertained—before selection of the best form of intervention in each case. Conservative versus surgical management depends on the type and severity of fracture as well as the specific short- and long-term needs of the athlete.

Distal Radial Fractures

The most common fractures of the wrist involve the distal radius and carpal scaphoid. Colles' fracture (dorsal angulation) and Smith's fracture (volar angulation) involve the distal radius. These injuries are casted differently, and one must not mistake one for the other. Whereas Colles' and Smith's fractures are common in the general population, they do not occur frequently in athletes. Galeazzi's fracture, involving fracture of the distal to middle third of the radius with distal radioulnar dislocation, has been discussed earlier in this chapter.

In adolescent athletes, a fall on the outstretched hand may result in a shearing injury through the distal radial epiphysis. This type of trauma typically gives rise to a Salter-Harris Type II injury with dorsal metaphyseal fracture. In younger athletes, ages 8 through 12, a pure Salter Type I epiphyseal separation is typical; the radial epiphysis displaces either volar or dorsal with minimal medial or lateral shift. The lateral radiograph is most useful for diagnosis of this injury, with particular attention to the pronator quadratus sign, a dark shadow on the lateral forearm radiograph representing a shift in the fat plane overlying the pronator quadratus muscle (99). This is similar to the changes in the anterior and posterior fad pads at the elbow in the presence of elbow fracture. Even fresh, undisplaced distal radial and ulnar fractures will be accompanied by a positive radiographic pronator quadratus sign in 98% of cases (100). This sign is present when anterior displacement of the pronator quadratus shadow is 7 mm or more

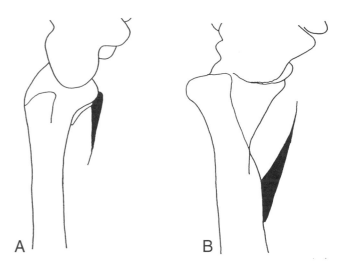

Figure 12.39. The pronator quadratus sign. **A.** Normal wrist. **B.** Abnormal sign with anterior displacement and separation from the distal edge of the radius. (Reprinted with permission from Sasaki Y, Sugioka S. The pronator quadratus sign: its classification and diagnostic usefulness for injury and inflammation of the wrist. J Hand Surg 1989;14:80–83.)

and when the distal edge of this shadow is significantly separated from the volar lip of the radius. When present, an underlying bone or joint injury should be suspected (Fig. 12.39A and B illustrates the normal and abnormal pronator quadratus signs).

Radial styloid fractures may lead to a suspicion of significant radiocarpal ligamentous disruptions and associated carpal instability. The injury is produced by avulsive force transmitted through the palmar extrinsic ligaments with potential tearing of the intrinsic scapholunate or lunotriquetral ligaments.

Physical examination in distal radial fractures reveals pain, tenderness, and swelling locally. Radiographs confirm the diagnosis. Displaced fractures are usually treated successfully with closed reduction and immobilization. Stable radial styloid fractures are often reduced by ulnar deviation of the wrist and hand. However, scapholunate/lunotriquetral dissociations are frequent, and the needs of the athlete may require that rigid internal fixation be performed to allow for restoration of stability.

Simple nondisplaced and reduced fractures of the radial styloid may heal rapidly within 4 to 6 weeks of immobilization. The athlete may return to competition after 3 to 4 weeks with protection of the injury in many cases, depending on the sport. A soft cast is used for protection during competition and practice, and a hard cast may be used off the playing field. The location of injury may prevent ball-handling athletes from participation until the injury is fully rehabilitated.

Scaphoid Fractures

The scaphoid is the most commonly fractured carpal bone. The mechanism of injury is usually forced hyperextension of an ulnarly deviated wrist on an outstretched hand (98). The athlete presents with pain and tenderness with loss of concavity of the anatomical snuffbox. Wrist range of motion is decreased by pain and swelling.

Scaphoid fractures may not become radiographically apparent for 2 to 6 weeks posttrauma. Diagnosis can be confirmed at 2 weeks with technetium bone scan. Because the major artery supplying the scaphoid enters at the scaphoid waist, the risk of ischemic necrosis and nonunion increases as the fracture line occurs more proximally. Radiographs should be performed every 2 weeks during the course of management to assess changes that reveal fracture (in the absence of a bone scan), evidence of osteonecrosis and nonunion, and evidence of proper healing.

The classic management of cast immobilization until either healing occurs or until nonunion is documented (e.g., 3 to 6 months) is not appropriate for most high-performance athletes. Stable nondisplaced fractures may be managed by short-arm thumb spica cast immobilization or functional bracing until healing occurs (usually within 6 to 8 weeks). In non–ball-handling contact sports, less rigid orthotics or silicone casts may be used for competition, with rigid casts being used for practice. In crucial situations, associated ligamentous injuries may be evaluated arthroscopically, and open or arthroscopically assisted internal fixation can be used. After rigid fixation of stable injuries (e.g., transverse waist fractures), return to competitive play may begin once 80% of the rehabilitation goals have been attained (Fig. 12.38). In mild cases this can be as early as 1 week posttrauma, assuming that an appropriate short-arm thumb spica orthosis is worn and risks are adequately explained to the athlete (101).

Unstable scaphoid injuries such as oblique fractures, proximal or distal pole fractures, or displaced fractures may require anatomical alignment and internal stabilization (e.g., internal compression screw fixation) to obtain a reasonably rapid return to competition and to avoid secondary carpal instability, nonunion, excessive stiffness, or arthritis (98).

Freeland (102) found that when tenderness was absent at both the anatomical snuffbox and the scaphoid tubercle, there was virtually no chance of scaphoid fracture. These patients require symptomatic treatment only. However, it is recommended that all other causes of wrist pain be excluded through appropriate diagnostic evaluation.

The scaphoid compression test is useful to determine clinically when fracture union has occurred in scaphoid waist fractures. It can be performed even while the patient is in a cast (Fig. 12.40) (103).

Fractures of the Hook of the Hamate

Fractures of the hook of the hamate often occur during sporting activities such as golf (nondominant hand), racket sports, and baseball (nondominant hand). This injury results from a direct blow to the hypothenar eminence and is often difficult to identify on routine PA and lateral views of the wrist (16). On a PA view the hamate may appear sclerotic, or the cortical margins may

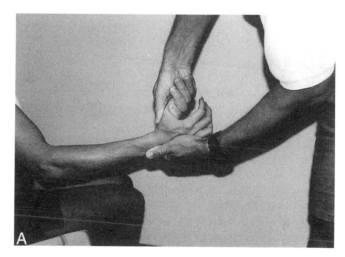

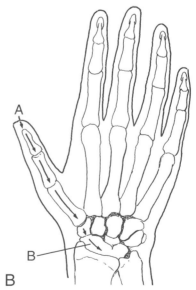

Figure 12.40. The scaphoid compression test. **A.** Compression is applied along the long axis of the first metacarpal into the scaphoid. **B.** Compressive force is transmitted to the scaphoid.

be poorly defined or absent. The carpal tunnel view usually reveals the fracture. In some cases, lateral views or CT may be required to confirm the diagnosis.

Hamate hook fractures produce localized palpatory tenderness in the hypothenar region. Range of motion is usually noncontributory. Loss of grip strength is common, and concomitant ulnar nerve compression may be present.

The fracture may be treated conservatively by cast immobilization for 4 to 6 weeks. However, these fractures most commonly present as chronic nonunions because of late diagnosis; therefore, operative intervention is often necessary, involving excision of the fracture fragment or the entire hook. Rehabilitation usually progresses rapidly, with return to competition 4 to 6 weeks after surgery.

Boxer's Fracture

Fractures of the neck of the fifth metacarpal are common. The injury was originally coined as a result of the frequency with which fifth metacarpal fractures occurred in street boxing. The mechanism of trauma is usually abrupt impact loading through the long axis of the metacarpal (Fig. 12.37).

History of trauma and location of pain laterally with edema are clues to diagnosis, which is confirmed by radiographs. These fractures are generally easy to reduce. Patient comfort may be increased in severely angulated fractures using an ulnar nerve block. Pressure under the metacarpal head with downward pressure on the metacarpal shaft usually restores satisfactory alignment. Malrotation must also be corrected. With angulations in excess of 60°, percutaneous K-wire fixation may be necessary.

Closed reduction of a boxer's fracture is maintained using a well-molded plaster splint. Anterior and posterior 3-inch plaster splints carefully molded on the volar side of the metacarpal neck with downward pressure on the dorsum of the metacarpal shaft provide the best external fixation.

Postreduction radiographs must be reviewed carefully to be sure that no more than 20° angulation remains. Radiographs must be repeated weekly for the first 4 weeks to check that reduction has been maintained. After 4 weeks of plaster cast immobilization, a fabricated orthosis can give adequate protection and should be continued for 12 weeks (101).

Athletes who must continue to participate in their sport or reenter their sport quickly will require K-wire fixation, otherwise, excessive angulation with malunion may develop.

Fractures to the neck of the fourth metacarpal are treated the same as those to the fifth metacarpal. However, literature indicates that fractures to the neck of the second and third metacarpals require surgical reduction to minimize volar angulation, preserving optimal hand function. Prominent metacarpal heads directed volarly into the palm can impair gripping maneuvers. The second and third metacarpals are rigid with very little motion at the carpometacarpal junction; as a result, angulation at the metacarpal necks is poorly tolerated.

Bennett's Fracture

Bennett's fracture is an articular fracture of the proximal end of the first metacarpal (101). The fracture fragment is the volar ulnar portion of the articular surface. The deep volar carpal ligament attached to the fragment holds it in place. The pull of the abductor pollicis longus tendon inserted at the base of the metacarpal shaft displaces the metacarpal shaft proximally.

Treatment of Bennett's fracture involves reduction of the shaft of the metacarpal to the stationary fracture fragment and holding it in position until bone healing occurs. Reduction is accomplished by long axis traction coupled with pronation and abduction of the base of the metacarpal. Because this fracture is often unstable, two small K-wires are usually placed percutaneously through the base of the first metacarpal and into the adjacent carpals or into the second metacarpal. The K-wires do not need to go into the fracture fragment.

A thumb spica cast is used from 10 days to 14 weeks, depending on the security of fixation. Range of motion exercises for the thumb should be started at 10 days unless the carpometacarpal joint has been pinned. A thumb spica orthosis should be worn for protection during activities, including sports, for 12 weeks.

Gamekeeper's Thumb (Skier's Thumb)

Campbell coined the term gamekeeper's thumb in 1955 because of the high incidence of this injury among English gamekeepers (104). It consists of a partial or complete rupture of the ulnar collateral ligament at the MPJ of the thumb. This injury is common in football and is produced by a fall on an outstretched hand. Athletic equipment, such as ski poles, lacrosse sticks, and hockey sticks, also contribute to its incidence.

The athlete with an ulnar collateral ligament avulsion will complain of pain in the first web space with weakened pinch on using the thumb.

Clinical examination will confirm pinch weakness and will usually reveal swelling along the ulnar border of the first metacarpal. Acute injuries will be accompanied by local palpatory tenderness.

To distinguish partial from complete tears, the MPJ should be stressed in both flexed and extended positions. By comparing stability with the opposite thumb, if ligamentous laxity is at least 30° greater on the involved side, a complete tear should be suspected. Instability may occur to a lesser degree with partial tears.

Radiographs may show a displaced, rotated chip of bone where the ulnar collateral ligament avulsed from its attachment at the proximal phalanx. If a chip fracture is noted, it almost always indicates compete rupture of the ligament.

Partial tears can be managed with a thumb spica cast worn for 3 weeks. The cast should then be replaced by a volar splint, which is removed periodically throughout the day to allow the athlete to perform active exercises of the thumb and wrist. Because stability of the thumb is necessary for functional use, splinting should be continued until 6 weeks posttrauma.

Indications for surgical repair include gross instability, presence of interposed soft tissue, and intraarticular, displaced, or rotated fractures. Prognosis for surgical repair of acute injuries is better than for prognosis of chronic injuries.

Metacarpal Fractures

Metacarpal fractures may result from a fall or contact between athletes. These injuries often involve dorsal crushing blows, resulting in significant edema throughout the dorsal aspect of the hand. Proper immobilization with 60°–70° of metacarpophalangeal flexion will prevent an extension contracture from developing. The effects of flexion immobilization are counteracted by an early extension exercise program beginning after 3 weeks. The athlete should extend the metacarpophalangeal joint while simultaneously flexing the interphalangeal joint.

Metacarpal fractures are more stable than phalangeal fractures because of additional support from surrounding bones and muscles.

Metacarpal shaft fractures may be classified as transverse, oblique, or comminuted with varying sizes of butterfly fragments. Reduction of short oblique and transverse fractures is often impeded by entrapment of interposing muscle. If this is the case, open reduction may be required. Any shortening of the fracture must be corrected to restore and maintain hand function.

Conservative management with closed reduction and immobilization is appropriate for most cases. In general, active motion is not initiated until at least 3 weeks postinjury. Protective splinting continues for several more weeks as dictated by radiograph findings.

Phalangeal Fractures

Phalangeal fractures may be either nonarticular or articular. Nonarticular phalanageal fractures will be discussed by location. The majority of proximal phalangeal fractures are spiral or oblique fractures that tend to shorten. If displaced, these fractures are unstable because of axial traction exerted by the tendons crossing the injury. The traction used in reducing these fractures is not maintained by external fixation alone. However, closed reduction with percutaneous K-wire fixation is often successful for these fractures.

The less frequently encountered transverse fracture to the proximal end of the proximal phalanx presents with volar angulation and may be difficult to reduce. Maximally flexing the proximal fragment will tighten the collateral ligaments of the (metacarpophalangeal) joint and stabilize this fragment. Using traction and flexion, the fracture may then be reduced. If the fracture is unstable, K-wire fixation is required.

Transverse fractures of the middle phalanx are angulated palmarly and must be reduced and held with the adjacent joints in flexion. These fractures can be treated adequately with external splinting unless they are unstable. With instability, percutaneous K-wire fixation is again used. The dense cortical bone of the diaphysis of the middle phalanx takes 12 weeks or more to heal (105). External splinting should continue for 6 weeks before starting range of motion exercises. Protection during activity is recommended for 3 or 4 months until the fracture is well healed.

Articular fractures of the phalanges are common in sports. Fractures at the distal ends of the proximal and middle phalanges are often long oblique fractures involving one or both condyles. The fracture fragment displaces proximally, resulting in angulation at the joint. Again, because of axial traction from tendons, reduction can only be maintained by percutaneous K-wire fixation. Open reduction is often needed in these cases to obtain adequate compression (106).

For athletic participation in phalangeal fractures, external immobilization should continue for 12 weeks. Joint stiffness is a frequent complication of articular fractures, and tendon adhesions frequently complicate proximal phalangeal fractures. Early range of motion is possible when stable internal fixation has been obtained (e.g., 7 to 10 days postinjury); this helps to minimize adhesions and joint stiffness. Once full stability of the fracture site is obtained, gentle mobilization or manipulation may be added to range of motion exercise to enhance range of motion and lyse adhesions.

PIP joint injuries are common in sports because fingers are frequently "jammed," resulting in a sore, swollen, and stiff joint. This may often involve a fracture-subluxation of the PIP joint. The fracture is usually recognized, but the dorsal subluxation may be overlooked if the radiographs are not carefully evaluated (101).

The subluxation is reduced by combined axial traction with passive flexion. However, the joint will resubluxate if the patient reextends the finger. This can be prevented by incorporating a dorsal extension block splint that prevents extension beyond 45°–60° but allows the patient to flex the joint actively. Active flexion exercises should also be encouraged. The patient's condition is followed weekly with repeat radiographs and, if indicated, by allowing 10 additional degrees of extension each week. By the end of 4 to 6 weeks full extension is gained without recurrent subluxation. After this point, the patient should continue rigorous flexion and extension exercises to regain full motion.

For participation in sports, the joint is immobilized at 40°–60° flexion and protected in this position. For some sports, an orthosis will be required that incorporates the hand, wrist, and forearm. The joint should be protected in this manner for 12 weeks.

DISLOCATIONS AND INSTABILITIES OF THE WRIST

Wrist Dislocations, Sprains, and Related Carpal Instabilities

Carpal dislocations include dislocations of the lunate, perilunar dislocations, and fracture-dislocations. These injuries are now widely accepted as different stages of the same injury pattern (107). However, these injuries are uncommon, accounting for less than 10% of all carpal injuries. Carpal dislocation is most commonly seen in the 20- to 35-year-old age-group and results from high impact. These injuries usually accompany a fall onto an outstretched hand from a building or ladder, from motor vehicle trauma, or during sports (108). The mechanism of injury involves wrist extension with ulnar deviation and fixed forearm supination.

Examination will reveal severe pain. Lunate dislocations occur volarly and are occasionally accompanied by scaphoid fractures. Because of the proximity of the median nerve, there is a potential for significant compressive neuropathy. This injury may also compress tendons within the carpal tunnel. Inspection reveals disruption of the normal volar contour of the wrist. Radiographs confirm the diagnosis. Closed reduction with 2 to 6 weeks of cast immobilization are normally provided. Rehabilitation must not stress the ligaments injured as a result of this dislocation, and activities that place the wrist into extension and ulnar deviation under axial loading must be avoided.

Distal (radio)ulnar dislocations, although infrequent, are overlooked in up to 50% of cases (109). The radius dislocates relative to the ulna, but these injuries are described in terms of the ulna's position (volar or dorsal) relative to the radius (e.g., dorsal or volar dislocation or subluxation of the ulna). Examination will reveal pain, swelling, and limited motion, particularly in pronation or supination of the forearm. Radiographs may show the injury, but faulty radiographic positioning can significantly alter the relationship of the distal end of the radius and ulna. Therefore, the forearm should be placed in neutral rotation with complete superimposition of the four metacarpals. A CT scan may be required to confirm the diagnosis. CT is a preferred modality because it can be performed with the patient's wrist immobilized in plaster.

Conservative treatment of dorsal dislocations/subluxations of the distal ulna consists of a long-arm cast used with the forearm in supination. Volar dislocations/subluxation of distal ulna require long-arm cast immobilization with the forearm in pronation.

In a reported case of volar distal ulnar dislocation involving a female body builder, Francobandiera et al. (110) reported an associated tear of the TFCC, and there was associated median neuropathy. Closed anatomical reduction with cast immobilization may be attempted unless associated soft tissue lesions necessitate surgical intervention.

Other carpal dislocations will be associated with a history of high-impact trauma, local tenderness, and deformity detected by plain radiography or CT scanning. As noted previously, all dislocations of the carpus are rare in sports and otherwise. Anatomical reduction and immobilization should be provided after excluding neuropathy and other soft tissue injuries (especially instabilities) in the wrist. Prognosis is determined more by the associated soft tissue injuries than by the carpal derangement itself (111).

Carpal bossing is the presence of a dorsal bony prominence ("carpal boss") that occurs more commonly at the third carpometacarpal joint and occasionally at the second carpometacarpal joint. Gunther (88) states that the cause is unknown. However, Beckenbaugh (94) asserts that it is caused by subtle dorsal subluxations or fracture subluxations of these joints. Others have postulated that bossing is caused by abnormalities of the ossification center in the styloid process of the third metacarpal base, with formation of a complete or partial os styloidium.

Injuries of the carpometacarpal joints occur from forced volar flexion of the hand and wrist, and sprains and dorsal fracture subluxations are often misdiagnosed. Because these injuries are common, careful examination technique of the carpometacarpal joints is described here. The examiner carefully supports the metacarpals with one hand and applies direct pressure with the palpating thumb of the opposite hand to the bases of the second through fourth metacarpals just proximal to their metaphyses. Tenderness implies sprain with or without a fracture of the carpometacarpal joint. Ligamentous instability of the joint is confirmed by supporting the metacarpals over their shafts and pressing distally over the metacarpal heads in a palmar and dorsal direction. This maneuver is known as the Linscheid test (Fig. 12.38) and will reproduce pain localized by the patient to the carpometacarpal joint.

Carpal bossing noted incidentally on examination is painful in less than half of patients. It may be associated with ganglion formation.

Injuries of the TFCC and ulnar collateral ligament provide an important challenge to the physician and need to be recognized and understood. The TFCC has three major functions: it cushions the ulnar carpus, stabilizes the distal radioulnar joint, and stabilizes the ulnar carpus. The loads borne by the ulnar carpus change as the forearm moves through supination and pronation. Supination produces a relatively negative ulnar variance (biomechanical shortening of the ulna relative to the radius, and hence an increase in ulnocarpal joint space), and pronation results in relatively positive ulnar variance. Positive ulnar variance is thought to be an etiologic factor in the production of degenerative TFCC lesions (87) and in athletic trauma to the TFCC (112).

Traumatic tears or perforations of the TFCC and its related structures usually result from a fall on the pronated outstretched wrist and forearm, from an acute rotational injury to the forearm, or from an axial load and distraction injury to the ulnar border of the forearm.

Clinically, the athlete presents with pain at the dorsal distal radioulnar joint that is sometimes localized to the ulnar side of the wrist. The pain is aggravated by active or resisted pronation or supination of the forearm. Passive forearm movements, if painful, suggest distal radioulnar subluxation or dislocation rather than a TFCC lesion. There may be an audible or palpable click, which is generally painful if present. Usually there is palpatory pain localized to the ulnocarpal area. This area is then compressed and distracted to evaluate the meniscus homolog, articular disc, and ulnar collateral ligament. TFCC lesions will be painful on compression only, whereas collateral ligament injuries will be painful with distraction, with radial deviation of the wrist, and with transverse palpation of the ligament itself at some point along its course. The diagnosis is confirmed preferably by high-field MRI examination but also by triple-injection arthrography or arthroscopy. Comparative studies show that MRI is at least equivalent to arthroscopy in the diagnosis of lesions of the TFCC (112), although at least one study clearly notes the superiority of arthroscopy in visualizing the cartilaginous portion of the lesion (113). Plain radiography is also important, however, for determining the presence of positive ulnar variance.

Conservative treatment involves rest or modification of activity, physiotherapeutic modalities, strengthening, and antiinflammatory measures. If pain persists and the diagnosis is confirmed through MRI, immobilization and complete cessation of activity should be provided for 6 weeks. If the condition continues to be nonresponsive or if it returns when activity is resumed, surgical excision of the tear is warranted, especially if the athlete wishes to continue competition long term.

Ulnar collateral ligament injuries without TFCC lesions are managed conservatively with pain control modalities, ultrasound, restrengthening, and gradual return to the sport.

Carpal instabilities are increasingly recognized as an important component of wrist injury. A generic diagnosis of wrist sprain is no longer appropriate. With careful history and examination, a specific diagnosis is usually evident. Only when a specific diagnosis is identified can proper clinical understanding and effective treatment be achieved.

Midcarpal instability involves a dissociation or subluxation of the capitate and the hamate on the lunate and triquetrum, respectively. This is secondary to loss of capsular ligament integrity and results in abnormal laxity between the proximal and distal row of carpals toward the ulnar side of the wrist. VISI and DISI patterns of instability describe the direction in which the lunate rotates, and the proximal row of carpals collapses due to laxity. In VISI, the distal aspect of the lunate rotates volarly, whereas in the DISI pattern, the distal aspect of the lunate rotates dorsally. These changes can be observed on a neutral lateral wrist radiograph. The radiographic angles used to determine these instabilities (e.g., scapholunate and capitolunate angles) have been described elsewhere in this chapter and appear in Figure 36A. VISI is present when the scapholunate angle is less than 30° or when the capitolunate angle is greater than 30° (114).

In VISI, patients present with vague ulnar pain and often have a painful, audible click, clunk, or snap during motion. This clunk is actually the midcarpal joint reducing. Clicking is elicited on examination by passively pronating the forearm and ulnarly deviating the wrist, and may be facilitated by the use of axial compression. The tenderness produced during reduction is localized to the capitolunate and triquetrohamate joints. Remember that clicks are only significant if they reproduce the patient's clinical symptoms; loose-jointed individuals may have painless clicks produced by passive manipulation. A VISI pattern may be present at rest (e.g., static instability), but videofluoroscopy may also reveal a concurrent DISI pattern with ulnar deviation from the neutral position. Definitive diagnosis of dynamic VISI pattern instability may require direct observation of midcarpal instability by videofluoroscopy.

Conservative treatment includes splinting (e.g., cock-up wrist splint) and pain control modalities. Surgical measures (ligamentous reconstruction or intercarpal arthrodesis) have been offered when conservative measures fail. However, the long-term results of ligamentous reconstruction, especially in athletes, have been poor (115). Furthermore, intercarpal arthrodesis results in a 50% decrease in motion, which is usually unacceptable for the competitive athlete (98). Thus, the midcarpal instability problem is best managed conservatively.

Whereas VISI involves instability of extrinsic carpal ligaments, DISI involves laxity of the scapholunate ligament, an intrinsic ligament of the wrist. DISI is the most common pattern of carpal instability and may progress to involve instabilities of other perilunar joints. It is present when the scapholunate angle is greater than 80° and may be present when this angle is between 60° and 80° (114). This pattern of instability is associated with unstable scaphoid fractures,

degenerative intercarpal arthrosis, and, in severe injuries, scapholunate dissociation (98). Early diagnosis before permanent attenuation of ligamentous tissue (if possible) is important to prevent progressive loss of internal wrist support, debilitating pain, and arthritis.

Rupture of the scapholunate ligament (e.g., scapholunate dissociation) will allow the scaphoid and lunate bones to rotate independently of one another (e.g., rotary subluxation of the scaphoid). The lunate rotates in a DISI pattern, whereas the scaphoid can be seen to rotate volarly on the neutral lateral roentgenogram. These injuries generally result from a fall or a direct blow on the ulnarly deviated and dorsiflexed wrist. In addition to DISI instability, radiographs will show widening of the scapholunate interval on the PA view. A measurement of 2 to 4 mm must accompany symptoms to be diagnostic. A joint space widening over 4 mm is confirmatory evidence of scapholunate ligament injury (116).

Scapholunate (DISI) instability produces pain and a feeling of weakness in the wrist, often associated with a palpable click. There is almost always palpatory tenderness at the anatomical snuffbox, and a click or sensation of "giving" may be produced with firm pressure here. Moving from the dorsal pole of the lunate, the examining thumb can be slid radially where a distinct sulcus may be felt while flexing and extending the patient's wrist. Continued pressure in this sulcus will allow slight ballottement of the dorsal pole of the scaphoid. If subtle fullness or completely localized tenderness is found, this suggests an occult dorsal ganglion or scaphoid impaction fracture. (94) From a differential diagnostic standpoint, when tenderness is found in this sulcus and in the snuffbox, scapholunate injury is present. If the sulcus is tender but the snuffbox is not, an occult dorsal ganglion is more likely than scapholunate injury.

In the competitive athlete it is important to make an early, definitive diagnosis when scapholunate dissociation is suspected. This is a potentially severe injury for an athlete. Completely disrupted scapholunate ligaments may be confirmed by MRI or arthroscopy. According to Koman et al. (98), closed treatment and simple cast immobilization is "almost certainly inadequate initial treatment" of complete scapholunate dissociations. These authors recommend closed reduction and percutaneous fixation or open reduction with ligamentous repair and pin fixation. Fixation is maintained for 4 to 6 weeks, and immobilization after this continues for another 6 to 8 weeks by short-arm cast. Full recovery generally requires

3 to 6 months, and return to full activity may never be possible, particularly in athletes whose sport requires heavy lifting or repeated forced loading of the wrist in dorsiflexion.

Lunotriquetral ligament tears may occur as an isolated injury or as part of a complex injury. This ligamentous injury is important to consider separately because it is, according to Weber (93), the most common injury affecting the ulnar side of the carpus. It can be produced by relatively small forces directed to the dorsum of the wrist including sudden axial loading of the extended wrist, twisting injuries during golf or bowling, or impact to the dorsum of the hand with the wrist flexed.

Patients with this injury complain of clicking within the wrist and loss of grip strength. The click is reproduced by axially loading the wrist while moving it passively through radial and ulnar deviation. Wrist range of motion is preserved. There is no visible swelling. There is point tenderness over the lunotriquetral joint. Ballottement of this joint will consistently produce pain. Pronation and supination of the forearm passively will not produce pain, but resisted pronation and supination will usually be painful. In the case of an isolated injury, no VISI patterns are demonstrated. The diagnosis is confirmed by wrist arthrography. There may be associated lesions of the TFCC.

Suggested treatments in the literature include cast immobilization for at least 6 weeks, ligament repair, ligament reconstruction, capitate-hamate-lunate-triquetral fusion, and lunotriquetral fusion. No single treatment has been uniformly successful (117).

An isolated tear of the lunotriquetral ligament must be differentiated specifically from ulnar impingement syndrome (UIS), which involves TFCC tearing, chondromalacia of the distal ulna and proximal lunate, and a tear of the ligament. Technetium 99m bone scanning will reveal the presence of chondromalacia. An MRI will show the TFCC tear. Clinically, the onset of symptoms in UIS is associated with minor repetitive trauma. It may follow a fracture of the radius with some radial shortening (and hence the advent of positive ulnar variance). Even considering these factors, differentiating between these two conditions may be difficult.

DISLOCATIONS OF THE HAND

MP Joint

Thumb MPJ dislocations are common in athletes. Dislocations of the MPJ excluding the thumb are rare, but most frequently involve the fifth digit. Metacarpophalangeal dislocations are classified into two types: simple (reducible) or complex (nonreducible through closed techniques). High-risk groups for thumb MPJ dislocation include football offensive linemen, stick and racket sports players, and snow skiers. If the ulnar or radial collateral ligaments of the thumb MPJ are injured, significant long-term functional impairment may result.

Thumb MPJ dislocations are usually obvious on inspection. Examination should be postponed until after radiographs of the injured thumb have been obtained. If the radiographs are normal, the clinical examination should include a determination of the point(s) of maximum tenderness. Pain over the collateral ligaments versus pain over the volar plate may suggest differing treatment alternatives. Collateral ligament instability is then assessed with the thumb MPJ in full flexion. This joint position allows accurate, selective assessment of these ligaments. Complete collateral ligament tears are determined by the absence of an end point on radial or ulnar stress examination of the joint. Complete tears require operative repair to reestablish the stability of the joint.

Mild acute sprains of the thumb metacarpophalangeal collateral ligaments can be managed with thumb spica taping or check-rein taping. Hand-based plastic splints can also be used.

After thumb metacarpophalangeal dislocation, with or without collateral ligament injury, joint enlargement, restriction of motion, and aching are common and may be permanent. However, functional impairment is usually slight due to the mobility of the interphalangeal and carpometacarpal joints of the thumb.

In conjunction with metacarpophalangeal dislocations, attenuation or rupture of the deep transverse metacarpal ligaments can occur after punching objects such as a volleyball or an opponent. This gives rise to volar subluxation of the involved digit. Due to associated soft tissue swelling, this injury is rarely diagnosed in the acute stage. When the deep transverse metacarpal ligaments are injured severely enough to require treatment, physical examination will reveal tenderness on anterior-posterior translation of two adjacent MP joint, or subluxation and deformity will be visible. Cast immobilization at 70°–90° flexion for 4 to 6 weeks is beneficial. Volar subluxation is frequently not symptomatic, and operative reconstruction is rarely necessary.

DIP Joint

Dislocations of the DIP joint are usually sustained when the extended distal phalanx is impacted by a ball, helmet, bases, walls, or the ground. Dislocations with gross deformity of a DIP joint often invite attempts at closed reduction by the athlete or others on the sidelines. However, radiographs before reduction are valuable in determining the presence of fracture-dislocation and for guiding appropriate treatment.

Dislocations without fracture are reduced with longitudinal traction and careful deliberate reversal of the deformity. Postreduction stability is assessed clinically, and alignment of joint surfaces is confirmed with radiographs. Immobilization of the DIP joint in 0°–20° of flexion for 10 to 21 days will usually provide effective treatment (118).

PIP Joint

The PIP joint dislocation is caused by impact loading, and the joint may dislocate in any plane. This is the most common athletic injury in the hand. Torquing the digit during wrestling or when caught in a football jersey has also given rise to a PIP dislocation. As with DIP joint dislocations, the temptation to reduce these injuries on the playing field should be avoided because the specific postinjury treatment required depends on an exact assessment of the injury sustained.

Volar PIP joint dislocations occur in conjunction with central extensor slip disruption. After concentric reduction (see below), continuous splinting is required for 3 to 6 weeks to prevent the development of a boutonnière deformity. After 3 to 6 weeks, continued splinting using plastic or aluminum devices during activity is recommended for an additional 4 to 6 weeks. Active DIP joint motion should be encouraged during this period.

Dorsal PIP dislocations occur more frequently than volar dislocations. Closed reduction techniques for both of these injuries involves exaggeration of the deformity, gentle longitudinal traction, and careful sliding of the concave-convex articular surfaces through their flexion-extension motion arc into the reduced position. High-velocity longitudinal traction is strongly discouraged because this may entrap soft tissue, such as the volar plate, in between the joint surfaces. A closed dorsal PIP dislocation that can be reduced in this fashion does not require operative intervention. If a concentric, well-aligned joint cannot be achieved by closed reduction, surgical methods are required. Athletes need to be apprised of the potential problems of joint enlargement and stiffness that can be present indefinitely, depending on the magnitude of injury.

PIP joint dislocations are very unforgiving, seldom returning to full alignment and complete range of motion. Chronic volar plate instability is uncommon, but may be present in wrestlers or other athletes who have not received adequate care while continuing with their hand-intensive sports. Recurrent dorsal dislocation of the PIP joint due to attenuation or rupture of the volar plate is rare (119).

TENDON INJURIES

Injuries to tendons can produce painful loss of mobility in athletes. Fortunately, these injuries have an excellent prognosis if they are accurately diagnosed and appropriately treated. Inflammation of the tendons in the wrist and forearm usually occurs where these tendons pass through synovially lined structures such as the flexor or extensor tendon sheaths.

Tendon Injuries of the Wrist and Lower Forearm

Stenosing tenosynovitis of the abductor pollicis longus and extensor pollicis brevis tendons (de Quervain's disease) as they pass through the first dorsal compartment was first described by de Quervain in 1895 (120). Athletes with this malady will report a history of repetitive wrist motion in ulnar deviation (e.g., racket sports). The chief complaint is pain overlying the radial styloid. The classic triad of clinical findings includes local swelling, tenderness just proximal to the tip of the radial styloid, and a positive Finkelstein's test. This test is performed by combining thumb flexion and full adduction with passive ulnar deviation of the wrist. Differential diagnosis in the athlete should include scaphoid fracture, flexor carpi radialis tendinitis, and intraarticular fractures or arthritis of the trapeziometacarpal joint. History alone will differentiate these conditions from de Quervain's tenosynovitis.

It is important to differentiate clinically which tendon or tendons are involved; specific transverse friction massage may be used to great advantage in quickly resolving this problem. Although the abductor pollicis longus and extensor pollicis brevis are classically described, the extensor pollicis longus—occupying its own synovial sheath—may be the offending tendon. Discrete point tenderness will be felt at the point of injury, and resisted testing the specific tendons will reveal which contribute most to the pain.

Acute conservative treatment involves rest, immobilization of the thumb in severe cases, and modalities such as pulsed ultrasound and ice. When there is no pain at rest and a progressive reduction of pain on resisted testing, gentle transverse friction massage is instituted. The athlete may be shown how to perform this procedure once daily between office visits. Resolution usually takes approximately 2 to 3 weeks. In difficult or chronic cases, injections of local anesthetic or steroid preparations have been used with good results.

Pain at the dorsal aspect of the distal ulna or ulnar carpus may be due to traumatic subluxation of the extensor carpi ulnaris tendon from its sheath. The best way to examine for this is to position the patient's forearm vertically with the wrist in neutral position. The examiner then moves the forearm passively through supination and pronation. Near full supination, the extensor carpi ulnaris tendon will become visible; with further supination and wrist flexion, a distinct snap can be felt if the extensor retinaculum has been ruptured. This will always be painful and may be associated with local swelling and palpatory tenderness. This is a commonly missed injury. Conservative treatment is long-arm cast immobilization with the forearm positioned in full supination.

Simple tendinitis of the extensor carpi ulnaris without subluxation may also occur. It is manifested by pain and swelling just distal to the ulnar head and may be exacerbated by resisted wrist extension and ulnar deviation. Ice, ultrasound, and gentle transverse friction massage provide effective treatment.

The abductor pollicis longus and extensor pollicis brevis tendons traverse the radial wrist extensors superficially at a point that is 4 to 6 cm proximal to Lister's tubercle. Pain, swelling, and sometimes snapping of the tendons in this area is known as intersection syndrome (121). This syndrome is thought to be caused by friction. This may give rise to an adventitious bursa or produce an inflammatory peritendinitis. Intersection syndrome must be differentiated from de Quervain's tenosynovitis.

In general, intersection syndrome can be managed conservatively with ice, ultrasound, transverse friction, and neuromuscular massage therapy locally. A cock-up wrist splint is useful in many cases. Surgical intervention is rarely necessary. A posttreatment exercise program emphasizing forearm flexibility and strength is recommended.

Aside from de Quervain's tenosynovitis and extensor pollicis longus tendinitis described above, there are four other sites of dorsal tendinitis at the wrist and forearm. These are illustrated in Figure 12.41. Extensor carpi ulnaris tendinitis and intersection syndrome have been considered previously. Here we will discuss tendinitis of the extensor digiti minimi at the distal extensor reti-

naculum, and extensor indicis proprius tendinitis at the proximal border of the extensor retinaculum.

Both extensor indicis proprius syndrome and extensor digiti minimi tendinitis are uncommon. Ritter and Inglis first described the extensor indicis proprius syndrome in 1969 (122). Both injuries involve vigorous, repetitive use of the wrist and present with pain and swelling over the involved tendon. Conservative treatment includes a regimen of rest, ice, ultrasound, and transverse friction massage, as for the other tendon injuries of the wrist.

Volar tendinitis may also develop at the wrist. Volar tendons that are subject to inflammation include the flexor carpi ulnaris, flexor carpi radialis, and digital flexor tendons where they pass through the carpal tunnel. Flexor carpi radialis tendinitis is rare in athletes and will not be considered here (123).

Flexor carpi ulnaris tendinitis is often bilateral and results from chronic repetitive trauma. This condition must be distinguished from pisotriquetral arthritis and instability in athletes who use rackets. In flexor carpi ulnaris tendinitis, pain is exacerbated by resisted wrist flexion. In pisotriquetral instability there may be painful resisted wrist flexion, but there will also be tenderness and occasional crepitation when the pisiform is passively translocated radially and ulnarly on the flat surface of the triquetrum. Flexor carpi ulnaris tendinitis is treated conservatively with rest, splint immobilization with the wrist in slight flexion, and physiotherapeutics for pain and in-

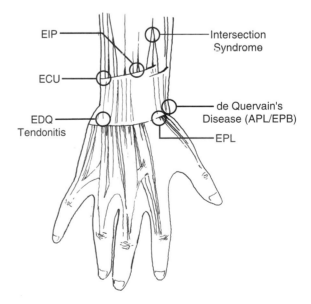

Figure 12.41. Common sites of tenderness involving the extensor tendons of the wrist, fingers, and thumb.

flammation. Conversely, pisotriquetral arthritis with instability may require surgical excision of the pisiform.

Digital flexor tendinitis manifests as stabbing or burning pain proximal to the carpal tunnel, which may extend up the forearm. This condition may result from acute wrist hyperextension injury or from repetitive use. Median neuropathy may coexist. Clinical examination will reveal tenderness and swelling just proximal to the wrist flexor creases. Electrodiagnostic studies are usually normal. Treatment is conservative and similar to that of flexor carpi ulnaris tendinitis.

Tendon Injuries of the Hand

Acute mallet finger, or rupture of the extensor tendon to the distal phalanx, is the most common closed tendon injury in the hand. It is caused by impact to the tip of the finger. It usually occurs in ball-handling sports where the athlete is required to catch. The ball forces the DIP joint abruptly into flexion, rupturing the tendon and sometimes avulsing bone from the proximodorsal aspect of the distal phalanx as well. Occasionally, the PIP joint maintains a position of hyperextension due to laxity of the volar plate and subsequent imbalance between the extensor and sublimus tendon.

On examination, there is exquisite tenderness over the dorsal aspect of the joint and a typical mallet finger appearance (Fig. 12.40). The distal joint can be extended passively but not actively. The nailbed is often involved in acute injuries, and this may require surgical intervention to facilitate healing.

McCue and Mayer (124) describe five patterns of mallet finger.

1. Fibers of the extensor mechanism are stretched without complete rupture.
2. The extensor tendon may rupture or avulse from the dorsal base without bony involvement.
3. The tendon avulsion may include a small bony attachment.
4. A true fracture is present with significant involvement of the articular surface.
5. A fracture-dislocation of the epiphyseal plate is seen only in children.

The first three patterns can be treated successfully with early splinting with the DIP joint in extension but not hyperextension. Immobilization should continue for 9 weeks, with periodic checkups to monitor the condition of the skin and change the type of splint if necessary. After 9 weeks the splint may be removed to initiate ac-

tive exercises. Aside from exercise activity, the splint should be worn for 3 more weeks. If, after this time, extension at the DIP joint is not maintained, splint usage should continue until it can be maintained.

During the healing phase, athletes are allowed to participate in sports providing that adequate protection is maintained. Ball handlers may require a dorsal splint to function better.

Avulsion of the flexor digitorum profundus typically occurs in football when a tackler grabs an opponent's jersey and sustains forced extension of the finger while he is actively flexing—hence the common designation of jersey finger. This injury most commonly affects the ring finger.

The athlete feels sudden pain in the distal phalanx at onset. The DIP joint will not flex, but this is often initially attributed to soft tissue swelling and tenderness. A small bony fragment may accompany the avulsion.

There is a consensus among physicians that surgical reattachment of the profundus tendon is the treatment of choice. However, athletes may choose to delay this until the end of the season, and in such cases a conservative program of exercises and physiotherapeutic modalities will maintain mobility and flexibility.

After surgical repair has been performed and there has been a 3-week postoperative rest period, active associated exercises for the profundus and superficialis tendons are essential to prevent tendon adherence. The uninjured hand can be used to isolate flexion movements first at the DIP joint, then at the PIP joint.

Boutonnière deformity is the second most common closed tendon injury in the hand. Despite this, early diagnosis of this injury is difficult. Boutonnèire deformity is produced by blunt trauma to the dorsal aspect of the PIP joint or acute flexion of this joint against active resistance. The typical appearance of boutonnière deformity is seen in Figure 12.42.

The injury involves a buttonhole-like split in the extensor hood of the middle phalanx caused by (1) disruption of the central slip of the extensor tendon, and (2) a tear in the triangular ligament (Fig. 12.43). This results in a flexed PIP joint with hyperextension of the DIP joint. After injury the PIP joint assumes a fixed flexion angulation of 15°–30°. The inability of active extension at this joint is often erroneously attributed to joint swelling and pain. If improperly diagnosed, the finger is often splinted to allow slight finger flexion for comfort. Unfortunately, this position (although more comfortable) will ultimately lead to further deformity; hence, accurate diagnosis is imperative.

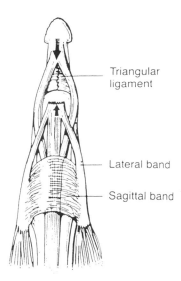

Figure 12.42. In an established boutonnière deformity, flexion deformity of the proximal interphalangeal joint is caused by loss of active extension through the central slip, plus the deforming force of the lateral bands, which now pass volar to the axis of the proximal interphalangeal joint. Intrinsic muscle pull through the lateral bands leads to hyperextension of the distal interphalangeal joint. (Reprinted with permission from DeLee JC, Drez DD. Orthopaedic sports medicine: principles and practice. Philadelphia: WB Saunders, 1994:956.)

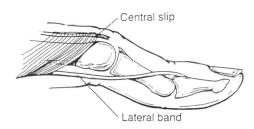

Figure 12.43. Boutonnière deformity is caused by disruption of the central slip of the extensor tendon (short arrow) and tearing of the triangular ligament (long arrow), which in time allows the lateral bands to slip below the axis of the PIP joint. (Reprinted with permission from DeLee JC, Drez DD. Orthopaedic sports medicine: principles and practice. Philadelphia: WB Saunders, 1994;956.)

In acute treatment the PIP joint should be splinted in continuous full extension; the DIP joint should be left free to allow active flexion and passive flexion exercise. The splint should be used for 6 weeks. The athlete is allowed to participate in sports provided he or she is comfortable with the splint and not exposed to situations that could potentially lead to further injury.

Damage to the proximal membranous portion of the volar plate may give rise to a boutonnière appearance, but the extensor hood is intact. This injury is known as a pseudoboutonnière deformity. It is usually created by a hyperextension or twisting injury to the PIP joint.

On examination of pseudoboutonnière deformity a flexion contracture of the PIP joint will be noted. Passive extension of the PIP joint is more resistant than in typical boutonnière deformity. There will be slight hyperextension of the DIP joint.

Static splinting of the PIP joint in extension is maintained for 6 to 8 weeks with this injury, after which active exercises should be initiated. Athletes are allowed to participate in sports with adequate protection. Splinting should be maintained until complete pain-free motion has been restored.

Trigger finger is a condition caused by repeated trauma to the flexor tendon sheath, which can result in inflammation and swelling that restricts the normal gliding of the tendons within their sheath. A small nodule already present in the flexor tendon may be impinged at either the proximal or distal ends of the sheath, giving rise to a snapping sensation or a locking of the finger in flexion or extension.

Trigger finger is treated conservatively by rest with splinting, then progressive range of motion. In some instances cortisone has been injected into the sheath with good success. If the problem persists, surgical intervention may be required.

NERVE COMPRESSION SYNDROMES: WRIST

Nerve entrapment syndromes in the wrist and hand in athletes primarily involve mechanical compression due to repetitive loading or trauma. Rettig (125) posits that the primary lesion of entrapment neuropathies in athletes is vascular compromise (e.g., vasa nervosum) of a segment of nerve. Anoxia of the nerve results in edema that may augment the effects of the initial compression. If compression persists over months, proliferation of fibroblasts will eventually lead to intraneural scarring.

Median Neuropathy

Carpal tunnel syndrome is the most common compression neuropathy at the wrist in athletes. Any sports-related activity that involves repetitive wrist movements and grasping may be associated with this disorder, but it is particularly common in weight lifters.

Clinical features include paresthesia or dysesthesia of the thumb, index, and middle fingers with subjective or objective grip strength weakness. Opponens pollicis weakness is a diagnostic hallmark. Tinel's sign may be positive over the volar wrist, and Phalen's test is usually positive as well.

Myofascial trigger points in the supinator and ECRB can accompany or mimic this syndrome.

These muscles should be examined. Confirmatory evidence is the presence of prolonged median nerve latencies across the wrist through nerve conduction studies.

The presence of forearm or brachial pain that is worse at night is sometimes overlooked. This may be associated with noticeable wrist symptoms, but this again is a common finding in carpal tunnel syndrome.

Treatment consists of cessation of athletic activity and the use of a cock-up wrist splint. It is important for the athlete to wear the splint at night. Neuromuscular massage therapy helps to decongest myofascial involvement at the forearm and may expedite recovery. In acute cases, application of an ice cup or ice pack will minimize pain and inflammation. Electrical stimulation is only indicated in cases of persistent edema or pain (126).

Retinacular release surgery has been used in refractory cases, sometimes with good effect. The author believes that unsuccessful surgeries are often the result of an inaccurate or incomplete diagnosis, typically with failure to identify myofascial trigger points or compressive median neuropathies (e.g., pronator teres syndrome or anterior interosseous nerve syndrome) elsewhere in the upper extremity.

Cyclist's palsy involves palmar neuropathy noted almost exclusively in avid or competitive bicyclists. It does not involve exclusively median neuropathy but is considered here as a separate entity because of its prevalence in sports medicine practice.

Jackson (127) studied 20 cyclists, each of whom rode more than 100 miles weekly; 9 of these 20 cyclists were found to have hand or finger numbness during cycling. These symptoms resolved completely after the ride. Electrodiagnosis was carried out in all cyclists, and in no case was there a positive study. Seven of the cyclists had discomfort that was consistent with a peripheral nerve distribution: four had median nerve involvement and three had ulnar nerve involvement. Jackson concluded that hand position was the causative factor in the development of palmar neuropathies.

The treatment of cyclist's palsy involves simply changing the bicycle to ensure proper fit, changing riding technique to include frequently varying hand positions, and advocating properly padded gloves and handlebars. Cessation of activity for a time in severe cases may also be required.

Ulnar Neuropathy

Guyon's canal syndrome is a compressive neuropathy of the ulnar nerve as it passes through Guyon's canal. It develops primarily in bicyclists but can also result from falls on extended wrists and can accompany other ulnar carpal traumas. In cyclists, this disorder usually occurs as a result of prolonged gripping of the handlebars over long periods (hours to days).

Patients present with paresthesias in the ulnar nerve distribution with a particular complaint of pain in the fifth finger. Examination reveals tenderness over Guyon's canal. Tinel's sign will evoke radiating symptoms into the fifth finger, reproducing the chief complaint. Grip strength may be reduced because 40% of grip is supplied by ulnar-innervated musculature in the hand. The adductor pollicis muscle is ulnar-innervated and, when weak, elicits Froment's sign, wherein the flexor pollicis is substituted for the weak adductor pollicis. The first dorsal interosseous muscle is also innervated by the ulnar nerve and may test weak. Two-point discrimination may be increased in an ulnar-nerve distribution. Allen's test will differentiate nerve compression from a vascular problem such as hypothenar hammer syndrome. The cubital tunnel should be evaluated to exclude compression at this site. TFCC tears may coexist with Guyon's canal syndrome, and examination should extend to the evaluation of this structure.

Treatment includes cessation from the offending activity, splint immobilization, and ice therapy. If symptoms do not diminish rapidly, a baseline and serial EMG can help monitor progress over several weeks or months. If motor deficit persists, serious consideration must be given to decompression of Guyon's canal.

Radial Neuropathy

Wartenberg's syndrome (cheiralgia paresthetica) is compression of the superficial branch of the radial nerve at the dorsoradial aspect of the wrist and can give rise to pain and paresthesias over the dorsoradial aspect of the hand and thumb. This was originally described by Wartenberg in 1932 (128). In athletes, this syndrome is produced by repetitive pronation, supination, and ulnar deviation movements that produce traction or shearing of the superficial branch of the radial nerve. Wrist bands in racket sports actually potentiate this injury, which has also been called handcuff neuropathy when present in those so adorned (129).

Conservative treatment with splinting in forearm supination is recommended if the problem is 6 to 12 months old. More acute injuries benefit from rest, ice, splinting, and appropriate padding during athletic competition (129).

NERVE COMPRESSION SYNDROMES: HAND

Bowler's Thumb (Perineural Neuritis of Ulnar Digital Nerve)

Bowler's thumb is the most common injury involving a digital nerve in the hand in athletes. This syndrome involves repeated compressive trauma of the ulnar digital nerve of the thumb, resulting from the thumb hole of the bowling ball. Perineural fibrosis ensues, reducing the mobility of the nerve and enhancing further compressive forces. Compression may also occur directly to the digital nerve in the web space of the thumb as this space is stretched over the surface of the bowling ball during grip.

The bowler will present with paresthesias along the ulnar aspect of the thumb and in many cases with pain. Examination may reveal swelling or thickening over the base of the thumb at its ulnar and volar aspects, and in advanced cases the fibrotic nerve tissue may be detected as palpable, tender cord of tissue. Tinel's sign over the area is positive. There is no diminution of motor function, although decreased exertion during grip is produced by pain. Two-point discrimination is usually normal but may be increased.

Treatment in the acute stage involves discontinuation of the offending activity, ice, and symptomatic relief with modalities. The thumb hole can be enlarged and finger holes can be drilled closer to the thumb hole. In advanced cases a molded plastic thumb guard can be used during bowling to prevent compression. Symptoms will reduce using the thumb guard, but it may take up to 6 months for full resolution.

Digital Nerve Neuropathy

Branches of the median nerve supply the skin of the index and middle fingers and half of the ring finger as extensions of the median sensory fibers. These interdigital nerves in the palm may be compressed, especially with repetitive trauma to the palm. One reported case in the literature describes this entity in a 16-year-old cheerleader (130). Compression can also occur from phalangeal fracture or inflammation of the MPJ or tendon. Presenting symptoms include pain in one or two fingers exacerbated by lateral hyperextension of the affected digits, and tenderness and dysesthesia over the palmar surfaces between the metacarpals. Abnormal median sensory potentials may be noted with nerve conduction studies. Symptoms abate with cessation of the offending activity.

VASCULAR SYNDROMES

Vascular syndromes usually result from repetitive trauma to the palmar aspect of the hand and wrist, although they occasionally may be associated with a single traumatic event. The injured structures are superficial, and athletes who use their palms to decelerate balls and absorb forces are predisposed to injury of the vasculature.

Examination involves careful history and physical examination with the addition of some special tests. Anamnesis should focus on mechanisms of repeated blunt trauma but should not overlook hand pallor with cold exposure (e.g., Raynaud's), history of smoking (Berger's disease), and other nontraumatic, potentially etiologic factors. Initial inspection should screen for areas of pallor, cyanosis, trophic ischemic changes, and ulcerations at the tip of the digits. Palpation for pulsatile masses is performed in search of aneurysms. Soft, compressible masses may represent hemangioma. Arteriovenous fistula will manifest as a palpable mass with a fluid thrill. Tenderness in a palpable vascular mass suggests thrombosis. Complete examination of the upper extremity pulses beginning at the subclavian artery, together with comparative blood pressure measurements, will complete the vascular examination.

Allen's test is performed by compressing both ulnar and radial arteries and having the patient tightly grip his or her hand repetitively. The patient then relaxes the hand and one of the vessels is released. The hand should blush within 5 seconds or less. A positive test indicates disease or decreased blood flow in the released artery. The test is repeated and the other artery is released. Allen's test should always be performed bilaterally for comparison.

A digital Allen's test has been described in which a similar procedure is performed at the radial and ulnar digital arteries of each digit, looking for blushing of the digit. This can isolate areas of decreased blood flow. Doppler scanning, plethysmography, ultrasound and imaging, and cold testing are also noninvasive methods of assessing blood flow to the hand.

Hypothenar Hammer Syndrome

Hypothenar hammer syndrome has been described in conjunction with judo, karate, lacrosse, hockey, and falls on the athletic field of play. It is caused by either repetitive trauma or a single traumatic episode. It involves damage to the ulnar artery at the area of trauma in the ulnar aspect of the palm. Ulnar artery thrombosis occurs when there is damage only to the intima of the artery. True aneurysm of the ulnar artery results from fusiform swelling of all layers of the arterial wall. A false aneurysm is caused by rupture of the vessel arterial wall with extravasation, organization, and encapsulation of the resulting hematoma (125). Finally, vasospasm of the distal ulnar vessels may occur as a consequence of increased sympathetic tone after injury to the vessel wall.

In hypothenar hammer syndrome, the patient experiences pain and coldness in the fingers secondary to ischemia from ulnar artery thrombosis, aneurysmal dilatation with compromised distal flow, or sympathetic vasospasm as described above. There may be radiation of symptoms into the forearm when repetitive impact loading is the offending activity. Rest pain and night pain are only present in advanced cases and are frequently associated with distal ulcerations of the skin from ischemia.

Ulnar artery aneurysm may present with vascular, neuropathic, or combined symptoms; the ulnar nerve lies in close relation to the artery and expansion of the artery may compress the nerve. The diagnosis of Guyon's canal syndrome has already been described. With concomitant ulnar artery aneurysm, Allen's test will be positive. A negative Tinel's sign at Guyon's canal indicates primary vascular involvement even when neurologic symptoms are present. Examination will include evaluation of pulses, palpation for thrills, and auscultation of the palm for bruits.

Conservative treatment involves rest from the offending activity and observation unless severe ischemic changes are noted. When symptoms are not severe, the use of increased padding in a baseball or handball glove may be all that is necessary to prevent the advancement of symptoms.

Sympathetic vasospasm is common in the baseball pitcher's index finger from local stimulation of the digital sympathetics secondary to digital pressure. Conservative treatment with rest is a advocated. In severe cases vasodilator medications or sympathetic blocks have been advocated.

Repetitive Trauma Lesions and Digital Ischemia

Repetitive palmar concussion is unavoidable for handball players and baseball players. Circulatory problems that result include multiple areas of decreased perfusion of the hands and digits due to vascular injury and subsequent occlusion and narrowing of the digital arteries. Considering that the palms of a baseball catcher must decelerate between 150 and 200 pitches per game (many of which exceed velocities of 90

mph), it is not surprising that less than one half of professional catchers have normal circulation to the left index finger (131). However, circulation is improved through the habitual use of protective padding such as a thick golf or handball glove worn under the catcher's mitt. In a study of handball players, Buckout and Warner (132) found decreased perfusion with thermography in 17 of 22 athletes. The temperature of players' hands were significantly lower than those of a control group. Accumulated playing time was associated with more diminished perfusion.

Conservative management of digital vessel compromise in these athletes involves the incorporation of protective padding into play at all times. If severe, the activity should be discontinued for a time in conjunction with splinting. Return to the sport must always follow appropriate functional progression to prevent reinjury.

OTHER SYNDROMES

Ganglion Cysts

Ganglion cysts have been mentioned above in conjunction with a variety of wrist disorders as a differential diagnostic consideration. Despite its frequent occurrence, its cause is unknown. The dorsal wrist ganglion has been shown to arise from the scapholunate ligament (133), and its palmar counterpart arises from either the scaphotrapezial or radioscaphoid joints (134). A recent study (135) proposes that wrist ganglia are a secondary manifestation of underlying periscaphoid ligamentous injury. When painful wrist symptoms persist after operative excision of the ganglion, underlying static or dynamic scaphoid instability should be suspected. In such an instance, scapholunate dissociation may be present together with DISI pattern instability.

A ganglion cyst inside Guyon's canal can give rise to the ulnar neuropathy of a Guyon's canal syndrome.

Carpal ganglia that are symptomatic are not always palpable. As noted previously, occult wrist ganglions are common. They are diagnosed by exclusion. The patient presenting with an occult ganglion will characteristically describe a vague, intermittent wrist pain aggravated by use (e.g., waxing and waning pattern). Dorsal wrist pain is reproduced by maximum wrist extension with overpressure. Radiographs are negative. Dorsal wrist pain is well localized on palpation, usually to the scapholunate junction.

Anecdotal reports of successful smashing of a dorsal ganglion cyst using a book or other flat object must be discarded. The ganglion cyst is more complex and may signify other pathology within the wrist. Bombastic rupture of the cyst may ignore or create more serious problems, especially in the highly competitive athlete whose wrist and hand function must be preserved carefully. Certainly, this treatment cannot be considered conservative. Furthermore, it is obvious that painful occult ganglia cannot be smashed.

Careful evaluation for all related pathologies is essential. Surgical excision is the treatment most recommended in the sports medicine literature.

Subungual Hematoma

A blood blister under the fingernail or toenail is common. Pressure builds under the nail as the fluid volume of the hematoma increases. Pain from this can hinder full participation in sports. Although sharp hypodermic needles have been recommended to bore through the nail (thereby releasing the hematoma), the pressure required to bore the nail is time-consuming and painful in severe cases. The time-honored method of using the red-hot end of a paper clip is still, in the author's opinion, the most rapid and effective method of releasing pressure under the nail. Several holes can be made, depending on the size of the nail and the underlying hematoma. Care should be taken to clean the nail thoroughly after this procedure is completed. Antibiotic ointment has also been recommended for a few days afterward.

References

1. Yocum YA. Non-operative treatment of elbow problems. Clin Sports Med 1989;8:439–451.
2. Haraldsson S. On osteochondrosis deformans juvenilis capituli humeri including investigation of intra-osseous vasculature in distal humerus. Acta Orthop Scand Suppl 1959;suppl:38.
3. Boyd HB. Tennis elbow. J Bone Joint Surg AM 1973;55:1183–1187.
4. Conrad RW. Tennis elbow: its course, natural history, conservative and surgical management. J Bone Joint Surg 1973;55:1177.
5. Cyriax J. Textbook of orthopaedic medicine. Baltimore: Williams & Wilkins, 1969;1:307–318.
6. Goldie I. Epicondylitis lateralis humeri. Acta Chir Scand 1964; 339(Suppl):3–119.
7. Nirschl RD. Tennis elbow. Orthop Clin North Am 1973;4:787.
8. Stoeckart R, Vleeming A, Snijders CJ. Anatomy of the extensor carpi radialis brevis muscle related to tennis elbow. Clin Biomech 1989;4:210–212.
9. Moore KL. Clinically oriented anatomy. Baltimore: Williams & Wilkins, 1980;827.
10. Kessel L, Rang M. Supracondylar spur of the humerus. J Bone Joint Surg Br 1966;48:765–769.
11. Wilbourn AJ. Electrodiagnostic testing of neurologic injuries in athletes. Clin Sports Med 1990;9:229–245.
12. Hershman E, Wilbourn AJ, Bergfeld JA. Acute brachial neuropathy in athletes. Am J Sports Med 1989;17:655–659.
13. Mills GP. The treatment of tennis elbow. Br Med J 1928;1:12–13.
14. Roles NC, Maudsley RH. Radial tunnel syndrome: resistant tennis elbow as a nerve entrapment. J Bone Joint Surg 1972;54:499–508.
15. Greenspan A, Norman A. The radial head, capitellum view: useful technique in elbow trauma. AJR 1982;138:1186–1188.
16. Kerr R. Diagnostic imaging of upper extremity trauma. Radiol Clin North Am 1989;27:891–908.
17. Blane CE, Kling TF, Andrews JC, et al. Arthrography in the posttraumatic elbow in children. AJR 1984;143:17–21.
18. Singson RD, Feldman F. Rosenberg ZS. Elbow joint: assessment with double-contrast CT arthrography. Radiology 1986;160:167–173.
19. Hudson TM. Elbow arthrography. Radiol Clin North Am 1981;19:227–241.
20. Rogers LF. Radiology of skeletal trauma. New York: Churchill Livingstone, 1982.
21. Franklin PD, Dunlop RW, Whitelaw G, et al. CT of the normal and traumatized elbow. J Comput Assist Tomogr 1988;12:817.
22. Blickman JG, Dunlop RW, Sanzone CF, et al. Is CT useful in the traumatized pediatric elbow? Pediatr Radiol 1990;20:184–185.
23. Hoffer PB, Genant HK. Radionuclide joint imaging. Semin Nucl Med 1976;6:121–137.
24. Moore TM, Klein JP, Patzakis MJ, et al. Results of compression plating of closed Galeazzi fracture. J Bone Joint Surg Am 1985;67:1015–1021.
25. Hughston JC. Fracture of the distal radial shaft: mistakes in management. J Bone Joint Surg Am 1957;39:249–264.
26. Dolan JB, Dell PC. Distal ulnar fracture: a reverse Galeazzi fracture. Surg Rounds Orthop 1987;1:45–47.
27. Watson JT. Fractures of the forearm and elbow. Clin Sports Med 1990;9:59–83.
28. Bado JL. The Monteggia lesion. Clin Orthop 1967;50:71–86.
29. Sarmiento A, Kinman PB, Murphy RB, et al. Treatment of ulnar fractures by functional bracing. J Bone Joint Surg Am 1976;58:1104–1107.
30. Pollock F, Pankovich AM, Prieto JJ, et al. The isolated fracture of the ulnar shaft. J Bone Joint Surg Am 1983;65:339–342.
31. Kvidera D, Dedegana L. Stress fracture of the olecranon: report of two cases and review of literature. Orthop Rev 1983;12:113–116.
32. Torg JS, Moyer RA. Non-union of a stress fracture through the olecranonepiphyseal plate observed in an adolescent baseball pitcher. J Bone Joint Surg Am 1977;59:264–265.
33. Wilkerson RD, Johns JC. Non-union of an olecranon stress fracture in an adolescent gymnast: a case report. Am J Sports Med 1990;18:432–434.
34. Hunter IY, O'Connor GA. Traction apophysitis of the olecranon. Am J Sports Med 1980;8:51.
35. Michelli I. Traction apophysitis. Clin Sports Med 1987;6:389.
36. Kovach J, Baker B, Mosher J. Fracture separation of the olecranon ossification center in adults. Am J. Sports Med 1985; 13:105-113.
37. Arie GB. Biomechanical analysis of the javelin throw. Track Field Q Rev 1980;80:9.
38. Hulkko A, Orava S, Nikula P. Stress fractures of the olecranon in javelin throwers. Int J Sports Med 1986;7:210–213.
39. Waris W. Elbow injuries of javelin-throwers. Acta Chir Scand 1946;93:563–573.
40. Hurley JA. Complicated elbow fractures. Clin Sports Med 1990;9:39–57.
41. Mason JA, Shutkin NM. Immediate active motion treatment for fractures of the head and neck of the radius. Surg Gynecol Obstet 1943;76:731–737.
42. Mason ML. Some observations on fractures of the head of the radius with a review of 100 cases. Br J Surg 1954;42:123–132.

43. Shmueli G, Herold HZ. Compression screwing of displaced fractures of the head of the radius. J Bone Joint Surg Br 1981;63:535–538.

44. Thompson DJ. Comparison of flexion versus extension splinting in the treatment of Mason type I radial head and neck fractures. J Orthop Trauma 1988;2:117–119.

45. Miller KG, Drennan DB, Mavlahn DJ. Treatment of displaced segmental radial head fractures. J Bone Joint Surg Am 1984;63:712–717.

46. Weseley MS, Barenfield PA, Eisenstein HL. Closed treatment of isolated radial head fractures. J Trauma 1983; 23:36–39.

47. Millis MB, Siner I, Hall JE. Supracondylar fractures of the humerus in children: further experience with a study in orthopedic decision-making. Clin Orthop 1988; 188:90–97.

48. Rockwood CA, Wilkins KE, King RE. Fractures in children. 2nd ed. Philadelphia: JB Lippincott, 1984;3.

49. Milch H. Fractures and fracture dislocation of the humeral condyles. J Trauma 1964;4:592–607.

50. Riseborough EJ, Radin FL. Intercondylar fractures of the humerus in adults: a comparison of operative and nonoperative treatment in twenty-nine cases. J Bone Joint Surg Am 1969;51:130–141.

51. Grana WA, Rashkin A. Pitcher's elbow in adolescents. Am J Sports 1980;8:333–336.

52. Papavasihous V. Fracture-separation of the medial epicondylar epiphysis of the elbow joint. Clin Orthop 1982; 171:172.

53. Siske TD. Fractures of the upper extremity. In: Campbell's operative orthopedics. St. Louis: CV Mosby, 1986.

54. Woods GW, Tullos HS. Elbow instability and medial epicondyle fractures. Am J Sports Med 1977;5:23–30.

55. Panner HJ. A peculiar affection of the capitulum humeri resembling Calvé-Perthes disease of the hip. Acta Radiol 1929;10:234.

56. Josefson PO, Gentz C, Johnell O, et al. Surgical versus non-surgical treatment of ligamentous injury following dislocation of the elbow joint. J Bone Joint Surg Am 1987;69:605–608.

57. Boe S, Holst-Nielsen F. Intra-articular entrapment of the median nerve after dislocation of the elbow. J Hand Surg (Br) 1987;12:356–358.

58. Hotchkiss RN. Common disorders of the elbow in athletes and musicians. Hand Clin 1990;6:507–515.

59. Greene CP. The curve ball and the elbow. In: Zarins B, Andrews JR, Carson WG, eds. Injuries to the throwing arm. Philadelphia: WB Saunders, 1985:38–39.

60. Anderson TE, Ciocek J. Specific rehabilitation programs for the throwing athlete. AAOS Instr Course Lect 1989; 38:487–491.

61. Jobe FW, Stark H, Lombardo SJ. Reconstruction of the ulnar collateral ligament in athletes. J Bone Joint Surg Am 1986;68:1158–1163.

62. Woo CC. Traumatic radial head subluxation in young children: a case report and literature review. J Manipulative Physiol Ther 1987;10:191–200.

63. McVay CB. Surgical anatomy. 6th ed. Philadelphia: WB Saunders, 1984;2:1063–1064.

64. Schafer RC, Faye LJ. Motion palpation and chiropractic technic. 2nd ed. Huntington Beach: MPI, 1990:357–359.

65. Mennell J McM. Joint pain. Boston: Little, Brown & Co., 1964:32–90.

66. Duke JB, Tessler RH, Dell PC. Manipulation of the stiff elbow with patient under anesthesia. J Hand Surg (Am) 1991;16:19—24.

67. Goldie I. Epicondylitis lateralis. Acta Chir Scand 1964; 339(Suppl):104–109.

68. Briggs CA, Elliot BG. Lateral epicondylitis: a review of structures associated with tennis elbow. Anat Clin 1985; 7:149–153.

69. Wadsworth TG. Tennis elbow: conservative, surgical, and manipulative treatment. Br Med J 1987;249: 621–624.

70. Kamien M. A rational management of tennis elbow. Sports Med 1990;9:173–191.

71. Dijs H, Mortier G, Driessens M, et al. A retrospective study of the conservative treatment of tennis-elbow. Acta Belg Med Phys 1990;13:73–77.

72. Lundeberg T, Haker E, Thomas M. Effect of laser versus placebo in tennis elbow. Scand J Rehabil Med 1987;19:135–138.

73. Struthers J. On some points in the abnormal anatomy of the arm. Foreign Med Chir Rev 1854;14:170.

74. Jobe FW, Fanton GS. Nerve injuries. In: The elbow and its disorders. Philadelphia: WB Saunders, 1985: 497–501.

75. Buehler MJ, Thayer DT. The elbow flexion test: a clinical test for the cubital tunnel syndrome. Clin Orthop 1986;233:213–216.

76. Upton ARM, McComas AJ. The double crush and nerve entrapment syndromes. Lancet 1973;2:359–362.

77. Dole WA. Thoracic outlet compression syndrome. Arch Surg 1982;117:1437–1445.

78. Jones J. Pitfalls in the management of cubital tunnel syndrome. Orthop Rev 1989;28:36–44.

79. Dellon AL. Review of treatment results for ulnar nerve entrapment at the elbow. J Hand Surg Am 1989;14: 688–700.

80. Royle SG, Burke D. Ulna neuropathy after elbow injury in children. J Pediatr Orthop 1990;10:495–496.

81. Posner MA. Compressive neuropathies of the median and radial nerves. Clin Sports Med 1990;9:343–361.

82. Miller-Breslow A, Terrono A, Millender LH. Nonoperative treatment of anterior interosseous nerve paralysis. J Hand Surg Am 1990;15:493–496.

83. Spinner M. The arcade of and its relationship to posterior interosseous nerve paralysis. J Bone Joint Surg Br 1968;50:809–812.

84. Travell J, Simons D. Myofascial pain and dysfunction: the trigger point manual. Baltimore: Williams & Wilkins, 1983:155.

85. Stevenson TR, Smith DJ. Cuts and scrapes of knees and elbows. Postgrad Med 1989;85:361–365.

86. Hursh LM. Numbers and types of sports injuries. JAMA 1967;199:167.

87. Palmer AK. Triangular fibrocartilage complex lesions: classification. J Hand Surg (Am) 1989;14:594–606.

88. Gunther SF. The carpometacarpal joints. Orthop Clin North Am 1984;15:259.

89. Moran CA. Anatomy of the hand. Phys Ther 1989;69: 1007–1013.

90. Mayfield JK. Wrist ligamentous anatomy and pathogenesis of carpal instability. Orthop Clin North Am 1984; 15:209–216.

91. Mayfield JK, Williams WJ, Erdman AG, et al. Biomechanical properties of human carpal ligaments. Orthop Trans 1979;3:143.

92. Mayfield JK, Johnson RP, Kilcoyne RE. The ligaments of the human wrist and their functional significance. Anat Rec 1976;186:417–428.

93. Weber ER. Concepts governing the rotational shift of the intercalated segment of the carpus. Orthop Clin North Am 1984;15:193–207.

94. Beckenbaugh RD. Evaluation and management of the painful wrist following injury: An approach to carpal instability. Orthop Clin North Am 1984;15:289–306.

95. Jones LA. The assessment of hand function: a critical review of techniques. J Hand Surg (Am) 1989;14: 221–228.

96. Linn MR, Mann FA, Gilula LA. Imaging the symptomatic wrist. Orthop Clin North Am 1990;21:515–543.

97. Giuliani G, Poppi M, Pozzati EP et al. Ulnar neuropathy due to a carpal ganglion: The diagnostic contribution of CT. Neurology 1990;40:1001–1002.

98. Koman LA, Mooney JF, Poehling GG. Fractures and ligamentous injuries of the wrist. Hand Clin 1990;6: 477–491.

99. Sasaki Y, Sugioka S. The pronator quadratus sign: its classification and diagnostic usefulness for injury and inflammation of the wrist. J Hand Surg (Br) 1989;14: 80–83.

100. MacEwan DW. Changes due to trauma in the fat plane overlying the pronator quadratus muscle: a radiologic sign. Radiology 1964;82:879–886.

101. Culver JE. Sports-related fractures of the hand and wrist. Clin Sports Med 1990;9:85–109.

102. Freeland P. Scaphoid tubercle tenderness: a better indicator of scaphoid fractures? Arch Emerg Med 1989;6: 46–50.

103. Chen SC. The scaphoid compression test. J Hand Surg (Br) 1989;14:323–325.

104. Campbell CS. Gamekeeper's thumb. J Bone Joint Surg Br 1955;37:148–149.

105. Moberg E. The use of traction treatment for fractures of phalanges and metacarpals. Acta Chir Scand 1950;99: 341–352.

106. Stark HH. Troublesome fractures and dislocations of the hand. AAOS Instr Course Lect 1970;19:130–149.

107. Green DP, OBrien GT. Classification and management of carpal dislocations. Clin Orthop 1980;149:55.

108. Lewis DC, Johnson SR. Spontaneous dislocation of the lunate in a weightlifter. Injury: Br J Accident Surg 1990;21:252–253.

109. Rainey RK, Plautsch ML. Traumatic dislocation of the distal radioulnar joint. Orthopedics 1985;8:896–900.

110. Francobandiera C, Maffulli N, Lepore L. Distal radioulnar joint dislocation, ulna volar in a female body builder. Med Sci Sports Exerc 1990;22:155–158.

111. Garcia-Elias M, Dobyns JH, Cooney WP, et al. Traumatic axial dislocations of the carpus. J Hand Surg (Am) 1989;14:446–457.

112. Mandelbaum BR, Bartolozzi AR, Davic CA, et al. Wrist pain syndrome in the gymnast. Am J Sports Med 1989;17:305–317.

113. Cerofolini E, Luchetti R, Pederzini L, et al. MR evaluation of triangular fibrocartilage complex tears in the wrist: comparison with arthrography and arthroscopy. J Comp Assist Tom 1990;14:963–967.

114. Gilula LA, Weeks PM. Posttraumatic ligamentous instabilities of the wrist. Radiology 1978;129:641–651.

115. Bryan RS, Dobyns JH. Fractures of the carpal bones other than lunate and navicular. Hand Clin 1987;3:135.

116. Barry MS, Kettner NW, Pierre-Jerome C. Carpal instability: Pathomechanics and contemporary imaging. Chiro Sports Med 1991;5:38–44.

117. Pin PG, Young L, Gilula LA, et al. Management of chronic lunotriquetral ligament tears. J Hand Surg (Am) 1989;14:77–83.

118. Hankin FM, Peel SM. Sport-related fractures and dislocations in the hand. Hand Clin 1990;6:429–453.

119. Palmer AK, Linscheid RL. Chronic recurrent dislocations of the proximal interphalangeal joint of the finger. J Hand Surg 1978;3:95–97.

120. de Quervain F. Ueber eine form von chronischer tendovaginitis. Correspondenz-Blatt Fur Schweizer Aerzte 1895;25:389–394.

121. Grundberg AB, Reagan DS. Pathologic anatomy of the forearm: intersection syndrome. J Hand Surg (Am) 1985;10:299–302.

122. Ritter MA, Inglis AE. The extensor indicis proprius syndrome. J Bone Joint Surg Am 1969;51:1645.

123. Stern PJ. Tendinitis, overuse syndromes, and tendon injuries. Hand Clin 1990;6:467–476.

124. McCue FC, Mayer V. Rehabilitation of common athletic injuries of the hand and wrist. Clin Sports Med 1989;8: 731–776.

125. Rettig AC. Neurovascular injuries in the wrists and hands of athletes. Clin Sports Med 1990;9:389–417.

126. Wolf SL. Electrotherapy. New York: Churchill Livingstone, 1981:179–182.

127. Jackson DL. Electrodiagnostic studies of the median and ulnar nerves in cyclists. Phys Sportsmed 1989;17:137–148.

128. Wartenberg R. Cheiralgia paraesthetic (isolierte neuritis des Ramus superficialis nervi radialis). Z Ges Neurol Psychiatry 1932;141:145–155.

129. Dorfman LJ, Jayram AR. Handcuff neuropathy. JAMA 1978;239:957.

130. Shields RW Jr, Jacobs IB. Medial palmar digital neuropathy in a cheerleader. Arch Phys Med Rehabil 1986; 67:824–826.

131. Lowrey CW, Chadwick RO, Waltman EN. Digital vessel trauma from repetitive impact in baseball catchers. J Hand Surg 1976;1:236–238.

132. Buckout BC, Warner MA. Digital perfusion of handball players. Am J Sports Med 1980;8:206–207.

133. Angelides AC, Wallace PF. The dorsal ganglion of the wrist: its pathogenesis, gross anatomy, and surgical treatment. J Hand Surg 1976;1:228–335.

134. Carstam N, Eiken O, Andren L. Osteoarthritis of the trapezioscaphoid joint. Acta Orthop Scand 1968;39:354–358.

135. Watson HK, Rogers WD, Ashmead D. Reevaluation of the cause of the wrist ganglion. J Hand Surg Am 1989; 14:812–817.

Athletic Injuries of the Pelvis, Hip, and Thigh

Stephen M. Perle

Most of the forces generated to walk or run are created by muscles that have their origin or insertion on the femur or pelvic bones (1, 2). The resulting forces are translated into motion at the acetabulum and, to a lesser degree, at the sacroiliac joint. This alone makes the pelvis, hips, and thighs very important areas in sports medicine. This chapter reviews mechanisms of sports injuries in these areas and reviews the features of a full clinical evaluation.

CLINICAL EVALUATION

History

AGE

Age is an important factor in the diagnosis of athletic injuries of this region because of susceptibility to certain problems at certain ages.

Hip joint pain in a young boy should always bring Legg-Calvé-Perthes disease (ages 3 to 12) and a slipped femoral capital epiphysis (ages 10 to 15) into the differential diagnosis (3). However, a slipped femoral capital epiphysis can present with symptoms referable exclusively to the knee (4). Osteochondritis dissecans is a possible cause of unilateral hip pain. Bilateral hip pains with no known trauma that may be associated with a fever and fatigue suggest the possibility of juvenile rheumatoid arthritis (younger than age 16) (3).

Alternatively, in the older athlete (ages 20 to 60), hip pain with no known trauma is more likely to be the result of rheumatoid arthritis (3) or degenerative joint disease (DJD) (3). However, DJD may only be an incidental finding on a radiograph and may not really contribute to the patient's symptoms (5–7).

Deep bone pain raises suspicions of neoplastic growths, both benign and malignant. Benign neoplasia commonly seen in this region are simple bone cyst (ages 3 to 14 with symptoms only after fracture), aneurysmal bone cyst (ages 5 to 20), giant cell tumor (ages 20 to 40), and osteoid osteoma (ages 10 to 25). Osteosarcoma (ages 10 to 25) and Ewing's sarcoma (ages 10 to 25) are the most likely cancers that may present in an adolescent complaining of bone pain. In the older athlete (older than 40), metastatic bone tumors are the most likely type of malignancy to present with deep bone pain (3).

Lower back and leg pain may suggest ankylosing spondylitis (ages 15 to 35) and osteitis condensans ilii (ages 20 to 40), usually seen in adults (3). DJD (in those 40 and older) (3) of the sacroiliac joint can also present with lower back and leg pain (8).

Finally, children (ages 3 to 10) with pain of muscle origin at secondary epiphyses are opened to the suspicion of osteochondrosis. Typical locations include iliac crest, ischial apophysis, ischiopubic synchondrosis, symphysis pubis, femur, and greater trochanter (3).

GENDER

There are differences in injury rates between males and females for certain types of injuries and certain body parts.

Women have a higher risk for stress fracture (9) due to lower bone density (10). Pelvic stress fractures are much more common in women, and this may be due to the fact that the female pelvis is smaller and less dense than the male pelvis (10–12). Women are more prone to musculotendinous problems around the hip, such as trochanteric bursitis and iliotibial tendinitis due to increased Q angles associated with the wider female pelvis (10–13). Except in the sport of waterskiing, the female athlete's genitalia are much less prone to injury than the male's (14).

In children, boys tend to have a higher rate of injury due to increased participation in higher risk sports (15). Additionally, some of the disease entities mentioned above in relation to age have a gender predilection (Table 13.1).

HISTORICAL FACTORS

Many patients will present with a reinjury or with what they may believe is a new problem but is either a recurrent problem or a direct or indirect result of a previous injury (16). This is par-

Table 13.1.   Gender and Age Incidence of Conditions (3)

Condition	Gender	Age
Legg-Calvé-Perthes disease	5:1 ♂:♀	3–12
Juvenile rheumatoid arthritis	Systemic-1:1 ♂:♀, polyarticular-1:2 ♂:♀ monoarticular-1:3 ♂:♀	<16
Rheumatoid arthritis	<Age 40 1:3 ♂:♀ >Age 40 1:1 ♂:♀	20–60
Primary degenerative joint disease	♂:♀ 1:10	>40
Simple (unicameral) bone cyst	♂:♀ 2:1	3–14
Aneurysmal bone cyst	65% of cases ♀	5–20
Giant cell tumor	♂:♀ 2:3 Malignant type ♂:♀ 3:1	20–40
Osteoid osteoma	♂:♀ 2:1	10–25
Osteogenic sarcoma	♂:♀ 2:1	10–25
Ewing's sarcoma	♂:♀ 1:2	10–25
Metastatic bone tumors		>40
Osteochondroses	♂>♀	3–10
Ankylosing spondylitis	♂:♀ 10:1	15–35
Osteitis condensans ilii	♂:♀ 1:9 Mostly multiparous females	20–40
Reiter's syndrome	♂:♀ 50:1	18–40

ticularly true in females, as girlhood injuries are often not properly rehabilitated because girls are "too fragile and God will heal it" (17). Therefore, it is important to discover the history of both sports-related and non–sports-related injuries.

Physical Examination of the Pelvis, Hip, and Thigh

INSPECTION

Posture

Levels of the anterior superior iliac spine (ASIS) and posterior superior iliac spine (PSIS) and greater trochanters should be checked. Is the athlete hyperlordotic, hypolordotic, or normolordotic? Owing to uneven weight distribution from leg length differences, the long leg side is prone to overuse injuries due to increased forces at foot-plant (18).

Gait

Is it antalgic? Patients should be watched while doing their sporting-type movements, that is, running, jumping, race walking, cutting, swinging, kicking, clubbing, or batting. Is there any obvious rotation of the hips or aberrant movement? It should be determined if the abnormal movements are a compensation due to the injury or "normal" and a cause of injury (18).

Inflammation

Obvious signs of inflammation (tumor, rubor, calor, dolor), swelling, redness, and ecchymosis as well as apparent muscle tone (visible signs of spasm or atrophy) should be checked. The Q angle should be measured (18).

Table 13.2.   Orthopedic Tests of the Pelvis, Hip, and Thigh (19–21)

Allis' sign	Minor's sign
Approximation test	Nachlas' test
Belt test	Nachlas' knee flexion test
Ely's test	Neri's bowing test
Erichsen's test	Ober test
Freiberg's sign	Paces sign
Gaenslen's test	Patrick's Fabere test
Gapping test	Piedallu's sign
Gauvain's sign	Piriformis myofascitis test
Gillis' test	Sacral apex pressure (prone springing) test
Goldthwait's test	Sacroiliac-lumbosacral differential test
Hibb's test	
Hip abduction stress test	
Internal femoral torsion signs	Sacroiliac rocking (knee-to-shoulder) test
Kemp's test	
Laquerre's test	Smith-Peterson test
Lasegue's differential sign	Squish test
Lasegue's test	
Lewin's standing test	Thoracolumbar range of motion
Lewin-Gaenslen test	Toe-to-mouth test
Mazion's step-flex test	Trendelenburg test
Mennell's test	Yeoman's test

PALPATION

The region should be palpated, feeling for muscle tone, myofascial trigger points, areas of tenderness, and areas of increased or decreased temperature (18).

ORTHOPEDIC TESTS

A complete discussion of how to perform and the meaning of orthopedic tests is out of the purview of this text. Table 13.2 (19–21) lists the orthopedic tests that pertain to this region of the body.

RANGES OF MOTION

Hip

Passive and active range of motion (ROM) of the hip joint should be checked, as should bilateral symmetry in ROM (18).

A decreased active ROM due to pain with a normal passive ROM suggests a dysfunction in the prime mover in the restricted range. Pain on passive ROM in the opposite direction is confirmation. Pain on isometric contraction of the prime mover is further confirmation of a muscular dysfunction—either an acute or chronic strain or tear or a myofascial trigger point of the prime mover (22, 23).

Loss of bilateral symmetry can be the cause or the result of the patient's complaint.

Thoracolumbar

This ROM should also be examined because sacroiliac dysfunction can affect this (24).

JOINT PLAY EXAMINATION

Sacroiliac

The examiner should check for parallel sway. This is done by the examiner's placing thumbs on both the patient's PSIS with the patient's legs parallel. The patient laterally flexes to the left and right. The examiner should check to see that an imaginary line connecting PSIS remains parallel to the floor. If not, this is suggestive of sacroiliac joint dysfunction requiring manipulation (24). The Gillet test (Fig. 13.1) should be performed to deter-

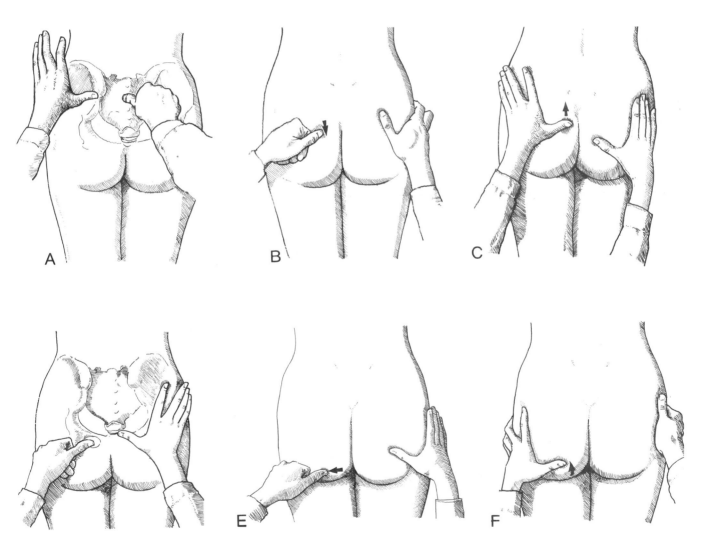

Figure 13.1. Gillet test. **A–C.** The right thumb contacts the second sacral tubercle, and the left thumb contacts the left PSIS. **B.** The patient flexes the left hip greater than 90°. The PSIS should move before S2; if not, there is left upper sacroiliac joint flexion restriction. **C.** The patient flexes the right hip greater than 90°. The PSIS should move before S2; if not, there is left upper sacroiliac joint extension restriction. **D–E.** The right thumb contacts the second sacral tubercle, and the left thumb contacts the left ischial tuberosity. **E.** The patient flexes the left hip greater than 90°. The ischial tuberosity should move before S2; if not, there is left lower sacroiliac joint flexion restriction. **F.** The patient flexes the right hip greater than 90°. The ischial tuberosity should move before S2; if not, there is left lower sacroiliac joint extension restriction. Repeat as above to right sacroiliac, switching right and left above.

mine what specific sacroiliac joint restriction needs manipulation (24, 25).

Hip

There are nine different motions in the joint play examination of the hip. They are as follows.

1. Long-axis extension (Fig. 13.2).
2. Extension (Fig. 13.3).
3. Flexion (Fig. 13.4).
4. Posteroanterior (PA) glide (Fig. 13.5).
5. Posterior joint play (Fig. 13.6).
6. External rotation (Fig. 13.7).
7. Internal rotation (Fig. 13.8).
8. Flexion-adduction (Fig. 13.9).
9. Lateral distraction (Fig.13.10) (26–29).

NEUROLOGIC TESTS

The only applicable neurologic tests are tests of sensation, motor strength, and proprioception sense in the hip (30). However, other neurologic tests such as the patellar reflex or cerebellar

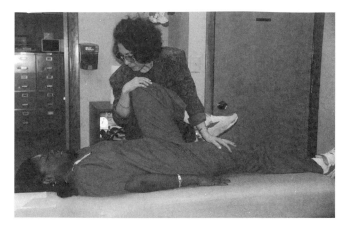

Figure 13.4. Hip flexion joint play. The examiner flexes the patient's hip maximally.

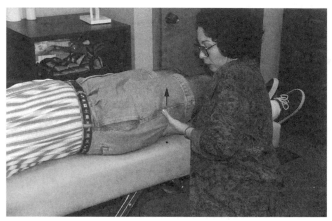

Figure 13.5. Hip PA glide joint play. The examiner applies an anteriorly directed force at the hip joint.

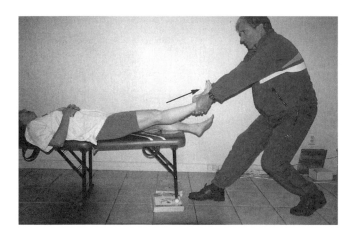

Figure 13.2. Hip long axis extension joint play. The patient's ischial tuberosity is on the cephalad edge of the pelvic section of the table. The examiner assesses joint play in the hip while pulling the long axis.

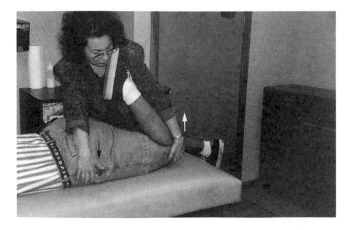

Figure 13.3. Hip extension joint play. The examiner extends the contralateral thigh while pushing anteriorly with the heel of the hand at the joint.

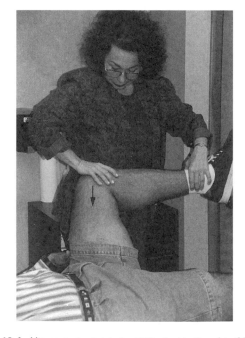

Figure 13.6. Hip posterior joint play. With the hip flexed to 90°, the examiner pushes along the femur posteriorly.

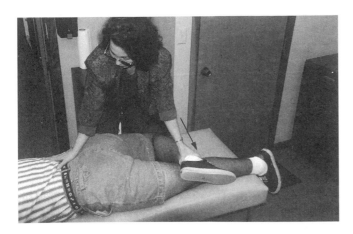

Figure 13.7. Hip external rotation joint play. The examiner externally rotates the hip by pushing on the lower leg (if the patient has a patent knee) with the patient prone.

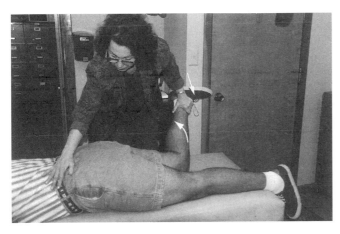

Figure 13.8. Hip internal rotation joint play. The examiner internally rotates the hip by pushing on the lower leg (if the patient has a patent knee) with the patient prone.

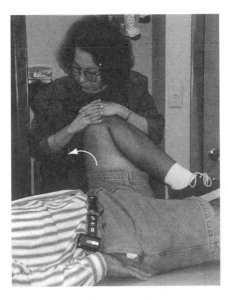

Figure 13.9. Hip flexion-adduction joint play. Force is directed posteriorly through the femur, while the femur is moved in an arc from 90° of flexion to 140° and into full adduction.

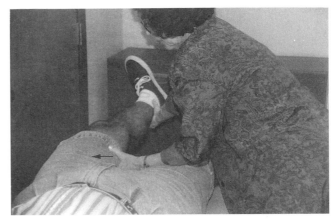

Figure 13.10. Hip lateral distraction joint play. The examiner pushes the femur from medial to lateral.

tests may be rendered abnormal when joint and muscle dysfunction is present.

DIAGNOSIS BY SELECTIVE TENSION

The concept of diagnosis by selective tension was developed by Cyriax (31). It has been refined and made more accessible by Hammer (32). For a more detailed discussion please refer to either text.

Diagnostic Imaging

RADIOGRAPHY

Standard plain film views of the region include anteroposterior (AP) pelvis, AP lateral sacrum, AP and lateral coccyx, AP hip and frog leg view, AP and lateral femur (3). Other more specialized studies will be discussed with the appropriate conditions.

Laboratory Assessment

Laboratory assessment is only indicated when there is a suspicion that the athlete's condition is the result of an underlying systemic disease. An example would be the ordering of a rheumatoid panel of blood tests if an arthritic disease process is suspected.

Physiologic Tests

ELECTRONEURODIAGNOSTIC STUDIES

These are only needed if there is a suspicion that a nerve has been injured, as in meralgia paresthetica (30) or disc herniation.

MUSCLE TESTING

Manual Muscle Testing

Muscle testing is a useful diagnostic procedure that can help determine which specific muscle the athlete has injured. The injured muscle may still test as +3, but if the athlete complains of pain, it is probably still involved. Manual muscle testing also differentiates between ligamentous and tendinous injuries. Ligament injuries will not be tender during a manual muscle test (18).

Mechanical Muscle Testing

Muscle testing using any of the various instruments on the market will provide the physician and athlete with a quantitative assessment of the extent of injury and the progress of rehabilitation. This can be done by comparing injured with uninjured sides. Also, the athlete can be compared with normative ratios of strength of antagonist muscles (33, 34). Devices that test throughout the full ROM would seem to be most appropriate for a thorough assessment of degree of injury and status of rehabilitation; tests of isometric strength are joint-angle specific and therefore provide limited information about the entire ROM (35).

ABSORPTIOMETRY

In patients who have multiple stress fractures or multiple occurrences of stress fractures, absorptiometry is a useful tool to determine absolute bone density. This will let the physician decide if the stress fractures are the result of an early case of osteoporosis or the result of some type of training error (36).

SPECIFIC INJURIES

Stress Fractures/Stress Reaction

TERMINOLOGY

Stress fractures were first described in the medical literature as march fractures by Briethaupt in 1855, who found them in Prussian army recruits (37). The medical literature shows a trend toward new terminology in relation to the condition commonly referred to as a stress fracture. The new term is stress reaction, coined by Jackson et al. (38). This replaces stress fracture to describe a condition in which plain film radiographs are normal but there is a positive bone scan (9, 38, 39). One might think of stress reactions as a bone strain, analogous to a muscle strain (40). A stress fracture is then a microfracture seen on plain film radiographs and on bone scan (9, 38, 39). In this chapter, the term stress reaction will be used to describe this condition whether or not there is plain film evidence of a fracture.

PELVIS

Mechanism of Injuries

A few authors have proposed that pelvic stress reactions, as opposed to stress reactions in other bones, are the result of tensile forces associated with running rather than compressive forces. The alternating phases of running with adductors, extensors, and flexors pulling on the pubic ramus create the tensile stress that results in pelvic stress reactions (11, 41, 42). The added stress of changes in training (added mileage or hill training), surface, or shoes (41); errors in training (40); or leg length differences (43) may be the proximate cause for the stress reaction.

Clinical Features

Wachsmuth reported the first case of a pubic stress fracture in three military recruits in 1937. Stress reactions of the pubic arch in athletes, however, were not reported until 1978 (40, 43). Pelvic stress reactions are not common, with a reported incidence of 0.3 to 2.4% of all stress reactions, but the frequency is increasing (44–47). They are seen more often in women than in men (11, 12, 46, 48). The new prevalence of these stress reactions is believed to be due to the increased number of women participating in jogging and marathon racing (43) and the increased number of runners overall (9). Running is the largest single cause of stress reactions (40). Among runners, pelvic stress reactions occur most often to the noncompetitive recreational runner (46) and account for only 1.25% of all runners' stress reactions (45). Pelvic stress reactions often occur in athletes participating in jumping sports, such as basketball (49), but also in hockey (50), bowling, and gymnastics (51).

The patient's history is important in making an accurate diagnosis, with particular attention paid to changes in training, running surface, and running shoes (40, 41). The athlete will usually relate a history of pain after activity (41), which may be a dull ache (52). The pain is typically relieved by rest, but premature resumption of activity can lead to early and intense recurrence of pain. Stress reaction commonly causes the athlete to limp (41). Micheli suggests that a stress reaction must be suspected in any athlete who has activity-related, persistent pain (53). Many athletes will have what Noakes et al. have termed the positive standing sign—that is, they cannot stand unsupported or have discomfort or frank pain on the affected side while pulling on their pants (52). The symptoms are usually local to the area of the stress reaction but can spread to the inguinal, peroneal, or adductor regions (41), buttocks (43), anterior hip, or anterior thigh (54).

Most pelvic stress reactions occur at the junction of the ischium and the inferior pubic ramus (41, 45). Marymount et al. reported on four young athletes with unusual location for stress reaction—the sacroiliac joint. Three patients were teenagers and one was 10 years of age. All had pain on extension at the iliac apophysis or sacroiliac joint, which caused changes in the athlete's gait. These children participated in the shot put, sprints, tennis, gymnastics, or ballet (39). There is also a case report of a 50-year-old runner with stress reaction of the sacroiliac joint referring pain to the buttocks (51).

Typically, pain is produced during contraction of any muscles in the area of the stress reaction (41, 42, 44). There is also excruciating deep bone pain on palpation over the site of the stress reaction (41, 42, 52). The symptoms of a pelvic stress reaction can frequently mimic the symptoms of other running-related problems such as adductor muscle strains, adductor tendinitis, trochanteric bursitis, tenoperiostitis of the hamstrings, DJD, referred pain from the lumbar spine or the sacroiliac joints (41), muscle tears in the groin and hamstring, osteitis pubis, and avulsion fractures of the adductor or hamstring muscles (43, 45).

Testing Strategy

Radiographs taken soon after the development of a pelvic stress reaction generally show no signs (9, 41, 52). Radiographs that are taken late in the natural history of stress reaction can show callus formation that may resemble osteosarcoma (41).

Radiographs are much less sensitive, specific, and accurate in diagnosing stress reactions than bone scans (55, 56). Therefore, it has been suggested by Matheson et al. (40) that technetium-99m bone scan should be the only imaging modality used (Fig. 13.11). Patients who have multiple stress reactions or a history of repeated stress reactions should have their bone density measured. The best test is dual beam absorptiometry (36).

The differential diagnosis of pelvic stress reaction should be strongly considered in any female runner who presents with pain in and around the pelvic girdle, anterior thigh, groin, or hip that is brought on by activity and relieved by rest (54).

Milgrom et al. (57) reported the case of an Israeli soldier who had 13 different sites of stress reaction. This case is of interest because some of his stress reactions healed during the time he was training and developing more stress reactions. This and other cases of multiple sites of stress reactions in a single athlete suggest that full body bone scans, rather than regional scans, may be indicated for all suspected cases of stress reaction (56).

In juveniles, bone scans are not helpful in differentiating stress reaction or fracture from infection, malignancy, or osteoid osteoma, as all these conditions will have positive findings when scanned. Systemic signs of fever, leukocytosis, and lethargy should help make the diagnosis of infection. Malignant conditions may be differentiated from stress fracture by tomograms or serial radiographs over a 6-week period (58).

Treatment

The basis of treatment of a pelvic stress reaction is rest (43, 52). However, stress reactions

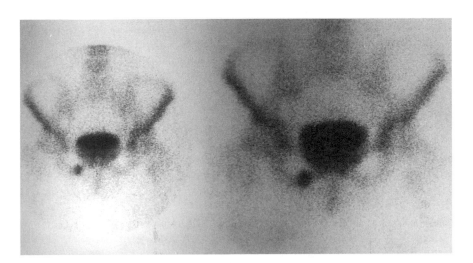

Figure 13.11. Pelvic stress reaction. Technetium-99m bone scan shows a hot spot in the inferior pubic ramus in a female long-distance runner. (Courtesy of Jerry Lubliner, M.D.)

and fractures have been known to heal while the athlete continues to train vigorously (57). This fact brings into doubt most theories for the causes of stress reaction/fracture. Even so, rest is still the treatment of choice. It is rare that rest will require more than the cessation of weight-bearing exercise (called "relative rest"). Some cases will require the use of crutches for a short period (43). In addition, Mills et al. have demonstrated that microcrystalline hydroxyapatite will speed the healing of fractures (59). This type of supplement might then be indicated in the treatment of stress reactions. There are rare occasions when a pelvic stress reaction progresses to become a complete fracture (43). Delayed union can also occur in pelvic stress fractures when the athlete continues to train (60).

Generally, the athlete can and should continue some sort of exercise program during the resting phase of the treatment to maintain cardiovascular fitness. The athlete may ride an exercise bicycle, swim, walk, or run in a pool or use a nonjarring exercise like the cross-country skiing simulator (Nordic track). One of the safest exercises is an upper body ergometer (60, 61). Pain is unfortunately the only guide to determine the appropriateness of a particular exercise (62).

Rehabilitation

The only consideration in rehabilitation is that the athlete must return gradually to the normal training regimen. Too rapid resumption of training can result in a new stress reaction/fracture (60).

Prognosis

Generally, cases of pelvic stress fracture/reaction will require 2 or months of rest to resolve (46, 52).

Prevention

Because it is generally accepted that pelvic stress reactions are the result of avulsive forces (11, 41, 42), these forces should be minimized. Janda has shown that the hamstrings, quadriceps, tensor fascia lata, short adductors, and iliopsoas have a tendency toward muscle tightness. This pathophysiologic condition must be addressed as part of a program of prevention for pelvic stress reactions (63, 64). According to Mennell, muscles that cross a joint that lacks normal joint play will become hypertonic (28). Logically, these joints should be manipulated to restore normal joint play and thereby reduce the hypertonicity (65–67). In addition, muscles that harbor myofascial trigger points are also tight

and should be treated appropriately to remove the trigger points (68).

Prevention for all athletes should also include a proper training schedule—one that does not put excessive stress on the athlete's body too quickly. In addition, for female athletes, prevention must include maintenance of bone density by avoiding behaviors that contribute to calcium loss, such as excessive intake of animal protein, insufficient calcium intake (69, 70), or excessive phosphorus (69) or alcohol intake (70). Studies have shown that oral microcrystalline hydroxyapatite can increase, or prevent further loss of, bone density in osteoporotic patients, even after menopause (71–73), in the presence of some disease states (74–76) and with the use of corticosteroids (75–77).

FEMORAL

Mechanism of Injury

The first reported case of a femoral stress reaction was described by Blecher in 1905 (78). Like pelvic stress reactions, femoral stress reactions are thought to be the result of training errors, poor running form, changing running shoes, or changing running surface (36). As opposed to pelvic stress reactions, it is the compressive forces that cause femoral stress reactions (11). During walking, these forces in the femur are 6.4 times body weight; during running, these forces are estimated to be 10 to 20 times body weight (79). As a result, femoral stress reactions are associated with jumping sports (49), which have obviously greater compressive forces. Stress reactions of the femoral neck are associated with hockey (50), ballet, long-distance running, and gymnastics (51), whereas stress reactions in the femoral shaft are most associated with long-distance running (51). Subtrochanteric stress reactions may be due to avulsive forces on the insertion of the vastus medialis or adductor brevis muscles (36).

Femoral stress reactions are more prevalent among older athletes (40) and are among the most common locations for stress reactions among female athletes (80).

Stress reactions/fractures have a higher incidence in the femur than in the pelvis. There is no agreement in the literature as to the most common location for femoral stress reactions (9, 36, 45–47, 58, 60, 81). The incidences have been reported to range from 2% to 34% (9, 36, 44, 80) for all locations of femoral stress reactions, 1.3% to 2.4% for stress reactions of the femoral neck (44, 46), and 1.7% to 3.8% for the femoral shaft (44, 46, 47).

The 34% figure is from studies done by the Israeli army. This very high incidence is believed to be due to a different testing strategy used by the Israelis, who used bone scans rather than plain film radiography, for an initial imaging modality. This was due to their finding that between 33% and 69% of all femoral stress reactions are asymptomatic (9) and 50% will never show any changes on plain film radiography (60). This gives further evidence to the assertion that a hot spot on a bone scan, signifying a stress reaction, may simply be evidence that the bone was strained from overuse or misuse, similar to soft tissue strain etiology.

Clinical Features

The predominant symptom in femoral neck stress reactions is groin pain, but pain referral to the anterior thigh or knee may be present (78, 79, 82). The pain tends to be characterized as achy and is not well localized (44, 79). This pain may be present only with weight-bearing and result in an antalgic gait. The athlete will usually be pain-free when resting, and symptoms will worsen with increased activity (44, 78, 82). Symptoms may include an aching hip on the first steps after resting (78, 79). There may be pain and/or a limitation of the extreme ranges of hip motion, especially internal rotation (79, 82, 83) or flexion (79). The athlete should be questioned carefully about symptoms in both legs as bilateral femoral stress reactions have been reported (57, 82, 84). Patients are very often asymptomatic (9, 82) and present only after complete fracture (82).

There is sometimes tenderness over the anterior aspect of the hip (40, 79, 82). Pain can often be elicited by percussion over the greater trochanter with a fist (79, 82). A cavus foot is a common finding in patients with femoral stress reactions (40).

Stress fractures of the femoral neck have been categorized by Burrow as transverse and compressive. The compressive type is characterized by a small crack on the inferior surface of the femoral neck. It is the more common type in the pediatric or adolescent patient and rarely needs any treatment. Conversely, the transverse type shows initially a haze of internal callus and then a minute crack on the superior surface of the femoral neck. There is often pain and limping (85). Most importantly, however, this type will very often progress to a complete fracture with displacement and should, when first diagnosed, be considered a surgical emergency and referred for reduction and internal fixation (60, 79, 82, 85).

Diagnosis of stress reactions of the femoral shaft is more difficult because of a lack of symptoms and physical examination findings. There is usually a complete pain-free ROM around both the hip and knee. Athletes will complain of mild deep thigh soreness, usually of insidious onset (60, 86).

Pain can sometimes be elicited by "bending" the femur or by hanging the leg over a table with support only halfway along the thigh (83). Johnson et al. have dubbed this test the fulcrum test. It is performed by having the athlete sit on a table with the lower leg hanging off the edge of the table. The examiner places one forearm under the affected thigh. The examiner's free hand is placed on the athlete's knee, and downward pressure is applied. A positive test produces pain, usually sharp and possibly apprehension. The location of the stress reaction is positively correlated with the location along the femur where the test is positive (87). These athletes are often misdiagnosed as having quadriceps strain (86), muscle cramps, or charley horse (79).

Testing Strategy

Initial physical examination in suspected cases should include the fulcrum test (87). Plain radiographs may demonstrate femoral stress fracture (46), but 33% will have no findings early in the condition and 50% with positive findings on bone scan will never show radiographic evidence of the stress reaction. Plain film radiography is, however, more specific for stress fracture than bone scans (60), although a stress reaction may be confused with the appearance of osteogenic sarcoma (58) or a femoral neck osteoid osteoma (85). If there is no demonstrable stress fracture on radiographs and a high degree of suspicion for stress reactions exists, then technetium bone scan should be performed (58).

The reader is referred back to the paragraph regarding diagnosing stress fractures in children in the section on pelvic stress fractures.

Treatment

Except as mentioned above, for the transverse type of femoral neck stress fracture (which should be considered a surgical emergency), treatment is to avoid excessive stress to the bone by using crutches if needed or simply avoiding vigorous activity that will bring on symptoms and delay healing (83, 85). The use of microcrystalline hydroxyapatite nutritional supplement as discussed previously may also aid in treatment (59).

Rehabilitation

Because less stress is applied to the femur (as opposed to the pelvis) by muscular action alone, athletes with femoral stress fractures generally can continue their training on a bicycle or in a pool. They too are governed by symptoms but are less likely to need to use an upper body ergometer to maintain cardiovascular fitness (60).

Prognosis

The average case will resolve in 8 weeks (40), but many will require more than 2 months (46).

Prevention

As stated previously, subtrochanteric stress fractures are thought to be the result of avulsive forces from the vastus medialis and adductor brevis muscle (36), and this site is considered by some to be the most common site for femoral shaft stress fractures (60). Janda has shown that muscle tightness of both the short adductors and the quadriceps is common (63, 64). Prevention of this type of stress reaction should center on proper stretching of the involved muscles. Muscles that harbor myofascial trigger points will also be tight (68). These trigger points must be treated. In addition, Mennell has stated that muscles that cross a joint that does not have normal joint play motions will become hypertonic (65–67). The previously discussed guidelines concerning preventive training schedules also apply in this case.

SACRUM

Stress reactions of the sacrum are rare. They may present with pain that radiates to the groin or gluteal region. Definitive diagnosis can be made by technetium bone scan. Treatment should be protected weight bearing (88).

Fractures

PELVIC

Mechanism of Injuries

Fractures of the pelvis are rare in the athletic setting (89–91) and are generally only seen as a result of major trauma from automobile and motorcycle-racing accidents (11). They are also seen in equestrian events, rodeo (11), skiing (91), and mountain climbing (86). Few fractures of the iliac wing due to direct trauma have been reported in tackle football (92).

Clinical Features

Generally, after pelvic fracture, the patient is unable to bear weight. A typical mechanism of injury is an anterior to posterior force, a laterally directed blow over the buttock, or shear forces from a fall (11). Usually, fractures of the pelvis are in multiple sites (93) except in children (92). There may be a history of inability to void, numbness, tingling, or weakness in the lower extremity. The patient should be evaluated for intraabdominal bleeding (11).

Types of Pelvic Fractures

Pelvic fractures are classified as stable or unstable. A stable fracture is a fracture of one site, usually the inferior or superior ischial ramus, and does not disrupt the hemipelvis. An unstable fracture indicates more than one fracture site (92, 94). These fractures are often associated with sacroiliac dislocation or fracture near this joint. They are also associated with disruption of the pubic symphysis or a fracture of the pubic ramus. However, pubic dislocation is more common than pubic fracture (95).

Testing Strategy

Any patient that presents with extreme pain in the pelvis after major trauma should have AP, lateral, and oblique radiographic views of the pelvis performed (92). Inlet and outlet views may be helpful (11). Bone scanning is not called for in cases of isolated pelvic fracture (94). Computed tomography (CT) scanning may be helpful in diagnosing major pelvic trauma. Evaluation should begin with inspection. There may be large hematomas over the flank or posteriorly over the sacroiliac joint. Scrotal hematomas are also seen. There may be internal rotation or shortening of one limb. The pelvic ring should be palpated to determine areas of tenderness. The pelvis can be compressed or forced outward at the ASIS to determine instability (11). In cases of disruption of the pelvic ring, evidence of complications (such as ruptured bladder and urethra and retroperitoneal hemorrhage) is rare (86, 95).

Treatment

Goals in treatment are to prevent significant deformity and malunion. Stable fractures can be treated by refraining from weight bearing. Unstable fractures must by fixated by either open or closed methods (86).

Prognosis

Stable pelvic fractures generally require 6 to 8 weeks to become relatively solid so that partial weight bearing may occur. Unstable fractures may require 3 months of bed rest (11).

FEMORAL FRACTURES

Mechanism of Injuries

Femoral fractures are not common (96) but are seen in skiers (91), usually as a result of collision (97). Fractures of the femoral neck are rare in children (98).

Treatment

Femoral fractures were formerly routinely treated with open reduction and internal fixation. Using the newer closed intermedullary rod or nail, the patient can walk using crutches in a day or so and then leave the hospital in 3 to 4 days (91, 99). Supracondylar fractures also need open reduction and internal fixation (100).

Rehabilitation

In patients with an intermedullary nail or rod, isometric quadriceps exercises can be started as soon as pain permits. This is followed by straight leg raising exercises. Aggressive rehabilitation will allow the athlete to return to sports more quickly (91, 101).

Prognosis

Athletes with intermedullary nailing and rehabilitation can often return to contact sports as early as 6 to 12 months after the fracture (100, 101).

AVULSION FRACTURES

Mechanism of Injuries

Avulsion fractures are usually caused by sudden muscle tension across an open apophysis (102, 103), which is the weakest part of the skeleton (104). This muscle tension can be produced either by a concentric or a eccentric contraction used to accelerate or decelerate the body (102, 103), or an uncoordinated movement (104). They can result from excessive passive stretching, such as a dancer doing a split or a first baseman stretching to tag the bag (102, 103). Avulsion fractures are usually the result of a tight musculotendinous unit (53). In children and adolescents, the tendon is stronger than the bone; therefore, avulsion fractures result instead of tendon ruptures (104, 105). Explosive muscular effort with a cold muscle may also cause avulsion (106).

Avulsion fractures are infrequently due to direct trauma (103, 104). The most common locations for avulsion fractures are the anterior inferior iliac spine (AIIS) (92) and the ischial tuberosity (92, 104). Locations and causes of avulsion fractures in the pelvic hip and thigh are summarized in Table 13.3 (4, 45, 53, 80, 92, 98, 103, 104, 106–108). An infrequent site of avulsion fracture is the sacral apophyseal ring, with only 30 cases reported (106).

Clinical Features

Avulsion fractures are usually seen in the teenage athlete (98, 108). The athlete will complain of sudden sharp pain that started while using the affected limb (98, 104, 108). They will usually present to a doctor 24 to 48 hours after the injury (108), although half of affected athletes will be

Table 13.3. Locations and Causes of Avulsion Fractures

Apophysis	Muscle	Sports
Lesser trochanter	Iliopsoas (107)	Running (108), football, basketball (103)
Iliac crest	Transverse abdominis, external and internal oblique abdominal	Skating and running (103)
Iliac crest	Iliotibial band (ITB) (103)	
Anterior inferior iliac spine (AIIS)	Rectus femoris (107)	Soccer, hurdling, field hockey, running (103), and gymnastics (53)
Ischial tuberosity	Hamstrings (107) and adductors	Jumping, running, baseball, figure skating, basketball and hockey (45), and cheerleading (4, 103)
Anterior superior iliac spine (ASIS)	Sartorius (107)	Football, bicycle racing, track, softball (103), weight training (80), and gymnastics (53)
Greater trochanter	Hips abductors (98), gluteus medius (104)	
Sacral apophyseal ring		Soccer (106)
Pubic bone	Adductor muscles (92), pectineus (106)	Power lifting (squat) (106)

able to maintain normal activity (104). Avulsion fractures of the lesser trochanter of the femur will often cause the athlete to start and then stop running. They will have trouble flexing the hip to walk up stairs and have a limp (108). Avulsion of the sacral apophyseal ring has presented with low back pain and sciatica-like pain giving the appearance of a herniated nucleus pulposus (109).

Clinical Evaluation

There usually is localized tenderness, crepitus, or a hematoma. Sometimes an avulsed fragment can be palpated (Fig. 13.12). There is also usually a restriction of ROM around the hip due to muscle spasm or pain (104, 108). The athlete will have pain on resisted motion using the affected muscle (108). Avulsion of the AIIS appears to be less painful than avulsion of the ASIS (104). An athlete with an avulsion of the sacral apophyseal ring may have a restriction of lumbosacral flexion and extension, tenderness in the buttocks, a positive straight leg raise (SLR) test with pain all the way into the calf but normal deep tendon reflexes (DTR), and sensory and motor function (106).

Testing Strategy

Careful review of radiographs is needed, and bilateral views are often required to make a diagnosis (98). CT scan is the best test for sacral apophyseal ring avulsion. Radiographs in this case can be normal, and myelogram can show indentation at a disc without defect or shift of the nerve root (106). Biopsy should be avoided because mitoses present in the healing callus may lead to an erroneous diagnosis of neoplasia (104).

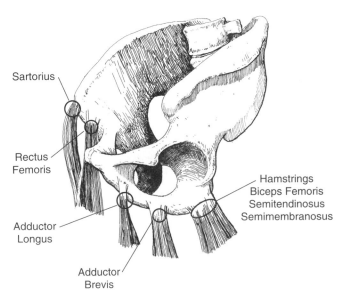

Figure 13.12. Sites of avulsion fractures.

Sartorius

Rectus Femoris

Adductor Longus

Adductor Brevis

Hamstrings
Biceps Femoris
Semitendinosus
Semimembranosus

Differential Diagnosis

Avulsion fractures need to be differentiated from strains of the muscle whose bony attachment is involved. They also can give the appearance of an inguinal hernia, lymphadenitis, phlebitis, and even epididymitis (98). Sacral apophyseal ring avulsion needs to be differentiated from a herniated nucleus pulposus (106).

Treatment

Treatment is symptomatic. Bed rest or the use of crutches is prescribed as needed for 1 to 2 weeks. The patient can then walk but will often show a limp for 2 to 3 weeks. In 6 to 8 weeks after injury, the patient can resume activity as tolerated (102, 104, 107, 108). Surgical excision should be performed on sacral apophysis avulsion fractures if nonsurgical symptomatic care is ineffective after several weeks (106).

Prognosis

Generally, the prognosis with only symptomatic treatment is excellent (102, 104, 107, 108). These athletes become asymptomatic despite a possible persistent radiographic deformity (104).

Prevention

It is not viable to ask athletes to give less than their all to their sport as a means to prevent avulsion fractures. The only viable preventive measure is to eliminate muscle tightness, whether that tightness is due to joint dysfunction (65–67) or muscle tightness as defined by Janda (63, 64) or tightness from myofascial trigger points (68).

Joint Injury

DEGENERATIVE JOINT DISEASE

Mechanism of Injuries

Secondary DJD is known to be a result of congenital joint abnormalities, any disease that alters the normal structure and function of the joint, or acute or chronic trauma to the hyaline cartilage or surrounding tissues (110–112). It is commonly believed that primary DJD is the result of wear and tear of joints (110, 113). However, studies have shown that there is no correlation between long-distance running and the later development of DJD (5, 110, 111, 114–116). Actually, the major research model for DJD is immobilization of a joint (75, 117–119), and immobilization has been shown to cause DJD (120). Lack of wear and tear (no load) has been shown to cause DJD in the hip (121). Janda has proposed that primary DJD is the result of abnormal movement patterns that overstress the joint involved (63, 122, 123). Examination for faulty movement patterns will be presented below.

Clinical Features

DJD has eight essential radiologic signs: asymmetrical distribution, nonuniform loss of joint space, osteophytes, subchondral sclerosis, subchondral cysts, intraarticular loose bodies, intraarticular deformity, and joint subluxation (3). However, only 25 to 30% of subjects with DJD as evidenced by radiographs are clinically symptomatic (5).

Treatment

Aspirin and nonsteroidal antiinflammatory drugs (NSAIDs) are considered to be the drugs of choice for the pain and inflammation associated with DJD (124). There is a growing amount of evidence that NSAIDs (aspirin included) as a class of drugs may interfere with the metabolism of cartilage (75, 117, 125–132) and may even accelerate the degeneration of the joint (132–139). Thus, it would seem imprudent to use these medications in patients with DJD. Because intermittent loading of joints has been shown to stimulate regeneration of cartilage (140), weight-bearing exercise might help in the treatment of DJD. Some authors have suggested that manipulation is beneficial in the treatment of symptoms associated with DJD (141, 142) and may even prevent the condition (143). In addition, the correction of faulty movement patterns may also be a beneficial treatment (63, 122, 123).

Prevention

Given the suggested role of abnormal movement patterns in the development of DJD, these patterns need to be examined for and corrected when present (63, 122, 123). Considering the role that immobilization and abnormal movement play in the pathogenesis of DJD, manipulation should also be considered in a program of prevention of DJD (63, 117–119, 122, 123, 143, 144). Intermittent loading of joints has been shown to stimulate regeneration of cartilage (140); therefore, exercise involving weight bearing should help in preventing DJD.

PUBIC SYMPHYSITIS/OSTEITIS PUBIS

Mechanism of Injuries

It has been suggested that pubic symphysitis is a precursor or subtle variant of osteitis pubis (145). As a result, these conditions will be discussed together. The first reported case of osteitis pubis was after surgery in 1924 (146). Most cases seemed to develop after urogenital surgery (147); however, cases have been reported in athletes who participate in hockey (50, 145), race walking (145, 147), soccer (14, 145, 148), rugby, karate, cricket, cycling, wrestling, running (145), and basketball (149). It has been suggested that pubic symphysitis develops in runners due to strenuous conditioning of the abdominals and adductor muscles (145). Avascular necrosis of the pubic synchondrosis is one proposed mechanism for osteitis pubis (147). Cases in athletes have been known to develop after strenuous exertion or after an infected blister on the ankle (147). However, the patient may have no history of any injury (148).

Clinical Features

Groin pain may develop suddenly or gradually, in a localized or diffuse distribution, and it may be sharp or dull. The athlete may have bilateral or unilateral symptoms (150). The patient may have pyrexia, transient dysuria and restricted abduction, and external rotation (147). Symptoms are worsened by activity and relieved by rest (148, 150) and may be severe enough to stop the athlete from participating in his or her sport (150). The pain is often in the suprapubic region extending into the lower abdomen (148). Pain may radiate down the thigh (148), along the adductors and into the groin, testes (14, 145, 150), perineum, hip, or sacrum (150). The following may worsen symptoms: pivoting on one leg, kicking a ball, sprinting, jumping, suddenly changing direction, climbing stairs (148), and performing abdominal crunches and straight leg raises (145). The patient may notice clicking in the pubes when getting out of a chair, turning over in bed, or walking on uneven ground (148). In rare cases, pain may refer into the bladder, provoking tenesmus (150). The number of cases appears to be on the rise (150).

Clinical Evaluation

There may be a painful restriction of hip motions (147), especially abduction and external rotation (147, 150). The pain usually occurs with both passive and active motions of the hip (150). Often, there is pain on resisted adduction (14).

Radiographic examination should include AP, lateral, and oblique views of the pubes and symphysis (150). Four weeks after onset of symp-

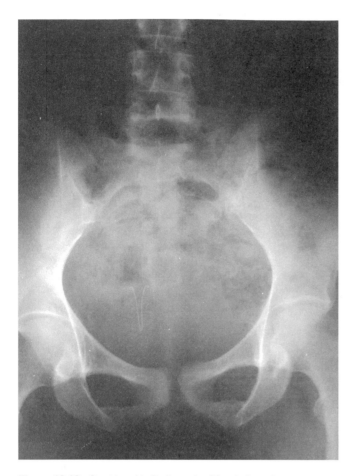

Figure 13.13. Osteitis pubis. Radiograph of female long-distance runner. Initial diagnosis was adductor muscle strain. Note the widening and irregularity of the symphysis. The original diagnosis by the radiologist was osteomyelitis. (There is also an IUD in place.)

toms, radiographs often show irregularity of the symphyseal margins (147, 148), accompanied by widening of the cleft (147, 148) and sometimes instability (148). These radiographic changes remain after symptoms have resolved (147). However, in a study of professional soccer players, it was found that 76% of players without groin symptoms and 81% of those with symptoms had radiologic abnormalities of the pubic symphysis (148). In long-standing cases, myositis ossificans may be found in the adductor longus and brevis as well as the obturator internus and externus near to the bony insertions (150). Sacroiliac joints are often involved and should be checked for dysfunction (148).

Testing Strategy

Technetium bone scan may be valuable in making an accurate, early diagnosis (145). Radiographs of the pelvis will usually be diagnostic 4 weeks after the onset of symptoms (147, 148) (Figs. 13.13, 13.14, and 13.15).

Differential Diagnosis

Pubic symphysitis cases are difficult to diagnose due to the vague lower abdominal and pelvic symptoms (145). They are most often misdiagnosed as adductor muscle strain (145). However, this has also been confused with inguinal hernia; prostatitis; orchitis; groin pull (149); urolithiasis (150, 151); acute rheumatism (147); muscle strain; osteomyelitis; ankylosing spondylitis; rheumatoid arthritis; Reiter's syndrome; hyperparathyroidism; primary and metastatic tumors (145); direct, indirect, femoral, or Littre's hernia; prostatitis; epididymitis; deferentitis; ureter stones; varicocele; and hydrocele (150).

Treatment

In the acute stage, local pressure and ice for 30 minutes to 1 hour may be helpful (150). Pubic symphysitis has been treated by eliminating aggravating activities for 2 weeks to 3 months, NSAIDs (14, 145, 148), and local injections of cortisone (145). Smodlaka, however, specifically does not recommend the use of cortisone (150).

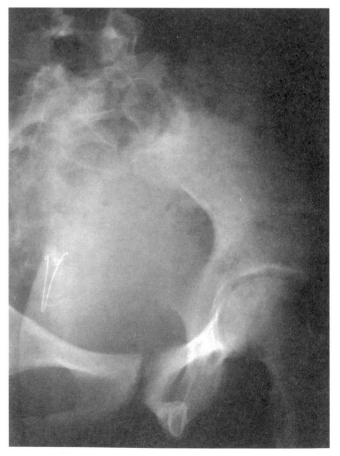

Figure 13.14. Osteitis pubis. Oblique radiograph of same patient as in Fig. 13.15. On this view, the irregularity of the symphysis is more apparent.

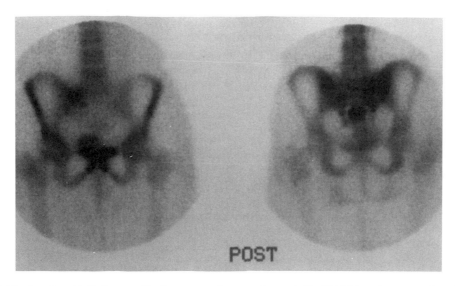

Figure 13.15. Osteitis pubis. Technetium-99m bone scan of same patient as in Fig. 13.14. Note the increased uptake at the pubes and the superior and inferior pubic rami bilaterally. (Courtesy of Jerry Lubliner, M.D.)

Bed rest may be called for (145, 148). Manipulation (14) or mobilization (150) of the hip can be helpful. Heat, particularly moist heat, is best in the chronic stages. Bicycling has been used successfully to maintain fitness in these cases (145). If the condition is unresponsive to conservative treatment, surgical treatment involves curettage of the synchondrosis (147). Sometimes fusion is performed; however, this can lead to more problems due to transmission of forces to the rest of the pelvis (14).

Prognosis

Two weeks to 3 months (145, 147) healing time is common, but healing can take several years (152).

Prevention

Smodlaka recommends stretching and strengthening all groin muscles (150).

Gonadal Trauma

MALE—TESTICULAR/PENILE

The male genitalia are seldom injured during sports activity (153). The penis is very mobile when not erect and therefore rarely injured (153). Lacerations of the penis have been caused by direct soccer kicks (14), and direct blows are known to cause vascular injuries and potency problems (153). Diagnosis is made by a retrograde urethrogram performed with a mixture of radiopaque contrast media and sterile water-soluble jelly. This condition is treated by primary repair or insertion of transcutaneous suprapubic catheter (153).

Bicycler's penis results from pressure of the bicycle seat on the pudendal nerve (154). This can cause paresthesia and numbness in the perineum and phallus after a long ride. There may be transient urinary retention or decreased force of voiding. The condition resolves itself with no apparent sequelae after a hiatus from cycling (153). This condition can be eliminated or elevated by altering the angle of the bicycle seat (153) or by using a seat with a longitudinal furrow (154).

Mild testicular trauma can lead to extreme pain, spasm, and discomfort. This can usually be alleviated dramatically by the following procedure. The athlete should be told first what will be done. The athlete is then lifted approximately 6 inches off the ground and dropped. The impact appears to stop the spasm of the cremasteric muscles (155).

Trauma to the testes may lead to a serious injury. If the injured testis feels similar to the uninjured side except for mild swelling (156), it can usually be treated by bed rest and the application of an ice pack wrapped in a towel. This will usually alleviate much of the pain (153, 156). If a swelling that cannot be transilluminated continues or if there is extreme pain, the patient should be referred to a urologist (153). Early (within 3 days of injury) surgical intervention in cases of traumatic hematocele shows that there is a much greater chance to save the testicle (156).

FEMALE

Injuries to female gonadal organs of the pelvis are rare. Vaginal and rectal douches have been reported in inexperienced water-skiers. The typical history is that the female had difficulty standing on the skis and her buttocks or perineum dipped into the water. Water entering the vagina with great force can cause internal lacerations and lead to salpingitis, infertility, peritonitis, and abortion. Rectal injuries from a forceful water douche while skiing have also been reported. Therefore, it is recommended that both men and women wear wetsuits to prevent injury during waterskiing (157, 158).

Joint Sprain/Strain

HIP

Mechanism of Injuries

The hip is one of the most stable joints anatomically but is susceptible to injury when in the flexed position (159). Hip sprains are uncommon sports injuries (90, 160, 161), accounting for less than 4% of all sprains and 1% of all injuries (161). In children and adolescents, injury is more likely to the proximal femoral epiphysis than to the joint. In adults, injury to the muscles is more likely than to the joint (162). The injury is usually the result of severe twisting (163).

Clinical Features

A sprained hip often refers pain to the medial aspect of the knee (162) or to the lower back (164).

Clinical Evaluation

Injury to the hip joint should result in a positive Patrick's Fabere test (162).

Testing Strategy

Radiographs should be taken to rule out fracture (163).

Treatment

The patient should rest and support walking with crutches until walking is no longer painful. Then the athlete should progress to rehabilitation of the muscles, ROM, and proprioception around the joint (163).

SACROILIAC

Mechanism of Injuries

Sacroiliac sprains may be the result of trauma as seen in football, soccer, rugby, hockey, basketball, and baseball. They may also be due to repetitive strain to the joint that is found when running with a short leg (165). Janda reports that sacroiliac sprain is so often associated with

piriformis spasm that it is difficult determining which came first (166). Repetitive strain is seen in long-distance runners, hurdlers, jumpers, football and soccer players, ballet dancers, golfers, and bowlers. Symptoms from sacroiliac sprains resulting from repetitive strain will be gradual in onset (167). Hypomobility (joint dysfunction) of one sacroiliac joint puts more stress on the contralateral joint and can therefore cause or predispose that joint to a sprain/strain.

Clinical Features

Sacroiliac sprains may cause the following symptoms: low back pain in the distribution of the thoracolumbar paravertebral musculature, pain in the gluteal region, pain in the muscles of the thigh, knee pain, hip pain, and even headache or neck pain (168). Fickel reports a case of sacroiliac sprain causing a lateral snapping hip (168).

Testing Strategy

The Gillet test has been shown to be a reliable test for sacroiliac joint dysfunction (169).

Differential Diagnosis

This should include chordoma, ankylosing spondylitis, or sacroiliitis and should be ruled out by appropriate imaging studies (165). According to Travell and Simmons, a very rare myofascial trigger point in the soleus may refer deep pain to the ipsilateral sacroiliac joint (170). This author has found this trigger point to be more common among athletes than in the general population. In patients with no other cause for PSIS pain and tenderness, treatment of this soleus trigger point often will eliminate the symptoms.

Treatment

Manipulation of a hypermobile joint is contraindicated. Treatment should include using a support to restrict motion in the affected joint (167). If one joint is hypermobile but the other is hypomobile (dysfunction), the restricted joint should be manipulated. Manipulation is used as a means of correcting the dysfunction in the sacroiliac joint (168).

Joint Dysfunction

MECHANISM OF INJURIES

Joint dysfunction in the pelvis and hip can occur from intrinsic or extrinsic trauma, as described elsewhere in this chapter.

this condition (173,
efined by Janda may
(63, 64). If complete
ws alteration of mus-
deep tendon reflexes,
esonance imaging (MRI)
rule out lumbar disc le-
canal stenosis (173).

ts that may be involved in
eralgia paresthetica include
nsor fascia lata, quadratus
psoas, pectineus, sartorius,
(174). Other conditions to in-
tial diagnosis include trochan-
), inguinal lymphadenopathy,
ps, Legg-Calvé-Perthes disease,
, intermittent claudication (30),
, central or lateral canal stenosis,
r systemic disease (173).

), Kadel et al. (30), and Stites (175)
successful treatment of this condi-
iropractic manipulation. Unrespon-
may require weight loss, exercises
he lumbar lordosis, local injections of
anesthetic, iontophoresis, phonophore-
ns-cutaneous electrical nerve stimula-
S) (30).

Muscle Injuries

CTOR

nism of Injuries

ductor muscle strains are common in run-
activities that include cutting (rapid change
irection) (177) such as football and soccer
8). They are also common in ice hockey (50).

erential Diagnosis

ith chronic adductor strains, inguinal hernia
pelvic lesions should be ruled out with clini-
valuation and imaging studies (177).

ment

hafer reports that manipulation of sacroiliac
lysfunction in athletes with groin strains of-
rovides immediate relief of pain (179).
verse friction massage (TFM) as described

HAMSTRINGS

Mechanism of Injuries

Studies have shown that hamstring injuries account for 1 to 11% of all injuries (181–187) and 32% of all muscle strains in runners (183). They are also common in soccer players (188). It is generally accepted that strains, pulls, or ruptures of the hamstrings are due to tight muscles that may not have been adequately stretched or warmed-up before exercise (34, 177, 189–195). However, Wiktorsson-Möller et al. found that warming up and/or massage were not as effective in increasing hip ROM as stretching alone (196). In addition, as noted in Chapter 1, adequate studies have not proven conclusively that stretching and warm-up prevent muscle strains (189); thus, it cannot be stated conclusively that tight muscles cause hamstring injury.

An imbalance between the quadriceps and the hamstrings has also been implicated as a cause of hamstring strains (34, 192). However, there is no agreement about what a normal hamstring to quadriceps strength ratio should be (197–199). As the velocity increases, this ratio does approach unity (1:1) (197, 199). Burkett has shown that if a hamstring is weaker by 10% or more than the hamstring in the other leg, or if the quadriceps to hamstring ratio is less than 2:1, there is an increased risk of a hamstring strain/pull (33). In addition, Heiser et al. found that athletes with this same imbalance were likely to reinjure the hamstring (34).

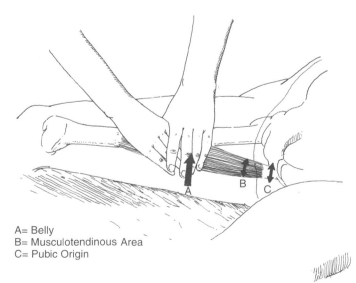

A= Belly
B= Musculotendinous Area
C= Pubic Origin

Figure 13.16. Adductor transverse friction massage.

CLINICAL FEATURES

Pain and symptoms of joint dysf¬
play the sudden onset and sha¬
characteristic of all joint dys¬

HIP

Clinical Evaluation

Joint dysfunction in the hip is ⟨
following directions (26).

- Long-axis extension.
- Flexion.
- Flexion-adduction.
- Lateral distraction.
- Extension.
- PA glide.
- Posterior joint play.
- External rotation.
- Internal rotation (26–29).

Schafer and Faye recommend using the Patrick's Fabere test as a screening for hip dysfunction. If there is a loss of ROM and the resistance is springy, the authors suggest treatment be directed toward the muscles. If the endplay is harder, then treatment (unless contraindicated) should be manipulation of the hip joint (26).

Treatment

Manipulation is the treatment of choice for joint dysfunction. Manipulation is accomplished by adding an impulse at the end point of joint play assessment (26–29).

SACROILIAC

Mechanism of Injuries

Sacroiliac dysfunction, like sacroiliac sprains, can be the result of trauma (falls) or repetitive stress of the joint (167). It is common among runners (171).

Clinical Features

The patient may complain of pain over the sacroiliac joint near the PSIS. Symptoms may be referred to the leg, groin, over the greater trochanter, posterior thigh to the knee, and occasionally to the lateral or posterior calf to ankle, foot, and toes (167, 172).

Testing Strategy

The Gillet test has been shown to be a reliable method of determining sacroiliac joint dysfunction (169).

myofascial trigger points, giv
of myofascial trigger points
tightness (68) and therefore o
or to mimic the symptoms o
174). Muscle shortening as
also be an etiologic factor
neurologic examination sh
cle strength or diminished
CT scanning or magnetic
should be performed to
sion or central or lateral

Differential Diagnosis

Specific trigger poin
what appears to be m
gluteus, piriformis,
lumborum (173), ili
and rectus femoris
clude in the differe
teric bursitis (17
ruptured quadric
thrombosis (174
lumbar disc lesio
and neoplastic o

ι
1,
gar.
caus
(e.g., ι

Clinical F⟨

Typical ⟨
(174), burn⟨
esthesia, and
lateral femora⟨
sory function ⟨
have any motor .
may report that sy⟨
ing up stairs, wear⟨
and/or standing (30,
acerbate (173) or allevi⟨

Clinical Evaluation

These patients may sh
touch sensation over the anι
173). Pressure over the inguin
reproduce symptoms in the tι
mography may show an area of ⟨
the distribution of the lateral femι
nerve (175).

Testing Strategy

Because meralgia paresthetica has re
to chiropractic care, motion palpation ex
tion of the spine and pelvis is require⟨
173–175). The patient should be examin⟨

Treatment

Ferezy (17⟨
all reported
tion with c⟨
sive cases
to reduce ⟨
steroids or
sis, or tra
tion (TEN

ADDU⟨

Mecha⟨

Ad⟨
ning⟨
of ⟨
(17

Injuries to muscle are most common during the eccentric phase of contraction, which occurs in the hamstrings while decelerating the swing phase leg (177, 200) or the leg after kicking a ball (188). During deceleration, the hamstrings and the gluteus maximus muscles increase their activity by 30 to 50% over concentric contraction (200). However, during eccentric contraction, less muscle fibers are firing, meaning more load per fiber (200)—hence the damage to the muscle. Delayed onset muscle soreness (DOMS), the pain the occurs 1 to 2 days after training, is considered to be the result of eccentric muscle contraction (201–203).

Running by itself is known to produce tight, weak hamstrings (53). Lewit has noted that joint dysfunction at the L4/5, L5/S1, and sacroiliac joints will produce spasm of the hamstrings (204). Janda has shown that chronic tightness in the psoas muscle leads to reciprocal inhibition of the glutei muscles, a pseudoparesis (67). This places more stress on the hamstrings to both accelerate and decelerate the thigh. According to Janda, hamstrings (like the other postural muscles) are prone to chronic tightness (64, 67, 123). With the added requirements of replacing the function of gluteus maximus and the inherent weakness in the hamstrings from their own tightness, we see further reason for hamstring injury.

Static stretching, as advocated by many authors, has been thought to be the best form of stretching (202, 205–209). However, it should be kept in mind that the muscle spindle functions to allow the nervous system to maintain joint position and prevent changes in muscle length (210). With this in mind, it seems that static stretching seeks to train the nervous system to ignore the muscle spindle and thereby allow a greater stretch (211). This "training" would appear to be counterproductive, in that it would make injuring a muscle easier, having diminished the protective action of the muscle spindle. This may be another mechanism behind chronic hamstring injuries (205, 212, 213).

Athletes who have experienced hamstring strains are prone to repeated strains (195). In addition, an athlete occasionally injures a hamstring by traumatically overstretching the muscle, as when a first baseman performs a split while trying to tag the bag before the runner does (212).

Clinical Features

In mild cases, the muscle does not hurt until the athlete cools down. The athlete may say in moderate or severe cases that he or she felt the muscle pop or tear. There is usually immediate pain and disability (191). The pain is usually local but may radiate up and down the thigh (21).

Clinical Evaluation

There is often pain or ecchymosis around the involved hamstring (214) that will eventually gravitate to the knee (212). Diagnosis by selective tension (215) will show probable pain on resisted hip extension (216) and on resisted knee flexion (214, 216) (tested with the leg in internal, external, and neutral rotation) (216). There might also be pain on passive straight leg raise (21, 214, 216) or hip flexion (216). The examiner should palpate the muscle to feel for a gap from torn muscle fibers (191). Patients with chronic hamstring strains should have their lower back examined for spondylolisthesis and possible herniated nucleus pulposus (177).

Grading

Most injuries are grade 1 and 2. Grade 3 injuries are rare and might require surgical repair to restore function (177). The muscle is best palpated with 15° of flexion. The patient then attempts contraction and points to the site of pain. In grade 1 injuries, there is a mild injury with a small area of pain and no palpatory defect in the muscle. For grade 2 injuries, the area of pain expands but there is still no palpatory defect in the muscle (180, 212). Grade 3 injuries are severe, with a large area of pain. There is often quick swelling and a definite palpatory gap in the muscle (177).

Testing Strategy

Piriformis syndrome can be ruled out via Paces sign or Freiberg's sign (21). MRI (217) or ultrasound (218) may be used to determine the extent of injury.

Differential Diagnosis

Sciatica (216), posterior thigh compartment syndrome (21, 219), piriformis syndrome (21), scar tissue from previous tears (21), pubic symphysitis (145), myofascial trigger points in the piriformis and/or gluteus minimus muscles (220), and myofascial trigger points in the hamstring muscles themselves (221) should be ruled out. In pediatric and adolescent athletes, avulsion fractures of the ischial tuberosity must be suspected and ruled out via radiographs (4, 45, 107). Lumbar facet syndrome may cause hamstring spasm and give the appearance of primary hamstring injury (222).

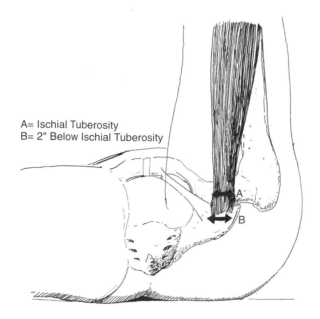

A= Ischial Tuberosity
B= 2" Below Ischial Tuberosity

Figure 13.17. Hamstring transverse friction massage (at proximal attachment).

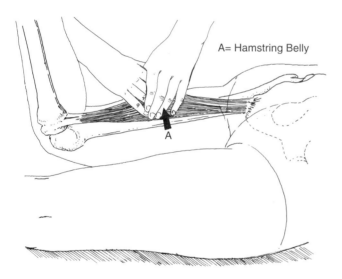

A= Hamstring Belly

Figure 13.18. Hamstring transverse friction massage (in muscle belly).

Treatment

Rest, ice, compression, and elevation (RICE) therapy is always the first treatment (34, 177, 223). The use of ice has been shown to reduce healing time (223). After 3 days, the athlete can start to do isokinetics at high speeds. The athlete's maximum torque is compared with baseline data after the fifth day. When peak torque is 70% of baseline at 60°/sec, the athlete is allowed to jog. Athletes return to action when their peak torque is 95% of baseline at 60°/sec and they have good agility (34).

NSAIDs have been suggested as appropriate for the treatment of acute muscle strains (177, 224). However, their appropriateness in the man-

agement of acute soft tissue injury has been brought into question as a result of research. A study has shown that NSAIDs delay the regeneration of muscle while simultaneously causing analgesia, which allows early motion (225). They may also have a negative effect during the proliferative phase of healing by slowing DNA synthesis (226), and their clinical effectiveness has not been demonstrated (227).

Cibulka et al. have shown that manipulation of sacroiliac joint dysfunction in athletes with hamstring strains significantly increases muscle strength in the involved hamstring (214). To prevent chronic disability due to scar tissue cross-linkage and speed recovery, light TFM may be used at the site of injury (Figs. 13.17 and 13.18) (180, 228).

In cases in which overstretch was the cause for the hamstring injury, there is a possibility of myositis ossificans developing (229, 230).

Rehabilitation

The daily adjustable progressive resistive exercise (DAPRE) technique has been shown to result in impressive gains in strength after injury (Tables 13.4 and 13.5) (231).

Prognosis

Mild or superficial injuries heal in a matter of days to a week. More severe or deeper injuries will require 1 week to 1 month to heal (34, 98, 191).

Table 13.4. Daily Adjustable Progressive Resistive Exercise (DAPRE) Technique (231)

Set	Portion of Working Weight Used	No. of Repetitions
1	$\frac{1}{2}$	10
2	$\frac{3}{4}$	6
3	Full	Maximum[a]
4	Adjusted	Maximum[b]

[a]Number of repetitions performed during the third set is used to determine the adjusted working weight for the fourth set according to the guidelines in Table 13.5.
[b]Number of repetitions performed during the fourth set is used to determine the adjusted working weight for the next day according to the guidelines in Table 13.5.

Table 13.5. General Guidelines for Adjustment of Working Weight (231)

No. of Repetitions Performed During Set	Adjustment to Working Weight for Fourth Set[a]	Adjustment to Working Weight for Next Day[b]
0–2	Decrease 5–10 lb and perform set over	Decrease 5–10 lb and perform set over
3–4	Decrease 0–5 lb	Keep the same
5–7	Keep the same	Increase 5–10 lb
8–12	Increase 5–10 lb	Increase 5–15 lb
≥13	Increase 10–15 lb	Increase 1–20 lb

[a]The number of repetitions performed during the third set is used to determine the adjusted working weight for the fourth set according to the guidelines in Table 13.4.
[b]The number of repetitions performed during the fourth set is used to determine the adjusted working weight for the next day according to the guidelines in Table 13.4.

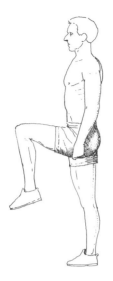

Figure 13.19. Hamstring dynamic range of motion. Quadriceps are contracted to stretch the hamstrings while maintaining normal pelvic position. Exercise is repeated 5 to 15 times.

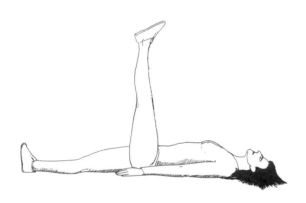

Figure 13.20. Hamstring dynamic range of motion. Quadriceps are contracted to stretch the hamstrings while maintaining normal pelvic position. Exercise is repeated 5 to 15 times.

Prevention

Correction of the factors discussed above that possibly predispose to hamstring injuries should be considered to prevent injury or reinjury. Manipulation of any sacroiliac joint dysfunction may help prevent hamstring strain (214).

Stretching of the hamstrings (34, 177, 190–192, 194, 195, 232, 233), preferably by dynamic range of motion (DROM) exercises (Figs. 13.19 and 13.20), may be helpful in preventing injury (202, 212, 213, 234). Studies on rabbits have shown that isometrically preconditioned muscles require more stretch and force to be torn (233). Because isometric contraction is part of DROM exercises, there appears to be good reason for using this type of exercise as a warm-up and stretch. Research has been equivocal on whether static stretching reduces the risk of injury (213). Although postfacilitative (fast) stretching (after

Janda) will restore normal function to a shortened hyperexcitable muscle (64, 67, 123), there does not appear to be any research on influence of this type of therapy on preventing hamstring injuries. Rehabilitative exercises should aim to restore hamstring to quadriceps ratios and balance between hamstrings on both sides of the athlete's body (34, 192).

QUADRICEPS

Mechanism of Injuries

Rectus femoris muscle strains are common in running, jumping, and kicking activities (177). Clinical features, clinical evaluation, grading, and management are similar to those previously discussed. TFM as described in Chapter 1 should also be implemented appropriately (Fig 13.21) (180).

COMPARTMENT SYNDROME

Compartment syndrome usually refers to a condition of the lower leg (see Chapter 16) (235, 236). The first reported case of posterior thigh compartment syndrome was reported in 1982 by Raether and Lutter (219). The athlete was a nationally ranked distance runner who complained

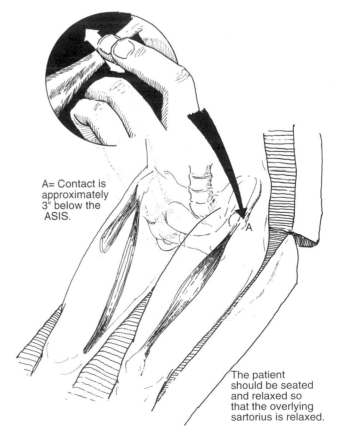

A= Contact is approximately 3" below the ASIS.

The patient should be seated and relaxed so that the overlying sartorius is relaxed.

Figure 13.21. Rectus femoris transverse friction massage.

of "lifeless" legs, hamstring tightness, weakness after 2 to 4 miles of running (120 to 140 miles per week was usual), and uncharacteristic aching after hard running. There was a pressure reading of 32 mm Hg before and after running. The athlete was treated conservatively for 6 months and finally had a fasciotomy, resulting in complete resolution of complaints (219).

PIRIFORMIS SYNDROME

Mechanism of Injuries

Piriformis syndrome is the compression or irritation of the sciatic nerve by a contracted or stretched piriformis muscle (230). Travell and Simmons (237) suggest piriformis syndrome is the result of three conditions: nerve and vascular entrapment by the piriformis muscle at the sciatic foramen, referral of myofascial pain from myofascial trigger points in the piriformis, and sacroiliac dysfunction. In athletes, the most likely causes are direct trauma to the buttocks and overstress of the piriformis muscle due to hyperpronation of the foot (237).

Clinical Features

The patient may complain of pain in the low back, groin, perineum, buttock, hip, posterior thigh and leg, foot, and rectum during defecation. Women may complain of dyspareunia, and men may complain of impotence (237). This condition is seen often in runners (171, 238).

Clinical Evaluation

Piriformis syndrome is diagnosed by Paces sign, which is pain on resisted abduction and external rotation of the thigh, or Freiberg's sign, which is forced internal rotation of the extended thigh (21). A myofascial trigger point in the piriformis can be identified by palpation of a taut band and by eliciting tenderness of the trigger point by external palpation (237).

Differential Diagnosis

The syndrome is easily confused with the symptoms of a herniated intervertebral disc and lumbar facet syndrome. If bilateral, spinal stenosis should be considered.

Treatment

Standard treatment of myofascial trigger points (i.e., stretch and spray, postisometric relaxation, ultrasound, ischemic compression, and injection) should be effective in these cases (237). In addition, manipulation of any associated sacroiliac joint hypomobility (dysfunction) is indicated (237). Another popular treatment is operative transection of the piriformis muscle (230, 239, 240). In some cases, it seems that minimal attempts at appropriate treatment of myofascial trigger points were attempted unsuccessfully before surgery (239, 240). These cases might have responded if more effective conservative care were instituted before seeking surgical consultation.

Rehabilitation

The piriformis should be strengthened to prevent recurrence.

Prevention

The predisposing hyperpronation should be corrected, and prehabilitation of the piriformis should be implemented (237). Normal sacroiliac mobility should be maintained (241).

Contusions

QUADRICEPS—MYOSITIS OSSIFICANS

Mechanism of Injuries

Myositis ossificans is the development of heterotrophic soft tissue calcification usually thought to be the result of contusion type of trauma (3, 242) (a charley horse (243)), although only 40 to 60% of cases report a history of trauma (242). In the lower extremity, this usually occurs in the quadriceps muscle (244) but has been reported in the hamstrings (242, 245) and around the greater trochanter and iliac wing (246). Most cases follow trauma from contact sports such as football (247), wrestling (246), soccer, and rugby or from falls from a bicycle (248). Stretching (242) and manipulation under anesthesia for adhesions of the knee (229) also have resulted in myositis ossificans. Repeated trauma results in an increased chance that this condition will result (243, 249). Most authors believe that improper treatment, that is, the use of vigorous (243, 250–252) or light massage (243, 248), stretching (243, 248, 250, 251, 253), and physical therapy (250) will increase the likelihood that a muscle contusion will progress to myositis ossificans.

Clinical Features

After injury there will be increasing pain in the thigh and limitation of knee flexion (248). Sometimes the diagnosis of myositis ossificans is not made until a completely ossified myositis ossificans from a previous injury is reinjured and fractures or as an incidental finding on a radiograph (248).

Clinical Evaluation

Palpation shortly after injury will usually find an acutely tender indurated mass with a limitation of knee ROM (248). After development of bone, palpation shows a tender bony mass that may be associated with muscle atrophy and significant limitation of ROM (250). Ryan et al. found that the risk factors for the development of myositis ossificans from a quadriceps contusion are knee flexion of less than 120°, injury that occurred while playing football, previous quadriceps injury, delay in treatment of longer than 3 days, and ipsilateral knee effusion (254).

Testing Strategy

Kirkpatrick and Koman (255) suggest that ultrasonic imaging may be the best modality for an early diagnosis of myositis ossificans. Besides being cheap, noninvasive, and fast, it is relatively precise in showing an image of the soft tissue changes that are precursors to myositis ossificans. Also, these changes will show up on ultrasound before any changes seen on angiography, bone scan, plain film radiography, and CT scanning. Ultrasound is highly sensitive in the detection of calcific deposits in soft tissues (256). Ellis and Frank (248) report that the earliest evidence on plain film appeared on the 11th day after injury and the latest at 6 weeks. The initial appearance is a fine, lacy radiopacity that later becomes a cloudy ossification (3). The first signs of faint calcification show up within 2 to 6 weeks after onset of symptoms (257). Sequential radiographs will show a mass that is very radiopaque at its margins and more radiolucent in the center (3). After maturation of the myositis ossificans heterotrophic bone, usually at 10 to 13 weeks, CT scans show mature cortical bone shell around a lucent center (229, 257). They will also usually show a rim of mineralization around the lesion after 4 to 6 weeks (257). The appearance of myositis ossificans on MRI is such that it may be confused with malignancy (257), although MRI will best demonstrate the extent of soft tissue abnormalities associated with the myositis ossificans (258).

Differential Diagnosis

Myositis ossificans has been misdiagnosed as a soft tissue sarcoma, resulting in amputation and radiation therapy. Histologically, these conditions can be difficult to differentiate but are easy to distinguish on CT. Periosteal osteosarcomas have dense centers with less well-defined margins that fade into the soft tissue and do not have a cortical shell. Ossification is rare in lipomas, but when it occurs it is deep in the lesion. Ossification may occur in hemangioma of muscle but it does so in a diffuse manner, giving a Swiss cheese appearance (242).

Treatment

It appears that even with "proper" treatment, some athletes who sustain quadriceps contusions will still develop myositis ossificans (254, 259, 260). (This then brings up the question of whether massage and physical therapy are actually so dangerous, but without compelling evidence these treatments should still be avoided.) In the acute stage, the contusion should be treated with ice, compression, and rest (250, 254). Ryan et al. (254) found a very low progression toward ossification with the protocol illustrated in Tables 13.6 and 13.7.

This protocol resulted in only 9% of contusions progressing into myositis ossificans (254). Surgery is indicated only when the bony mass has completely matured and the athlete has pain that is associated with muscular weakness and a significant loss of joint movement (250). Few cases will require surgery (254).

Prognosis

In one study, 36% of cases of myositis ossificans showed complete bone resorption (243). Athletes can usually return to play within 2 to 3

Table 13.6.   Inpatient Quadriceps Contusion Therapy (254)

Phase 1—Limit Hemorrhage	Phase 2—Restoration of **Pain-free** Motion
Rest: bed rest; ice: ice pack applied to injured area; compression: thigh-length support hose and bandage wrap entire thigh: elevation: hip and knee flexed to tolerance	Continuous passive motion; well-leg gravity-assisted motion: supine and prone active knee flexion; isometric quadriceps contraction; ice, crutch ambulation, bandage wrap
Advance to next phase when:	
Comfortable; **pain-free** at rest; stabilized thigh girth	**Pain-free** passive range of motion 0°-90°; good quadriceps control; crutch ambulation with patient weight bearing to tolerance and negotiating steps After completion, continue to Phase 2 as outpatient (see Table 13.7)

Table 13.7.   Outpatient Quadriceps Contusion Therapy (254)[a]

Phase 1—Limit Hemorrhage	Phase 2—Restoration of **Pain-Free** Motion	Phase 3—Functional Rehabilitation Strength and Endurance
Rest: weight bearing to tolerance, crutch ambulation if limp present; ice: ice massage for 10 min; cold pack/cool whirlpool for 20 min; compression: bandage wrap entire thigh (occasional use: long-leg support hose, conform taping); elevation: hip and knee flexed to tolerance; isometric quadriceps contraction <10 reps	Ice or cool whirlpool, 15–20 min; isometric quadriceps exercises, 15–20 min; supine and prone active flexion; well-leg gravity-assisted motion; static cycle: minimum resistance; discard: 1) crutches when range of motion >90°, no limp, good quadriceps control, and pain-free, with flexed weight bearing gait; 2) bandage, when thigh girth reduced to equivalent of uninjured thigh	**Always pain-free.** Static cycle with increasing resistance; Cybex; swim; walk; jog (pool and surface); run.
	Advance to next stage when:	
Comfortable, **pain-free** at rest; stabilized thigh girth	>120° **pain-free** active knee motion; equal thigh girth bilaterally	Full active range of motion; full squat; **pain-free** all activities; wear thigh girdle with thick pad 3 to 6 months for all contact sports.

[a]Mild and moderate treat daily/severe treat twice daily.

weeks of injury and few have residual loss of ROM (250, 254).

Prevention

The best prevention for myositis ossificans of the anterior thigh is adequate protection from trauma (261) and proper treatment as outlined above. Educating athletes and coaches is crucial (259), since Ryan et al. found that a delay in treatment for 3 days was a significant risk factor for the progression of a contusion to myositis ossificans (254).

HIP POINTER

Mechanism of Injuries

A hip pointer is a contusion of the iliac crest (262) and is the most common of all hip injuries (200). It is commonly the result of impact with a helmet, knee, elbow, artificial turf (263), goal post, hockey boards, or hockey or lacrosse stick (103). This injury affects the insertion of the abdominals and oblique muscles (263) and may cause some tearing of muscle fibers along the iliac crest (200).

Clinical Features

These are exceptionally painful injuries (103, 200, 263). The athlete may have pain when walking, coughing, sneezing (200), or performing many everyday movements. The area will often become discolored from ecchymosis (200, 263).

Clinical Evaluation

Radiographs are required to rule out epiphyseal avulsion fracture (103) and fracture with or without displacement of the iliac crest (263).

Treatment

Initial treatment should include RICE therapy (103, 200, 263). Aspiration is not recommended. Local injections of lidocaine have been used, as well as oral analgesics and antiinflammatories to reduce discomfort (263). After 72 hours, ice massage should be used with an elastic wrap in between ice massage treatments. Contrast baths should be started once swelling, ecchymosis, and soreness are gone. No further treatment is required when the athlete is pain free (200, 263). Appropriate padding will help to prevent reinjury (200, 263). If there has been displacement of the iliac crest, surgery may be required (263).

Rehabilitation

Rehabilitation is accomplished by strengthening the abdominal musculature and restoring ROM (263).

Prognosis

Most cases resolve in 4 to 6 weeks. However, if there has been a displacement of the iliac crest, recovery may take 8 months (263).

Prevention

Adequate protective padding is the only prevention (200, 263).

Snapping Hip

ANTERIOR

Mechanism of Injuries

This type of snapping hip occurs when the iliopsoas tendon snaps over the iliopectineal prominence (eminence), which is located just superior to the acetabulum (Fig. 13.22) (264, 265). This condition is often the result of a tight iliopsoas (265–267). It has also been suggested that this condition in dancers is the result of a capsular or section phenomenon due to the wide ROM in the dancer's hip. This increased ROM allows a partial subluxation of the joint (53, 159, 268), with iliofemoral ligaments moving over the femoral head, and the iliopsoas tendon moving over the lesser trochanter (159). Anterior snapping hip has been seen in male and female runners (266) and occurs often in female dancers (53, 266, 268) and gymnasts (53, 267). It is often painless (268) but may be secondary to some injury to the hip (264). In dancers, it may be due to improper technique; changing technique has been known to correct the problem (268). Gymnasts have noticed this condition associated with some maneuvers done on the uneven parallel bars (267).

Clinical Features

There is an audible snapping sound (264, 266) when the hip is moved into extension (265, 266) or into flexion (264).

Clinical Evaluation

Usually this snapping can be felt while palpating in the inguinal region as the athlete

moves the hip (265–267). There may be tenderness at the pelvic brim as the iliopsoas tendon crosses (267). Bursography with cineradiography (266) or arthrogram (264) often will show the snapping of the iliopsoas tendon associated with the motion of the hip and the sound production (264, 266).

Treatment

Schaberg found that although rest did reduce the symptoms, it did not completely resolve the condition (266). Suggested treatments include stretching of the iliopsoas and adductors (267), ultrasound, deep heat, strengthening the hip extensors and adductors (53), and changing dance technique (268). Surgery may be required to correct this condition (53, 264, 266).

Prognosis

Weiker et al. have reported that the condition will resolve in 6 to 8 weeks with stretching of the adductors and iliopsoas (267).

LATERAL

Mechanism of Injuries

This type of snapping hip occurs when the iliotibial band (ITB) snaps over the greater trochan-

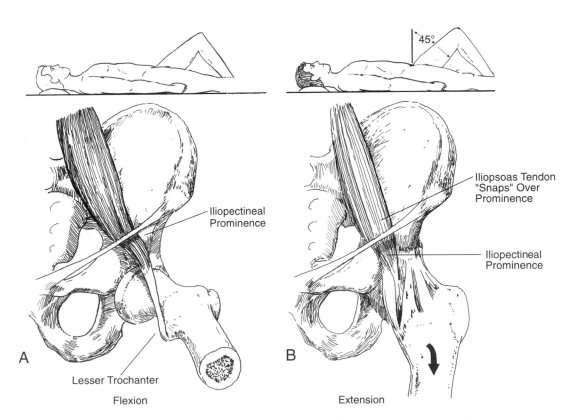

Figure 13.22. Anterior snapping hip. Snapping is felt as the psoas muscle "snaps" over the iliopectineal prominence as the hip is flexed (**A**) and extended (**B**).

ter of the femur (Fig. 13.23) (265, 269, 270). This condition is usually the result of a tight ITB (265, 268, 269) and is usually painless (266, 268, 270, 271). However, this may be part of an ITB syndrome (ITB friction syndrome, ITB tendinitis), with the patient complaining of pain at the origin of the tensor fascia lata, lateral aspect of the knee, lateral femoral epicondyle, and insertion of the ITB (272). It has also been suggested that snapping hip can be the result of the gluteus medius muscle catching against the edge of the greater trochanter (159, 271, 273). Fickel (168) has reported one case in which a snapping hip was caused by a sacroiliac joint sprain. An increased Q angle predisposes to snapping hip (270) and is therefore more common in women, due to their greater Q angle (274, 275). During hip flexion, the ITB moves anteriorly to the greater trochanter; during extension, it moves posteriorly (270). Sometimes the athlete will complain that his or her hip is "going out of place" when it snaps (265).

Clinical Features

The snap usually occurs when the athlete moves the thigh between flexion and extension (265). The snapping hip is often associated with no discomfort (168, 265, 268, 270). In some cases, the patient may complain of discomfort from an associated trochanteric bursitis (276, 277) or tendinitis of the tensor fascia lata (168, 271). Pain can radiate to the lateral thigh or buttocks (276). This condition is common in hurdlers (278), run-

ners (276), dancers (53, 265, 268, 278), and gymnasts (53, 278). There may be tenderness to palpation over the greater trochanter (276). Snapping hip has been shown to be associated with joint dysfunction in both the sacroiliac joints (168, 270) and the acetabulum (270). Patients may have myofascial trigger points in quadratus lumborum (270); gluteus minimus (168, 270), maximus (168), and medius; and tensor fascia lata muscles (270, 279). Faulty muscle firing orders can be found in snapping hip syndrome both in hip abduction and hip extension (270). Mennell points out that ITB tightness can also result from Achilles' tendon problems, and any leg length discrepancy must be corrected (280).

Clinical Evaluation

The patient commonly has a positive Ober's test (269, 270, 281). The snap is not always heard, but can usually be felt by palpating over the greater trochanter while the patient does the motion that causes the snap (265, 270, 282). Sometimes the snapping can be auscultated (168).

Treatment

Stretching the ITB is the number one treatment (265, 268, 272, 276, 279, 283). Treatment of associated trigger points either by spray and stretch (270) or by ischemic compression/Nimmo's receptor-tonus method have been found helpful in these cases (168, 279). Manipulation of the sacroiliac joint has been reported to be an effective treatment (168, 270). It is important that

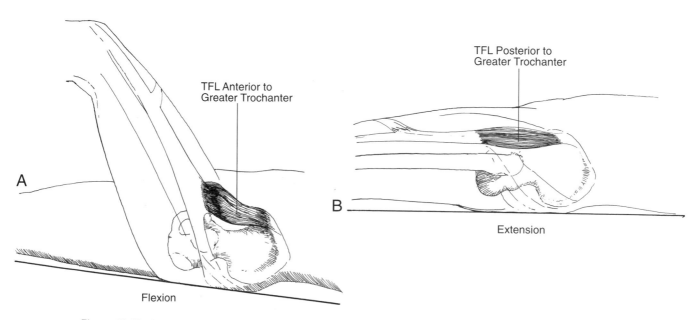

Figure 13.23. Lateral snapping hip. Snapping is felt as the iliotibial band snaps over the greater trochanter of the femur as the hip is flexed (**A**) and extended (**B**).

normal muscle firing orders are restored (270). This can be effected by correcting joint dysfunction and muscle tightness or through proprioceptive reeducation exercises (241). NSAIDs have been suggested for the treatment of this condition (268, 272, 276), but this may be unwise considering the possible inhibitory effect these drugs have on the healing of soft tissue (225, 226) and given their lack of proven clinical efficacy (227). In cases unresponsive to conservative treatment, surgical intervention has been helpful (53, 276, 282, 284).

Rehabilitation

Exercises to strengthen the hip abductors and extensors are important (53, 265).

Iliotibial Band Syndrome

Mechanism of Injuries

Iliotibial band (ITB) syndrome is generally described as a condition that occurs when the ITB rubs against the lateral femoral epicondyle, resulting in inflammation (86, 265). The author's clinical experience has shown that in many cases of ITB syndrome, the patient also has tenderness at both the origin and insertion of the ITB (i.e., ASIS and Gerdy's tubercle, respectively) and over the greater trochanter. Trochanteric bursitis, too, is considered a separate condition. The author has also found that further palpation will elicit tenderness at all the above-named locations associated with the ITB, but this is a less common presentation. Garrick and Webb (272) also discuss ITB syndrome as being a more pan-thigh syndrome. Because inflammation at all four areas mentioned may have the same cause (86, 282, 285–287), in reality these are all manifestations of the same syndrome. Treatment of all manifestations of this syndrome will be covered separately, but all parts of the syndrome should be considered when treating athletes with any one of these presenting complaints.

Tendon Injury—Tendinitis/Tendinosis

TERMINOLOGY

Historically, tendinitis is the diagnosis given nearly all painful tendon structures, their synovial sheaths, and adjacent bursae. Almost any painful tissue has been assumed to be inflamed because of the disproportionate role that pain plays in inflammation. However, histopathologic studies have distinguished between acute traumatic inflammatory response and insidious chronic tendon degeneration. The latter condition is termed tendinosis. Just as osteoarthritis has been renamed osteoarthrosis or DJD due to the lack of inflammation, many cases previously diagnosed as tendinitis should now properly be called tendinosis (288).

Mechanism of Injuries

Tendinitis is caused by the tendon being subjected to greater tensile stress than it can effectively absorb. This results in microtears (289). Actual rupture of tendons does not usually occur without previous disease (105). Leadbetter suggests that tendinitis is not the result of microtrauma, but of macrotrauma. Microtrauma, usually from overuse, is more causally related to degeneration of the tendon (i.e., tendinosis), which may result in spontaneous tendon rupture (288).

Clinical Features

Tendinitis of the gluteus medius muscle occurs usually at the insertion but can occur in the origin. Symptoms may be similar to trochanteric bursitis. Psoas may develop a tendinitis at its insertion on the lesser trochanter or near the musculotendinous junction (180). The author has found this commonly associated with an anterior "snapping" hip syndrome (see above) and muscle tightness of the psoas (see below). Rectus femoris may develop a tendinitis at the origin. Because the rectus femoris is a weak hip flexor, the patient may have pain with hip flexion and/or knee extension (180). Hamstring tendinitis has been described at the ischial tuberosity that refers pain to the posterior thigh. This condition usually causes pain while sitting, running quickly, and stretching the hamstrings (21).

Clinical Evaluation

Tendinitis/tendinosis will definitely produce pain on resistive testing of the muscle involved and may produce pain on passive stretch of the same muscle (180). See Table 13.8 (216) for appropriate tests. MRI may be the best test to differentiate tendinosis from tendinitis (290).

Treatment

Ice should be applied for 15 minutes every 1 to 2 hours in acute cases of tendinitis. In chronic cases, ice should be used after any activity that irritates the tendon (289). TFM is essential in the treatment of tendinitis (180). Because of the traumatic hyperemia that TFM causes, it may be useful in tendinosis.

Stanish (289) describes an eccentric exercise program for the treatment, rehabilitation, and prevention of tendon injuries (i.e., tendinitis and tendinosis) (Table 13.9). The program is begun only when it can be accomplished without pain. Progression to the successive stages in the exercise program is only when pain or discomfort is limited to the last set of 10 repetitions. If there is no pain in the last set, there is insufficient loading of the tendon to result in any increase in the tendon's strength and therefore no benefit.

Bursitis

TROCHANTERIC

Mechanism of Injuries

Trochanteric bursitis, by itself, is a relatively uncommon injury (2.4% of all runner injuries) (16). This condition is more common in women due to

Table 13.8.   Hip Function Diagnosis of Lesions (216)

Tests	Osteo-arthritis	Trochan-teric Bursitis	Iliopec-tineal & Iliopsoas Bursitis	Ischio-gluteal Bursitis	Adductor Tendi-nitis	Gluteus Medius Tendi-nitis	Upper Rectus Tendi-nitis	Ilio-psoas Tendi-nitis	Upper Ham-string Tendi-nitis	Piri-formis Syn-drome	Loose Bodies	Osteitis Pubis
Passive Flexion (140°)	L+/−	+/−(1)	+	+/−			+/−	+/−(1)	+/−L		Springy Block +/−	+
Passive Extension (30°)	L+/−	+/−	+/−				+/−	+/−				
Passive Abduction (50°)	L+/−	+/−			+/−							+
Passive Adduction (30°)	+/−	+/−				+/−						
Passive Medial Rotation (40°)	L+/−	+/−	+/−			+/−	+/−			+/−		
Passive Lateral Rotation (60°)		+/−	+/−			+/−	+/−				Springy Block +/−	
Resisted Flexion			+					+				
Resisted Extension		+/−		+					+			
Resisted Adduction					+							+
Resisted Abduction		+/−				+						
Resisted Medial Rotation		+/−										
Resisted Lateral Rotation		+/−								+		
Resisted Knee Extension							+					
Resisted Knee Flexion				+/−					+			
Joint Play Evaluation (1) passive flexion with adduction												

+: pain; +/−: possible pain; L: possible limited range of motion. (From Hammer WI. The hip and thigh. In: Hammer WI, ed. Functional soft tissue examination and treatment by manual methods: the extremities. Gaithersburg, MD: Aspen Publishers, 1991:117.)

Table 13.9. Eccentric Exercise Program for Tendon Injuries

Stretch
  Static stretch
    Hold 15 to 30 seconds
    Repeat 3 to 5 times
Eccentric exercise
  Three sets of 10 repetitions
  Progression:
    Days 1 and 2: slow
    Days 3 to 5: moderate
    Days 6 and 7: fast
  Increase external resistance; after day 7, repeat cycle
Stretch, as before exercise
Ice: crushed ice or ice massage applied to tender or painful area for 5 to
  10 minutes

After Stanish WD, Curwin S, Rubinovich M. Tendinitis: the analysis and treatment for running. Clin Sports Med 1985;4:593–609.

their wider pelvis (10, 13). As mentioned previously, trochanteric bursitis has the same cause as ITB syndrome: training error (abrupt increase in mileage, speed work, or hill running), shortened tensor fascia lata muscle, cross-over gait, limb length discrepancy, hyperpronation or hypersupination of the foot, quadriceps insufficiency (272), direct trauma to the greater trochanter (98, 272), and/or running on a canted road (282).

Clinical Features

The pain from trochanteric bursitis may be local or radiate down the thigh to the lateral knee (282, 291) or into the buttocks (282). Symptoms may be worsened by walking on stairs, squatting, walking, and side lying on the affected side (291).

Clinical Evaluation

There is tenderness to palpation over the greater trochanter (276). The patient's symptoms can usually be recreated by the physician putting his or her hand over the greater trochanter and having the athlete move the thigh through the running motion (282). According to Hammer (180), the following tests may be positive in cases of trochanteric bursitis: pain on passive hip flexion with adduction; passive medial or lateral rotation and passive abduction; pain on resisted hip extension, abduction, and medial and lateral rotation; positive Ober's test; and pain on resisted testing of the tensor fasciae latae. The following signs have been seen in nonathletes and may be present: positive Ober's test, low back spasm, atrophy of the thigh or leg, pain with hyperextension of the hip, tight hamstrings, leg hyperesthesia, limp, scoliosis, or shortening of the lower extremity (13). Radiographs are usually normal (291).

Differential Diagnosis

Trochanteric bursitis should be differentiated from acetabular pain, sciatic nerve root irritation (284), meralgia paresthetica, herniated disc (291), and myofascial trigger points in the tensor fascia lata (291).

Treatment

Conservative management should include the use of cryotherapy, TFM (in chronic cases) (284), moist heat, ultrasound (284), and antiinflammatory medications (282, 284). Sometimes crutches are needed to relieve symptoms early in treatment (98). It has been suggested that only 5% of cases are unresponsive to conservative therapy and require surgery (284).

Prognosis

Clancy (282) found that subacute and chronic cases resolved in 6 to 10 weeks or 6 to 8 weeks if surgery was performed.

CLINICAL ENTITIES THAT CAN CAUSE OTHER PROBLEMS

Muscle Tightness (Janda)

In the region of the pelvis, hip, and thigh, the muscles that usually develop muscle tightness are psoas (Figs. 13.24–13.27), rectus femoris (Figs. 13.24, 13.28–13.30), tensor fascia lata (Figs. 13.31–13.33), hamstrings (Figs. 13.34–13.36), piriformis (Figs. 13.37–13.39), and short hip adductors (Figs. 13.40–13.42) (63).

Text continued on page 351.

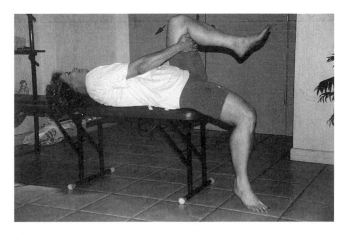

Figure 13.24. Normal modified Thomas test. The patient lies with the hips at the edge of a high table. The thigh on the side to be tested is allowed to hang off the table. The contralateral hip is maximally flexed. Note the alignment of the thigh and leg. The thigh is in line with the body and below the level of the table, and the leg is vertical.

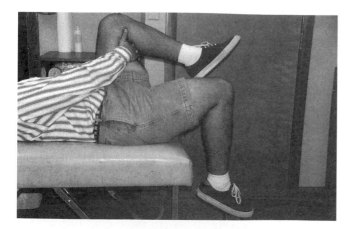

Figure 13.25. Muscle tightness—psoas. Hip flexion above the level of the table demonstrates possible muscle tightness of the psoas on the right. Diagnosis is confirmed by the examiner attempting to extend the hanging thigh, feeling for endfeel. Normal muscle will continue to give while shortened muscle will have an abrupt endfeel.

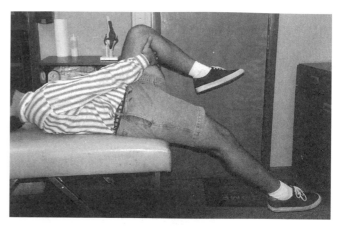

Figure 13.28. Muscle tightness—rectus femoris. Note that the knee is extended so that the leg is not vertical. Diagnosis is confirmed by the examiner attempting to extend the hanging thigh and flex the knee, feeling for endfeel. Normal muscle will continue to give while shortened muscle will have an abrupt endfeel.

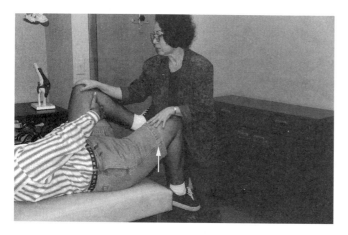

Figure 13.26. Psoas postfacilitation stretch : contraction. Patient contracts the psoas with maximal effort in the midrange of motion for 10 seconds.

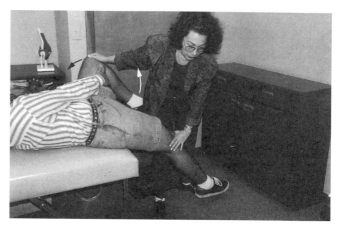

Figure 13.29. Rectus femoris postfacilitation stretch : contraction. Patient contracts the rectus femoris (trying to extend the knee) with maximal effort in the midrange of motion for 10 seconds.

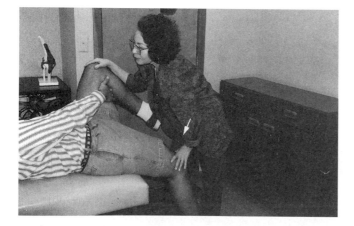

Figure 13.27. Psoas postfacilitation stretch : stretch. After contraction, the patient rapidly stops contraction and the examiner rapidly stretches the muscle by pushing the thigh toward the ground. The muscle should not be forced but should be stretched only as far as it allows. The stretch is held for 10 seconds. Then the examiner flexes the hip and holds the thigh for 20 seconds. The sequence in Figs. 13.26 and 13.27 is repeated 3 to 5 times as needed.

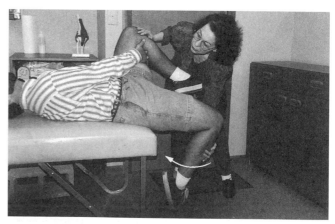

Figure 13.30. Rectus femoris postfacilitation stretch : stretch. After contraction, the patient rapidly stops contraction and the examiner rapidly stretches the muscle by flexing the knee and extending the hip. The muscle should not be forced but should be stretched only as far as it allows. The stretch is held for 10 seconds. Then the examiner flexes the hip, extends the knee, and holds the leg for 20 seconds. The sequence in Figs. 13.29 and 13.30 is repeated 3 to 5 times as needed.

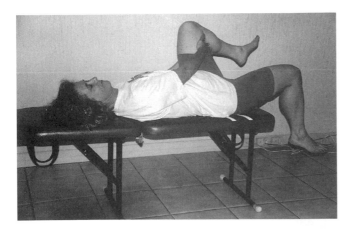

Figure 13.31. Muscle tightness—tensor fascia lata. Same position as Figure 13.25. Hip is held in flexion above the level of the table and slight abduction, demonstrating possible muscle tightness of the tensor fascia lata on the right. Diagnosis is confirmed by the examiner attempting to extend and adduct the hanging thigh, feeling for endfeel. Normal muscle will continue to give while shortened muscle will have an abrupt endfeel.

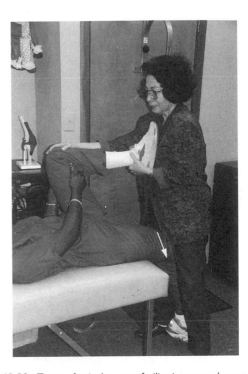

Figure 13.33. Tensor fascia lata postfacilitation stretch-stretch. After contraction, the patient rapidly stops contraction and the examiner rapidly stretches the muscle. This is accomplished by the examiner straightening his or her own hip and knee. The muscle should not be forced but should be stretched only as far as it allows. The stretch is held for 10 seconds. Then the examiner flexes the hip and holds the thigh for 20 seconds. The sequence in Figs. 13.32 and 13.33 is repeated 3 to 5 times as needed.

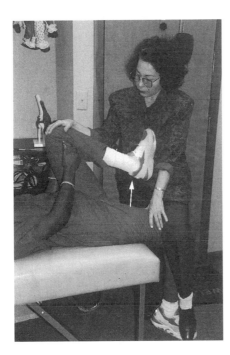

Figure 13.32. Tensor fascia lata postfacilitation stretch-contraction. Patient contracts the tensor fascia lata, attempting to abduct and flex the hip with maximal effort in the midrange of motion for 10 seconds.

Muscle Dyssynergy (Bad Firing Order)

HIP EXTENSION

The normal muscle firing order for hip extension is as follows.

1. Hamstrings then glutei (or vice versa).
2. Contralateral lumbar erector spinae.
3. Ipsilateral lumbar erector spinae.
4. Contralateral thoracic erector spinae.
5. Ipsilateral thoracic erector spinae (63).

Text continued on page 353.

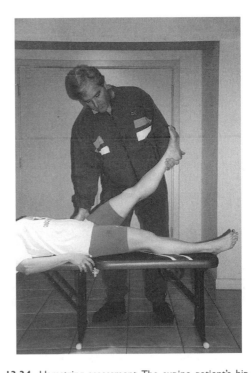

Figure 13.34. Hamstring assessment. The supine patient's hip is flexed with the knee extended. Normal range of motion is 70° before pelvic motion. The examiner should attempt to flex the hip, feeling for endfeel. Normal muscle will continue to give while shortened muscle will have an abrupt endfeel.

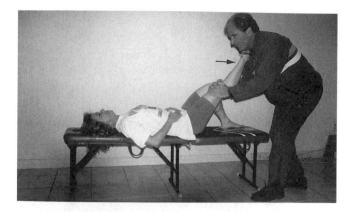

Figure 13.35. Hamstring postfacilitation stretch : contraction. Patient contracts the hamstring with maximal effort in the midrange of motion for 10 seconds.

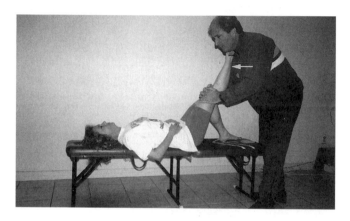

Figure 13.36. Hamstring postfacilitation stretch : stretch. After contraction, the patient rapidly stops contraction and the examiner rapidly stretches the muscle. The examiner will need to maintain knee extension during the stretch. The muscle should not be forced but should be stretched only as far as it allows. The stretch is held for 10 seconds. Then the examiner extends the hip (to approximately 30° of hip flexion) and holds the thigh for 20 seconds. The sequence in Figs. 13.35 and 13.36 is repeated 3 to 5 times as needed.

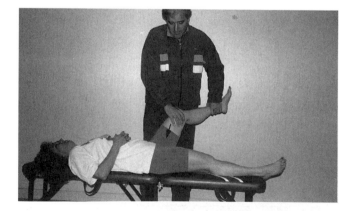

Figure 13.37. Piriformis assessment. With the patient supine, the examiner flexes the hip to 60°. The examiner pulls the thigh into maximal adduction and pushes posteriorly through the femur (this keeps the patient's pelvis on the table) and then internally rotates the hip by pushing on the lower leg, feeling for endfeel. Normal muscle will continue to give while shortened muscle will have an abrupt endfeel. The examiner may also stand on the contralateral side to perform this test.

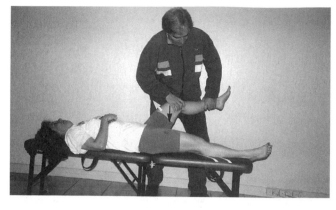

Figure 13.38. Piriformis postfacilitation stretch : contraction. Patient contracts the piriformis, attempting to externally rotate the hip with maximal effort in the midrange of motion for 10 seconds.

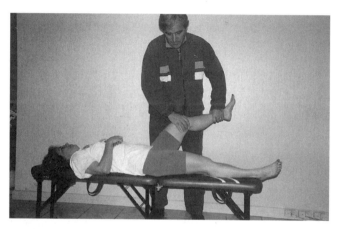

Figure 13.39. Piriformis postfacilitation stretch : stretch. After contraction, the patient rapidly stops contraction and the examiner rapidly stretches the muscle. The muscle should not be forced but should be stretched only as far as it allows. The stretch is held for 10 seconds. Then the examiner externally rotates the hip and holds the leg for 20 seconds. The sequence in Figs. 13.38 and 13.39 is repeated 3 to 5 times as needed.

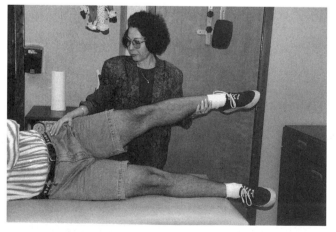

Figure 13.40. Short adductors assessment. The examiner attempts to abduct the hip, contacting the patient's distal femur while stabilizing the pelvis, feeling for endfeel. Normal muscle will continue to give while shortened muscle will have an abrupt endfeel. Normal muscle should abduct 40° before any pelvic motion.

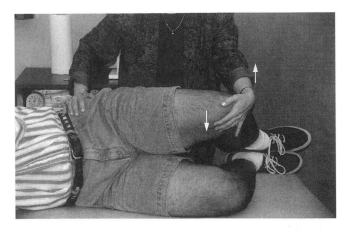

Figure 13.41. Short adductors postfacilitation stretch: contraction. Patient contracts the adductors, attempting to pull the thigh toward the ground with maximal effort in the midrange of motion for 10 seconds.

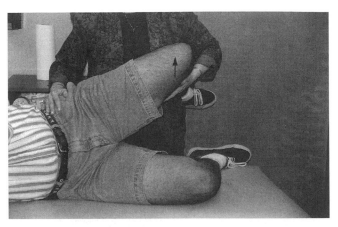

Figure 13.42. Short adductors postfacilitation stretch: stretch. After contraction, the patient rapidly stops contraction and the examiner rapidly stretches the muscle by abducting the hip while stabilizing the pelvis. The muscle should not be forced but should be stretched only as far as it allow. The stretch is held for 10 seconds. Then the examiner adducts the hip to a few degrees to abduction and holds the thigh for 20 seconds. The sequence in Figs. 13.41 and 13.42 is repeated 3 to 5 times as needed.

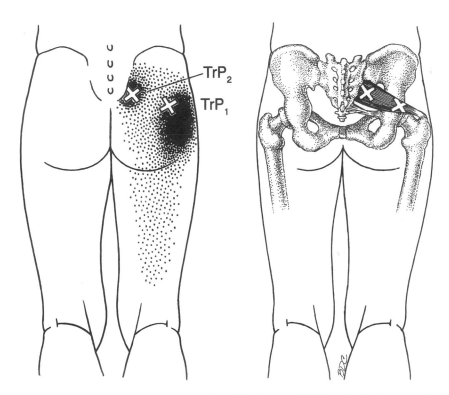

Figure 13.43. Piriformis myofascial trigger points. (From Travell JG, Simmons DG. Vol. 1: Myofascial pain and dysfunction: the trigger point manual. The lower extremities. Baltimore: Williams & Wilkins, 1992:2:186–214.)

HIP ABDUCTION

The normal muscle firing order for hip abduction is as follows.

1. Glutei.
2. Tensor fascia lata.
3. Quadratus lumborum (64).

Myofascial Trigger Points

Myofascial trigger points in the piriformis (Figs. 13.43 and 13.44), psoas (Figs. 13.45 and 13.46), quadratus lumborum (Figs. 13.47 and 13.48), and glutei (Figs. 13.49 and 13.50) are common, but are often misdiagnosed causes of

Text continued on page 355.

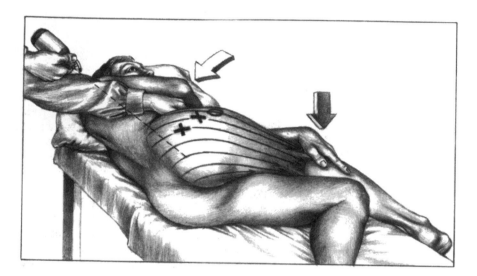

Figure 13.44. Spray and stretch of piriformis myofascial trigger points.

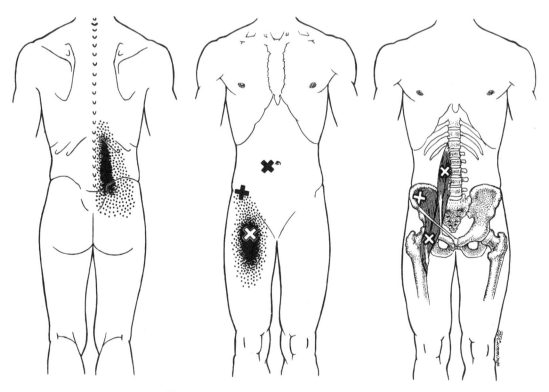

Figure 13.45. Psoas myofascial trigger points.

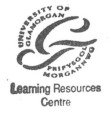

lower back pain that may radiate into the thigh (anterior, posterior, and lateral) and beyond (171, 270, 292, 293). Other muscles of the thigh and hip are prone to myofascial trigger points that can cause pain, discomfort, and other symptoms that may be caused by or attributed to athletic injuries. It is suggested that the reader consult Travell and Simmons for details (292).

Erector Spinae—Sacrotuberous Ligament Reflex

The pathologic erector spinae reflex may be associated with pelvic dysfunction (228, 294,

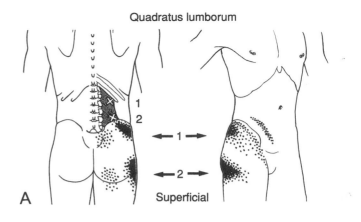

Quadratus lumborum

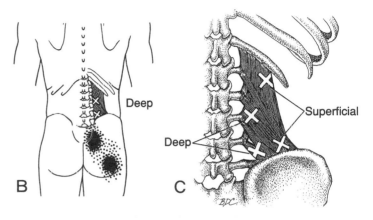

Figure 13.47. Quadratus lumborum myofascial trigger points.

295). This reflex, which the author believes should be termed pathophysiologic, is elicited by plucking from medial to lateral the erector spinae in the T5-T11 region. If present, there is a weak to a pronounced contraction of the erector spinae in the thoracic region, possibly extending to the entire erector and sometimes into the leg and/or neck. Sometimes the contraction is elicited in the erector spinae contralateral to the one being plucked (228, 294). Patients who exhibit this reflex will have increased tension and tenderness in their erector spinae. They also have positive tests of pelvic dysfunction (see above discussion of pelvic dysfunction) and a unilaterally positive Patrick's Fabere test (294, 295). The patient will have a tender sacrotuberous ligament on the ipsilateral side of the positive test (228, 294, 295).

Patients with this positive reflex may have a varied symptom picture. They may have one-sided, low back pain that is aggravated by sitting and walking down stairs. In long-standing cases, the patient may have neck pain or headaches or even tenderness in the pelvic or-

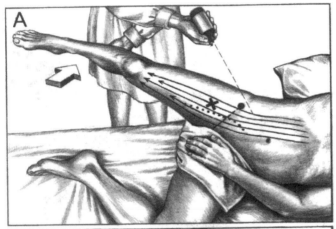

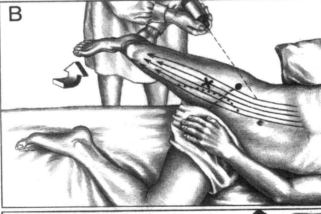

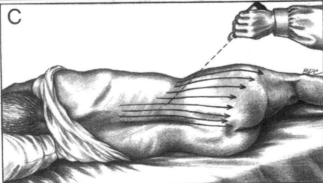

Figure 13.46. Spray and stretch of psoas myofascial trigger points.

Text continued on page 357.

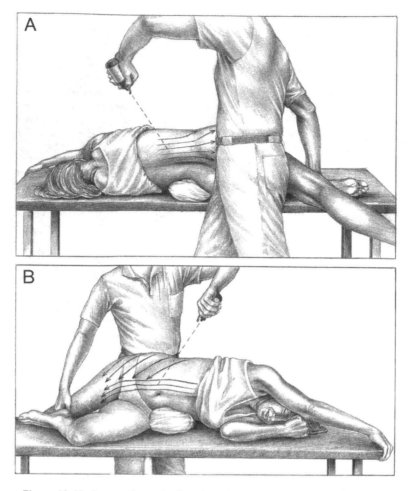

Figure 13.48. Spray and stretch of quadratus lumborum myofascial trigger points.

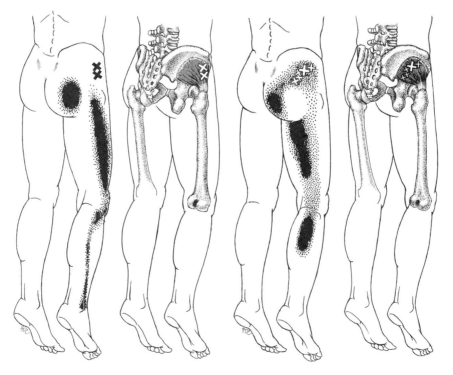

Figure 13.49. Gluteus minimus myofascial trigger points.

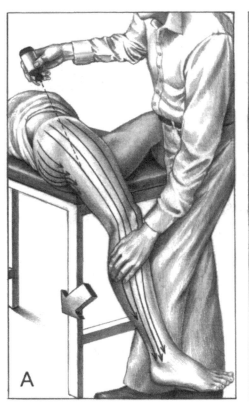
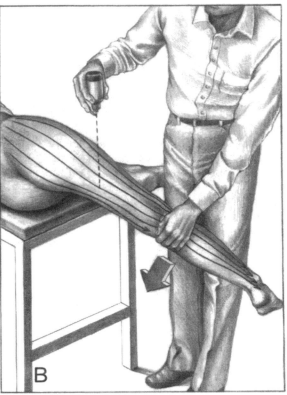

Figure 13.50. Spray and stretch of gluteus minimus myofascial trigger points.

gans, dysmenorrhea, dyspareunia, and/or an urge to defecate (295).

Suggested treatment of this condition includes intrarectal pressure on the erector spinae on the ipsilateral side of the positive reflex (295). The procedure as described by Midttun and Bojsen-Møller (295), although done intrarectally, has some similarity to the Logan Basic contact, familiar to chiropractic physicians (296). Silverstolpe (294) has suggested that treatment can be accomplished successfully by massage of the sacrotuberous ligament externally and continuously for 1 to 3 minutes until the patient reports that there is no more pain. After successful treatment, the reflex cannot be elicited (228, 294, 295). In the author's clinical experience, the patient will often experience a dramatic reduction in muscle tension in the erector spinae.

References

1. Clarke H. Muscular strength and endurance in man. Englewood Cliffs, NJ: Prentice-Hall, 1966:139.
2. Brunnstrom S. Clinical kinesiology. 3rd ed. Philadelphia: FA Davis, 1972:320–322.
3. Yochum T, Rowe L. Essentials of skeletal radiology. Baltimore: Williams & Wilkins, 1987.
4. Collins HR. Epiphyseal injuries in athletes. Cleve Clin Q 1979;42:285–295.
5. Lane N, Bloch D, Jones H, et al. Long-distance running, bone density, and osteoarthritis. JAMA 1986;255:1147–1151.
6. Lewit K. Manipulative therapy in rehabilitation of the motor system. London: Butterworth, 1985:10–11.
7. Mennell JM. Joint pain: diagnosis and treatment using manipulative techniques. Boston: Little, Brown & Co., 1964;26:157–159.
8. Yeoman W. The relation of arthritis of the sacro-iliac joint to sciatica. Lancet 1928;2:1119–1122.
9. Jones BH, Harris JM, Vihn TN, et al. Exercise-induced stress fractures and stress reactions of bone: epidemiology, etiology, and classification. In: Pandolf KB, ed. Exercise and sport science reviews. Baltimore: Williams & Wilkins, 1989;17:379–422.
10. Wilkerson LA. The female athlete. Am Fam Physician 1984;29:233–237.
11. Kellam JF. Fracture of the pelvis and femur. In: Torg JS, Welsh RP, Shephard RJ, eds. Current therapy in sports medicine. 2nd ed. Philadelphia: B.C. Decker, 1990:310–316.
12. Hunter LY. The female athlete. Med Times 1981;109:48–57.
13. Gordon EJ. Trochanteric bursitis and tendinitis. Clin Orthop 1961;20:193–202.
14. Williams JGP. A colour atlas of injury in sport. London: Wolfe Medical Publications, Ltd., 1980:82–89.
15. Watson AWS. Sports injuries during one academic year in 6799 Irish school children. Am J Sports Med 1984;12:65–71.
16. Marti B, Vader JP, Minder CE, et al. On the epidemiology of running injuries, the 1984 Bern Grand-Prix study. Am J Sports Med 1988;16:285–294.
17. Haycock CE. The female athlete—past and present. J Am Med Wom Assoc 1976;31:350–352.
18. Cyriax J. Diagnosis of soft tissue lesions. 8th ed. Textbook of orthopaedic medicine, vol 1. Philadelphia: Baillière Tindall, 1982:43–69.
19. Hoppenfeld S. Physical examination of the spine and extremities. New York: Appleton-Century-Crofts, 1976:143–169.

20. Magee DJ. Orthopedic physical assessment. Philadelphia: WB Saunders, 1987:219–265.
21. Puranen J, Orava S. The hamstring syndrome: a new diagnosis of gluteal sciatic pain. Am J Sports Med 1988;16:517–521.
22. Magee DJ. Orthopedic physical assessment. Philadelphia: WB Saunders, 1987:8–13.
23. Travell JG, Simons DG. Myofascial pain and dysfunction: the trigger point manual. Baltimore: Williams & Wilkins, 1983:52.
24. Schafer RC, Faye LJ. Motion palpation and chiropractic technique—principles of dynamic chiropractic. Huntington Beach, CA: Motion Palpation Institute, 1989:261–263.
25. Mierau DR, Cassidy JD, Hamin T, et al. Sacroiliac joint dysfunction and low back pain in school aged children. J Manipulative Physiol Ther 1984;7:81–84.
26. Schafer RC, Faye LJ. Motion palpation and chiropractic technique—principles of dynamic chiropractic. Huntington Beach, CA: Motion Palpation Institute, 1989:241–292, 382–385.
27. Magee DJ. Orthopedic physical assessment. Philadelphia: WB Saunders, 1987:256–257.
28. Mennell JM. Joint pain, diagnosis and treatment using manipulative techniques. Boston: Little, Brown & Co., 1964:130–133.
29. Gale PA. Joint mobilization. In: Hammer WI, ed. Functional soft tissue examination and treatment by manual methods: the extremities. Gaithersburg, MD: Aspen Publishers, 1990:210–212.
30. Kadel RE, Godbey WD, Davis BP. Conservative and chiropractic treatment of meralgia paresthetica: review and case report. J Manipulative Physiol Ther 1982;5(2):73–88.
31. Cyriax J. Diagnosis of soft tissue lesions. 8th ed. Textbook of orthopaedic medicine, vol 1. Philadelphia: Baillière Tindall, 1982.
32. Hammer WI, ed. Functional soft tissue examination and treatment by manual methods: the extremities. Gaithersburg, MD: Aspen Publishers, 1991.
33. Burkett LN. Causative factors in hamstring strains. Med Sci Sports Exerc 1970;2:39–42.
34. Heiser TM, Weber J, Sullivan G, et al. Prophylaxis and management of hamstring muscle injuries in intercollegiate football players. Am J Sports Med 1984;12:368–370.
35. Fleck SJ, Kraemer WJ. Designing resistance training programs. Champaign, IL: Human Kinetics, 1987:16–20.
36. Sartoris DJ, Resnick D. Osteoporosis: update on densiometric techniques. J Musculoskel Med 1989;6:108–123.
37. Butler JE, Brown SL, McConnell BG. Subtrochanteric stress fractures in runners. Am J Sports Med 1982;10:228–232.
38. Jackson DW, Wiltse LL, Dingeman RD, et al. Stress reactions involving the pars interarticularis in young athletes. Am J Sports Med 1981;9:304–312.
39. Marymount JV, Lynch MA, Henning CE. Exercise-related stress reaction of the sacroiliac joint: an unusual cause of low back pain in athletes. Am J Sports Med 1986;14:320–323.
40. Matheson GO, Clement DB, McKenzie DC, et al. Stress fractures in athletes: a study of 320 cases. Am J Sports Med 1987;15:46–58.
41. Latshaw RF, Katner TR, Kalenak A, et al. A pelvic stress fracture in a female jogger: a case report. Am J Sports Med 1981;9:54–56.
42. Selakovich W, Love L. Stress fractures of the pubic ramus. J Bone Joint Surg Am 1954;63:573–576.
43. Pavlov H, Nelson TL, Warren RF, et al. Stress fractures of the pubic ramus: a report of twelve cases. J Bone Joint Surg Am 1982;64:1020–1025.
44. Hallel T, Amit S, Segal D. Fatigue fractures of tibial and femoral shaft in soldiers. Clin Orthop 1976;118:35–43.
45. Tehranzadeh J, Kurth LA, Elyaderani MK, et al. Combined pelvis stress fracture and avulsion of the adductor longus in a middle distance runner. Am J Sports Med 1982;10:108–111.
46. Hulkko A, Orava S. Stress fractures in athletes. Int J Sports Med 1987;8:221–226.
47. Orava S, Hulkko A. Delayed unions and nonunions of stress fractures in athletes. 1988;16:378–382.
48. Cox JS, Lenz HW. Women in sports: the Naval Academy experience. Am J Sports Med 1979;7:355–360.
49. Walter NE, Wolf MD. Stress fractures in young athletes. Am J Sports Med 1977;5:165–169.
50. Sim FH, Simonet WT, Scott SG. Ice hockey injuries: causes, treatment and prevention. J Musculoskel Med 1989;6:15–44.
51. Fink-Bennett DM, Benson MT. Unusual exercise-related stress fractures: two case reports. Clin Nucl Med 1984;9:430–434.
52. Noakes TD, Smith JA, Lindenberg G, et al. Pelvic stress fractures in long distance runners. Am J Sports Med 1985;13:120–123.
53. Micheli LJ. Overuse injuries in children's sports: the growth factor. Orthop Clin North Am 1983;14:337–360.
54. Thorne DA, Datz FL. Pelvic stress fractures in female runners. Clin Nucl Med 1986;11:828–829.
55. Giladi M, Ziv Y, Aharonson Z, et al. Comparison between radiography, bone scan and ultrasound in the diagnosis of stress fractures. Mil Med 1984;149:459–461.
56. Prather JL, Nusynowitz ML, Snowdy HA, et al. Scintigraphic findings in stress fracture. J Bone Joint Surg Am 1977;59:869–874.
57. Milgrom C, Chisin R, Giladi M, et al. Multiple stress fractures: a longitudinal study of a soldier with 13 lesions. Clin Orthop 1985;192:174–179.
58. Branch HE. March fracture of the femur. J Bone Joint Surg 1944;26:387–391.
59. Mills TJ, Davis H, Broadhurst BW. The use of a whole bone extract in the treatment of fractures. Manitoba Med Rev 1965;45:92–96.
60. Hershman EB, Mailly T. Stress fractures. Clin Sports Med 1990;9:183–214.
61. Spain J. Prehabilitation. Clin Sports Med 1985;4:575–585.
62. McBryde AM. Stress fractures in runners. Clin Sports Med 1985;4:737–752.
63. Janda V. Pain in the locomotor system—a broad approach. In: Glasgow EF, Twomey LT, Scull ER, et al. eds. Aspects of manipulative therapy. 2nd ed. New York: Churchill Livingstone, 1985:148–151.
64. Jull GA, Janda V. Muscles and motor control in low back pain: assessment and management. In: Twomey LT, Taylor JR, eds. Physical therapy of the low back. New York: Churchill Livingstone, 1987:253–278.
65. Mennell JM. Joint pain: diagnosis and treatment using manipulative techniques. Boston: Little, Brown & Co., 1964:4.
66. Mennell JM. Back pain: diagnosis and treatment using manipulative techniques. Boston: Little, Brown & Co., 1960:9.
67. Janda V. Muscle weakness and inhibition (pseudoparesis) in back pain syndromes. In: Grieve GP, ed. Modern manual therapy of the vertebral column. New York: Churchill Livingstone, 1986:197–201.
68. Travell JG, Simons DG. Myofascial pain and dysfunction: the trigger point manual. Baltimore: Williams & Wilkins, 1983:16.
69. Jowsey J. Osteoporosis. In: Nelson CL, Dwyer AP, eds. The aging musculoskeletal system. Lexington, MA: The Collamore Press, 1984:75–90.
70. Werbach MR. Nutritional influences on illness: a sourcebook of clinical research. 2nd ed. Tarzana, CA: Third Line Press, 1993:331–333.
71. Dixon ASJ. Non-hormonal treatment of osteoporosis. Br J Med 1983;286:999–1000.

72. Durance RA, Parsons V, Atkins CJ, et al. Treatment of osteoporotic patients: a trail of calcium supplements (Ossopan) and ashed bone. Clin Trials J 1973;3:67–73.

73. Windsor ACM, Misra DP, Loudon JM, et al. The effect of whole-bone extract on 47Ca absorption on the elderly. Ageing 1973;2:230–234.

74. Epstein O, Kato Y, Dick R, et al. Vitamin D, hydroxyapatite, and calcium gluconate in treatment of cortical bone thinning in postmenopausal women with primary biliary cirrhosis. Am J Clin Nutr 1982;36:426–430.

75. Stellon A, Davies A, Webb A, et al. Microcrystalline hydroxyapatite compound in the prevention of bone loss in corticosteroid-treated patients with chronic active hepatitis. Postgrad Med J 1985;61:791–796.

76. Nilsen KH, Jyason MIV, Dixon ASJ. Microcrystalline calcium hydroxyapatite compound in corticosteroid-treated rheumatoid patients: a controlled study. Br Med J 1978;October:1124.

77. Pines A, Raafat H, Lynn AH, et al. Clinical trial of microcrystalline hydroxyapatite compound ("Ossopan") in the prevention of osteoporosis due to corticosteroid therapy. Curr Med Res Opin 1984;8:734–742.

78. Blickenstaff LD, Morris JM. Fatigue fracture of the femoral neck. J Bone Joint Surg Am 1966;48:1031–1047.

79. Lombardo SJ, Benson DW. Stress fractures of the femur in runners. Am J Sports Med 1982;10:219–227.

80. Kowal DM. Nature and causes of injuries in women resulting from an endurance training program. Am J Sports Med 1980;8:265–269.

81. Orava S, Puranen J, Ala-Ketola L. Stress fractures caused by physical exercise. Acta Orthop Scand 1978;49:19–27.

82. Hajek MR, Noble HB. Stress fractures of the femoral neck in joggers. Am J Sports Med 1982;10:112–116.

83. Masters S, Fricker P, Purdam C. Stress fractures of the femoral shaft—four case studies. Br J Sports Med 1986;20:14–16.

84. Blatz DJ. Bilateral femoral and tibial shaft stress fractures in a runner. Am J Sports Med 1981;9:322–325.

85. Devas MB. Stress fractures of the femoral neck. J Bone Joint Surg Br 1965;47:728–738.

86. Hershman EB, Lombardo J, Bergfeld JA. Femoral shaft stress fractures. Clin Sports Med 1990;9:111–119.

87. Johnson A, Weiss C, Wheeler D. Stress fractures of the femoral shaft in athletes—more common than expected: a new clinical test. Am J Sports Med 1994;22:248–256.

88. Atwell EA, Jackson DW. Stress fractures of the sacrum in runners: two case reports. Am J Sports Med 1991;19:531–533.

89. Whiteside JA, Fleagle SB, Kalenak A. Fractures and refractures in intercollegiate athletes: an eleven-year experience. Am J Sports Med 1981;9:369–377.

90. Shively RA, Grana WA, Ellis D. High school sports injuries. Phys Sportsmed 1981;9:46–50.

91. Kristiansen TK, Johnson RJ. Fractures in the skiing athlete. Clin Sports Med 1990;9:215–224.

92. Rubenstein JD. Radiographic assessment of pelvic trauma. J Can Assoc Radiol 1983;34:228–236.

93. Gertzbein SD, Chenoweth DR. Occult injuries of the pelvic ring. Clin Orthop 1977;128:202–207.

94. Nutton RW, Pinder IM, Williams D. Detection of sacroiliac injury by bone scanning in fractures of the pelvis and its clinical significance. Injury 1982;13:473–477.

95. Holdsworth FW. Dislocation and fracture-dislocation of the pelvis. J Bone Joint Surg 1948;30:461.

96. Bass AL. Injuries of the leg in football and ballet. Proc Roy Soc Med 1967;60:527–530.

97. Yvars MF, Kanner HR. Ski fractures of the femur. Am J Sports Med 1984;12:386–390.

98. Craig CL. Hip injuries in children and adolescents. Orthop Clin North Am 1980;11:743–754.

99. Key J, Jarvis G, Johnson D, et al. Leg injuries. In: Subotnick SI, ed. Sports medicine of the lower extremity. New York: Churchill Livingstone, 1989:293.

100. Cohn SL, Sotta RP, Bergfeld JA. Fractures about the knee in sports. Clin Sports Med 1990;9:121–139.

101. Marder RA, Chapman MW. Principles of management of fractures in sports. Clin Sports Med 1990;9:1–11.

102. Metzmaker JN, Pappas AM. Avulsion fractures of the pelvis. Am J Sports Med 1985;13:349–358.

103. Tehranzadeh J, Serafini AN, Pais MJ. Avulsion and stress injuries of the musculoskeletal system. New York: S. Karger, 1989:24–33.

104. Fernbach SK, Wilkenson RH. Avulsion injuries of the pelvis and proximal femur. AJR 1981;137:581–584.

105. McMaster PE. Tendon and muscle ruptures: clinical and experimental studies on the causes and location of subcutaneous ruptures. J Bone Joint Surg 1933;15:705–722.

106. Hyde TE, Danbert RJ. Avulsion of the pectineus muscle in weight lifting. Chiro Sports Med 1987;1:144–149.

107. Salter RB, Harris WR. Injuries involving the epiphyseal plate. J Bone Joint Surg Am 1963;45:587–621.

108. Dimon JH III. Isolated fractures of the lesser trochanter of the femur. Clin Orthop 1972;82:144–148.

109. Fujita K, Shinmei M, Hashimoto K, et al. Posterior dislocation of the sacral apophyseal ring: a case report. Am J Sports Med 1986;14:243–245.

110. Berkow R, ed. The Merck manual of diagnosis and therapy. 15th ed. Rahway, NJ: Merck Sharp & Dohme Research Laboratories, 1987:1258–1259.

111. Oka M, Hatanpaa S. Degenerative hip disease in adolescent athletes. Med Sci Sports Exerc 1976;8:77–80.

112. Mankin HJ. The reaction of articular cartilage to injury and osteoarthritis. N Engl J Med 1974;291:1285–1292.

113. Sokoloff L. Current concepts of the pathogenesis of osteoarthritis. In: Nelson CL, Dwyer AP, eds. The aging musculoskeletal system: physiological and pathological problems. Lexington, MA: The Collamore Press, 1984:113–120.

114. Sohn RS, Michelli LJ. The effect of running on the pathogenesis of osteoarthritis of the hips and knees. Clin Orthop 1985;198:106–109.

115. Panush RS, Schmidt C, Caldwell JR, et al. Is running associated with degenerative joint disease? JAMA 1986;255:1151–1154.

116. Eichner ER. An epidemiologic perspective: does running cause osteoarthritis? Phys Sportsmed 1989;17:53–54, 147–149.

117. Palmonski MJ, Colyer RA, Brandt KD. Joint motion in the absence of normal loading does not maintain normal articular cartilage. Arthritis Rheum 1980;23:325–334.

118. Palmonski MJ, Brandt KD. Running inhibits the reversal of atrophic changes in canine knee cartilage after removal of a leg cast. Arthritis Rheum 1981;24:1329–1337.

119. Palmonski M, Perricone E, Brandt E. Development and reversal of a proteoglycan aggregation defect in normal canine knee cartilage after immobilization. Arthritis Rheum 1979;22:508–517.

120. Navarro AH, Sutton JD. Osteoarthritis IX: biomechanical factors, prevention and nonpharmacologic management. Md Med J 1985;34:591–594.

121. Bullough P, Goodfellow J, O'Connor J. The relationship between degenerative changes and load-bearing in the human hip. J Bone Joint Surg Br 1973;55:746–758.

122. Janda V. Muscles as a pathogenic factor in back pain. IFOMT Conference, Christchurch, New Zealand. 1980:1–20.

123. Janda V. Rational therapeutic approach of chronic back pain syndromes. Symposium on chronic back pain, rehabilitation and self help, Turku, Finland. 1985:69–74.

124. Berkow R, ed. The Merck manual of diagnosis and therapy. 15th ed. Rahway, NJ: Merck Sharp & Dohme Research Laboratories, 1987:1261.

125. Vidal Y, Plana RR, Cifarelli A, et al. Studies on the safety of a new non-steroidal anti-inflammatory drug: Protacine (CR 604). Arzneimittelforschung 1979;29:1126–1129.

126. Palmonski MJ. Effect of salicylate on proteoglycan metabolism in normal canine articular cartilage in vitro. Arthritis Rheum 1979;22:746–754.

127. Palmonski MJ, Brandt KD. In vivo effect of aspirin on canine osteoarthritic cartilage. Arthritis Rheum 1983; 26:994–1001.

128. Palmonski MJ, Brandt KD. Relationship between matrix proteoglycan content and the effects of salicylate and indomethacin on articular cartilage. Arthritis Rheum 1983;26:528–531.

129. Palmonski MJ, Brandt KD. Effects of salicylate and indomethacin on glycosaminoglycan and prostaglandin E2 synthesis in intact canine knee cartilage ex vivo. Arthritis Rheum 1984;27:398–403.

130. Palmonski MJ, Brandt KD. Effects of some nonsteroidal anti-inflammatory drugs on proteoglycan metabolism and organization in canine articular cartilage. Arthritis Rheum 1980;23:1010–1020.

131. Bollet AJ. Inhibition of glucosamine-6-PO4 synthesis by salicylate and other anti-inflammatory agents in vitro. Arthritis Rheum 1965;8:624–631.

132. McKenzie LS, Horsburgh BA, Ghosh P, et al. Osteoarthrosis: uncertain rationale for anti-inflammatory drug therapy. Lancet 1976;(April 24):908–909. Letter.

133. Coke H. Long-term indomethacin therapy of cox-arthrosis. Ann Rheum Dis 1967;26:346–347.

134. Newman NM, Ling RSM. Acetabular bone destruction related to non-steroidal anti-inflammatory drugs. Lancet 1985;(July 6):11–13.

135. Sudmann E, Bang G. Indomethacin-induced inhibition of haversian remodelling in rabbits. Acta Orthop Scand 1979;50:621–627.

136. Törnkvist H, Lindholm TS, Netz P, et al. Effect of ibuprofen and indomethacin on bone metabolism reflected in bone strength. Clin Orthop Rel Res 1984;187:255–259.

137. Doherty M, Holt M, MacMillan P, et al. A reappraisal of "analgesic hip." Ann Rheum Dis 1986;45:272–276.

138. Rashad S, Revell R, Hemingwas A, et al. Effect of non-steroidal anti-inflammatory drugs on the course of osteoarthritis. Lancet 1989;(September 2):519–522.

139. Milner JC. Osteoarthritis of the hip and indomethacin. J Bone Joint Surg Br 1972;54:752. Letter.

140. Gustavsen R. Training therapy: prophylaxis and rehabilitation. New York: Thieme Inc., 1985:49.

141. Mennell JM. Joint pain: diagnosis and treatment using manipulative techniques. Boston: Little, Brown & Co., 1964:157–159.

142. Gatterman MI. Chiropractic management of spine related disorders. Baltimore: Williams & Wilkins, 1990:151t.

143. Lewit K. Manipulative therapy in rehabilitation of the motor system. London: Butterworth, 1985:28–29.

144. Palmonski MJ, Brandt KD. Aspirin aggravates the degeneration of canine joint cartilage caused by immobilization. Arthritis Rheum 1982;25:1333–1342.

145. Koch RA, Jackson DW. Pubic symphysitis in runners: a report of two cases. Am J Sports Med 1981;9:62–63.

146. Beer E. Periostitis of the symphysis and descending rami of the pubes following suprapubic operations. Int J Med Surg 1924;37:224–225.

147. Howse AJG. Osteitis pubis in an Olympic road-walker. Proc Royal Soc Med 1964;57:88–90.

148. Harris NH, Murray RO. Lesions of the symphysis in athletes. Br Med J 1974;4:211–214.

149. Pearson RL. Case report: osteitis pubis in a basketball player. Phys Sportsmed 1988;16:69–70.

150. Smodlaka VN. Groin pain in soccer players. Phys Sports Med 1980;8:57–61.

151. Kulund D. The injured athlete. 2nd ed. Philadelphia: JB Lippincott, 1988:423.

152. Pyle LA. Osteitis pubis in an athlete. J Am Coll Health Assoc 1975;23:238–239.

153. York JP. Sports and the male genitourinary system: genital injuries and sexually transmitted diseases. Phys Sportsmed 1990;18:92–96, 98–100.

154. Kulund DN. The injured athlete. Philadelphia: JB Lippincott, 1982:343.

155. Roy S, Irvin R. Sports medicine: prevention, evaluation, management and rehabilitation. Englewood Cliffs, NJ: Prentice-Hall, 1983:291.

156. Briner WW, Howe WB, Jain RK. Case conference: scrotal injury in a high school football player—surgical exploration vs diagnostic testing. Phys Sportsmed 1990; 18:64–68.

157. Morton DC. Gynaecological complications of water-skiing. Med J Aust 1970;1:1256–1257.

158. Tweedale PG. Gynecological hazards of water-skiing. Can Med Assoc J 1973;108:20–21. Letter to the editor.

159. Wheeler LP. Common musculoskeletal dance injuries. Chiro Sports Med 1987;1:17–23.

160. Garfinkel D, Talbot AA, Clarizio M, et al. Medical problems on a professional baseball team. Phys Sportsmed 1981;9:85–93.

161. DeHaven KE, Lintner DM. Athletic injuries: comparison by age, sport and gender. Am J Sports Med 1986;14: 218–224.

162. Schafer RC. Chiropractic management of sports and recreational injuries. Baltimore: Williams & Wilkins, 1982:462–463.

163. Anonymous. Athletic training and sports medicine. 2nd ed. Park Ridge, IL: American Academy of Orthopaedic Surgeons, 1991:305.

164. Lewit K. Manipulative therapy in rehabilitation of the motor system. London: Butterworth, 1985:135.

165. Triano JJ, Hyde T. Manipulation. Spine: State of the Art Reviews. 1990;4:446–453.

166. Janda V. The relationship of hip joint musculature to the pathogenesis of low back pain. International Conference on Manipulative Therapy, Perth, Western Australia. 1983:28–31.

167. Gatterman MI. Chiropractic management of spine related disorders. Baltimore: Williams & Wilkins, 1990: 114–124.

168. Fickel TE. "Snapping hip" and sacroiliac sprain: example of cause-effect relationship. J Manipulative Physiol Ther 1989;12:290–392.

169. Herzog W, Read LJ, Conway PJW, et al. Reliability of motion palpation procedures to detect sacroiliac joint fixations. J Manipulative Physiol Ther 1989;12:86–92.

170. Travell JG, Simmons DG. Myofascial pain and dysfunction: the trigger point manual. the lower extremities. Baltimore: Williams & Wilkins, 1992;2:429.

171. Perle SM. Runner's pelvis. Chiropract J 1989;(Feb):13.

172. Kirkaldy-Willis WH. The site and nature of the lesion. In: Kirkaldy-Willis WH, ed. Managing low back pain. 2nd ed. New York: Churchill Livingstone, 1988:135–137.

173. Ferezy JS. Chiropractic management of meralgia paresthetica: a case report. Chiro Tech 1989;1:52–56.

174. Radler M, Rossen J. Femoral nerve entrapment syndrome: treatment with chiropractic manipulation. Am Chiro 1984;(July):7, 8, 13.

175. Stites JS. Meralgia paresthetica: a case report. Res Forum 1986;(Winter):55–58.

176. Little H. Trochanteric bursitis: a common cause of pelvic girdle pain. Can Med Assoc J 1979;120:456–458.

177. Baker BE. Current concepts in the diagnosis and treatment of musculotendinous injuries. Med Sci Sports Exerc 1984;16:323–327.

178. Estwanik JJ, Sloane B, Rosenberg MA. Groin strain and other possible causes of groin pain. Phys Sportsmed 1990;18:54–58, 60, 65.

179. Schafer RC. Chiropractic management of sports and recreational injuries. Baltimore: Williams & Wilkins, 1982:454.

180. Hammer WI. The hip and thigh. In: Hammer WI, ed. Functional soft tissue examination and treatment by manual methods: the extremities. Gaithersburg, MD: Aspen Publishers, 1991:105–122.

181. Collins K, Wagner M, Peterson K, et al. Overuse injuries in triathletes: a study of the 1986 Seafair Triathlon. Am J Sports Med 1989;17:675–680.

182. Maughan RJ, Miller JDB. Incidence of training-related injuries among marathon runners. Br J Sports Med 1983;17:162–165.

183. Brubaker CE, James SL. Injuries to runners. Sports Med 1974;2:189–198.

184. Jacobs SJ, Berson BL. Injuries to runners: a study of entrants to a 10,000 meter race. Am J Sports Med 1986;14:151–155.

185. Watson MD, DiMartino PP. Incidence of injuries in high school track and field athletes and its relation to performance ability. Am J Sports Med 1987;15:251–254.

186. Canale ST, Cantler ED, Sisk TD, et al. A chronicle of injuries of an American intercollegiate football team. Am J Sports Med 1981;9:384–389.

187. Kretsch A, Grogan R, Duras P, et al. 1980 Melbourne marathon study. Med J Aust 1984;141:809–814.

188. Geiringer SR. The biomechanics of running. J Back Musculoskel Rehabil 1995;5:273–279.

189. Garrett W Jr. Muscle injuries: clinical and basic aspects. Med Sci Sports Exerc 1990;22:436–443.

190. Desiderio VG. Hamstring injuries. In: Taylor PM, Taylor DK, eds. Conquering athletic injuries. Champaign, IL: Leisure Press, 1988:144–145.

191. Kulund DN. The injured athlete. 2nd ed. Philadelphia: JB Lippincott, 1988:421–433.

192. Roy S, Irvin I. Sports medicine: prevention, evaluation, management and rehabilitation. Englewood Cliffs, NJ: Prentice-Hall, 1983:303–305.

193. MacLennan W, Hall M, Timothy J, et al. Is weakness in old age due to muscle wasting? Age Ageing 1980;9:188–192.

194. Schafer RC. Chiropractic management of sports and recreational injuries. Baltimore: Williams & Wilkins, 1982:468–470.

195. Agre JC. Hamstring injuries: proposed aetiological factors, prevention, and treatment. Sports Med 1985;2:21–33.

196. Wiktorsson-Möller M, Öberg B, Ekstrand J, et al. Effects of warming up, massage and stretching on range of motion and muscle strength in the lower extremity. Am J Sports Med 1983;11:249–252.

197. Burnie J. Factors affecting selected reciprocal muscle group ratios in preadolescents. J Sports Med 1987;8:40–45.

198. Tabin GC, Gregg J, Bonci T. Predictive leg strength values in immediately prepubescent and postpubescent athletes. Am J Sports Med 1985;13:387–389.

199. Gillian TB, Sady SP, Freedson PS, et al. Isokinetic torque levels for high school football players. Arch Phys Med Rehabil 1979;60:110–114.

200. Adelaar RS. The practical biomechanics of running. Am J Sports Med 1986;14:497–500.

201. Stauber WT. Eccentric action of muscles: physiology, injury and adaptation. In: Pandolf KB, ed. Exercise and sports sciences reviews. Baltimore: Williams & Wilkins, 1989;17:157–185.

202. Mora J. Dynamic stretching: a kinder, gentler method of stretching. Triathlete 1990;84:28, 30–31.

203. McArdle WD, Katch FI, Katch VL. Exercise physiology energy, nutrition and human performance. Philadelphia: Lea & Febiger, 1986:392–397.

204. Lewit K. Manipulative therapy in rehabilitation of the motor system. London: Butterworth, 1985:309.

205. Alter MJ. Science of stretching. Champaign, IL: Human Kinetics, 1988.

206. Anderson B. Stretching. Bolinas, CA: Shelter, 1980.

207. Roy S, Irvin I. Sports medicine: prevention, evaluation, management and rehabilitation. Englewood Cliffs, NJ: Prentice-Hall, 1983:40.

208. Taylor PM, Braun KA. Stretching exercises. In: Taylor PM, Taylor DK, eds. Conquering athletic injuries. Champaign, IL: Leisure Press, 1988:195–205.

209. Kulund DN. The injured athlete. Philadelphia: JB Lippincott, 1982:166.

210. Harris DA, Henneman E. Feedback signals from muscle and their efferent control. In: Mountcastle VB, ed. Medical physiology. 14th ed. St. Louis: CV Mosby, 1980:703–717.

211. Schultz P. Flexibility: day of the static stretch. Phys Sports Med 1979;7:109–117.

212. Perle SM, Murphy DR. Clinicians notebook: hamstring strains (pulls). Chiro Sports Med 1991;5:29–30.

213. Murphy DR. A critical look at static stretching: are we doing our patients harm? Chiro Sports Med 1991;5:67–70.

214. Cibulka MT, Rose SJ, Delitto A, et al. Hamstring strain treated by mobilizing the sacroiliac joint. Phys Ther 1986;66:1220–1223.

215. Cyriax J. Diagnosis of soft tissue lesions. 8th ed. Textbook of orthopaedic medicine, vol 1. Philadelphia: Baillière Tindall, 1982:49–51.

216. Hammer WI. The hip and thigh. In: Hammer WI, ed. Functional soft tissue examination and treatment by manual methods: the extremities. Gaithersburg, MD: Aspen Publishers, 1991:117.

217. Sartoris D, Bronzinsky S, Resnick D. MRI's role in assessing musculoskeletal disorders. J Musculoskel Med 1987;4:12–26.

218. Nosaka K, Clarkson PM. Muscle damage following repeated bouts of high force eccentric exercise. Med Sci Sports Exerc 1995;27:1263–1269.

219. Raether P, Lutter L. Recurrent compartment syndrome in the posterior thigh: report of a case. Am J Sports Med 1982;10:40–42.

220. Simmons D. Myofascial pain syndrome due to trigger points. IRMA monograph series no. 1. International Rehabilitation Medicine Association, 1987:25–27.

221. Travell J, Simmons D. Myofascial pain and dysfunction: the trigger point manual. the lower extremities. Baltimore: Williams & Wilkins, 1992;2:325.

222. Peters R. Facet syndrome. Eur J Chiro 1984;32:85–102.

223. Wilkerson G. Inflammation in connective tissue: etiology and management. Athletic Training 1985;21:298–301.

224. Weiker G. Getting a leg up can be a pain. Sportcare & Fitness 1988;1:16–23.

225. Almekinders L, Gilber J. Healing of experimental muscle strains and the effects of nonsteroidal anti-inflammatory medication. Am J Sports Med 1986;14:303–308.

226. Almekinders LC, Baynes AJ, Bracey LW. An in vitro investigation into the effects of repetitive motion and nonsteroidal antiinflammatory medication on human tendon fibroblasts. Am J Sports Med 1995;23:119–123.

227. Weiler J. Medical modifiers of sports injury: the use of nonsteroidal anti-inflammatory drugs (NSAIDs) in sports soft-tissue injury. Clin Sports Med 1992;11:625–644.

228. Skoglund CR. Neurophysiological aspects on the pathological erector spinae reflex in cases of mechanical pelvic dysfunction. J Man Med 1989;4:29–30.

229. Ivey M. Myositis ossificans of the thigh following manipulation of the knee. Clin Orthop 1985;198:102–105.

230. Jankiewicz JJ, Hennrikus WL, Houkom JA. The appearance of the piriformis muscle syndrome in computed tomography and magnetic resonance imaging: a case report and review of the literature. Clin Orthop Rel Res 1991;262:205–209.

231. Knight KL. Guidelines for rehabilitation of sports injuries. Clin Sports Med 1985;4:405–416.

232. Garrick JG, Webb DR. Sports injuries: diagnosis and management. Philadelphia: WB Saunders, 1990:182.

233. Safran MR, Garrett WE, Seaber AV, et al. The role of warmup in muscular injury prevention. Am J Sports Med 1988;16:123–129.

234. Dominquez RH, Gajda R. Total body training. New York: Warner Books, 1982.

235. Garrick JG, Webb DR. Sports injuries: diagnosis and management. Philadelphia: WB Saunders, 1990:264.

236. Roy S, Irvin R. Sports medicine: prevention, evaluation, management, and rehabilitation. Englewood Cliffs, NJ: Prentice-Hall, 1983:435–437.

237. Travell JG, Simmons DG. Myofascial pain and dysfunction: the trigger point manual. The lower extremities. Baltimore: Williams & Wilkins, 1992;2:186–214.

238. Myers KP, Thomas R, Barker T. Sciatica of muscular origin in a recreational runner: a case report. Chiro Sports Med 1991;5:31–33.

239. Vandertop WP, Bosma NJ. The piriformis syndrome: a case report. J Bone Joint Surg Am 1991;73:1095–1096.

240. Park HW, Jahng JS, Lee WH. Piriformis syndrome: a case report. Yonsei Med J 1991;32:64–68.

241. Liebenson C. Active muscular relaxation techniques: part II. Clinical application. J Manipulative Physiol Ther 1990;13:2–6.

242. Zeanah W, Hudson T. Myositis ossificans, radiological evaluation of two cases with diagnostic computed tomograms. Clin Orthop 1982;168:187–191.

243. Thorndike A. Myositis ossificans traumatica. J Bone Joint Surg 1940;22:315–323.

244. Anonymous. Athletic training and sports medicine. 2nd ed. Park Ridge, IL: American Academy of Orthopaedic Surgeons, 1991:307–308.

245. Snook GA. Injuries in intercollegiate wrestling: a 5-year study. Am J Sports Med 1982;10:142–144.

246. Tong VYW, Howe J. Traumatic myositis ossificans. J Chiro 1983;20:91–92.

247. Matlin P. The appearance of bone scans following fractures including immediate and long-term studies. J Nucl Med 1979;20:1227–1231.

248. Ellis M, Frank HG. Myositis ossificans traumatica: with reference to the quadriceps femoris muscle. J Trauma 1966;6:724–738.

249. Key J, Jarvis G, Johnson D, et al. Leg injuries. In: Subotnick SI, ed. Sports medicine of the lower extremity. New York: Churchill Livingstone, 1989:309.

250. Lipscomb AB, Thomas ED, Johnson RK. Treatment of myositis ossificans traumatica in athletes. Am J Sports Med 1976;4:111–120.

251. Anato NA. Myositis of the hip in a professional soccer player: a case report. Am J Sports Med 1988;16:82–83.

252. Garrick JG, Webb DR. Sports injuries: diagnosis and management. Philadelphia: WB Saunders, 1990:192.

253. Garrick JG, Webb DR. Sports Injuries: diagnosis and management. Philadelphia: WB Saunders, 1990:193.

254. Ryan JB, Wheeler JH, Hopkinson WJ, et al. Quadriceps contusions: West Point update. Am J Sports Med 1991;19:299–304.

255. Kirkpatrick JS, Koman LA. The role of ultrasound in the early diagnosis of myositis ossificans: a case report. Am J Sports Med 1987;15:179–181.

256. Fornage BD, Eftekhari F. Sonographic diagnosis of myositis ossificans. J Ultrasound Med 1989;8:463–466.

257. Kransdorf MJ, Meis JM, Jelinek JS. Myositis ossificans: MR appearance with radiologic-pathologic correlation. AJR 1991;157:1243–1248.

258. Ehara S, Nakasato T, Tamakawa Y, et al. MRI of myositis ossificans circumscripta. Clin Imaging 1991;15:130–134.

259. Rothwell AG. Quadriceps hematoma: a prospective clinical study. Clin Orthop Rel Res 1982;171:97–103.

260. Jackson DW, Feagin JA. Quadriceps contusions in young athletes. J Bone Joint Surg Am 1973;55:95–105.

261. Key J, Johnson D, Jarvis G, et al. Knee and thigh injuries. In: Subotnick SI, ed. Sports medicine of the lower extremity. New York: Churchill Livingstone, 1989:309.

262. Anonymous. Athletic training and sports medicine. 2nd ed. Park Ridge, IL: American Academy of Orthopaedic Surgeons, 1991.

263. Key J, Johnson D, Jarvis G, et al. Hip, pelvis and low back injuries. In: Subotnick SI, ed. Sports medicine of the lower extremity. New York: Churchill Livingstone, 1989:313–314.

264. Lyons JC, Peterson LFA. The snapping iliopsoas tendon. Mayo Clin Proc 1984;59:327–329.

265. Sammarco GJ. The dancer's hip. Clin Sports Med 1983;2:485–498.

266. Schaberg JE, Harper MC, Allen WC. The snapping hip syndrome. Am J Sports Med 1984;12:361–365.

267. Weiker GG. Musculoskeletal problems and the gymnast. In: Grana WA, Lombardo JA, Sharkey BJ, et al. eds. Advances in sports medicine and fitness. Chicago: Year Book, 1989;2:194.

268. Reid DC, Burnham RS, Saboe LA, et al. Lower extremity flexibility patterns in classical ballet dancers and their correlation to lateral hip and knee injuries. Am J Sports Med 1987;15:347–352.

269. Ober FR. Back strain and sciatica. JAMA 1934;104:1580–1583.

270. DeFranca GG. The snapping hip syndrome: a case study. Chiro Sports Med 1988;2:8–11.

271. Hoppenfeld S. Physical examination of the spine and extremities. New York: Appleton-Century-Crofts, 1976:151.

272. Garrick JG, Webb DR. Sports injuries: diagnosis and management. Philadelphia: WB Saunders, 1990:186–192.

273. Cyriax J. Diagnosis of soft tissue lesions. 8th ed. Textbook of orthopaedic medicine, vol 1. Philadelphia: Baillière Tindall, 1982:61.

274. Magee DJ. Orthopedic physical assessment. Philadelphia: WB Saunders, 1987:296.

275. Kaplan PE, Tanner ED. Musculoskeletal pain and disability. East Norwalk, CT: Appleton & Lange, 1989:173.

276. Zoltan DJ, Clancy WG. A new operative approach to snapping hip and refractory trochanteric bursitis in athletes. Am J Sports Med 1986;14:201–204.

277. Desiderio VG. Hip bursitis (hip tendinitis). In: Taylor PM, Taylor DK, eds. Conquering athletic injuries. Champaign, IL: Leisure Press, 1988:141–142.

278. Arnheim DD. Essentials of athletic training. St. Louis: Times Mirror/Mosby College Publishing, 1987:254.

279. Schneider MJ. Snapping hip syndrome in a marathon runner: treatment by manual trigger point therapy: a case study. Chiro Sports Med 1990;4:54–58.

280. Mennell JM. Back pain. Boston: Little, Brown & Co., 1960:165.

281. Hoppenfeld S. Physical examination of the spine and extremities. New York: Appleton-Century-Crofts, 1976:167.

282. Clancy WG. Runners' injuries: part two. evaluation and treatment of specific injuries. Am J Sports Med 1980;8:287–289. Symposium.

283. Stanish WD. Overuse injuries in athletes: a perspective. Med Sci Sports Exerc 1984;16:1–7.

284. Brooker AF. The surgical approach to refractory trochanteric bursitis. Johns Hopkins Med J 1979;134:98–100.

285. Anonymous. Athletic training and sports medicine. 2nd ed. Park Ridge, IL: American Academy of Orthopaedic Surgeons, 1991:371.

286. Wiltse LL, Frantz CH. Non-suppurative osteitis pubis in the female. J Bone Joint Surg Am 1956;38:500–516.

287. Subotnick SI. Clinical biomechanics. In: Subotnick SI, ed. Sports medicine of the lower extremity. New York: Churchill Livingstone, 1989:165.

288. Leadbetter W. Cell-matrix response in tendon injury. Clin Sports Med 1992;11:533–578.

289. Stanish WD, Curwin S, Rubinovich M. Tendinitis: the analysis and treatment for running. Clin Sports Med 1985;4:593–609.

290. Pope C. Radiologic evaluation of tendon injuries. Clin Sports Med 1992;11:579–599.

291. Little H. Trochanteric bursitis: a common cause of pelvic girdle pain. Can Med Assoc J 1979;120:456–458.

292. Travell JG, Simmons DG. Myofascial pain and dysfunction: the trigger point manual. the lower extremities. Baltimore: Williams & Wilkins, 1992;2:217–226.

293. De Franca GG, Levine LJ. Case report: the quadratus lumborum and low back pain. J Manipulative Physiol Ther 1991;14:142–149.
294. Silverstolpe L. A pathological erector spinae reflex—a new sign of mechanical pelvis dysfunction: proposal of treatment. J Man Med 1989;4:28. Brief communication.
295. Midttun A, Bojsen-Møller F. The sacrotuberous ligament pain syndrome. In: Grieve GP, ed. Modern manual therapy of the vertebral column. New York: Churchill Livingstone, 1986:590–602.
296. Logan VF, Murray FM, eds. Textbook of Logan basic methods. Chesterfield, MO: L.B.M., Inc., 1950.

The Knee

Thomas A. Souza

The knee is a functional marvel. Although appearing as a simple hinge joint, the knee has an intricate network of ligaments that mechanically and neurologically govern the function of the joint, resulting in subtle combinations of movement not readily apparent visually. Although attempts at synthesizing these components have led to amazing advances, it is unlikely that any artificial device will fully supplement loss of any key structures in or around the knee.

An investigation into the components of the knee complex is warranted before attempts at evaluation and determination of treatment and rehabilitation approaches are made. Paramount in the understanding of any individual joint is the concept of kinesiologic linkage: the dependency on biomechanical factors in other joints above and below. Any approach to evaluation or treatment must consider this linkage, particularly with the athlete. Therefore, the following discussion is primarily directed at the knee; an understanding of how the knee participates with other joints in primary movements such as walking, running, or cycling is crucial to full understanding.

FUNCTIONAL ANATOMY

Osteology

Investigation of the bony architecture reveals clues to the functional requirements and capacities of the knee. The shape and angulation of bone dictate movement restrictions and possibilities. There is an inherent instability of the knee if only the bony restraints are considered. This places an enormous demand on soft tissue performance.

The distal femur is composed of two bulbous condyles (Fig. 14.1). The medial condyle extends slightly more distal than the lateral, which results in a femoral angulation of approximately 10° medially (1). The condyles extend posteriorly with an increasing radius and are convex, yet slightly flattened, which results in more contact area with the tibia. The shapes of the condyles

differ, with the medial being shorter anterior to posterior and angled slightly medial. The lateral is sagittally oriented and longer than the medial as well as extending farther anteriorly. This extension helps prevent lateral dislocation of the patella. This structural difference also establishes a locking mechanism for the knee in full extension, as will be discussed later.

In between the two condyles is a depression called the trochlear (intercondylar) groove. It provides bony tracking and stabilization for the patella. As the femur moves with flexion and extension of the knee, the patella—relative to the femur—glides through this groove.

Epicondyles are present on both femoral condyles. The lateral epicondyle may be an area of irritation from the iliotibial band (ITB) (2). Superior to the medial epicondyle is the adductor tubercle, which is often a site of pain due to strains of the adductor magnus and vastus medialis obliquus (VMO) muscles that attach here (3). The medial epicondyle is the femoral insertion for the medial collateral ligament and is often painful or tender when there is a sprain.

The proximal tibia consists of two large, superiorly flattened condyles that articulate with the femoral condyles (Fig. 14.2). The medial condyle is concave, whereas the lateral is slightly convex. This difference is equalized by the concavity effect of the lateral meniscus (1). The condyles extend back posteriorly, overhanging the shaft of the tibia, providing a broad support for the femoral condyles as they move into flexion. The tibial condyles are also angled downward posteriorly approximately 5°–10° (1). Between the condyles on the superior surface are two small bony stalactites referred to as intercondylar eminences (also referred to as spines or tubercles). There are no ligamentous or bony attachments to these areas as one might expect (4). It appears that they serve as blockage to lateral translation and therefore may fracture. Medial tibial spine fractures in children seem to occur most often

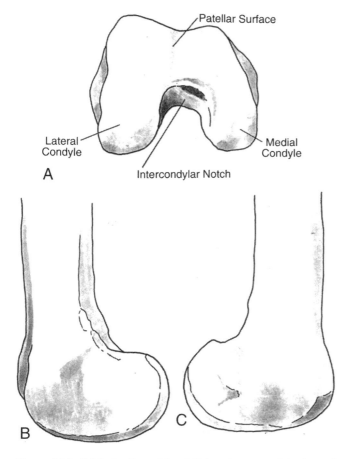

Figure 14.1. **A** Inferior, **B** medial, and **C** lateral aspects of the femoral condyles. (Reprinted with permission from Hertling D, Kessler RM. Management of common musculoskeletal disorders. 2nd ed. Philadelphia: Harper & Row, 1990:395.)

with bicycle accidents in which a blow to the anterior thigh is applied by ground contact with the knee flexed (5). The tibial tubercles mark the axis of rotation for the knee, according to Walker (6). Posterolateral, there is an articular facet on the tibia for the head of the fibula.

The patella is the largest sesamoid bone in the body. It is triangular, with the apex pointing inferiorly. The posterior surface is covered with the thickest hyaline cartilage in the body (4). The articular surface is divided into lateral, medial, and odd facets. The lateral and medial facets are divided by the median ridge, the thickest area of cartilage. This ridge is often where chondromalacia begins (7).

Ligaments

The knee is statically supported by a group of ligaments that are both distinct from and also thickenings of the investing capsule and fascia. The oversimplified concept of the knee supported externally by two collateral ligaments and internally by the cruciates is misleading. With the un-

derstanding that the static control of the knee is composed of an intertwining of a complex network of layered ligamentous supports, the naive concept of a simple hinge-joint with independent components is converted to a more functional concept of joined interdependence. Proprioceptive coordination is paramount. When damage occurs, injury to only one structure is less conceivable.

Gruber et al. (8) and Solomonow et al. (9) have noted reflexes related to the ligaments of the knee. When stimulated, there is reflex contraction of supporting musculature. It is believed that this crucial role should be preserved as much as possible during surgery. In particular, with cruciate surgery, the recommended approach is to preserve as much as possible of the residual "stump" as opposed to attaining a "clean" joint, allowing the remaining proprioceptive input to help in controlling stabilization of the knee.

The capsule surrounds the knee joint extending from above the condyles down to the menisci.

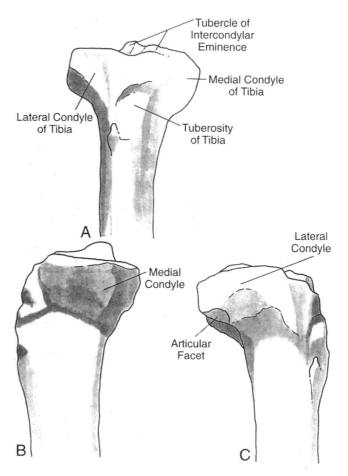

Figure 14.2. Bony anatomy of the **A** anterior, **B** medial, and **C** lateral aspects of the tibia. (Reprinted with permission from Hertling D, Kessler RM. Management of common musculoskeletal disorders. 2nd ed. Philadelphia: Harper & Row, 1990:396.)

The lower extension of the capsule from the meniscus to the tibia is referred to as the coronary ligament (4). Joint line tenderness may indicate damage to either the coronary ligament or meniscus. Further testing is needed to differentiate. Damage to any of these structures tends to shift responsibility to the dynamic support provided by the muscles.

MEDIAL STABILIZATION

Static medial support is provided by two major structures, the medial capsular ligament and the tibial (medial) collateral ligament (MCL). These are sometimes referred to as the deep and superficial medial collateral ligaments, respectively. The deep ligament is a thickening of the capsule and is divided into three sections. The posterior section is often referred to separately as the posterior oblique ligament. This distinction is important because this section is thought to serve as a major stabilizer preventing valgus and medial rotary instability. The deep capsular ligament is at-

tached to the meniscus and is therefore more likely to be involved with meniscus injury and vice versa. Special consideration must be given to the posterior oblique ligament when rehabilitation of the knee includes knee extension. It may be overstretched from 60°–90° (10). The MCL is a secondary stabilizer for anterior posterior knee movement assisting the anterior cruciate (11).

The MCL is long, extending from the medial epicondyle to 4 to 7 cm below the joint line. The tibial attachment is actually below the pes anserine insertion (Fig. 14.3). The MCL prevents excessive external rotation and abduction of the tibia on the femur. Even in flexion some of the anterior fibers remain taut, providing some stabilization.

LATERAL STABILIZATION

Unlike the medial side, the superficial ligament—referred to as the lateral (fibular) collateral ligament (LCL)—is not attached to the meniscus. The lateral collateral is separated from the menis-

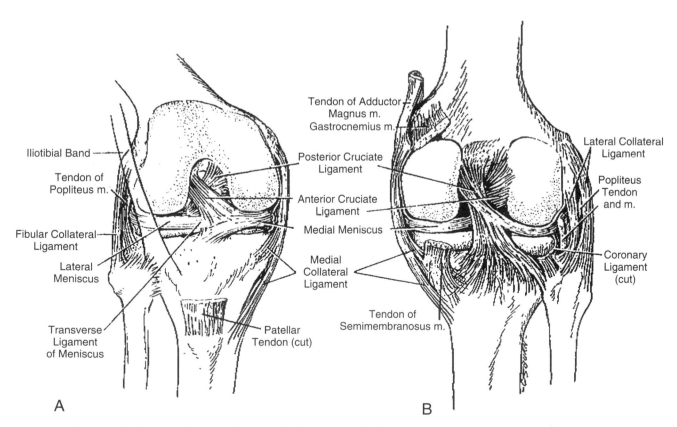

Figure 14.3. Anatomic drawings of the knee. **A.** Anterior view. Patellar tendon is sectioned and the patella reflected upward. Knee flexed. Note that the cruciate ligament rises in front of anterior tibial spine, not from it. Note also that the medial meniscus is firmly attached to the medial collateral ligament. **B.** Posterior view. Knee extended. Note that the posterior ligament has been removed. The two layers of the medial collateral ligament are shown diagrammatically, as is the tibial portion of the lateral collateral ligament. The posterior cruciate ligament rises behind the tibia, not on its upper surface. Observe the femoral attachment of the anterior cruciate ligament at the back of the notch. (Reprinted with permission from O'Donoghue DH, Treatment of injuries to athletes. 4th ed. Philadelphia: WB Saunders, 1984:477.)

cus by the tendon of the popliteus muscle. A small bursa often exists between the popliteus tendon and the LCL. The LCL is much shorter than the medial side ligaments, with insertions at the lateral condyle of the femur and superior head of the fibula (Fig. 14.3). It is taut (like the medial ligament) on outward rotation of the tibia. In addition, it provides varus support in extension and adduction of the tibia on the femur. It is injured less often than the medial due to its freedom from the lateral meniscus and the fact that contact injury is usually from the outside of the knee, causing a compression force rather than a stretch.

ANTERIOR-POSTERIOR STABILIZATION— CRUCIATE LIGAMENTS

The cruciates are crucial for providing support and guidance of rotational movement. They increasingly cross with internal rotation of the tibia and uncross with external rotation (Fig. 14.4) (12). The cruciates are named according to their tibial attachments. An easy reminder is to cross the fingers (index under the middle). The middle finger represents the anterior cruciate, and the index finger represents the posterior cruciate.

Anterior Cruciate

The anterior cruciate ligament (ACL) is intraarticular yet extrasynovial; it is covered by a tent of synovium (13). It is approximately the size of the little finger. Insertions are at the anterior intercondylar area of the tibia, from which it spirals posteriorly and laterally to insert on the medial aspect of the lateral femoral condyle in a vertical orientation (Fig. 14.5). The ACL is usually described as containing three coiled bundles. The anterior fibers are tight on extension, whereas in flexion the posterior fibers are tight (14). The anterior fibers attaching to the tibia rotate to become the medial fiber attachment on the femur. This unique design allows a part of the ligament to be taut through most ranges of motion—an engineering feat hard to imitate.

The ACL is tightest in the extremes of flexion and extension. In midflexion it tightens with internal rotation. Through its connection with the meniscus, the ACL helps guide rotational movement, in particular, the "screw-home" mechanism in the last few degrees of knee extension. In addition, it serves the stabilization functions mentioned above, preventing hyperextension, forward movement of

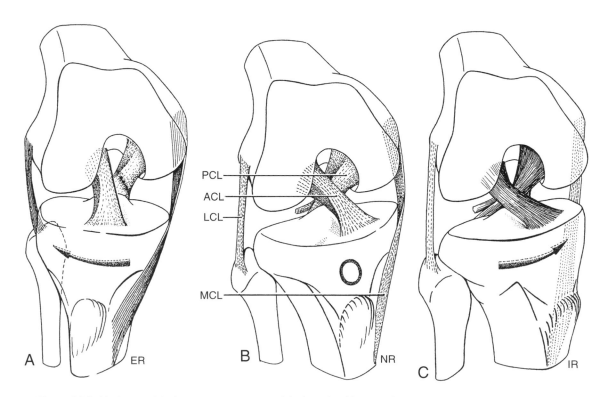

Figure 14.4. Mechanics of the ligamentous structures of the knee. In addition to their synergistic functions, the cruciate and collateral ligaments also exercise a basic antagonistic function during rotation. **A.** In external rotation, it is the collateral ligaments that tighten and inhibit excessive rotation by becoming crossed in space. **B.** In the neutral position, none of the four ligaments is under unusual tension. **C.** In internal rotation, the collateral ligaments become more vertical and lax, while the cruciates become coiled around each other and come under strong tension. (Reprinted with permission from Muller W. The knee: form, function, and ligament reconstruction. New York: Springer-Verlag, 1983:67.)

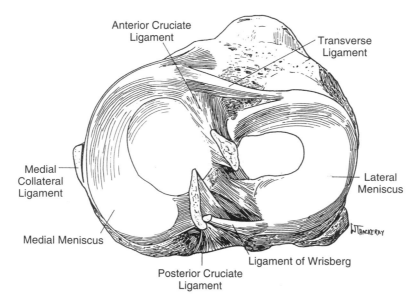

Figure 14.5. The tibial plateau. Note the shape and attachments of the medial and lateral menisci. (Reprinted with permission from Nicholas JA, Hershman EB, eds. The lower extremity and spine in sports medicine. St. Louis: CV Mosby, 1986;687.)

the tibia on the femur in flexion, and internal rotation. It is suggested that external rotation is prevented by the wrapping of the ACL around the medial side of the lateral femoral condyle (15).

Posterior Cruciate

The posterior cruciate ligament (PCL) is much broader, approximately the size of a thumb. It too is intraarticular and extrasynovial. The course of the fibers runs from the posterior intercondylar area anteromedial to the lateral aspect of the medial femoral condyle to the intercondylar notch (Fig. 14.5). Twisting like the ACL, the posterior fibers on the tibia become the lateral fibers on the femur. Recently, Kennedy et al. discovered a number of proprioceptive fibers in the ligament, suggesting an important afferent function that was previously only suspected (16).

Functionally, the PCL prevents backward movement of the tibia on the femur. Dynamically, this is supported by the popliteus and hamstring muscles. The PCL also prevents excessive internal rotation of the tibia, a function it shares with its anterior counterpart.

Additional posterior support is provided by the posterior capsule and a thickening referred to as the popliteal oblique ligament. Dynamically, they are reinforced by the semimembranosus muscle. Laterally, the arcuate ligament (an extension of the capsule) lends some support through its attachment to the styloid process of the fibula and the connection with the superficial fibers of the popliteus.

Blood supply to the cruciates is mainly from the middle genicular artery (17). There is some supply from the terminal branches of the inferior genicular artery. Orientation of the vessels is parallel to the collagen fibers of the ligaments. Clinically, it is important to note that adult damage to the anterior cruciate is often a midsubstance tear that severs the vascular supply entirely due to the above mentioned orientation.

Branches of the tibial nerve supply the cruciates, serving primarily a vasomotor function. Recently, fibers separate from the vasculature lying within the ligament have been identified (18). This lends some credence to the belief that the cruciates serve a proprioceptive function in addition to their stability role.

PATELLAR STABILITY

A combination of static and dynamic supports helps track the patella through flexion and extension of the knee. The ligamentous (static) component is relatively symmetrical. That is, most named structures have a lateral and medial element. The structure of this support is layered, with the most superficial referred to as the arciform layer (19). It lies anterior to the patellar tendon and posterior to the prepatellar bursa. The arciform layer bridges one of the major support structures—the medial and lateral retinaculi. The retinaculi are fascial extensions of the vastus muscles, enveloping and binding the patella. The patellotibial ligaments (medial and lateral) are condensations of the retinaculum in the interme-

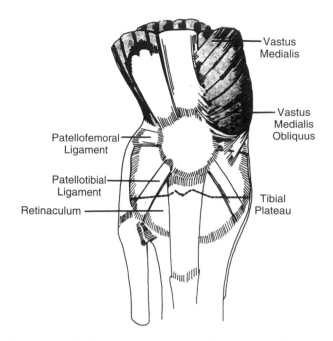

Figure 14.6. Medial and lateral patellotibial ligaments are oblique condensations of the retinacula. (Reprinted with permission from Hughston JC, Walsh WM, Puddu G. Patellar subluxation and dislocation. Philadelphia: WB Saunders, 1984:10.)

Table 14.1. Patellar Stability

Ligamentous (Static)	Muscular (Dynamic)
Superficial—arciform layer	Quadriceps tendon plus the fascial extensions of the vasti muscles (retinaculi)
Intermediate—patellotibial ligaments	
Deep—patellofemoral ligaments	

diate layer. In the deep layer, the condensations are the patellofemoral ligaments (Fig. 14.6) (Table 14.1) (19).

The patellofemoral ligaments are usually thin and provide little support except when vastus medialis dysplasia is present. As always, when one structure fails to perform a function, a secondary structure is usually available. Yet, in this case, the backup support lacks dynamic control. In contrast, the patellotibial ligaments have no dynamic backup; therefore, they are—out of necessity—more functional. Centrally, the patellar tendon or ligament provides sagittal stability.

Dynamic support is directed through the quadriceps tendon and, as mentioned previously, the fascial extensions (retinaculi) of the vastus muscles. The retinaculi and patellar tendon have been demonstrated to have a high density of free nerve endings that are theorized to perform a mechanoreceptor/reflex function in stability of the patella (20). Disruption of these structures with a lateral release or other forms of surgery

may seriously compromise the stability of the patella –the exact opposite intention of these surgeries.

Much attention has been focused on the section of the vastus medialis referred to as the VMO (21). It serves a crucial function in tracking of the patella, in particular, through the last degrees of knee extension. Additionally, there is a lateral counterpart from the vastus lateralis. Specific muscle functions will be discussed later.

Menisci

The menisci are structures that help deepen the articulation of the femoral condyles with the tibia. This tends to add static support and help decrease joint reaction forces to the tibia. Together they are wedge-shaped and thicker in the periphery. Centrally, they do not extend over the entire joint surface (Fig. 14.5). Although originally called semilunar cartilages, they have no cartilage and develop embryologically from the same tissue as the cruciates (4). The medial meniscus is more C shaped and larger, corresponding to the larger medial femoral condyle. Attachments to the deeper portions of the MCL fix the meniscus and restrict much movement. The lateral meniscus is normally more oval, and smaller, and is not firmly attached to the LCL, allowing more movement. Both menisci have tibial attachments referred to as anterior and posterior horns. These are close to the tibial insertions for the cruciates. Several ligaments acting together join meniscus to meniscus, meniscus to cruciates, and meniscus to bone (Fig. 14.5). They are as follows.

1. Coronary ligament—the inferior connection of the investing capsule.
2. Transverse ligament (Winslow)—connects the anterior horns of the medial and lateral meniscus.
3. Barkow's ligament—connects the posterior horn of the lateral meniscus to the anterior horn of the medial meniscus.
4. Meniscofemoral ligaments (named in relation to PCL)—connect the lateral meniscus to the medial femoral condyle.
   A. Anterior meniscofemoral—ligament of Humphrey.
   B. Posterior meniscofemoral—ligament of Wrisberg.
5. Meniscopatellar ligaments—connect the patella with the anterior menisci.

The meniscofemoral, transverse, and Barlow's ligaments are not consistently demonstrable in all dissections (22).

Through these connections, the menisci move during femoral-tibial motion. During flexion and extension they move with the tibia, moving anterior on extension via the meniscopatellar attachments (Fig. 14.7) and posterior on flexion via the popliteus attachment to the lateral meniscus and the extension of the semimembranosus attachment to the medial meniscus (23). They follow the femur during rotational movement. This is apparent if one actively internally rotates the tibia while palpating the medial joint line—the meniscus is felt to bulge. On external rotation, a depression is felt over the joint line, indicating retraction. The limit of motion of the lateral meniscus is approximately 10 mm; for the medial meniscus, only 2 mm (24).

Controversy about the exact functional capacities of the menisci still exists. Last emphasizes that one of the main functions is rotation (4). He uses the example of the fruit bat, which is the only mammal without menisci or a popliteus muscle. This bat is unable to rotate the knee. Certainly, the intimate connections with the cruciates help substantiate this theory on a more functional basis. It seems appropriate to use an analogy of the menisci as tracks for the femoral condyles, guided by the cruciates. This figure-eight description by Helfet (25) is crucial to the understanding of interdependent relationships and the effects of damage or removal of any elements (Fig. 14.8).

The weight-bearing function of the menisci is probably not one of direct contact. Due to the menisci's ability to spread a thin film of synovial

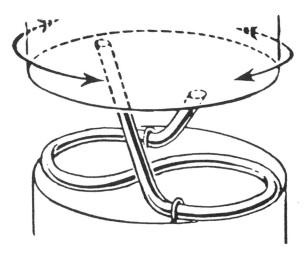

Figure 14.8. The figure-eight description of meniscal function. The anatomic arrangement and continuity of the cruciates with the semilunar cartilage suggest that the function of guiding rotation is shared in this figure-eight manner. (Reprinted with permission from Helfet AJ. Disorders of the knee. 2nd ed. Philadelphia: JB Lippincott, 1982, 105.)

fluid, irritating direct surface contact with the femoral condyles is prevented. (The menisci are not covered with synovial membrane.) Any disruption of this normal oiling process, such as sudden direct compression combined with rotation, allows tearing of the meniscus.

The medial and lateral genicular arteries supply the meniscus (26). With a spoke-like configuration, the branches of these arteries extend in a radial fashion from the periphery toward the center of each meniscus. The extent of supply seems limited to between 10% and 30% of the width of the meniscus (27). This is an important consideration in prognosis of repair with peripheral tears. Also, the extent of blood supply is greater in the younger individual.

Muscles

The muscles of the knee must serve a number of simultaneous functions. These include tracking of the patella, deceleration/acceleration of the leg, flexion/extension of the knee, and varus/valgus stability. As with all muscular supported structures, the knee may rely on secondary functions of particular muscles when primary muscles or ligaments are damaged. Because some muscles originate from the pelvis or insert at the foot/ankle, a kinematic interrelationship exists that must always be considered with evaluation and rehabilitation.

QUADRICEPS

The quadriceps is the largest muscle mass in the body made up of four distinct sections: rec-

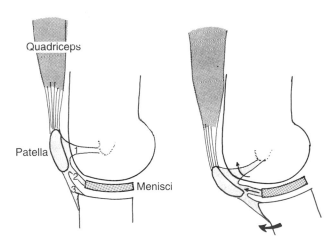

Figure 14.7. Meniscal movement during femoral tibial motion. The quadriceps extend over the anterior knee joint with three ligamentous extensions: 1: the epicondylopatellar part attaches to the epicondylar eminence of the femur and guides rotation of the patella; 2: the meniscopatellar attaches to and pulls the meniscus forward during knee extension; and 3: the infrapatellar tendon, which attaches to the tibial tubercle and extends the tibia on the femur. (Reprinted with permission from Caillet R. Knee pain and disability. 2nd ed. Philadelphia: FA Davis, 1983:17.)

Quadriceps

Patella

Menisci

tus femoris, vastus lateralis, vastus intermedius, and vastus medialis. It performs in several ways.

- Extension of the knee, a function of the group as a whole.
- Flexion of the hip, a secondary function of the rectus femoris only.
- Tracking of the patella, a function of the oblique sections of the vastus medialis and lateralis (including their fascial extension— the retinaculum).

Through the imbedded sesamoid bone, the patella, the combined insertions of the quadriceps gain a mechanical advantage of leverage on the tibia. The quadriceps are also important in the stability needed when the posterior cruciate has been damaged. The nerve supply to all four muscles is the posterior division of the femoral nerve, L2–L4.

Rectus Femoris

The rectus femoris is the most superficial of the quads. It is a thin muscle originating from the anterior inferior iliac spine and inserts into the patella. This attachment provides a stabilizing effect on the pelvis and secondarily may assist in hip flexion. With extension of the hip, the rectus femoris is stretched. This allows a more powerful contraction of the muscle with simultaneous extension of the knee.

Vastus Intermedius

Like all the vasti muscles, the vastus intermedius originates off the femur, thereby only crossing one joint—the knee. It is the deeper, more bulky section lying close to the anterior shaft of the femur. A small muscle, the articularis genu, arises beneath the vastus intermedius to insert into the suprapatellar pouch and medial plica (if present). Not part of the quadriceps per se, the articularis genu serves a coordinated function of pulling the suprapatellar pouch/plica out of the way on extension of the knee, avoiding impingement by the patella (28).

Vastus Lateralis/Medius

The vastus lateralis and medius form the outer borders of the quadriceps group. As mentioned previously, their insertions into the patella have several orientations. The oblique orientation seems to serve a tracking function. In particular, the VMO seems crucial in preventing lateral migration of the patella during flexion/extension. An intimate connection with the adductor magnus at the adductor tubercle again points out the interrelationship common to many knee structures.

Much attention has been paid to this section of the vastus medialis (21). It was once believed that it was the first muscle to atrophy with immobilization of the knee. However, it has been found that simply due to its superficial (and therefore visible) location, it is a more easily monitored sign of generalized quadriceps atrophy (21).

Another misconception was that the VMO was the main muscle contracting through the last 15° of knee extension. It has been demonstrated that all the quadriceps group contracts through this range; however, it appears that the VMO is crucial for medial stability of the patella throughout this range of motion (21).

Although it would appear that the quadriceps would cause an anterior displacement of the tibia in relation to the femur, new research indicates that this is position dependent (29). In other words, from 30° to full extension there was an anterior displacement of approximately 6 mm, whereas flexion of 80° and beyond caused a small posterior displacement of 1.5 mm. Additionally, loading of the quadriceps distally caused internal rotation from 0°–90°, whereas a small amount of external rotation occurred from 90°–120° of flexion. This information will be important to clinical decision making in rehabilitation of the anterior cruciate-deficient knee.

HAMSTRINGS

The hamstrings are a group of three muscles that arise from the ischial tuberosity. They include the semimembranosus, semitendinosus, and biceps femoris. Like the quadriceps, they serve several functions including the following.

- Flexion of the knee.
- Deceleration of the leg.
- Some rotational abilities in flexion.
- Extension of the hip (when the knee is extended).
- Stability functions with knee extension.

The hamstrings are an indispensable component of conservative management of ACL-associated instability, preventing forward movement of the tibia on the femur.

The hamstrings' nerve supply is from the tibial portion of the sciatic nerve, L5-S1. The only exception is the short head of the biceps femoris, which receives its innervation from the common peroneal nerve—still L5-S1. An interesting association exists with the adductor magnus muscle. This muscle is composed of both flexor and adductor components. There is no fascial septum separating it from the hamstrings. It too is supplied by the tibial portion of the sciatic nerve.

Semimembranosus

The semimembranosus is the largest of the hamstrings. It fans out to a broad insertion into the posteromedial knee. The several insertion points include the following.

- The oblique popliteal ligament.
- The posterior capsule and medial meniscus.
- The medial tibia.

This insertional buttressing helps dynamically support the posteromedial knee against rotational forces and, in addition, pulls the medial meniscus slightly posterior during knee flexion (30).

Semitendinosus

The semitendinosus, as the name implies, is more tendon-like with an insertion on the medial tibia with two other muscles referred to as the pes anserine group. These include the sartorius and gracilis. Together they act to stabilize the knee medially in extension. In flexion, they act to rotate the tibia medially.

Biceps Femoris

As this name implies, the biceps femoris has two heads: the short and long. The long head originates off the ischial tuberosity with the other hamstring group. The short head originates off the lateral femur. The insertion is functionally important, fanning out to insert at the following.

- The posterior head of the fibula.
- The lateral upper tibia.
- The LCL and posterior capsule.

The attachment to the tibia allows some minor lateral rotation function. The collateral ligament and capsular attachment allow a tightening of these structures providing dynamic stability in flexion (31).

POPLITEUS

The popliteus has a muscular attachment on the posterior surface of the proximal tibia. Spiralling forward there are two insertions: one to the lateral meniscus and a femoral attachment on the anterior lateral condyle that is tendinous. The course of this tendon runs between the LCL and the lateral meniscus (Fig. 14.9). It is surrounded by a sheet of synovial tissue and creates an access through the capsule, although remaining extraarticular (26). There is some disagreement as to which is actually the origin and insertion of this muscle. However, the issue seems academic when considering its actions.

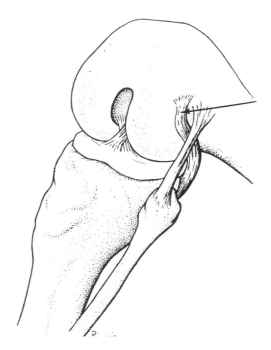

Figure 14.9. The anatomical course of the popliteus tendon. Note the most common location of tenderness in popliteus tendinitis. (Reprinted with permission from Nicholas JA, Hershman EB, eds. The lower extremity and spine in sports medicine. St. Louis: CV Mosby, 1986:1000.)

- Internal rotation of the tibia (or external rotation of the femur).
- Retraction of the lateral meniscus during knee flexion.
- Prevention of anterior displacement of the femur on the tibia.
- A lateral stabilizing function in extension.

Last believes that the popliteus is the key to unlocking of the screw-home mechanism (4). To initiate unlocking, the popliteus in concert with the hamstrings provide internal rotation and flexion, respectively. The attachment to the meniscus seems crucial in preventing pinching between the femur and tibia during flexion of the knee.

Warren et al. believe the popliteus to act as both a muscle and a ligament (26). When the muscle fibers are pulled distally, internal rotation of the tibia occurs (muscular action). When the tendinous fibers are pulled proximally, there is no apparent movement (ligament function for stabilization). This latter effect seems important in stabilization with the PCL on downhill walking or running.

ITB

The ITB is a tendinous extension of the combined insertions of the tensor fascia latae and the gluteus maximus. Originating from the anterior superior iliac spine, the band narrows as it follows a path down the lateral thigh (similar to a pant seam) to insert at Gerdy's tubercle on the proximal tibia. It also shares fascial extensions with the vastus lateralis, biceps femoris, LCL, and patellar retinaculum (Fig. 14.3).

Its importance lies in its changing function as it passes anterior or posterior to the lateral epicondyle. The epicondyle marks the point at which the ITB changes function from a flexor to an extensor of the knee. This occurs at approximately 30° of flexion. As it passes posterior to the axis of rotation, it becomes a flexor; as it passes anterior, it becomes an extensor. This change of function becomes crucial in the understanding of the pivot shift phenomenon found with rotary instability of the knee (as will be described later). Constant rubbing over the lateral epicondyle by a tight ITB may result in the classic ITB syndrome (2).

PES ANSERINE

The pes anserine (goose foot) group of muscles is a combination of three distinct origins with one common insertion. The muscles are the semitendinosus, sartorius, and gracilis. The strongest is the semitendinosus (part of the hamstring trio) that originates off the ischial tuberosity. The gracilis arises from the pubis; the sartorius from the anterior superior iliac spine. They all insert in a conjoined tendon on the proximal medial tibia slightly superolateral to the insertion of the MCL.

In concert, they act as flexors of the knee; when flexed, they act as internal rotators. They are described by Last as "guy ropes" from the tibia to the pelvis. He makes the observation that the sartorius and gracilis are weak as muscles per se and their functions are redundant. Yet their widely spaced origins on the pelvis are mechanically suited for stability (4). Chiropractically, this observation has been clinically noted and used when examining the pelvis.

The insertion point on the tibia is cushioned by a bursa; therefore, it may be the sight of a localized bursitis (pes anserine bursitis).

GASTROCNEMIUS

The gastrocnemius is the only muscle of the triceps surae group to cross the knee joint. Part of the combined tendinous insertion into the calcaneus, the gastrocnemius originates with two heads onto the posterior surface of the lateral and medial condyles of the femur, providing dynamic posterior stability to the knee. Like many muscles of the knee, the attachments are often cushioned by bursa that may become inflamed.

Bursa

There are numerous bursae around the knee placed strategically at points of friction. Some are isolated; others communicate with the joint capsule with some variation. In general, the suprapatellar pouch behind the patella, semimembranosus, and popliteus may connect with the joint capsule. This implies that joint swelling may extend into these areas (Fig. 14.10).

Infrapatellar Fat Pad

The infrapatellar fat pad is a mobile structure located at the distal end of the patella and extending down to the tibia behind the patellar ligament (Fig. 14.10). It moves with flexion and extension through attachments to the quadriceps. On flexion, it fills the intercondylar notch; on extension, it covers the trochlear surface of the femur. It is theorized that the fat pad lubricates the femoral surfaces during its movement (1).

Helfet believes that adhesions between the fat pad and meniscus are a common cause of knee stiffness with meniscus tears or dashboard injuries (25). Hoffa's syndrome is a condition that occurs in girls and women during their menstrual period. Fluid accumulation in the bursa leads to painful distention.

Plica

A plica is a redundant fold of synovium that failed to mature with the rest of the knee. The result is a shortened tissue that may become symptomatic when traumatized or when it physically binds down the patella. There are several types of plica. The most common is the medial shelf plica, which is found in up to 60% of the population (32). The medial shelf plica extends from the superior patella down to the infrapatellar fat pad in association with the patellar tendon (Fig. 14.11).

BIOMECHANICS

From a cursory observation it would appear that the knee functions as a simple hinge joint, allowing flexion and extension only. Within the hinge concept lies an error in visual assumption. Knee movement is also a combination of sliding/gliding plus rotation. All these combined movement patterns are outlined by the bony architecture and orchestrated by the internal guid-

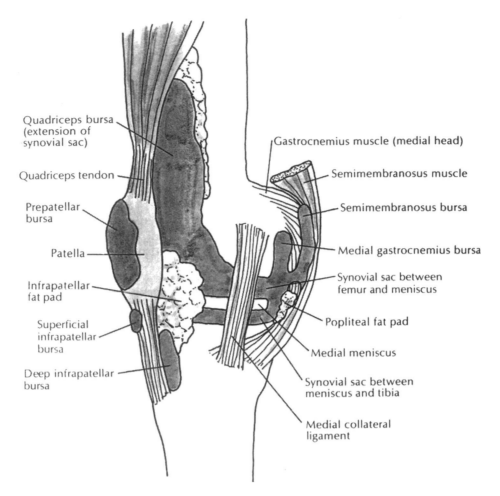

Figure 14.10. Bursae and synovia of the knee from the medial aspect. (Reprinted with permission from Hertling D, Kessler RM. Management of common musculoskeletal disorders. 2nd ed. Philadelphia: Harper & Row, 1990:305.)

ance of the cruciate/meniscus complex. Outside forces are statically resisted and dynamically adjusted by the musculotendinous/ligamentous system.

There are several questions that need to be answered when attempting to grasp the complexity of knee biomechanics.

- What are the active and passive ranges of motion?
- What are the osseous and soft tissue restraints to the extremes of these motions (Table 14.2)?
- What are the dynamic requirements placed on these structures during ambulation?
- What are the actions of internal structures during ambulation?
- What are the reactive forces being applied during movement?

These are questions concerning normal knee mechanics. In addition, pathomechanics of the knee must be understood to promote rational decision making in the treatment and prevention of

knee disorders. This includes the results of absent or damaged structures on other tissues, normal movement patterns, and joint-reactive forces. Clinically, it is important to understand these relationships when using testing procedures. One should ask, "What are the rationale and accuracy of the procedure?"

Range of motion of the knee is determined by active and passive elements. Although all six movements are possible passively, active abduction/adduction is not. It is essentially an accessory movement. In full extension or 0° of flexion, other complementary movements of adduction/abduction and internal/external rotation are not possible actively or passively. As flexion progresses, passive abduction/adduction increase to a few degrees until approximately 30° (33). Beyond this point soft tissue restriction prevents movement. In general, adduction (varus) is usually more accessible than abduction (valgus) due to the relative laxity of the LCL.

Rotation increases as the knee flexes to 120°. At approximately 90° of flexion external rotation

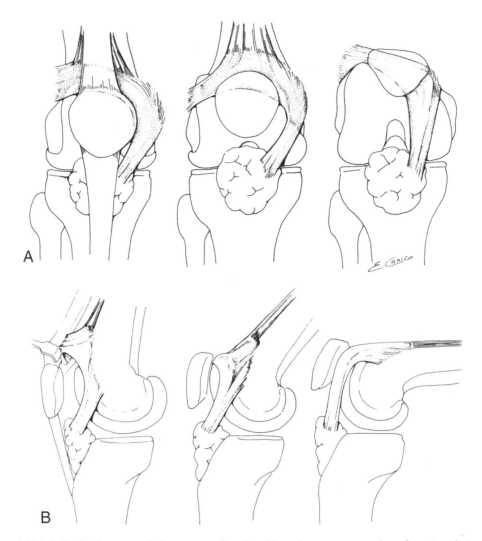

Figure 14.11 A–B. Configuration of the suprapatellar plica. Note the movement and configuration during flexion. (Reprinted with permission from Henry JH. Diagnosis of anterior knee pain. Clin Sports Med 1989;8;188.)

Table 14.2. Soft Tissue Restraints to Knee Movement

Movement	Soft Tissue Restriction
Extension	ACL, PCL, posterior capsule, anterior horns of menisci, and passive hamstrings
Flexion	ACL, PCL, posterior horns of menisci, passive quads
Adduction	LCL, posterolateral capsule (includes arcuate complex)
	Secondarily: ACL, PCL, and medial meniscus
Abduction	MCL, posteromedial capsule
	Secondarily: ACL, PCL, and lateral meniscus
Internal rotation	ACL on the PCL, LCL, posterolateral capsule (includes arcuate complex and menisci)
External rotation	MCL, posteromedial capsule, and menisci

ACL, anterior cruciate ligament; PCL, posterior cruciate ligament; LCL, lateral collateral ligament; MCL, medial collateral ligament.

ranges to approximately 45°, whereas internal rotation is less—approximately 30°. Continued flexion may increase the amount of available rotation 5°–10°. Beyond 120°, soft tissue restriction causes a decrease of rotational ability (Table 14.3) (32).

Full flexion is approximately 140°. Usually 10°–20° of passive increase over active is possible. At this extreme of flexion, the knee becomes less mobile, decreasing the available adduction/abduction and rotational movements.

Descriptions of movement between the tibia and femur are not constant. During the first 20° of flexion a rolling (sometimes called rocking) motion occurs. This is in part due to the unlocking of the knee from full extension. Beyond 20° of flexion, the movement is more of a sliding (sometimes called gliding) motion. When two bones rotate in relation to each other, there is a microsecond when one point does not move. This is referred to as the instant center of rotation. A rolling motion occurs when the instant center and contact point coincide. A sliding movement occurs when the instant center does not coincide with the point of contact but lies at the intersection of lines drawn perpendicular to

two moving reference points (Fig. 14.12). This has been evaluated taking a series of lateral knee radiographs at 10° increments of flexion (32). Using a marking system, the instant center is found and its movement sketched. Abnormal movement may be observed in patients with internal derangement where the knee moves

Table 14.3. Available Movements Based on Knee Position

Movement	Amount of Motion Based on Knee Position
Flexion	0°–140° actively; 10° more with passive assistance.
Abduction/adduction	None available at full extension. A few degrees of passive movement is available passively at 30° knee flexion. This decreases with increased knee flexion.
Internal rotation	None available in full extension; 30° are available at 90° knee flexion. This may increase 5°–10° as the knee reaches 120°. Beyond this there is a decrease.
External rotation	None available in full extension; 45° are available at 90° knee flexion. This may increase 5°–10° as the knee reaches 120°. Beyond this there is a decrease.

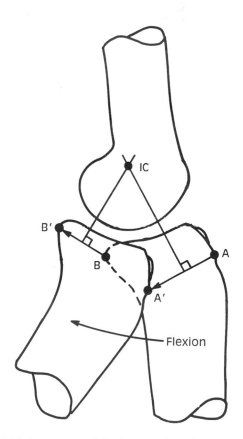

Figure 14.12. Instant center (IC) of rotation during knee motion. The instant center of rotation is located at the intersection of perpendicular bisectors of lines connecting two displaced points on the tibia as the knee flexes. Here, points A and B move to A′ and B′, respectively. (Reprinted with permission from Nicholas JA, Hershman EB, eds. The lower extremity and spine in sports medicine. St. Louis: CV Mosby, 1986:735.)

around a displaced instant center causing stretching of soft tissue restraints. Caution must be used to guarantee no rotation occurs during the radiograph series.

Having addressed the raw mechanics of flexion/extension, it is important to review the intricate internal cooperations of the soft tissue elements. At full extension, there is an osseous lock that prevents movement. The cruciates are essentially unlocked while the mechanically advantaged peripheral structures, such as the collateral ligaments and supporting muscles, are under passive tension. Initiating flexion, the popliteus unlocks the knee imparting internal rotation with subsequent crossing of the cruciates (stabilization shifting centrally). The menisci move posteriorly with the help of the retracting arms of popliteus and semimembranosus.

WALKING AND RUNNING

An approach to the understanding of knee mechanics must include a review of the basics of walking and running. Gait is usually divided between weight-bearing and non–weight-bearing events. Weight-bearing is usually divided into three basic phases: heel strike, stance, and toe-off. This accounts for the walking sequence and 75% of running in most individuals. Non–weight-bearing is simply referred to as the swing phase. More divisions may be used depending on the detail desired. Unfortunately, the terminology is not consistent among authors when describing these events.

At heel strike, the tibia is slightly externally rotated and the knee is close to full extension. This provides a firm base of support for the transfer of weight onto one leg. Immediately after heel strike, as the stance phase begins, there is internal rotation of the tibia as the knee flexes to absorb the stress from ground-reactive forces. The external and internal rotation of the tibia is directly related to subtalar motion at the ankle. The ankle is a firm support with subtalar supination slightly before and at the instant of heel strike (34). During the stance phase, the foot adapts to weight-bearing surfaces and absorbs the resultant force; it unlocks into a flexible structure. The entire lower extremity, beginning with the pelvis and ending at the tibia, internally rotates during this phase. The rotation and translation occurring in the lower extremity are parallel, yet the degree of movement increases distally. For example, translation at the pelvis is greater than at the knee, which is greater than at the ankle (35). This integration is crucial to the function of all the cogs in the kinematic wheel.

At approximately 25% of the stance phase, weight is shifting laterally. As the subtalar joint approaches neutral, the tibia and femur approach neutral rotation. At 50% of the stance phase, neutral rotation of the knee is attained. Weight distribution continues laterally as the subtalar joint supinates. The tibia and femur externally rotate and the leg extends for toe-off. Again, the lower extremity has shifted to a locked position, providing a firm base for propulsion at toe-off.

Muscularly, the events at the knee are a reflection of a semicircular distribution of stresses applied to the medial knee throughout the stance phase of the gait cycle. If one were to observe an individual from above, it would be apparent that the knee describes a half-circle in the transverse plane. This is self-apparent when ascending steps.

At heel strike, stress is applied to the postero-medial corner of the knee. Muscular support is provided by the gluteus maximus and medius, the quadriceps and hamstrings, and the tibialis anterior. During the stance phase the stress is distributed medially. This is balanced by the adductors, quadriceps, hamstrings, and gluteus medius. At toe-off, the forces are directed anteromedially and the muscular support is from the triceps surae, peronei, and tensor fascia latae (36).

The swing phase is not a totally passive event. At the beginning, the short head of the biceps, gracilis, and sartorius contracts. The middle of the swing phase is essentially mechanical. At the end of the swing phase there is contraction of the quadriceps to extend the leg for heel strike, with the hamstrings acting as a brake to this action. The abductors pull the leg outward to provide a more neutral contact at heel strike.

BICYCLING

Bicycling is often used in the rehabilitation of knee disorders. Biomechanically, the patello-femoral joint reaction forces are reduced 5 times compared with walking or running (37). This is due to lack of loading in the seated position. Although not weight-bearing, it is still possible to overstrain medial or lateral elements of the musculature by toeing-in or out excessively. Pedaling speed has no apparent effect on patellofemoral reaction forces; however, seat height and pedal resistance do (37). When the knee is fully extended or when a posterior foot position is used, there is an increased stress to the ACL. Decreased saddle height increases patellofemoral compression.

Pathomechanics

PIVOT SHIFT PHENOMENON

When internal integrity is lost in the knee joint, a biomechanical consequence is clinically evident with the patient history and on specific testing. The rotary stability of the knee is maintained through a combination of ligamentous and muscular coassistance. The central modulators are the cruciates. When this system is unbalanced, abnormal rotary movement occurs with the proprioceptive interpretation of instability. A shifting is perceived by the patient, almost as if the knee goes in and out of place. This sensation is due to the pull of the quadriceps during extension of the knee, causing anterior subluxation of the tibia on the femur (with ACL damage), and reduction caused by the pull of the hamstrings on flexion. Rotary movement occurs due to the lack of peripheral support from the capsule and ligamentous systems in the medial or lateral sectors of the knee. Clinically, this phenomenon is reproduced by a passive movement of the knee. The ITB acts to cause rotary movement (through passive pull) due to its lateral attachment at the proximal tibia. Therefore, during extension of the knee, the ITB passively pulls the tibia into anterolateral subluxation; with flexion, the tibia is reduced into neutral (38). This movement is often visible and certainly palpable as excessive motion at the lateral tibia with ACL deficiency.

ABNORMAL QUADRICEPS ANGLE

The angle of pull of the quadriceps on the tibia is referred to as the quadriceps (Q) angle. This is measured by following a line taken from the anterior-superior iliac spine through the patella. A line taken from the tibial tuberosity is extended through the patella. The point of intersection describes the Q angle (Fig. 14.13). Normals for males and females are not standardized. However, females in general have a larger angle. General agreement is that a Q angle beyond 20° is likely to be a cause of abnormal patellar tracking (39). A change as small as from a 10° to 15° Q angle increases patellofemoral joint reaction forces 50% (40). In addition, an increased angle indicates a shift of stresses medially at the tibiofemoral joint. This results in chronic stretching of soft tissue elements such as the capsule, ligaments, and muscular structures.

There are a number of biomechanical predispositions to an increased Q angle. Anteversion of the hip, tibial torsion, and pronation are the most common causes. Muscularly, weakness of the external rotators and abductors may be a factor (41).

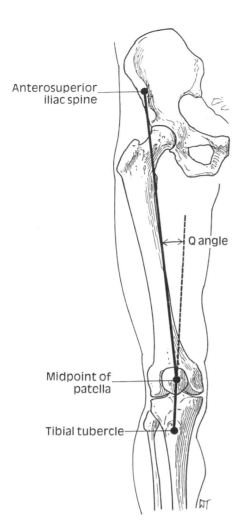

Anterosuperior iliac spine

Q angle

Midpoint of patella

Tibial tubercle

Figure 14.13. The quadriceps (Q) angle. (Reprinted with permission from Nicholas JA, Hershman EB, eds. The lower extremity and spine in sports medicine. St. Louis: CV Mosby, 1986:676.)

HISTORY AND EXAMINATION

History

The weighted importance of a good history can never be overstated. Suspicions raised lead to paths of questioning untraveled by the less inquiring and experienced examiner. This may result in unnecessary testing or treatment procedures. Questions that must be asked include the following.

1. What type of onset (traumatic/nontraumatic, overuse, other)?
2. If traumatic, what was the mechanism of injury (activity, direction of force application) (Table 14.4)?
3. If overuse, what activity is the possible cause (any change in routine of sports activity)?
4. If swelling has/had occurred (Table 14.5)?
   A. Location (localized = bursa or ligament; diffuse = intraarticular).
   B. Timing (immediate [within 6 hours] = hemorrhagic; delayed [more than 6 hours] = likelihood of synovial irritation).
5. Was a pop heard at the time of injury (most likely ACL; also meniscus tears and subluxating patella are possible)?
6. Has the knee locked (most likely due to a meniscus tear or any intraarticular obstruction such as osteochondritis dissecans or torn ACL)? Note: true locking is painful, and movement in either flexion or extension is not possible.
7. Is there any sense of instability (meniscus or cruciates are commonly involved)?
   A. During what activities does it occur (running, cutting, climbing stairs, squatting)?

Table 14.4. Relationship Between Direction of Force and Structures Damaged

Force Applied	Damage	Example
Varus or valgus (no rotation)	Collateral ligament Epiphyseal fracture Patellar dislocation/subluxation	Block to the outside of the knee (example of valgus force; most common)
Varus or valgus (with rotation)	Collaterals + cruciates Collaterals + patellar dislocation/subluxation Meniscus test	Fall or blocked while cutting
Blow or fall on patella	Patellar fracture Patellar cartilage damage Pinched suprapatellar pouch Infrapatellar fat pad or plica	Dashboard injury
Anterior blow to tibia (knee flexed)	Posterior cruciate	Fall on flexed knee
Anterior blow to tibia or hyperextension	ACL, then PCL	Land from a jump with a straight leg
Deceleration (noncontact)	ACL	Sudden stop to change direction
Rotation with compression (noncontact)	Meniscus	Foot is fixed while tibia and femur rotate in opposite direction as in cutting

ACL, anterior cruciate ligament; PCL, posterior cruciate ligament.

Table 14.5. Common Historical Complaints

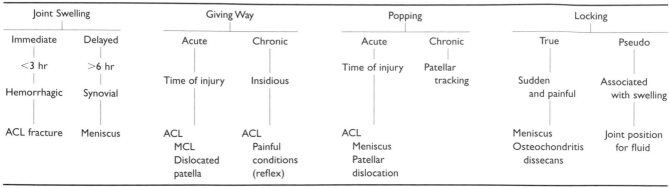

Joint Swelling		Giving Way		Popping		Locking	
Immediate	Delayed	Acute	Chronic	Acute	Chronic	True	Pseudo
<3 hr	>6 hr			Time of injury	Patellar tracking	Sudden and painful	Associated with swelling
Hemorrhagic	Synovial	Time of injury	Insidious				
ACL fracture	Meniscus	ACL MCL Dislocated patella	ACL Painful conditions (reflex)	ACL Meniscus Patellar dislocation		Meniscus Osteochondritis dissecans	Joint position for fluid

ACL, anterior cruciate ligament; MCL, medial collateral ligament.

B. Was it slow in developing or immediately after injury?

C. Any maneuvers used by the patient to compensate?

8. Any previous injuries or surgeries of either knee?

9. Any diagnosis of present or previous injury?

10. Standard pain questions (quality, frequency, aggravated by, relieved by, radiation, positionally related)?

Recently there has been a switch to weighting a functional examination as high or higher than the objective evaluation found with orthopedic testing. Several functional evaluations have been developed that provide a rather accurate assessment of the capabilities of the athlete after rehabilitation or surgery. Two of the most commonly used include the Lysholm and Cincinnati knee scoring questionnaires (42). Although different scores are generated with the same patient using each questionnaire, they serve as important estimates of functional ability.

Directed by this historical jigsaw puzzle, the examiner should be able to construct a partial image of the potential problem. A full perspective is completed by the examination results.

Observation

Observation of the exposed lower extremity should focus on a lack of symmetry between the well and involved leg. Standard inclusion of atrophy, scars, bruises, swelling, and bony deformities should be sought. Significant structural possibilities include the following.

1. Pronation/supination.
2. Genu valgus/varus.
3. Tibial torsion.
4. Orientation of the patellae.
5. Femoral anteversion/retroversion.

Table 14.6. Postural Observation for the Knee

Position	Structure	Abnormality
Standing		
Anterior view	Tibia	Tibial torsion
		Internal (foot points in)
		External (foot points out)
	Knee	Genu varum (bowlegged)
		Genu valgum (knock-kneed)
	Patellae	Squinting patellae
	Iliac crests	Unleveling (best palpated)
Lateral view	Knee	Genu recurvatum
	Patellae	Patella alta (camelback)
Posterior view	Feet	Pronation/Supination
Seated	Tibia	Tibial torsion (viewed from above)
	Patellae	Patella alta (frog-eyed appearance)
	Knee	VMO atrophy (best determined with resisted extension)

VMO, vastus medialis obliques.

Again, a lack of symmetry is a visual clue to the possibility of predisposition. Bilateral abnormalities are usually more subtle and not as likely to produce unilateral symptoms. Using the above structural excessive conditions, the examiner may attempt correlation with the presenting complaint and subsequent examination findings. Discussed as separate structural abnormalities, it is important to understand their common coexistence. A summary of these observations is presented on a view perspective (anterior, posterior, and lateral) in Table 14.6.

PRONATION/SUPINATION

Excesses of pronation and supination affect the knee by shifting weight medially or laterally. This is due to the internal rotation associated with pronation and the external rotation associated with supination. Determination of this problem is discussed in Chapter 15 in more detail. However, a posterior view of the standing patient will usually reveal bowing of the Achilles tendon. Medial bowing indicates pronation; lateral bowing indicates supination. Observation in the neutral subtalar position and the navicular drop test (43) are also helpful.

GENU VARUM/VALGUS/RECURVATUM

Genu varum is commonly referred to as a bow-legged appearance. Viewed from anterior, the space between the legs is excessive. This appearance is often due to or associated with tibia varum. Genu valgum is commonly referred to as knock-kneed. A small amount of valgus is normal in the adult.

Genu recurvatum or hyperextension of the knee is visible from a lateral view. This is an indication of lax ligaments, particularly the posterior capsule. A small amount of hyperextension is common in young girls. In adults, it is important to observe whether there is an excessive lumbar lordosis. This is often associated with a compensatory hyperextension of the knee.

TIBIAL TORSION

Tibial torsion is a rotational tibial shaft deformity. It is a structural defect and is not to be equated with an accessory movement abnormality of an internally or externally rotated tibia. Tibial torsion may be determined by positioning the standing patient so that the patellae are facing straight forward. With lateral (external) tibial torsion, the feet will point outward more than a few degrees. With medial (internal) tibial torsion, they point inward (44). This same displacement of the feet may be observed in the seated patient with the legs hanging off the table. Viewed from above, the bowing of the tibia and associated foot displacement are seen. Lateral tibial torsion is associated with genu valgum and medial tibial torsion with genu varum.

Another method of determining torsion is to measure the intramalleolar angle. Normally, the lateral malleolus lies posterior to the medial malleolus, forming an angle of approximately 15°. By placing one finger on the medial malleolus and one finger anterior to the lateral malleolus, a straight line should be formed between the fingers. When internal tibial torsion is present, the lateral malleolus will be anterior to this line.

FEMORAL TORSION (ANTEVERSION/RETROVERSION)

Femoral torsion is the angle between the shaft of the femur and the condyles. Anteversion essentially causes a medial torquing, increasing the valgus angle at the knee and reducing available external rotation of the femur. The opposite compensations may be found with retroversion. The Craig test (45) is used to determine the amount of anteversion and retroversion as described in Chapter 13.

ORIENTATION OF THE PATELLAE

Viewed anteriorly, it is important to observe whether one or both patella point medially (squinting patellae) or laterally in the standing patient. This same observation can be made in the seated patient.

Patella alta, or a high-riding patella, may be observed in the seated patient as a frog-eyed appearance. In the standing or supine patient, it may appear as a camelback sign in which two humps are visible from a lateral view (Fig. 14.14). The top hump is the patella; the lower hump is the infrapatellar fat pad. Measurement by the Insall-Salvati method is made on a lateral view of the knee. The distance between the inferior pole of the patella and the tibial tuberosity (length of the patellar tendon) is measured and should form a ratio of 1:2 with the length of the patella (46).

PALPATION

Palpation coupled with a good history serve to focus the examiner's attention initially on a limited number of possibilities. Considerations

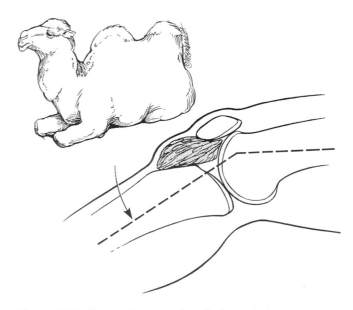

Figure 14.14. The camelback sign of patella alta. As the knee approaches extension, the enlarged fat pad becomes prominent. The prominence of the fat pad and the high patella produce two humps—the camelback sign. (Reprinted with permission from Nicholas JA, Hershman EB, eds. The lower extremity and spine in sports medicine. St. Louis: CV Mosby, 1986;1021.)

should include tenderness, swelling, nodules, and temperature.

TENDERNESS

Areas of tenderness are either the direct result of trauma or are suggestive of specific tissue strain. Muscles are often tender along their tendons and at their insertions. Some common areas of point tenderness include the following (Fig. 14.15).

1. Adductor tubercle—attachment for the vastus medialis obliquus, adductor longus, medial retinaculum, and plica.
2. Medial femoral condyle—the superior surface is where the MCL inserts.
3. Medial proximal tibia—a hand's width below the joint line is the insertion of the pes anserine muscles and slightly distal, the insertion of the MCL.

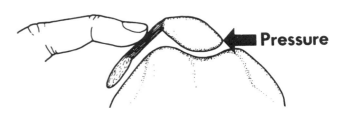

Figure 14.16. Examination of the lateral retinaculum. (Reprinted with permission from Fulkerson J. Awareness of the retinaculum in evaluating patellofemoral pain. Am J Sports Med 1982;10:147.)

4. Joint line—usually indicates sprain of the coronary ligament with possible involvement of the meniscus.
5. Patellar tendon—either patellar tendinitis (jumper's knee) or infrapatellar bursitis are possible (tenderness either side of the patellar tendon in the joint line indicates fat pad irritation).
6. Inferior pole of the patella—indicates either patellar tendinitis or Sinding-Larsen-Johansson disease.
7. Tibial tuberosity—indicates Osgood-Schlatter disease (either old or new).
8. Gerdy's tubercle (lateral proximal tibia)—insertion point for the ITB.
9. Anterior to the femoral attachment of the LCL—area of insertion for the popliteus.
10. Lateral epicondyle—area rubbed by tight ITB.
11. Either side of the patella—areas of the retinaculum; to palpate, press patella medially in the extended, relaxed leg. Palpate under the medial border of patella. Reverse for the lateral (Fulkerson method) (Fig. 14.16) (47).

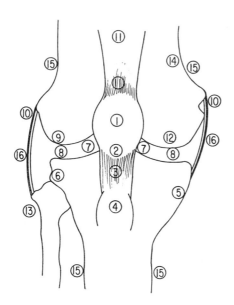

Figure 14.15. Localization of swelling and/or tenderness in various painful knee syndromes.

1. Patella: dislocation, chondromalacia, prepatellar bursitis or neuralgia.
2. Jumper's knee, Sinding-Larsen-Johansson disease.
3. Patellar tendinitis, infrapatellar bursitis.
4. Osgood-Schlatter's disease.
5. Pes anserine bursitis.
6. Iliotibial band insertion.
7. Fat pads, degenerative arthritis.
8. Meniscal tears or cysts, intraarticular foreign bodies, degenerative arthritis.
9. Popliteus tendinitis.
10. Pellegrini-Stieda syndrome, collateral ligament syndromes.
11. Quadriceps tendinitis strain or rupture, suprapatellar bursitis.
12. Aseptic necrosis of femoral condyle (medial).
13. Peroneal nerve.
14. Saphenous nerve.
15. Osteoarthropathy.
16. Collateral ligament strains, tears, ruptures.

(Reprinted with permission from Reilly BM. Practical strategies in outpatient medicine. Philadelphia: WB Saunders, 1991:236.)

SWELLING

It is important to differentiate swelling on the historical questions of both onset and location. In most cases, bursal swelling is localized whereas intraarticular swelling is diffuse. The exception to this generalization is when a bursa communicates with the joint, as occurs with the suprapatellar pouch and semimembranosus bursa. The feel of the swelling is important in differentiating sanguineous from synovial origin. When there is a hemorrhagic swelling, the skin feels quite tense, doughy, and is usually warm. Synovial swelling is not significantly warmer and has a less thickened feel—boggy.

A firm localized swelling at the joint line that is more apparent on standing may represent a meniscal cyst. A localized swelling that appears medially on contraction of the hamstrings may indicate a small fascial herniation. Posteriorly, medial joint line swelling is often due to the semimembranosus bursa (this was referred to in the past as a Baker's cyst). Tests for swelling will be discussed in the specific testing section.

Neurologic Testing

The primary goal of neurologic testing of the knee is to determine if lumbar nerve root involvement is a factor or whether peripheral nerve entrapment or damage is the cause of a pain or numbness complaint. Standard testing involves deep tendon reflex evaluation via the patellar tendon for the L4 nerve root, sensory evaluation with a pinwheel to determine if objective changes are evident in a dermatomal or peripheral nerve pattern, and muscle testing to determine neurologic causes of weakness.

Orthopedic Testing

Physical examination of the knee should be performed as soon as possible after injury. On-the-field evaluation is preferred before the disguises of swelling and muscle spasm are present. If significant swelling or muscle spasm is present (and a serious injury can be ruled out by history and radiographs—a difficult task), then one may adopt a cautious wait-and-see attitude while addressing the patient's pain needs and allow the swelling to decrease, thus permitting proper evaluation. If serious damage (especially to a ligament) cannot be ruled out, then referral for aspiration and/or examination under anesthesia may be necessary.

Examination should proceed with several perspectives in mind. Regionally, one should approach the problem from a viewpoint of limiting possibilities based on location. This is developed from the history and palpation findings. Further modification is made based on the suspected tissue involvement in that location (specific disorder). For example, a patient with joint line pain would be tested specifically for a meniscus tear (the most likely possibility); however, the tenderness is often due to a sprain of the coronary ligament. This sprain may be isolated or in association with a meniscus tear. Negative or equivocal findings would point (through a process of elimination) toward an isolated coronary ligament sprain.

There is usually a hierarchy of concerns when examining the knee. It is important in on-the-field examination to check neurologic and vascular integrity. Fracture may be determined if obvious; however, radiographs are usually required. In evaluating the knee joint itself, begin with testing for stability. Ligament evaluation is crucial in many cases due to the limited grace period for surgical repair of total ruptures (3 to 5 days) (48). The patient should also be evaluated for another potentially serious condition, patellar subluxation. Next, progression is usually to the meniscus. Although serious, meniscus damage rarely demands immediate surgery (unless complicated by ligamentous involvement).

If trauma is not involved, a sequence of an examination optimizing patient comfort and minimizing multiple changes of position should be used. The preceding hierarchy may still be used followed by testing for overuse and/or malalignment problems. Completion of the examination involves functional assessment including muscle testing and activity performance.

It must be appreciated that there are often several descriptions of how to perform a specific orthopedic test. In addition, the accuracy of many of the tests has not been documented sufficiently. When performing orthopedic tests, one should be cautious when describing a test result as positive when there is doubt in the examiner's mind. Interpretively, it is more communicative to describe the response to the test or describe it as a "soft positive."

LIGAMENT STABILITY TESTS

Ligament testing evaluates stability. The outer ligaments provide resistance to adduction/abduction forces and secondarily rotation. The cruciates provide resistance to posterior/anterior forces and rotation. Isolated ligament testing is difficult due to the orientation of the surrounding musculature. In full extension, for example, many of the more peripheral muscles buttress the collateral ligament system. This also provides a clue to the seriousness of an injury when instability is perceived.

It is crucial to test the healthy leg first (if one exists) as a comparison. To some degree, ligament laxity may be normal for a particular individual. This is particularly true in tall individuals, younger patients, and female patients.

Ligament injury has been divided into three grades. Grade 1 injury indicates minor damage with no instability. Grade 2 indicates more significant damage with some degree of laxity perceived; however, there is enough integrity left to prevent full opening of the joint. Grade 3 injury indicates total rupture with loss of restraint and ensuing instability. In reality there are subgrades of these major categories and the distinction is not always so evident. In particular, it is important to consider the addition of a grade beyond grade 3 that would indicate total rupture of the tested ligament plus injury to other soft tissue restraints. For example, when a full rupture of the MCL occurs, it may be complicated by injury to the PCL and capsule.

Varus/Valgus Testing at 0° and 30° (Fig. 14.17 A and B).

The collateral ligaments are stressed by varus and valgus forces. Application of varus forces tests

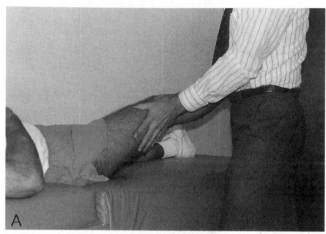

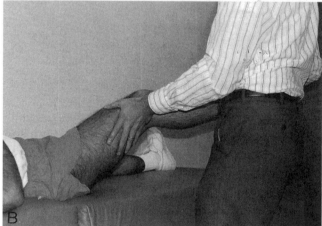

Figure 14.17. Varus and valgus test. **A.** 0°. **B.** 30° of flexion.

the lateral collateral; valgus forces test the medial collateral. The sequence to testing is to begin in 0° of flexion (full extension). Even a small amount of flexion will fool the examiner into perceiving instability. For example, most chiropractic tables have a slight slant toward the foot of the table. This adds a small degree of flexion and makes full extension testing inaccurate. To guarantee full extension, lift the patient's leg and ask him or her to relax completely. Stabilize at the ankle and apply a medially (valgus) or laterally (varus) directed force to the knee (Fig. 14.17). If opening of the joint is observed visually or tactilely, a minimum of a third-degree tear (full rupture) is found (48). This is because the knee is usually locked osseously and further held solid by soft tissues. If isolated damage to this collateral ligament system is present, other structures will still prevent instability. Therefore, opening in full extension implies that not only is damage to the collateral ligament present, but also the cruciates, capsule, and possibly muscles in that area are also damaged (Table 14.7). If instability is found, there is no need to proceed to the second portion. Remember to test the uninvolved leg to determine the degree of individual inherent laxity. A loose joint congenitally may cause the laxity to be overestimated.

If full extension is stable, progress to test with the knee flexed at 20°–30°. At this position of flexion, the posterior capsule and posterior cruciate are more relaxed compared with full extension. Again, a varus or valgus force is applied being careful to take out any hip rotation that may lead to a false-positive interpretation (motion occurring at the hip, not at the knee). Leaving the thigh on the examining table while allowing the knee to flex off the table also assures a more relaxed position. Further isolation may be accomplished by externally rotating the knee, which takes the stress off the cruciates and places it on

Table 14.7.   Collateral Ligament Instability Testing

Position	Response	Structures Involved
Valgus stress		
With full extension	Laxity	MCL plus one or both cruciates
20°–30° flexion	Laxity (no endfeel)	Isolated MCL rupture (if test in full extension is negative)
	Laxity (some endfeel)	Second-degree sprain of MCL
	No laxity but painful	First-degree sprain of MCL
Varus stress		
With full extension	Laxity	LCL rupture plus posterior cruciate
20°–30° flexion	Laxity (no endfeel)	Isolated LC rupture (if test in full extension is negative)
	Laxity (endfeel)	Second-degree sprain of LCL
	No laxity but painful	First-degree sprain of LCL

Note: It is crucial to compare findings with the healthy leg. Also, if the test result is positive for laxity in full extension, do not progress to the second position. General grading is based on millimeters of laxity; 1+ = 5 mm, 2+ = 10 mm, 3+ = 15 mm, 4+ = 20 mm. Anything greater than 1+ is considered abnormal.
MCL, medial collateral ligament; LCL, lateral collateral ligament.

the collaterals (49). There are a few "positive" possibilities.

1. If no endfeel is felt, a third-degree tear is present (plus possibly other structures) (Table 14.7).
2. If an endfeel is felt yet instability is still perceived, a second-degree tear is present.
3. If no instability is felt yet pain is produced, a first-degree tear is present.

Stress radiographs may also be used to detect instability; however, their use is rarely indicated. One exception is in the adolescent in whom a differential diagnosis between ligament damage and epiphyseal damage is needed (50). If stress radiographs are taken while testing in full extension, the following graded system is used for quantification:

- Grade 1 = 5-mm opening
- Grade 2 = up to 10-mm opening
- Grade 3 = greater than 10-mm opening

Anterior/Posterior (Straight) Instability Testing

Testing for the integrity of the cruciates involves first assessing straight anterior/posterior and posterior/anterior stability. Testing for straight instability is done with a series of maneuvers or, more recently, with an instrument such as the KT-1000 (Medimetric, San Diego, CA) or Genucom (51). These devices are considered more accurate, and the results more consistently reproducible than in manual testing. It is common for the patient complaining of instability to be able to reproduce the sensation and actual subluxation by specific positioning. This voluntary approach is often revealing. In chronic cases, more active-resistive testing will be more rewarding than the following passive tests (49). Manual testing is accomplished first with the anterior cruciate through the use of two standard tests: Lachman's and anterior drawer.

Lachman's (52) (Fig. 14.18)

The examiner stabilizes the femur with one hand. The knee is flexed to between full extension and 20°. The leg is slightly rotated externally. The other hand then pulls forward on the proximal tibia. The advantage of Lachman's is that hamstring muscle spasm or meniscus blocking (found with the drawer test) are not positionally effective restrictors. Attention must be paid to the discovery of a pseudo-Lachman's found with MCL rupture.

The standard Lachman's described above is not always possible due to patient position at the

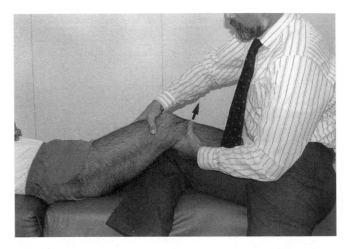

Figure 14.18. Lachman's test. The leg is slightly rotated externally, stabilized with the upper hand in 0°–20° flexion, and the pull on the proximal tibia is forward.

time of injury or the size of the athlete's leg. Alternative positions include the following.

A. Lachman's may be performed with the examiner seated at the end of the table and the patient's lower leg unsupported by the end of the table. The examiner supports the knee over his or her knee with 30° of flexion. From this position, the femur is stabilized and an anterior force imparted to the tibia (Fig 14.19A).
B. Stable Lachman's may be performed by allowing the heel to rest on the table with the knee flexed to approximately 30°. From this position, the anterior tibial pull is performed with distal femoral stabilization (Fig. 14.19B).
C. Side-supported Lachman's may be performed with the examiner on the side of the table supporting the knee between his or her arm and side, with the knee flexed to approximately 30°. The Lachman's is performed from this position (Fig. 14.19C).
D. Prone Lachman's is performed with the patient face down (53). The examiner's hand is placed under the distal femur and pulled posteriorly while the other hand pushes anteriorly. The advantage of this position is the assistance of gravity and the fact that the size of the femur is not a limiting factor if the examiner's hands are small (Fig. 14.19D).
E. No-touch Lachman's is performed with the patient supine (54). The headward hand is placed under the involved knee and onto the uninvolved distal femur, lifting the leg into 30° flexion. The patient then attempts active extension against gravity (Fig. 14.19E). The examiner palpates and/or watches for anterior displacement of the femur.

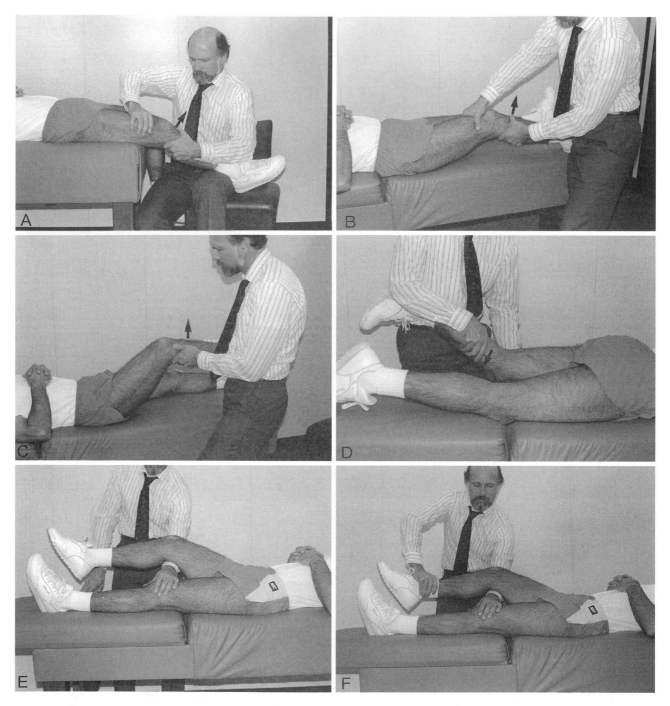

Figure 14.19. Variations of Lachman's test. **A.** Lower leg unsupported. **B.** Stable Lachman's with lower leg supported. **C.** Side-supported Lachman's. **D.** Prone Lachman's. **E.** No-touch Lachman's. **F.** Dynamic Lachman's.

F. Dynamic Lachman's or active Lachman's is the same position as the no-touch Lachman's; however, the examiner resists the attempt of the patient into active extension (Fig. 14.19F) (55).

Anterior Drawer (48)

The supine patient is positioned with the hip flexed to 45° and the knee at 90°. The examiner stabilizes the leg by sitting on the foot of the in-

volved leg. With thumbs palpating the joint line and tibial plateau, the examiner (using full body weight) pulls anteriorly by leaning backward (Fig. 14.20). The disadvantage of this patient position is the biomechanical advantage of the hamstrings, which are often in spasm in the acute setting. In addition, at 90° of knee flexion, the meniscus may act as a door wedge preventing anterior movement (possible false-positive) (Fig. 14.21). In the chronic ACL-deficient knee, gradual capsular laxity develops allowing detection by the anterior drawer test. Caution must be used in misinterpreting a test result as positive when a posterior cruciate tear is present. PCL tears allow sagging posteriorly in this position; as the examiner pulls forward, the knee is actually being drawn back into a neutral position. This mistake may be avoided by observing the tibial tubercle of the involved leg to determine if it is as far anterior as the healthy leg. A flattening of this normal prominence is a clue to PCL damage. This is referred to as the posterior sag sign or the gravity drawer test.

This sag sign is also visible with the patient's hips flexed to 90° and the ankles supported by

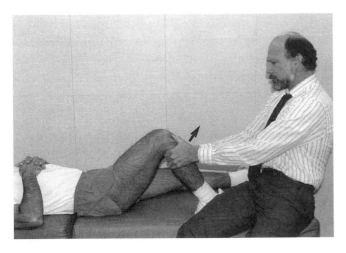

Figure 14.20. Anterior drawer test. The examiner should use a good amount of body weight to perform this test.

the examiner (Fig. 14.22). Gravity is then acting perpendicular to the tibia, which may be more sensitive for posterior laxity. Again, the reference points are the tibial tuberosities. By adding pressure posteriorly, the test may be made more sensitive and is sometimes referred to as the Godfrey test (56).

With the patient placed in the standard drawer position, resistance may be applied to the patient's attempt at active extension (Fig. 14.23). A variation on the performance of the drawer test is to position the patient with the knee and hip flexed 90°, with the examiner pulling the tibia upward against gravity (Fig. 14.24). Another variation is to perform the drawer test with the patient seated at the end of the table. The examiner pulls forward on the dependent tibia (Fig. 14.25).

As with collateral testing, a sequence of testing is preferred. This sequence is based on accuracy rather than severity. It has been demonstrated that Lachman's is more accurate, especially in an acute setting (52). Movement anteriorly of more than 6 mm is considered generally abnormal.

Next, the posterior cruciate is tested with the same positioning as with the anterior drawer. The difference is that a posterior force is applied to the tibia. Often the test is not necessary due to the sag sign mentioned above.

Anterolateral/Anteromedial Rotary Instability Testing

When the ACL is damaged, it is rare that isolated tears occur. With multiple tissue damage, more than straight instability results. This rotary

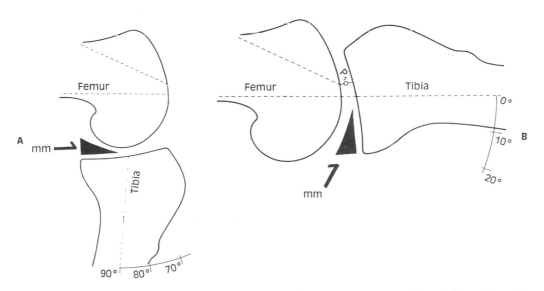

Figure 14.21. If the anterior drawer sign is performed at **(A)** 90° of flexion, the posterior horn of the medial meniscus (mm) abuts against the round surface of the medial femoral condyle. This "door stopper" effect can cause a negative test result even if the anterior cruciate ligament is torn. When testing in **(B)** relative extension, a comparatively flat weight-bearing surface of the femur allows the tibia to subluxate forward in relation to the femur if the anterior cruciate ligament is torn (Lachman test). (Reprinted with permission from Torg JS, Conrad W, Kalen V. Am J Sports Med 1976;4:84.)

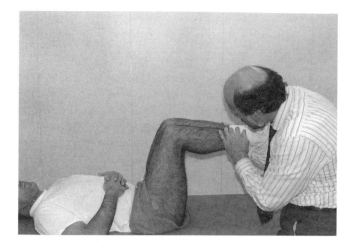

Figure 14.22. The sag sign. The normal prominence of the tibial tubercle is absent when posterior cruciate laxity is present.

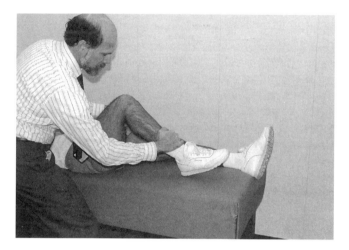

Figure 14.23. Testing of active extension in the drawer testing position.

instability is assessed via two types of testing procedures. The first type uses rotation and forward pull to stress the suspected structures. The second involves the pivot shift phenomenon. Testing for the pivot shift phenomenon assumes the knee to be in subluxation anteriorly when positioned less than 20°–30° of flexion. After this degree of flexion, the tibia is assumed to have returned to neutral. This is due, at least in part, to the pull of the ITB. As the knee passes 20°–30°, the ITB pulls the tibia forward into subluxation. The reverse occurs as the knee flexes beyond this position. Following is a description of the many tests used.

1. Slocum's (57). Essentially, Slocum's is a modification of the anterior drawer test. By rotating the knee 30° medially and pulling forward, the examiner may detect anterolateral instability. Rotation externally 15° and pulling forward tests anteromedial instabil-

ity. Care must be taken not to exceed the degrees of rotation given. False-negative results may be found with this excess due to stabilization by other structures.

2. Flexion-rotation drawer test (by Noyes et al.) (58). This is similar to a posterior drawer test but with the knee flexed to 20°–30°. With the leg stabilized by the side of the examiner, the femur is allowed to drop posteriorly in relation to the tibia. With the knee subluxated anteriorly, the examiner slowly pushes the tibia posteriorly in an effort to reduce the anterior subluxation. Alternate pushing and releasing should make evident rotary movement (occurring around the PCL) visible as the femur rotates medially and laterally.

3. Crossover test (38) (Fig. 14.26). The crossover test is an attempt to reproduce the patient's perception of instability while walk-

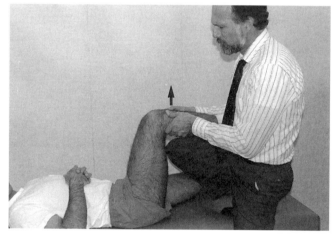

Figure 14.24. Anterior drawer test performed with knee and hip flexed to 90°.

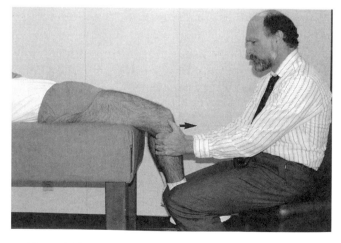

Figure 14.25. Anterior drawer test with unsupported lower leg.

applied while maintaining the medial rotation and anterior push on the fibular head. At approximately 20°–30°, a reduction of the tibia posteriorly will be felt. This is a test for anterolateral instability.

2. Modified pivot shift test (60). A recent group of investigators found that hip position had a dramatic effect on the sensitivity of the standard pivot shift test. Briefly, they found that with the hip abducted and the leg externally rotated, many arthroscopically documented rotary instabilities were detected that were not found with the standard test. The finding of increased sensitivity with the tibia externally rotated was later confirmed by Noyes et al. (61). The increase in sensitivity is based on the suggestion that with the leg internally rotated, the passive stretch from the ITB—which assists with pivot shift maneuvers—is diminished. In other words, some tension is needed in the ITB to cause subluxation or reduction of the tibia. Too much tension (caused by adduction of the hip or internal rotation of the tibia) may stabilize the tibia and therefore prevent subluxation.

3. Slocum's pivot shift test (Fig. 14.28) (62). The supine patient turns on his or her side to approximately 30° with the involved side down. With the leg extended, medial rotation and a valgus force are applied. The examiner's thumb applies a posterior to anterior force on the fibular head. As the knee is flexed, a reduction of the tibia will be appreciated at approximately 20°–30°.

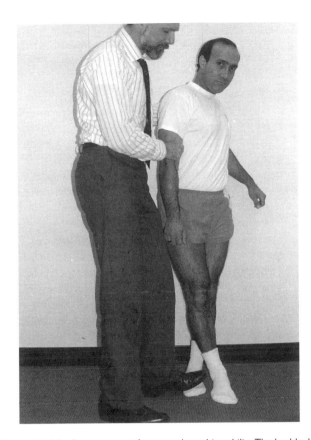

Figure 14.26. Crossover test for anterolateral instability. The healthy leg is crossed in front of the involved leg. With the physician gently stabilizing the foot on the involved leg, the patient is instructed to rotate the torso away from the involved side and then contract the involved quadriceps. A subluxation will be perceived by the patient.

ing. The standing patient crosses the healthy foot in front of the involved leg. The examiner stabilizes the involved foot by stepping on it cautiously. The patient is instructed to rotate the torso away from the involved side and then contract the quadriceps of that leg. A subluxation will be felt by the patient and indicates anterolateral rotary instability.

PIVOT SHIFT TESTS

Pivot shift tests are dependent on the integrity of the ITB. False-negative results may then occur. The following tests start with the knee in a subluxated position of extension.

1. Lateral pivot shift (MacIntosh) (59) (Fig. 14.27). The supine patient's hip is flexed to 20° with slight medial rotation. The examiner supports the leg at the calcaneus while the other hand flexes the leg to approximately 5° while pressing on the fibular head. This should cause subluxation of the tibia. As the knee is flexed, a valgus force is

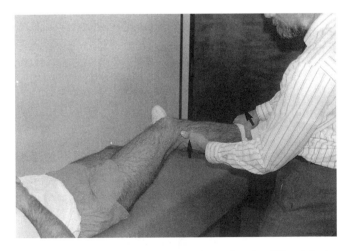

Figure 14.27. Lateral pivot shift test. The hip is flexed to 20° and the leg internally rotated. The leg is supported at the calcaneus while the other hand flexes the leg to approximately 5° while pressing on the fibular head. As the knee is flexed, a valgus force should be applied while the internal rotation of the leg is maintained.

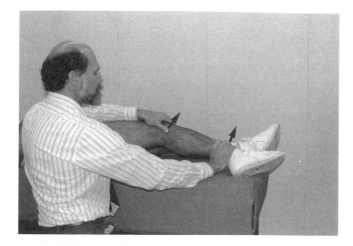

Figure 4.28. Slocum's pivot shift test. The supine patient turns 30° toward the uninvolved side. Medial rotation and valgus force are applied to the extended leg, and a posterior to anterior pressure is directed to the fibular head by the examiner. As the knee is flexed, a reduction of the tibia will be felt.

The following tests start with the knee in a reduced position of flexion.

1. Losee test (63). The patient lies supine while the examiner stabilizes the leg against his or her abdomen. The leg is flexed to 30° and externally rotated. A valgus force is applied with the thumb hooked behind the fibular head. At this point the tibia is in a reduced position. As the leg is extended, the tibia is allowed to rotate medially. As full extension is approached, a clunk sensation will be perceived by the examiner and the patient, indicating anterolateral subluxation.

2. Hughston jerk test (64). The patient is supine with the hip flexed to 45°. The knee is flexed to 90°. While extending the leg, the examiner applies a medial/valgus force. At approximately 30°, the tibia will jerk forward into subluxation. According to the test description, further extension will allow the tibia to reduce spontaneously. This test is not as accurate as other pivot shift tests (65).

Posterolateral and Posteromedial Rotary Instability Testing

As with testing for anterolateral/medial instability, the examiner may test by rotary means. In other words, by using the combination of the drawer test coupled with internal and external rotation (such as the Slocum test used for anterior rotary instability), the examiner may detect the posterior counterpart. Therefore, the examiner may position the patient for the drawer test. With internal rotation and a posterior force, the

examiner may detect movement indicative of posteromedial instability. With an external rotation/posterior force coupling, posterolateral instability is detectable. This test may be performed in either the supine or seated position. Other tests include the following.

1. Reverse Lachman's (Fig. 14.29). With the patient lying prone, the examiner flexes the knee to approximately 20°–30°. Supporting the femur, the examiner exerts a posterior force on the tibia in an attempt to detect abnormal movement.

2. Reverse pivot shift test (66). Using the same principles as the pivot shift maneuver, the supine patient's involved leg is lifted with support at the calcaneus. This is supported against the examiner's pelvis. The leg is flexed to approximately 80° and then externally rotated. This position should subluxate the tibia posterolaterally. The leg is then allowed to extend while the examiner imparts a valgus force. Near full extension the tibia will reduce into a neutral position.

3. Recurvatum test (Fig. 14.30) (67). The supine patient is relaxed with the knees extended. The examiner lifts the leg from the toes and observes movement of the tibial tuberosities. The affected knee should go into hyperextension on the lateral side of the tibia. The knee will appear to be in a varus orientation relative to the healthy leg. This is a test for posterolateral instability.

4. Dynamic posterior shift test (Fig. 14.31) (68). The patient's hip is flexed to almost 90° and maintained in this position while the examiner passively extends the knee. Gravity plus the tightening effect of the hamstrings will cause the tibia to subluxate

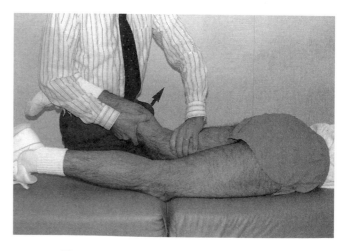

Figure 14.29. Reverse (or prone) Lachman's test.

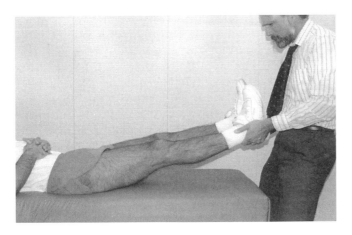

Figure 14.30. Recurvatum test for posterolateral instability. The affected knee should go into hyperextension on the lateral side of the tibia and will appear in a varus orientation relative to the healthy leg.

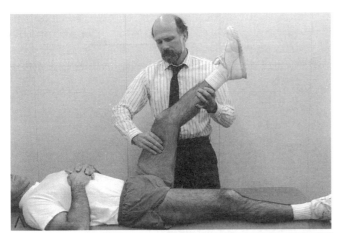

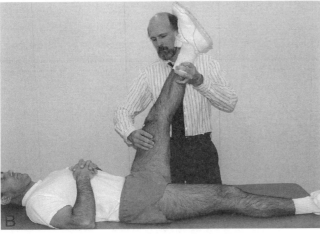

Figure 14.31. Dynamic posterior shift test. **A.** and **B.** The patient's hip is maintained at almost 90° flexion while the examiner passively extends the knee.

posteriorly in knees with posterior laxity. Continuing to extend the knee, near full extension, the knee will suddenly jerk or clunk into reduction. The patient may feel a reproduction of the instability sensation during the maneuver. Another active test is to have the patient sit with the knees off the end of the table. The examiner resists knee flexion and observes for posterior movement at the tibia (Fig. 14.32).

MENISCUS TESTING

There are several approaches to testing the meniscus. They are as follows.

1. Compress a torn meniscus posteriorly and cause a clicking or grinding sensation (or sound) (e.g., McMurray's).
2. Determine whether full extension is possible or blocked by a meniscus tear (e.g., Helfet's).
3. Monitor joint line signs such as tenderness, retraction of the meniscus, migration of pain during flexion/extension, and detection of meniscal cysts.

Following are the most commonly used tests.

COMPRESSION TESTS

1. McMurray's (Fig. 14.33) (69). As originally described by McMurray, the examiner flexes the knee to the buttocks and rotates it internally and externally, palpating the joint line for grinding or clicking. Generally, a click indicates a displaced meniscal tear (longitudinal tear). Grinding with pain points more toward a horizontal tear. There is some disagreement about the second portion of the test. Some authors describe extending the leg from the first position with a valgus force coupled with internal rotation; other authors insist on external rotation. The other disagreement is with what the test indicates.

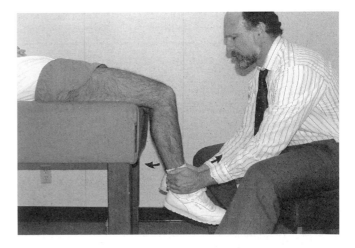

Figure 14.32. Resisted knee flexion of the unsupported lower leg. The examiner watches for posterior movement of the tibia.

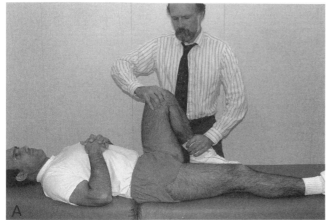

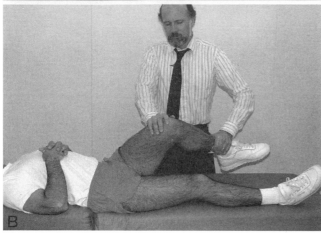

Figure 14.33. McMurray's test. **A.** Starting position. **B.** Extension of the leg with valgus force and internal rotation.

Does internal rotation/valgus identify a medial or lateral tear? Extending the leg with a varus force has been coupled with either internal or external rotation. The author's suggestion is to perform all the variants and determine the pain/click or grind location. Using this information coupled with other indicators such as joint line tenderness should help. Remember, compression tests like McMurray's are sensitive to tears in the posterior and middle portions of the meniscus. Moreover, compression sufficient to cause a positive is absent from 90° of flexion to full extension. Clicking past this point is almost always patellar in origin. Snapping or clicking of the hip is commonly misinterpreted as originating in the knee. The patient can be asked if unsure.

2. Apley's (Fig. 14.34). The prone patient's knee is flexed to 90°. The examiner applies pressure through the heel of the involved leg while compressing proximally, with internal and external rotation. If pain is produced, a posterior tear is suggested. Additionally, if

distracting the knee relieves the pain, more weight is given to the test. The author suggests padding the thigh slightly above the patella to avoid creating a false-positive result from patellar grinding. Davies and Larson (70) have suggested that by testing with increasing amounts of extension, anterior tears of the meniscus might be detected if pressure by the examiner continues through the long axis of the tibia.

3. Medial-lateral grind test (Fig. 14.35) (71). This new test is described by Anderson and Lipscomb. Essentially a compression test, the examiner grasps the lower leg of the supine patient and stabilizes it against his or her side while using the other hand to palpate the joint line. The leg is flexed to 45° while applying a valgus force, then extended while imparting a varus force. This combination produces a circular motion of the knee when viewed from above. A positive test result is indicated by grinding at the joint line.

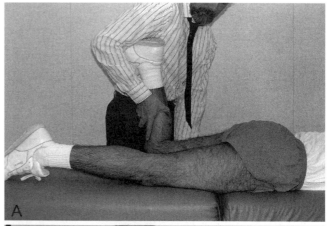

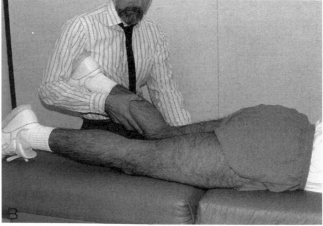

Figure 14.34. Apley's compression test. **A.** Traditional position. **B.** Testing with increasing amounts of extension may reveal anterior tears of the meniscus.

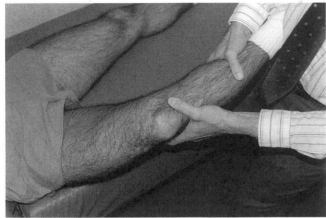

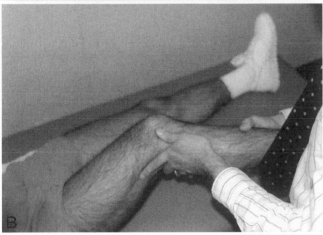

Figure 14.35. Medial-lateral grind test. **A.** Varus force is applied during flexion. **B.** Valgus force is applied during extension.

Additional maneuvers that may compress the meniscus and cause pain are a full squat and duck walking. While squatting, the pain is usually at the bottom of the squat where the compression is greatest (as opposed to during the squat, which could indicate chondromalacia and other patellofemoral disorders). Duck walking is not recommended due to the possibility of increasing damage and/or symptoms.

TESTS FOR BLOCKED EXTENSION

1. Helfet test (Fig. 14.36) (25). Normally, with the knee flexed, the tibial tuberosity is in line with the midline of the patella. In extension, because of the external rotation of the screw-home mechanism, the tibial tuberosity is in alignment with the lateral third of the patella. This may be tested by marking the tibial tuberosity and central patella and observing flexion and extension. If positive, the tibial tuberosity will fail to migrate laterally indicating internal blockage. Usually this is meniscal but could also

indicate cruciate damage. Helfet also describes a test in which a block to extension is observed. Then the examiner passively flexes the knee and forcibly internally and externally rotates the tibia. This reduction test is positive when a click is heard on rotation and the patient is able to extend the leg fully.

2. Bounce home test. Supporting the supine patient's heel, the examiner flexes the knee and then allows it to extend passively. If full extension is not reached or a springy or rubbery endfeel is perceived, a meniscus tear is the suspected cause.

JOINT LINE SIGNS

Although most examiner's palpate the anterior joint line for tenderness, it has been demonstrated that the more frequent location for a medial meniscus tear is medially or posteromedially at the joint line. Anterior joint line pain could in-

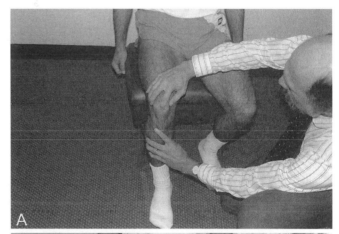

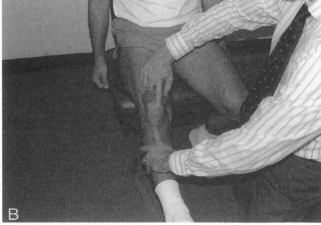

Figure 14.36. Helfet test. **A.** In flexion, the tibial tubercle should line up with the midline of the patella. **B.** In the normal knee, the tibial tubercle migrates laterally during extension. Failure to migrate indicates blocked extension.

dicate either a meniscus tear or only a coronary ligament sprain. The following tests are extensions of the joint line tenderness observation.

1. Steinman's test (49). Joint line tenderness is a common finding with meniscal involvement. This test couples this observation with the recognition that the meniscus moves posteriorly on flexion and anteriorly on extension. While palpating the joint line, the examiner asks the patient if the pain or tenderness migrates. If so, it is important to determine if it follows the above pattern of migration—posteriorly on flexion and anteriorly on extension. It is possible to have an overlap finding over the MCL, making distinction difficult.

2. Retracting meniscus test. Again, with the recognition of mobility of the meniscus, the examiner may determine by rotation of the leg and foot whether movement is felt. The patient is usually seated or may lie supine. The knee must be flexed to 90° to access the joint line properly. While palpating the joint line anterior to the MCL, the lower leg and foot are passively rotated internally and externally. A normal feel would be slight bulging at the joint line on internal rotation while a small depression would appear on external rotation (assuming there is no intraarticular swelling). The bulging is believed to be the meniscus moving anterior with internal rotation. If a depression is not felt with external rotation, a meniscus tear blocking rotation is suspected (or joint line swelling is considered as a possibility).

PATELLAR TESTING

In addition to the numerous structural assessments and measurements that are needed in evaluating the patella, some specific testing is usually indicated. The principle is based on compression of the posterior surface of the patella with either production of crepitus or pain. Also it is important to test for stability of the patella with the apprehension test or VMO coordination test.

1. Patellar inhibition test (patellar grind test, Clarke's test). There are many variations of this testing approach. Essentially, it is based on pressing the patella distally while the patient lies supine with the knee extended and relaxed. The grind test simply presses the patella posteriorly in the same patient position. Clarke's is a combination of approaches, holding the patella distally and then having the patient contract the quadriceps. It is important to flex the leg 5°–10° before performing the test. In full extension, the suprapatellar pouch may be pinched, producing a a false-positive examination finding. These test results are positive in patients with chondromalacia patellae; however, results may be positive with other patellofemoral problems.

2. Waldron's test (72). As the patella moves (relative to the femur) through flexion and extension of the knee, different portions are in contact with the femur. This test attempts to identify which part of the patella is involved, in particular with chondromalacia. Clinically, this directs any restrictions to specific ranges of motions when exercising. The standing patient is asked to complete a full squat. If pain is felt at a particular part of the range of motion, the examiner has a clue as to which part of the posterior surface is involved. The examiner may palpate the patella during the movement, noting any tracking deviations or crepitus. This too may be a helpful clue.

3. Apprehension test. This stability test attempts to displace the patella laterally to determine a tendency toward subluxation or dislocation. The supine patient is positioned first with the knee at 30°. The examiner then slowly attempts to displace the patella outwardly while watching the patient's reaction. If subluxation is anticipated by the patient, he or she will often attempt to stop the examiner by grabbing for the knee, contracting the quadriceps, or simply looking apprehensive. The test may be repeated in full extension if negative at 30°.

4. VMO coordination test (Fig. 14.37). With the patient supine, the examiner places his or her fist under the patient's knee. The patient then attempts to extend the knee slowly without pressing down or lifting away from the examiner's fist. The patient should be reminded to extend as fully as possible. The indication of tracking instability is the lack of coordinated full extension. In other words, the patient either has difficulty smoothly accomplishing extension or recruits either the extensors or flexors of the hip to accomplish extension. This has been suggested as a test for VMO function not on the basis of strength but more importantly on synchronized action. This may be a subtle indicator of dysfunction of the VMO that may result in patellar pain.

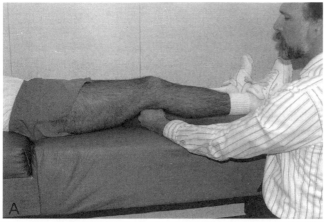

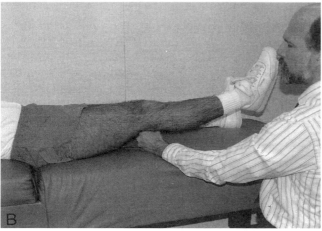

Figure 14.37. Vastus medialis obliquus (VMO) coordination test. **A.** Starting position. **B.** The patient is instructed to extend the leg smoothly, without pressing down on or lifting away from the examiner's fist.

PLICA TESTS

A plica may be detected indirectly by its possible effect on patellar tracking as the following tests indicate.

1. Hughston plica test (45). The examiner stabilizes the lower leg against his or her side and uses the other hand to push the patella medially while palpating the medial femoral condyle near the joint line. The leg is passively flexed and extended while maintaining the medial force and simultaneously palpating. If snapping or clicking occurs under the examiner's fingers, a plica is possible.
2. Plica stutter test (45). The seated patient relaxes the legs while the examiner palpates the patella (medial side). The patient extends the lower leg while the examiner notes any stuttering of patellar tracking. This usually occurs at approximately 45°–60° of flexion.

Additionally, if the plica rides over the condyle with resultant erosion, palpation of the lateral-anterior aspect of the medial condyle with the knee flexed beyond 90° may reveal tenderness. Palpation of the plica itself may be possible medial to the patellar tendon; however, distinction from other structures is difficult.

ITB TESTS

Tests for the ITB attempt to compress the band over the lateral epicondyle of the femur through stretching or direct pressure.

1. Modified Ober's (Fig. 14.38). Originally Ober's test was developed to detect a contracture of the abductors of the hip. Modification helps detect tightness of the ITB and possible irritation at the lateral epicondyle. The patient lies on his or her side with the affected side up. The bottom leg is bent and flexed toward the chest to eliminate inter-

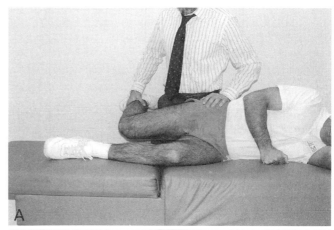

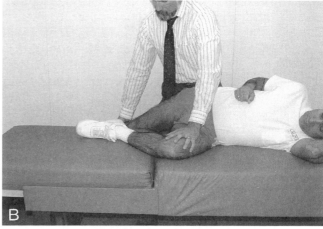

Figure 14.38. Modified Ober's test. **A.** Starting position. Note the forward flexion of uninvolved leg to eliminate interference. **B.** The involved leg is extended and allowed to drape over the table, while the examiner stabilizes the pelvis. Pain at the lateral epicondyle and inability to go below the edge of the table are indications of iliotibial band involvement.

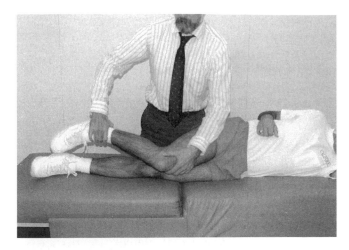

Figure 14.39. Noble's test. The leg is flexed and extended while exerting pressure over the lateral epicondyle. In a positive test, pain is usually elicited at 20°–30° degrees of flexion as the iliotibial band passes over the lateral epicondyle.

ference. The top leg (suspected knee) is extended. With the patient close to the edge of the table, the examiner stabilizes the pelvis and allows the leg to drape over the edge of the table as far as possible. Positive reactions include:

A. pain over the lateral epicondyle, Gerdy's tubercle, or greater trochanter of the femur;

B   inability of the leg to adduct appreciably over the edge of the table indicating tightness of the ITB.

2. Noble's (Fig. 14.39). Noble's test involves placing the patient on the unaffected side. The affected knee is flexed and extended while the examiner exerts direct pressure over the lateral epicondyle. Tenderness should be elicited at approximately 20°–30° as the band passes over the epicondyle. This sometimes appears as a painful arc where, although not tender at full extension or moderate flexion, tenderness appears in the above mentioned range.

WILSON'S TEST FOR OSTEOCHONDRITIS DISSECANS (73)

With the patient seated and knees relaxed, the examiner internally rotates the lower leg. The patient is asked to extend the leg while the examiner maintains the internal rotation. At approximately 30° the patient will experience pain (usually medial). The patient is then asked to rotate the leg externally and continue extension. Pain should diminish or disappear if a classic osteochondritis dissecans is present.

TESTS FOR SWELLING

Tests for intraarticular swelling are often unnecessary due to the obvious visual appearance. However, in subtle cases in which only a small amount of fluid exists in excess or when differentiating between suprapatellar swelling and joint swelling is not possible, testing may help (45).

1. Stroke test. To determine small intraarticular effusion, the stroke test is performed. While stroking proximally on the medial side of the knee joint, the other hand strokes distally on the lateral side. If an excess of fluid is present, a small bulge or palpable wave will appear medially.

2. Fluctuation test. In an attempt to create a wave of fluid, the examiner presses first over the suprapatellar area with the palm of one hand and then presses below the patella with the other. The examiner is sensitive to fluid fluctuating proximally and distally with the maneuver.

3. Ballottement test. A test that, at best, determines large amounts of effusion is the ballottement test. The examiner flexes or extends the leg until uncomfortable. The intent is to feel a floating of the patella on tapping the patella.

Accessory Movement Testing

Orthopedic tests assess gross movement, at best. However, accessory movement is subtle and not under voluntary control by the patient. In other words, it is attained through passive movement at the end of a range of motion. For the knee, it is important to test three main joints: the tibiofemoral, patello-femoral, and tibiofibular. There are numerous descriptions by Mennel (74), Faye (75), Corrigan and Maitland (76), and others that involve a variety of approaches. The common idea is to determine blockage to passive end-range movement at the joint. A normal feel should be springy and involve a small but perceptible amount of movement (less than that felt with instability). A generalized approach will be presented here. Further techniques may be found in the works of the above authors (74, 77).

Anterior/Posterior Glide

Anterior/posterior glide of the tibiofemoral joint is tested with the examiner supporting the calf of the supine patient. While palpating the joint line, the examiner imparts an anterior to posterior force (Fig 14.40). Posterior/anterior glide is performed with the patient prone. The ankle of the patient is supported by the shoulder of the examiner. The examiner interlocks the fingers behind the popliteal fossa and pulls with a posterior to anterior directed force (Fig 14.41).

Side Gliding

Slide gliding into abduction or adduction is performed on the supine patient with one hand cupped around the tibia and the other hand around the femur. Then a scissors action is imparted with the knee in a few degrees of flexion.

Movement of the Tibiofibular Joint

Movement of the tibiofibular joint is best assessed with the supine patient's knee bent to

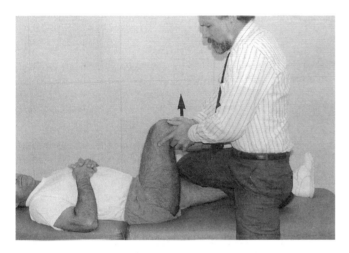

Figure 14.40. Testing for anterior/posterior glide. The patient's calf is supported, and an anterior to posterior force is applied while palpating the joint line for glide.

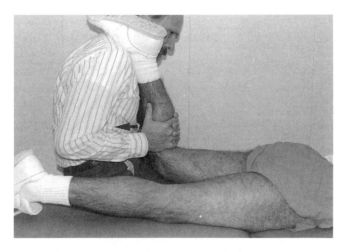

Figure 14.41. Testing for posterior/anterior glide. With the patient prone and the ankle supported by the shoulder of the examiner, the examiner interlocks the fingers behind the popliteal fossa and pulls with a posterior to anterior force.

90%. The examiner grasps hold of the fibular head and pulls anterior and posterior.

Patellar Movement

Patellar movement is tested with the patient supine. The knee is extended and relaxed. The examiner then passively moves the patella in a superior, inferior, medial, and lateral direction, determining any blockage to movement.

Muscle Testing

Testing of muscles should include an assessment of strength and an evaluation of tightness. This requires testing isometrically in various ranges and stretching in the extremes of movement. If possible, testing with isokinetic equipment is helpful in establishing baselines for comparison and monitoring rehabilitative progress. Normals should be based on the healthy leg counterparts and not mathematically determined. Care must be taken in determining functional capacity with isolated testing, given that many sports-related activities are complicated patterns of movement currently inaccessible to quantitative measurement.

Manual muscle testing is rather nonspecific and should be used as a gross assessment of strength. The reproduction of the patient's complaint, indicating a specific muscle, is more valuable.

Recently, there has been a surge of interest in the use of a hand-held dynamometer (HHD). The HHD measures force output and not direct strength. The examiner places the HHD on the extremity at an appropriate position (the more distal, the more accurate)—making sure to stabilize the device—and asks the patient to exert a maximal force for 3 seconds. Intertester reliability seems highest in the upper extremity and lowest in the lower extremity, with the exception of the hip flexors (78).

Measurements

Measurements are generally used to determine the extent of effusion in acute cases and the amount of atrophy in chronic cases. Taken bilaterally and measured in centimeters, several locations are used. Although not standard, it is important to be consistent with the same patient. Recommended points are as follows.

1. At the joint line.
2. Above the patella:
   A. 4 cm (for vastus medialis).
   B. 8 to 10 cm (for general quadriceps).

3. Below the patella at the tibial tubercle (for triceps surae).
4. Leg length measurement (determination of true versus apparent)

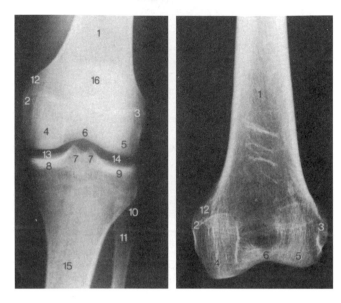

Figure 14.42. Standard anteroposterior (AP) radiographs of the knee with relevant anatomy. (Reprinted with permission from Yochum TR, Rowe LJ. Essentials of skeletal radiology. Baltimore: Williams & Wilkins, 1987:48.)

Diagnostic Imaging

RADIOGRAPHIC EVALUATION

Radiographic evaluation provides a limited amount of information, some of it being indirect evidence of underlying soft tissue pathology. With the advances in computed tomography (CT) scans, bony pathologies such as fractures are better demonstrated than with plain radiographs.

Standard views include anteroposterior and lateral. Specialized views include tunnel, tangential, and stress views.

1. Anteroposterior (AP) (Fig. 14.42). Although routinely and specifically used in acute cases, the AP view is taken with the patient lying with the knee extended. If any loss of joint space is to be determined, the AP view is best taken in a standing position. Additionally, it is important to look for the lateral capsular sign in acute cases in which internal derangement, such as an anterior cruciate tear, may occur (79).
2. Lateral (Fig. 14.43). The lateral view is taken with the knee at 30° of flexion and is usually taken in the lateral recumbent po-

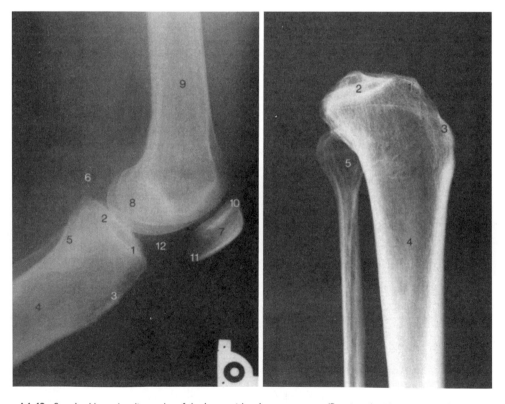

Figure 14.43. Standard lateral radiographs of the knee with relevant anatomy. (Reprinted with permission from Yochum TR, Rowe LJ. Essentials of skeletal radiology. Baltimore: Williams & Wilkins, 1987:50.)

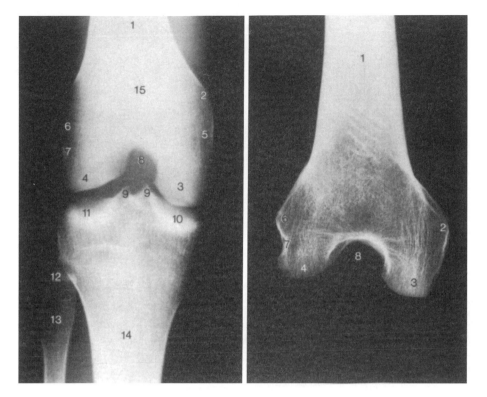

Figure 14.44. Standard tunnel (intercondylar) radiograph of the knee with relevant anatomy. (Reprinted with permission from Yochum TR, Rowe LJ. Essentials of skeletal radiology. Baltimore: Williams & Wilkins, 1987:5.)

sition. One measurement that is used is to determine patella alta or baja. This is based on a measurement of the patellar tendon length and the patella length. If the patellar tendon length exceeds 1 cm, patella alta is suspected; the reverse is true for patella baja (80).

3. Tunnel (Fig. 14.44). The tunnel view is taken posteroanterior at different degrees of flexion. Pathology that is visible includes osteochondritis dissecans and osteochondral fractures.

4. Tangential. A number of tangential views are available, for example:
   A. Sunrise view.
   B. Hughston view.
   C. Merchant view.
   D. Lauren view.

   The most common is the sunrise view. The intention of these views is to visualize the patellofemoral articulation more completely. The posterior surface of the patella is visible, as is the relationship between the patella and the trochlear surface of the femur (Table 14.8).

5. Stress. Essentially, stress views are radiographic evaluations of stability tests. For example, in evaluating collateral ligament damage, a varus or valgus stress is applied at both 0° and 30° of flexion while a radiograph is taken. With cruciate damage, an anterior or posterior drawer test is performed with radiographic documentation. These views are rarely necessary, except in the adolescent in whom epiphyseal damage needs to be differentiated from collateral ligament damage (48).

ARTHROGRAPHY

With the current surge of arthroscopic repair, arthrography has diminished in use. This has occurred even though several studies have shown the superiority of arthrography over arthroscopy with many meniscal lesions (81, 82). Each technique has its limits.

- Arthrography is not as accurate with central ridge and lateral compartment pathology.
- Arthroscopy is limited in the viewing of posterior and peripheral meniscus tears.

The advantage of arthrography is its cost, low morbidity, and accuracy. Arthroscopy's main advantage is if pathology is evident, surgical correction may be performed immediately.

Table 14.8.   Radiographic Findings: Tangential View

Tangential View	Knee Flexion	Technique and Position	Measurements	Miscellaneous
Hughston	55 degrees	Prone position. Beam directed cephalad and inferior, 45 degrees from vertical.	1) Sulcus angle (118°) 2) Patella index AB / XB−XA NL Male 15 Female 17	—Patellar dislocation —Osteochondral fracture —Soft tissue calcification (fold dislocated patella or fracture) Patellar subluxation Patellar tilt Increased medial joint space Apex of patella lateral to apex of femoral sulcus Lateral patella edge lateral to femoral condyle
Merchant	45 degrees	Supine position. Beam directed caudal and inferior, 30 degrees from vertical.	1) Sulcus angle (138°) 2) Congruence angle Med. −6° Lat.	Hypoplastic lateral femoral condyle (usually proximal) —Patellofemoral osteophytes —Subchondral trabeculae orientation (increase or decrease) —Patellar configuration (Wiberg-Baugart)
Laurin	20 degrees	Sitting position. Beam directed cephalad and superior, 160 degrees from vertical.	1) Lateral patellofemoral angle NL ABNL ABNL 2) Patellofemoral index Ratio A/B Med. Lat. Normal = 1.6 or less	I II/III II IV III Jagerhul

From Carson WG, James SL, Larson RL, et al. Patellofemoral disorders—physical and radiographic examination: part II. Clin Orthop 1984;185:178–186.

MAGNETIC RESONANCE IMAGING

Magnetic resonance imaging (MRI) can be used to detect a number of knee lesions including the following.

1. Meniscus tears.
2. Cruciate tears.
3. Collateral ligament tears.
4. Infection.
5. Bone infarct.
6. Bone marrow infiltration.
7. The patellar tendon.
8. Soft tissue tumors.

The patient is supine with the leg externally rotated between 10° and 15°. A surface quadrature coil is necessary to increase the signal-to-noise ratio. Both sagittal and coronal images are considered routine with thickness slices between 3 and 5 mm. Slice thicknesses as small as 1.5 mm are obtainable with two new techniques: fast low-angle shot (FLASH) and gradient-recalled acquisition in the steady state (GRASS) (83, 84).

For meniscus tears a sagittal, spin-echo, T1-weighted image is commonly used. Coronal views are also used and may identify common tears such as the bucket handle, parrot-beak, and the variant, discoid meniscus. The meniscus usually has a low-intensity (dark) image on MRI. Tears usually have a higher signal intensity (lighter), probably due to fluid content. Care must be taken to avoid misinterpreting several normal structures as pathology, including the transverse ligament, popliteus tendon, lateral inferior geniculate artery, and concavity of the outer portion of the meniscus (85).

The cruciate ligaments are also low-intensity images. If on viewing several sagittal images, the ACL is not seen, it is assumed that it is torn. The posterior is assumed to be torn when the low-intensity image is interrupted. If the image is widened or the intensity is increased, swelling is likely indicating damage.

4

Specific Conditions

The following is a discussion of specific knee disorders with some suggestions on treatment and rehabilitation. Further suggestions are given in Chapter 4. Table 14.9 summarizes common knee conditions, their examination findings, and treatment.

Cruciate Ligament Injury

The anterior cruciate is damaged much more frequently than the posterior. Due to its stabilizing functions preventing anterior displacement of the tibia on the femur and possible prevention of internal rotation, the ACL is damaged by both:

1. Outward forces (contact or noncontact) causing:
   A. Valgus plus rotation.
   B. Excessive anterior/posterior movement.
2. Internal forces caused by overcontraction of the quadriceps (noncontact).

Examples of common historical presentations include the following.

1. An athlete tackled from the side while the foot is on the ground.
2. A basketball player who hyperextends on landing (usually on an opponent's foot).
3. Sudden deceleration when attempting to cut (quadriceps pull).

Hyperextension and deceleration injuries are more likely to produce isolated injury to the ACL. Contact injuries usually result in multiple tissue damage (86). In the past it was assumed that when contact involved a valgus stress with internal rotation of the leg, a terrible triad of ACL, MCL, and medial meniscus damage resulted. Recently, it has been demonstrated that it is more common to have a triad of ACL, MCL, and lateral meniscus (87). Apparently, the MCL acts to protect the medial meniscus, not aid in its tearing as previously believed.

In the acute presentation, the patient will report an injury that may have caused an audible pop. There is usually immediate swelling (within 3 hours) indicating a hemarthrosis (88). Additionally, the person may report instability. This latter complaint is far more common in the chronic ACL-deficient patient and may be the only complaint.

If left untreated, the natural course for isolated tears of the ACL is to resolve gradually with a de-

Table 14.9. Knee Disorders

Disorder	Signs and Symptoms	Positive Tests	Treatment	Avoid
Patellofemoral arthralgia	Peripatellar pain Movie sign Painful crepitus	Clark's Waldron's Retinacular test	Correct pronation Strengthen VMO Stretch lateral structures	Flex/ext through crepitus ROM
Iliotibial band syndrome	Lateral knee pain	Ober's Noble's	Stretch ITB Correct pronation Rotational adjustment	Downhill running Side-posture adjustment
Popliteus tendinitis	Lateral knee pain and behind LCL	Resisted int. rotation	Correct pronation Cross-friction massage Isometric int. rotation	Downhill walking or running
Osgood-Schlatter's	Tender tibial tubercle Tight quads Patella alta	Resisted extension	Stretch quads Bracing	Excessive running and jumping
Bursitis	Localized swelling and tenderness	Compression	Ice Pulsed ultrasound	Pressure Overuse
Superior tibiofibular subluxation	Lateral knee pain with instability	Instability at 30°	Fibular head adjustment (support may be needed)	Ankle sprains Excessive hamstring exercise (biceps femoris)
Anterior cruciate tear	Pop at injury Immediate swelling Laxity	Lachman's Drawer Pivot shift MRI or arthroscopy	Strengthen hamstrings and knee rotators Bracing	Quad isotonic exercise initially
Collateral ligament	Tenderness over ligament Possible laxity	Stability test at 0° and 30°	Strengthen muscle support Functional bracing	Knee extension from 30°–0°
Meniscus tear	Joint line tenderness Swelling Locking Giving way	McMurray's Med-lat grind test Apley's MRI or arthroscopy	1. Acute pain relief 2. Adjust carefully 3. Refer if signs and symptoms continue	Squatting and rotational stress in early rehabilitation
Osteochondritis dissecans	Anterior knee pain Possible locking	Wilson's Tunnel view on radiograph	Possible surgery	Blow to anterior knee

VMO, vastus medialis obliques; ROM, range of motion; ITB, iliotibial band; LCL, lateral collateral ligament; MRI, magnetic resonance imaging.

crease of swelling and pain. The future for this patient is usually one of gradual onset of instability and repeated bouts of swelling and sometimes pain.

Testing of the ACL should begin with Lachman's test in the acute setting. Hamstring spasm and meniscal blocking are eliminated in this position. Additionally, the knee should be tested for rotary instability using one of the many pivot-shift maneuvers. Use of the drawer test is recommended; however, its sensitivity in acute settings is not equal to that in chronic cases in which capsular laxity will help to expose the underlying ACL deficiency.

Radiographic evaluation is usually unremarkable unless sufficient damage to other structures has occurred. This is sometimes evident through observation of the lateral capsular sign on a routine anteroposterior view. A small chip of bone, often off the lateral tibial plateau, is visible. MRI has demonstrated an associated osseous injury in a large percentage of ACL tears.

Treatment of ACL tears is dependent on several reasonings (4).

1. Isolated tears are more responsive to conservative care than complicated tears.
2. Complicated tears (acute rotary instability) deserve orthopedic consult with possible surgical consequences.
3. Age- and activity-related criteria are used to determine need and quality of stability.

Conservative treatment should be reserved for chronic ACL deficiency (in particular in the older, less athletic individual) and acute tears with resolved swelling. Treatment is directed at substituting other structures for the laxity lost by the ACL. Dynamically, this may be replaced by strengthening of the hamstrings to the level of the strength of the healthy leg quadriceps. This helps prevent anterior displacement of the tibia. Strengthening of the gastrocnemius may serve a similar purpose. Conversely, it is crucial to avoid quadriceps extension exercises initially, substituting isometrics to prevent atrophy. Ihara and Nakayama demonstrated the effectiveness of proprioceptive training through the use of balance boards (89). The seated patient is required to attempt stabilization while the therapist displaces a platform on casters. The casters are located at only two corners. This is followed by the patient's use of a wobble board. Other approaches focusing on proprioceptive training are advocated using various proprioceptive neuromuscular facilitation (PNF) techniques. Usually a contract-relax technique is used to facilitate the hamstrings at 30° flexion with the patient prone (90).

Functional exercises with elastic tubing are used to decrease shear forces. These include seated extension against elastic tubing resistance (Fig. 14.45) and quad half-squats against the resistance of tubing (Fig. 14.46). Sport cord running is a variation of elastic tubing exercise in which the athlete runs against the resistance of the tubing fixed by a partner (Fig. 14.47) or stationary object such as a pole or tree. The joint reaction forces are less than with unresisted running.

Isokinetic testing has recently revealed a deficit of thigh muscle strength with old grade 2 sprains (91). This deficit was significant at higher speeds, especially with flexion. The authors recommend high-speed isokinetic rehabilitation to address this issue.

Caution should be used with any knee extension exercises with the load placed distal on the leg, such as exercise machines for knee extension. Although cycling is an excellent non–weight-bearing exercise for the knee, caution should be used when rehabilitating an ACL knee. Increased saddle height leads to more shear force.

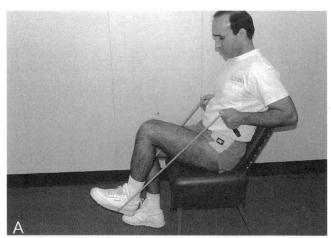
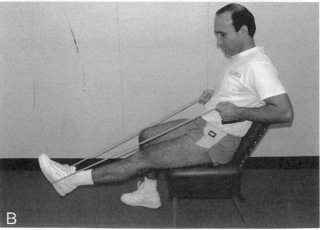

Figure 14.45. A and **B.** Seated extension with elastic tubing.

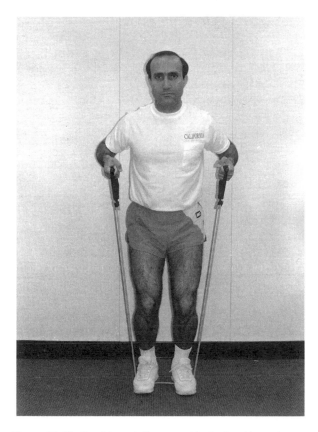

Figure 14.46. Quadriceps half squats with elastic tubing resistance.

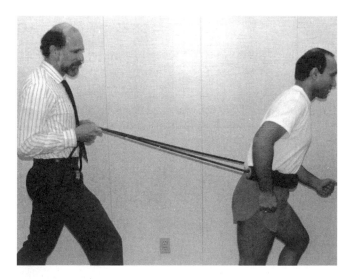

Figure 14.47. Running against elastic tubing resistance.

A midsaddle height coupled with an anterior foot position on the pedal decreases ACL stress (92). Exercise may temporarily increase knee laxity. This tendency does not occur in power lifters performing squats, but does in basketball players and recreational runners (93).

Functional bracing is recommended to protect against future injury for those attempting to avoid surgery yet still participate in sports and for those who have had surgery. Although there are a myriad of braces to choose from, the general principle of the brace is to prevent hyperextension and limit rotatory movement while simultaneously offering some protection to an outside valgus-directed force. The prototype brace is the Lennox-Hill (Lennox Hill Brace Co., Long Island City, NY). Newer, lighter models include the CTI (Innovation Sports, Irvine, CA) and Townsend (Townsend Inc., Bakersfield, CA) among others.

A posterior cruciate tear is less common. It usually is caused by an anterior blow to the tibia with the knee in a flexed position. Other injuries include severe hyperextension and severe collateral ligament injuries.

Swelling is usually less severe due to rupture of the capsule with escape of any fluid produced. Testing should include observation with the patient supine and the knee flexed to 90°. Depression of the tibial tubercle compared with the healthy leg is a common finding. Other tests are described in the section under testing.

Rehabilitation focuses on strengthening the quadriceps with deemphasis of the hamstrings. Surgical repair is usually not as successful as for ACL injury and usually leaves some degree of laxity.

Collateral Ligament Injury

The majority of collateral ligament injuries occur on the medial side. There are several predispositions.

1. There is a normal slight valgus orientation of the knee.
2. During weight-bearing (the stance phase) the tibia internally rotates, increasing medial stress.
3. Many contact injuries involve a valgus force.

The severity of injury may vary from a simple acute or chronic first-degree sprain, such as breaststroker's knee (94), or one that is associated with chronic pronation to total rupture (third-degree tear). Patient presentation is dependent on severity and will therefore vary from minor medial knee pain to gross instability.

Palpation of the collaterals should be performed in the Hardy position (95). This is accomplished by placing the ankle of the injured leg over the knee of the uninvolved leg. This tightens the collateral ligaments bringing them out in relief. Tenderness is often found at the femoral insertion point on the condyle. Joint line tenderness and swelling are also possible.

Testing should include a valgus challenge for medial tears first performed at full extension, then at 20°–30° flexion. Instability at full extension indicates a complicated full tear including involvement of the posterior cruciate. This is a referable case. If negative, testing at 30° is performed. If gross instability is found, an isolated total rupture is likely. Instability, but with an endfeel, indicates a second-degree tear. When there is no instability but pain is produced with these maneuvers and passive internal rotation, a first-degree tear is likely.

Third-degree tears coupled with cruciate involvement must be referred for treatment within 3 to 5 days. Surgical repair after this point has a disappointing success rate (41). Isolated third-degree tears have been treated conservatively with a long-leg cast for several weeks followed by a proper rehabilitative program (96). The outcome of isolated third-degree tears treated conservatively has been documented as satisfactory (97, 98).

Second-degree tears should be placed in a helical brace for 2 to 3 weeks while the patient concomitantly performs sitting exercises for the knee musculature. This should be followed by a graduated rehabilitative program over 2 to 3 months. Although asymptomatic and apparently functional, ligaments do not attain nearly full strength recovery for as long as 1 year (99).

Rehabilitation of first-degree tears involves eliminating any chronic causative activity of predisposition such as pronation. Use of a medial heel wedge is helpful, as is pelvic adjusting. Strengthening of the medial rotators and adductors beginning with isometrics and proceeding to isotonic cable or tubing exercises is appropriate and helpful.

Meniscus Injury

Meniscus damage is common in sports as either an isolated entity or combined with cruciate or collateral injury. Some sports (e.g., soccer) have a higher incidence of meniscus injury compared with football, in which ligamentous injury predominates (39).

Injury causes two distinct types of lesions.

1. Peripheral detachment.
2. Tears (two general types):
   A. Horizontal tears.
   B. Vertical (longitudinal) tears.

The determination of which type of injury occurs seems dependent on age-related changes in the articular cartilage (39). If, for example, the articular cartilage is degenerated and hardened, a horizontal tear is more likely, especially with rotational injury. The same mechanism of injury in a much younger individual may produce a vertical tear or cause no damage at all. Meniscus injury in the preadolescent and adolescent is relatively uncommon (100).

Predisposition to meniscus injury is present with the following.

1. The medial meniscus, which is predisposed due to its relative lack of mobility (compared with the lateral).
2. Older individuals (due to articular cartilage degeneration).
3. The individual with preexisting anterior cruciate or capsular damage.
4. The lateral meniscus when a discoid meniscus is present (101) (an abnormal variant).

Damage may occur in either a contact or noncontact manner. Several common scenarios are as follows.

1. The athlete is hit from the outside, causing a valgus-directed force coupled with rotation of the knee (contact injury).
2. When the foot is fixed to the ground (as with cleats) and the knee rotates externally relative to the femur (usually medial meniscus damage).
3. In any situation in which the knee is prevented from externally rotating through the last few degrees of extension (blocked screw-home mechanism; distributes force to meniscus); this may occur when simply rising quickly from a squatting position.

The athlete usually reports a history of trauma followed by knee pain and swelling. Due to the relative sparsity of meniscal vasculature, the patient will report a slow onset of swelling—after 3 to 6 hours (indication of synovial irritation). Depending on the magnitude of extrameniscal damage, signs and symptoms may vary. Swelling is often the only sign and is sometimes not present at all (especially in isolated small tears). In acute injuries, the patient may report a locking or giving way sensation. In addition, with some meniscus tears, a pop is heard by the patient. The patient may not seek medical attention until long after the injury. The common presentation in the chronic situation is recurrent bouts of swelling, locking, and/or giving way. Again, during the asymptomatic phase, damage may still be occurring to the articular cartilage (102).

Testing for meniscus tears is often not possible in the acute setting due to the requirement of full flexion for compression tests of the knee. If any swelling is present or there is a block to flexion by a torn meniscus (usually posterior horn), tests like McMurray's are impossible. If surgical repair is necessary, there is no immediate requirement for referral (unless cruciate or collateral ligament damage is suspected). Therefore, it is recommended to focus on reduction of swelling to provide a testable knee. Garrick and Webb (103) even suggest that testing with an acute tear may cause more damage. They suggest a less-compressive test. Flexing the knee to 90°, the leg is allowed to drop medially (opening up the medial joint space). The hip is abducted and the leg extended. Lack of pain with this maneuver is supposed to rule out a medial meniscus tear.

The vertical (e.g., bucket handle) tear is commonly found in the middle or posterior meniscus. This type of tear will be detected by compression maneuvers (squatting) or testing (McMurray's). The test result is positive when a painful click is produced. A grinding or grating sensation is more common with testing of horizontal tears.

Anderson and Lipscomb determined that the sensitivity of meniscus testing is minimal when each test is graded separately. However, they found that at least one of three tests was positive in 79% of arthroscopically demonstrable meniscus tears (71). These are as follows.

1. Joint line tenderness (Steinman's test).
2. McMurray's.
3. Medial-lateral grind test.

Petersen and Frankel believe that the Helfet test, which demonstrates loss of external rotation of the tibia on full extension, is extremely sensitive (33).

Radiographic evaluation is essentially normal unless degenerative changes associated with chronic tears are evident. This is best seen on an anterior knee radiograph taken during weight-bearing. Damage is demonstrated by loss of the normal joint space (usually medial).

When equivocal, two rational approaches should be considered. First is referral for MRI for a more definitive confirmation. Second is conservative treatment while waiting to determine whether recurrent swelling, locking, or giving way appears. If so, referral for orthopedic consultation is requisite.

Conservative management of meniscus tears is controversial. If joint line tenderness is present, yet the history and other examination findings are unequivocally negative, it is likely that a coronary (capsular) ligament sprain is the cause. Treatment usually involves cross-friction massage followed by icing for 2 to 3 weeks (104).

Stable vertical tears occurring in the periphery of the meniscus may be treated conservatively (105). If a small tear is suspected, conservative treatment may involve adjusting the knee to restore normal accessory motion and bracing for 2 to 3 weeks, while the patient maintains a strict isometric program. This will prevent the often observed sign of quadriceps atrophy following meniscal injury. After this initial phase, a generalized knee program should be prescribed.

Helfet has observed that in an attempt to unlock their knees or decrease pain, patients often adjust their knees by quick extension (25). He also observed that chronic tears may be asymptomatic while causing significant articular damage (102). Coupling these two concepts, it is important for the treating doctor to recognize the effectiveness of adjusting the knee in restoring motion and decreasing pain. However, reduction of symptoms does not indicate a curative effect on the already existing damage and certainly does not guarantee prevention of future articular damage. Referral is warranted if a patient responds well to conservative care but has an increasing frequency of recurrent bouts of signs or symptoms.

Surgical treatment of small peripheral tears in adults is usually with arthroscopic repair. Younger athletes may be treated conservatively. Larger vertical tears are treated, as much as possible, with a partial meniscectomy performed arthroscopically.

Decision-making with the treatment of significant tears may be a double-edged sword. If a total meniscectomy is performed, the individual will be predisposed to early degenerative changes and arthritis. If treated conservatively, the same consequences are likely.

Patellofemoral Disorders

The patellofemoral apparatus includes the quadriceps attachment to the patella, the patella, and the patellar tendon. Disorders generally fall into three categories.

1. Extensor disorders (e.g., patellar tendinitis, Osgood-Schlatter's, Sinding-Larsen-Johansson).
2. Intrinsic patellar disorders (e.g., chondromalacia, bipartite patella, fracture).
3. Tracking or malalignment disorders (e.g., patellofemoral arthralgia, subluxating or dislocating patella, or many of the disorders from 1 and 2).

EXTENSOR DISORDERS

Extensor disorders are caused by overuse or strain of the quadriceps insertion into the superior patella, patellar tendon, or insertions of the patellar tendon into the inferior pole of the patella or tibial tuberosity. Testing and differentiation are usually accomplished by a combination of a history involving excessive running or jumping coupled with the following physical examination findings.

1. Pain produced on resisted extension of the knee (it is important to test knee extension in various ranges of motion).
2. Pain localization by the patient or tenderness localization produced by resisted extension.
    A. Slightly above patella—quadriceps tendinitis.
    B. Superior or inferior pole of the patella—Sinding-Larsen-Johansson in the adolescent, patellar tendinitis in the adult or adolescent.
    C. Patellar tendon—patellar tendinitis (jumper's knee) or bursitis.
    D. Tibial tuberosity—Osgood-Schlatter's or patellar tendinitis.

Further differentiation is made by patient age. Sinding-Larsen-Johannson and Osgood-Schlatter's occur in the adolescent, usually between the ages of 9 and 13. These conditions are often included under the umbrella classification of osteochondrosis. The damage is caused by excessive pull on apophyseal centers that have not undergone ossification. A significant finding with Osgood-Schlatter's is a tender enlarged tibial tuberosity. Radiographs are rarely indicated with these disorders. There are rare occasions when an avulsion occurs at the tibial tuberosity (106). Clinically, the clue to this possibility is persistent tibial tuberosity pain at rest.

Treatment of the extensor disorders is a generalized approach of modification of the causative activity, ice after activity, and a daily routine of gradual stretching for the quadriceps and other knee musculature. Use of the Osgood-Schlatter brace may be helpful. It is not recommended that the young athlete be suspended from all physical activity unless pain is continuously present at rest or the patient is noncompliant with activity modifications.

FRACTURE VERSUS BIPARTITE PATELLA

Fracture of the patella is uncommon (45). When it does occur, there will be a history of direct trauma to the patella. Diagnosis is suggested by the history coupled with patellar pain. Radiographs are needed for confirmation. The patella may fracture either horizontally or in multiple fragments.

Bipartite patella are unfused portions of the patella, usually in the superior-lateral pole, which are generally asymptomatic. Trauma or sports activity requiring excessive running or jumping may initiate symptoms. Clinically, this is more common in males and often is bilateral. Radiographs taken of the patella anteroposteriorly and tangentially are helpful. If differentiation between a fracture and bipartite is difficult, bilateral views may provide the answer.

MALALIGNMENT DISORDERS

Malalignment of the patellofemoral mechanism may result in a plethora of problems. The predisposition to malalignment may cause dislocation/subluxation of the patella, resulting in a combination of soft tissue damage and osteochondral fracture. Insidiously, malalignment develops into a peripatellar pain syndrome due to soft tissue involvement (patellofemoral arthralgia) or actual cartilage degeneration of the patella (chondromalacia). Clinically, the differentiation between only soft tissue or cartilage degeneration is difficult.

The common denominator with malalignment disorders is an abnormal positioning or tracking of the patella. The underlying predispositions are numerous.

1. Structural or functional problems possibly resulting in an increased Q angle:
    A. Anteversion of the hip.
    B. Genu varum/valgum.
    C. Tibial torsion.
    D. Pronation.
    E. Weak external rotators of the hip (piriformis) and abductors (gluteus medius) (107).
2. Osseous abnormalities of the femur or patella:
    A. Underdeveloped lateral femoral condyle.
    B. Abnormally shaped patella (e.g., thin median ridge).
    C. Shallow trochlear (intercondylar) groove.
3. Patella alta (high-riding) or baja (low-riding).
4. Muscular imbalance.
    A. Weakened medial structures (VMO).
    B. Tight lateral structures (ITB vastus lateralis).

PATELLAR DISLOCATION AND SUBLUXATION

Patellar dislocation is not always due to malalignment. It is possible for the athlete to dislocate the patella by planting the foot in a flexed position while attempting to cut to the opposite direction. A valgus force is then created while the quadriceps are contracting strongly. Complications are common and numerous. Many of the soft tissue stabilizing structures for the patella are torn, such as the medial retinaculum, VMO, or even the quadriceps tendon. Other damage includes articular cartilage damage to the patella or femoral condyle (this often occurs when the patella relocates, hitting the lateral femoral condyle). Osteochondral fractures may also occur in the same setting, particularly in younger athletes.

Historical description by the patient is usually that they felt their knee go out of place (or back in place during reduction). Other signs and symptoms are variable depending on the number of damaged structures; however, medial knee pain and swelling are common.

If there is sufficient swelling to disguise the displaced patella and/or reduction has occurred, the examiner may initially miss the diagnosis. In the acute setting, the displacement is readily apparent. Reduction is accomplished by carefully extending the knee. If unsuccessful, mild medial pressure is added. No other attempts should be made if the above maneuvers do not succeed. In all the above scenarios, whether reduction has occurred or not, the knee should be packed in ice, splinted, and the patient sent for radiographs and treatment.

Treatment involves immobilization in a cylinder cast for 4 to 6 weeks. Patellar stabilization braces should be worn during activity. The vastus medialis obliquus should be facilitated and strengthened.

Patellar subluxation is similar in presentation and often impossible to differentiate from spontaneous reduction of a dislocated patella. With spontaneous reduction there is usually an immediate hemarthrosis. Subluxation is common in those who have had dislocation in the past and in those who have damaged patellar restraining tissues and allowed them to heal elongated. Testing should include the apprehension test first at 30°, then at full extension if negative.

PATELLOFEMORAL ARTHRALGIA

By far, the most common nontraumatic cause of knee pain is patellofemoral arthralgia (PFA) (108). The literature is full of aliases such as runner's knee, medial retinaculitis, patellar malalignment syndrome, and others (109). In prearthroscopic times, this purely soft tissue disorder was usually misdiagnosed as chondromalacia patella (110). Clinically, it is difficult to differentiate between the two disorders. Many of the tests for chondromalacia may be positive with PFA. Absolute response to conservative care points away from the diagnosis of chondromalacia.

The onset of pain is usually gradual. The location is either patellar or peripatellar (medial, lateral, inferior). Occasionally, the pain is referred to the posterior knee. One of the most common complaints is pain ascending or descending stairs. As the disorder progresses, the patient will complain of stiffness and pain on rising from a prolonged seated position. This is referred to as the movie or theater sign (this is also positive with osteoarthritis and chondromalacia) (111).

Observational clues would classically consist of the miserable malalignment group, which includes femoral anteversion, medial squinting of the patella, genu recurvatum, tibia varum, and compensatory pronation. More commonly, only one or two of these abnormalities are seen. These and other problems like patella alta require observation in both the seated and standing positions.

Tenderness is often found at the retinaculum using the Fulkerson test (47). Additional sites of tenderness include the insertion of the VMO and ITB. The following tests may be positive.

1. Patellar grind or Clarke's.
2. Waldron's.
3. Displacement of the patella medially with the knee at 30° flexion.
4. VMO coordination test.
5. Modified Ober's.

Radiographic evaluation would be helpful only in detecting underlying abnormalities of the patella or femur. These are usually apparent with one of several specialized tangential views (Table 14.8).

Treatment pivots around correction of the soft tissue contributors to malalignment. This includes the following.

1. Stretching of the lateral musculature and the ITB.
2. Strengthening of the VMO may begin with the VMO test performed with a towel (this is often preceded or simultaneously combined with an isometric contraction of the adductors due to common insertion at the adductor tubercle, which results in a more efficient contraction).
3. Pronation support consisting of:
   A. Temporary use of taping or a medial heel wedge to determine effectiveness of an orthotic.
   B. Change to a running shoe with pronation support and firm heel counter.
   C. Orthotics.

4. Stretching of tight musculature that may increase compressive forces on the patella.
    A. Quadriceps/hamstrings.
    B. Triceps surae.

Focus on the VMO is based on the observed reversal of normal timing order between the vastus lateralis and medialis obliques in patients with extensor mechanism dysfunction (112).

ILIOTIBIAL BAND SYNDROME

The ITB is often tight in athletes. A study of flexibility in dancers revealed a high incidence of tight lateral structures (113). When tight, the ITB will grate over the lateral epicondyle of the femur at approximately 30° of flexion, causing irritation. Therefore, repetitive flexion and extension activities such as running are the main causes. Sedentary individuals are not immune. A prolonged seated position effectively shortens the ITB so that any repetitive activity such as walking or running may initiate lateral knee pain.

Found more commonly in runners, the patient with ITB will usually report a gradual onset of lateral knee pain over a few weeks. Initially tolerable, the pain often becomes disabling. They may report a strange sound similar to a creak produced when rubbing a finger over a wet balloon (114). Downhill running will often be the historical variable that initiated onset.

Tenderness is located at one of several points: Gerdy's tubercle, the lateral epicondyle, and occasionally the greater trochanter. Clinical differentiation is usually a simple matter of testing the patient for a tight ITB (modified Ober's) or adding compression over the lateral epicondyle (Noble's). Asking the patient to stand full weight-bearing on the involved side and flex the leg to 30° will often reproduce the pain.

Treatment involves restriction of any inciting activity such as running, while gradually stretching the ITB using a PNF technique such as hold-relax. A technique that is safe and effective is to have the supine patient cross the bent healthy leg over the involved leg. Using the healthy ankle as resistance, the patient uses a 15 to 25% isometric contraction into abduction for 8 to 10 seconds and then relaxes. Using the healthy leg, the patient pushes the involved leg into a new position of stretch. Side posture adjusting on the involved side is not recommended during the first 2 weeks of treatment. Sudden stretching, as may occur in side posture adjusting, may initiate a reflex tightening and irritation.

Popliteus Tendinitis

Popliteus tendinitis is similar to the ITB syndrome in its lateral location. The popliteus is strained when its functions of stability for the anterior movement of the femur or internal rotation of the tibia are strained. This occurs often in downhill walking or running when the femur is forced forward against the resistance of the PCL and popliteus.

The pain location with popliteus tendinitis is usually at the insertion point anterior to the femoral insertion of the LCL. Tenderness along its tendinous course behind the LCL is also a possible finding. Testing involves resistance to active internal rotation of the tibia. Additionally, Corrigan and Maitland (76) describe a test in which the supine patient is in a figure-four position. The examiner resists the patient's attempt at knee flexion while palpating behind the LCL. This maneuver should increase tenderness or create pain behind the LCL (76). Finally, a weight-bearing test similar to that for the ITB syndrome is used. The patient performs the same maneuver as described above but with internal rotation of the leg at 30°. The internal rotation supposedly distinguishes between popliteus and ITB involvement (115).

Treatment should include application of ice and rest from the inciting activity. Cross-friction massage is suggested by Cyriax and Cyriax; it is usually performed over the tendon of the muscle (116).

Proximal Tibiofibular Subluxation

The tibiofibular articulation moves superior and inferior during these movements of the ankle through the connection with the interosseous membrane between the tibia and fibula. Subluxation is most often due to a sudden dorsiflexion (or plantar flexion) injury to the ankle. Therefore, the patient may not report a knee injury but instead an ankle sprain/strain.

Subluxation of the proximal tibiofibular joint is being highlighted due to the possibility of irritation to the common peroneal nerve. A radiating lateral leg pain similar to nerve root irritation may occur.

Subluxation is suspected when the patient is unable to bear full weight on the affected leg at 30° of flexion without a sense of instability. A confirmation may be made by asking the patient to then support the posterior fibular area with the foot of the healthy leg or the examiner's hand. If this decreases or eliminates the sense of instability, a subluxation is likely (Fig. 14.48) (25). Motion palpation (accessory motion) should be per-

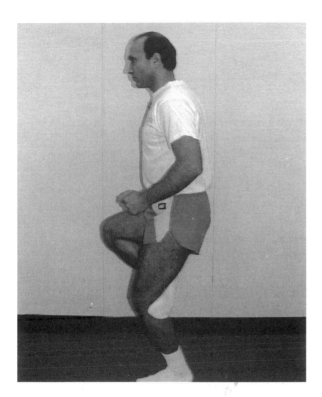

Figure 14.48. Testing for subluxation of the proximal tibiofibular joint. Subluxation is suspected if the patient reports a feeling of instability when bearing full weight on the affected leg at 30° of knee flexion.

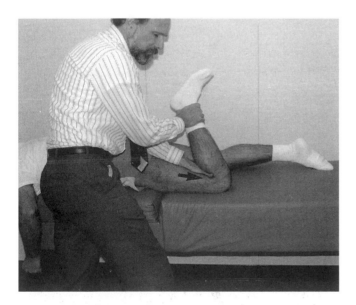

Figure 14.49. Setup for adjusting the fibular head from posterior to anterior.

formed in an attempt to correlate with the above findings and help dictate the direction of force application.

Adjusting the fibular head (usually from posterior to anterior) is the treatment of choice in most cases. Figure 14.49 demonstrates the setup. If the treatment is successful, yet the problem is re-

current, it may be necessary to support the area with a brace and ask the patient to use crutches for a few days after the adjustment.

Bursitis

Bursitis is a common event in contact sports. Direct trauma to a bursa will usually cause a discrete swelling. Although found in multiple locations around the knee, the swellings are all generally treated the same, including protection from subsequent trauma and attempts to decrease swelling with ice and (cautiously) pulsed ultrasound. Recurrent bouts of swelling are common and may require surgical excision. The bursa does grow back within approximately 6 months. A point to keep in mind is that when the suprapatellar pouch is irritated, it may swell to a large size (to 12 inches above the patella).

Osteochondritis Dissecans

Osteochondritis dissecans is a disorder in which a portion of the femoral condyle (usually the posterolateral area of the medial condyle) forms a separate loose fragment. This may potentially interfere with movement, locking the joint like a "marble in the gears." There are several suspected causes such as trauma, disturbance of blood supply, or genetic factors. Divided into two groups (younger than 15 years of age and older than 15), it appears that the younger group does not have a traumatic cause. It often occurs bilaterally and may be asymptomatic if the defect has not become an actual loose body. Testing includes both the Wilson test and palpation of the femoral condyle with the knee flexed beyond 90°. Radiographic evaluation must include a tunnel view. There is a normal variant that will eventually ossify and not produce symptomatology (39).

In the older group (older than 15 years of age), trauma is more likely the cause; therefore, it is bilateral less often. Diagnosis again is with Wilson's test, femoral condyle palpation, and radiographs. Treatment is more often surgical with this group, and the condition seems to worsen as the person ages.

General Treatment and Rehabilitation

Treatment of acute presentations focuses on pain relief, swelling prevention/reduction, and support (if needed). An additional concern in the subacute phase is prevention of atrophy. With resolution of pain/swelling, attention is shifted to prevention of recurrence with appropriate rehabilitation. Bracing may be desired for possible prevention or functional support.

Standard approaches to pain relief (such as ice, analgesics, rest elevation, and TENS) are helpful. Yet the majority of retraining will be delayed until at least 90% range of motion, in particular extension, is restored. Suggestions for increasing soft tissue restriction to full range of motion are given by the author (117). Caution must be used in attempting to increase range of motion. Mechanical blockage from internal derangement may appear similar to soft tissue restriction. Pain (as opposed to a stretching sensation) produced with these maneuvers is an indicator to stop and further assess the possibility of more serious damage.

A generalized exercise program beginning with a preliminary facilitation phase is presented in Tables 14.10 and 14.11. Goals must be met in each phase before progressing, thus assuring a gradual return to full activity. The preliminary phase emphasizes isometrics and straight leg raises during which range of motion is increased. Progressing through elastic tubing exercise, followed by machine-resistive training, the athlete

Table 14.10. Knee Rehabilitation: Initial Phase—Performed 3 Times a Day

Type	Muscles	Sets[a]	Repetitions	Contraction	Rest
Quad setting (isometrics)	Quads/hamstrings	1–2	10–12	8 sec	3–5 sec
SLR supine (with setting)	Quads/psoas	2–3	10–12	3 sec	3–5 sec
	Vastus medialis				
	Biceps femoris				
Side lying					
Abduction	Gluteus medius	"	"	"	"
	Peroneals				
Adduction	Adductors				
Prone	Gluteals/spinal extensors	"	"	"	"
Stretch (use PNF)	Gastroc/soleus	5	10–20	8–10 sec	5 sec
	Hamstrings				
	Tensor fascia lata				
	Quadriceps				
	Adductors				

[a]A rest period of 1–3 min between sets is recommended.

Table 14.11. General Knee Exercise Program

Exercise/Stretch	Activity	Amount
Beginning phase—begun when patient has 90% ROM; no joint irritation		
Stretch	PNF stretch for hams, ITB, and gastrocnemius	3–5 sets, 10–20 reps
Isometrics	Performed every 20°	1–2 sets, 10–12 reps
SLR with weights	Supine, prone, sidelying	2–3 sets, 10–12 reps
Functional work	Shallow knee bends, lunges, step-downs	2–3 sets, 10–12 reps
Isotonic exercise (with elastic tubing or pulley)	Knee extension, flexion, abd/add, int/ext rot.	Based on PRE or DAPRE
Aerobic exercise	Healthy leg bicycling and rowing, upper body work	30 min at target heart rate for aerobic work
Intermediate phase—begun when patient has 75% strength and endurance of healthy leg; continue the stretch, functional work, and aerobic exercise and add the following		
Isotonics (use universal or Nautilus)	Knee and hip work (accentuate eccentrics)	Based on PRE or DAPRE
Sport cord training	⅓ Knee bends, forward/backward run	Average: 3 sets, 20 reps
PNF diagonals	Emphasize flexion/extension, int/ext rot.	Several sets to fatigue
Proprioceptive work	Wobble or balance board using both legs	Average: 5 sets; 3–5 min
Advanced phase—begun when patient has 90% of strength and endurance of healthy leg; continue stretch and proprioceptive work; continue above isotonic work if isokinetic is not available		
Isokinetics	Knee extension/flexion patterns	10–20 reps, at multiple speeds (emphasize fast)
PNF (sport specific)	Patterns imitate patient's sport pattern	Several sets to fatigue
Agility drills	Figure-eights	5–10 sets for total of 45 min
	Cutting maneuvers	
	Cariocas	
	Rope jumping	
	Side-to-side jumping	

ROM, range of motion; PNF, proprioceptive neuromuscular facilitation; ITB, iliotibial band.

Table 14.12.   Knee Bracing

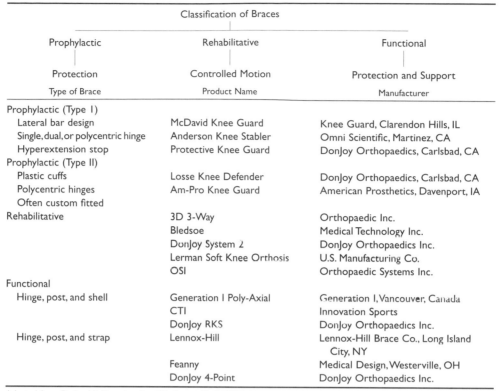

	Classification of Braces	
Prophylactic	Rehabilitative	Functional
Protection	Controlled Motion	Protection and Support
Type of Brace	Product Name	Manufacturer
Prophylactic (Type I)		
Lateral bar design	McDavid Knee Guard	Knee Guard, Clarendon Hills, IL
Single, dual, or polycentric hinge	Anderson Knee Stabler	Omni Scientific, Martinez, CA
Hyperextension stop	Protective Knee Guard	DonJoy Orthopaedics, Carlsbad, CA
Prophylactic (Type II)		
Plastic cuffs	Losse Knee Defender	DonJoy Orthopaedics, Carlsbad, CA
Polycentric hinges	Am-Pro Knee Guard	American Prosthetics, Davenport, IA
Often custom fitted		
Rehabilitative	3D 3-Way	Orthopaedic Inc.
	Bledsoe	Medical Technology Inc.
	DonJoy System 2	DonJoy Orthopaedics Inc.
	Lerman Soft Knee Orthosis	U.S. Manufacturing Co.
	OSI	Orthopaedic Systems Inc.
Functional		
Hinge, post, and shell	Generation I Poly-Axial	Generation I, Vancouver, Canada
	CTI	Innovation Sports
	DonJoy RKS	DonJoy Orthopaedics Inc.
Hinge, post, and strap	Lennox-Hill	Lennox-Hill Brace Co., Long Island City, NY
	Feanny	Medical Design, Westerville, OH
	DonJoy 4-Point	DonJoy Orthopaedics Inc.

Adapted from Paulos LE. Knee bracing. Clin Sports Med 1990;9:4.
Patellar braces attempt to decrease patellar forces and/or control tracking through various devices such as:
• Cho-Pat (infrapatellar strap).
• Knee sleeves with patellar "holes" with and without straps.
• Knee sleeve with horseshoe guidance.
Specialized braces for Osgood-Schlatter's such as the Shultz Osgood Schlatter Brace.

should maintain aerobic capacity in preparation for the advanced phase. This final phase should focus on agility skills and sport-specific activities. Specific restrictions include the following.

1. Avoidance of knee extension exercises in the range of motion where crepitus or pain is present with all knee disorders, particularly patellofemoral problems.
2. Initial avoidance of knee extension exercise should be prescribed for patients with ACL involvement. Eventually, some extension may be allowed; however, it should never be through terminal extension.
3. The PCL-deficient patient should avoid hamstring-resistive exercise. Hyperextension should also be avoided.
4. Full squats should be avoided in suspected cases of meniscus tears.
5. Specific restraints should be dictated by an orthopedic surgeon based on the specific type of surgery performed.

Knee Bracing

The controversy about knee bracing is likely to be long lived. Initial hopes were that bracing could provide substantial protection and control of instability, yet no conclusive evidence demonstrating support for these concepts has been found. Secondary considerations were given to proprioceptive theories of the benefits of bracing. This too has not been adequately substantiated. Without convincing research confirmation, athletes still seem impressed with the performance of bracing and often insist on its use.

In 1984, the American Academy of Orthopedic Surgeons (AAOS) Sports Medicine Committee categorized bracing into three broad categories.

1. Prophylactic—intended to provide protection from valgus (or varus) forces in an attempt to prevent injury or reinjury to the collateral ligaments (mainly MCL).
2. Rehabilitative—intended to control motion within restricted ranges during recovery from surgery or injury.
3. Functional—intended to control instability and provide protection concomitantly. Used mainly in ACL-deficient knees.

A list of popular braces in each category is given in Table 14.12.

Selection of bracing should include the following considerations.

1. Cost—universal-type bracing (off-the-shelf) is often less expensive but less durable and protective in many instances.
2. Fit—custom-fitted bracing is generally more stable; however, slippage is a problem even with this type. It must also be remembered that if the brace is fitted before full rehabilitation, the size of the leg may increase.
3. Comfort—in particular with functional bracing, elastic straps are more comfortable than rigid ones but are less effective.
4. Material—lighter weight materials are also more comfortable, yet the trade-off is in durability and effectiveness. Lighter metals bend more easily, offering less protection. Light composite materials may be more brittle and also may be prone to fatigue cracks.
5. Generalized function—functional braces may be dynamic (applying a preload to prevent excessive motion usually through strapping) or stable; function is essentially stressed only when excessive motion occurs.
6. Hinge type—single, dual, and polycentric hinges may be unilateral or bilateral. Inherently, the brace with the most control is the bilateral hinge brace with a rigid shell and condylar pads that better control position.

SUMMARY

The knee is one of the most commonly injured areas in sports. Injury may occur through several mechanisms. In addition to overuse injury, the knee is particularly vulnerable to contact injury due to its natural exposure. Many injuries are difficult to evaluate in the acute setting due to accompanying swelling or pain. Therefore, on-the-field evaluation is crucial before the severity of the injury is camouflaged by pseudostability. Conservative management is preferable in most knee disorders with some exceptions.

- Ligament ruptures with additional tissue involvement (i.e., muscles, capsule, subchondral bone).
- Meniscus tears that are the source of unresolving signs and symptoms.
- Fractures, tumors, or infections.

It is crucial for the examiner to have the skills necessary to determine the need for referral in these cases.

References

1. Hertling D, Kessler RM. Management of common musculoskeletal disorders. 2nd ed. New York: Harper & Row, 1990.
2. Noble CA. The iliotibial band friction syndrome in runners. Am J Sports Med 1980;4:232–234.
3. Bose K, Kamgasumtherman R, Osman MBH. Vastus medialis oblique: an anatomic and physiologic study. Orthopaedics 1980;3:880–883.
4. Last RJ. Anatomy: regional and applied. 6th ed. New York: Churchill Livingstone, 1978:139–204.
5. Nichols JN, Tehranzadeh J. A review of tibial spine fractures in bicycle injury. Am J Sports Med 1987;15:172.
6. Walker PS. Human joints and their artificial replacements. Springfield, IL: Charles C. Thomas, 1977:39.
7. Goodfellow J, Hungerford DS, Woods C. Patello-femoral joint mechanics and pathology: chondromalacia patellae. J Bone Joint Surg Br 1976;58:291.
8. Gruber J Wolter D, Lerse W. Der vordere Kneuzbandreflex (LCA-Reflex). Unfaitchrung 1986;89:551.
9. Solomonow M, Barata R, Zhou BH, et al. The synergistic action of the anterior cruciate ligament and thigh muscles in maintaining joint stability. Am J Sports Med 1987;15:207.
10. Montgomery JB, Steadman JR. Rehabilitation of the injured knee. Clin Sports Med 1985;4:333–343.
11. Zarins B, Boyle J. Knee ligament injuries. In: Nicholas JA, Hershman EB (eds). The lower extremity and spine in sports medicine. St. Louis: CV Mosby, 1986;1:929.
12. Baker CL, Norwood LA, Hughston JC. Acute combined posterior and posterolateral instability of the knee. Am J Sports Med 1984;12:204.
13. Noyes FR, et al. Arthroscopy in acute traumatic hemarthrosis of the knee-incidence of anterior cruciate tears and other injuries. J Bone Joint Surg Am 1980;62:687–695.
14. Norwood LA Jr, Cross MJ. Anterior cruciate ligament: functional anatomy of its bundles in rotary instabilities. Am J Sports Med 1979;7:23–26.
15. Kulund DN. The injured athlete. Philadelphia: JB Lippincott, 1982:384–385.
16. Kennedy JC, et al. Nerve supply of the human knee and its functional importance. Am J Sports Med 1986;14:309–315.
17. Arnoczky SP. Anatomy of the anterior cruciate ligament. Clin Orthop 1983;172:19.
18. Kennedy JC, Weisberg HW, Wilson AS. The anatomy and function of the anterior cruciate ligament as determined by clinical and morphological studies. J Bone Joint Surg Am 1974;56:223.
19. Terry GC. The anatomy of the extensor mechanism. In: Henry JH, ed. Patellofemoral problems. Clin Sports Med 1989;8:163–177.
20. Beidert RM, Stauffer E, Friederich NF. Occurrence of free nerve endings in the soft tissue of the knee joint: a histologic investigation. Am J Sports Med 1992;20:430.
21. Lieb FJ, Perry J. Quadriceps function: an anatomical and mechanical study using amputated limbs. J Bone Joint Surg Am 1968;50:1535–1548.
22. Heller L, Langman J. The meniscofemoral ligaments of the human knee. J Bone Joint Surg Br 1964;46:307.
23. Oretorp B, Risberg B. Studies of the fine structure of the medial meniscus and ligaments and their anatomical relations to the human knee. Medical Dissertations 63, Linkoping University, Sweden, 1978.
24. Barantigan OC, Voshell AF. The mechanics of the ligaments and the menisci of the knee joint. J Bone Joint Surg 1941;23:44–66.
25. Helfet AJ. Disorders of the knee. 2nd ed. Philadelphia: JB Lippincott, 1982:104–116.
26. Warren R, Arnoczky SP, Wickiewiez TL. Anatomy of the knee. In: Nicholas JA, Hershman EB, eds. The lower extremity and spine in sports medicine. St. Louis: CV Mosby, 1986;657–694.
27. Arnoczky SP, Warren RF. Microvasculature of the meniscus and its response to injury: an experimental study in the dog. Am J Sports Med 1983;11:131–141.
28. Fox JM. Injuries to the thigh. In: Nicholas JA, Hershman EB, eds. The lower extremity and spine in sports medicine. St. Louis: CV Mosby, 1986;1092.

29. Hirokawa S, Solomonow M, Lu Y, et al: Anterior-posterior displacement of the tibia elicited by quadriceps contraction. Am J Sports Med 1992;20:299.

30. Johnson RJ, Pope MH. Functional anatomy of the meniscus: symposium on reconstruction of the knee. AAOS. St. Louis: CV Mosby, 1978:3.

31. Marshall JL, Girgis FG, Zelko RR. The biceps femoris tendon and its functional significance. J Bone Joint Surg Am 1972;54:1444.

32. Jackson RW, et al. The pathologic medial shelf. Orthop Clin North Am 1982;13:307.

33. Petersen L, Frankel VH. Biomechanics of the knee in athletes. In: Nicholas JA, Hershman EB, eds. The lower extremity and spine in sports medicine. St. Louis: CV Mosby, 1986;695–727.

34. Mann RA. Biomechanics of running. In: Nicholas JA, Hershman EB, eds. The lower extremity and spine in sports medicine. St. Louis: CV Mosby, 1986:396–411.

35. Levens AS, Inman VT, Blosser JA. Transverse rotation of the segments of the lower extremity in locomotion. J Bone Joint Surg Am 1948;30:859.

36. Mann RA, Moran GT, Dougherty SE. Comparative electromyography of the lower extremity in jogging, running, and sprinting. Am J Sports Med 1986;14:501–510.

37. Ericson MO, Nisell R. Patellofemoral joint forces during ergometric cycling. Phys Ther 1987;67:1365–1369.

38. Jacob RP, Staubi HU, Deland JT. Grading the pivot shift: objective tests with implications for treatment. J Bone Joint Surg Br 1987;69:294–299.

39. Roy S, Irwin R. Sports medicine. Englewood Cliffs, NJ: Prentice-Hall, 1983;316.

40. Minns RJ, Birnie AJM, Abermethy PJ. A stress analysis of the patella and how it relates to patellar articular cartilage lesions. J Biomech 1979;12:699–711.

41. Beckman M, Craig R, Lehman RC. Rehabilitation of patellofemoral dysfunction in the athlete. In: Lehman RC, ed. Rehabilitation Clin Sports Med 1989;8:844.

42. Bollen S, Seedhom BB. A comparison of the Lysholm and Cincinnati knee scoring questionnaires. Am J Sports Med 1991;19:189.

43. Brody DM. Running injuries. In: Nicholas JA, Hershman EB, eds. The lower extremity and spine in sports medicine. St. Louis: CV Mosby, 1986;1546–1548.

44. Staheli LT, Engel GM. Tibial torsion. Clin Orthop 1972; 86:183.

45. Magee DJ. Orthopedic physical assessment. Philadelphia: WB Saunders, 1987;266–313.

46. Insall J, Salvati E. Patella position in the normal knee joint. Radiology 1971;101:101–104.

47. Fulkerson JP. Evaluation of the peripatellar soft tissues and retinaculum in patients with patellofemoral pain. In: Henry JH, ed. Patellofemoral problems. Clin Sports Med 1989;8:197–202.

48. O'Donoghue DH. Treatment of injuries in athletes. 3rd ed. Philadelphia: WB Saunders, 1976;575.

49. Strobel M, Stedfeld HW. Diagnostic Evaluation of the Knee. Berlin: Springer-Verlag, 1990.

50. Kennedy JC. The injured adolescent knee. Baltimore: Williams & Wilkins, 1979.

51. Anderson AF, Snyder RB, Federspeil CF, et al. Instrumented evaluation of knee laxity: a comparison of five arthrometers. Am J Sports Med 1992;20:135.

52. Jonsson TB, Althoff L. Clinical diagnosis of ruptures of the anterior cruciate ligament: a comparative study of the Lachman test and the anterior drawer sign. Am J Sports Med 1982;10:100.

53. Feagin JA. Principles of diagnosis and treatment. In: The crucial ligaments: diagnosis and treatment of ligamentous injuries about the knee. New York: Churchill Livingstone, 1988.

54. Cross MJ, Schmidt DR, Mackie IG. A no-touch test for the anterior cruciate ligament. J Bone Joint Surg Br 1987;69:300.

55. Wirth CJ, Artmann A. Diagnostische probleme bei frischen und veraltelen kreuzbandverletzugen des Kniegelenkes. Arch Orthop Unfallchir 1975;81:333.

56. Davies GJ, Malone T, Bassett FH. Knee examination. Phys Ther 1980;60:1565.

57. Slocum DB, Larson RL. Rotary instability of the knee. J Bone Joint Surg Am 1968;50:211.

58. Noyes FR, Butler DL, Grood ES, et al. Clinical paradoxes of anterior instability and a new test to detect its instability. Orthop Trans 1978;2:36.

59. Galway HR, Macintosh DL. The lateral pivot shift: a symptom and sign of anterior cruciate ligament insufficiency. Clin Orthop 1980;147:45.

60. Bach BR Jr, Warren RF, Wickiewicz TL. The pivot shift phenomenon: results and description of a modified clinical test for anterior cruciate ligament insufficiency. Am J Sports Med 1988;16:571–576.

61. Noyes FR, Grood ES, Cummings JF, et al. An analysis of the pivot shift phenomenon: the knee motions and subluxations induced by different examiners. Am J Sports Med 1991;19:148.

62. Slocum DB, James SL, Larson RL, et al. A clinical test for anterolateral instability of the knee. Clin Orthop 1976;118:63.

63. Losee RE, Ennis TRJ, Southwick WO. Anterior subluxation of the lateral tibial plateau: a diagnostic test and operative review. J Bone Joint Surg Am 1978;60:1015.

64. Hughston JC, Walsh WM, Puddu G. Patellar subluxation and dislocation. Philadelphia: WB Saunders, 1984.

65. Muller W. The knee: form, function, and ligament reconstruction. New York: Springer-Verlag, 1983.

66. Jacob RP, Hassler H, Staeubli HU. Observations on rotary instability of the lateral compartment of the knee. Acta Orthop Scand Suppl 1981;52:1–32.

67. Hughston JC, Norwood LA. The posterolateral drawer test and external rotational recurvatum test for posterolateral instability of the knee. Clin Orthop 1980;147:82.

68. Shelbourne KD, Benedict F, McCarrol JR, et al. Dynamic posterior shift test: an adjuvant in evaluation of posterior tibial subluxation Am J Sports Med 1989;17:275.

69. McMurray TP. The semilunar cartilages. Br J Surg 1942;29:407.

70. Davies GJ, Larson R. Examining the knee. Phys Sports Med 1978;49–68.

71. Anderson AF, Lipscomb AB. Clinical diagnosis of meniscal tears: description of a new manipulative test. Am J Sports Med 1986;4:291–293.

72. Waldron VD. A test for chondromalacia patellae. Orthop Rev 1983;12:103.

73. Wilson JN. A diagnostic sign in osteochondritis dissecans of the knee. J Bone Joint Surg Am 1967;49: 477–480.

74. Mennel J McM. Joint pain. Boston: Little, Brown & Co., 1964.

75. Faye JL. Motion palpation of the spine. Huntington Beach, CA: Motion Palpation Institute, 1980.

76. Corrigan B, Maitland GD. Practical orthopaedic medicine. London: Butterworths, 1983:145.

77. Schafer RC, Faye LJ. Motion palpation and chiropractic technic: principles of dynamic chiropractic. Huntington Beach: MPI Institute, 1989.

78. McMahon LM, Burdett RG, Whitney SL. Effects of muscle group and placement site on reliability of hand-held dynamometry strength measurements. J Orthop Sports Phys Ther 1992;15:236.

79. Woods GW, Stanley RF, Tullos HS. Lateral capsular sign: x-ray clue to a significant knee instability. Am J Sports Med 1979;7:27–33.

80. Lancourt JE, Cristini JA. Patella alta and patella infera: their etiologic role in patellar dislocation, chondromalacia and apophysitis of the tibial tubercle. J Bone Joint Surg Am 1975;57:1112–1115.

81. Dumas JM, Edde DJ. Meniscal abnormalities: prospective correlation of double contrast arthrography and arthroscopy. Radiology 1986;160:453–456.

82. Thiju CJP. Accuracy of double contrast arthrography and arthroscopy of the knee joint. Skeletal Radiol 1982;8:182–192.

83. Spritzer C, Vogler J, Martinez S, et al. MR imaging of the knee: preliminary results with a 3D FT GRASS pulse sequence. AJR 1988;150:597–603.
84. Tyrrel R, Gluckert K, Pathria M, et al. Fast 3D imaging of the knee: comparison with arthroscopy. Radiology 1988;166:865–872.
85. Herman L, Beltram J. Pitfalls in MR imaging of the knee. Radiology 1988;167:775–781.
86. Kennedy JC, Fowler PJ. Medial and anterior instability of the knee. J Bone Joint Surg Am 1971;53:1257–1270.
87. Shelbourne KD, Nitz PA. The O'Donoghue triad revisited: Combined knee injuries involving anterior cruciate and medial collateral ligament tears. Am J Sports Med 1991;19:474.
88. De Haven KE. Diagnosis of acute knee injuries with hemarthrosis. Am J Sports Med 1980;8:9–14.
89. Ihara H, Nakayama A. Dynamic joint control training for knee ligament injuries. Am J Sports Med 1986;14:309–315.
90. Day RW, Wildermuth BP. Proprioceptive training in the rehabilitation of lower extremity injuries. Adv Sports Med Fitness 1988;1:241.
91. Kannus P, Jarvinen M, Johnson R et al. Function of the quadriceps and hamstring muscles in knees with chronic partial deficiency of the anterior cruciate ligament: Isometric and isokinetic evaluation. Am J Sports Med 1992;20:162.
92. Ericson MO, Nisell R. Tibiofemoral joint forces during ergometer cycling. Am J Sports Med 1986;14:285.
93. Steiner ME, Grana WA, Chillag K, et al. The effect of exercise on anterior-posterior knee laxity. Am J Sports Med 1986;14:24.
94. Vizsolyi P, Taunton J, Robertson G, et al. Breaststroker's knee. Am J Sports Med 1987;15:63–71.
95. Boland AI Jr. Soft tissue injuries of the knee. In: Nicholas JA, Hershman EB, eds. The lower extremity and spine in sports medicine. St. Louis: CV Mosby, 1986;999–1000.
96. Fetto JF, Marshall JL. Medial collateral ligament injuries of the knee: a rationale for treatment. Clin Orthop 1978;132:206–217.
97. Elsasser JC, Reynold FC, Omohundro JR. The nonoperative treatment of collateral ligament injuries of the knee in professional football players. J Bone Joint Surg Am 1974;56:1185.
98. Behrens F, Templeton J. Ligamentous injuries to the medial side of the knee: a one to ten-year follow up. J Bone Joint Surg Br 1980;62:127.
99. Noyes FR. Functional properties of knee ligaments and alterations induced by immobilization-a correlative biomechanical and histological study in primates. Clin Orthop 1977;123:210.
100. Busch MT. Meniscus injuries in children and adolescents. In: Singer KM, ed. Meniscal injuries. Clin Sports Med 1990;9:661.
101. Woods GW, Whelan JM. Discoid meniscus. In: Singer KM, ed. Meniscal injuries. Clin Sports Med 1990;9:695–706.
102. Helfet AJ. Osteoarthritis of the knee and its early arrest. AAOS Instr Course Lect 1971;20.
103. Garrick SG, Webb DR. Sports injuries: diagnosis and management. Philadelphia: WB Saunders, 1990.
104. Hammer WL. Meniscotibial (coronary) ligament sprain: diagnosis and treatment. Chiro Sports Med 1988;2:48–50.
105. Weiss C, Lundberg M, Maberg P, et al. Non-operative treatment of meniscal tears. J Bone Joint Surg Am 1989;71:811–822.
106. Shmidt DR, Henry JH. Stress injuries of the adolescent extensor mechanism. In: Henry JH, ed. Patellofemoral problems. Clin Sports Med. 1989;8:352–354.
107. Beckman M, Craig R, Lehman RC. Rehabilitation of patellofemoral dysfunction in the athlete. In: Lehman RC, ed. Rehabil Clin Sports Med 1989;8:844.
108. Henry JH. The patellofemoral joint. In: Nicholas JA, Hershman EB, eds. The lower extremity and spine in sports medicine. St. Louis: CV Mosby, 1986:1013.
109. Pretorius DM, Noakes TD, Irving G, et al. Runner's knee: what is it and how effective is conservative management? Phys Sports Med 1986;14:71–81.
110. Lund F, Nilsson BE. Arthroscopy of the patellofemoral joint. Acta Orthop Scand 1980;51:297–302.
111. Insall J, Falvo KA, Wise DW. Chondromalacia patellae: a prospective study. J Bone Joint Surg Am 1976;58:1–8.
112. Voight ML, Weider DL. Comparative reflex response times of vastus medialis obliques and vastus lateralis in normal subjects and subjects with extensor mechanism dysfunction: an electromyographic study. Am J Sports Med 1991;19:131.
113. Reid DC, Burnham RS. Lower extremity flexibility patterns of classical ballet dancers and their correlation to lateral hip and knee injuries. Am J Sports Med 1987;15:347–352.
114. Renne JW. The iliotibial band friction syndrome. J Bone Joint Surg Am 1975;57:1110–1111.
115. Apple DF. End-stage running problems. Clin Sports Med 1985;4:661.
116. Cyriax JH, Cyriax PJ. Illustrated manual of orthopaedic medicine. London: Butterworths, 1983:103–104.
117. Souza TA. Treatment of common knee disorders: general principles. Chiro Sports Med 1990;4:81–92.

Biomechanics of the Foot and Ankle

Thomas C. Michaud

To appreciate fully the pathophysiology associated with the majority of sports-related lower extremity injuries, the practitioner must possess a thorough understanding of the various joint and muscle interactions associated with locomotion. Given the extremes in ground-reactive forces associated with even routine activity, for example, the average person takes 10,000 to 15,000 steps daily (1), with each foot absorbing the equivalent of nearly 640 metric tons (2), it becomes easy to see how even subtle biomechanical abnormalities might produce chronic injury.

Because of the complexity of articular interactions, this chapter begins with a review of static and dynamic anatomy of the foot and ankle. This information is followed with a discussion of first normal and then abnormal motions associated with the gait cycle. Various parameters necessary for ideal motions are outlined, and then methods of treatment—including manipulation, stretches, exercises, and orthotics—are discussed.

ANATOMY

The foot and ankle contain 28 bones with 55 articulations (3) that function synchronously to allow for a variety of activities during the different phases of gait. During early stance phase, the foot dissipates ground-reactive force associated with heel strike and becomes a mobile adapter necessary to accommodate discrepancies in terrain; during late stance phase, the foot becomes a rigid lever arm necessary to transfer body weight from rearfoot to forefoot after heel lift occurs. The foot accomplishes these diverse actions by means of complex movement patterns around the ankle, subtalar, midtarsal, and first ray axes. The following section reviews the primary articulations of the foot and ankle with regard to location of axes and motions available. This is followed by a discussion of the mechanical advantage afforded individual muscles of the lower extremity, as determined by their angle of approach and distance from each of the various axes.

Ankle Joint

Also known as the talocrural joint, the ankle joint is the articulation between the talar trochlea and the distal tibia and fibula. According to Subotnick (3), the average axis of motion for this joint lies approximately 10° to the transverse plane and 17° to the frontal plane (Fig. 15.1). Notice that this axis approximates the bisection of the distal malleoli. Because of its proximity to the transverse and frontal planes, this axis typically allows for almost pure dorsiflexion/plantarflexion. Inman et al. (4) note that the ankle axis may deviate by as much as 23° from the transverse plane and that the added range of adduction/abduction associated with this higher axis plays an important role in absorbing the rotational motions of the shank. Root et al. (5) believe that such large variation in the location of this axis is relatively uncommon and is usually found only in individuals possessing limited ranges of subtalar motion during the early years of skeletal growth. The authors state the unusually high axis results from a functional adaptation of bone as the ankle attempts to compensate for the limited subtalar motion by developing a supinatory/pronatory axis.

Regardless of the position of its axis of motion, plantarflexion around this axis is limited by tension created in the surrounding soft tissues (particularly by the anterior talofibular ligament) and by an osseous block produced when the posterior tubercle of the talus contacts the posterior margin of the articular surface of the tibia (6). Motion in the direction of dorsiflexion is limited primarily by tension in the triceps surae musculature and the posterior restraining ligaments, i.e., the posterior deltoid and the posterior talofibular ligaments. Also, because the talus is wider anteriorly, ankle dorsiflexion may also be restricted by a bony block when the wider aspects of the talus come into contact with the articular surfaces of the distal tibia and fibula. The clinical significance of a premature osseous block will be discussed later in this chapter.

Subtalar Joint

The subtalar joint is located between the talus and calcaneus. Although rarely mentioned, individual variation in the development of this joint may result in the formation of one, two, or three separate articulations. Bruckner (7), in his study of 32 cadaveric subtalar joints, noted that 20 specimens had two distinct articulations (with slight variation between each one); the remaining 12 had three separate articulations. Motion in the subtalar joints possessing three articulations is limited by osseous block/joint incongruence, whereas motion in the more mobile double and single facet configurations is limited by muscular/ligamentous restraining mechanisms.

Motion in the average subtalar joint occurs around an axis that lies 42° to the transverse plane and 16° to the sagittal plane (Fig. 15.2) (5). The position of this axis allows for triplanar motion with almost equal amounts of frontal (eversion/inversion) and transverse (adduction/abduction) plane motion. Because the axis lies so close to the sagittal plane, only limited amounts of dorsiflexion/plantarflexion are possible.

Just as there is much individual variation in the shape of the subtalar articulations, there is also much variation in the location of the axis of motion. Numerous investigators (8–10) have noted positional variation in the subtalar joint axis ranging from 20° to 68.5° from the transverse plane and 4° to 47° from the sagittal plane. In practice, the approximate position of the subtalar joint axis can be determined by comparing the range of rearfoot inversion/eversion with the range of tibial rotations as the standing patient pronates and supinates the

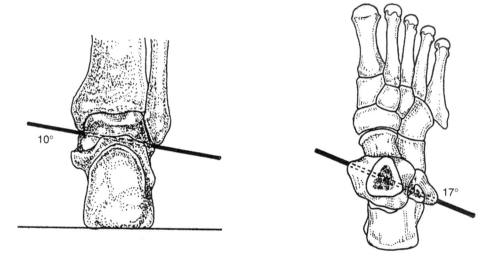

Figure 15.1. Axis of motion for the ankle joint.

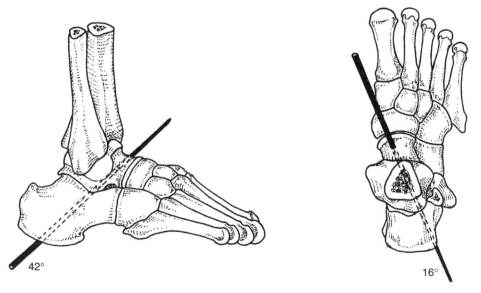

Figure 15.2. Axis of motion for the subtalar joint.

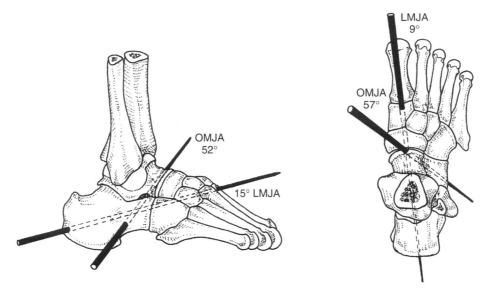

Figure 15.3. The midtarsal joint axes of motion: oblique midtarsal joint axis (OMJA) and longitudinal midtarsal joint axis (LMJA).

subtalar joint. If the axis lies 45° to the transverse plane, every 1° of rearfoot motion will produce 1° of tibial rotation. If the axis is positioned near 70° to the transverse plane, the amount of tibial rotation will greatly exceed rearfoot motion (e.g., 2° of rearfoot eversion will be accompanied by 8° of internal tibial rotation). Conversely, if the axis lies close to 20°, the rearfoot motion will greatly exceed tibial rotation (e.g., 10° of rearfoot eversion will be accompanied by only 2° of tibial rotation). The location of the subtalar joint axis is clinically significant; a high axis could be responsible for chronic injury to structures proximal to the subtalar joint, whereas a low axis could be responsible for chronic injury to structures distal to the subtalar joint.

Midtarsal Joint

The midtarsal joint consists of the combined articulations between the talonavicular and calcaneocuboid joints. These joints function as a unit to allow for triplanar motion that occurs around two distinct axes: the oblique midtarsal joint axis and the longitudinal midtarsal joint axis (11). Although individual variation exists, the oblique midtarsal joint axis lies 52° to the transverse plane and 57° to the sagittal plane, whereas the longitudinal midtarsal joint axis lies 15° from the transverse plane and 9° from the sagittal plane (Fig. 15.3) (8).

The location of the oblique midtarsal joint axis allows for large amounts of sagittal and transverse plane motion (dorsiflexion/plantarflexion and abduction/adduction, respectively) with relatively small amounts of frontal plane motion (inversion/eversion). The longitudinal midtarsal joint, because of its close proximity to the trans-

verse and sagittal planes, allows for almost pure inversion/eversion.

The midtarsal joint is similar to a triarticulated subtalar joint in that it has an osseous locking mechanism to prevent excessive motion (12). Although movement in the direction of supination is resisted by soft tissue restraining mechanisms, movement in the direction of pronation comes to an abrupt halt when the superoproximal border of the pronating cuboid comes into contact with the dorsal border of the overhanging calcaneus. Further midtarsal pronation is prevented by tension in the various restraining ligaments (primarily the long and short plantar ligaments, calcaneonavicular ligament, and bifurcate ligament) (Fig. 15.4). Midtarsal pronation beyond this point is not possible without overwhelming the restraining ligaments and subluxing the calcaneocuboid joint (5). As with the subtalar joint locking mechanism, the midtarsal locking mechanism is a uniquely human trait that allows for improved bipedal ambulation (8).

First Ray

The first ray is a functional unit consisting of the medial cuneiform and the first metatarsal. First ray motion occurs around an axis that lies approximately 45° to both the frontal and sagittal planes (Fig. 15.5). The location of this axis allows for relatively equal amounts of dorsiflexion/plantarflexion and inversion/eversion. Because the axis lies so close to the transverse plane, the range of adduction/abduction is clinically insignificant.

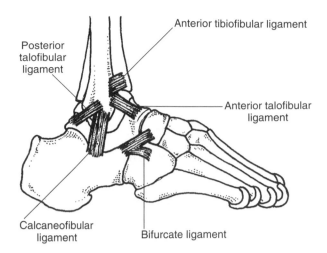

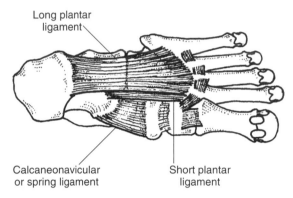

Figure 15.4. The midtarsal restraining ligaments.

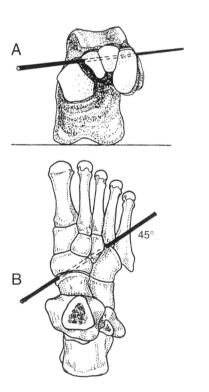

Figure 15.5. Axis of motion for the first ray.

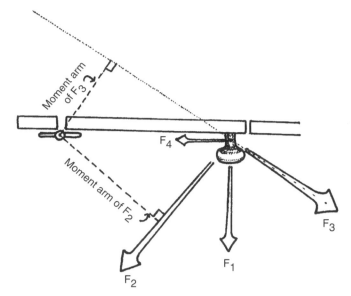

Figure 15.6. Door hinge analogy.

MUSCLE FUNCTION

Although the location of the various axes is determined by the shape of the articular surfaces (11), movement around these axes is determined by the combined interactions of all forces acting on the body (the most common forces being muscular, gravitational, inertial, frictional, and ground-reactive forces). To appreciate how these forces produce motion (or resist motion), it is important to understand that all forces possess magnitude, direction, a line of application, and a point of application. A force will most effectively produce motion when its line of application occurs in a plane perpendicular to the joint's axis of motion and when the perpendicular distance between this line of action and the axis of motion is greatest, That is, when it has the longest lever arm. This concept is best demonstrated using a door and hinge analogy (Fig. 15.6). If forces F1 through F4 (which are applied by a rope tied to the door handle) were equal in magnitude, F1 would have the greatest moment (moment refers to the tendency, or measure of tendency, to produce motion) followed by F2 and F3. F4, regardless of its magnitude, would be unable to move the door because its line of action passes directly through the axis of motion.

Figure 15.6 also serves to demonstrate how one force can produce two distinct actions. Notice that if one were to attempt to open the door by pulling along line F2, part of the force would go into opening the door and part of the force would go into compressing the hinge. This represents an important concept regarding the application of forces in the body. When a force is applied perpendicular to an axis, the force may be resolved into rotational and nonrotational components; the nonrotational component will either compress or distract the joint surfaces. Whereas the rotational component is important because it is responsible for producing motion around an axis, the compressive component is also important because it may be responsible for stabilizing a joint. For example, as heel lift occurs to initiate the propulsive period of gait, various muscles and ligaments must work together to create the strong compressive forces necessary to stabilize the osseous structures as vertical forces reach their highest levels. Failure to generate sufficient compressive forces would allow the bony structures to shift as vertical forces peaked.

So far the discussion has considered only forces that are applied perpendicular to the axis of motion. As one might suspect, forces in the body are not so cooperative as to align themselves perpendicularly to a joint's axis. When a force's line of action deviates from perpendicular (as it most frequently does), determining the rotational and nonrotational components requires first resolving the line of action into forces acting perpendicular to the axis and forces acting parallel to the axis. Figure 15.7 illustrates the same door pictured previously; however, now force Fl is angled 30° superiorly to the perpendicular plane of the axis. This force can now be resolved into what is termed a normal component

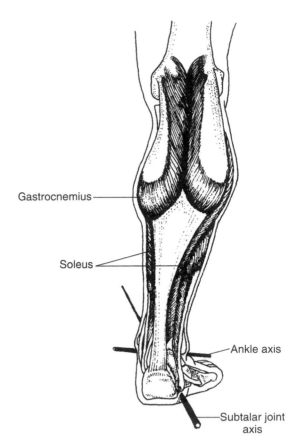

Figure 15.8. Gastrocnemius/soleus. These muscles are strong plantarflexors of the foot around the ankle joint axis and moderately strong supinators of the subtalar joint.

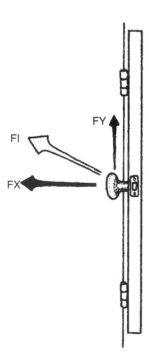

Figure 15.7. Door hinge analogy.

(Fx), which is applied perpendicularly to the axis and possesses rotational and nonrotational components, and a tangential or shearing component (Fy), which is applied parallel to the axis and is typically unable to produce motion without subluxing or dislocating the joint. Fortunately, the shearing component of force is usually resisted by bony/ligamentous restraining mechanisms and/or the pull of antagonistic muscles.

This information regarding the different components of force can be applied to the muscular system in that the ability of a muscle to produce motion at a particular joint is dependent on the length of its lever arm (which may be increased via sesamoid bones) and the angle in which it approaches the axis (which can be improved or made more perpendicular with the help of various pulleys, i.e., the retinacular sheath, peroneal tubercle, sustentaculum tali, etc). Figures 15.8 to 15.13 demonstrate the relationships among various muscles and axes of the foot and ankle. The actions described in the legends refer only to concentric contractions; eccentric contractions would produce the opposite effect.

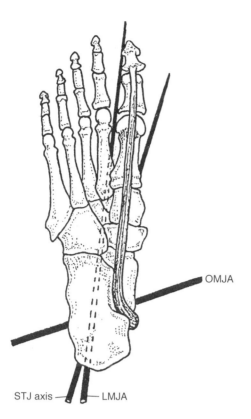

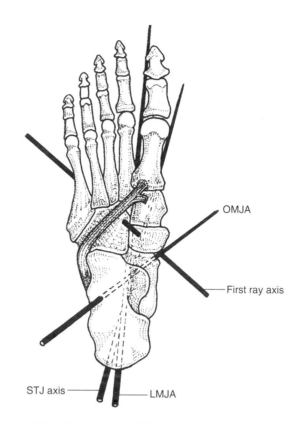

Figure 15.9. Flexor hallucis longus. This muscle is a strong plantarflexor of the ankle joint but, because it crosses the subtalar joint axis at an angle less than perpendicular, it is only a weak subtalar joint supinator.

Figure 15.11. Peroneus longus. When the cuboid is stable, this muscle is a strong plantarflexor of the first ray and pronator of the forefoot around the longitudinal midtarsal joint axis. It is a weak ankle joint plantarflexor and a moderately strong subtalar joint pronator.

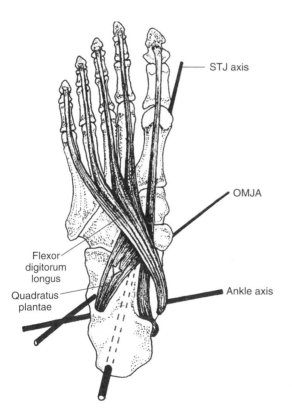

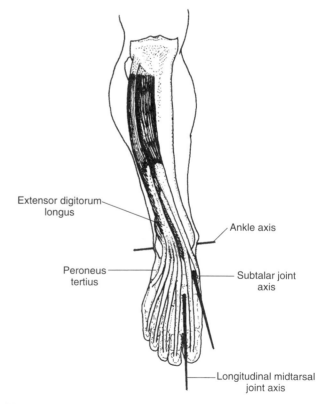

Figure 15.10. Flexor digitorum longus is a strong ankle joint plantarflexor, a moderate subtalar joint supinator, and a very strong supinator of the forefoot around the oblique midtarsal joint.

Figure 15.12. Extensor digitorum longus. This muscle is a strong plantarflexor of the ankle joint. Because its tendon passes laterally to both the subtalar and longitudinal midtarsal joint axes, it is a moderate pronator of the forefoot around these axes.

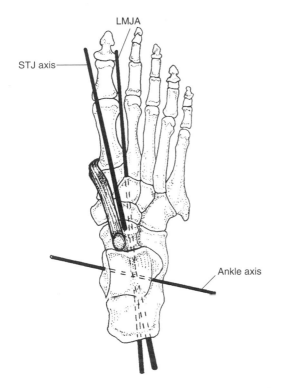

Figure 15.13. Tibialis anterior. Because its tendon passes so close to the oblique midtarsal joint axis, it is unable to affect motion around this axis. It is, however, a strong dorsiflexor of the first ray and a moderately strong supinator of the forefoot around the longitudinal midtarsal joint axis. It is a slightly weaker supinator of the subtalar joint.

IDEAL MOTIONS DURING THE GAIT CYCLE

The gait cycle is the basic reference in the description of human locomotion. One full gait cycle consists of the time between successive ipsilateral heel strikes: it begins when the heel initially makes ground contact and ends the moment the same heel strikes the ground with the next step (4). Each gait cycle is divided into stance and swing phases that typically occupy 62% and 38% of the gait cycle, respectively (Fig. 15.14) (4, 5).

When walking, the gait cycle lasts approximately 1 second. As a result, stance phase occurs in approximately 0.6 second and swing phase in 0.4 second. For a better description of the various kinetic interactions occurring during the stance phase, this portion of the gait cycle has been subdivided into contact, midstance, and propulsive periods (Fig. 15.15). The timing and primary events associated with each portion of the gait cycle are discussed in the following sections.

Contact Period

Without doubt, this period is the most clinically significant because when virtually all shock

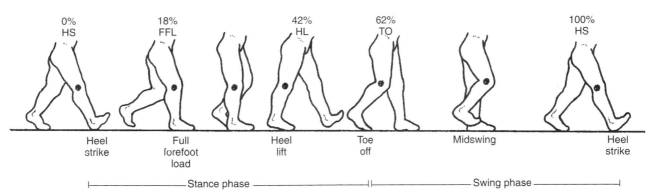

Figure 15.14. Gait cycle of the right leg. Stance phase begins at heel strike and ends when the great toe leaves the ground. Swing phase continues until the heel again strikes the ground. The length of stride refers to the distance between successive ipsilateral heel strikes. Inman et al. (4) mention that the average stride length is approximately 0.8 times body height and the average cadence is approximately 115 steps per minute. The author emphasizes that there is significant individual variation, in that each person seems to choose a gait pattern that is metabolically most efficient.

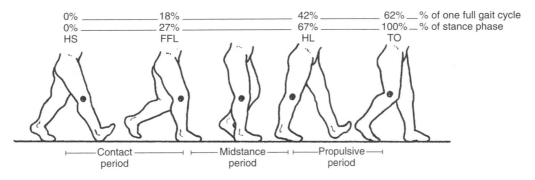

Figure 15.15. The various periods of stance phase.

absorption occurs. Considering that the average person takes 10,000 to 15,000 steps daily (1), absorbing between 1 and 3 times body weight each time heel strike occurs (2), the importance of the contact period shock-absorbing mechanisms cannot be understated.

The contact period begins with heel strike and ends with full forefoot load (Fig. 15.15). As the foot proceeds through its contact period, a combination of ground-reactive forces (which are initially applied to the posterolateral heel) and inertial forces (the pelvis and lower extremity continue their internal rotation that began during early swing phase) cause the ankle to plantarflex and the subtalar joint to pronate. Plantarflexion of the ankle is resisted by eccentric contraction of the anterior compartment muscu-

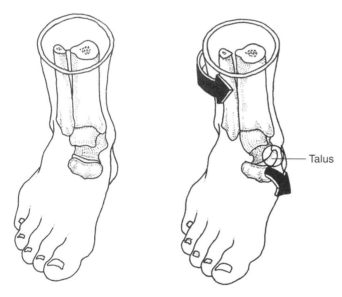

Figure 15.16. Talar motions during the contact period.

lature (13). These muscles play an important role in absorbing shock; they smoothly lower the forefoot to the ground, thereby minimizing trauma to the plantar soft tissues. Radin and Paul (14) state that joint motion controlled by muscles lengthening under tension is the primary kinematic process responsible for shock absorption.

Throughout the contact period, the subtalar joint is pronating from the slightly supinated position present at heel strike; the calcaneus is inverted approximately 2° during heel strike (15). As the subtalar joint pronates, the talus moves into an adducted and plantarflexed position (Fig. 15.16), which allows for shock absorption via two distinct mechanisms. First, talar plantarflexion allows for shock absorption as it results in a lowering of the ankle mortise, which produces a cushioning effect during heel strike and the early contact period. Second, talar adduction is also responsible for shock absorption as it produces an obligatory internal rotation of the tibia that acts to unlock the extended knee. This allows eccentric contraction of the quadriceps to absorb shock as the knee flexes. Subotnick (15) claims that the subtalar joint must pronate a minimum of 6° to dampen vertical forces effectively.

In addition to its role in shock absorption, subtalar joint pronation is also essential for surface adaptation, because it allows for an added range of midtarsal motion by improving the alignment of the talonavicular and calcaneocuboid axes (Fig. 15.17). Phillips and Phillips (16) demonstrated that this parallelism of axes produces an additional 11.6° of midtarsal motion. This added range of motion allows for deflection of the medial longitudinal arch that is essential for shock ab-

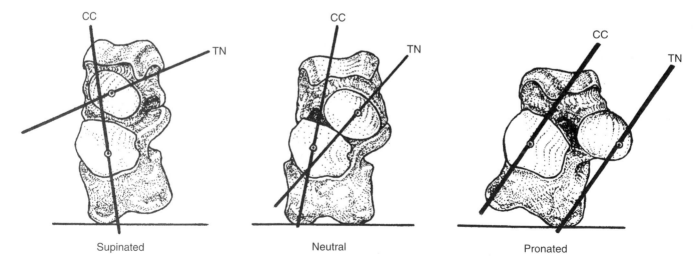

Supinated	Neutral	Pronated

Figure 15.17. Anterior view of the right talus and calcaneus. Note the parallelism of the talonavicular and calcaneocuboid joint axes as the subtalar joint pronates.

sorption and surface adaptation. Ker et al. (17) also note that deflection of the arch provides a natural energy return mechanism, in which approximately 17 J of energy are stored in the stretched muscles and ligaments of the arch (primarily the plantar fascia, long and short plantar ligaments, and spring ligament). This energy is returned during the latter half of stance in the form of elastic recoil. The authors liken this to a bouncing rubber ball and claim that enough strain energy is stored in the arch to make running more efficient.

Midstance Period

Midstance period begins at full forefoot load and ends at heel lift. It is the longest period, occupying 40% of stance phase and lasting approximately 0.24 second (18). Throughout this period, the foot is attempting to convert itself from the mobile adapter necessary for the contact period to the rigid lever arm needed for the propulsive period (19). It partially accomplishes this task by taking advantage of the forward momentum of the contralateral lower extremity; the forward momentum of the swing phase leg externally rotates the pelvis (white arrow in Fig. 15.18), which then externally rotates the weight-bearing leg (black arrow in Fig. 15.18). Because the leg and talus behave as a closed kinetic chain during midstance, external rotation of the weight-bearing leg causes the talus to abduct, which in turn supinates the subtalar joint. This motion helps stabilize the tarsals by decreasing the parallelism of the midtarsal joint axes. All these actions are assisted by various muscular interactions that will be discussed in more detail at the end of this section.

By the end of midstance, the subtalar joint should have supinated back to its neutral position; i.e., the head of the talus should be directly behind the navicular. For this to occur, the midtarsal joint must possess an adequate range of eversion around its longitudinal axis. To understand why this midtarsal motion is necessary, picture the following events. As the subtalar joint is supinating, the entire foot is inverting. Because body weight maintains the medial foot on the ground, inversion of the rearfoot (subtalar supination) can occur only if the medial aspect of the forefoot plantarflexes while the lateral aspect of the forefoot dorsiflexes (Fig. 15.19). This motion occurs around the longitudinal midtarsal joint axis and constitutes eversion around that axis.

Ideally, the midtarsal joint will allow only enough motion for the rearfoot to reach vertical. At that time, the forefoot will (it is hoped) "lock" against the rearfoot, as the superior border of the

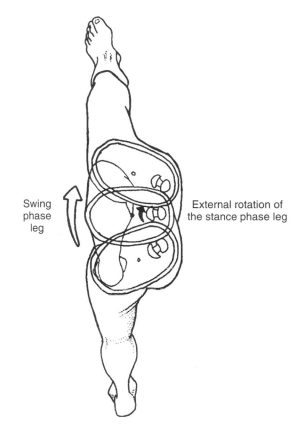

Figure 15.18. Forward motion of the swing phase leg (white arrow) externally rotates the stance leg (black arrow), which in turn allows for supination of the subtalar joint.

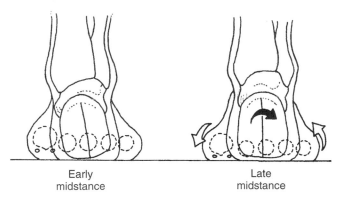

Early midstance   Late midstance

Figure 15.19. Posterior view of right foot. The forefoot compensates for subtalar joint supination by everting around the longitudinal midtarsal joint axis.

pronating cuboid comes into contact with the dorsal border of the overhanging calcaneus (12). This sudden approximation of the calcaneocuboid joint represents an osseous locking mechanism that is maintained by tensing various restraining ligaments. Continued motion, either subtalar joint supination or midtarsal joint pronation, is not possible without overwhelming the restraining ligaments and subluxating the calcaneocuboid joint (5).

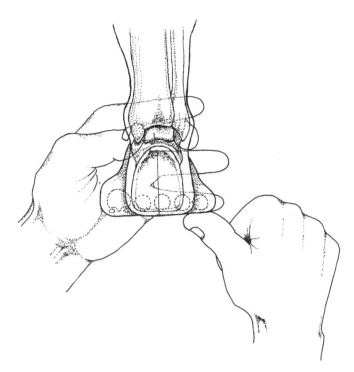

Figure 15.20. Identifying the midtarsal joint locking position. One hand maintains the head of the talus directly behind the navicular, while the opposite thumb dorsiflexes the fourth and fifth metatarsal heads to the point of firm resistance. Ideally, all the metatarsal heads will rest on the same transverse plane and the plantar forefoot should parallel the plantar rearfoot.

The osseous locking of the forefoot against the rearfoot at the calcaneocuboid joint is a prerequisite for normal gait, because it minimizes muscular strain by allowing for a smooth transfer of accelerational forces through a locked lateral column (11). Basmajian and Deluca (13) state that muscles should be considered only as a dynamic reserve for stabilization because they cannot provide the support afforded by a well-designed skeletal system. Failure of the calcaneocuboid to lock into its close-packed position would result in a shifting of the tarsals, as vertical forces are transferred from rearfoot to forefoot after heel lift occurs; the foot would behave as a flexible lever arm, which is ineffective in the transfer of forces.

Clinically, the locking position of the calcaneocuboid joint is determined easily by placing the subtalar joint of the prone patient in a neutral position and applying firm dorsiflexion force to the fourth and fifth metatarsal heads (Fig. 15.20). This dorsiflexion force duplicates the application of ground-reactive force during terminal midstance and gives the examiner an accurate picture of the forefoot-to-rearfoot relationship present when the midtarsal locking mechanism engages. As mentioned, the calcaneocuboid joint will ideally lock when the sagittal bisection of the rearfoot is perpendicular to the ground or, as in

this case, when the plantar forefoot is parallel to the plantar rearfoot. This locking position, in addition to stabilizing the forefoot against the rearfoot, also serves to improve the functional alignment between the Achilles tendon and the calcaneus and protects against lateral instability of the ankle mortise by decreasing dependence on the lateral compartment musculature (20).

Propulsive Period

The propulsive period begins the moment heel lift occurs and ends with toe-off. This period occupies the final 33% of stance phase and lasts approximately 0.2 second. Although it appears to be a simple process, there are many actions responsible for producing heel lift. First, the forward momentum of the torso displaces the center of mass directly over the forefoot, thereby minimizing the vertical forces responsible for maintaining ground contact at the heel. Second, the continued contraction of the soleus and deep posterior compartment muscles acts to limit the range of ankle dorsiflexion by decelerating the forward momentum of the proximal tibia. This action allows the forward momentum of the center of mass to be applied directly toward lifting the heel. Third, the gastrocnemius muscle plays a particularly important role by simultaneously flexing the knee while plantarflexing the ankle. These combined actions serve to lift the knee upward and forward, which allows for an improved range of heel lift while also assisting with hip flexion. Because of this, the gastrocnemius indirectly allows for improved ground clearance during swing phase.

After the heel has left the ground, the foot must safely channel large amounts of vertical forces through locked and stable articulations. As stated by Root et al. (5), if the proximal articulations are not stabilized against the distal articulations, they will be placed into motion (and potentially injured) by forces acting on the foot. The foot is able to protect itself by again taking advantage of the external shank rotation supplied by the forward momentum of the opposite swing phase leg. Because the closed kinetic chain ends at the metatarsal heads after heel lift occurs, the continued external leg rotation will produce mild supination around the subtalar joint axis (ground-reactive forces no longer maintain the calcaneus in a fixed position, so it is free to move with the rotating talus). It also produces significant supination around the oblique midtarsal axis; the entire rearfoot pivots medially as it abducts and dorsiflexes around the oblique midtarsal joint axis (Fig. 15.21). Note that in Figure 15.21 the external leg rotation creates a screw-like motion at the midfoot that greatly increases arch height, thereby converting the foot into a rigid lever.

Supination around the oblique axis of the midtarsal joint is aided by contraction of the intrinsic muscles originating from the medial calcaneus (particularly abductor hallucis). It is also aided by what is known as the windlass effect of the plantar fascia—dorsiflexion of the toes after heel lift draws the plantar fascia around the metatarsal heads, which acts to pull the anterior and posterior pillars of the longitudinal arch together (Fig. 15.22). This approximation of the rearfoot and forefoot allows for continued supination around the oblique midtarsal joint axis with its concomitant increase in arch height.

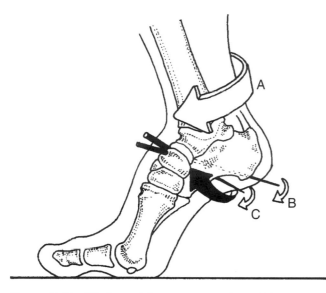

Figure 15.21. (A) External leg rotation produces slight supination around the **(B)** subtalar axis and significant supination of the forefoot around the **(C)** oblique midtarsal joint axis. These motions increase arch height (black arrow), thereby stabilizing articulations of the foot.

Although considerable stability is afforded by the increased arch height, the foot could not be considered a rigid lever were it not for the continued forefoot pronation around the longitudinal midtarsal joint axis. During early propulsion, the calcaneocuboid locking mechanism is maintained by forceful contraction of the soleus muscle, which is simultaneously plantarflexing the ankle and inverting the subtalar joint. Whereas ankle plantarflexion allows for a forward acceleration of body mass, subtalar joint inversion allows ground-reactive forces to dorsiflex the fourth and fifth metatarsals, thereby locking the lateral column. The effectiveness of the soleus muscle to maintain the midtarsal locking mechanism is only temporary. Early in propulsion, the range of ankle plantarflexion places the soleus muscle in such a shortened position that it is unable to generate sufficient force to invert the calcaneus; therefore, it can no longer maintain the midtarsal locking mechanism via ground-reactive forces (5). At this time, the continued forceful contraction of peroneus longus (which passes beneath the cuboid in the peroneal groove) acts to dorsiflex and evert the cuboid, thereby maintaining the close-packed position of the calcaneocuboid joint.

An important consideration regarding the propulsive period function of the lateral column is that because the fourth and fifth metatarsals are shorter than the remaining metatarsals, the lateral column is unable to maintain ground contact during mid and late propulsion. Therefore, it is unable to assist with the forward acceleration of body mass during these portions of the propulsive period. Locking of the calcaneocuboid joint at this time continues to serve a purpose—it af-

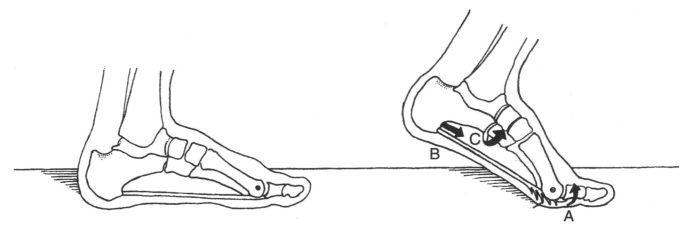

Figure 15.22. The windlass effect of the plantar fascia. **A.** During the propulsive period ground-reactive forces dorsiflex the toes, thereby pulling the plantar fascia around the metatarsal heads. **B.** This action results in the approximation of rearfoot and forefoot and assists with increasing the **(C)** height of the medial longitudinal arch. (Adapted from Newel SG. Conservative treatment of plantar fasciitis. Phys Sportsmed 1977;5:68–73.

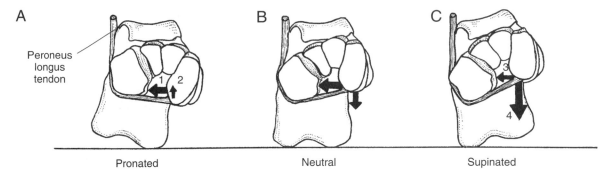

Figure 15.23. The effect of subtalar positioning on peroneus longus function. **A.** When the subtalar joint is pronated, the peroneus longus tendon creates a mild dorsiflexion force around the first ray axis. **B.** As the subtalar joint moves into its neutral position, peroneus longus exerts a mild plantarflexion force around the first ray axis. **C.** This plantarflexion force exponentially increases as the subtalar joint supinates.

fords peroneus longus and brevis an effective lever arm as they now function to direct body weight medially toward the opposite foot by everting the entire lateral column. This medial shift of body weight is necessary to maintain a straight gait pattern and to allow the final transfer of vertical forces to occur off the medial forefoot, which is better equipped to handle these forces as the first metatarsal is twice as wide and four times as strong as any of the other metatarsals (21). Because of its passage under the cuboid and eventual insertion into the base of the first metatarsal and medial cuneiform, peroneus longus has the interesting ability to transfer body weight medially while simultaneously stabilizing the medial forefoot so it may better tolerate these forces. This stabilizing action is related to the improved angle of approach afforded the peroneal tendon as the subtalar joint is supinating (Fig. 15.23).

The improved ability of peroneus longus to function as a first ray plantarflexor is extremely important during the propulsive period. The increased arch height, coupled with the normal parabolic curve of the metatarsal heads, necessitates that the first ray plantarflex actively to maintain ground contact. In addition to the importance of maintaining ground contact to resist ground-reactive forces, active plantarflexion of the first metatarsal also allows for the dorsal-posterior shifting of the first metatarsophalangeal joint's transverse axis. This is necessary for the hallux to reach its required range of 65° dorsiflexion (Fig. 15.24).

The combined actions of peroneus longus as an evertor of the lateral column and a plantar flexor of the first ray allow for what Bojsen-Moller (12) refers to as a high-gear push-off. By everting the lateral column, peroneus longus allows the final transfer of body weight to occur through

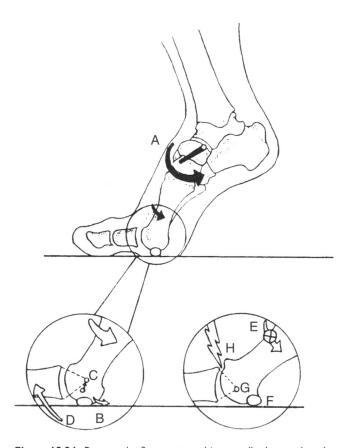

Figure 15.24. Because the first metatarsal is normally shorter than the second metatarsal, it must actively plantarflex to maintain ground contact during the propulsive period **(A).** As the first metatarsal plantarflexes, the metatarsal head glides posteriorly along the sesamoids **(B),** which allows for a dorsal-posterior shift of the transverse axis of the first metatarsophalangeal joint **(C).** This new axis allows for an unrestrained range of hallux dorsiflexion **(D).** Failure of the first metatarsal to plantarflex during propulsion **(E)** inhibits the posterior glide of the metatarsal head on its sesamoid **(F),** which in turn prevents the dorsal posterior shift of the transverse axis. The hallux is now forced to dorsiflex around the original axis **(G).** This results in a "jamming" of the dorsal cartilage **(H)** with characteristic resorption of subchondral bone and dorsal lipping of the first metatarsal head.

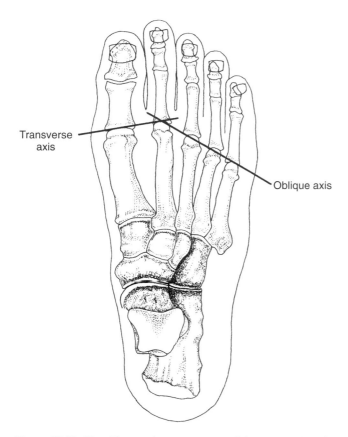

Figure 15.25. The oblique and transverse axes of the metatarsal heads.

the transverse axis of the metatarsal heads (Fig. 15.25). Use of the transverse axis supplies the ankle plantarflexors with a longer and more effective lever arm for accelerating body mass forward. Failure of peroneus longus to evert the lateral column would allow for continued supination of the subtalar joint, with the final push-off occurring as a rolling action through the oblique axis of the metatarsal heads. Because the oblique axis has a shorter lever arm to the ankle axis, it allows for a less-efficient propulsion referred to as a low-gear push-off. Bojsen-Moller (12) states that use of the transverse axis via peroneus longus contraction represents the final evolutionary change in the process of producing a fast, efficient propulsion.

During the final portion of the propulsive period, the foot will ideally be supinated around the oblique midtarsal and subtalar joint axes (although the subtalar joint is actively pronating from this supinated position secondary to peroneal eversion of the lateral column) and pronated around the longitudinal midtarsal joint axis. The longitudinal midtarsal joint axis is maintained in a pronated position during late propulsion as extensor digitorum longus and peroneus tertius are vigorously contracting in prepa-

ration for the swing phase of gait. The final transfer of forces should occur through the hallux, which has been stabilized throughout the propulsive period by contraction of the flexor hallucis longus. The entire lower extremity has continued to rotate externally throughout propulsion and into the swing phase of gait (5).

Swing Phase

The swing phase, which begins at toe-off and ends at heel strike, occupies 38% of one full gait cycle and lasts approximately 0.4 second. There are two primary functions of the foot and ankle during this phase. The first is to allow enough dorsiflexion for the forefoot to clear the ground by midswing. The second is to position the articulations so the supporting musculature may more effectively dampen impact forces as the next heel strike occurs.

Ground clearance of the forefoot is accomplished by forceful contraction of the muscles that flex the knee and hip and by the anterior compartment musculature (which, as mentioned, begins contracting during late propulsion in preparation for swing phase). Because the ankle reaches its maximally plantarflexed position of 20° shortly after toe-off, the anterior compartment muscles have less than 0.2 second to overcome inertial forces and dorsiflex the forefoot into a safe position by midswing. Because extensor digitorum longus and peroneus tertius are the first anterior compartment muscles to contract (5), the foot (in addition to dorsiflexing at the ankle) will immediately pronate around the oblique midtarsal and subtalar axes. These muscles possess significant lever arms for pronating these axes (Fig. 15.12). The dorsiflexion components of these pronatory motions assist with ankle dorsiflexion to allow for improved ground clearance.

Almost immediately after extensor digitorum longus and peroneus tertius contract, tibialis anterior and extensor hallucis longus begin contracting, thereby significantly increasing the dorsiflexion movement created at the ankle. Root et al. (5) claim that extensor hallucis longus is the strongest ankle dorsiflexor during early swing phase. Tibialis anterior, by virtue of its insertion on the first metatarsal and medial cuneiform, also acts to improve ground clearance by dorsiflexing the first ray during early swing phase.

By the time midswing has occurred, the ankle is dorsiflexed to a near neutral position, the subtalar and midtarsal joints are pronated (the midtarsal joint is pronated around both axes), and the first ray is dorsiflexed and inverted. These combined actions, when coupled with knee and hip flexion, allow for maximum amounts of ground clearance.

Shortly after the forefoot has cleared the ground, muscles of the swing leg have a relatively quiet period when motion is maintained by inertial forces generated during propulsion and early swing (13). Just before heel strike, the anterior compartment muscles simultaneously contract in anticipation of dampening the impact forces associated with the contact period. Because of their relationships with the various axes, tibialis anterior and extensor digitorum longus produce mild dorsiflexion at the ankle, with tibialis anterior significantly inverting the forefoot while extensor digitorum longus and peroneus tertius assist with ankle dorsiflexion and pronation of the forefoot around the oblique midtarsal joint axis. By positioning the foot with the ankle dorsiflexed, the forefoot inverted, and the subtalar joint slightly supinated, the pre-tensed muscles of the foot and leg are now prepared to dampen the ground-reactive forces associated with stance phase effectively. With sprint running and anticipated falls, other shock-absorbing muscles (gastrocnemius, vastus lateralis, gluteus maximus) become hyperactive before heel strike as they pre-tense in an attempt to dampen the perceived

increase in ground-reactive forces more effectively (Figs. 15.26–15.28) (22).

PARAMETERS NECESSARY FOR IDEAL FUNCTION

For the previously described movement patterns to occur, several parameters for the norm must exist.

1. The lower tibia should be straight ($\pm 2°$).
2. When the subtalar joint is held in its neutral position, the vertical bisection of the rearfoot should parallel the vertical bisection of the lower leg ($\pm 2°$).
3. The calcaneocuboid joint should lock with the vertical bisection of the rearfoot perpendicular to the plantar surface of the forefoot.
4. The ankle, with the subtalar joint maintained in its neutral position, must dorsiflex a minimum of $10°$.

The first three criteria are readily evaluated simply by placing the subtalar joint of the prone patient in its neutral position and applying a firm dorsiflexion force beneath the fourth and fifth metatarsal heads. This locks the calcaneocuboid joint and duplicates the position the foot will be in before heel lift; the forefoot is stabilized against

Text continued on page 432.

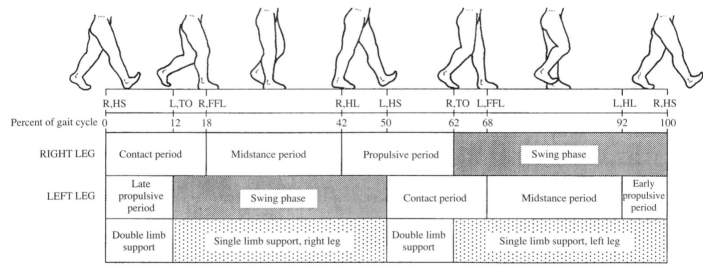

L–Left
R–Right
HS–Heel strike
FFL–Full forefoot load
HL–Heel lift
TO–Toe off

Figure 15.26. The feet simultaneously contact the ground twice during one full gait cycle: from 0 to 12% and from 50 to 62% (the first and last 12% of stance phase). These percentages are far from constant; the time spent in double-limb support decreases drastically as the individual's speed increases. In running, there is no double-limb support and each single-limb support stance phase is followed by a brief airborne period in which neither foot contacts the ground (10). (Adapted from Murphy PC, Baxter DE. Nerve entrapment of the foot and ankle in runners. Clin Sports Med 1985;4:753–763.)

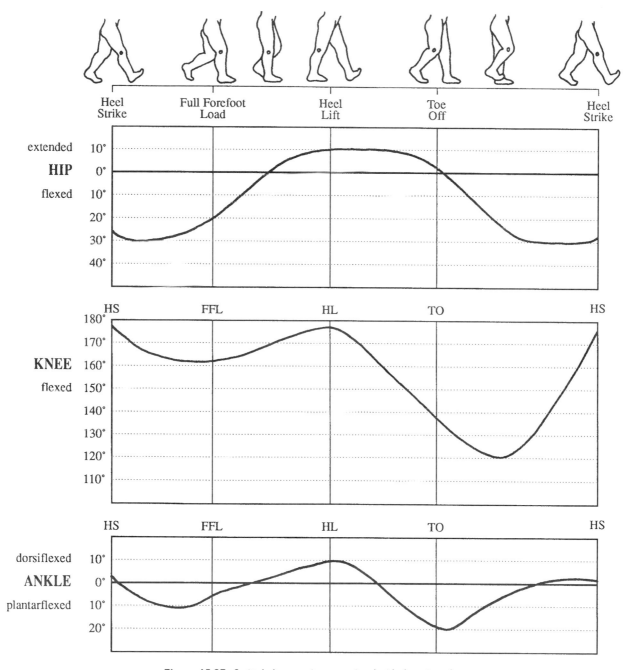

Figure 15.27. Sagittal plane motions associated with the gait cycle.

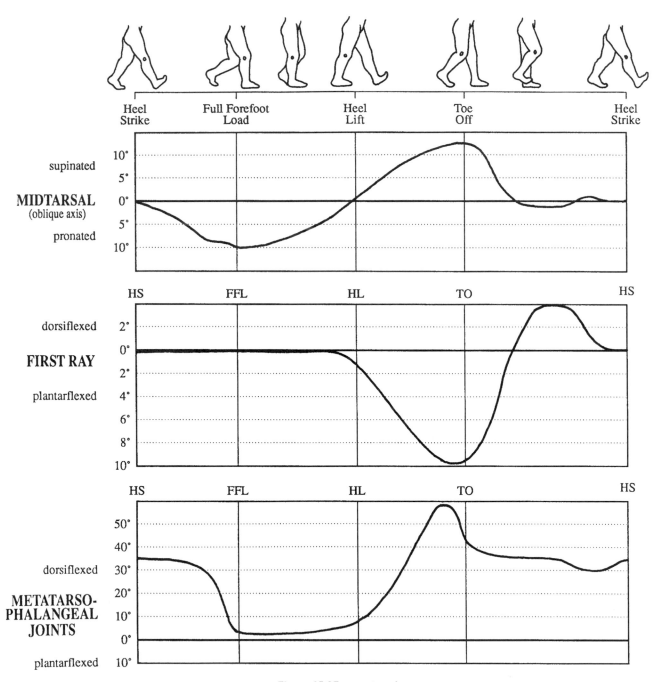

Figure 15.27—continued

The excessive internal tibial rotation may also be responsible for medial knee injury, as the medial tibial plateau is forced into rapid posterior glide beneath the medial femoral condyle. This movement strains the medial meniscus, the me- dial joint capsule, and may produce chronic pes anserine bursitis. (Lutter (31) was able to relate 77% of 213 knee injuries to faulty mechanics of the foot.) Most authorities believe that excessive subtalar pronation most frequently produces me-

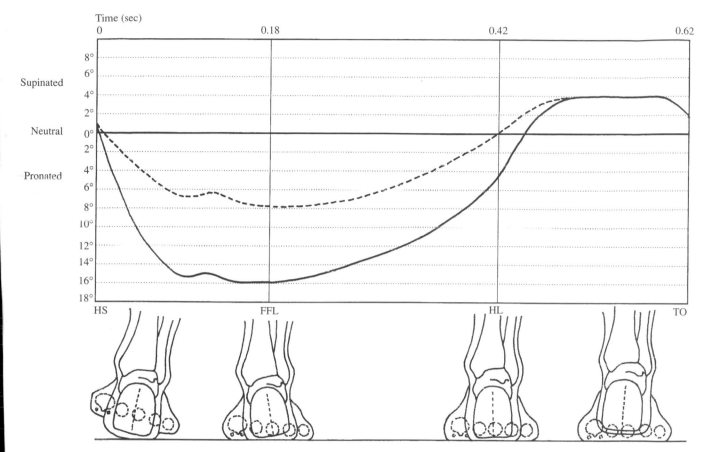

Figure 15.30. Stance phase motions with a rearfoot varus deformity (solid line).

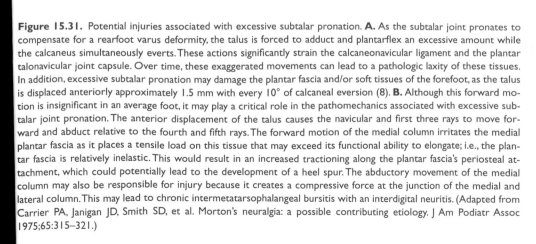

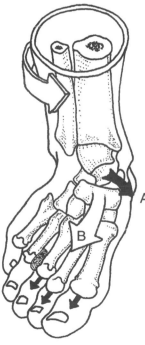

Figure 15.31. Potential injuries associated with excessive subtalar pronation. **A.** As the subtalar joint pronates to compensate for a rearfoot varus deformity, the talus is forced to adduct and plantarflex an excessive amount while the calcaneus simultaneously everts. These actions significantly strain the calcaneonavicular ligament and the plantar talonavicular joint capsule. Over time, these exaggerated movements can lead to a pathologic laxity of these tissues. In addition, excessive subtalar pronation may damage the plantar fascia and/or soft tissues of the forefoot, as the talus is displaced anteriorly approximately 1.5 mm with every 10° of calcaneal eversion (8). **B.** Although this forward mo- tion is insignificant in an average foot, it may play a critical role in the pathomechanics associated with excessive sub- talar joint pronation. The anterior displacement of the talus causes the navicular and first three rays to move for- ward and abduct relative to the fourth and fifth rays. The forward motion of the medial column irritates the medial plantar fascia as it places a tensile load on this tissue that may exceed its functional ability to elongate; i.e., the plan- tar fascia is relatively inelastic. This would result in an increased tractioning along the plantar fascia's periosteal at- tachment, which could potentially lead to the development of a heel spur. The abductory movement of the medial column may also be responsible for injury because it creates a compressive force at the junction of the medial and lateral column. This may lead to chronic intermetatarsophalangeal bursitis with an interdigital neuritis. (Adapted from Carrier PA, Janigan JD, Smith SD, et al. Morton's neuralgia: a possible contributing etiology. J Am Podiatr Assoc 1975;65:315–321.)

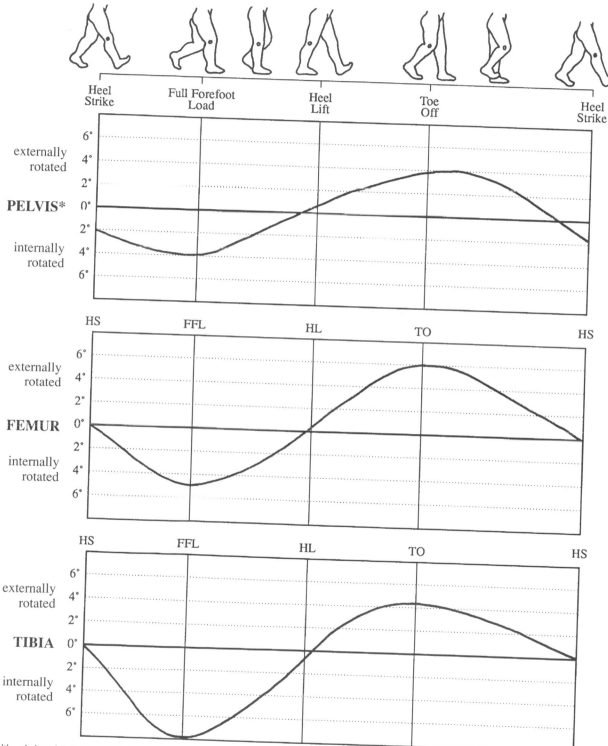

*Although the pelvis in this graph is internally rotated only 2° at heel-strike, as higher speeds of locomotion are reached the pelvis may be maximally inter- nally rotated at heel-strike, thereby allowing for an increased length of stride. Note the ipsilateral rotation of the pelvis is countered by contralateral rotation of the torso with the shift in motion occurring at about the eighth thoracic vertebra.

Figure 15.28. Transverse plane motions associated with the gait cycle.

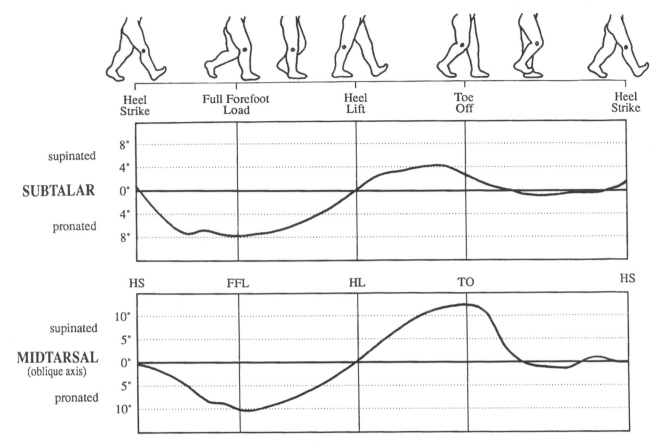

Figure 15.28—continued

the rearfoot and the subtalar joint is in its midline position. The ideal alignment pattern is illustrated in Figure 15.20.

ABNORMAL MOTIONS DURING THE GAIT CYCLE

As expected, whenever there are specific guidelines identifying a norm, there are bound to be situations in which individuals deviate from these parameters. In fact, individual variation in the shape of the articular surfaces and/or defects in the triplanar development of the osseous structures make deviation from one or more of these outlined parameters the rule rather than the exception. As will be demonstrated, departure from any one of these parameters will result in some type of biomechanical malfunction. The following section will review the pathomechanics associated with deviation from each of the described parameters.

Alignment of the Subtalar Joint and Lower Leg

By far, the most common deviation from the norm is the rearfoot varus deformity. This rep-

resents an osseous malformation in which the tibia has formed in a bowed position and/or the subtalar joint has formed in such a way that the calcaneus is excessively inverted when the subtalar joint is maintained in its neutral position (Fig. 15.29).

Because the rearfoot varus foot type represents the combined degrees of tibiofibular varum and subtalar varum, deformity greater than the ideal of 4° (a 2° variance for subtalar varum plus the 2° variance for tibiofibular varum) is extremely common. In one epidemiologic study of various foot types, McPoil et al. (23) found a rearfoot varus deformity exceeding 4° in 98.3% of the individuals measured. Because of this, it is more appropriate to refer to a straight lower leg as ideal rather than the norm.

The etiology of this deformity is related to a failure of the tibia and/or calcaneus to straighten from the bowed positions present during infancy (24). Because the heel is maintained in an inverted position, initial ground contact occurs along the posterolateral edge of the calcaneus. To compensate for this deformity, the subtalar joint must pronate excessively just to bring the medial condyle of the calcaneus to the ground

(Fig. 15.30). The degree of subtalar joint pronation is directly related to the degree of the deformity, e.g., a person with an 8° tibiofibular varum coupled with a 4° subtalar varum must pronate 12° for the medial heel to make ground contact. Unfortunately, this fairly large range of subtalar pronation does not represent the final range of subtalar pronation during the contact period. Because the forefoot remains inverted around the longitudinal midtarsal joint axis during contact (this position is maintained by eccentric contraction of tibialis anterior), the subtalar joint must continue to pronate an additional 6°–8° to bring the medial forefoot to the ground.

The rearfoot varus deformity produces dysfunction of the subtalar joint primarily during the contact period, as this joint most often returns to a stable position by late midstance/early propulsion (Fig. 15.30). This contact period pronation may still be responsible for a wide variety of injuries, partly because the overall range of motion is so large and, more importantly, because the subtalar joint reaches its peak angular displacement during the first 50% of the contact period (25). Recent research has demonstrated that the angular velocity of subtalar pronation may play a primary role in the development of various injuries (26). Because the subtalar joint acts as a directional torque

transmitter converting frontal plane motion of calcaneus into axial rotation of the shank lower extremity (27), the tibia in this situatio internally rotate 20° in 0.08 second. (The tibi rotate even more if a high subtalar joint a present.) The rapid, sometimes extreme rar motion associated with subtalar compensati a rearfoot varus deformity is capable of gene tremendous amounts of torque. These forces be dampened effectively within fractions of ond, thousands of times a day, if the individu remain injury free. Examples of possible al dysfunction associated with rearfoot varus mity are illustrated in Figure 15.31.

In addition to producing various injuries foot, excessive subtalar pronation may sponsible for a wide range of injuries alc kinetic chain. For example, it has been mented that excessive subtalar prona causally related to shin splints (28) (shin being defined as pain along the medial di thirds of the tibia). Also, Matheson et have demonstrated that excessive subta nation predisposes to lower tibial stre tures. This is possibly because the dist with its relatively low polar moment o (30), is unable to tolerate the increased t strains associated with excessive talar ad

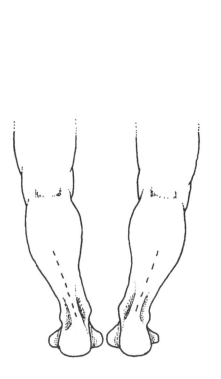

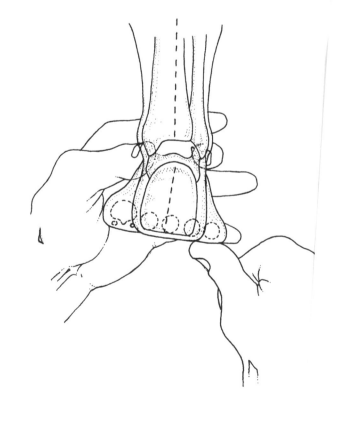

Figure 15.29. Tibial and subtalar varum.

dial knee injury (32). However, in a study of 100 cases of iliotibial band friction syndrome, Noble (28) concluded that excessive subtalar joint pronation was a significant etiologic factor in the development of that injury. Apparently, the excessive internal tibial rotation "drags" the distal iliotibial band over the lateral femoral epicondyle, thereby predisposing to this friction syndrome.

One final point of interest relates to retropatellar pain with excessive subtalar joint pronation. Although most authorities (33) state that excessive pronation increases the quadriceps (Q) angle, thereby predisposing to retropatellar arthralgia, this is only true during static stance when the cruciate ligaments maintain the extended knee in a locked position. When the knee is flexed (as it is during the contact period), the tibia internally rotates further than the femur, thereby decreasing the Q angle (34). This may be troublesome. Huberti and Hayes (35) demonstrated that a reduction in the Q angle will, approximately 50% of the time, result in a reduction of pressure beneath the lateral patella facet with a redistribution of this pressure elsewhere (thereby increasing the potential for chondromalacia at these points). Perhaps this is why Kegerreis (34) states that excessive subtalar joint pronation is as causally related to the plical band syndrome as an increased Q angle is related to extensor mechanism dysfunction.

To prevent injury, persons with rearfoot varus deformity require strong, well-coordinated muscles so they may smoothly decelerate the range of subtalar pronation. If the excessive pronation does produce an injury, it may be necessary to fabricate a foot orthosis with the heel posted in varus (Fig. 15.32). The post basically acts to bring the surface to the patient's medial foot, rather than forcing the patient to pronate to bring the medial foot to the ground. The ability of the varus post to control subtalar motions has been demonstrated by Cavanaugh et al. (25). By using high-speed cinematography and force plate analysis, the authors were able to demonstrate that the addition of a varus post not only decreased the overall range of subtalar pronation, but also produced a significant reduction in the angular velocity in which pronation occurred. In addition, the force plate analysis revealed a significant decrease in medial shear forces at the time of initial ground contact. Mann (27) theorized that use of a medial support would bring about a decrease in eversion of the calcaneus and internal rotation of the tibia. The author emphasized that altering the transverse plane motion of the tibia may correct clinical symptoms at the knee and hip.

The observation that varus posts decrease the range and speed of subtalar pronation has been

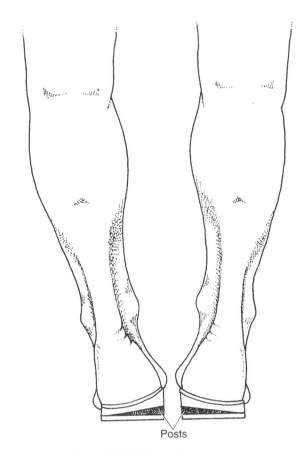

Posts

Figure 15.32. The rearfoot varus post.

supported by other investigators (36–38). Smart et al. (39) were so impressed with the ability of the varus wedge to control the range of subtalar motion that they recommended use of a 12-mm wedge in all casual and athletic shoe wear.

In addition to the control afforded by the varus post, subtalar joint motion can also be controlled by adequately supporting the medial longitudinal arch. Clarke et al. (37) state that supporting the arch is an effective method for reducing pronation. Also, the degree of subtalar pronation present during the contact period may be lessened by having the patient wear motion control sneakers with a duo-density midsole and by avoiding sneakers with a large lateral flare.

Alignment of the Rearfoot and Forefoot

As mentioned, the calcaneocuboid joint should lock into its close-packed position with the vertical bisection of the rearfoot perpendicular to the plantar surface of the forefoot. Unfortunately, this is not always the case. Individual variation in the triplanar ontogeny of the tarsals may allow the plantar forefoot to be maintained in either an inverted or everted position when the calcaneocuboid locking mechanism is engaged. If the plantar forefoot locks in an inverted position relative to the plantar

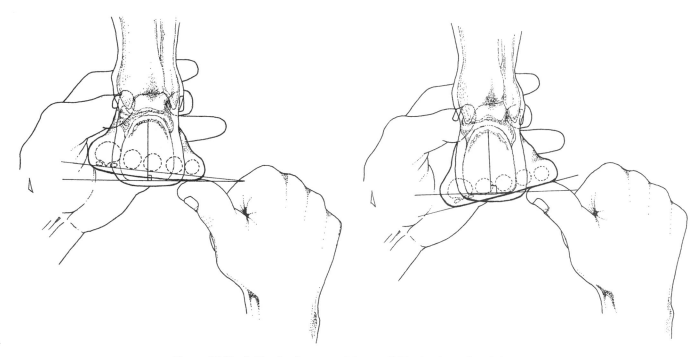

Figure 15.33. A. The forefoot varus deformity. **B.** The forefoot valgus deformity.

rearfoot, it is referred to as a forefoot varus position (Fig. 15.33A). Conversely, if the plantar forefoot locks in an everted position, it is referred to as a forefoot valgus deformity (Fig. 15.33B).

Forefoot Varus

Although the forefoot varus deformity is less common than the forefoot valgus, in that the forefoot varus is present in less than 9% of the population (23), an individual with this deformity is frequently seen in a clinical setting because the forefoot varus is responsible for many knee, hip, and pelvic disorders. Straus (40) originally described this deformity in 1927, attributing it to a failure of the talar neck to derotate from its infantile inverted position. Although most authorities continue to blame talar neck derotation as the cause of this deformity, McPoil et al. (41) recently disproved this theory, suggesting that it results from osseous abnormality of the midtarsal joint, not variation in the talar head or neck.

To compensate for the constantly inverted position of the forefoot, the subtalar joint is forced to pronate through extreme ranges just to bring the medial forefoot to the ground (Fig. 15.34). This exaggerated range of subtalar pronation causes the talus to shift medially relative to the calcaneus, which in turn supplies body weight with a much more effective lever arm for maintaining the subtalar joint in a pronated position. This creates a vicious cycle, in that the range of subtalar pronation necessary to compensate for

the forefoot deformity during contact period allows body weight to maintain this pronated position throughout midstance and early propulsion.

The increased range of subtalar pronation present during the contact period predisposes to the same types of injuries seen with a rearfoot varus deformity. However, continued subtalar joint pronation throughout midstance and propulsion makes this deformity particularly destructive, as it disallows locking of the calcaneocuboid joint and creates a series of conflicting motions between the knee and talus. Because the talus is held in an adducted position by the pronated subtalar joint (this position is maintained by the superimposed body weight), the external rotational moment created by the swing phase leg is unable to generate a force strong enough to abduct the talus. Therefore, the torsional forces associated with this external rotational moment must be stored temporarily in the stance phase lower extremity. The release of these stored torsional forces is frequently evidenced by a sudden "abductory twist" of the rearfoot the moment heel lift occurs. That is, because ground-reactive forces no longer maintain the plantar heel, the entire rearfoot is free to snap medially, as though released from a loaded spring. Clearly, the development of such torsional forces has the potential to do much damage. Because a chain is most likely to give at its weakest link, the prolonged application of these forces will most likely produce a pathologic laxity of the involved joint capsules, particularly the knee.

Coplan (42) demonstrated that individuals who pronate excessively display significantly greater ranges of tibiofemoral rotation, particularly as the knee approaches full extension (its normal position of function as torsional strains peak during late midstance). In her study, which was done about weight bearing, the mean range of tibial rotation when the knee was flexed 5° was 11.4° for the normal group and 18.5° for the pronating group. The author speculated that the opposing rotary torques present during the late midstance period produced laxity of the structures that normally limit knee rotation.

Whereas subtalar pronation during the midstance period predisposes to injury because of conflicting movement patterns between the leg and talus, continued subtalar pronation through the propulsive period may be even more destructive. This is because it maintains a parallelism of the midtarsal axes. The continued parallelism of these axes essentially produces an unlocking of the articulations at a time when maximum stability is needed. This results in plastic deformity of the ligaments that limit midtarsal motion, which in turn allows for even greater ranges of subtalar joint pronation and concomitant cal-

caneal eversion. Glancy (43) theorizes that prolonged calcaneal eversion will create permanent elongation of the subtalar supinators, which eventually limits the ability of these muscles to store elastic energy during early stance phase. As a result, these muscles are unable to return the pronated subtalar joint to its neutral position and a cycle of excessive subtalar pronation, soft tissue elongation, muscular dysfunction, and continued subtalar pronation is perpetuated. This cycle may eventually end with subluxation of the unstable articulations.

For several reasons, the chronically everted heel associated with the forefoot varus may predispose to a variety of injuries. For example, prolonged calcaneal eversion is considered an etiologic factor in the development of tarsal tunnel syndrome (44, 45). This is because it may compress various branches of the calcaneal nerves at several sites. The medial and lateral plantar nerves may be compressed against the sharp fascial edge of the abductor hallucis muscle (46), whereas branches of the lateral plantar nerve and the nerve to abductor digiti quinti may be compressed between the plantar aponeurosis, intrinsic foot muscles, and the calcaneus (47).

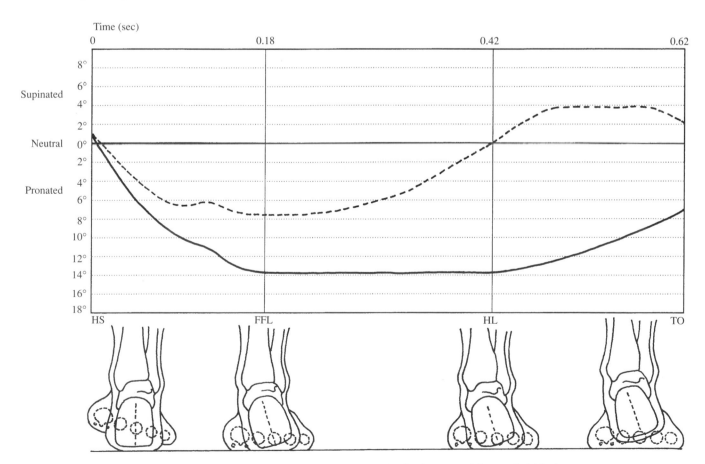

Figure 15.34. Stance phase subtalar joint motions with a forefoot varus deformity (solid line).

A valgus heel may also produce injury to the plantar fascia as the adducted talus inhibits normal propulsive period supination around the oblique midtarsal joint axis (Fig. 15.21). This negates the approximation of the anterior and posterior pillars associated with the windlass mechanism, and the tensile strain developed in the plantar fascia is transferred into this tissue's periosteal attachment on the medial calcaneal tubercle. Over time, the prolonged tractioning may produce inflammatory erosive changes with proliferation of new bone, i.e., calcaneal spur formation (48, 49).

Possibly the most important factor limiting propulsive period stability in the forefoot varus deformity is the inability of peroneus longus to stabilize the first ray when the subtalar joint is pronated. As previously mentioned, subtalar pronation alters the angle of approach afforded peroneus longus to the first ray axis, making it ineffective as a first ray plantarflexor (Fig. 15.23). Because ground-reactive forces are normally transferred to the medial forefoot during propulsion, the first metatarsal must be stabilized effectively by a mechanically efficient peroneus longus if it is to resist application of these forces. Failure of peroneus longus to stabilize the first ray will result in a dorsal shifting of the first metatarsal as ground-reactive forces are applied (Fig. 15.35). This eventually leads to the formation of a hypermobile first ray that is unable to assist with the transfer of forces during propulsion. As a result, greater amounts of pressure are borne by the second, third, and fourth metatarsal heads; this is frequently evidenced by diffuse callus formation beneath these metatarsal heads. Root et al. (5) mention that propulsive period pronation of the subtalar joint (with the associated shifting of the hypermobile first ray) will predispose the first metatarsophalangeal joint to different deformities depending on the alignment of the metatarsals. If

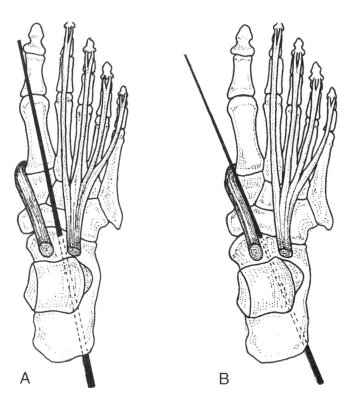

Figure 15.36. A. When the subtalar joint is in its neutral position, the tibialis anterior tendon has a significant lever arm to supinate the subtalar joint. **B.** When the subtalar joint is pronated, the tibialis anterior is unable to control subtalar motion. The improved lever arm afforded extensor digitorum longus allows this muscle to maintain the subtalar joint in a pronated position throughout swing phase (10, 46).

metatarsus rectus is present, the metatarsophalangeal joint is prone to developing hallux limitus; if metatarsus adductus is present, the metatarsophalangeal joint is prone to developing hallux abductovalgus. The reader is referred to other sources for detailed discussion of the pathomechanics associated with these deformities (5, 50).

A final consideration in the pathomechanics of the forefoot varus deformity relates to the inability of the tibialis anterior muscle to resupinate an excessively pronated subtalar joint during late swing phase. Because subtalar pronation shifts the subtalar joint's axis of motion closer to the insertion of tibialis anterior (Fig. 15.36), this muscle is frequently unable to supinate the subtalar joint in time for the next heel strike. As a result, heel strike occurs with the calcaneus progressively more everted. Subotnick (15) states that failure to negotiate a phasically sound subtalar resupination during late swing phase will result in a loss of kinetic shock absorption, with eventual pronatory subluxation of the subtalar joint. The individual with a forefoot varus deformity may compensate for the lack of shock absorption by shortening the stride length (which lessens

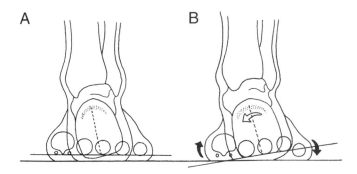

Figure 15.35. Without the stability associated with a mechanically efficient peroneus longus, the first ray is forced into a dorsiflexed and inverted position.

initial impact forces) and/or by striking the ground with the ankle in an excessively dorsiflexed position. (This position allows the anterior compartment muscles more time to assist with shock absorption as they decelerate the ankle through a larger range of plantarflexion.)

To treat the forefoot varus deformity properly, it is necessary to take a plaster impression that accurately captures the forefoot-to-rearfoot relationship with the foot maintained in its neutral position. (A full weight-bearing impression would be useless because the plantar forefoot and rearfoot shift to the same transverse plane makes proper treatment impossible.) A positive model is then made from the plaster impression and, after the appropriate changes are made to allow for soft tissue displacement, a shell (of whatever material the practitioner desires) is molded along the plantar contour. An angled wedge or post is then placed beneath the distal medial aspect of the orthotic shell, just proximal to the metatarsal heads. The post should be of sufficient height to bring the sagittal bisection of the rearfoot to vertical (Fig. 15.37).

By supporting the inverted forefoot, the post prevents pronatory compensation by the subtalar joint and allows the foot to enter the propulsive period with all of its articulations locked and stable. As with the rearfoot varus deformity, the orthotic does not change the osseous malposition—it merely accommodates the deformity by bringing a custom-molded surface to the neutral position foot.

In regard to controlling motion during terminal stance phase, there is a major shortcoming of the orthotic shell. Because it ends along the distal metatarsal shafts, it is only able to control motion during the contact and midstance periods when body weight is centered over the orthotic shell. It is for this reason that Glancy (43) states that "the foot and ankle complex is most vulnerable to injury and most difficult to control between heel lift and toe-off."

Because the normal progression of forces passes beyond the distal metatarsal shafts during the propulsive period (they are centered over the metatarsal heads and hallux), the orthotic shell and post become nonfunctional at a time when control is needed the most. Because of this, the subtalar joint is forced to pronate suddenly in an attempt to bring the medial forefoot to the ground. If a small forefoot varus deformity is present, the propulsive period pronation necessary to bring the medial forefoot to the ground typically does not produce injury because it is well-controlled by the mechanically efficient musculature. If, however, a large forefoot varus deformity is present (i.e., greater than 4°), the added range of propulsive period pronation may produce a significant shifting of the articulations that may be responsible for injuries such as intermetatarsal bursitis, interdigital neuritis, and bunion pain, to name a few.

The propulsive period pronation associated with a large forefoot varus deformity can be prevented with what is referred to as a compressible post to sulcus. This addition represents a continuation of the forefoot post beneath the metatarsal heads, ending at the sulcus (the base of the toes). This extension of the forefoot post is made from a flexible material (usually rubber or crepe), so as not to limit dorsiflexion at the metatarsophalangeal joints. The compressible post to sulcus is recommended for all forefoot deformities greater than 4°.

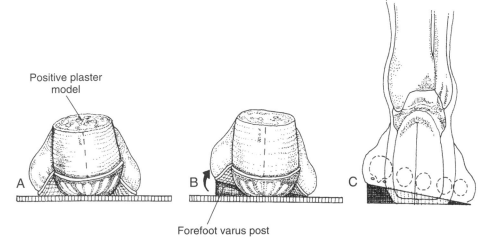

Figure 15.37. Posterior view of the right positive model. A forefoot varus post is placed under the medial forefoot, bringing the sagittal bisection of the rearfoot to vertical.

In addition to treatment with foot orthoses, the individual with a forefoot varus deformity should also be evaluated for proprioceptive deficits (observe closed-eye, single leg stance for 10 seconds). Because the forefoot varus often produces joint hypermobility (which detrimentally affects proprioceptive feedback), it may be necessary to reeducate the central nervous system with balance board exercises. Also, motion control sneakers with external heel stabilizers are recommended to support the rearfoot and prevent breakdown of the heel counter. Generic arch supports should be avoided when treating the forefoot varus deformity; this foot type typically lacks a medial arch both on and off weight bearing (51). The inappropriate use of an arch support may eventually damage the first metatarsophalangeal joint (5). It could also lead to a neuropraxia of the medial and lateral plantar nerves, as these nerves may be compressed between the arch support and the calcaneus (52).

As with all foot deformities, the individual articulations of the foot and ankle should be evaluated to determine the presence of joint dysfunction. As noted by Hiss (53), excessive rearfoot eversion may allow for displacement of one or more of the tarsals, which, despite the overall flexibility of the foot, can become locked in an abnormal position. The author uses an example of how a subluxed cuboid produces "tension" on the supporting ligaments and underlying quadratus plantae muscle to the point that the individual redistributes body weight medially, thereby damaging the first metatarsophalangeal joint. Hiss (53) also states that joint dysfunction in the first tarsometatarsal articulation (which is a common finding with a forefoot varus deformity) produces a significant decrease in proprioceptive awareness.

Forefoot Valgus

The forefoot valgus deformity is the most frequently seen frontal plane deformity of the forefoot. In their evaluation of 116 feet, McPoil et al. (23) noted that 44.8% presented with a forefoot valgus deformity. In another study of 552 feet, Burns (54) noted that 70% of all frontal plane deformities were in valgus. He also noted that this deformity was more likely to be larger than the forefoot varus. It should be noted that this was a symptomatic population.

The exact etiology of the forefoot valgus remains obscure, possibly because it is of multiple origins. It may simply represent a congenital anomaly in the calcaneocuboid joint that disallows the normal close-packed position. For example, in Bojsen-Moller's study of the calca-

neocuboid joint (12), 8% of the cuboids evaluated lacked a calcanean process, and the corresponding articular surface on the calcaneus was flat. The calcaneocuboid joint in this situation could allow for greater ranges of forefoot eversion (i.e., forefoot valgus), as the cuboid would be allowed to glide along the flattened surface of the calcaneus. (Normally, the calcanean process serves as a pivot that the cuboid will dorsiflex and evert around until its dorsal border contacts the overhanging calcaneus.) The calcaneocuboid joint lacking the calcanean process is classified in the plane variety (12), which allows for greater ranges of gliding motion compared with the concavoconvex type of configuration typically present.

What has become the most widely accepted theory regarding the development of the forefoot valgus deformity is described by Sgarlato (55) as developmental overrotation of the talar neck. Because the forefoot valgus deformity is not seen in children, it is believed that a period of transition is needed to transform the talar neck from the varus position present at birth to the valgus position by adulthood. Although the simplicity of this theory makes it tempting to accept, the work by McPoil et al. (41) has all but disproved this theory. In their study of anatomical abnormalities of the talus, the authors could find no correlation between the forefoot valgus deformity and the position of the talar neck. It is possible that postmortem changes in the foot could be responsible for error in their evaluations, but this is unlikely because this was a particularly well-planned study.

The final consideration regarding the etiology of the forefoot valgus deformity relates to the formation of a pes cavus foot; *Dorland's Medical Dictionary* defines pes cavus as "an exaggerated height of the longitudinal arch of the foot, present from birth or appearing later because of contractures or disturbed balance of muscles." Because the forefoot valgus deformity is often present in the cavus foot, possible etiologies for its formation should include those etiologies associated with the development of the cavus foot, namely congenital malformation, neuromuscular disorder, various idiopathic conditions (such as scarlet fever or diphtheria, which may produce a discrepancy in bone or muscle growth), and trauma.

Because the cavus foot typically possesses limited ranges of subtalar joint motion (56) and because the heel in the cavus foot is often maintained in a varus attitude (referred to as a cavovarus foot), it is possible that the forefoot valgus deformity merely represents a develop-

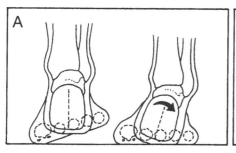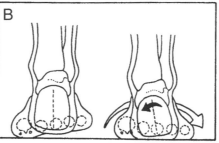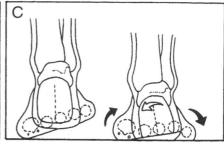

Figure 15.38. Patterns of compensation for the forefoot valgus deformity. If the forefoot deformity is rigid **(A)**, the subtalar joint must supinate to bring the lateral plantar forefoot to the ground. When a flexible forefoot valgus is present **(B)**, the plantar forefoot is able to make ground contact without affecting subtalar motions as long as the range of forefoot inversion is large enough to compensate for the forefoot valgus deformity. However, if the size of the deformity exceeds the range of inversion available around the longitudinal midtarsal joint axis **(C)**, the forefoot (in its attempt to make ground contact) will invert its full range around the longitudinal midtarsal joint axis (note the central metatarsals). The forefoot will then continue to compensate via pronation (dorsiflexion and inversion) around the first ray axis and supination (plantarflexion and eversion) around the fifth ray axis (arrows in C).

mental malformation necessary to compensate for the inverted and rigid rearfoot. It should be emphasized that the reverse of this situation may also be true, in that the inverted heel associated with the cavovarus foot may be secondary to the rigid and everted forefoot (57).

Regardless of the exact etiology, the forefoot valgus deformity may significantly alter biomechanics of the foot. The extent of the mechanical malfunction is dependent on the size of the deformity and the rigidity of the midfoot. Because of this, the deformity is divided into rigid and flexible subgroups to describe the compensatory pathomechanics associated with the forefoot valgus more accurately. The rigid forefoot valgus possesses limited ranges of midtarsal and first ray motion and is only able to bring the plantar forefoot to the ground via supination of the subtalar joint (Fig. 15.38A). The flexible forefoot valgus is able to bring the plantar forefoot to the ground via inversion around the longitudinal midtarsal joint axis and, if necessary, dorsiflexion and inversion of the first ray (Figs. 15.38B and C). In Burns' survey of various foot types (54), he found 70% of all forefoot valgus deformities to be flexible.

The pattern of compensation in a flexible forefoot valgus deformity is dependent on the range of motion available around the midtarsal joint (Figs. 15.38B and C). In some cases, the flexible forefoot valgus deformity may possess such large ranges of longitudinal midtarsal joint inversion that the subtalar joint is allowed to pronate excessively throughout all periods of the stance phase. Foot movements in this situation would be similar to those seen in a forefoot varus foot type.

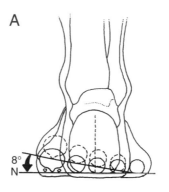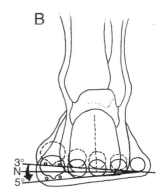

Figure 15.39. A. Normally, the forefoot can evert from its fully inverted position only until the plantar forefoot reaches horizontal (N). **B.** When a flexible forefoot valgus deformity is present, the plantar forefoot is able to evert beyond horizontal while the range of inversion remains limited. The overall range of motion remains the same.

The individual with an extremely flexible forefoot valgus may occasionally pronate through all periods of stance phase. However, a more common movement pattern is seen in individuals possessing normal or decreased ranges of longitudinal midtarsal joint axis inversion with increased ranges of longitudinal midtarsal axis eversion (Fig. 15.39).

During the contact period, the individual with this range of midtarsal motion could pronate the subtalar joint only until the forefoot reaches its fully inverted position, with motion occurring at both the longitudinal midtarsal joint axis and first ray axis (Fig. 15.40). At that time, the soft tissue restraining mechanisms that stabilize these axes would prevent continued subtalar joint motion.

During the midstance period, this foot can easily accomplish a phasically sound resupination of

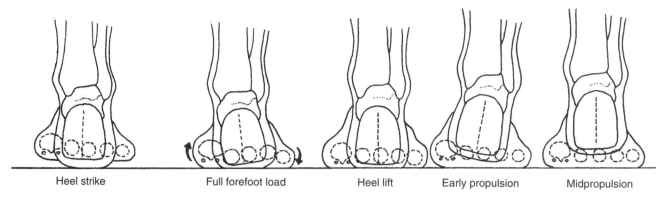

Figure 15.40. Motions with a flexible forefoot valgus deformity possessing limited ranges of longitudinal midtarsal joint axis inversion. The first ray at full forefoot load has dorsiflexed and inverted to allow the full range of subtalar pronation (normally the first ray does not move during the contact period).

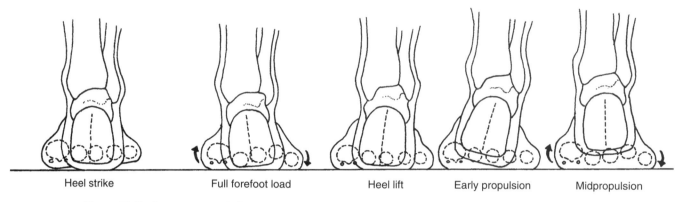

Figure 15.41. Foot motions with flexible forefoot valgus deformity greater than 6° (posterior view of the right foot).

the subtalar joint. However, because of the increased range of eversion available around the longitudinal midtarsal joint axis, the calcaneocuboid joint does not lock when the rearfoot reaches its vertical position during heel lift. If the range of available forefoot eversion is small (i.e., less than 6°), the individual may attempt to lock the lateral column during the propulsive period by inverting the rearfoot (see early propulsion in Fig. 15.40). Although this increased range of subtalar supination helps stabilize the articulations by bringing the calcaneocuboid joint into its close-packed position, it can be damaging because it creates a lateral instability capable of producing chronic inversion sprain of the ankle mortise (5, 20). To protect against this lateral instability, the individual will typically invert the forefoot around the longitudinal midtarsal joint and first ray axis (if necessary), thereby bringing the rearfoot back to its perpendicular position (see midpropulsion in Fig. 15.40).

Although these motions reestablish frontal plane stability of the ankle mortise, they may be destructive because they set the articulations of the midfoot and forefoot into motion as vertical

forces peak. This may lead to chronic bunion pain over the dorsomedial first and dorsolateral fifth metatarsal heads, as the adventitious bursae are sheared between the skin (which is maintained in a fixed position by shoe gear) and the rotating metatarsal heads. Also, inversion of the forefoot during propulsion prevents the normal plantarflexion motion of the first ray necessary for the dorsal-posterior shift in the first metatarsophalangeal joint's transverse axis (and may therefore be responsible for the development of hallux limitus or hallux abductovalgus). This will also lessen the ability of the first metatarsal head to resist ground-reactive forces (as is evidenced by a diffuse callus formation beneath the second and third metatarsal heads).

If the flexible forefoot valgus is greater than 6°, the excessive subtalar supination necessary to lock the calcaneocuboid joint may be evident as early as late midstance (Fig. 15.41). This premature subtalar supination increases the range of calcaneal inversion and external tibial rotation, which strains the peroneals (these muscles attempt to decelerate the exaggerated movements). As this foot enters its propulsive period, the individual initially protects against the lateral insta-bility by inverting the forefoot around the mid-tarsal and first ray axes. However, when a large forefoot valgus deformity is present, the amounts of forefoot inversion needed to bring the rearfoot to perpendicular often exceed the ranges of mo-tion available around these axes. This being the case, the continued range of calcaneal eversion necessary to bring the rearfoot back to vertical can only occur via sudden pronation of the sub-talar joint. This predisposes to injury because it unlocks all the articulations of the foot at a time when maximum stability is essential.

The flexible forefoot valgus deformity produces lateral instability with its associated dysfunction primarily during terminal stance phase. The rigid forefoot valgus deformity, regardless of its size, will produce postural dysfunction during all por-tions of stance phase (Fig. 15.42).

During the contact period, the individual pos-sessing a rigid forefoot valgus deformity will be able to pronate the subtalar joint only until the plantar forefoot makes ground contact. At that time, the subtalar joint is forced into rapid supina-tory compensation (referred to as the "supinatory rock"), as the rearfoot tips laterally to bring the plantar forefoot to the ground (see midcontact in Fig. 15.42). If this foot had been flexible, the first ray and midtarsal joint would have compensated for the forefoot valgus deformity by allowing the entire forefoot to invert. However, because this foot possesses such limited ranges of midtarsal and first ray motion, the lateral aspect of the plantar forefoot can only make ground contact if the sub-talar joint supinates.

Although the pattern of compensation illus-trated in Figure 15.42 is often described as clas-sic for a rigid forefoot valgus deformity (58), clin-ically it is rarely seen. More often, the individual with the forefoot deformity is able to avoid the supinatory rock by striking the ground with the rearfoot excessively inverted. This may be a learned response in which the subtalar joint is deliberately inverted beyond neutral in anticipa-tion of the supinatory rock. More commonly, it is the result of a combination rearfoot varus/fore-foot valgus deformity in which the degree of rear-foot varus is equal to or exceeds the degree of forefoot valgus. Although this movement pattern may be beneficial because it disallows supinatory compensation of the subtalar joint during the contact period (the subtalar rock would create conflicting movements between the talus and leg), it may also be detrimental in that the subta-lar joint continues to move through a limited range of motion. Because subtalar pronation is the body's primary shock-absorbing mecha-nism, the sudden termination of this motion early in the contact period requires the body to absorb relatively large amounts of force in a very short period. In this abrupt and jarring action, the normal vertical forces associated with the contact period and during walking, average 110% body weight (59), must now be absorbed in fractions of a second. This results in a greater force impulse being applied to the pos-terolateral heel and possibly transferred proxi-mally along the lateral aspect of the entire lower extremity. This may explain why individuals with cavus feet are more likely to suffer from femoral stress fracture (29), greater trochan-teric bursitis (32), and iliotibial band friction syndrome (31).

To minimize these destructive force impulses, many individuals with this forefoot deformity will strike the ground with the ankle in an excessively dorsiflexed position (15). In addition to delaying the initial contact of the plantar forefoot (which allows the subtalar joint to pronate for a longer period), the increased amount of ankle dorsiflex-ion affords the anterior compartment muscles more time to assist with shock absorption (they decelerate the ankle through greater ranges of plantarflexion). Unfortunately, although this pat-tern of compensation may improve the foot's abil-ity to absorb shock, it may also predispose to

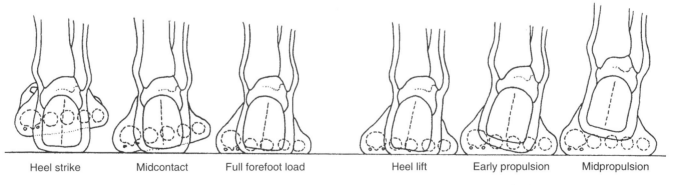

| Heel strike | Midcontact | Full forefoot load | Heel lift | Early propulsion | Midpropulsion |

Figure 15.42. Foot motions with a rigid forefoot valgus (posterior view of the right foot).

chronic myositis/periostitis of the anterior compartment tissues.

Whereas the rigid forefoot valgus deformity produces high-impact symptoms during the contact period, the midstance period motions are relatively normal. The exception is that the rearfoot is maintained in an excessively inverted position. Unfortunately, this may result in chronic tenosynovitis of the peroneus longus (which is tractioned behind the lateral malleolus). It may also be responsible for an entrapment neuropathy of the superficial peroneal nerve where this nerve pierces the fascia between the anterior and lateral compartments, approximately two thirds of the way down the leg (60). Cangialosi and Schall (60) claim that the excessive subtalar joint supination associated with the rigid forefoot valgus deformity creates a "tautness of the nerve against its fascial window" that provides the initial stimulus for a neuropathy. The authors mention that the clinical signs of this mononeuropathy may range from hyperesthesia to anesthesia along the distal lateral leg and dorsal foot. The authors also claim that palpation in the area where the nerve exits the fascial window may reveal a nodular fibrosis along the course of the nerve, and that compression at this point may exacerbate the pain along the nerve's sensory distribution.

As this foot enters its propulsive period, the subtalar joint is often unable to prevent lateral instability because of the typically limited range of subtalar eversion, which is often limited to 5° or less in a cavus foot (35). As a result, the subtalar joint remains supinated and the application of ground-reactive forces progresses from the lateral heel to the lateral forefoot. This is where the final transfer of force occurs around the oblique transverse metatarsal axis, not the transverse metatarsal axis (Fig. 15.43).

As mentioned earlier, Bojsen-Moller (12) refers to the use of the oblique metatarsal axis as a low-gear push-off because of the significantly shorter lever arm afforded this axis. The author was able to study the structural interactions associated with a low-gear push-off by using a large glass plate as a walking platform and then recording the various portions of the gait cycle with a high-speed camera. These photos revealed that with low-gear push-off, propulsion proceeded as a rolling action over the lateral part of the ball of the foot with the leg externally rotated, the rearfoot inverted, and the forefoot adducted. As the foot moves into its final stages of propulsion, continued ground contact at the lateral forefoot forces the lesser digits into an excessively dorsiflexed position. This predisposes to Morton's neuroma (61),

as dorsiflexion of the lesser toes tractions the interdigital nerve against the transverse ligament. Also, because the lesser digits are less firmly attached to the plantar fascia (12), dorsiflexion of the lesser toes is unable to produce a tightening of the plantar fascia and the stabilization afforded by the windlass mechanism is lost. This was demonstrated in Bojsen-Moller's recordings (12), in that during low-gear push-off (although the medial arch became high), neither the plantar fascia nor peroneus longus could be seen to tense under the skin. Also, the author emphasized that throughout low-gear push-off, the rearfoot remains inverted; thus, the postaxial fibular edge is exposed to large vertical forces. It seems likely that this lateral displacement of vertical forces predisposes to fibular and lateral knee injuries.

Regardless of whether the forefoot valgus deformity is flexible or rigid, the goal of conservative treatment is to allow neutral position function of the subtalar joint. As with the forefoot varus deformity, this is best accomplished by taking an impression of the foot that accurately captures the forefoot-to-rearfoot relationship when the calcaneocuboid joint is locked and the talar head is maintained behind the navicular. A positive model is then made from this impression, and the appropriate changes are made to allow for soft tissue displacement on weight-bearing and for the lowering of the medial longitudinal arch necessary for shock absorption. After these changes have been made, an orthotic shell is molded along the plantar surface, ending just proximal to the metatarsal heads. An angled wedge or post is then added to the plantar anterolateral shell, bringing the bisection of the rearfoot to a vertical position (Fig. 15.44).

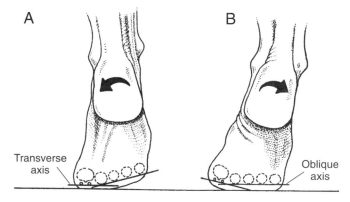

Figure 15.43. A. Ideally, the subtalar joint pronates during late propulsion, allowing the final push-off to occur around the transverse metatarsal axis. **B.** When a rigid forefoot valgus deformity is present, the rigid and inverted rearfoot is unable to pronate through the range necessary to access the transverse metatarsal axis. The foot is forced to roll off its oblique metatarsal axis.

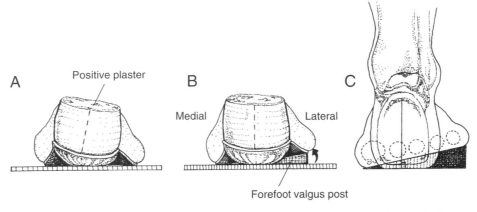

Figure 15.44. A–C. Posterior view of the right positive model. A forefoot valgus post is placed under the lateral forefoot, bringing the sagittal bisection of the rearfoot to vertical.

This post should never exceed 15° because shoe fit becomes a problem and the distal lateral shell may dig into the shaft of the fifth metatarsal. When a large post angle is necessary, the posting should be extended under the metatarsal heads to allow for continued control throughout the propulsive period. Without this extension, the foot with a large forefoot valgus deformity (i.e., greater than 4°) would tip laterally during early propulsion. This could result in continued symptomatology as propulsive period forces continue to be transferred along the post-axial fibular border.

When a flexible forefoot valgus deformity is present, the shell of the orthotic (specifically, the calcaneal incline angle) will limit excessive subtalar pronation, whereas the forefoot post will prevent lateral instability. Schoenhaus and Jay (58) claim that if initiated early, use of a functional orthotic will prevent severe hallux abductovalgus and bunion formation.

When the forefoot valgus deformity is rigid, the forefoot post is invaluable during propulsion. It assists in the development of a high-gear push-off by shifting the progression of forces medially through the transverse axis of the metatarsal heads. Use of the high-gear push-off will improve the windlass effect of the plantar fascia, displace the transfer of vertical forces away from the post-axial fibular border, and minimize stretching of the more lateral interdigital nerves as the lesser toes dorsiflex through smaller ranges. The forefoot post will also be effective during the contact period; it prevents excessive subtalar supination. This allows for a more equal distribution of ground-reactive forces across the metatarsal heads, which lessens the potential for painful plantar calluses.

It must be stressed that even though the forefoot valgus post prevents excessive rearfoot in-

version during the contact period, it is unable to provide the continued range of subtalar pronation necessary for adequate shock absorption. This is because the forefoot post should only be large enough to bring the subtalar joint to its neutral position. Although overposting the lateral forefoot to increase the range of subtalar pronation would be beneficial during the contact period because it would improve the foot's ability to absorb shock, it would be detrimental during early propulsion because it would forcefully maintain the subtalar joint in a pronated position as vertical forces peak. This could eventually lead to plastic deformity of the spring ligament, chronic medial Achilles peritendinitis, and/or chronic strain of the soleus muscle, which fires vigorously during propulsion in an attempt to reestablish subtalar neutrality by inverting the entire foot up and over the oversized post.

The only way the individual with a rigid forefoot valgus deformity can properly absorb shock is if the subtalar joint possesses adequate ranges of pronation. Because this motion is frequently limited in these persons, many high-impact symptoms will continue despite proper use of the forefoot post. It is for this reason that several authors claim that rigid foot types respond less favorably to orthotic therapies (62, 63). However, the rigidity of the foot does not necessitate a poor prognosis. By vigorously manipulating the fibrotic articulations, the individual is often able to resume a symptom-free life style. Hiss (53) notes that even slight increases in joint mobility often produce dramatic reductions in pain. It must be stressed that when a limited range of subtalar pronation is present bilaterally and/or the joint's end play lacks the normal feel associated with joint dysfunction, it should be suspected that the limited range of motion is the result of a triarticulated subtalar joint, which makes manipulation a contraindication.

Even if increasing the range of subtalar pronation is not possible, the symptomatology associated with a rigid forefoot valgus may still be lessened by simply inserting shock-absorbing material under the heel, recommending sneakers with well-cushioned midsoles, and/or instructing the individual to walk with shorter strides. McKenzie et al. (32) advocate that individuals with cavus feet should wear slip-lasted, curve-lasted shoes with softer ethylene vinyl acetate (EVA) midsoles. Also, to minimize patient frustration with a treatment program, these individuals should be informed that they are typically slow healers. In one study relating certain foot types to knee injuries in runners, Lutter (64) noted that cavus-related injuries required 85 days before full return to running was possible, whereas the pronation-related injuries required only 46 days.

Ankle Dorsiflexion

With the subtalar joint maintained in neutral, the ankle must be able to dorsiflex a minimum of 10° for walking and 25° for jogging (65); even greater ranges are necessary for speed walking.

During stance phase, the ankle reaches its maximally dorsiflexed position just before heel lift (Fig. 15.45). The greater the range of hip extension during late midstance (as with running and speed walking), the greater the range of ankle dorsiflexion necessary to compensate. If the ankle is unable to move through the range needed to compensate for hip extension, the foot will attempt to supply the remaining range by

pronating the subtalar joint. This action tilts the oblique midtarsal joint axis into a more horizontal position, which allows for greater amounts of forefoot dorsiflexion (Fig. 15.46). Although this movement allows for increased amounts of forefoot dorsiflexion, it may be damaging in that it unlocks the articulations during propulsion and prevents locking of the calcaneocuboid joint. It also inhibits the approximation of the anterior and posterior pillars, as the windlass mechanism becomes nonfunctional (which greatly stresses the plantar fascia as the origin and insertion of this tissue are moving in opposite directions).

If for any reason the subtalar and midtarsal joints are unable to compensate fully for a limited range of ankle dorsiflexion, the individual will be

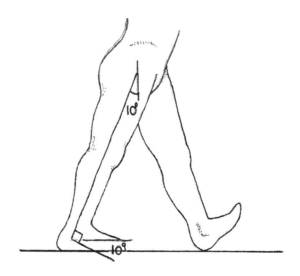

Figure 15.45. The range of ankle dorsiflexion should equal the range of hip extension.

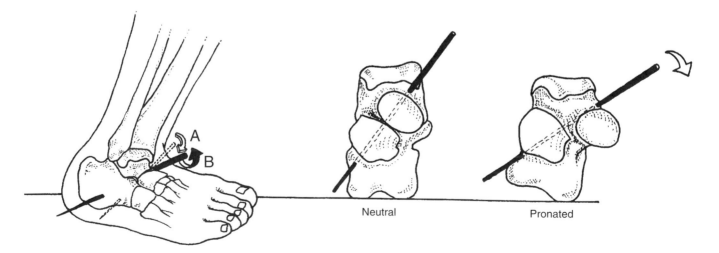

Figure 15.46. A. Normally, the oblique midtarsal joint axis lies 52° to the transverse plane and allows for relatively large ranges of forefoot abduction. **B.** When a limited range of ankle dorsiflexion is present, pronation of the subtalar joint will shift the oblique midtarsal joint axis into a more horizontal position, which allows the forefoot to dorsiflex around this axis.

Neutral   Pronated

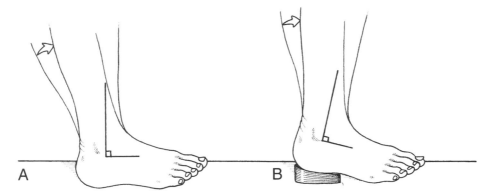

Figure 15.47. Use of a heel lift significantly increases the range of available ankle dorsiflexion.

predisposed to a metatarsal stress syndrome. The inertial forces associated with forward progression of the body will forcefully drive the heads of the longest metatarsals into the ground. Also, a restriction in ankle dorsiflexion may damage the anterior talotibial articulation; the leading edge of the anterior inferior tibia is often forced to collide into the sulcus on the dorsal talar neck (66).

If there is only a slight limitation in ankle dorsiflexion, the distal tibiofibular articulation will attempt to accommodate the talar sulcus by gapping anteriorly; that is, this articulation may gap as much as 1.5 mm anteriorly (67). However, the ability of this syndesmotic joint to accommodate the talar neck is limited at best. Over time, the repeated contact between the talar neck and distal tibia results in a bony reaction with the eventual formation of an impingement exostosis (66). O'Donoghue (66) states that "this reaction has an adverse rather than protective effect [in that] the more bone that is piled up, the more easily impingement occurs, and so a vicious cycle is formed resulting in gradually increased disability." The author notes that the pain associated with the impingement exostosis is readily exacerbated by activities that increase the demands for ankle dorsiflexion, such as fast running, walking up hills, and prolonged squatting.

Treatment of a limited range of ankle dorsiflexion varies. If the range is limited by muscular contracture, various static and dynamic stretches should be performed with the rearfoot maintained in an inverted position to prevent midtarsal compensation. (This maintains integrity of the medial arch by locking the midtarsal joint.) If the range is limited by joint dysfunction, manipulation is the treatment of choice. If the range of ankle dorsiflexion is limited by bony restriction (such as an impingement exostosis or a congenitally wide anterior talus),

restoration of ankle dorsiflexion is not possible and conservative treatment dictates that a heel lift be used to prevent damaging the medial longitudinal arch (Fig. 15.47).

It should be emphasized that decreased ankle dorsiflexion, by itself, is not treated with a foot orthotic. If an orthotic is prescribed to control the propulsive period pronation associated with a limited range of ankle dorsiflexion, iatrogenic injury might result. The midtarsals would collide into the arch of the orthotic as they attempt to compensate for the impaired ankle motion. If there are structural deformities in addition to a decreased range of ankle dorsiflexion, a posted orthotic may be used, but only in conjunction with a heel lift and a slight lowering of the medial arch.

Summary

Although these described parameters represent only a few of the more commonly seen deformities responsible for foot and ankle dysfunction, it is hoped that they give the reader a sense of how structural and/or kinetic variations may go on to produce abnormal movement patterns. By coupling the manual skills necessary to treat hypomobile articulations with an understanding of how foot orthoses may control excessive motion, the practitioner has the ability to favorably modify lower extremity movement patterns in a wide range of situations. This is invaluable in the prevention and treatment of sports-related injuries.

References

1. Bojsen-Moller F. Anatomy of the forefoot, normal and pathologic. Clin Orthop 1979;142:10.
2. Magee D. Orthopedic physical assessment. Philadelphia: WB Saunders, 1987:317.
3. Subotnick S. Normal biomechanics. In: Subotnick S, ed. Sports medicine of the lower extremity. New York: Churchill Livingstone, 1989:140.

4. Inman VT, Ralston JH, Todd F. Human walking. Baltimore: Williams & Wilkins, 1981.

5. Root MC, Orion WP, Weed JH. Normal and abnormal function of the foot. Los Angeles: Clinical Biomechanics, 1977.

6. Lambrinudi C. New operation on drop foot. Br J Surg 1927;15:193–200.

7. Bruckner J. Variations in the human subtalar joint. J Orthop Sports Phys Ther 1987;8:489–494.

8. Manter JT. Movements of the subtalar and transverse tarsal joints. Anat Rec 1941;80:397–409.

9. Green DR, Whitney AK, Walters P. Subtalar joint motions. J Am Podiatry Assoc 1979;69:83.

10. Root ML, Weed JH, Sgarlato TE, et al. Axis of motion of the subtalar joint. J Am Podiatry Assoc 1966;56:149.

11. Hicks JH. The mechanics of the foot. J Anat 1954;88:25–31.

12. Bojsen-Moller F. Calcaneocuboid joint and stability of the longitudinal arch of the foot at high and low gear push-off. J Anat 1979;129:165–176.

13. Basmajian JV, Deluca CJ. Muscles alive their functions revealed by electromyography. 5th. ed. Baltimore: Williams & Wilkins, 1985;377.

14. Radin EL, Paul IL. Does cartilage compliance reduce skeletal impact loads: the relative force-alternating properties of articular cartilage, synovial fluid, periarticular soft tissues and bone. Arthritis Rheum 1970;197.

15. Subotnick SI. Biomechanics of the subtalar and midtarsal joints. J Am Podiatry Assoc 1975;65:756–764.

16. Phillips RD, Phillips RL. Quantitative analysis of the locking position of the midtarsal joint. J Am Podiatry Assoc 1983;73:518–522.

17. Ker RF, Bennett MB, Bibby SR, et al. The spring in the arch of the human foot. Nature 1987;325:147–149.

18. Scranton PE, et al. Support phase kinematics of the foot. In: Bateman JE, Trott AW, eds. The foot and ankle. New York: Brian C. Decker, 1980.

19. Hunt GC. Examination of lower extremity dysfunction. In: Gould JA, Davies GJ, eds. Orthopaedic and sports physical therapy. St. Louis: CV Mosby, 1985:408–436.

20. Michaud TC. Aberrancy of the midtarsal locking mechanism as a causative factor in recurrent ankle sprains. J Manipulative Physiol Ther 1989;12:135–141.

21. Hutton WC, Dhanedran M. The mechanics of normal and hallux valgus feet, a quantitative study. Clin Orthop 1981;157:7–13.

22. Mero A, Komi P. Electromyographic activity in sprinting at speeds ranging from sub-maximal to supra-maximal. Med Sci Sports Exerc 1987;19:266–274.

23. McPoil TG, Knecht HG, Schuit D. A survey of foot types in normal females between the ages of 18 and 30 years. J Orthop Sports Phys Ther 1988;9:406–409.

24. Hlavac H. Compensated forefoot varus. J Am Podiatry Assoc 1970;60:229–233.

25. Cavanaugh PR. The shoe-ground interface in running. In: Mack RP, ed. Symposium on the foot and leg in running sports. St. Louis: CV Mosby, 1982:30–44.

26. Messier SP, Pittala KA. Etiologic factors associated with selected running injuries. MSSE 1988;20:501–505.

27. Mann RA. Biomechanics of running. In: Mack RP, ed. Symposium on the foot and leg in running sports. St. Louis: CV Mosby, 1982:1–29.

28. Noble CA. Iliotibial band friction syndrome in runners. Am J Sports Med 1980;8:232–234.

29. Matheson GO, et al. Stress fractures in athletes: a study of 320 cases. Am J Sports Med 1987;15:46–58.

30. Riegger C. Mechanical properties of bone. In: Gould JA, Davies GJ, eds. Orthopaedic and sports physical therapy. St. Louis: CV Mosby, 1985:3–49.

31. Lutter LD. Foot related knee problems in the long distance runner. Foot Ankle 1980;1:112–116.

32. McKenzie DC, Clement DB, Taunton JE. Running shoes, orthotics and injuries. Sports Med 1985;2:234–247.

33. D'Amico JC, Rubin M. The influence of foot orthoses on the quadriceps angle. J Am Podiatr Med Assoc 1986,76:337–339.

34. Kegerreis S, Malone T, Johnson F. The diagonal medial plica: an underestimated clinical entity. J Orthop Sports Phys Ther 1988;9:305–309.

35. Huberti HH, Hayes WC. Patellofemoral contact pressures. J Bone Joint Surg 1984;66:715–724. Abstract.

36. Bates BT, Osternig LR, Mason B, et al. Foot orthotic devices to modify selected aspects of lower extremity mechanics. Am J Sports Med 1979;7:338–342.

37. Clarke TE, Frederick EC, Hlavac HF. Effects of a soft orthotic device on rearfoot movement in running. Podiatr Sports Med 1983;1:20–23.

38. Novick A, Kelley DL. Position and movement changes of the foot with orthotic intervention during the loading response of gait. J Orthop Sports Phys Ther 1990;7:301–312.

39. Smart GW, Taunton JE, Clement DB. Achilles tendon disorders in runners: a review. Med Sci Sports Exerc 1980;12:231–243.

40. Straus WL. Growth of the human foot and its evolutionary significance. Contrib Embryol 1927;101:95.

41. McPoil T. Cameron JA, Adrian JF. Anatomical characteristics of the talus in relation to forefoot deformities. J Am Podiatr Med Assoc 1987;77:77–81.

42. Coplan JA. Rotational motion of the knee: a comparison of normal and pronating subjects. J Orthop Sports Phys Ther 1989;10:366–369.

43. Glancy J. Orthotic control of ground reaction forces during running: a preliminary report. Orthotics Prosthetics 1984;38:12–40.

44. Kopell P, Thompson WL. Peripheral entrapment neuropathies. Baltimore: Williams & Wilkins, 1963:32.

45. Kuritz HM, Sokoloff TH. Tarsal tunnel syndrome. J Am Podiatry Assoc 1975;65:830.

46. Murphy PC, Baxter DE. Nerve entrapment of the foot and ankle in runners. Clin Sports Med 1985;4:753–763.

47. Przylucki H, Jones CL. Entrapment neuropathy of the muscle branch of lateral plantar nerve: a cause of heel pain. J Am Podiatry Assoc 1981;71:119–124.

48. Neale D, Hooper G, Clowes C, et al. Adult foot disorder. In: Neale D, ed. Common foot disorders, diagnosis and management: a general clinical guide. Edinburgh: Churchill Livingstone, 1981:56–57.

49. Newell SG. Conservative treatment of plantar fasciitis. Phys Sportsmed 1977;5:68–73.

50. Michaud TC. Pathomechanics and treatment of hallux limitus: a case report. Chiro Sports Med 1988;2:55–60.

51. Spencer AM. Practical podiatric orthopedic procedures. Cleveland: Ohio College of Podiatric Medicine, 1978.

52. Waller JF. Hindfoot and midfoot problems of the runner. In: Mack RP, ed. Symposium on the foot and leg in running sports. St. Louis: CV Mosby, 1982:71.

53. Hiss JM. Functional foot disorders. Los Angeles: The Oxford Press, 1949.

54. Burns MF. Non-weightbearing cast impressions for the construction of orthotic devices. J Am Podiatry Assoc 1977;67:790–795.

55. Sgarlato TE. A compendium of podiatric biomechanics. San Francisco: California College of Podiatric Medicine, 1971.

56. Lutter LD. Cavus foot in runners. Foot Ankle 1981;1:225–228.

57. Lariviere JY, Miladi L, Dubousset JF, et al. Medial pes cavus in children: a study of failures following Dwyer's procedure. Revue de Chirurgie Orthopedique 1985;71:563–573.

58. Schoenhaus HD, Jay RM. Cavus deformities, conservative management. J Am Podiatry Assoc 1980;70:235–238.

59. Katoh Y, Chao EYS, Laughman RK, et al. Biomechanical analysis of foot function during gait and clinical applications. Clin Orthop 1983;177:23–33.

60. Cangialosi CP, Schall SJ. The biomechanical aspects of anterior tarsal tunnel syndrome. J Am Podiatry Assoc 1980;70:291–292.
61. Carrier PA, Janigan JD, Smith SD, et al. Morton's neuralgia: a possible contributing etiology. J Am Podiatry Assoc 1975;65:315–321.
62. Bordelon RL. Surgical and conservative foot care. Thorofare, NJ: Slack, 1988:179.
63. D'Ambrosia R, Drez D. Prevention and treatment of running injuries. Thorofare, NJ: Slack, 1982.
64. Lutter LD. Orthopedic management of runners in the foot and ankle. In: Batemen JE, Trott AW, eds. The foot and ankle. New York: Thieme-Stratton, 1980.
65. Scranton PE, et al. Forces under the foot: a study of walking, jogging and sprinting: force distribution under normal and abnormal foot. In: Batement JE, Trott AW, eds. The foot and ankle. New York: Thieme-Stratton, 1980.
66. O'Donoghue DII. Impingcmcnt cxostosis of the talus and tibia. J Bone Joint Surg 1957;39:835–852.
67. Close JR. Some applications of the functional anatomy of the ankle joint. J Bone Joint Surg 1956;38:761–781.

Injuries of the Leg, Ankle, and Foot

Ted L. Forcum

REGIONAL FUNCTIONAL ANATOMY

To treat injuries of the lower extremity effectively, one must first have a general understanding of the functional anatomy of this region. Most sports, with the exception of swimming, require a closed kinetic chain activity throughout this region. With the foot and ankle acting as the base of this chain, they can have a significant effect on how the body performs, not only through the lower extremities, but also into the upper quadrant.

The foot and ankle are composed of 28 bones and 55 articulations that allow for shock absorption, propulsion, and mobile adaptation to uneven surfaces. This region bears the weight of the entire body and a great deal of force is transmitted through it, which may further complicate treatment and recovery processes.

Functional Anatomy of the Leg

The lower leg is supported by 2 bones and 13 muscles. The tibia, the larger of the two bones, bears approximately five sixths of the body's weight. The fibula bears approximately one sixth of the body's weight. The fibula is attached laterally to the tibia, via a facetal articulation both proximally and distally. The proximal head of the fibula has a facet on the superior surface that articulates with the tibia just inferior to the lateral tibial plateau. The common peroneal nerve courses just posterior to the head of the fibula, where it wraps anteriorly and divides into the deep peroneal nerve and the superficial peroneal nerve. The distal facet of the fibula articulates with the tibia and the lateral facet of the dome of the talus. This distal end, the lateral malleolus, forms the lateral portion of the ankle mortise joint. The fibula's medial border forms a sharp edge where the attachment of the interosseous membrane unites the tibia and fibula, dividing the anterior compartment of the leg from the deep posterior compartment. There are four distinct compartments to the lower leg, divided by the tibia, fibula, and its strong fascial membranes.

These compartments are the anterior, lateral, posterior, and deep posterior.

Anterior Crural Compartment

The anterior crural compartment houses the tibialis anterior, extensor digitorum longus, peroneus tertius, and extensor hallucis longus muscles (Fig. 16.1). It also contains the deep peroneal nerve and the anterior tibial vessels (1).

The tibialis anterior originates at the lateral tibial condyle and the upper two thirds of the lateral tibia, attaching to the intermembranous septum. It courses anteriorly down the leg and medially across the foot, attaching to the plantar medial cuneiform and the base of the first metatarsal. The tibialis anterior acts to dorsiflex and invert the foot.

The tibialis anterior's eccentric action of controlling plantarflexion of the foot subsequent to heel strike during gait is clinically important. As with all the muscles in the anterior compartment, it is innervated by the deep peroneal nerve. The extensor hallucis longus originates in the midhalf of the anterior fibula and the interosseous membrane, coursing anteriorly down the leg and medially across the foot. It attaches to the distal phalanx of the great toe, allowing for extension of the great toe and dorsiflexion of the foot with some lateral rotation of the forefoot.

The extensor digitorum longus originates at the lateral tibial condyle, the upper three fourths of the anterior fibula, and the interosseous membrane. It courses anteriorly down the leg and across the dorsum of the foot inserting at the middle and distal phalanges of the second through fifth toes. This muscle acts to extend the phalanges and assist in dorsiflexion (2).

The peroneus tertius originates at the distal anterior fibula and intermuscular septum. It courses laterally to the base of the fifth metatarsal. Its insertion is known to be variable and primarily acts to evert the foot and assist in dorsiflexion.

The tendons of the anterior compartment all possess a synovial sheath that surrounds the

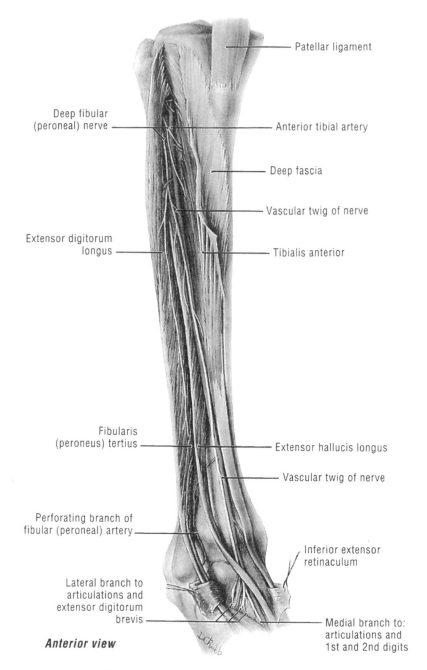

Patellar ligament

Deep fibular (peroneal) nerve

Anterior tibial artery

Deep fascia

Vascular twig of nerve

Extensor digitorum longus

Tibialis anterior

Fibularis (peroneus) tertius

Extensor hallucis longus

Vascular twig of nerve

Perforating branch of fibular (peroneal) artery

Inferior extensor retinaculum

Lateral branch to articulations and extensor digitorum brevis

Medial branch to: articulations and 1st and 2nd digits

Anterior view

Figure 16.1. Anatomy of the anterior crural compartment. (Reprinted with permission from Agur AR. Grant's atlas of anatomy. 9th ed. Baltimore: Williams & Wilkins, 1991.)

tendons in the region of the ankle mortise. The tendons are bound by a superior retinaculum proximal to the malleoli and an inferior extensor retinaculum. These retinaculi prevent tendon bowing during active dorsiflexion of the foot.

Lateral Crural Compartment

The lateral compartment is bordered by the anterior crural intermuscular septum anteriorly, with the fibula medially, and with the posterior crural intermuscular septum posteriorly. The lateral compartment houses two muscles, the peroneus longus and the peroneus brevis. Both of

these muscles act to plantarflex the ankle and evert the foot. They are supplied by the superficial peroneal nerve, a branch of the common peroneal nerve (2).

The peroneus longus originates at the lateral tibial condyle and the head and upper two thirds of the lateral fibula. The muscle courses laterally down the leg with its tendon arcing posteriorly around the lateral malleolus, diving inferiorly around the cuboid bone to insert on the medial cuneiform and the base of the first metatarsal. This muscle provides foot eversion and some eversion and plantarflexion of the first ray.

Because of the oblique angle with which the peroneus longus attaches to the base of the first metatarsal, it is important in the maintenance of the medial transverse and lateral longitudinal arches.

The peroneus brevis originates from the distal one third of the fibula and courses laterally down the leg, with this tendon arcing posteriorly to the lateral malleolus attaching to the styloid process and the superior base of the fifth metatarsal. The peroneus longus and the peroneus brevis occupy a common synovial sheath that passes posteriorly to the lateral malleoli (using it as a pulley) and inferiorly to the peroneal trochlea or tubercle. The peroneus brevis appears to be much less involved in this process. The belly of the peroneus brevis lies deep to the peroneus longus.

The two muscles of the lateral compartment are supplied by the superficial peroneal nerve. These fibers originate from the L5-S1 nerve roots. The superficial peroneal nerve courses from a posterior to anterior position as it wraps around the neck of the fibula, then descends inferiorly down the anterior crural intermuscular septum (Fig. 16.2). The nerve penetrates the deep fascia to be-

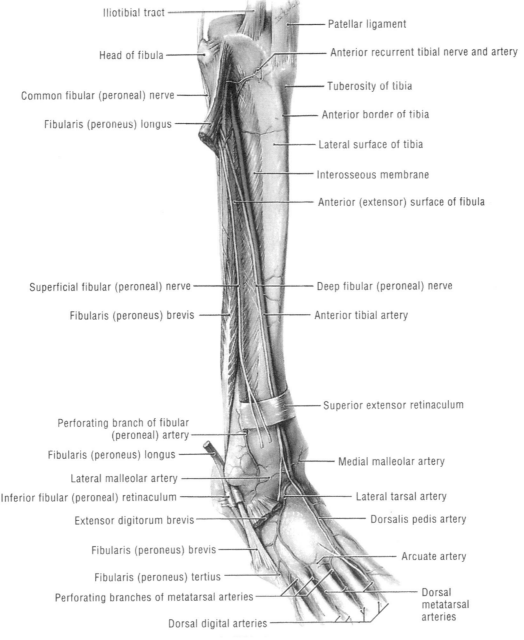

Figure 16.2. Anatomy of the lateral crural compartment. (Reprinted with permission from Agur AR. Grant's atlas of anatomy. 9th ed. Baltimore: Williams & Wilkins, 1991.)

come superficial in the distal one third of the leg. There it supplies sensation to the skin on the lower part of the leg, dorsum of the foot, and the toes, with the exception of the first interdigital web.

There are no primary arteries of the lateral compartment. Vasculature is fed into the compartment via branches from the posterior tibial artery.

Superficial Posterior Crural Compartments

The posterior crural compartment, divided into two groups of structures by the transverse crural intermuscular septum, functionally acts as two distinct compartments. The superficial posterior compartment contains four muscles: the gastrocnemius, soleus, plantaris, and popliteus. The muscles from this group provide 80% of the plantarflexion force at the ankle. The popliteus, however, does not cross the ankle joint; rather, it crosses the knee. The popliteus originates from the lateral femoral condyle and popliteal ligament to insert on the posterior tibia. This muscle is innervated by the medial or interior popliteal nerve, a branch of the tibial nerve that originates from the L4-5 and S1-3 nerve roots. Its primary action is to flex the knee and medially rotate the tibia.

Moving more superficially, the soleus originates from the head and upper one third of the fibula, middle third of the medial tibia, and the intermuscular septum (Fig. 16.3). The soleus shares its attachment to the middle posterior calcaneus with the gastrocnemius.

The plantaris muscle lies between the gastrocnemius and soleus, running obliquely from its origin at the lateral supracondylar line of the femur to the medial posterior aspect of the calcaneus as part of the medial Achilles tendon. The muscle is relatively short and its size will vary considerably. The plantaris is a muscle of disputed significance and may be absent within the general population.

The gastrocnemius is composed of two heads, the medial and lateral. They originate from the lateral and medial femoral condyle, respectively. Both the soleus and the gastrocnemius act to plantarflex the foot; however, the gastrocnemius crosses the knee joint and therefore also assists with knee flexion. Both the gastrocnemius and soleus are innervated by the medial popliteal nerve, a branch of the tibial nerve.

Deep Posterior Crural Compartment

The deep posterior compartment, commonly referred to as the medial compartment, is composed of three muscles (sometimes referred to as Tom, Dick, and Harry): the tibialis posterior, flexor

digitorum longus, and flexor hallucis longus (Fig. 16.4). Some texts will refer to the popliteus as being part of the deep compartment, rather than the superficial compartment (2).

The tibialis posterior is a muscle of great clinical significance. It originates in the posterior lateral tibia, upper two thirds of the medial fibula, and intermuscular septum. The muscle lies deep within the leg, and its tendon pulleys around the medial malleolus to attach to the navicular tubercle, plantar cuneiforms, and base of the second, third, and fourth metatarsals. The tibialis posterior can have up to eight insertions on the plantar aspect of the foot. This muscle acts to plantarflex the ankle and invert the foot, thereby maintaining the medial longitudinal arch and eccentrically controlling pronation (1).

The tibialis posterior, along with all the muscles of the deep posterior compartment, is innervated by the medial or internal popliteal nerve. The medial popliteal nerve is a branch of the tibial nerve, which is derived from the L4, L5, and S1-3 nerve roots.

The flexor digitorum longus originates from the middle three fifths of the posterior tibia and the intermuscular septum. It courses medially across the ankle, posterior to the medial malleolus, to attach to the distal phalanges of the second through fifth toes. This muscle acts to flex the toes, plantarflex the foot, and invert the ankle.

The flexor hallucis longus originates from the distal one third of the posterior fibula and the interosseous membrane. It inserts at the distal phalanx of the hallux to create flexion of the great toe. All these tendons possess a synovial sheath and are bound at the ankle by the flexor retinaculum.

Functional Anatomy of the Ankle and Foot

The functional anatomy and biomechanics of the ankle and foot are discussed in detail in Chapter 15. However, some specific anatomical features of clinical relevance will be discussed individually with each appropriate condition.

Sensory Innervation of the Lower Leg, Ankle, and Foot

The dermatomes of the lower leg, ankle, and foot are derived from the L3-S2 nerve roots (Fig. 16.5). The L3 dermatome descends across the anterior thigh to the medial aspect of the proximal leg to midcalf. The L4 dermatome descends the anterior leg, across the patella medially, to the medial malleolus and the medial aspect of the foot, providing sensation through the medial half of the hallux. The L5 dermatome descends ante-

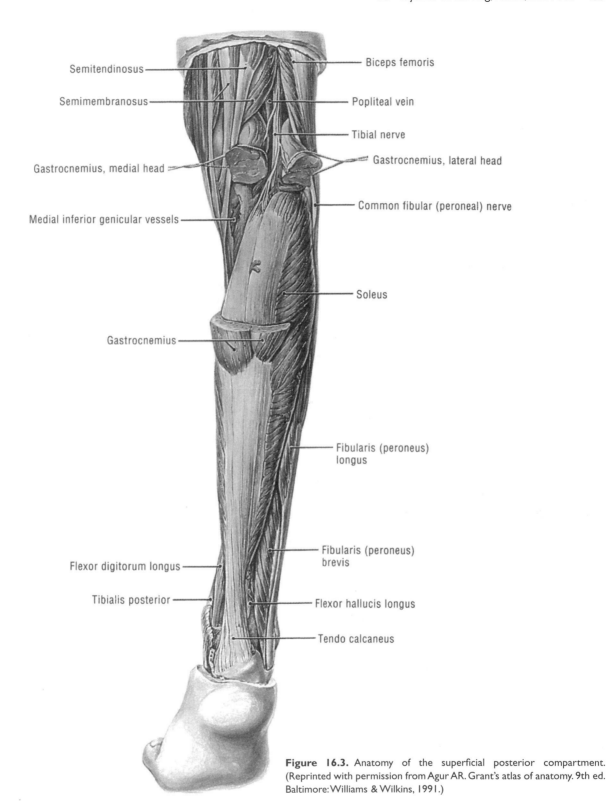

Semitendinosus

Semimembranosus

Gastrocnemius, medial head

Medial inferior genicular vessels

Gastrocnemius

Flexor digitorum longus

Tibialis posterior

Biceps femoris

Popliteal vein

Tibial nerve

Gastrocnemius, lateral head

Common fibular (peroneal) nerve

Soleus

Fibularis (peroneus) longus

Fibularis (peroneus) brevis

Flexor hallucis longus

Tendo calcaneus

Figure 16.3. Anatomy of the superficial posterior compartment. (Reprinted with permission from Agur AR. Grant's atlas of anatomy. 9th ed. Baltimore: Williams & Wilkins, 1991.)

rior laterally to the anterior aspect of the ankle and the dorsum of the foot, providing sensation to the lateral half of the hallux to the fourth phalanx. It also provides sensation to the lateral plantar aspect of the heel, plantar aspect of the lateral foot, and the fourth digit through lateral aspect of the

hallux. The S1 dermatome descends the postero-lateral leg, providing sensation to the lateral foot excluding the heel. The S2 dermatome descends the midline of the lower leg, providing sensation to the posterior and medial aspect of the leg calcaneus and medial arch (3, 4).

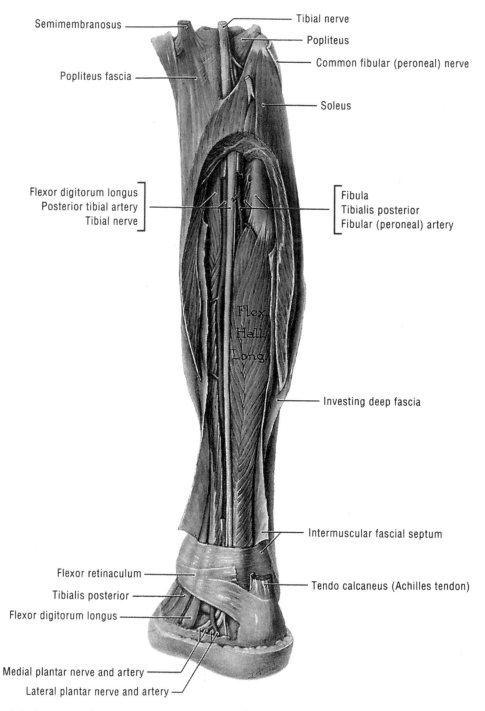

Semimembranosus

Popliteus fascia

Flexor digitorum longus
Posterior tibial artery
Tibial nerve

Flex.
Hall.
Long.

Flexor retinaculum

Tibialis posterior

Flexor digitorum longus

Medial plantar nerve and artery

Lateral plantar nerve and artery

Tibial nerve

Popliteus

Common fibular (peroneal) nerve

Soleus

Fibula
Tibialis posterior
Fibular (peroneal) artery

Investing deep fascia

Intermuscular fascial septum

Tendo calcaneus (Achilles tendon)

Figure 16.4. Anatomy of the deep posterior compartment. (Reprinted with permission from Agur AR. Grant's atlas of anatomy. 9th ed. Baltimore: Williams & Wilkins, 1991.)

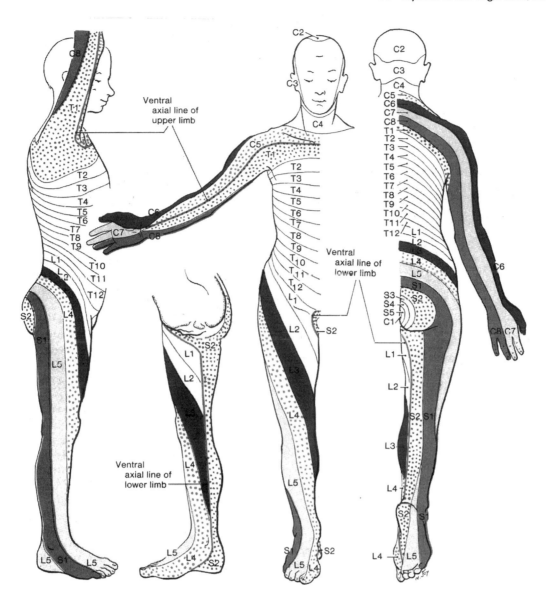

Figure 16.5. Dermatomes of the lower extremity. (Reprinted with permission from Moore KL. Clinically oriented anatomy. 2nd ed. Baltimore: Williams & Wilkins, 1985.)

Dermatomal and trigger point pain referral should be considered when pain extends into the lower leg, ankle, and foot without objective or provoking clinical findings within this region.

INJURIES OF THE LOWER LEG, FOOT, AND ANKLE

Compartment Syndromes of the Leg

As discussed previously, the leg is divided into four compartments that are divided by bony and fascial elements (Fig. 16.6). Some authors believe that the tibialis posterior muscle may be considered a fifth compartment bound by an additional fascial layer (5). Likewise, the foot is divided into fascial compartments and may range from four to six individual compartments.

All these compartments may develop a compartment syndrome, a condition of elevated intercompartmental pressure. With exercise, muscular volume may increase 20%. In compartment syndrome, the fascial layers do not allow for accommodation of the additional volume. The result is the collapse of the venous return system and neurocompression.

The most common cause of compartment syndrome is overexertion by those unaccustomed to a particular level of exercise.

Acute Compartment Syndrome

Acute compartment syndrome is a medical emergency requiring immediate surgical fascial release to reduce intercompartmental compression, thus preventing permanent neurologic and

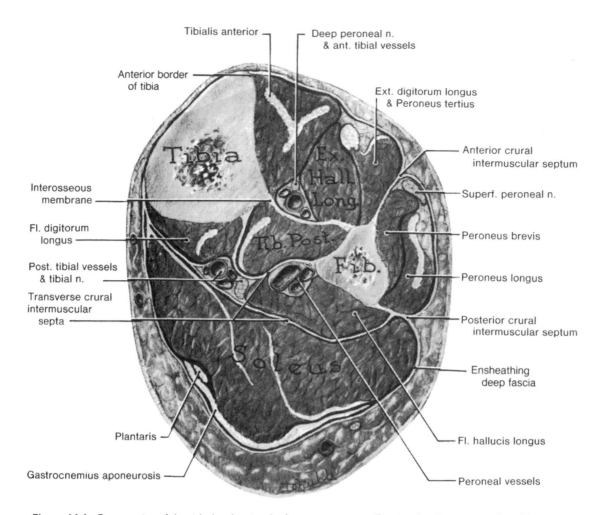

Tibialis anterior

Anterior border of tibia

Deep peroneal n. & ant. tibial vessels

Ext. digitorum longus & Peroneus tertius

Anterior crural intermuscular septum

Superf. peroneal n.

Interosseous membrane

Fl. digitorum longus

Peroneus brevis

Peroneus longus

Post. tibial vessels & tibial n.

Transverse crural intermuscular septa

Posterior crural intermuscular septum

Ensheathing deep fascia

Plantaris

Gastrocnemius aponeurosis

Fl. hallucis longus

Peroneal vessels

Figure 16.6. Cross-section of the right leg showing the four compartments. (Reprinted with permission from Moore KL. Clinically oriented anatomy. 2nd ed. Baltimore: Williams & Wilkins, 1985.)

muscular damage. Acute compartment syndrome may result from seemingly minor injury or overexertion (6). The injury may not even be in direct proximity of the compartment involved. For example, there have been reported cases of compartment syndrome after oral maxillofacial surgery (7). Prolonged compression may also cause an acute onset of compartment syndrome (8), such as the use of pneumatic antishock trousers after surgery or for the treatment of hypovolemic shock (9, 10). Compartment syndrome has even been observed after a person falls asleep on the involved extremity (11). Exercise-induced acute compartment syndrome usually presents unilaterally. A bilateral presentation is typically associated with a pre-existing medical condition (12).

Chronic Compartment Syndrome

Chronic compartment syndrome typically affects young people (13 to 30 years of age) who are engaged in endurance sports (13). However, it is also common in sports such as karate, volleyball, and soccer.

Although history and clinical findings alone are sufficient to establish a diagnosis of chronic compartment syndrome, diagnostic confirmation should use slit catheter readings of intracompartmental pressures. One or more of the following intramuscular pressures would be considered diagnostic of chronic compartment syndrome in the lower leg: a preexercise pressure greater than 15 mm Hg, a 1-minute postexercise pressure greater than 30 mm Hg, and a 5-minute postexercise pressure greater than 20 mm Hg (14). The pressure recordings in the deep posterior compartment may depend on which muscle is involved and may vary from the above-mentioned readings (15).

In compartment syndromes, pain increases as the level of exercise exertion progresses. This is unlike a tendinitis, in which pain may occur initially but will decrease as the muscles warm up. Symptoms are often characterized by numbness or tingling in the nerve that traverses through that particular compartment. Typically, symptoms are alleviated promptly with the conclusion of exercise. Symptoms may be affected by sudden weather changes, particularly a high-pressure front followed by a low-pressure front. The reduced external pressure may produce a relative increase of pressure within a compartment with poor venous drainage.

In-office evaluation may be fairly unremarkable; however, evaluation immediately after exercise may demonstrate a reduction of pulse from the artery descending from the compartment of the leg (usually the dorsal pedal or the posterior tibial artery). Fullness and firmness within the muscular compartment may be present on palpation. An electromyography (EMG) study may note a reduction of nerve conduction through the nerves of the compartment. Within the anterior compartment, the compression of the deep peroneal nerve may create muscular paralysis of the tibialis anterior and a drop foot with a steppage gait.

Approximately 45% of those with chronic compartment syndrome are found to have a muscular herniation (14). Such syndromes may also be characterized histologically by an accumulation of intermyofibrillar lipid globules (16).

Compartment syndromes are most commonly found in the anterior and deep posterior compartments, followed by the lateral and superficial compartments. Seventy-five percent of these cases occur bilaterally.

Deep posterior compartment syndromes demonstrate pain on stretching and resistance postexercise; there may be a diminished posterior tibial pulse, which should raise concern for the onset of an acute compartment syndrome. Sensory changes may be noted on the sole of the foot and, rarely, into the toes (17). Deep posterior compartment syndrome can be categorized as a Type III medial tibial stress syndrome.

Anterior compartment syndrome may demonstrate weakness of the toe extensors and foot dorsiflexors, and pain may be produced on stretching these structures. The dorsal pedal pulse may be diminished. The affected nerve is the deep peroneal, which distributes sensation to the dorsum of the foot. Compression within the anterior compartment of the leg will distinctly cause paresthesia at the web space between the first and second toes (18, 19).

If the superficial posterior compartment is affected, the athlete may demonstrate pain on resisted plantarflexion and dorsiflexion stretching of the ankle. The sural nerve may become depressed, creating sensory changes in the lateral foot (17).

Syndromes in the lateral compartment may demonstrate weakness, with eversion and pain on stretching into ankle inversion. The nerve involved is the superficial peroneal nerve, which may create sensory changes within the dorsum of the foot and toes.

Arterial entrapment syndrome should be considered as a differential diagnosis when compartment syndrome is suspected. The most common arterial entrapment syndrome in young athletes is entrapment of the popliteal artery by the medial head of the gastrocnemius or the soleal fascia. A family history of occlusive vascular disease and the presence of atrophic changes in skin and nail beds should be evaluated.

Conservative treatment of chronic compartment syndrome should begin with training modification. The hydrostatic pressure of deep water training may be beneficial for maintaining aerobic fitness. Biomechanics, training surfaces, and footwear should be assessed. The use of hot and cold therapies with stretching may be useful, as may therapeutic modalities such as ultrasound. Massage may reduce vascular congestion and myofascial restrictions. Joint mobility should be assessed at the proximal and distal fibula. If motion restriction occurs in these segments, manipulation and/or mobilization is indicated to allow for bony expansion of the compartment.

Despite extensive conservative efforts, surgical referral may be necessary for fascial release (20). Compartmental pressures in excess of 30 to 35 mm Hg suggest the need for surgical fascial release. Fasciotomy relieves pain and provides good results in approximately 60% of cases (18).

Fascial Hernia

Fascial hernias are often caused by compartment compression syndromes or blunt trauma. The most common site is within the anterior compartment, where a defect of the overlying fascia allows the underlying musculature to bulge through. This bulging may increase with exercise or with increased compartmental pressure. Such hernias are often asymptomatic. However, when this bulging causes symptoms, it is usually during activity. When at rest, a defect may be palpable through the fascia.

Conservative treatment of a fascial hernia may involve therapeutic modalities for temporary relief. A counterpressure pad may be devised by cutting a felt or foam pad and securing it with tape over the defect in an attempt to prevent further bulging (21). Surgical closure of this hernia rarely provides favorable results, and in many cases may actually exacerbate the symptoms, particularly in those cases that are secondary to compartment syndrome.

Vascular Occlusions

THROMBOPHLEBITIS

The most common site for venous thrombosis is in the pelvis and legs. Prolonged pressure over the popliteal fossa and/or the calf when inactive increases the likelihood of thrombophlebitis. Venous thrombosis may also occur subsequent to a severe injury, when the injured individual must remain still for an extended period. Cramping of the calf is the most noted symptom. Signs may demonstrate erythema and swelling along the course of the vein. Pain may be reproduced by dorsiflexion of the foot while compression is applied to the calf, such as in Homans' sign or Moses' test (22). Claudication may occur after prolonged periods of sitting, such as during travel. Symptoms may mimic those of a Baker's cyst or gastrocnemius rupture. Estrogen therapy or other conditions that may affect blood vessel clotting may be contributory. The diagnosis should be confirmed by venogram and prompt referral for anticoagulant therapy. Massage is contraindicated with this condition, out of a concern for dislodging the embolism. Wearing support stockings or wrapping with an Ace bandage from the foot to the groin may be useful in assisting venous circulation. Signs of embolism and thrombosis may include respiratory stress or chest pain (23).

POPLITEAL ARTERY ENTRAPMENT SYNDROME

Popliteal artery entrapment syndrome is an uncommon yet significant condition that causes intermittent claudication. The symptoms present as calf muscle cramping and early fatigue. Occasionally, there may be paresthesia on the plantar surfaces of the foot. These symptoms are expedited by running on an incline or by repeated jumping. The vessels may be impinged by a cyst or a fibrous tissue strand. More commonly, compression will occur by compression entrapment of one of the heads of the gastrocnemius (usually the medial), soleus, or plantaris (24). Anatomical variations in the course of the popliteal artery may contribute to a predisposition for this condition.

Clinical presentation is usually accompanied by a history of intermittent claudication in a nonatherosclerotic individual. Symptoms are usually unilateral in young athletes, but may present bilaterally. Posterior tibial and dorsal pedal pulses may be reduced, particularly with active plantarflexion or forced dorsiflexion. Doppler testing, angiographic magnetic resonance imaging (MRI), or angiographic radiographs may be useful to define the blood flow pattern. A patient may be able to run without difficulty, but walking will generally exacerbate symptoms.

This condition, when the symptoms are mild or when it is detected early, may respond to a significant reduction of offending activities, along with therapeutic modalities to relax the plantarflexors followed by general stretching. However, with advanced symptoms, surgical decompression may be necessary because repeated compression can lead to an embolism or thrombosis within the artery and the potential loss of the limb.

DORSAL PEDAL ARTERY ENTRAPMENT

Dorsal pedal artery entrapment is fairly common (Fig. 16.7), but rarely results in severe or permanent injury. Entrapment is usually secondary to improper footwear, especially ski boots, in-line

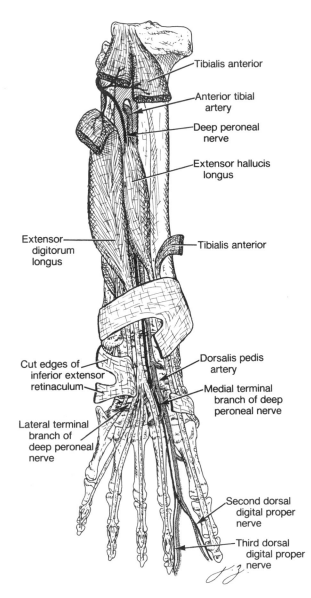

Figure 16.7. Anatomy of the dorsal foot. Note common areas of dorsal pedal artery entrapment at the retinaculum and near the first metatarsocuneiform joint. (Reprinted with permission from Draves DJ. Anatomy of the lower extremity. Baltimore: Williams & Wilkins, 1986.)

skates, and shoes that have a low instep. Most commonly, this entrapment is the result of shoelaces that are tied too tightly. Symptoms are a generalized numbness, tingling, and occasionally throbbing over the dorsum of the foot. These symptoms are normally relieved by simply loosening the shoelaces or creating pressure relief over the dorsum of the foot. If symptoms are prolonged, this condition should be differentiated from entrapment of the medial dorsal cutaneous nerve.

NERVE ENTRAPMENT SYNDROMES

Neuropathies of the lower extremities are infrequent (Fig. 16.8). However, it is likely that many of these cases are undiagnosed; under static examination, the athlete may be asymptomatic. Therefore, examination may require the demonstration of a functional activity or active provocation of compression. Peripheral neuropathies should be of initial concern when evaluating a diabetic patient or a patient with a history of alcohol abuse. Other metabolic processes may be a factor in these cases (25). Additionally, a double crush syndrome or pain from a more proximal origin must be ruled out for successful treatment.

Peripheral nerve injuries, particularly to the peroneal nerve and the tibial nerve, are often associated with ankle inversion sprains (26). In grade 2 inversion sprains, EMG studies show that the peroneal nerve is impaired 17% of the time, whereas the tibial nerve is impaired in 10% of cases. In grade 3 sprains, the peroneal nerve is involved in 86% of cases, whereas the tibial nerve is involved in 83% (17). In many cases, these individuals will appear clinically normal. However, such subclinical conditions may contribute to functional instability and early reinjury. Therefore, careful functional retesting of ankle inversion sprains may be necessary before return to activity. These individuals will likely require a prolonged rehabilitation process to allow for maximal functional stability.

SUPERFICIAL PERONEAL NERVE ENTRAPMENT

Neurapraxia of the superficial peroneal nerve may occur as a result of plantarflexion and inversion of the ankle, as well as direct impact such as in karate or soccer. Other causes may involve a tethering of the nerve at the fibular neck and distally as the nerve exits the fascia (27). Compression may occur at the origin of the peroneus longus muscle. At this point, the peroneal nerve emerges deep to the muscle. With an inversion force, the muscle compresses the peroneal nerve against the bone. With full inversion, the nerve should be allowed to move 5 to 8 mm (Fig. 16.9) (23).

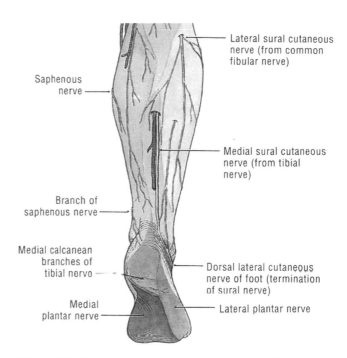

Figure 16.8. Cutaneous nerves and sensory patterns of the lower extremity. (Reprinted with permission from Agur AR. Grant's atlas of anatomy. 9th ed. Baltimore: Williams & Wilkins, 1991.)

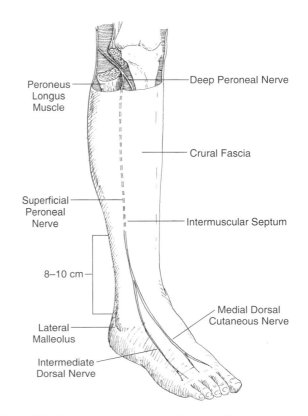

Figure 16.9. The most common course of the superficial peroneal nerve. The common peroneal nerve crosses deep to the peroneus longus inferior to the head of the fibula, where it divides into the deep peroneal and superficial peroneal nerve. Compression at this point may cause entrapment neuropathy. The superficial peroneal nerve pierces the deep fascia 8 to 10 cm proximal to the lateral malleolus. Fascia herniation or nerve stenosis commonly occurs at this point. (Adapted from Oloff LM. Musculoskeletal disorders of the lower extremities. Philadelphia: WB Saunders, 1994.)

Occasionally, these symptoms may result from hypermobility of the tibiofibular joint, particularly at the head of the fibula. At this point, stabilization with wrap or tape may be helpful for reducing motion. Manipulation to restore balanced motion may also be helpful.

The most common location for superficial peroneal nerve entrapment is at the site where the nerve exits the deep fascia of the lateral compartment, approximately 8 to 10 cm proximal to the anterior ankle joint (28). Symptoms may include sharp, burning pain along the nerve's distribution. With extreme compression, motor function of the peroneus brevis and longus may be impaired. Symptoms may be provoked by plantarflexion and inversion maneuvers of the ankle. Digital compression over the nerve, primarily at its fascial exit, may also reproduce symptoms. Typically, sensory changes will occur over the distal leg, dorsum of the foot, and dorsal aspect of the first four toes, with the exception of the first web space.

The superficial peroneal nerve and its branches are often irritated by footwear; therefore, an evaluation for localized pressure is necessary. Ski boots may require modification or a change from a front-entry boot to a rear-entry boot. With cycling, a change from toe-clip pedals to clipless pedals may be required, as the dorsal strap can cause nerve compression on the foot. In general, most neurapraxias respond to conservative measures (29). However, decompression and release of the fascia are occasionally necessary.

Therapeutic modalities may be helpful in these cases, along with massage, ice, and heat therapy. Heel lifts may reduce tension on the nerve. Should joint instability exist in the ankle, ankle bracing should be provided, being careful not to cause further impingement by any compressive strapping.

Nutritionally, vitamins B_6 and E may be helpful for increasing peripheral circulation and reducing neuritis pain.

MEDIAL DORSAL CUTANEOUS NERVE ENTRAPMENT

The medial dorsal cutaneous nerve is a branch of the superficial peroneal nerve. It is most frequently entrapped as it passes over the first metatarsal cuneiform joint (30). Footwear is the most common cause of compression at the anterior aspect of the ankle, frequently called anterior tarsal tunnel syndrome, or over the first metatarsal cuneiform joint, traditionally referred to as vamp pain. Hypermobility of the first ray may create a dorsal exostosis at the metatarsal cuneiform joint. This exostosis frequently will create direct impingement of the nerve between the spur and the footwear. A plantarflexed position of the first ray may also contribute to medial dorsal cutaneous nerve entrapment.

Treatment in these situations should involve footwear modifications. At the ankle, avoiding lacing through the last eyelet or using a pulley or heel lock lacing system may be adequate to relieve symptoms. At the first metatarsal cuneiform joint, applying a doughnut pad made of foam or felt may provide adequate pressure relief. Additional pressure relief may be achieved by skipping the eyelets adjacent to the first metatarsal cuneiform junction. In the case of a boot, local stretching or a cutout may be necessary. These neurapraxias also respond well to other conservative measures such as manipulation, mobilization, ultrasound, electrotherapeutics, and ice therapies.

INTERMEDIATE DORSAL CUTANEOUS NERVE ENTRAPMENT

The intermediate dorsal cutaneous nerve is rarely involved, but may occasionally be aggravated by footwear or a direct blow to the anterior ankle or the dorsal lateral foot over Lisfranc's joint. Injury to this branch may be provoked further during forefoot inversion. The medial dorsal cutaneous nerve and the intermediate dorsal cutaneous nerve are frequently entrapped secondary to surgical procedures to the dorsum of the midfoot (26).

The intermediate dorsal cutaneous nerve generally responds well to the same conservative measures described for the medial dorsal cutaneous nerve.

SAPHENOUS NERVE ENTRAPMENT

The saphenous nerve courses inferiorly down the leg adjacent to the saphenous vein. It is rarely entrapped in most sports, but it may be involved in direct trauma in sports such as football, soccer, and karate. Progressive genu valgum may also contribute to tractioning of the saphenous nerve. More commonly, the nerve sustains a contusion at the anterior medial ankle or is entrapped at the first metatarsal cuneiform joint by footwear or an exostosis. Complications of Achilles tendon surgery also may impair the saphenous nerve.

The saphenous nerve may also be provoked by applying a valgus stretch to the knee while simultaneously plantarflexing the foot and everting the forefoot. An identifying sign for saphenous nerve entrapment is pain on direct palpation of the nerve along its course to the base of the first metatarsal (Fig. 16.10) (23).

DEEP PERONEAL NERVE ENTRAPMENT

The deep peroneal nerve bifurcates from the common peroneal nerve, along with the superficial peroneal nerve, near the head of the fibula and penetrates deep to the peroneus longus muscle. Therefore, similar to the superficial peroneal nerve, it too can have entrapment syndromes resulting from mechanical irritation or compression in this region (Fig. 16.11). The deep peroneal nerve provides motor fibers to the muscles of the anterior compartment and therefore is also known as the anterior tibial nerve. It provides sensation to a very small region: the medial half of the second toe, lateral side of the first toe, and intervening web space. Neurapraxia may result from an anterior compartment syndrome, fascial herniation, or direct trauma. Nerve entrapment or compression at the proximal origin may result in a drop foot from paralysis of the anterior compartment (31).

The deep peroneal nerve passes deep to the superior and inferior extensor retinaculum. Entrapment in this area is often called the anterior tarsal tunnel syndrome. Compression in this area may result from a direct blow or a severe ankle sprain. Shoes may also cause mechanical encroachment, in which case avoiding lacing through the last eyelet or using a pulley or heel lock system of lacing should be used. Therapeutic modalities are ef-

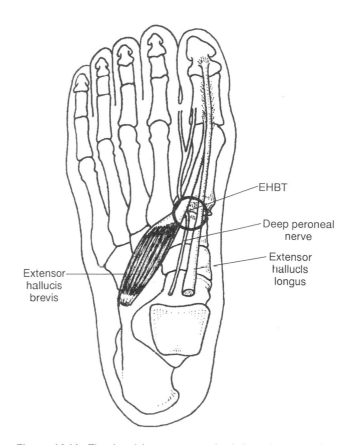

Figure 16.11. The dorsal base exostosis (circled area) may produce tenosynovitis of the extensor hallucis longus and/or brevis and may result in entrapment neuropathy of the deep peroneal nerve where it passes beneath the extensor hallucis brevis tendon. (Reprinted with permission from Michaud TC. Foot orthoses and other forms of conservative foot care. Baltimore: Williams & Wilkins, 1993.)

fective in this area for reducing inflammation under the retinaculum, provided that the causative or aggravating factors have been eliminated.

An anterior talar fracture may cause mechanical irritation to the deep peroneal nerve, which is pinned down by the extensor retinaculum against the anterior talus.

Compression of this nerve in the foot may occur at the first and second metatarsal cuneiform joints. In this region, the nerve passes deep to the extensor hallucis brevis tendon and may be aggravated by hyperplantarflexion of the hallux (Fig. 16.11). Compression of this nerve may be further aggravated by a dorsal exostosis of either the first or second metatarsal cuneiform joint (30). Direct trauma to the nerve in this region may result from lacing of footwear or by direct impact, such as when someone steps on the foot.

The patient may present early with numbness over the dorsum of the foot or in the web space of the first and second toes. With progression, the web space may develop a burning sensation. With proximal entrapment, weakness of the an-

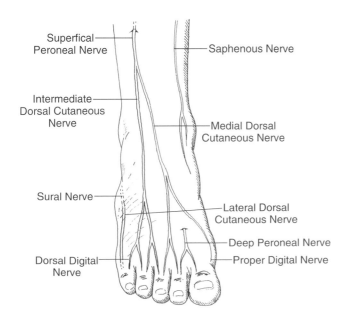

Figure 16.10. Typical nerve distribution of the dorsum of the foot. (Adapted from Oloff LM. Musculoskeletal disorders of the lower extremities. Philadelphia: WB Saunders, 1994.)

terior tibialis and extensor musculature may be evident. A foot drop may appear in severe cases. Tractioning of the nerve by plantarflexion and inversion of the foot may re-create or exacerbate symptoms. Distal entrapments may demonstrate a positive Tinel's sign at the anterior ankle and dorsal metatarsal cuneiform joints. EMG and nerve conduction velocity studies may be helpful for localizing entrapment levels.

Entrapment at the extensor retinaculum responds well to distal tibiofibular manipulation and mobilization, as well as ankle joint manipulation. Therapeutic modalities are also effective for reducing inflammatory irritations of this region. Eliminating mechanical stresses, including those from footwear, may be necessary. Optimizing biomechanics, such as controlling overpronation, may also be helpful. This is especially true for entrapment at the dorsal metatarsal cuneiform joints. At this juncture, a pressure relief pad or donut may be helpful, as well as avoiding the laces that cross these structures. Midtarsal and metatarsal cuneiform manipulation may provide relief.

Nutritionally, vitamins B_6 and E may be helpful for increasing peripheral circulation and reducing neuritis pain.

SURAL AND LATERAL DORSAL CUTANEOUS NERVE ENTRAPMENT

Sural nerve entrapments are rare. The sural nerve courses down the posterior compartment between the medial and lateral heads of the gastrocnemius. At the distal musculotendinous region of the gastrocnemius, the nerve descends superficially, coursing laterally halfway between the fibula and the Achilles tendon. The nerve then progresses distally to form the lateral dorsal cutaneous nerve along the dorsal lateral foot (Fig. 16.12) (17).

The sural nerve provides sensation to the lateral foot. Neurapraxia may result from direct trauma to the nerve in the calf or prolonged compression of the nerve. Fracture of an os peroneum, the fifth metatarsal, or of the fibula have been reported to cause sural neuritis (32). These symptoms may be secondary to postsurgical complications of the Achilles tendon or lateral foot (33). The sural nerve has communicating branches to the intermediate dorsal cutaneous nerve. These branches cross over the anterior calcaneus and sinus tarsus. Therefore, neuritis in this region may be confused with sinus tarsus syndrome. Signs of sural nerve involvement are sensory changes along the distribution of the

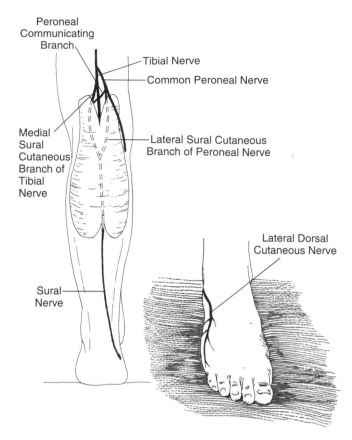

Figure 16.12. Distribution of the sural nerve in the posterior leg. It may be located posterior to the lateral malleolus or over the calcaneus by the peroneal tubercle, where the nerve is now designated the lateral dorsal cutaneous nerve. (Adapted from Reid DC. Sports injury assessment and rehabilitation. New York: Churchill Livingstone, 1992.)

nerve. Provocative stretching of the nerve may include dorsiflexion and/or plantarflexion of the ankle with inversion of the foot.

Conservative treatment may incorporate the use of a heel lift to reduce traction on the sural nerve. Massage to the calf and Achilles tendon may reduce adhesive scarring that can irritate the sural nerve. Other therapeutic modalities may prove useful, depending on the location of entrapment. On occasion, subluxation of the cuboid bone may aggravate the lateral dorsal cutaneous nerve. In such instances, manipulation will prove beneficial.

Nutritionally, vitamins B_6 and E may be helpful for increasing peripheral circulation and reducing neuritis pain.

POSTERIOR TIBIAL NERVE ENTRAPMENT AND MEDIAL TARSAL TUNNEL SYNDROME

The most common site of posterior tibial nerve compression is in the medial fibroosseous tarsal tunnel, which is created by the confluence of the calcaneus and medial malleolus and is enclosed by the flexor retinaculum (Fig. 16.13) (34). Compression of the posterior tibial nerve can occur as a result of compartment syndrome of the deep posterior compartment. Compression has been reported secondary to a Baker's cyst (35), hemorrhage in the popliteal fossa (36), and secondary to complications of postsurgical fixation of the tibia (37, 38).

The medial tarsal tunnel is divided into four channels, which follow the mnemonic, "Tom, Dick, ANd Harry." Tom represents the tibialis posterior. Dick represents the flexor digitorum longus. AN represents the posterior tibial artery and nerve. Harry represents the flexor hallucis longus. This mnemonic describes the anatomical relationships of these structures in the channel going from proximal to distal.

In 98% of individuals, the posterior tibial nerve will divide into its terminal branches within the tarsal tunnel. These branches are the medial plantar nerve and the lateral plantar nerve. The medial calcaneal nerve is somewhat variable, having been found to branch off the posterior tibial nerve or the lateral plantar nerve, and also may branch either within the tarsal tunnel or proximal to it.

Tarsal tunnel syndrome may have a variety of causes. In athletes, a ganglion or posttraumatic synovial cyst may cause pressure inside the canal. In these cases, symptoms may be intermittent and associated with swelling with activity.

Trauma can occur within the tarsal tunnel via direct impact, secondary to ankle sprains, tight calves, or fracture of the calcaneus. On occasion, tarsal tunnel syndrome may be a postsurgical complication of the Achilles tendon or first ray

surgery. Venous engorgement may also cause nerve compression; however, nerve compression may also cause venous engorgement, thereby perpetuating compression within the tarsal tunnel (17, 39).

Overpronation or a valgus heel is considered the most common cause of microtraumatic medial tarsal tunnel syndrome. With ankle eversion, the flexor retinaculum is pulled taught, increasing compression within the compartment.

Clinically, tarsal tunnel syndrome presents itself with burning paresthesia in the plantar aspect of the foot and medial ankle. Often there may be a sensation of an impending arch cramp. Plantar numbness and tingling are common symptoms. These pains and paresthesias are usually aggravated with activity and generally worsen at night.

On examination, Tinel's sign over the flexor retinaculum will be positive. Edema may be evident posterior to the medial malleolus. Occasionally, vibration perception and two-point discrimination over the plantar aspect of the foot will be depressed. Hammer toes may be a late complication of tarsal tunnel syndrome. In general, symptoms generally present themselves insidiously. Gender proves to be unrelated to this condition, except with children and adolescents. In this population, the condition appears to be more prevalent in females.

EMG and nerve conduction studies are essential for definitive diagnosis; however, they are positive in only 65% of patients with clinical tarsal tunnel syndrome.

Conservative treatment begins with activity modification. In the runner, reducing mileage and

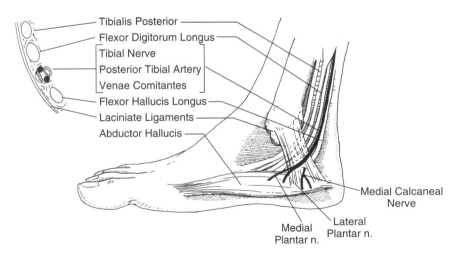

Figure 16.13. Anatomy of the medial tarsal tunnel. Note the branching of the medial and lateral plantar nerves as they course deep to the abductor hallucis. The medial calcaneal branch pierces the flexor retinaculum. (Adapted from Oloff LM. Musculoskeletal disorders of the lower extremities. Philadelphia: WB Saunders, 1994.)

moving to a flat, soft surface for training is beneficial. Most physiotherapeutic modalities designed to reduce inflammation will prove effective in this area (40). Manipulation and mobilization of the ankle mortise and subtalar joint into inversion to restore normal joint inversion mechanics and reduce tension on the flexor retinaculum should be applied as indicated. Taping the calcaneus into an inverted position may yield symptomatic relief. Footwear designed for pronation control and functional biomechanical orthotics may prove necessary for long-term support and prevention of recurrence. For those individuals with vascular insufficiencies or edema, wearing support stockings may be necessary.

Nutritionally, vitamins B_6 and E may be helpful for increasing peripheral circulation and reducing neuritis pain.

MEDIAL CALCANEAL NERVE COMPRESSION AND HEEL NEUROMAS

Repeated trauma directly to the medial calcaneal branch of the posterior tibial nerve is frequent among long-distance runners (Figs. 16.13 and 16.14). Continued microtrauma may lead to the formation of a neuroma (41). Entrapment may also occur postsurgically as a result of a medial plantar approach for plantar fascial release or heel spur excision (42). Most often, this condition is related to excessive pronation (43).

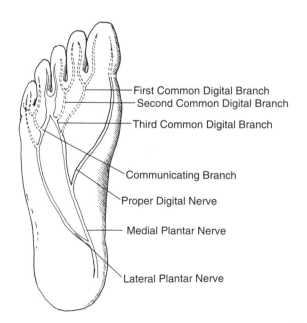

—First Common Digital Branch
—Second Common Digital Branch
—Third Common Digital Branch

—Communicating Branch
—Proper Digital Nerve
—Medial Plantar Nerve
—Lateral Plantar Nerve

Figure 16.14. Typical nerve distribution on the sole of the foot. Note the neuroma depicted on the third common digital branch. (Adapted from Oloff LM. Musculoskeletal disorders of the lower extremities. Philadelphia: WB Saunders, 1994.)

At onset, symptoms are experienced only during activity and primarily at heel strike. Generally, the pain is mild and felt only as burning or tingling along the medial border of the heel. With progression, pain may radiate laterally and posteriorly over the heel and into the ankle. On occasion, a neuroma may be palpable in the plantar medial aspect of the heel.

Other conservative treatment begins with training modifications such as moving the athlete to softer surfaces with a reduction of long-, slow-distance miles. The patient will often be asymptomatic during faster training, when the runner moves more toward the midfoot and forefoot on footstrike. This will help differentiate this condition from plantar fasciitis. The use of antipronation footwear along with soft ethylene vinyl acetate or viscoelastic material for varus wedging at the calcaneus may allow for pain-free training. However, this wedge may need a pressure cutout at the site where the medial calcaneal nerve dips under the medial calcaneus. Taping the calcaneal fat pad from a lateral to medial position may also be helpful. Other conservative treatment includes ice and physiotherapeutic modalities for the reduction of inflammation and scarring. Nutritionally, vitamins B_6 and E may be helpful for increasing peripheral circulation and reducing neuritis pain.

The majority of heel pain cases respond to conservative care management over a course of several weeks or months (44).

MEDIAL PLANTAR NERVE ENTRAPMENT

The medial plantar nerve may become compressed within the tarsal tunnel or at the origin of the adductor hallucis muscle (Fig. 16.13). Occasionally, this nerve will pierce through the adductor hallucis muscle as it courses along the plantar medial aspect of the foot. An accessory or hypertrophic adductor hallucis muscle may entrap this nerve by pinning it against the calcaneus. In such situations, symptoms may begin as numbness and tingling into the plantarmedial forefoot (toes one through three) and the medial aspect of the fourth toe. These symptoms usually begin at the great toe and progress laterally. With progression of the condition, burning pain may appear, as well as a cramping sensation within the arch (23).

Treatment should be similar to care for tarsal tunnel syndrome. In addition, taping the great toe into an abducted position may create a temporary reduction of compression of this nerve against the calcaneus from the adductor hallucis muscle.

LATERAL PLANTAR NERVE ENTRAPMENT

The lateral plantar nerve may become entrapped within the tarsal tunnel or under the fibrous origin of the plantar aponeurosis. Entrapment may occur secondary to plantar fasciitis. Symptoms will include numbness, tingling, and burning pain into the lateral plantar aspect of the foot (45).

Conservative treatment should be similar to the approach used for treatment of medial tarsal tunnel syndrome. In addition, low dye strapping may provide a benefit.

PLANTAR DIGITAL NERVE ENTRAPMENT AND MORTON'S NEUROMA

The plantar digital nerves are the terminal branches of the lateral and medial plantar nerves. These nerves are often entrapped by a variety of soft tissue structures at the level of the deep transverse intermetatarsal ligament, where the nerve courses inferiorly and becomes trapped between the metatarsal heads and other soft tissue structures. Such is the case with Morton's neuroma. The term neuroma is a misnomer in that there is a peripheral thickening, most commonly of the third common plantar digital nerve, rather than a true neoplasm of the cells of the nervous system (23). A related condition, known as Joplin's neuroma, is the compression of the proper digital nerve over the medial aspect of the first metatarsal and hallux, frequently involving the sesamoid apparatus.

Causative factors may relate to footgear that is too short or too tight. Systemic disease, infection, direct trauma, and altered biomechanics may also be causative factors.

Symptoms are variable. Patients may describe symptoms as an electric shock, fullness, lump sensation, or hot, burning jab on the bottom of the foot or between the toes. Frequently, light touch is intolerable and even the weight of bed sheets on the foot can be painful. Pain is generally increased with activity and weight bearing. Occasionally, symptoms may increase at night. Sullivan's sign, i.e., splaying of the involved toes, may be present (Fig. 16.15).

Pain is often produced by the lateral squeeze test, in which the forefoot is compressed side to side. Mulder's test involves both side-to-side squeezing and dorsal-to-plantar intermetatarsal pressure. Both of these tests reproduce painful symptoms. High-resolution ultrasonography and MRI are both useful for imaging digital nerve entrapments or neuromas. These procedures have limitations, however, and false-negative results

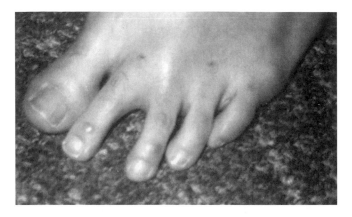

Figure 16.15. Sullivan's sign of the second and third toes secondary to a second interdigital neuroma. Note the splaying of the toes. (Courtesy of T.L. Forcum.)

are frequent. Sensory nerve conduction tests may also aid in diagnostic conclusions.

Interdigital neuritis predominates in women 78% of the time. This may implicate aggravation by high-heeled shoes and shoes with narrow toe boxes. The most common occurrence is in the third web space, followed by the second, and at much less frequency the first; the fourth web space is the least common. Painful burning and aching into the plantar foot occur in approximately 90% of patients, with radiation into the affected toes approximately 65% of the time (23).

Conservative treatment should begin with the use of a metatarsal bar, metatarsal pad, or neuroma plug placed proximal to the second to fourth metatarsal phalangeal joints. Therapeutic modalities should be used through the interdigital space to reduce inflammation and scarring along the course of a nerve. Frequently, manipulation of the metatarsal phalangeal joint and intermetatarsal joints will restore normal biomechanics and reduce symptomatology. Overpronation should be controlled to reduce torsional strain on the intermetatarsal joints, and a functional biomechanical orthotic may be indicated. Shoes with a wide forefoot are a necessity for recovery. Wearing high-heeled shoes and shoes with a pointed toe must be avoided for any chance of recovery. Nutritionally, vitamins B_6 and E may be helpful for increasing peripheral circulation and reducing neuritis pain.

Musculotendinous Injuries

MUSCULAR STRAINS

Muscular strains are among the most common injuries in athletics. Contractile force or overstretching causes excessive tensile forces within the muscle and thus fibrous disruption. Most strains occur at the musculotendinous junction.

However, strains can occur anywhere within muscular tissue. Sprinting and court sports such as tennis and basketball are the most common causes of muscular strain due to the requirements of sudden acceleration.

Muscular strains can occur during eccentric and concentric contractions. In the lower leg, many motions are controlled eccentrically for shock absorption and maintenance of balance. Eccentric contractions rely on a strong muscular contraction while the muscle itself is forcefully lengthened. This produces a great amount of force throughout the muscle-tendon unit and hence a great potential for injury. Strains in this region can occur from a single muscular contraction or overstretch, or from repetitive overuse forces that produce an accumulative effect of fatigue failure of the muscle-tendon unit.

Strains are classified as follows (21, 23).

1. First-degree strains (Type I) are mild muscular pulls caused by a stretch injury to a portion of the muscular unit. There is an estimated disruption of less than 5% of the muscular fibers. On examination, localized pain and swelling may be minimal or absent. Type 1 muscular strains are the most common. They usually allow the patient to ambulate; however, the patient may need the assistance of a compression sleeve or tape.

2. Second-degree strains (Type II strain) are moderate muscle pulls caused by trauma resulting from an excessive stretch or violent contraction. There is moderate hemorrhage and swelling. A significant degree of function is lost, and muscular spasm is present. Localized swelling (and possibly ecchymosis) indicates that the perimysium and fascia remain intact; this is often referred to as a Type 2A strain. Disruption of the perimysium and fascia are often evidenced by a diffuse edema ecchymosis and may be referred to as a Type 2B strain. The pain is generally more diffuse with second-degree strains, and a palpatory defect may be noted. Laboratory studies may help differentiate a second-degree strain; muscle enzymes are elevated, with maximal levels occurring 2 to 3 days after injury.

   Second-degree strains are treated similarly to first-degree strains, with the exception that soft tissue massage is avoided during the acute stages to reduce the risk of worsening the tear. Type 2 strains also require non–weight-bearing with crutches for ambulation.

3. Third-degree strains (Type III) are severe, with complete disruption of either the muscle or tendon. A palpable defect is usually present. This condition is characterized by ecchymosis, hematoma, loss of muscle function, diffuse edema and tenderness, spasm, and severe pain. With poor approximation, surgical repair is required. MRI or ultrasound may be useful for determining the extent of injury and degree of approximation (46).

TENDON INJURIES

Acute and chronic tendon disruption are common in the foot and ankle. A large number of tendons in this region support the entire body weight and provide shock absorption and propulsion. Tendons generally repair slowly because of their limited blood supply. There is both an internal and an external blood supply to the tendon. The internal system traverses the endotenon. The external system is derived from muscular branches on one end and periosteal branches at its insertion end. The paratenon supplies blood to the middle one third of the tendon. The tendons of the anterior, deep posterior, and lateral compartments all possess a sheath that serves to lubricate the tendon as it passes through the retinaculum or changes directions around a bony prominence. The sheath contains two layers of highly vascularized tissue, which passes nutritional supply on to the tendon.

The paratenon is a loose areolar tissue. Both the tendinous sheath and paratenon assist in the glide motion of the tendon through surrounding tissues. Many of the chronic problems with tendon disruption occur because of fibrous adhesions to the surrounding tissues. This prevents the normal gliding motion of the tendon and creates chronic inflammation.

Tendinitis is the most common tendon injury in athletics. When the injury includes the tendon sheath apparatus, the term tenosynovitis is used. When no tendon sheath is involved, the term peritendinitis is sometimes used. In general, these injuries can be divided into three types: peritendinitis crepitans, chronic tenosynovitis, and stenosing tenosynovitis (21, 23).

Peritendinitis is a localized swelling and disruption that occurs at the muscular tendinous junction. Pain is frequently elicited with resisted motion and overstretching. The most common cause of this injury is overuse. This injury responds well to conservative treatment, including physiotherapeutics, transverse friction massage, and taping. Auscultation may reveal crepitus with movement.

Chronic tenosynovitis responds well to conservative treatment. Localized swelling often occurs within the synovial sheath, and pain is usually elicited during both resisted motion and passive overstretching. Because the sheath is lined by synovial tissue, it is also subject to those diseases involving the synovium, such as rheumatoid arthritis, Reiter's disease, and other seronegative disorders.

Stenosing tenosynovitis occurs when adhesions form between the tendon and the tendon sheath, or between the entire tendon apparatus and surrounding tissue. These adhesions prevent the tendon from gliding freely. The tendon may undergo deterioration to the point of rupture. Conservative care leads to variable results based on severity. Tenography is a type of radiography in which contrast medium is injected into the tendon sheath proximally. The contrast flow medium flows distally and may show interruptions at the point of stenosis. This procedure can often prove therapeutic. The injection of large volumes of fluid into the synovial space provides pressure to stretch or break adhesions.

MRI is the most effective imaging technique for evaluating muscular and tendinous defects. It is often useful in acute and chronic cases. However, this imaging technique has cost limitations. Ultrasonography has advantages in terms of cost. Ultrasonography has continued to progress over the years and prove valuable in diagnosing partial and total tendon disruptions at a much lower cost than MRI.

MUSCULOTENDINOUS INJURIES OF THE ANTERIOR COMPARTMENT

Tibialis Anterior Musculotendinous Disruption

Musculotendinous strains of the tibialis anterior, extensor digitorum longus, extensor hallucis longus, and peroneus tertius are common. The individual muscle involved may be isolated by individual muscle testing and stretching.

Muscle testing of the tibialis anterior can be performed by placing the foot in a dorsiflexed and inverted position while maintaining toe flexion. The practitioner applies resistance by pulling the foot in a plantarflexed direction. Isolated stretching of the tibialis anterior is performed by extending the toes while pulling the foot in a plantarflexed direction and everting the foot. Pain in these motions and pain along the course of the muscle and tendon indicate involvement. Palpable tenderness will often be noted in the proximal aspect of the muscle belly and along the course of the tendon near the extensor retinaculum and its insertion.

Extensor Digitorum Longus Musculotendinous Disruption

The extensor digitorum longus courses laterally to the tibialis anterior, often eliciting pain within the muscle belly or along the course of the tendons, particularly at the extensor retinaculum and over the midfoot. Pain may be elicited by resisted muscle testing of the extensor digitorum longus with the foot in neutral and the toes extended. The concomitant resistance of both toe plantarflexion and foot plantarflexion is applied. Overstretching of the extensor digitorum longus can be produced by plantarflexing the toes, followed by plantarflexion of the foot. Pain with palpation, muscle testing, and overstretching is indicative of disruption in this muscle.

Extensor Hallucis Longus Musculotendinous Disruption

The extensor hallucis longus is also tested by eliciting painful resistance, stretching, and palpation. Its muscle belly lies deep to the tibialis anterior and extensor digitorum longus, originating from the middle half of the anterior surface of the fibula and interosseous membrane. Palpation is often assisted by active dorsiflexion of the great toe. Resisted muscle testing is performed by extending the great toe while dorsiflexing and inverting the foot. Resistance is achieved by applying a plantarflexed flexion resistance to the great toe. Overstretching of this muscle can be performed by plantarflexing the great toe, followed by eversion and plantarflexion of the foot. The extensor hallucis longus is frequently involved in runners who overpronate, particularly those with a large forefoot varus deviation or midtarsal dysfunction as described in Chapter 15. With these individuals, the extensor hallucis longus eccentrically controls the lowering of the forefoot to the ground from heel strike to foot flat. With a forefoot varus deviation, the extensor hallucis longus must exert this controlling force over a greater range of motion.

Peroneus Tertius Musculotendinous Disruption

The peroneus tertius may be palpated along the distal one third of the anterior surface of the fibula. It inserts along the dorsal base of the fifth metatarsal, with its tendon running with those of the extensor digitorum longus. This muscle is often involved with inversion sprains, particularly those with a strong plantarflexion component. Other common mechanisms of injury may include karate side kicks or overuse with a hackey sack.

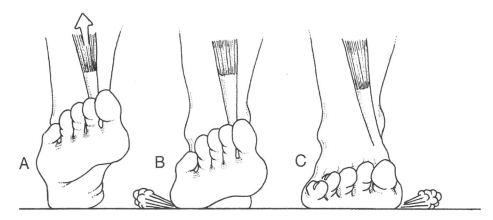

Figure 16.16. Ankle plantar flexion during the early and midcontact period is resisted by eccentric contraction of the anterior compartment muscles (arrow in **A**). This resistance is accentuated with downhill running and overpronation. When this occurs, anterior compartment musculotendinous injury may result. Approximately 40% of the way through contact period **(B)**, the fifth metatarsal head strikes the ground. The forefoot is then smoothly loaded from lateral to medial, with the entire forefoot making ground contact approximately 70% of the way through the contact period **(C)**. (Reprinted with permission from Michaud TC. Foot orthoses and other forms of conservative foot care. Baltimore: Williams & Wilkins, 1993.)

All the muscles of the anterior compartment are innervated by the deep peroneal nerve. The anterior tibialis is primarily controlled by fibers derived from the L4 neurologic level, whereas the extensor hallucis longus, extensor digitorum longus, and peroneus tertius derive more of their control from the L5 nerve root level.

Injury to the L4 nerve root can cause a paralysis of the tibialis anterior, resulting in a foot drop. This condition is noted by a slapping noise as the foot strikes the ground. This is because of poor eccentric control of lowering the foot as the heel strikes. Also, the individual must elevate the involved leg sufficiently to prevent drag of the toe on the ground and thus develops a steppage gait.

Injuries to the anterior compartment may involve one or all of the muscles within the compartment, but the anterior tibialis is most commonly involved. Anterior "shin splints" are extremely common in runners, particularly those who overstride or run with a forward body lean. This requires excessive dorsiflexion to clear the foot over the ground. This dorsiflexion then has to be controlled by the muscles of the anterior compartment from heel strike to foot flat (Fig. 16.16). Such repetitive eccentric control will often lead to an overuse disruption of the musculotendinous fibers of this compartment.

Repetitive isometric and concentric contractions of the muscles of the anterior compartment are required during activities such as snowshoeing and cycling with the use of toe clips. These muscles are used to raise the foot and toes during the swing phase of snowshoeing and during the active lifting phase in cycling, while moving the pedal from the position of seven-o'clock to one-o'clock.

Frequently, these muscles will also be irritated by footwear. Improper fit or lacing may irritate the tendons as they pass over the dorsum of the foot and in the region of the anterior ankle as the tendon passes underneath the extensor retinaculum. Irritation at the ankle is often derived from either the laces being too tight and/or the eyelet of the shoe being positioned too far proximally and posterior for the instep of the patient. This irritation may be eliminated by either skipping the last eyelet of the shoe or, in cases in which this creates heel slippage, using a pulley lacing system. When pronation is the aggravating factor, low dye taping of the foot may be beneficial along with use of an antipronation shoe and functional biomechanical orthotic.

During acute strains, short leg splinting may be necessary, maintaining the foot and ankle in a neutral position. Often, a compressive sleeve over the anterior compartment may reduce symptoms. Care must be taken to ensure that sequelae of multiple acute anterior compartments strains or chronic strain do not develop into an anterior compartment syndrome. During contact sports, adequate padding should be provided to ensure that contusions do not add to the already existing inflammatory process. As with most tendinitis and muscular strains, conservative management uses ice, particularly ice massage in the acute stages. Ultrasound and electrical muscular stimulation, along with massage and other therapeutic procedures and modalities, will augment the recovery process. Muscular rehabilitation is necessary, beginning with isometric resistance of dorsiflexion followed by concentric resistance and eccentric contractions.

MUSCULOTENDINOUS INJURIES OF THE LATERAL COMPARTMENT

The peroneus longus originates from the lateral tibial condyle, head, and upper two thirds of the lateral fibula to insert on the medial cuneiform and the base of the first metatarsal. Its primary task is the plantarflexion and eversion of the foot and the plantarflexion of the first ray. Excessive strain on this muscle-tendon complex can cause compression of the common peroneal nerve as it crosses deep to the muscle near its origin. This further compromises the muscle via neurologic weakness, as the muscles of the lateral compartment are innervated by the superficial peroneal nerve.

Muscular strain of this area commonly occurs in those individuals who underpronate; active contraction of the peroneal musculature is required to stabilize the foot. This can also occur when using footwear that is excessively worn on the lateral aspect. Peroneal tendinitis may occur secondary to chronic ankle sprains. At times, these sprains will rupture the inferior peroneal retinaculum and a portion of the superior peroneal retinaculum. This may lead to chronic subluxation of the peroneal tendons and a tethering of the tendon over the lateral malleolus (47). An accessory bone, the os peroneum or os fibulare, will also frequently create symptoms within the peroneal tendon (48). With severe ankle sprains, the peroneus brevis may be involved, fracturing the styloid of the fifth metatarsal. This may, however, be confused with malunion of the secondary ossification center or an accessory bone, the os

vesalianum. Avulsion fracture of the fifth metatarsal lies transverse to the long axis of the shaft, whereas the secondary ossification center is transverse.

Peroneal tendinitis from overuse may develop from cycling with the use of toe clips or clipless pedals, rollerblading, and repetitive impact on the ends of a sliderboard.

In tenosynovitis of the peroneal tendons, one usually cannot distinguish between the peroneus longus and the peroneus brevis because they share a common synovial sheath. Peroneus longus tendinitis in the midfoot may occur secondary to overuse or acute trauma. Frequently, this tendon pathology will occur from subluxation of the cuboid, which alters the mechanical forces that the peroneus longus exerts on the first cuneiform and first metatarsal.

Pain may be provoked along the course of the muscle or tendon, as well as with overstretching the muscle-tendon unit by placing the foot in dorsiflexion and inversion. Pain may also be produced by muscle testing of the peroneal structures through resisted eversion while the foot is placed in plantarflexion.

Treatment of lateral compartment strains should emphasize the causal relationship. Those caused by subluxation of the cuboid are best treated with manipulation of the cuboid in an inferior to superior direction, followed by support of the cuboid with a plantar cuboid pad and footwear to prevent overpronation. Shoes that are broken down laterally should be replaced, and individuals who underpronate should use a curved last shoe with a flexible midsole (Fig. 16.17). Strain secondary to an inversion sprain can be treated with the use of ankle bracing and taping, such as an Aircast or active ankle support. The use of a valgus wedge may be helpful during the treat-

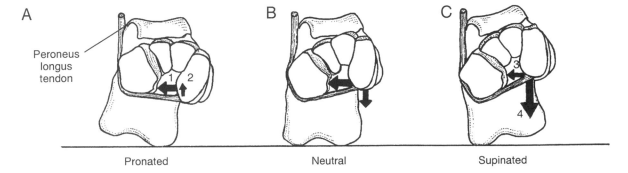

Figure 16.17. The effect of subtalar position on peroneus longus function. With excessive overpronation or underpronation (oversupination of the foot), forces transmitted through the peroneal tendon are altered and thus may result in musculotendinous disruption. (Reprinted with permission from Michaud TC. Foot orthoses and other forms of conservative foot care. Baltimore: Williams & Wilkins, 1993.)

ment of acute peroneal tendinitis. Rehabilitation should be emphasized for proprioceptive and muscular strength to prevent chronic inversion sprains.

MUSCULOTENDINOUS INJURIES OF THE DEEP POSTERIOR COMPARTMENT

Muscular tendon strain of the structures of the deep posterior compartment are common, particularly in those who overpronate.

Tibialis Posterior Musculotendinous Disruption

The tibialis posterior originates from the lateral portion of the posterior tibia and the upper two thirds of the medial fibula to insert into five different locations within the midfoot (Fig. 16.18). Posterior tibial dysfunction can occur from overuse (most commonly overpronation) or acute trauma. A rapid eversion and dorsiflexion force is usually the insulting mechanism for acute disruption of the posterior tibialis unit.

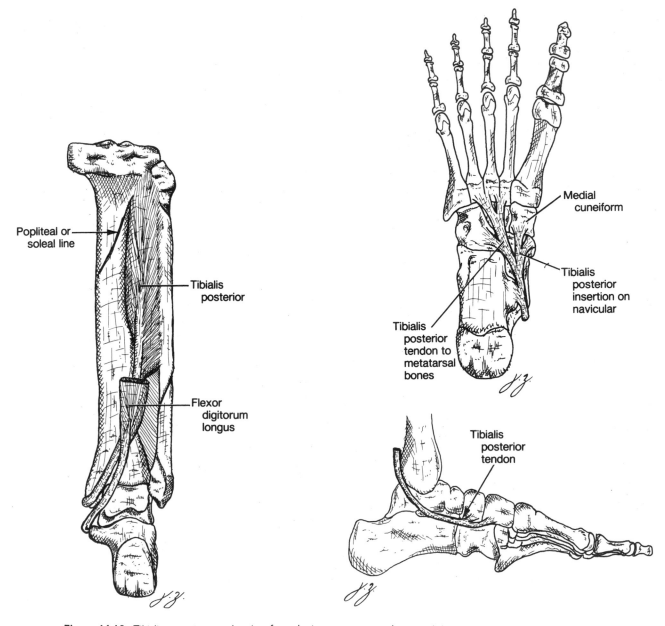

Figure 16.18. Tibialis posterior muscle arises from the interosseous membrane and the adjoining tibia and fibula to insert into the tuberosity of the navicular bone and slips to adjacent bones and the bases of the second, third, and fourth metatarsal bones. (Reprinted with permission from Draves DJ. Anatomy of the lower extremity. Baltimore: Williams & Wilkins, 1986.)

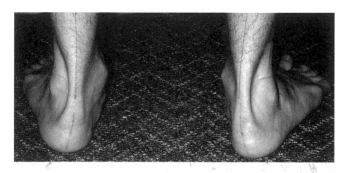

Figure 16.19. "Too many toes" sign is demonstrated by the visualization of too many toes laterally deviated on weight bearing, with tibialis posterior disruption or overpronation. (Courtesy of T.L. Forcum.)

Stage One. Tibialis posterior dysfunction has been categorized in three stages (49). With stage one there is peritendinitis or tendon degeneration with only mild/moderate symptoms of aching along the medial aspect of the ankle. Symptoms are exacerbated with training and generally develop gradually over time.

On examination, swelling may be evident in the posterior medial ankle. In the standing posture, the rearfoot and forefoot alignment is often unremarkable. Asking the patient to perform a single heel raise test may demonstrate some discomfort and early signs of weakness. The patient will be unable to raise the heel completely or will be incapable of locking the hindfoot by everting.

Stage Two. Stage two, a continued degeneration from stage one, is often associated with systemic disorders such as rheumatic disease. This stage demonstrates an elongation of the tibialis posterior tendon with progressive muscular weakness. This is evident by a significant abnormality of the patient's ability to perform a single leg heel raise. Generally, symptoms at this point have been present from several months to several years. Symptoms may be present at rest and through the entire length of the tibialis posterior tendon. On stance, the calcaneus is notably everted and the forefoot may be abducted. Evaluation of the patient in a comfortable standing stance will demonstrate this abduction by visualization of a great number of the toes. This sign is called the "too many toes" sign (Fig. 16.19).

Radiographs in this stage may demonstrate subluxation of the navicular from the head of the talus and divergence of the long axis of the talus with that of the long axis of the calcaneus. Disruption of the tibialis posterior tendon may be evident on MRI or ultrasonography.

Stage Three. Stage three of tibialis posterior disruption is rupture of the tendon and hindfoot deformity and stiffness. Rupture almost exclusively terminates any active lifestyle. Acute rupture may occur in individuals with predisposed tendinosis; however, it generally occurs with progressive tendinous degeneration. With complete rupture, a rigid flat foot develops with progressive rearfoot eversion. As this progresses, posterior impingement in the hindfoot often occurs. Stage three tendon disruptions are beyond the scope of conservative management (17).

Treatment of tibialis posterior muscular tendinous disruption should consist of functional biomechanical orthotics with the use of antipronation shoes. Functional taping to restrict eversion and pronation may be of particular benefit during the acute stages. Postexercise icing along with stretching and strengthening exercises of involved muscle are important.

The tibialis posterior is considered to be a postural muscle prone to tightening and fatigue. This will often produce a reflex inhibition of the antagonist, which further adds to lower extremity dysfunction and instability. Thus, during rehabilitative phases, appropriate proprioceptive exercises should be performed (Figs. 16.20 and 16.21). Strengthening can begin with isometric contraction. The resistance should be applied while the patient is actively inverting and plantarflexing the foot. Resisted concentric range of motion can be performed using surgical tubing or a weight strapped around the midfoot while the patient is in the side-lying position and actively inverting and plantarflexing the foot against gravity. In the later stages of rehabilitation, plyometric resistance can be developed by having the patient perform a single leg hop while inverting the foot during the float phase.

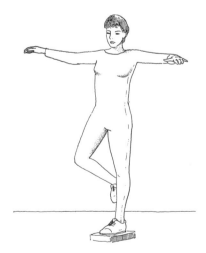

Figure 16.20. The patient stands on one foot on a dense piece of foam, beginning with the eyes open. After 1 minute of standing has been successfully completed without touching the other foot to the ground for balance, the patient advances to performing this activity with the eyes closed.

Flexor Digitorum Longus Musculotendinous Disruption

Flexor digitorum longus involvement may be associated with overpronation syndrome or a sudden increase of jumping or acceleration events. As the flexor digitorum longus becomes active, predominantly in propulsion, irritation may develop while performing interval training or sprints. Sports such as dancing, ballet, karate, and jumping sports may provide predisposition to injury of this muscle. Palpatory tenderness may be noted along the course of the muscle or along its lengthy tendon, primarily in the region of the midfoot. The use of similar taping and therapeutic methods, as described for the tibialis posterior, are effective for treatment of disruptions, along with the use of a toe crest pad to help decrease overuse of the muscle during toe-off phase.

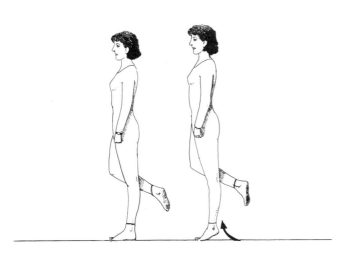

Figure 16.21. Standing unilateral heel raise not only strengthens the deep and superficial compartments, but also provides a proprioceptive challenge.

Flexor Hallucis Longus Musculotendinous Disruption

The flexor hallucis longus muscle-tendon unit may be disrupted by sports similar to those that disrupt the flexor digitorum longus. This muscle is particularly vulnerable during ballet when the athlete is performing en pointe. Irritation of this tendon may further occur during hyperextension injury of the first metatarsal phalangeal joint, such as in turf toe.

If overuse is the cause of origin, functional biomechanical orthotics and antipronation footwear are indicated. During the acute stage, the use of a rocker bottom sole or a rigid plate in the forefoot of a shoe may be helpful in reducing muscular activity of the flexor hallucis longus. Functional taping restricting dorsiflexion and foot pronation, such as a hallux lock and low dye taping, is particularly successful during early return to competition.

As with the flexor digitorum longus, rehabilitation exercises should incorporate toe flexion with foot plantarflexion and inversion. Such exercises may consist of picking up marbles, quarters, or socks (Fig. 16.22).

MUSCULOTENDINOUS INJURIES OF THE SUPERFICIAL POSTERIOR COMPARTMENT

Gastrocnemius Strain

One of the most common strains of the lower extremity involves the musculotendinous junction of the gastrocnemius. Repetitive eccentric loading is usually responsible for these injuries; however, an acute injury may develop as a result of a sudden acceleration when the calf is in a somewhat stretched position. This is the case in "tennis leg." There is some debate about whether tennis leg represents a rupture of the plantaris or

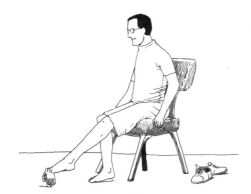

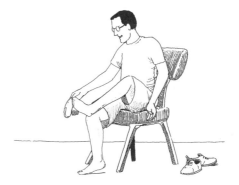

Figure 16.22. The sock pickup exercise strengthens the flexor digitorum longus and the other muscles of the deep posterior compartment and intrinsic foot muscle.

whether it is a second- or third-degree injury to the gastrocnemius musculotendinous junction. Regardless, tennis leg occurs suddenly with a sharp localized pain in the calf. Most patients describe a sensation of being struck in the back of the leg and possibly hearing a snap. Tennis leg most commonly affects the medial head of the gastrocnemius, particularly in Type 3 ruptures. This generally occurs subsequent to a sudden knee extension while the foot is dorsiflexed, or when the foot is caused to dorsiflex while the knee is in extension. A middle-aged athlete is most commonly affected by this condition. Ecchymosis and swelling are frequently present, particularly in those injuries in which a large amount of muscle is torn. Often, tennis leg is preceded by symptoms in the musculotendinous junction. Thus, prior musculotendinous degeneration may predispose the athlete to such ruptures.

Disruption of the medial head of the gastrocnemius muscle has frequently been misdiagnosed as thrombophlebitis (50).

At onset, rest, ice, compression, and elevation (RICE) therapy should be instituted immediately. Non–weight-bearing with crutches should be maintained in second- or third-degree injury. First-degree strains should use limited weight bearing and a heel lift, bilaterally, to reduce tension on the gastrocnemius. Strengthening and stretching along with Achilles stretching should be instituted at the earliest tolerable time.

Second-degree gastrocnemius strains may require the use of a short leg cast or splint. In more severe cases, a long leg cast with the knee held at 60° of flexion and the foot at 10°–15° of plantarflexion may be necessary to proximate the tissues. Third-degree strains may require surgical reattachment of the separated ends.

A patient who has sustained such a strain of the gastrocnemius is likely to strain the opposite leg. This is possibly due to compensation for (or continuation of) the same musculotendinous degenerative pattern.

Achilles Tendinitis

Achilles tendinitis is a common overuse syndrome that is often associated with foot pathomechanics such as underpronation and overpronation. Symptoms may progress insidiously from stiffness to pain and restricted motion. Symptoms may often develop after an overexertion effort and gradually progress thereafter. The condition is most common in the middle-aged athlete between 30 and 50 years of age; however, it

can be just as debilitating in the younger athlete. The most common location of tendinitis in the Achilles tendon is approximately 2 cm proximal to the superior margin of the calcaneus.

In running, 5.3 to 10 times the body weight is transmitted through this structure from contraction of the triceps surae. Tendinous disruption may involve the mesotenon, in which case the condition is known as peritendinitis (tenosynovitis). The mesotenon carries most of the blood supply to the midportion of the Achilles tendon. As a result, secondary changes in the tendon may occur as a result of vascular compromise.

Primary pathology of the Achilles tendon itself is usually the result of repetitive mechanical stress and microtearing. This usually occurs 2 to 6 cm above the insertion of the Achilles tendon, where its vascular supply is most limited (51). Tendinous degeneration or tendinitis may lead to bleeding with cyst formation, mucinoid degeneration, or calcification.

There are several causative factors for Achilles tendinitis. Varus deformities of the rearfoot and forefoot with functional overpronation create additional torque across the Achilles tendon, particularly its medial aspect (52). Because a majority of the pull of the triceps surae is on the medial side of the calcaneus, the Achilles tendon is additionally active in the control of overpronation and stabilization of the subtalar joint. Improper footwear may add to this stress by providing direct pressure irritation to the tendon or improper biomechanical control. Furthermore, shock absorption is an important factor. Excessively worn shoes and/or thinning of the calcaneal fat pad increases the shock-wave amplitude through the Achilles tendon on heel strike. To compensate, the soleus muscle increases its activity 40% to 60%, further increasing the load on the Achilles tendon. Other training errors such as running excessively on a cambered road, interval training, hill training, and a sudden increase in mileage are causative factors. Systemic diseases such as gout and rheumatoid arthritis may further complicate this condition.

Examination may elicit a thickened or swollen tendon. The exact site of maximum tenderness should be determined. Crepitation may often be palpated by passively dorsiflexing the ankle while firmly palpating over the nodularity of the tendon. Dorsiflexion may be limited, particularly with the knee extended. Performance of a single leg heel raise may reproduce pain and musculotendinous limitations.

Lateral radiographs may demonstrate soft tissue swelling, dystrophic calcification, or osteophytes. MRI may be necessary for further imaging, and ultrasonography can be helpful for further delineation of tendinous disruption (53).

Treatment should begin with RICE therapy. Appropriate training modifications should be made to reduce those aggravating factors that may perpetuate this condition. Footwear modifications may be indicated, such as the addition of heel lifts, bilaterally, to reduce stretch and muscular load across the Achilles tendon, or cutting away the heel counter to relieve pressure irritation. In addition, proper biomechanics of footwear must be evaluated to eliminate aggravating factors such as overpronation (52, 54). If footwear cannot control this feature, functional orthotics may be necessary. Those patients with Achilles tendinitis secondary to overpronation will demonstrate a point of maximal tenderness over the medial border of the tendon. During acute phases, partial weight bearing with crutches should be considered. Casting has shown limited success (55). Several sources discourage this form of treatment because it may predispose the tendon to chronicity via musculotendinous weakening from disuse. Some, however, favor the use of night splinting (particularly in acute situations) over a course of 3 to 6 weeks. Early pain-free range of motion must be stressed. As symptoms allow, eccentric exercises should be instituted to generate tendon hypertrophy.

In chronic cases, transverse friction massage may mobilize the peritenon and the tendon, thus allowing full range of motion. This is most effective when combined with an immediate follow-up of therapeutic modalities such as ice, ultrasound, microcurrent, and other therapies that limit inflammation.

Taping the foot in plantarflexion is useful during the early return to competition. Cortisone injections should be limited. There is a question of whether the risks of tendinous disruption or rupture that may occur after cortisone therapy outweigh any potential benefits that are thought to be transient and limited. Glycosaminoglycan polysulfate (GAGPS) has been shown to inhibit the formation of thrombin and fibrin. In chronic cases, hypertrophic scarring may be a limiting and aggravating factor in Achilles peritendinitis. Thus, GAGPS injections may be more applicable in chronic cases (23).

On rare occasions a tendon xanthoma may develop, invading the Achilles tendon at its insertion. This tumor is a benign, slow-growing mass containing cholesterol fat and a fibrous stroma, which frequently predisposes the Achilles tendon to disruption and even rupture. Although generally nonpainful, its known potential sequelae call for an appropriate surgical referral for excision (17).

Achilles Tendon Rupture

Achilles tendinitis is generally documented before Achilles rupture. There may be evidence of microscopic tearing, degeneration, and inflammation. This may present as local stabbing or prickling pain with sudden acceleration. These tendons may present with normal function, as 25% of intact fibers can allow for normal function of the Achilles tendon. A normal tendon can withstand forces of more than 2000 psi. These sites of tearing may be associated with a local zone of critical avascularization (52). This region is generally 2 to 6 cm above the calcaneus and generally coincides with the most common site of rupture. Predisposition to a rupture frequently follows a course of steroid injection. These injections are associated with reducing tensile strength and delaying normal healing of the tendon. Cysts within the tendon may also be associated with local steroid injection (55). Achilles tendon rupture is common several weeks after the injections. (Ten percent of steroidal tendon injections are said to lead to rupture.) Other risk factors for rupture include the presence of a tendon xanthoma or familial hyperlipidemia.

Thompson's test involves squeezing the calf while the patient is in a prone position. A positive test reveals little or no plantarflexion of the involved foot. It has an accuracy rate of 95% for diagnosis of an Achilles tendon rupture. High-resolution ultrasonography has an overall sensitivity rate of 96% in the detection of Achilles tendon pathology (56). It is recommended as a first-line approach in imaging of the Achilles tendon (53). MRI also elicits a high level of sensitivity for Achilles tendon pathology.

Ultrasonography is most useful for determining the effectiveness of conservative care. If the tendon ends approximate with plantarflexion, then conservative care should be attempted. The point at which tendon approximation occurs is a position in which the leg should be casted or splinted. The casting should involve either an above the knee or below the knee cast for 4 weeks. After this period, a new cast is applied with reduced plantarflexion. The total length of non–weight-bearing time is 4 to 8 weeks, after which a 2- to 3-mm heel lift should be used for an additional 4 weeks. Slow mobilization should take place with a gradual increase in strengthening exercises. Terminal exercises must include skipping, jumping, and rebounding activities to allow for hypertrophy of the tendon. There is some evidence suggesting that immobilization is unnecessary, and a brace or splint limiting dorsiflexion to neutral is sufficient.

There is a great deal of debate about the appropriate treatment of Achilles tendon ruptures. Conservative management of Achilles ruptures may result in a weaker tendon compared with surgical repair. However, complications of surgery may include wound healing problems with poor incision closure, particularly over the posterior aspect of the Achilles tendon. Infection is always a concern, as is excess scarring and sural nerve injury. If the diagnosis of rupture is delayed, surgical repair is the treatment of choice. Conservative treatment has been shown to restore tendon strength to 49% to 84% of that of the normal leg. Surgical treatment has been demonstrated to restore tendon strength from 71.2% to 101% of the nonoperated leg (17, 23, 42, 57).

Soleus Strain

Soleus strains usually occur in combination with gastrocnemius strains; however, the soleus may be involved extensively in medial tibial stress syndrome. In such situations, bone scans will demonstrate an uptake in the tibia correlating to the origin of the soleus. Such strains may occur more often in the long-distance runner. Examination will demonstrate symptoms while dorsiflexing the foot with the knee in a flexed position. A gastrocnemius strain may produce symptoms in this position; however, it will be less significant than while the knee is extended. As the soleus attaches medially onto the calcaneus, it has an important role in controlling the subtalar joint by limiting pronation. Treatment of soleus strains is similar to that of gastrocnemius strains. However, stretching and rehabilitative exercises are to be performed with the knee flexed.

Plantaris Musculotendinous Disruption

The plantaris originates from the supralateral femoral condyle and inserts on the medial aspect of the calcaneus. There is a great deal of controversy regarding the plantaris muscle and tennis leg. It was once thought that tennis leg, a condition caused by sudden acceleration and forceful dorsiflexion of the foot with extension of the knee, was a rupture of the plantaris muscle. Current thought is directed more toward the gastrocnemius as being primarily involved. The plantaris is considered rudimentary and insignificant by some. It does, however, attach to the lateral leg,

cross the knee joint, and attach to the medial aspect of the calcaneus. Thus, it may have some effect in controlling the subtalar joint and possibly medial rotation of the tibia.

MUSCULOTENDINOUS INJURIES OF THE DORSAL FOOT

Extensor Digitorum Brevis Disruption

The extensor digitorum brevis may be overstretched and strained in an ankle inversion sprain. On occasion, avulsion fracture may occur from the supralateral calcaneus.

Extensor Hallucis Brevis Disruption

The extensor hallucis brevis may be involved concomitantly with injury to the extensor hallucis longus. With muscular hypertonicity or tendinous disruption, entrapment of the deep peroneal nerve may occur as this muscle intersects between the first cuneiform metatarsal articulation (Fig. 16.11) (30).

MUSCULOTENDINOUS INJURIES OF THE PLANTAR FOOT

Abductor Hallucis Strain

First-degree musculotendinous strains of the abductor hallucis muscle have been seen. There are several potential causes of this injury: overuse, secondary to hallucis abducto valgus, direct trauma, and acute overstretching of the muscle-tendon unit during an activity such as soccer, karate, or wrestling. Compression neuropathy may often occur at the medial plantar nerve and is known as "jogger's foot." This condition occurs where the medial plantar nerve courses deep to the origin of the abductor hallucis. This nerve is compressed against the calcaneus as the nerve passes between the deep abductor fascia and the spring ligament (Fig. 16.23) (30).

Myofascial trigger points may be active in the abductor hallucis, with a trigger point located at the anteromedial calcaneus and active referral to the medial first metatarsal phalangeal joint (58).

Plantar Fasciitis and Heel Spurs

The plantar fascia, also known as the plantar aponeurosis, connects the calcaneal tubercle to the forefoot. The plantar fascia may become painful at the distal fibers (usually in the midfoot) or the proximal fibers near the insertion at the medial tubercle of the calcaneus. This condition is often referred to as "heel pain syndrome," and is

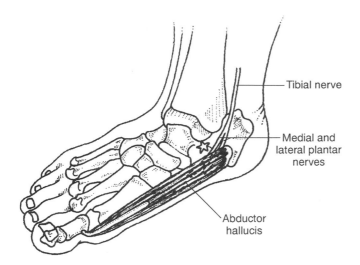

Figure 16.23. Calcaneal eversion and valgus hallux deviation may produce compression of the medial and lateral plantar nerves. (Reprinted with permission from Michaud TC. Foot orthoses and other forms of conservative foot care. Baltimore: Williams & Wilkins, 1993.)

differentiated from a variety of other syndromes, many of which occur concomitantly. The differential diagnosis should include calcaneal fat pad atrophy, calcaneal stress fracture, tarsal tunnel syndrome, entrapment of the medial calcaneal nerve, first sacral radiculopathy, and Sever's disease in 9- to 11-year-olds. Systemic arthritides may present with heel pain. Conditions such as rheumatoid arthritis, ankylosing spondylitis, Reiter's syndrome, and gout may be differentiated by what often appears radiologically as a large and fluffy calcaneal spur, as well as through further isolation via blood tests. Blood tests should consist of an erythrocyte sedimentation rate (ESR), rheumatoid factor, human leukocyte antigen B_{27} (HLA-B27), and uric acid.

Clinically, plantar fasciitis usually presents unilaterally, but it is common to have bilateral symptoms. Symptoms are generally worse in the morning with the first steps out of bed or with the first steps after prolonged sitting or non–weight-bearing. Symptoms are generally worsened after activity and prolonged weight bearing. Frequently, patients may present with secondary conditions related to antalgic position and gait. This antalgic posture consists of walking or standing on the lateral border of the foot. Symptoms may eventually progress to the inability to bear weight for more than a short period. Generally symptoms occur insidiously. However, acute conditions may occur as a result of a sudden increase in activity or a sudden resistance of dorsiflexion forces through the forefoot, particularly in the overweight athlete. The plantar fascia helps assist in the development

of the toe-off phase of gait. Propulsion is critical in this stage due to the windlass effect, whereby dorsiflexion of the first metatarsophalangeal joint elevates the medial longitudinal arch, locking the midfoot via tightening of the plantar fascia (28). This generates a more rigid foot for accentuating leverage for propulsion. Therefore, it is not surprising that jumping sports and other sports requiring rapid acceleration may cause acute plantar fasciitis to develop, whereas sports such as distance running may have a more insidious onset. The addition of hills and speed work as well as increased mileage may add to the onset of symptoms.

Distal plantar fasciitis will present with tenderness in the plantar fascia, particularly in the midfoot region. In these patients, dorsiflexion of the toes almost always exacerbates symptoms, particularly with the addition of ankle dorsiflexion. For these patients, symptoms are most notable in the propulsion phase and predominate in those individuals who have a pes cavus foot. These patients often respond best to orthotic control when a fascial groove is incorporated into the device and a well-cushioned top cover is used. Transverse friction massage and stretching may also be beneficial in the subacute and chronic phases.

Proximal plantar fasciitis frequently is asymptomatic with dorsiflexion of the toes. Palpation of the plantar fascia in the distal aspect of the forefoot and midfoot may be asymptomatic or present with minor symptoms. However, palpation of the origin of the plantar fascia at the medial calcaneal tubercle may result in exquisite pain. On palpation, this pain is usually knife-like, sharp, and often burning. Eighty percent of those with plantar fasciitis present with this type of symptom.

Proximal plantar fasciitis may occur secondary to a pes cavus or pes planus. Overpronation is a common precipitating factor, as are simple training errors. Plantarflexion of more than 60% may predispose an athlete to plantar fasciitis. This allows the runner more time in the propulsive phase of gait, which further dorsiflexes the first metatarsal phalangeal joint. In turn, the windlass effect is increased, creating greater stress within the plantar fascia (23).

Improper footwear may be a major cause of plantar fasciitis, both proximal and distal. Such footwear may allow excessive pronation or underpronation as well as impaired shock absorption. Excessive pronation elongates the plantar fascia during the midstance phase. Such elongation may be controlled by low dye taping and functional biomechanical orthotics to control forefoot and rearfoot deviations as well as any other mechanical deviations causing pronation. Recurrence of plantar fasciitis is high and primarily involves running sports.

No objective, reliable diagnostic test for plantar fasciitis is currently available because plantar fascia cannot be visualized effectively. Diagnosis should not be based on the radiographic finding of a heel spur (59). Heel spurs may be present in 50% to 75% of individuals with painful heels. On the nonpainful foot, these same spurs may be present 63% of the time. In the asymptomatic population, heel spurs may be present 10% to 30% of the time. Radiographs may be helpful, however, in revealing a fatigue fracture at the heel spur. This view should be performed as a 45° medial oblique view of the calcaneus (23). The presence of a spur by itself rarely correlates with the severity of symptoms or resistance to treatment. The plantar calcaneal spur is found deep to the fascia and is associated with traction and mechanical stress from the muscles of the first layer. However, when the spur is large, it can be associated with heel pain. This is more common in those conditions of systemic origin. Ultrasonography may have some use because the mean plantar fascia thickness is greater for persons with plantar fasciitis than for those without heel pain. More than 60% of symptomatic patients will demonstrate an increased uptake at the medial calcaneal tubercle with technetium-99 bone scans (17). This is nondiagnostic for plantar fasciitis or a calcaneal stress fracture because it most often represents periosteal traction at the medial calcaneal tubercle. Many believe that in 95% of cases, radiographs or bone scans are unnecessary.

Frequently, plantar fasciitis is associated with dysfunction of the plantarflexors of the foot. Conditions such as chronic Achilles tendinitis and trisurae strains may predispose the athlete to plantar fasciitis as a result of mechanical compensation.

Plantar fibromas may develop within the plantar fascia. These benign tumors are of unknown cause. Histologic study indicates a local chronic inflammatory process. These tumors are most commonly seen in middle-aged athletes but can be seen at any age. They present as a firm nodule within the plantar fascia. This nodule may be asymptomatic; however, it can present with pain during mechanical irritation.

The key to effective treatment of plantar fasciitis is aggressive conservative therapy and dedicated patient compliance. Achilles tendon stretching with the foot medially rotated and supinated is particularly useful in the acute stages. This position reduces tension on the plantar fascia. Increasing dorsiflexion at the ankle will help compensate and reduce the necessity for elongation of the plantar fascia. During the acute stages, unsupported stretching of the dorsiflexors and plantar fascia is not advised because it will frequently aggravate the condition. As the condition improves, nonsupported stretching of the plantarflexors can gradually be performed with the foot in neutral position. The use of heel lifts during the acute phases helps to decrease the angle of the hindfoot to the forefoot, thus shortening the origin and insertion of the plantar fascia. It is recommended that these heel lifts be used for only a short period because they also require additional dorsiflexion of the first metatarsal phalangeal joint at toe-off.

Treatment must concentrate not only on dorsiflexion of the ankle, but also on restoration of the full range of motion of dorsiflexion of the hallux at the metatarsal phalangeal joint. This combination is necessary to limit recurrence of the condition and/or compensatory conditions. Posterior night splints or casts have been shown to be effective for the reduction of symptoms, particularly morning stiffness (60).

Correction of abnormal biomechanics is essential, not only for recovery but also for prevention of recurrence. This correction may include the prescription of biomechanically controlled athletic footwear or the use of functional orthotics. Functional orthotics appear to be most effective after 6 to 8 weeks.

Manipulative treatment may be beneficial as a restoration of normal joint mechanics to reduce tension across the plantar fascia. Frequently, the calcaneus will demonstrate a restriction of anterior glide, dorsiflexion, abduction, and inversion. Additionally, mobilization and manipulation of the first ray are essential to ensure complete range of motion. During the acute phase, any midfoot manipulation should use a contact over the dorsum of the foot. Contacting the plantar aspect of the foot may be too painful to perform the procedure adequately. Plantar contact on the navicular and cuboid may be performed during the subacute and chronic stages, particularly in those conditions in which proximal plantar fasciitis occurs.

Concentrated stretching of the trisurae may be enhanced by applying hot packs to the calves while simultaneously icing the plantar fascia. These stretches should be performed several times per day. Icing the plantar fascia with the calf in the stretched position will further reduce

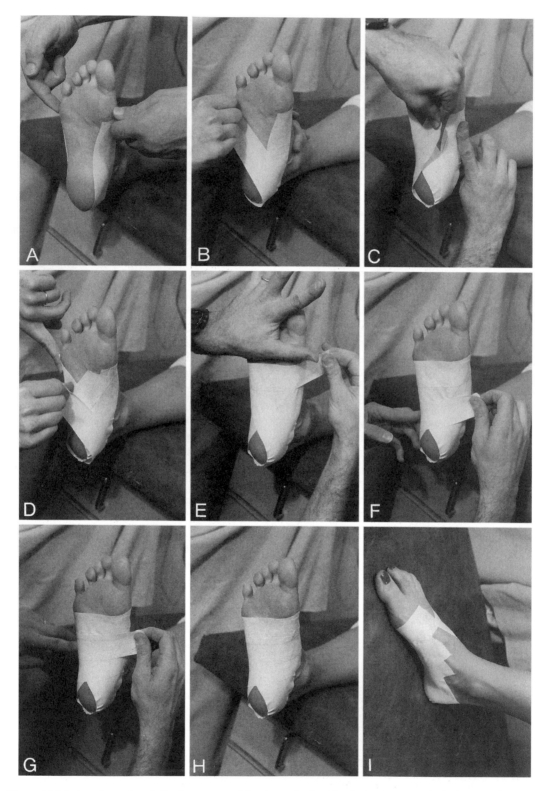

Figure 16.24. Low dye taping mimics the support of the plantar fascia and reduces pronation, which elongates the plantar fascia, creating irritation. **A.** Begin with a strip starting just proximal to the fifth metatarsal phalangeal joint (MPJ), wrapping posteriorly around the calcaneus, and ending just proximal to the first MPJ. **B.** The second strip runs from the fifth MPJ, around the heel, across the arch, and ends at the fifth MPJ again. **C.** The third strip runs from the first MPJ, around the heel, across the lateral arch, and ends at the first MPJ again. **D.** The fourth strip is the same as the second. More strips can be added with excessive weight or high-force activities. **E.** An anchor strip should be placed just proximal to the MPJ. Pressure should be applied to the forefoot to spread the metatarsals and prevent interdigital nerve impingement or metatarsalgia from excessive forefoot compression when the last strip of tape is placed. **F, G,** and **H.** Arch strips are placed from lateral to medial, beginning at the proximal foot and working distally. **I.** When weight bearing, the taped foot should feel snug. (Courtesy of T.L. Forcum.)

any complaints of the ice causing tightening to the plantar fascia. Frequently, these stretching therapies can be incorporated with other modalities such as ultrasound.

Therapeutic modalities such as ultrasound and electrical muscular stimulation may be effective in the reduction of pain and inflammation. The use of iontophoresis and phonophoresis should be evaluated closely; excessive callus formation on the plantar aspect of the foot may reduce the effectiveness of this therapy. Low dye strapping or taping of the foot is an essential part of successful treatment of plantar fasciitis (Fig. 16.24). It is important not to apply the tape too tightly in the forefoot region because weight bearing will spread the forefoot. Compression resulting from taping may cause a secondary irritation to the interdigital nerve or blistering.

Activity modification must occur, and secondary non–weight-bearing activities should be prescribed. Aerobic fitness can be maintained by deep-water running, cycling, and swimming (Fig. 16.25). Gradual introduction of nonimpact activities such as rowing or a stair stepper may be valuable for progressive reintroduction of the athlete to running activity. Use of a cross country ski machine in these stages may irritate plantar fasciitis due to the need for dorsiflexion of the first ray on propulsion. The athlete should be able to perform a single leg hop before returning to limited running activity.

Soft tissue massage of the plantar fascia is a

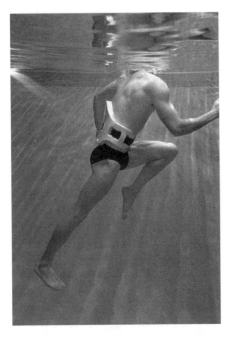

Figure 16.25. Deep-water running with the added buoyancy of an Aquajogger allows for non–weight-bearing cardiovascular exercise. (Courtesy of Excel Sports Science, Eugene, OR.)

required element along with stretching. The author recommends that the athlete perform a brief massage of the plantar fascia before getting out of bed in the morning, before any weight bearing and stretching. This massage can be performed adequately with the use of a golf ball, rolling the ball from the midfoot to the proximal aspect of the metatarsal phalangeal joints longitudinal to the foot. After performing several sweeps, medial to lateral rolls should be performed along the course of the plantar fascia, followed once again by longitudinal rolls. This massaging takes a short time, approximately 20 to 60 seconds, and should be performed any time there is prolonged non–weight-bearing on the foot. Transverse friction massage and myofascial release techniques can further enhance recovery.

Progressive resistance exercises are essential for returning the athlete to high performance. These exercises should begin with isometric toe curls, having the patient hold the contraction for 10 seconds, then repeat 6 to 10 times. This exercise is to be performed 1 to 3 times per day. Initially, some muscular cramping may occur, at which point the active contraction should be stopped. Reintroduction to the exercise should be limited to cramping tolerance. As strength develops, this exercise should progress to a continuous hold for 60 seconds without cramping. Concentric exercises should emphasize toe curling using a towel or an Archxerciser (Archxerciser, St. Louis, MO). Additional exercises should be performed for controlling biomechanics, such as strengthening exercises for the deep posterior compartment in those who overpronate. Strengthening exercises of the trisurae muscle group should be performed over a complete range of motion.

Final stage rehabilitation exercises must include proprioceptive exercises such as single leg stands with the eyes closed for 30 to 60 seconds (Fig. 16.15). Additionally, plyometric exercises will ensure optimal strength of the plantar fascia. Such exercises may consist of jumping rope or other hopping exercises.

Recovery from plantar fasciitis can be a slow process. A minimum of 6 months of conservative therapy should be completed before the consideration of surgery. Nine months of treatment twice a week is considered acceptable for this condition. Before any surgical referral, the competitive athlete should be informed of the surgical success rate of 60% to 80% for return to activity, as well as the fact that full return to high performance often is not possible. Surgical treatment of spurs will rarely improve the pain caused by plantar fasciitis.

Before surgical referral, care should be taken to confirm the original diagnosis. In addition, supporting diagnostic evidence (such as nerve conduction studies) should be gathered to rule out nerve entrapment, particularly of the first branch of the lateral plantar nerve and the medial plantar nerve. The previously mentioned laboratory tests should also be performed.

Medial Tibial Stress Syndrome

Medial tibial stress syndrome is a fasciitis and periostitis occurring along the medial aspect of the leg. This inflammation is due to tensile forces secondary to eccentric contraction of the muscles of the deep posterior and superficial posterior compartments. These forces are exerted on the fascial-periosteal attachment on the tibial crest where a stress reaction can occur. Bone scans have clearly demonstrated increased uptake at the origin of the soleus muscle. This may be secondary to foot pronation, which causes tensile forces to be distributed across the "soleus bridge." This bridge consists of the soleus muscle and deep fascia.

Medial tibial stress syndromes can be categorized as Type I, II, or III. Type I consists of a stress fracture and local stress reactions of the distal medial two thirds of the tibia. Discussion of this condition will be presented under stress fractures. Type II includes periostitis and fasciitis, which will be discussed in this section. Type III consists of a deep posterior compartment syndrome that was discussed earlier in compartment syndromes.

Type II medial tibial stress syndrome can be classified further into acute (less than 2 weeks), subacute (2 to 6 weeks), and chronic (more than 6 weeks) (17).

Symptoms are classified by severity as grades I through IV. Grade I demonstrates palpatory pain along the distal two thirds of the tibia with no symptoms otherwise. Pain is generally well localized; however, there is frequently a less severe region extending 3 cm distal and 5 cm proximal to the point of maximal pain. Grade II demonstrates pain primarily after running and at the onset of activity. Grade III will elicit pain both during and after activity. Grade IV demonstrates pain with walking and frequently low-grade discomfort during inactivity. Athletes may be unable to run.

Symptoms are frequently bilateral and generally develop insidiously. Because of the mild nature of onset, the athlete will frequently try to "run through it." Overuse is generally secondary to several contributing factors such as poor conditioning or sudden increases in training. Training on hard surfaces or worn footwear may further aggravate this condition, as soleal output is increased.

Many believe that poor running mechanics, such as accentuated toe-off, excessive crossover, and overpronation syndrome, are the primary causes of this condition. Improper footwear may contribute; a shoe with inappropriate forefoot flexibility may not allow for proper metatarsal phalangeal joint dorsiflexion, thus inhibiting the windlass effect. In addition, any shoe that excessively inhibits or augments pronation phase may make individuals susceptible to this condition.

Both pes cavus and pes planus will predispose athletes to medial tibial stress syndrome. Rigid pes cavus will impair normal shock absorption, adding additional stress to the tibia. Pes planus requires more output from the tibialis posterior and soleus, increasing fascial and periosteal strain. Muscular imbalances of the foot, such as those creating claw toe deformities, may require elevated activity from the flexor digitorum longus during the propulsive phase of gait.

Some believe that the periosteum may be disengaged traumatically from the bone by either ballistic avulsion or subperiosteal edema or hemorrhage. This theory has been supported by surgical findings.

Physical examination will demonstrate localized tenderness along the posteromedial tibia. Muscle testing of the lower extremity will be normal. Radiographs are usually negative, but occasional localized hypertrophy may be seen along the medial aspect of the tibia. Bone scans may be useful for differentiation from stress fracture. In the late phase, bone scans demonstrate diffuse longitudinal uptake, which indicates localized periostitis. Osteomyelitis should be an initial differential diagnosis along with stress fractures. Syphilis, although rare, may attack long bones and is more likely to do so in the young. Bony changes may occur 6 weeks to 15 months after the eruption of a chancre. Syphilitic periostitis may be characterized by nocturnal pain and may be relieved by movement. Radiographicaly, syphilis presents with a "sabre shin" deformity associated with a pseudo-bowing of the tibia from periosteal proliferation. Involvement is usually bilateral. Osteosarcoma and Ewing's sarcoma are rare, but should be considered because of their potential outcome. In addition, hypervitaminosis A and Paget's disease may also instigate periosteal changes.

Treatment should begin with rest. In mild cases, this may be in the form of training modifications such as reducing duration and intensity of activity. Fitness can be maintained by deep-water running or cycling. In severe cases, absolute rest including the use of crutches may be necessary. In the early phase of treatment, the reduction of inflammation and acute pain is the primary goal. An AirCast (AirCast, Newark, NJ) splint or Active Ankle Brace (BioMet, Warsaw, IN) may allow for reduced symptoms and modified training. Aggressive use of cryotherapy is recommended during this phase. Anti-inflammatory medication and nutritional elements will enhance this process further. Nutrition may be implicated in the etiology of medial tibial stress. One study found that 50% of athletes with shin soreness consume less than half the recommended dietary allowance of calcium (800 mg/day) (23).

Physiotherapy modalities such as interferential, diathermy, and ultrasound are all effective in the treatment of musculotendinous and periosteal injuries. Ultrasound has been shown to be particularly effective in accelerating bone healing. Pulsed ultrasound of 1 watt/cm² has been recommended. In the subacute phase, treatment focuses on preventing scar tissue and decreasing the tension along fascial planes. Application of moist heat followed by transverse friction massage may be helpful. Reduction of tensile forces can be achieved by taping the ankle in a fashion that would support the tibialis posterior and soleus. For some, the application of low dye strapping is sufficient to reduce tensile stress (Fig. 16.24); this would indicate the need or potential efficacy of foot orthoses. Functional biomechanical orthotics for the reduction of overpronation should be varus posted, using soft, nonacrylic posts and a shock-absorbing top cover.

Great attention should be paid to the athlete's footwear. Excessively worn footwear and footwear that does not sufficiently control the athlete's biomechanics should be replaced.

The next phase of treatment focuses on the strengthening of the muscle-bone interface. Initially, this should be achieved by stretching the soleus by dorsiflexing and everting the foot while the knee is flexed. Strengthening exercises should be prescribed after pain is controlled, beginning with isometric exercises and followed by eccentric and concentric exercises. Plyometric exercises should be prescribed in the final stages of rehabilitation. These exercises should focus on strengthening the soleus and the muscles of the deep posterior compartment. After the athlete can perform several one-leg hops without pain, plyometric exercises can be implemented. An effective plyometric exercise for this injury is the use of a one-legged hop or one-legged jump rope whereby the athlete inverts the foot during the jump phase.

The athlete should return to activity conscious of using accurate support and proper footwear and avoiding uneven and hard surfaces. Because cold weather may contribute to or aggravate this condition, long or midlength socks and elastic wrapping of the distal leg with a Molinpic self-grip tape (Cohepress reusable tape; Dome Publishing, Warwick, RI) may be helpful.

In rare cases in which conservative management is unsuccessful, surgical release of the soleus and/or cauterization of the periosteum may be necessary.

Capsular and Ligamentous Injuries of the Leg, Ankle, and Foot

ANKLE SPRAINS

Approximately 14% of athletic injuries are ankle sprains. This results in 10% to 20% of lost time in adolescent and professional athletes. It comprises approximately 25% of lost time in running and jumping sports (17). Ankle sprains constitute approximately half of the major injuries occurring in basketball. Although by nature the ankle joint is a stable mortise, chronic instability occurs in approximately 10% to 20% of patients after an acute ligament injury, irrespective of primary treatment (61). After 9 months, approximately 30% have residual complaints, and evaluation of the same group 6.5 years later showed that 39% had residual complaints (62). Such complaints interfere with daily living and sports activities.

Ninety-five percent of ankle sprains occur as a result of an inversion injury (17). This usually happens when the athlete is running straight and makes a sudden cut. These injuries are most likely to occur while the ankle is in plantarflexion, as the ankle mortise is in an unstable, loose-packed position. This is due to the shape of the talar dome, which is wider anteriorly, creating a close-packed position in dorsiflexion. Injuries in this position primarily injure the anterior talofibular ligament, the most commonly injured ligament of the body. When plantarflexion, inversion, and rotation are all present, injury occurs to the anterior talofibular ligament and the tibiofibular ligament. This is the most common mechanism of most ankle injuries. Pure inversion injuries are rare, but can occur when an athlete is coming down from a rebound, such as in basketball, and lands on another player's foot. Such injuries sprain the calcaneofibular ligament (Fig. 16.26). Injuries secondary to traumatic overpronation, abduction, eversion, and dorsiflexion will sprain the deltoid ligament. The deltoid ligament is fan-shaped and often will avulse the medial malleolus. This also frequently occurs secondary to a sudden change

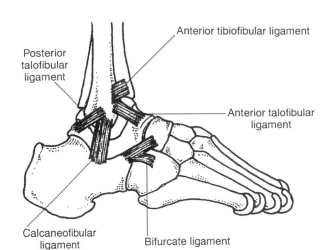

Figure 16.26. Lateral ligaments of the ankle. (Reprinted with permission from Michaud TC. Foot orthoses and other forms of conservative foot care. Baltimore: Williams & Wilkins, 1993.)

in direction or footing.

The mechanism of sprain will generally indicate which tissues will be involved in the injury. Dorsiflexion strains have a tendency to jam the talus into the ankle mortise because the anterior talus is wider than the posterior. This jamming under force separates the syndesmosis of the tibia and fibula, spraining the interosseous membrane and the anterior tibiofibular ligament. Osteochondral fractures of the talus may be associated with this injury. Frequently, an Achilles injury may overshadow an ankle sprain of this nature and the sprain may go untreated. Lack of treatment may lead to instability and chronicity (63). Plantarflexion sprains are usually coupled with inversion or eversion and the respective ligaments medially and laterally. Damage may occur to the anterior retinaculum and lateral posterior tubercle of the talus, particularly in those individuals with Stieda's process or os trigonum.

Several predisposing factors may precipitate recurring ankle sprains. Tight heel cords will predispose an athlete to ankle sprains simply by maintaining the ankle in an open, packed position. Contraction of the trisurae plantarflexes and inverts the rearfoot by the nature of its attachment medially on the calcaneus. This makes the ankle vulnerable to added forces, which may further invert the ankle.

Crossover gait can predispose the runner to inversion sprains by positioning the foot in an excessively supinated position as the heel strikes the ground. Thus, minimal additional force is necessary to invert the foot excessively at heel contact.

Peroneal proprioception and muscular strength are extremely important in the prevention of ankle sprains. The ability to feel or determine the ankle's position in space, and the capability of the muscle tissue to react quickly with significant strength, are crucial for prevention of inversion sprains. Proprioception can be improved through ankle rehabilitation exercises (64).

Shoes are an obvious source of predisposition. Excessively worn shoes that are broken down in the posterolateral portion predispose the foot to inversion sprains by placing the foot in an excessively inverted position at heel strike. Also, soccer-style shoes used during football may reduce the incidence of inversion sprains (21). Soccer cleats generally use a polyurethane sole with approximately 14 relatively flat, wide-based cleats. These cleats are much more stable than those on classic football style shoes. This allows for a more stable base, particularly on a well-maintained field. The use of a brace and/or taping along with a high-top shoe with wider diameter, lower height cleats can significantly reduce injury potential in an unstable ankle.

Shoes that are too narrow may additionally expose the ankle to inversion sprains as the additional width of the foot may bulge over the lateral edges of the sole, placing the foot in an inverted position and predisposing it to ankle sprains. Adequate footwear sizing is crucial for performance and the prevention of ankle injury.

Playing surfaces are another factor in ankle injuries. Uneven surfaces and potholes place the lower extremity in unpredictable situations. Frequently, the unsuspecting athlete is caught turning an ankle on a rock or pinecone on a completely smooth surface. It is possible that proprioceptive function is not stimulated while functioning over flat surfaces; thus, relatively small changes in terrain can have a significant impact on ankle instability.

Anatomical variations of the foot and ankle—such as tarsal coalition, rearfoot varus deformity, forefoot valgus deformity, or plantarflexed first ray—may be predisposing to chronic inversion sprains.

Ankle injuries are most common at the beginning of the athletic season, in the fourth quarter of play, and in the female athlete. The higher incidence of injury in the beginning of the season may point to fitness as a factor. Injury toward the end of competition may further indicate that fitness is a factor, as fatigue sets in late in the game (21, 23). Many women's athletic programs do not provide an adequate training base when compared with their male counterparts. However, this trend is changing as women's athletics are becoming more popular and levels of training are increased.

Classification of Ankle Sprains

Grade I. Ankle sprains are classified into three grades according to severity (17, 21). Although this classification scheme does not cover all situations, it is useful as a guideline for diagnosis and treatment. Grade I ankle sprains are mild, with recovery lasting approximately 1 to 2 weeks. This injury is a mild stretching of a single ligament, usually the anterior talofibular ligament. There is no resulting instability or functional instability. The athlete generally presents with normal gait, but an occasional slight limp may be noted. There is minimal functional loss; however, there is generally difficulty with hopping. Frequently, these individuals are capable of returning to activity with additional taping or bracing.

Examination demonstrates minimal swelling with no hemorrhage. There is point tenderness over the involved ligament, and functional testing is negative.

Grade II. Grade II or moderate ankle sprains may present with mild to moderate instability. This grade is generally indicative of a complete tear of the anterior talofibular ligament or a partial tear of the anterior talofibular ligament plus the calcaneofibular ligament. The athlete will present with a distinctive limp when walking, but will be capable of weight bearing. The athlete may need initial assistance off the field. The athlete is incapable of running, hopping, or performing a toe raise. Swelling is localized with moderate hemorrhage and will generally be isolated to the lateral ankle. The edema may reduce the definition of the Achilles tendon. Major tearing of the anterior talofibular ligament may result in an anterior drawer test that is positive; however, varus stressing should demonstrate a stable joint. In general, recovery will range from 2 to 6 weeks.

Grade III. Grade III sprains are severe and demonstrate both functional and structural instability. The athlete is incapable of bearing full body weight, and frequently even partial weight bearing is painful. There is almost a complete loss of range of motion. This injury is associated with tearing of both the anterior talofibular and calcaneofibular ligaments. There is a complete tear of the anterior capsule and tibiofibular ligament. Grade III injuries present with diffuse swelling throughout the ankle, leaving the Achilles tendon almost indistinct. Hemorrhage is evident, and tenderness will be diffuse both medially and laterally. The anterior drawer and varus stress tests will demonstrate pain and laxity. In general, return to activity will begin in 30 to 90 days.

History

In addition to the mechanism of injury, several questions should be asked to assess severity and differential diagnostic clues.

1. Can the athlete bear weight initially after the injury and did that ability change with the ensuing hours? The ability to walk is indicative of the severity level of the injury. However, with increasing inflammation and anxiety, walking may frequently become difficult. The inability to bear weight suggests a severe second- or third-degree injury.

2. A sound or sensation of a pop, snap, or crack may be accompanied by a severe sprain or fracture. History is significant because it indicates whether one is dealing with an acute injury or the aggravation of a chronic instability.

3. The rate of onset of swelling is of limited pertinence. However, the magnitude of swelling is generally indicative of the severity of injury. Rapid accumulation of swelling is usually representative of hemarthrosis.

4. Prior treatment should be assessed for expected outcome and appropriateness. Frequently, patients will present subsequent to self-treatment, treatment by an athletic trainer, or treatment prescribed by an emergency department. If recovery is not progressing as expected, this may indicate potential complicating sequelae.

5. The age of the athlete may influence diagnostic suspicion. Avulsion fractures are more commonly found in older patients (older than 55 years of age), whereas epiphyseal injuries are a primary concern in younger athletes.

6. Systemic diseases must be considered, particularly diabetes for the potential of diabetic neuropathy. Other systemic conditions such as arthritides or vascular disease will influence recovery.

7. Patient goals are always a primary concern. These goals will correlate with the aggressiveness of treatment provided and the intricacy of rehabilitation.

Palpation

A systematic approach to palpatory inspection

of the lower leg, foot, and ankle should be administered to evaluate the sprained ankle. Regardless of treatment, several sequelae may occur after an ankle sprain; however, most can be prevented through proper diagnosis and management.

Shortly after an injury, there is a "golden" period before the onset of inflammation. This is the ideal time to perform an examination because significant pain and swelling will not hamper the evaluation. With excessive swelling, complete examination may not be possible. In those cases, a follow-up examination 1 week after immobilization to evaluate local tenderness may be necessary. The examiner should work from proximal to distal, saving the suspected most tender points for last. This prevents patient pain and anxiety from impairing further examination. Palpation should begin at the neck of the fibula, moving down through the midshaft of the fibula to the lateral malleolus. Palpation should then assess the Achilles tendon and medial malleolus. Inspection of the foot should begin at the metatarsals, evaluating the base of the fifth metatarsal. Palpation of the navicular and cuboid should be performed, followed by palpation of the ankle ligaments, beginning at the deltoid ligament and the tendons of the medial compartment and proceeding to the peroneal tendons and the posterior talofibular ligament. If swelling is minimal, palpation of the lateral tubercle of the posterior talus is possible. Palpation of the bifurcate ligament and sinus tarsus should be followed by palpation of the anterior tibiofibular ligament and the anterior talofibular ligament.

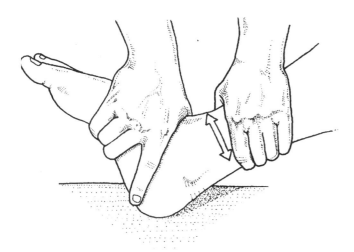

Figure 16.27. An alternative method of performing an anterior drawer test is to stabilize the foot and glide the tibia and fibula posterior. (Adapted from Michaud TC. Foot orthoses and other forms of conservative foot care. Baltimore: Williams & Wilkins, 1993.)

Orthopedic Tests for Ankle Ligament Instability

Orthopedic stress testing of the ankle should be performed bilaterally beginning with the non-injured leg. This process reduces patient anxiety and, it is hoped, will allow for better relaxation and increased accuracy of testing. The following tests should not be performed if there is obvious deformity of the ankle and if swelling occurred immediately after the injury. *Painful palpation over any bony surface or the inability to bear weight should preclude these tests until after radiographic examination can be achieved* (65).

Anterior Drawer Sign. The anterior drawer sign is the most significant test for ankle stability. The procedure is easy to perform by stabilizing the tibia and fibula. With the other hand, the ankle is held in a neutral to slightly plantarflexed position while grasping the calcaneus. A shear force is applied pulling the calcaneus and foot anteriorly (Fig. 16.27). A positive test is accompanied by anterior subluxation of the talus in the ankle mortise, which may present as a "clunk" (17). This test is also considered positive if excursion is more than 4 to 6 mm greater on the injured side than on the opposite side (66).

Inversion Sign (Varus Stress, Talar Tilt). Inversion testing with the ankle in neutral position assesses calcaneal fibular ligament integrity; with plantarflexion, it indicates anterior talofibular ligament integrity (21, 23, 42). This test is performed by stabilizing the distal leg, while inverting the rearfoot with the ankle at both neutral and moderate plantarflexion. Frequently, this test is accompanied by significant pain and a possible clunk (17). A spongy or indefinite endfeel may indicate complete rupture. This test may also be thought of as positive when, in the neutral position, more than 5° to 6° of motion are present on the injured side than on the noninjured side (Fig. 16.28).

Eversion Test (Valgus Stress). The eversion stress test is the exact opposite of the inversion stress test. This test assesses the structural integrity of the deltoid ligament (Fig. 16.28).

Side-to-Side Test. Side-to-side motion tests the integrity of the inferior tibiofibular ligaments and the interosseous membrane. A positive test is frequently associated with fracture. The ankle is held in neutral position without inverting or everting the calcaneus while the foot is sheared transversely. A soft endfeel and excessive glide are considered positive (17).

External Rotation Stress. External rotation stress testing maintains the ankle joint in neutral position while externally rotating the foot. This test is positive with disruption of the syndesmosis (67).

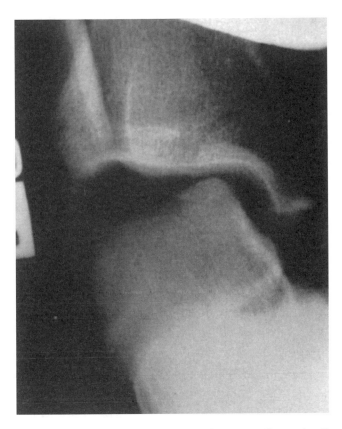

Figure 16.28. Inversion sign stress view showing significant talar tilt. (Reprinted with permission from McGlamry ED. Fundamentals of foot surgery. Baltimore: Williams & Wilkins, 1987.)

Squeeze Test. The squeeze test is performed by grasping the distal tibia and fibula and squeezing them together. The reduction of pain or excess excursion may indicate disruption of the syndesmosis (67).

Radiographic Examination

Ankle radiographs are necessary for any of the following indications.

1. Significant soft tissue swelling.
2. Palpatory tenderness over the malleoli.
3. Obvious deformity.
4. The inability to bear weight over four steps.
5. An individual older than 55 years of age (or younger than 12, according to some sources).

Obvious deformity and the inability to bear weight appear to be the most significant of these factors. Foot radiographs should be performed if there is pain in the midfoot or pain with bony palpation of the navicular, cuboid, or fifth metatarsal. Stress radiographs are rarely necessary during acute sprains; clinical examination adequately assesses ligament instability. Arthrogra-

phy may be useful to differentiate between a first- and second-grade ligament injury; however, this test should be performed shortly after the injury because clotting may seal capsular tears and prevent extravasation of the dyes. Tenography of the flexor hallucis longus and the peroneal sheath can be positive in as many as 25% of ankle sprains. A positive peroneal tenography indicates a tear of the calcaneal fibular ligament and a serious disruption of the ankle (Fig. 16.29) (65).

Sequelae of Ankle Sprains

Chronic sequelae of an ankle sprain are frequent. It is reported that 21% of individuals still have symptoms 9 years after an ankle sprain. Most of these symptoms can be related to ligamentous instability and the likely absence of proper rehabilitation (23). The most common sequelae are functional and ligamentous instability. The following potential sequelae of an ankle sprain will be addressed separately within this chapter.

1. Synovitis.
2. Anterior talar impingement.
3. Posterior impingement.
4. Sinus tarsus syndrome.
5. Subluxing peroneal tendons.
6. Lisfranc ligament instability.
7. Bifurcate ligament instability.
8. Cuboid subluxation.
9. Talar osteochondral lesion.
10. Posterior talus process fracture.
11. Fifth metatarsal styloid fracture.
12. Neurapraxia of the sural, superficial peroneal, and deep peroneal nerves.

Nerve injuries within the ankle occur at a high rate, particularly with grade III strains. Approximately 86% of grade III sprains involve peroneal nerve injury, whereas 83% involve the tibial nerve (17). Grade II ankle sprains are associated with a 17% concomitant injury to the peroneal nerve and 10% to the tibial nerve. Osteochondral lesions of the anterior talar dome are associated with 18% of inversion sprains. For many, recurring ankle sprains or their sequelae can be treated effectively by addressing the cause of aggravation. Structural variants that predispose to ankle sprains, such as a plantarflexed first ray or a rigid forefoot valgus, should be treated with a forefoot valgus posted orthotic or one that uses a first ray cutout.

Functional instability requires focus on rehabilitative strengthening and stretching, particularly of the calf, and development of proprioceptive skills. Mechanical instabilities secondary to

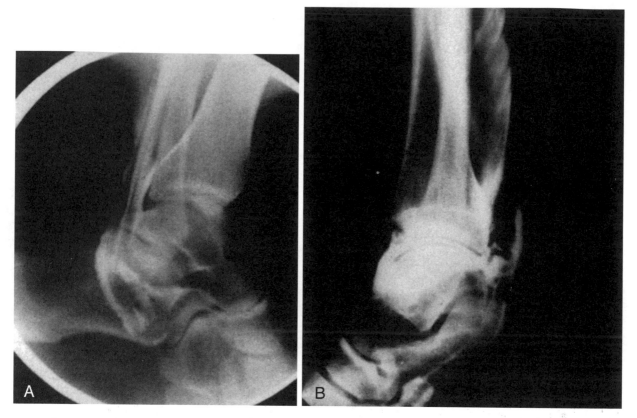

Figure 16.29. (A) Tenography of normal peroneal tendon and **(B)** peroneal tenogram demonstrating ruptured joint capsule and lateral collateral ligaments. (Reprinted with permission from McGlamry ED. Fundamentals of foot surgery. Baltimore: Williams & Wilkins, 1987.)

congenital hypermobility or ligamentous laxity may require taping or bracing for prevention of perpetuation or recurrence of symptoms. Subtalar joint instability associated with disruption of the talocalcaneal ligament and calcaneal fibular ligament may require the use of functional orthotics with a deep heel seat to stabilize the calcaneus and subtalar joint.

Frequently, sinus tarsus syndrome is perpetuated by the repetitive aggravation of overpronation secondary to ankle ligamentous instability. This condition may also respond to functional orthoses.

ON-FIELD ASSESSMENT OF ANKLE INJURY

When a significant ankle sprain occurs on the field, the athlete should be assisted off the field bearing no weight. Being in the spotlight on the playing field may increase the emotionality of the athlete during the assessment. Sideline evaluation may yield a more accurate determination. Cursory examination consisting of palpation should be performed to rule out gross deformity or obvious fracture. After this palpation, it should be determined whether the athlete can bear weight and take four consecutive steps. If the athlete is incapable of these four steps, radiographs are indicated. The shoe, sock, and any tape should be removed after weight-bearing determination and before proceeding with palpatory examination and orthopedic testing. The golden period should be used to perform anterior drawer and talar tilt before the onset of swelling. Should pain and swelling preclude examination, ice should be applied immediately.

In the case of a minor ankle sprain, in which the ankle demonstrates no instability or laxity on any of the orthopedic tests and there is minimal swelling, an assessment should be made regarding the capability of the athlete to perform before return to competition. First, the athlete must have the ability to walk without a limp. If the athlete is capable of ambulating without antalgia, a hop test can be performed. If the athlete can hop without pain, then the athlete should be evaluated for the ability to run forward and backward. With successful completion of those activities, along with figure-eight and side-to-side running without pain or a limp, the athlete can return to competition. The ankle should always be taped before the athlete returns to play in these cases (17, 21).

Treatment

Grade I Sprains. First-degree ankle sprains often require minimal or no treatment; however, misdiagnosis of a seemingly minor ankle sprain can cause sequelae of compensatory conditions or chronic recurrence secondary to instability. Even minor sprains should be assessed for structural and functional instability. With proper functional and structural stability, the athlete can often return to activity immediately or within a few days. Management should consist of icing the ankle after activity and stretching the gastrocnemius and soleus muscles frequently. Return to play should be accompanied by ankle taping.

Grade II Sprains. With significant instability and ligamentous rupture, surgical repair may be required. However, most second- and third-degree sprains respond appropriately to conservative management when there is adherence to a conscientious rehabilitation program. Following are the goals of such a treatment program.

1. Rapid reduction in inflammation.
2. Structural/ligamentous stabilization.
3. Early mobilization and restoration of range of motion.
4. Increased ability to bear weight.
5. Strength/muscular stabilization.
6. Increased functional stabilization and proprioception.
7. Gradual return to exercise and play.
8. Establishment of a home rehabilitation program.

The level of success in achieving these goals will be directly proportionate to the direct treatment of the isolated injuries, as well as the sport-specific functional stabilization program.

Control of Swelling. Regular and dedicated icing during the first 24 to 48 hours is crucial for the rapid reduction of inflammation. Because inflammation is the primary cause of pain subsequent to these injuries, the judicious use of ice is necessary. Ice should be applied as soon as possible after injury or exercise sessions. The maximum duration of cryotherapy should be 15 to 20 minutes, with 15 minutes being adequate to develop vasoconstriction. In the early stages, elevation and compression should be emphasized; gravity dependence may supersede the positive benefits of icing when the ankle is left below the heart. Therefore, the use of an ice bucket may be best left for the later stages of rehabilitation. Some authors believe that focal compression is more significant than frequency and duration of cryotherapy in enhancing the rate of recovery of inversion

ankle sprains (68). Clear evidence demonstrates the ineffectiveness of heat therapy, particularly in the early stages of rehabilitation.

Compression can be maintained by an open Gibney tape or tensor bandage. The use of an Air-Cast ankle icing unit or a vasopneumatic device to apply consistent compression over the injured tissue may further stimulate the reduction of soft tissue swelling (69).

Stabilization. Recommended stabilization can be achieved by athletic taping (70). However, this may be impractical due to cost or accessibility of skilled personnel to apply athletic taping. In severe cases, casting or the use of a short leg walking brace may be necessitated during the acute phase. Several ankle braces designed for inversion/eversion stabilization allow for plantar and dorsiflexion. For many, these braces are a more practical solution to stabilization than athletic taping. Such braces as the active ankle brace and the Air-Cast ankle brace allow for medial and lateral compression, which may be of further benefit with disruption of the syndesmosis. These braces clearly limit rotation and eversion/inversion motion without the fatigability of tape. Initially, tape will reduce range of motion by 30% to 50%. However, after 10 minutes of exercise, this control is diminished by 40% (17). Anterior drawer and talar tilt under stress radiography have demonstrated insignificant control with the use of athletic taping. However, those athletes who were taped demonstrated a significantly shorter reaction time. Thus, the efficacy of ankle taping may be restricted to the control of the extremes of ankle motion, and may help shorten reaction time of the peroneal muscles by affecting the proprioceptive function of the ankle (71).

Athletic taping is contraindicated in those athletes who have infections, eczema, open wounds, peripheral vascular disease, or peripheral neuropathy. Adhesive taping should be removed shortly after each practice session or athletic event. In the absence of a skilled health-care provider, tape should not be left on the athlete for more than 3 days.

Continuous taping can lead to an inequality of pressure and tension, particularly over contoured and uneven shapes of the ankle and foot. Strip taping or basket weaving has generally been assessed to provide the greatest level of strength and the highest level of continuity in applying compressive forces to the ankle (Fig. 16.30) (72).

Mobility. Early mobilization is essential for rapid recovery and the prevention of late residual symptoms and instability (73). Thirty percent of those who begin range of motion and weight-

SPECIFIC ANKLE REHABILITATION TAPING FOR: ISOLATED ANTERIOR TALO-FIBULAR LIGAMENT SPRAIN

Positioning: seated, with the calf supported and the foot held at a 90 degree angle

BASIC STRIPS	SUB-ACUTE: (beginning to weightbear) • activity depends on stage of healing • how much swelling? • weightbearing only if no pain	PROGRESSIVE STRIP ADAPTATIONS	
		FUNCTIONAL: (moderate to dynamic activity) • adequate support for individual ligament • enough mobility for moderate activity	RETURN TO SPORT: (training, then competition) • reinforced support • adaptations for specific needs of sport
BASIC PREPARATION: (clean, shave, spray) Prowrap anchors 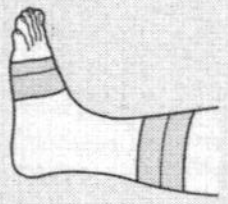	• if swelling is likely, use a **felt 'J'**-lateral side (bevel the edges) 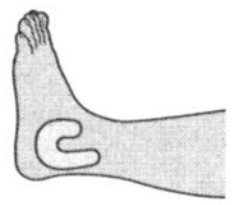	• if swelling persists, continue with **felt 'J'** • for increasing activity, use **heel and lace pads** 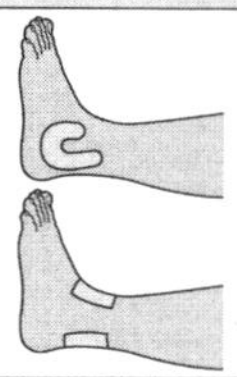	• **use heel & lace pads** 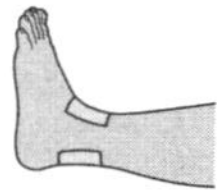
LATERAL SUPPORT: Stirrups 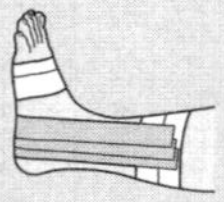	**modified basketweave** composed of: • **3 stirrups (vertical)** (start medially and pull up strongly on lateral side) • interlock stirrups with **2 horizontal strips** (strong lateral pull) 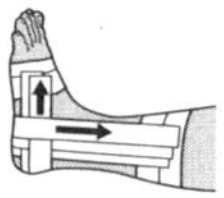	• continue with **modified basketweave** (extra pull on lateral side for both horizontal and vertical strips) 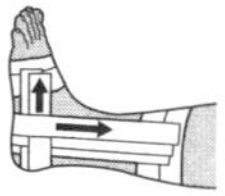	• continue with **modified basketweave** (extra pull particularly on lateral horizontal strips) • for more mobility, **fanned stirrups** can be used 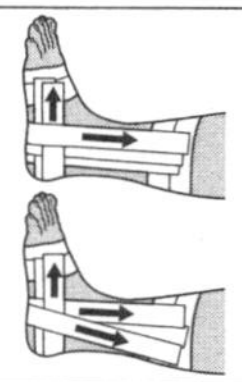
REINFORCEMENT: Ankle locks 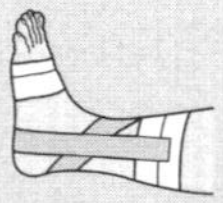	**lateral 'V' lock** with main tension pulling up on last component (posterior vertical strip) **medial 'V' lock** with main tension pulling from behind heel horizontally across medial malleolus 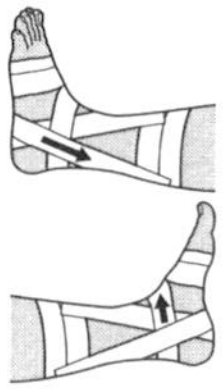	• continue with **l lateral V-lock** **l medial V-lock** 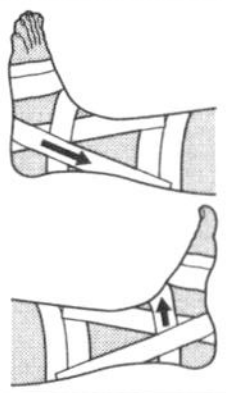	• continue with **lateral V-lock** **l medial V-lock** 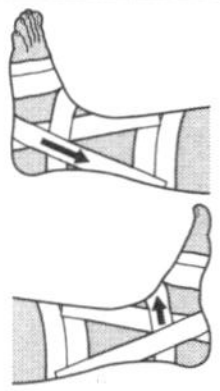
STABILIZATION: Figure-8 variations 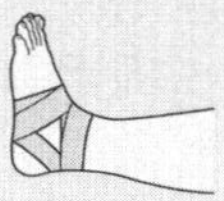	• **simple figure-8** (start medially and pull up strongly on lateral side) (ensure plantar flexion is restricted with this strip) 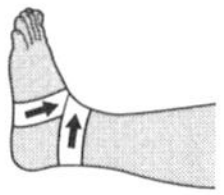	• **heel-locking figure-8** for added stability (always pull up strongly on lateral side) 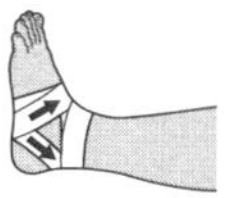	• continue with **heel-locking figure-8** or • if more plantar flexion needed for sport, use **reverse figure-8** (ensure that end-range plantar flexion is limited with previous locking strips or with closing figure-8) • if tight, rigid boots are necessary, omit this step 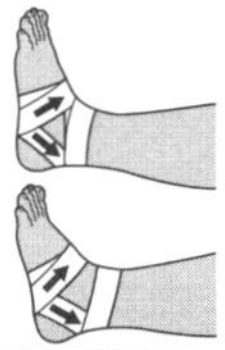
CLOSING-UP: Figure-8 variations 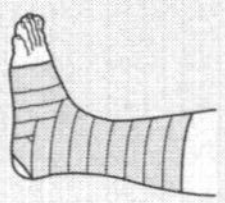	• add **felt heel-lift** for weightbearing 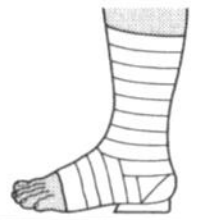	• **heel-lift** (optional) 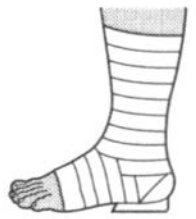	**Purpose:** *supports anterior talo-fibular ligament, prevents inversion, limits inward rotation of foot, end-range eversion and end-range plantar flexion, permits functional plantar flexion*

Figure 16.30. Ankle taping technique for a plantar flexion inversion sprain. (Reprinted with permission from Austin KA, Gwynn-Brett KA, Marshall SC. Illustrated guide to taping techniques. London: Mosby-Wolfe, 1994.)

bearing rehabilitation programs experience less pain at 3 weeks after injury than those who were immobilized in a plaster splint for 10 days.

Rehabilitation of Stable Ankle Sprains. Rehabilitation of grade II and stable grade III ankle sprains should consist of five stages (17).

Stage I. This first stage is the immediate management of the injury, consisting of isolating the cause of injury and diagnosing those structures involved. The primary goal of treatment at this stage is protecting the body part from further injury and minimizing hemorrhage and swelling. The immediate application of ice, compression, and elevation along with stabilization are essential. Stabilization may be accomplished with an open Gibney tape with a doughnut pad around the malleoli, a posterior splint, or other bracing. Gentle dorsiflexion and plantarflexion range of motion should be encouraged unless the injury is severe. Ice should be applied for 15 to 20 minutes every 1 to 1.5 hours. Light weight bearing should be encouraged, applying approximately 5% to 10% of body weight. This will help prevent calf shortening by positioning the foot in dorsiflexion and reducing active contraction of the gastrocnemius from non–weight-bearing use of crutches, where the knee is held in flexion and the ankle in plantarflexion.

Stage II. Stage II is the acute phase that primarily consists of inflammation lasting for several days. Those therapies associated with the reduction of inflammation are indicated during this phase of treatment. The use of intermittent pneumatic compression devices has been shown to reduce inflammation in the foot and ankle. Other modalities such as interferential therapy and H-wave may be helpful in reducing inflammation in this acute phase. Many believe that ice baths or whirlpools are necessary during this stage; however, gravitational dependence may actually increase edema. Active motion of the ankle may reduce this effect. In addition, cryokinetics may help break antalgic gate patterns. Cryokinetics begins with the application of ice or ice massage to the area until numbness occurs. This is followed by the athlete attempting to walk as normally as possible until discomfort develops. Many believe that this will reduce functional instabilities caused by improper muscular facilitation and antalgic gait. An athlete who is unable to walk without a limp subsequent to this icing is not ready for this type of therapy. Resisted isometric exercises should be applied after the athlete can apply 50% of body weight while using crutches. For a lateral ligament injury, the ankle should be moved into a position of eversion. Intrinsic foot

musculature can be exercised by performing toe curls isometrically with a towel on the floor or by picking up marbles or socks (Fig. 16.22).

If possible, these exercises should be performed with the leg in an elevated position. Cardiovascular fitness can be maintained by allowing the athlete to swim with the use of a pool buoy between the legs, taping and/or bracing the ankle before swimming, or aquajogging (Fig. 16.25). Many believe that this is the time to apply alternating hot and cold (contrast therapy) to reduce swelling rapidly.

Stage III. Stage III is the subacute stage that begins 2 to 7 days after injury. The goal of this stage is to continue to relieve pain and reduce inflammation but also to regain dorsiflexion. Continued use of therapeutic modalities to reduce inflammation and pain are helpful during this stage. Another primary goal of this stage is to increase weight bearing progressively. Passive range-of-motion exercises should be administered, limiting plantarflexion and emphasizing dorsiflexion. Stretching of both the soleus and gastrocnemius should be performed bilaterally.

Gluteus medius weakness frequently follows ankle sprains. Therefore, hip abduction exercises should be performed to regain gluteus medius strength. This can be performed in a side-lying position, elevating the leg to 30°, or with the use of surgical tubing.

With strength progression, the performance of heel raises should begin bilaterally, starting with a double leg heel raise with the patient holding onto the therapy table for balance and to accommodate partial weight bearing. This exercise should be repeated until the ankle becomes uncomfortable, at which time ice is reapplied. If the pain is aggravated by this exercise, lesser weight-bearing exercises can be performed by using surgical tubing. After the athlete is capable of performing 20 repetitions without pain, progression to heel raises without support should start. After successful completion of this exercise can be maintained without pain or aggravation, the athlete should progress to a single leg heel raise on the affected side while stabilizing the body by holding onto a table for balance. As with any exercise session, ice should be used afterward. The next progression is to perform a single leg raise without stabilization. Then heel raises should be performed on a slant board or stairs, allowing the heel to drop 3 to 5 cm. Toe walking and heel walking should be performed to develop proprioception and strength.

With continued recovery, the athlete should be requested to perform small hops for three to five

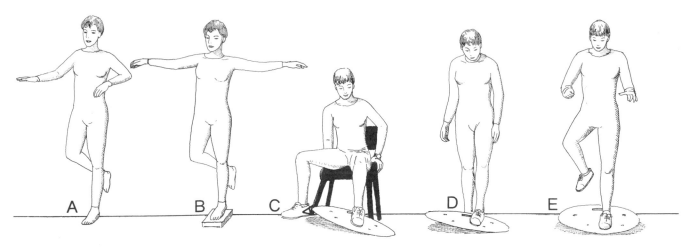

Figure 16.31. Proprioceptive exercises of progressively advancing challenge. **A** and **B** use open-chain kinetics; **C, D,** and **E** are closed-chain activities. Functional stability in athletics requires a great deal of proprioceptive skills.

repetitions. This achievement of functional stability and capacity to withstand forces several times the body weight indicates readiness to perform strengthening activities.

Stage IV. Stage IV is the continued progression of strengthening activities. The use of isokinetic or isotonic machines and/or exercises into inversion may be added. At this stage, inversion exercises can be performed without the fear of permanent lengthening or reinjury of the anterior talofibular ligament. The use of surgical tubing or sandbags can be instituted to exercise inversion/eversion and dorsiflexion. With continued progression, hopping and skipping are excellent activities to reestablish the proprioceptive and rebounding abilities of the foot. Emphasis in this stage should be on the addition of proprioceptive exercises using BAPS boards, rocker boards, tilt boards, and balance boards (Fig. 16.31). These proprioceptive exercises should be enhanced further by the addition of catching, passing, throwing, and dribbling a ball while trying to maintain balance. Increasingly difficult tasks are added gradually. In the early stages, ankle stabilization may be required for safe performance.

Mobilization and manipulation of the distal and proximal tibiofibular joint as well as the subtalar joint should be performed to prevent long-term fixations and joint dysfunction relating to long-term sequelae of ankle sprains. Ultrasound and other therapeutic modalities may be necessary in this phase to prevent chronic ligament or capsular thickening.

Heel walk and toe walk should be performed, followed by running on flat, even surfaces at a slow pace. Forward running should progress in

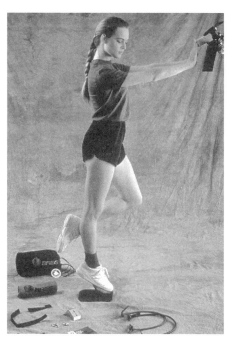

Figure 16.32. A Breg ankle rehabilitation kit provides for progressive range of motion, strengthening, and proprioceptive exercises. (Courtesy of Brian Moore.)

speed, and it is also helpful to use a treadmill that can incline. As forward running progresses, backward running should be instituted, followed by running curves, zigzags, and figure-eights. Jumping rope should begin with low-level hops on both feet, progressing in repetitions and hop height. Transition should be made to one-legged jump roping on the affected leg. At the end of this stage, the athlete should be able to perform wind sprints with the addition of 90° cuts and rapid decelerations.

Stage V. Stage V is the final rehabilitative phase, designed to return the athlete to full sport activity. Fartlek-style running is introduced, along with side-to-side jumping, sideways running, and crossover running. Sports-specific patterns should be performed to include primary athletic activities required in the athlete's sport. Complete muscular rehabilitation must be established before discharge, with the everters obtaining at least 80% of the strength of the inverters. Full dorsiflexion is essential for the establishment of normal gait patterns, and unrestricted joint play and motion patterns are necessary for restoration of arthrokinematics and proper articular congruity (Fig. 16.32).

Grade III Sprains. Conservative methods of treating the unstable ankle involve 3 to 6 weeks of immobilization in a short leg cast. Gradual weight bearing is instituted as tolerated after cast removal. Taping and bracing are also necessary subsequent to cast removal. At this point, stage III rehabilitation can begin. Surgery is indicated for acute injuries if a bony ossicle is dislodged into the joint space or if there is a large avulsion of the lateral malleolus. Osteochondral lesions of the talus also require surgical repair. Most studies that compare the effectiveness of surgery with conservative care generally compare surgical patients with patients who have received inadequate rehabilitation. Thus, clinical judgment must govern the indication for surgical referral. However, one study has shown that those nonsurgical patients who participated in an early mobilization program demonstrated more rapid return to work and activity than their surgical counterparts (17).

Posterior Ankle Impingement

Posterior impingement of the ankle can arise from either soft tissue or osseous structures. Pain is associated with plantarflexion or any activity whereby posterior glide of the calcaneus is forced. This may be associated with jumping, stopping, and cutting movements. This condition may be incapacitating, particularly for ballet dancers, soccer players, and runners.

Soft tissue impingement may result from synovitis or adhesions secondary to peroneal tendinitis or flexor hallucis longus tendinitis. Hypertrophy of the transverse tibial fibular ligament or a marsupial meniscus can also cause impingement (17, 21).

Bony impingement is due to elongation of the lateral process of the posterior talar tubercle (Fig. 16.33), a Stieda's process, or the presence of

an os trigonum, which is associated with incomplete fusion of a secondary ossification center. Fracture and/or stress fracture can also result from repetitive trauma or acute trauma to the lateral process of the posterior talus (74). Forced plantarflexion radiographs or bone scans may be necessary for this diagnosis. At 8 to 11 years of age, fusion generally occurs at the secondary ossification center of the lateral tubercle. In 3% to 11%, however, the center remains unfused, with 50% of unfused centers appearing bilaterally (17). Posterior talar compression may mimic Achilles tendinitis, peroneal tendinitis, or flexor hallucis longus tendinitis. Posterior impingement may be a sequela of an ankle sprain. The size of any bony abnormality is generally not associated with symptom severity but may result in limited range of motion. Pain may be provoked by placing the ankle in plantarflexion and forcefully gliding the calcaneus posteriorly into further plantarflexion. The pain is generally felt anterior to the Achilles tendon and posterior to the malleolus. Pain may be elicited by palpating the posterolateral talus between the Achilles tendon and peroneal tendons. Frequently, the patient will complain about discomfort when slipping on snug-fitting shoes or boots.

Conservative treatment is successful for this condition. Subtalar joint manipulation moving the calcaneus into dorsiflexion, anterior glide, and inversion creates nearly instantaneous relief of symptoms. Supporting this mobilized joint with low dye strapping helps maintain the anteriorly mobilized position of the calcaneus. Functional orthotics to support the calcaneal inclination angle may reduce plantarflexion of the calcaneus, and the concomitant reduction of

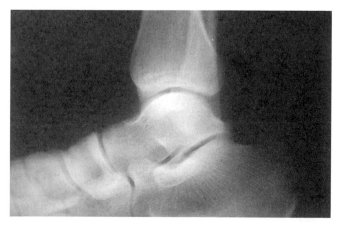

Figure 16.33. Elongated lateral process of the posterior talar tubercle, Stieda's process. (Courtesy of T.L. Forcum.)

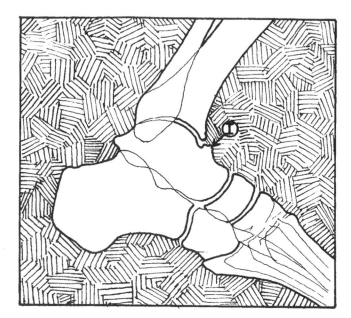

Figure 16.34. Anterior tibial spurring can cause impingement and reduced range of motion in dorsiflexion. (Reprinted with permission from Michaud TC. Foot orthoses and other forms of conservative foot care. Baltimore: Williams & Wilkins, 1993.)

overpronation will further reduce posterior glide of the calcaneus. Forceful stretching of the calves may aggravate this condition; tension from the stretch can impinge the calcaneus into the talus. However, high-frequency, low-intensity stretching is necessary to reduce low-grade constant compression. Reduced or modified weight bearing may be necessary, and activity such as aquajogging may be extremely useful during this period. Reminding the patient that loosening their shoelaces before putting on shoes will reduce repetitive irritation.

Posterior talar compression is frequently misdiagnosed. When properly diagnosed and treated, the athlete can return to unrestricted training in 1 to 4 weeks.

Anterior Talar Impingement Syndrome

Anterior talar impingement is related to osteophytes on the neck of the talus or the distal anterior tibia (Fig. 16.34). Symptoms are aggravated with dorsiflexion, which causes compression of these structures (75). Osteophytes generally form at the attachment sites of the joint capsule and may be related to traction spurring in runners and soccer players. Athletes that require prolonged ankle dorsiflexion under load, such as football linemen and rock climbers, may develop these osteophytes with painful dorsiflexion.

Conservative management relates to symptomatic treatment. Chronic impingement may lead to

capsulitis; therefore, interferential therapy to the ankle may be helpful. Ultrasound to the spurs may reduce inflammation and limit progression. Long axis distraction manipulation to the ankle joint itself generally provides significant relief. During acute phases, semi–weight-bearing activities, such as cycling, may be necessary.

Midfoot Sprains

Midfoot sprains are a frequent occurrence, secondary to inversion, eversion hyperplantarflexion, or torsion injury (76). This type of injury is common in such sports as soccer, karate, and beach volleyball. Other indirect mechanisms of injury involve plantarflexion or torsional injuries occurring as a result of foot stress associated with windsurfer toe straps or toe clips in cycling. Additional injuries may occur in ballet while en pointe or on tripping. Many of these injuries are often overlooked or considered insignificant. However, they may lead to degeneration, joint instability, or impingement. All these factors can affect athletic performance.

Bifurcate Ligament Sprain. The bifurcate ligament is composed of the dorsal calcaneocuboid and calcaneonavicular ligaments (Fig. 16.26). This is situated midway between the lateral malleolus and the base of the fifth metatarsal. Injury to this ligament is often secondary to inversion sprains, which may cause avulsion of the distal superior pole of the calcaneus. Proper diagnosis is made by noting tenderness and swelling over the ligament and aggravation by forefoot inversion. Treatment should be similar to that of an ankle sprain, with therapies directed specifically to that ligament. Transverse friction massage in subacute and chronic stages may be necessary. Manipulation of the cuboid and navicular may be indicated if subluxation or dysfunction is present. Additionally, bracing and taping may be necessary, as well as pressure relief padding for protection of the ligament from footgear. Temporary orthotics maybe useful for further stabilization. In chronic cases, a functional orthosis may be necessary to limit repetitive irritation from overpronation.

Dorsal Talonavicular, Cuneonavicular, and Tarsometatarsal Ligament Sprains. Dorsal foot ligament sprains are most commonly associated with hyperplantarflexion injuries. They can also be associated with direct trauma, such as in the case of impact from a karate kick or the dorsal foot being stepped on in basketball, volleyball, or football. It is also common in other sports such as soccer, cycling, windsurfing, and scuba diving.

Traumatic injury may result in avulsion fracture, but this may also frequently be associated with repetitive microtraumatic sprain. Such injuries may be further exacerbated by footgear, and laces must be skipped to avoid pressure over the injured structure. Isolation of the exact tarsal metatarsal ligament can be distinguished by plantarflexing each metatarsal independently. Thorough treatment and rehabilitation of this injury are necessary; altered kinematics of this articulation can cause degenerative spurring in the form of a dorsal exostosis. These exostoses are associated with neural impingement of the medial dorsal cutaneous nerve and the deep peroneal nerve, as discussed earlier in this chapter.

Treatment must involve pressure relief padding and alteration of footgear. Reduction of pathomechanics, such as overpronation, may require the temporary or permanent use of orthotics. Manipulation often achieves instantaneous relief; however, symptoms may return with improper rehabilitation and stabilization. Therapeutic modalities should be directed toward the specific ligament of involvement.

Plantar Midfoot Ligament Sprains. When disrupted, the calcaneal cuboid ligament (short plantar) and plantar calcaneonavicular ligament (spring) are often associated with subluxation of the cuboid (Fig. 16.35). Stabilization may require the use of taping and temporary orthotics, with a cuboid pad to reduce medial rotation and inferior displacement of the cuboid.

The plantar cuneonavicular and tarsometatarsal ligaments may further be strained by prolonged forefoot load or other pathomechanical patterns such as underpronation or overpronation. Proper treatment relies heavily on the use of low dye strapping and supportive exercises of the plantar fascia. For further treatment, see the section on plantar fasciitis.

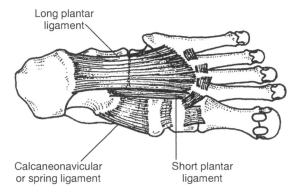

Figure 16.35. Ligamentous anatomy of the plantar foot. (Reprinted with permission from Michaud TC. Foot orthoses and other forms of conservative foot care. Baltimore: Williams & Wilkins, 1993.)

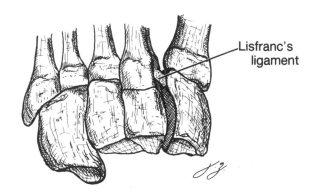

Figure 16.36. The attachment of the Lisfranc's ligament, the first or medial interosseous tarsometatarsal ligament. (Reprinted with permission from Draves DJ. Anatomy of the lower extremity. Baltimore: Williams & Wilkins, 1986.)

Lisfranc's Ligament Sprain. Rupture of Lisfranc's ligament results in separation of the first and second metatarsal bases (Fig. 16.36). This occurs in 1 per 50,000 to 60,000 people per year. Confirmation can best be obtained by comparing weight-bearing radiographs. The space between the first and second metatarsal bases will be widened 2 to 5 mm. The most common mechanism of injury to this structure involves a plantarflexed foot with axial loading and rotation, particularly external rotation. This pronation places Lisfranc's ligament under tension. With rupture, the use of a non–weight-bearing cast is appropriate. Internal fixation may be performed, but reports indicate that treatment methods and the severity of the diastasis have no effect on the final outcome of the condition. The average time before return to competition is estimated to be 14.5 weeks (23, 42, 77).

First Metatarsal Phalangeal Joint Sprain and Capsular Injury. Injuries to the first metatarsal phalangeal joint can be serious in athletes because these injuries interfere directly with propulsion and the windlass effect. Most injuries to the first metatarsal phalangeal joint result from hyperextension (hyperdorsiflexion) while the forefoot is planted and the heel is lifted. Hyperextension of the first metatarsal phalangeal joint (MPJ) is commonly referred to as turf toe as a result of its occurrence on artificial turf, particularly in football, baseball, and soccer. This injury is commonly associated with valgus stresses, particularly with excessively flexible shoes. This is especially true when the athlete is performing on hard surfaces such as artificial turf, tennis courts, and other similar surfaces. Excessively long shoes may be associated with hyperdorsiflexion sprains because the improper fit alters the flexion point of the shoe and creates an additional lever arm on toe-off to hyperextend the hallux.

Injuries may also occur as a result of hyper-plantarflexion where the toes are dragged across a surface and plantarflexed under the weight of the foot, referred to as "sand toe." This may occur in beach volleyball, gymnastics, and karate.

A frequent cause of first metatarsal phalangeal capsulitis may be from repetitive compression as a result of wearing a shoe that is too short. As the foot enters the pronation phase, the medial longitudinal arch lowers, elongating the total length of the foot. This causes the hallux to impact the front portion of the shoe, causing compression of the metatarsal phalangeal joint. This is further aggravated when excessive pronation occurs as the hallux is forced to dorsiflex under axial compression in an oblique plane, a direction in which the joint is not designed to move.

This condyloid joint allows for motion in multiple planes, but there is little motion in directions other than dorsiflexion and plantarflexion. In examining the joint, both active and passive motion should be assessed. There are approximately 30° of active plantarflexion and 50° of active extension. Passively, this may be increased to 70° to 90°. This joint should also be evaluated while the patient is standing. Range of motion will frequently be reduced dramatically in the dysfunctional foot in the unsupported weight-bearing position. However, significant changes often can be made to standing hallux extension by placing the rearfoot into neutral position.

Radiographs may differentiate bony articular changes. Arthrograms performed at the onset of injury may elucidate capsular integrity.

Examination may reveal exquisitely tender tissue surrounding the MPJ in acute cases. Swelling may create a hyperemic response similar to gout. Palpatory tenderness may be present over the plantar region of the metatarsal phalangeal joint. Differential diagnosis includes sesamoiditis, which should show tenderness on palpation over the sesamoids, particularly the medial. Other differentials include flexor hallucis longus or flexor hallucis brevis tendinitis. Gout can be differentiated via laboratory findings and history of onset. It is common for the sesamoids to be involved in hyperextension injuries to the extent of causing chondromalacia and even fracture. The long-term effects of turf toe may lead to hallux limitus or hallux rigidus. With extension there may be dorsal impingement and plantar plate avulsion.

Acute first metatarsal phalangeal sprains may require 2 to 12 weeks of time lost from activity. Early treatment should consist of those procedures and modalities that reduce inflammation. The patient should immediately be wearing a shoe that provides adequate length and rigidity. Additional rigidity to the forefoot may be applied by use of a steel spring or thermoplast cut in the shape of the insole. This material is then placed under the insole or sock liner to reduce motion of the first MPJ. Gentle early immobilization should be instituted, with emphasis on long axis oscillation, dorsal glide, and lateral glide. Tape should be applied, stabilizing the hallux. In the case of hyperextension injuries, the toe should be taped in a slight plantarflexion position. The insole of the athlete's shoe can be cut out under the distal hallux to accommodate this plantarflexion. In the case of hyperplantarflexion injuries, most shoe modifications are unnecessary, with the exception of placing a small pad under the distal hallux. Taping should be performed in neutral or a slight dorsiflexion. Rigid shoes still may be useful because excessive range of motion may cause capsular irritation and inflammation. As the inflammation decreases, manipulation techniques should play a major role in restoring normal joint mechanics and function. Strengthening exercises involving toe curls and toe extensions should be incorporated. Easy jogging can often be resumed before walking. Running has a lift-off phase that does not require dorsiflexion of the hallux. Walking, however, has a toe-off phase that requires further hallux dorsiflexion that may irritate the injured joint.

Hallux Limitus. Hallux limitus may be the result of chronic sequelae of sprains of the first MPJ or degenerative arthrosis secondary to microtrauma, acute trauma, or arthritic process. Both hallux limitus and rigidus may be associated with a long first metatarsal. Hallux limitus is hallmarked by the reduction of hallux dorsiflexion. This reduced dorsiflexion alters the normal gait patterns, which further accelerates this pathomechanical state. This may cause weight bearing on the lateral aspect of the foot and an adductory twist during the propulsive phase of gait. This twisting action allows for transfer of body over the forefoot.

Osteochondral spurring frequently causes a mechanical blocking of dorsiflexion (Fig. 16.37) (30). Frequently, these prominent lesions may become tender from direct compression of footgear over them. Conservative treatment must first address pain and joint function. Pain can be reduced with the reduction of inflammation. Ultrasound, icing after exercise bouts, and use of heat are often helpful in relieving symptoms. Activity modification must reduce acceleration, hill running, cutting, kicking, and kneeling activities. Shoes should be modified by the addition of a stiff metal or thermoplast insert as described with sprains of the first metatarsal phalangeal

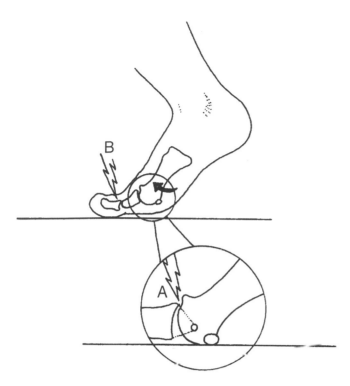

Figure 16.37. With hallux limitus, when the hallux reaches full dorsiflexion, the dorsal phalanx collides with the metatarsal head. (Reprinted with permission from Michaud TC. Foot orthoses and other forms of conservative foot care. Baltimore: Williams & Wilkins, 1993.)

joint (17). Shoes may further be modified by the application of a metatarsal bar or a rocker bottom sole. Shoes may also need to be modified to allow for toe box height; the toe box must be able to accommodate bony exostoses. As a temporary measure, this portion of the shoe may be cut away for pressure relief. With the reduction of pain, attention should focus on restoring normal biomechanics of the lower extremities. Functional orthoses may be useful for reducing excessive pronation, which causes oblique stresses across this joint. Mobilization and manipulation seem to maximize function and range of motion. The athlete should be taught to perform self-mobilization of the first MPJ, to be performed two to three times daily. Mobilization should emphasize long axis distraction and dorsal and plantar glide.

Hallux Rigidus. Hallux rigidus is the terminal progression of first metatarsal phalangeal joint degeneration—a nearly complete reduction of functional motion of the joint with osteophytosis. Conservative treatment amounts to symptomatic relief with use of therapeutic modalities. Manipulation should initially be avoided because it commonly aggravates this condition. Mobilization should be gentle. Athletic activities should not include those requiring forefoot propulsion, and

transition to activities such as rowing, cycling, and swimming should be encouraged. Conservative treatment is the same as that for hallux limitus. For a more aggressive approach, surgical treatment may be necessary. Complications in the young athlete include infection and wound inflammation. Other complications will vary, depending on the procedure used (17, 23).

Hallux Valgus. Hallux valgus is the lateral deviation of the great toe over 20°. The average deviation in adults is 15°. Although hallux valgus is a common condition (it appears in approximately 3% to 17% of the population), it rarely results from athletic injury (17). However, this condition is often irritated by athletic participation. In cases in which metatarsus primus varus is involved, the first metatarsal will deviate medially more than 10°. This lateral deviation of the first phalanx and the medial deviation of the metatarsal displace the sesamoids and also the flexor and extensor tendons. With progression, the abductor hallucis tendon is subluxed inferior to the MPJ, rendering it useless in the prevention of progression of this condition.

Factors that contribute to hallux valgus include wearing high-heeled shoes and shoes with pointed toes. Other factors include overpronation, arthritis, Achilles tendinitis, and previous metatarsal phalangeal trauma. With progressive degeneration and advanced deviation, the formation of a bunion occurs with subluxation and rotation of the first phalanx and the development of an adventitious bursa, medial to the first MPJ (Fig. 16.38). This bursa becomes irritated and inflamed with direct trauma and repetitive pressure.

Treatment of hallux valgus must begin with proper footwear. Footwear should provide ample room and motion control, particularly for prona-

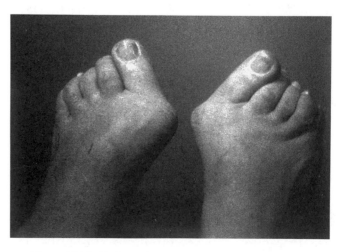

Figure 16.38. Marked hallux valgus. (Courtesy of T.L. Forcum.)

tion. During an acute exacerbation, a stainless steel spring or thermoplast in the forefoot to limit motion at the involved joint may be effective. Ice and ultrasound can help reduce local inflammation. Long-term treatment is geared toward prevention of exacerbation by limiting the progressive deviation of the phalanx and maintaining joint mobility. The use of splinting may reduce initial symptoms and reduce progression. Night splints have been found to be the most aggressive, whereas athletic taping is more practical for daytime and athletic use. Mobilization should be performed in the initial acute stages, followed by manipulation in the subacute and chronic stages. Long axis distraction with slight lateral glide or varus deviation is the direction of choice for mobilization and manipulation. If rotation has occurred at the phalanx, then counterrotation manipulation should follow. In mild conditions, EMS (particularly Russian stimulation) may be useful for stimulating the abductor hallucis muscle in an effort to strengthen and facilitate its activity to limit deviation progression. Occasionally, pressure relief padding such as a gel pad may be necessary. Cutting out the adjacent portions of the shoe may be indicated in the acute states. Footwear may need to be stretched to accommodate deformity. Footwear should have a high toe box and a low heel to reduce weight bearing onto the forefoot. It is important that no straps or medial supports on the shoe cross over this area. Should such supports cross over the adventitious bursa, irritation and inflammation may result, and these straps may require cutting or removal. Orthotics may be necessary to reduce overpronation. However, in view of space limitations, thoughtful prescription is necessary. With extensive degeneration and deviation of the hallux, few surgical procedures will allow the athlete to return to top performance (17).

Sesamoiditis. The sesamoid bones are two small ossicles housed in the flexor hallucis tendon that articulate with the plantar first metatarsal head in the region called the plantar plate. These sesamoids ossify at approximately age 10 in boys and age 8 in girls (17). A great number of variations occur in 10% to 33% of the population, the most common being a bipartite sesamoid (23). The sesamoids act as a fulcrum for the flexor hallucis brevis. This increases the mechanical advantage of this muscle in plantarflexing the great toe. Sesamoid pain may be the result of several conditions: bursitis, chondromalacia, osteoarthritis, stress fracture, traumatic impact, and crush fracture. These conditions should be differentiated from flexor hallucis longus tendinitis,

synovitis at the metatarsal phalangeal joint, and arthritides (78, 79).

The medial sesamoid is slightly more likely to be afflicted with these conditions. This may be secondary to overpronation or hallux valgus, which places this sesamoid in an altered weight-bearing pattern.

Chondromalacia occurs only on weight bearing or on localized palpation. Diagnosis can be made on clinical findings; however, skyline radiographs may be helpful in the advanced stages. Osteochondritis is also diagnosed based on radiographs, which demonstrate irregular trabecular patterns with a stippled appearance of the bones.

Presesamoid bursitis may be associated with systemic collagen disease. Palpation demonstrates a swelling that is soft and painful.

Trauma involving stress fracture may be differentiated via bone scan. More acute trauma causing fracture will be visualized on radiographs but may be difficult to distinguish from a bipartite sesamoid. With traumatic disruption, serial radiographs may demonstrate increased widening of the fracture, and bone scan will demonstrate a hot spot. This condition may be difficult to differentiate from turf toe. With traumatic disruption, injury to the plantar plate may occur. Such disruption may result in degenerative joint disease or avascular necrosis (Fig. 16.39) (80).

Treatment of sesamoiditis is similar to the treatment necessary for hallux limitus or first metatarsal phalangeal joint sprains, but should also use the following guidelines.

Sesamoid pain can be classified by grade (23). Grade I sesamoiditis elicits pain with activity and minimal pain on examination. This grade is easily treated with shoe modifications such as a dancer's pad and the use of antiinflammatory modalities.

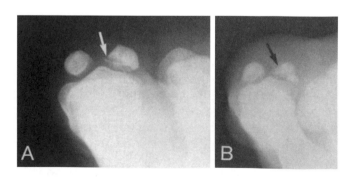

Figure 16.39. Hallux sesamoid bones: avascular necrosis. **A** and **B.** Observe the medial sesamoid, which is increased in density and exhibits a characteristic subchondral fracture. (Reprinted with permission from Yochum TR, Rowe LJ. Essentials of skeletal radiology. Baltimore: Williams & Wilkins, 1987;2.)

Grade II sesamoiditis elicits pain on all weight bearing and activity. Examination produces pain on palpation and passive dorsiflexion. Activity restriction and accommodative orthotics are necessary. In one study, 8 of 10 athletes with sesamoid pain were treated successfully with custom-fitted orthoses. The athlete may require selective restriction from weight-bearing activities for 2 to 6 weeks.

Grade III sesamoiditis demonstrates significant tenderness with palpation and antalgic weight bearing. Any range of motion elicits pain, particularly dorsiflexion. This patient requires non–weight-bearing and first metatarsal phalangeal immobilization. The use of crutches may be necessary for 1 to 2 weeks. Time lost from weight-bearing activities will exceed 6 weeks.

Lesser Toe Sprains and Capsular Injury (Metatarsalgia). Metatarsalgia refers to any condition that causes pain in the region of the metatarsals. However, pain caused by an interdigital neuroma is referred to specifically as Morton's neuroma (see section on interdigital nerve entrapment). There are several causes of metatarsalgia. A pes cavus foot along with a forefoot strike gait pattern predispose the athlete to this type of condition. Frequently there is fat pad atrophy, particularly in those athletes of advanced age. Trauma associated with metatarsalgia is usually related to landing on the forefoot from a jump. The most common cause of toe and metatarsal pain is simply stubbing a toe. Overuse injuries to the metatarsal region are common. They are normally associated with improper footwear providing inadequate forefoot cushioning or allowing for the pathomechanics of underpronation or overpronation. This is especially true with those athletes training on hard, unforgiving surfaces. This includes dancing or aerobics on a tile floor. A shoe with a narrowed toe box, especially one with an elevated heel, will displace compression and weight onto the forefoot. An athlete will often exhibit complaints of metatarsalgia during activity, although the perpetuating cause is an activity of daily living during which high-heeled shoes or shoes with inadequate forefoot cushioning are worn.

Other mechanical causes relate to a long and/or plantarflexed metatarsal. These metatarsals will show up radiographically with increased cortical thickening. A callus is generally present under the involved metatarsal head, indicating increased weight bearing. Calluses and plantar warts may cause—and be an indication of—altered shear forces or weight bearing through the metatarsal heads. Trimming or excising these structures can often lead to dramatic relief of symptoms. A common cause of metatarsalgia is related secondarily to a bunionectomy, whereby stresses are diverted onto the lesser metatarsals. Collagen vascular diseases may also attack this region, causing symptomatology. Muscular imbalances such as those causing claw toes, hammer toes, and equinus syndrome can lead to altered joint mechanics and increased weight-bearing across the metatarsal heads.

Freiberg's avascular necrosis of the metatarsal head, metatarsal stress fractures, Morton's neuroma, distal plantar fasciitis, tarsal tunnel syndrome, and plantar bursitis may be included in the list of possible diagnoses when evaluating metatarsalgia.

Patients with metatarsalgia generally present with insidious onset of symptoms unless trauma is the origin of this condition. Most patients will state that they feel better with shoes on rather than barefoot if appropriate footwear is worn. Metatarsalgia is classified in four grades (23).

Grade I presents with mild pain with activity. Treatment includes the use of therapeutic modalities, ice, metatarsal padding, shoe modifications, and possibly the use of an accommodating orthotic.

Grade II presents with moderate pain and some limitation of activities. In addition to the treatment provided for grade I, grade II patients require mobilization and/or manipulation of the metatarsal phalangeal joint. Partial weight bearing with the use of crutches may be necessary.

Grade III presents with moderate to severe pain with simple weight bearing. There is joint effusion and pain with joint distraction and compression. There may be pain with range of motion and sensitivity with squeezing. Several weeks of non–weight-bearing may be necessary in addition to the treatment provided in grade II. These patients may need the addition of a rocker bottom sole.

Grade IV is a subluxation or dislocation of the metatarsal phalangeal joints. In general, most of these patients require open reduction to reduce any deformities.

Hammer Toes and Claw Toes. Interphalangeal and metatarsophalangeal capsular contractions associated with intrinsic muscular imbalance can result in toe deformities.

Hammer toes involve the plantarflexed contracture of the proximal interphalangeal joint (PIP) with a slight dorsiflexed contracture of the metatarsophalangeal joint (Fig. 16.40) (17, 28, 58). Commonly, a callus is seen over the dorsal aspect of the PIP. Hammer toes are treated conservatively by the use of the toe crest pad or a hammer-toe (Budin's) splint. Footgear modifica-

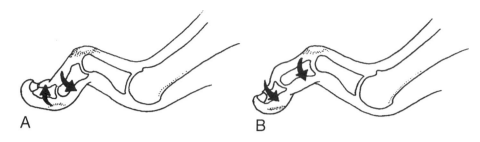

Figure 16.40. A. Hammer toe. **B.** Claw toe. (Reprinted with permission from Michaud TC. Foot orthoses and other forms of conservative foot care. Baltimore: Williams & Wilkins, 1993.)

tions may be necessary to prevent recalcitrant painful callus formation over the dorsal toes. In-office ultrasound and manipulation may be helpful along with a home, self-mobilization program. Treatment goals are primarily to prevent progression and reduce symptomatology in severe cases.

Claw toes generally are associated with a pes cavus foot and neurologic pathology (Fig. 16.40). Claw toes result from contractures and intrinsic muscular imbalances, to dorsiflex the metatarsal phalangeal joint and plantarflex the PIP and DIP joints. Conservative care for claw toes is less successful, but may reduce symptoms associated with painful corns and calluses. When symptoms are severe, capsular and extensor tendon lengthening may be necessary.

Associated with these conditions is the distal migration of the metatarsal cushion, the fat pad that protects the joint capsule of the metatarsal phalangeal joint. This distal migration leaves these joints vulnerable to impact injury and metatarsal phalangeal capsulitis.

Osteochondritis Dissecans of the Talar Dome

Osteochondritis dissecans of the talar dome accounts for approximately 0.9% of all fractures (17). However, many osteochondral fractures go unnoticed or are never properly diagnosed. This injury is probably more appropriately called a transchondral fracture or an osteochondral fracture because the condition is not an inflammatory process, as the "itis" suffix would imply. Osteochondral lesions primarily occur in the bone, followed by secondary cartilaginous proliferation or degeneration. It is estimated that 50% to 89% of osteochondral lesions occur secondary to trauma; however, most of these conditions are multifactorial. It is estimated that the majority of these injuries (71%) are secondary to inversion sprains. Causative trauma does not have to be significant; trivial insults that are frequently unnoticed may cause such disruptions. Osteochondritis is most common in the knee, ankle, elbow, and hip. This condition also tends to prevail in the young male, aged 10 to 20 years (80). These lesions are susceptible to osteonecrosis because the compressed or avulsed fragment of bone has

no soft tissue attachments and thus has a poor blood supply.

The patient usually presents with deep, achy pain that is aggravated by exercise. This is often accompanied by ankle swelling and occasionally crepitus or clicking. True locking or catching sensations may also occur with loose body formation. Occasionally, there will be joint line tenderness associated with these lesions. Most of these patients will present with limited range of motion, especially with dorsiflexion.

The medial aspect of the dome of the talus is the most common site of osteochondral lesions. These injuries most commonly occur during coupled plantarflexion, inversion, and rotation. These lesions often extend deep, measuring 2 to 5 mm, and occur most often in the central to posterior portions of the medial talar dome. Lateral lesions are more often shallow, measuring 1 to 2 mm, and are flake-like avulsions (80). These lesions are usually secondary to forceful inversion. Osteochondritis frequently goes undiagnosed, probably secondary to the fact that radiographs are often normal. Imaging is difficult because fragment sizes are small and the location may not allow for radiologic visualization. The internal oblique view may be helpful for talar dome observation. For evaluating the posteromedial aspect of the talar dome, overpenetrated views in a plantarflexed position will demonstrate this aspect of anatomy. Double contrast arthrography can be useful for elucidating loose bodies or fragmentation. Computed tomography (CT) scans are most helpful when slices are small and sagittal reconstructions are performed. CT is accurate 98% of the time and offers great assistance in localization (81). Bone scans are the most effective screening tool, with a sensitivity level of 99%. When evaluating the overlying cartilaginous tissue, MRI will provide the most accurate visualization.

In 1959, Berndt and Harty developed a classification system describing osteochondral lesions. This system was modified by Lomer et al. in 1993, when an additional stage was added (Fig. 16.41) (81).

Stage I lesions are a compression or impaction injury to the bony talus. This occurs secondary to impact from the fibula or tibia. Stage II is a partial or incomplete detachment of an osteochondral fragment. Stage III is a complete detachment of an osteochondral fragment, but with good apposition and alignment. Stage I, II, and III lesions are most often treated by immobilization and non–weight-bearing. Stage IV lesions are a complete fragmentation with displacement of the fragment into the joint space. The fifth stage of lesion is that described by Lomer et al., which is a radiolucent defect. Patients with the stage V radiolucent defect present with no catches, locking, or giving way. Fifty percent of these defects are not visualized on radiographs. Lomer et al. describe this lesion as being present in a higher than average age range. However, this may be due to the fact that the average time from injury to diagnosis is 36 months. It is theorized that stage V osteochondral lesions are sequelae of stage I, II, or III lesions that have undergone subsequent avascular necrosis. Histologically, the tissue found within this defect is a white, firm, fibrous tissue, nearly indistinguishable from articular cartilage (81).

As with any osteochondral lesion, the primary treatment goals are to reduce pain and to prevent progressive degeneration within the joint from osteochondral fragmentation. In girls up to age 11 and boys up to age 13, conservative care is recommended, using activity modification and mobilization. For stage I and II osteochondral lesions in 12-year-old girls and 14-year-old boys up to the age of 20, treatment is rest and protective devices providing ankle stabilization and shock absorption. With stage III, below the knee casting and non–weight-bearing for no more than 6 to 8 weeks is recommended. With those stage III injuries that do not respond to conservative care, stage IV in-

juries, and patients 20 years of age and older, surgical saucerization of small fragments and pinning of large fragments are recommended (23). In stage V lesions, conservative treatment and observation may be performed, but many questions remain regarding the efficacy of this treatment. Surgical treatment consists of drilling to the subchondral lesion and curettage. In one study of those undergoing surgery, 57% were unable to return to their sport. Four percent were able to return without limitations, and 39% returned with limitations (81).

STRESS FRACTURES OF THE LEG, ANKLE, AND FOOT

Stress fractures or fatigue fractures result from sustained microtrauma to bone that exceeds its ability to remodel. Microscopic defects develop at the site of maximum stress risers, where mechanical stress concentrates. In contrast to stress fractures, insufficiency fractures occur when normal stress is applied to abnormal bone. These fractures may be the result of rheumatoid arthritis or osteoporosis.

The distribution of stress fractures in the lower extremity is 34% to 50% in the tibia, 12% to 34% in the fibula, and 19% to 20% in the metatarsals with the second metatarsal being most common, followed by the third. Of stress fractures affecting the tarsal bones, the calcaneus and the navicular are the most common (17).

The incidence of stress fracture increases with various factors. Age is a determining factor. Frequency increases with progressive age until approximately age 36. Incidence increases further with postmenopausal women or those women

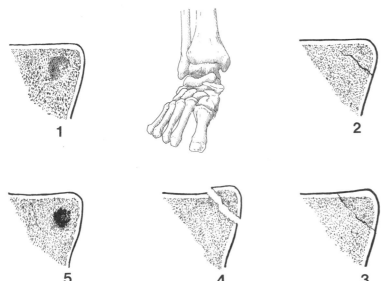

Figure 16.41. Classification of osteochondral lesions: (1) compression, (2) partially fractured but undisplaced, (3) completely fractured but undisplaced, (4) displaced fracture, (5) radiolucent (fibrous) defect. (Adapted from Loomer R, Fisher C, Lloyd-Smith R, et al. Osteochondral lesions of the talus. Am J Sports Med 1993;21:13–19.)

who are experiencing oligomenorrhea, amenor-rhea, low body fat, and other eating disorders. Stress fractures are approximately 10 times more frequent in the female athlete and 5 times more frequent in whites compared with blacks. Frequently, these injuries have delayed diagnoses because the athlete tends to train through them. Proper diagnosis may not be ascertained for up to 38 months.

There are two primary theories about the cause of stress fractures. The first theory is related to muscle fatigue secondary to repetitive overload. This fatigue reduces the ability of the soft tissues to absorb shock, thus increasing the forces onto the bony tissues. The second theory concerns the repetitive application of muscular overload forces and stress on the bony tissue. This may be associated with muscular imbalance or repetitive muscular overload. This theory may provide a rationale for the fact that non–weight-bearing bones also develop stress fractures (82).

The athlete with a stress fracture will generally present with localized pain and swelling. Pain is increased with weight bearing and decreased with rest. Symptoms generally develop insidiously, but symptoms may also occur with one excessive exertional effort. Percussion will generate pain, and the athlete will be unable to perform a one-legged hop as a result of pain. Pain may be associated with walking.

Other causative factors include excessive pronation or underpronation of the feet. Pes planus and pes cavus are associated with biomechanical malfunctions that reduce the body's ability to absorb shock. Hallux valgus and a Morton's foot are associated with increased transfer of weight onto the metatarsals during the push-off phase. Control of these biomechanical dysfunctions may be required for the prevention of recurrence and pain-free return to sports. In the case of athletes who wear track spikes or ballet slippers and who participate in gymnastics, low dye taping may be necessary for the reduction of foot pronation.

Imaging of stress fractures may be frustrating because radiographs are generally negative in the early and late phases. When applicable, antero-posterior (AP), lateral, and oblique views are recommended to try to achieve tangential visualization of the cortical bone to observe periosteal new bone, extracortical lucency, and endosteal new bone. These findings generally develop within weeks to months. Bone scans are highly sensitive for the detection of stress fractures, although they are very nonspecific. False-positive results are associated with stress reactions. False-negative re-

sults may be due to not obtaining an oblique view, particularly in the tibia. Bone scans will be positive within days and may stay positive for up to 1 year or more. The angiogram, blood pool, and delayed imaging portions of the triphasic bone scan will be positive in cases of soft tissue injury, whereas only the delayed image will be positive with a stress fracture.

Indications for bone scan imaging relate to the magnitude and duration of pain. If symptoms are progressive and intense and there is associated night pain, or the lesion is in an atypical location, bone scans are indicated. If the stress fractures are recurrent and there is a concern about osteoporosis, bone mineral content studies via single and dual photon absorptiometry are indicated. Single phase reveals cortical bone integrity whereas dual photon evaluates cancellous bone. CT is a useful alternative to plain films and bone scans, particularly in the tarsal navicular bone and the calcaneus. CT scan will best demonstrate bony details and also demonstrate bony repair more accurately. This may be more helpful in determining when the athlete can return to activity. MRI is also useful in confirming suspicion of stress fracture, but may be nonspecific in the early stages of stress fracture formation. MRI demonstrates the subtle changes in marrow edema and frequently demonstrates an area of involvement larger than that initially suspected (82).

Stress fractures are categorized by grades (23). Grade 0 is normal bone with equal osteoblastic and osteoclastic activity. Both plain films and bone scans are negative. Grade I is an asymptomatic stress reaction. These stress reactions are not visualized on plain films, but they do appear on bone scans. Grade II is associated with pain. CT scans may be the best imaging technique for this grade, although bone scans are usually positive. Plain films are still negative. Grade III stress fractures are associated with significant pain and are positive on both plain films and bone scans.

Stress fractures should be differentiated from stress reactions, tendinitis, periostitis, infection, and neoplasm. The primary neoplasms of concern are osteogenic sarcoma and osteoid osteoma.

Management of stress fractures should include the immediate application of rest, ice, compression, and elevation. With grade III stress fractures, the use of crutches for 1 to 2 weeks may be necessary, as well as immobilization with a cast or functional leg brace. Early active rest is advised to allow for bone healing to outpace the bone breakdown that occurs with disuse. During this stage, swimming and deep-water running allow for continued activity and the maintenance of cardiovascular fitness (Fig. 16.25). A gradual return to weight bearing may require partial weight bearing for an additional 1 to 2 weeks if pain is associated with full weight bearing. Crutches and braces should be used until full weight bearing and pain-free walking can be established. Complete immobilization is generally not indicated unless a visible crack in the bony cortex is seen on plain films. If this crack is evident on both cortices, stricter immobilization is necessary because such stress fractures may progress to an overt fracture. Pneumatic leg braces, such as an AirCast or an Active Ankle Brace, may help athletes with tibial and fibula stress fractures return to activity more quickly. One study demonstrated the return of the athlete to training after an average of 3.7 weeks and to competition in 5.3 weeks with these braces (82).

However, the most common problem with recurrent pain and delayed healing is an inadequate rest period. The repaired tissue is most vulnerable to reinjury in the first 4 weeks after reintroducing activity. After 2 weeks without ambulatory pain and complete rest, gradual reintroduction of activity can begin. This period varies for individual athletes and according to the area of injury. Delayed union or nonunion athletic stress fractures have a propensity to occur in the hallux sesamoids, midanterior tibial shaft, at the base of the fifth metatarsal, and in the tarsal navicular. A Finnish study has reported nonunion in up to 10% of cases (83). This has been related to late physician consultation and an inadequate rest period from intense physical activity.

Nutritional augmentation is recommended with the consumption of 1500 mg of calcium daily. This is especially important for amenorrheic women. Amenorrheic female athletes with decreased bone density may also benefit from estrogen therapy, especially if therapy is started early.

In those regions of bone where delayed recovery may be a potential complication or evident, electromagnetic field therapy may be indicated. This therapy has been shown to be effective in the treatment of overt nonunion fractures. It appears that dynamic magnetic fields are more effective than static magnetic fields for this recovery (84). Additional evidence has also provided support for the use of electrical bone stimulation and ultrasound therapy (23).

Training errors—especially errors of excessive duration, frequency, and intensity—are commonly associated with stress fractures. In addition, running on crowned roads can cause unequal distribution of weight. Leg length inequalities have shown an unequal distribution of weight through the lower extremities, which may further complicate recovery or be related to recurrence. When returning the athlete to activity, the 10% to 15% rule should apply. Increase intensity, duration, or frequency 10% to 15% weekly; only one variable should be increased at a time. A training log kept by the athlete, detailing mileage, terrain, intensity, diet, and associated pain, can be extremely helpful during follow-up visits.

Before return to competition, the athlete should obtain full pain-free range of motion. Strength of the associated musculature should be at least 90% of the strength of the contralateral limb. Physical examination should demonstrate a lack of point tenderness on percussion or palpation. There should be no increased warmth or swelling in the localized region. Functional mobility should be restored. A one-leg hop should be able to be performed without pain and with adequate balance. Aerobic and anaerobic capacity should be restored to the requirements of the activity before returning to competition (82).

Tibial and Fibular Stress Fractures

Tibial stress fractures can be considered a Type I medial tibial stress syndrome (17). They are usually a result of repetitive activity such as running, performing aerobics, and sprinting. The incidence of tibial stress fractures may be predictable. Those individuals with narrow-width tibias and a high degree of external hip rotation seem to be at greater risk. The tibia is the most common site of stress fracture in the lower extremity, followed by the fibula. The most common tibial site is approximately 12 to 15 cm proximal to the medial malleolus. Although tenderness may extend over a region of 6 to 8 cm, the fracture site is generally denoted by a pinpoint tenderness. Anterior midshaft stress fractures are the most difficult to manage because they have a higher frequency of delayed union, nonunion, and complete fracturing. Therefore, the rest period should be prolonged to 3 to 6 months in this area. If the repair process is not progressing with the use of conservative measures described above, surgical referral should be considered, wherein the fracture is excised and a bone graft applied. Tibial stress fractures typically respond to 8 to 10 weeks of active rest. The use of a stirrup brace, such as an AirCast or an Active Ankle Brace, has been shown to be extremely useful; such devices provide stabilization without the strict immobilization of a cast. Midtibial fractures require orthoses with a hinged ankle and complete non–weight-bearing. In the late phases of

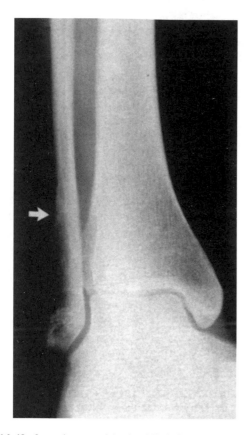

Figure 16.42. Stress fracture of the distal fibula. Periosteal new bone formation along with a radiolucent fracture line is seen in the distal diaphysis of the fibula. (Reprinted with permission from Yochum TR, Rowe LJ. Essentials of skeletal radiology. Baltimore: Williams & Wilkins, 1987;1.)

rehabilitation, the author recommends the use of Molinpic self-grip sports tape (Cohepress) to wrap the leg at and distal to the site of stress fracture on the distal tibia and fibula. This provides additional support as a compromise between the use of a functional brace and no support at all. Fibular stress fractures are generally associated with 6 to 8 weeks of active rest (Fig. 16.42).

Calcaneal Stress Fractures

Most stress fractures in the calcaneus are found in military recruits and long-distance runners. Twenty-seven percent of stress fractures are bilateral in soldiers.

In cancellous bones such as the calcaneus, a characteristic depression fracture usually occurs at the junction of the body and the posterior tubercle, perpendicular to the normal bony trabeculae. The bone tends to react to prevent fatigue failure by remodeling through the addition of trabeculae along the lines of stress. This requires up to 2 weeks. First, there must be the resorption of old trabeculae and then the laying down of new trabeculae.

Radiographically, the stress fracture will be

evidenced by endosteal cortical thickening followed by a radiolucent fracture line. The periosteal callus forms a linear transverse radiopaque line when viewed en face. The margins of the callus are hazy and poorly defined (80). The calcaneus is typical of this pattern. This should be differentiated from growth arrest lines, which are well defined.

Fractures of the calcaneus are the most common fractures of the tarsals and are usually caused by a jump or fall from a height. Secondarily, traumatic fractures are frequently associated with thoracolumbar compression fractures. In the case of fatigue fractures, the most common mechanism of injury is excessive repetitive stress. However, altered muscular imbalance may also be related. Hallux valgus, Morton's foot, and overpronation may provide additional predisposition. A high or low calcaneal inclination angle, osteoporosis, and aluminum-related bone disease may also be related to calcaneal stress fractures (85).

Examination may elicit palpatory pain and inflammation adjacent to the fracture site. Anvil heel compression test may produce some discomfort. This condition should be differentiated from retinaculitis, lateral or deep posterior compartment tenosynovitis, and posterior calcaneal subluxation or posterior ankle impingement.

The second most common site of stress fracture in the calcaneus is adjacent to the medial tuberosity, where calcaneal spur formation frequently occurs (17).

Navicular Stress Fracture

Navicular stress fractures are associated with a long delay in diagnosis, most likely radiographs are generally negative. Bone scans should be obtained with plantar and collimated views of the midfoot. However, false-negative results are common. CT scan may be more useful in formulating this diagnosis.

Delayed union or nonunion is also common with stress fractures of the tarsal navicular bone. This may be due to the frequency of delayed diagnosis or to the nature of the stress fracture itself.

Stress fractures of this region should be treated with non–weight-bearing cast immobilization for 8 weeks. This condition can have severe implications in athletes, not only due to the time away from training, but also due to the nonunion and displacement of the fracture which may lead to destabilization and a loss of functional integrity of the entire foot, thus impairing the entire lower kinetic chain. Displaced or non-union fractures should be treated with open reduction and internal fixation. At times this may require a bone graft. Appropriate supports should be maintained for the structure with the use of a functional orthotic and possibly the use of a scaphoid pad. Overpronation will aggravate this condition due to the excessive force output required by the tibialis posterior and anterior tibialis muscles. Thus, appropriate footwear is necessary (86).

Metatarsal Stress Fractures

Metatarsal stress fractures generally respond to 6 to 8 weeks of active rest. If two cortices are involved, non–weight-bearing is required to prevent overt fracture. Metatarsal stress fractures account for 19% to 20% of lower extremity stress fractures. The second metatarsal is most common (7% to 11%), followed by the third (7% to 8%) (Fig. 16.43), and the fourth and fifth (1% to 5%) (17). It is important to wear adequate footgear with proper stabilization and cushioning.

Sesamoid Stress Fractures

Sesamoid fracture and stress fracture may be

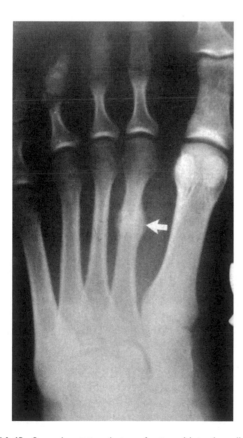

Figure 16.43. Second metatarsal stress fracture. Note the callus formation surrounding the mid-diaphysis. (Yochum TR, Rowe LJ. Essentials of skeletal radiology. Baltimore: Williams & Wilkins, 1987;1.)

difficult to distinguish from other first metatarsal phalangeal joint injuries such as flexor hallucis longus and flexor hallucis brevis tendinitis. It also may need to be differentiated from bipartite or multipartite sesamoids, avascular necrosis, or osteochondritis. Radiographs of the sesamoid should be performed with four views: anterior to posterior, lateral, oblique, and axial sesamoid. If differentiation between an overt fracture and a comminuted fracture is necessary, dorsiflexion stress views may be indicated. Dorsiflexion of the first metatarsal phalangeal joint will widen a fracture gap, whereas no widening will occur with bipartite or multipartite sesamoids.

During the acute phase when an obvious fracture line is evident, the athlete is treated with non–weight-bearing for 3 to 4 weeks with the hallux in a plantarflexed position. A soft metatarsal pad should be placed just proximal to the second through fourth metatarsal heads. The plantar portion of a weight-bearing cast should extend distally to support the toes. A weight-bearing cast should be worn for an additional 3 to 4 weeks. Those athletes with an acute stress fracture without an obvious fracture line may be treated with a functional leg brace or cast for 4 to 6 weeks. Chronic stress fractures of sesamoids should be treated with a weight-bearing cast for approximately 6 weeks. After this, an accommodative orthotic should be used in a shoe that has been modified by stiffening the sole and applying a metatarsal pad. At this point, rehabilitation similar to that described for turf toe or sesamoiditis should be provided, emphasizing the use of pulsed ultrasound therapy. Nonunion of hallux sesamoids is common; thus, aggressive rehabilitation should be provided (87).

ANKLE FRACTURES

Fractures of the ankle are frequently seen in association with ankle sprains. In the young athlete, oblique and comparison radiographs are frequently necessary to elucidate Salter Harris type alterations in the epiphyseal junctions.

Ankle fractures can be classified as malleolar, bimalleolar, and trimalleolar when the posterior aspect of the tibial plafond is involved (17).

Avulsion fracture of a small fragment of bone may indicate sparing of the ligament; however, if proper treatment and stabilization are not provided to allow for avulsion healing, this may represent significant instability. Small avulsion fragments from the tips of the malleolus often represent extra-articular structures and frequently are not symptomatic if nonunion occurs. Single malleolar fractures frequently are associated with ligamentous disruption of the opposing structures.

Fibular fractures can be classified by level of involvement: below the level of the joint, at the level of the joint, and above the level of the joint. The prognosis for these fractures becomes poorer as one moves from inferior to superior. Fractures above the level of the joint have the poorest prognosis. This leads to gross ankle mortise instability and interosseous membrane disruption. Frequently, there will be rotational malalignment along with widening of the ankle mortise with these fractures. When widening of the ankle mortise is increased 1 to 2 mm, the forces transmitted through the joint may be increased 30% to 40% (17).

Closed cast treatment is appropriate when fractures are not displaced or are successfully manipulated into good apposition, approximation, and alignment. However, great care must be taken to ensure that no widening occurs within the ankle mortise. Surgical reduction is indicated with excessive fracture displacement, ankle dislocation, and/or ankle mortise widening. This is also true if greater than one third of the joint surface is involved with fracture of the posterior malleolus of the tibia.

In the case of both surgical and nonsurgical treatment, the use of an ankle brace such as an AirCast or Active Ankle Brace is advisable. Rehabilitation after the cast has been removed should follow those steps described previously for a serious ankle sprain.

FRACTURES OF THE FOOT

Fractures of the foot account for approximately 10% of all fractures. These fractures may occur from direct blows to the foot, such as being stepped on or as a result of torsional stresses such as those occurring during an inversion sprain. Frequently, injury that does not entail a direct blow results in avulsive fracture (80).

Calcaneal Fractures. Calcaneal fractures can be divided in two ways: those that are interarticular versus extra-articular and those that are compressive versus avulsive. Extra-articular fractures comprise approximately 25% of calcaneal fractures and usually involve the medial calcaneal tubercle, anterior process, sustentaculum tali, or medial, lateral, or superior portions of the tuberosity.

Avulsion of the anterior process is the most common form of avulsive fracture of the calcaneus. The Achilles tendon inserts onto the posterior portion of the tuberosity of the calcaneus. When avulsion occurs to the superior portion of the tuberosity, known as a "beak" fracture, Achilles tendon avulsion may result.

When compression fracture of the calcaneus occurs, 10% of these are bilateral. An additional 10% are associated with thoracolumbar vertebral body or neural arch fracture. Calcaneal compression fractures may result from a fall or landing on the feet, such as when pole vaulters fail on an attempt and land on their feet with a relatively unprotected heel while wearing spiked track shoes. These fractures are frequently comminuted. With such fractures, the subtalar joint is usually involved, depressing the posterior facet of the calcaneus. In rare instances, a radiolucent fracture line will be seen. However, because of the crushed nature of the injury, such fracture lines are frequently not visualized.

Boehler's angle is formed by drawing a line from the superior posterior aspect of the tuberosity to the tip of the posterior facet, and a second line from the tip of the posterior facet through the superior margin of the anterior process. This angle normally measures 28°–40°. A positive Boehler's angle is less than 28° and indicates a depression fracture of the calcaneus (80). Bone scans, CT scans, and MRI may be helpful for further diagnostic conclusions (Fig. 16.44).

These fractures commonly present in older individuals with osteoporosis. Auto racing, aviation sports, sky diving, and rock climbing also will have a higher incidence of this type of fracture.

These fractures are associated with a high degree of late morbidity secondary to subtalar degeneration and degenerative changes to the calcaneal fat pad. Further widening of the heel may create impingement of the fibula. Such traumatic fractures are not easily treated and may be associated with secondary conditions such as tarsal tunnel syndrome.

Conservative treatment and operative treatment both have minimal success. Initial treatment of calcaneal fractures should be maintained by cast immobilization. Conservative treatment consists of the use of stable, well-cushioned footgear and the use of semirigid or soft orthoses to limit subtalar motion and provide optimal shock absorption. With calcaneal compression fractures, close observation of neurovascular structures must be maintained because they can easily be compromised by direct trauma or compression within the tarsal tunnels (88).

Talar Fractures

Talar fractures can be classified by anatomical locations, of the body, neck, or head. Talar body fractures, such as the osteochondral fractures discussed earlier in this chapter, result from inversion or eversion sprains of the ankle when direct contact is made between the talus and the

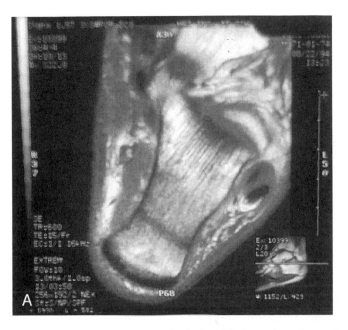 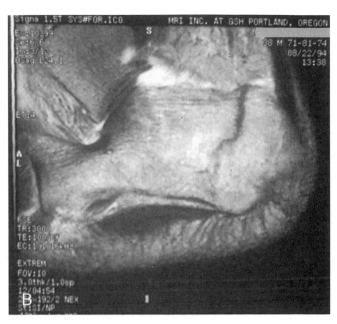

Figure 16.44. A and **B** show calcaneal stress fracture as noted on MRI. (Courtesy of T.L. Forcum.)

tibia or fibula.

Fractures of the talar neck are most often the result of an avulsion off the anterior surface. Vertical fractures can occur when compressive forces of the anterior tibia are forced downward through the neck of the talus. This may result from insults similar to those that create calcaneal fractures. World War I pilots who were forced to make crash-landings developed linear talar neck fractures that became known as "aviators fractures." Because there is poor collateral blood supply to the talus, due to the fact that 60% of the external surface of the talus is covered by articular cartilage, avascular necrosis is a common complication. The more anterior the neck fracture, the greater the likelihood for the development of avascular necrosis because the primary locations for portals of blood supply to the talus are at the sinus tarsus and tarsal canal.

Talar head fractures are less common. They are demonstrated by a linear fracture line anterior to the neck of the talus. These fractures can be managed conservatively if good alignment, apposition, and approximation are present (80).

MRI may be useful in the diagnosis of avascular necrosis, which is characterized by a decrease of the high signal associated with fat on a T1-weighted sequence.

Navicular Fractures

Avulsion fractures of the dorsal navicular bone are the most common type of fracture to occur secondary to plantarflexion and inversion sprains (86). Traumatic eversion may result in avulsion

of the medial tuberosity at the insertion of the tibialis posterior, and is often confused with an os tibiale externum, an accessory ossicle. Midbody navicular fractures are unusual; however, they may occur secondary to progression of a stress fracture. Such fractures require internal fixation for appropriate stabilization because delayed union and nonunion are common.

Cuneiform Fractures

Cuneiform fractures are rare. When they occur, they are frequently associated with tarsal metatarsal dislocation and disruption of Lisfranc's ligaments.

Cuboid Fractures

Cuboid fractures are rare. When fracture occurs, it appears most frequently on the lateral aspect. Such fractures may be confused with an os peroneum or os versalium.

Fractures of the Base of the Fifth Metatarsal

Avulsion Fracture of the Fifth Metatarsal. Avulsion fracture of the base of the fifth metatarsal often occurs secondary to inversion sprain, where the peroneus brevis muscle contracts to counteract the inversion forces, avulsing its insertion into the styloid of the fifth metatarsal. This condition is relatively common and can be successfully treated conservatively if the fragment is not excessively large or displaced. Treatments typically follow the course of that for the inversion sprain, and symptomatic progress is monitored. Care

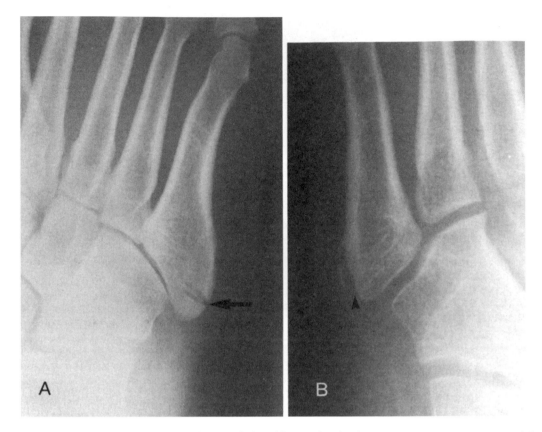

Figure 16.45. Jones' fracture versus normal variant. **A.** Jones' fracture has the characteristic transverse orientation of the fracture line on the base of the fifth metatarsal. **B.** The apophysis for the base of the fifth metatarsal is separated by a longitudinally oriented lucent cleft. (Reprinted with permission from Yochum TR, Rowe LJ. Essentials of skeletal radiology. Baltimore: Williams & Wilkins, 1987;1.)

should be taken to monitor the stabilization of this fragment; improper stabilization and rehabilitation may result in a large callus and painful bump. Once a painful bump is present, measures must be taken to provide pressure relief over the fifth styloid. Footwear may need to be stretched or cut out to accommodate this bump.

Avulsion fractures should not be confused with the normal apophysis of the base of the fifth metatarsal, which presents in a longitudinal orientation at the styloid of the fifth metatarsal (Fig. 16.45). Iselin's disease is an apophysitis of the base of the fifth metatarsal. This disease is seen in girls between the ages of 8 and 15 and in boys between the ages of 10 and 17. It is most commonly seen between the ages of 10 and 12. This condition is much like Osgood-Schlatter's disease. It is a self-limiting condition that should be treated symptomatically and must be differentiated from avulsion of the base of the fifth metatarsal (17).

Jones' (Dancer's) Fracture. A Jones' or dancer's fracture is a transverse fracture of the proximal diaphysis of the fifth metatarsal. This is a serious injury for the competitive athlete because its ten-

dency toward delayed union or nonunion is notorious and the fracture is slow to heal. Fracture may result from overuse, stress fracture progression, or indirect trauma. These fractures usually result from the confluence of axial loading of the forefoot and overload of the fifth ray, along with the tensile forces from the peroneus brevis insertion.

With early and proper treatment, conservative means of therapy should have approximately an 80% or higher success rate. This treatment requires early recognition, particularly in those cases where chronic stress overload is occurring. Proper treatment consists of a non–weight-bearing cast to be worn below the knee for approximately 8 weeks. At 4 weeks, this cast should be removed for evaluation of tenderness and evidence of union. After 8 weeks, if union appears to be delayed, electrical bone stimulation is recommended. Clinical union generally occurs within 10 to 14 weeks but may occur as early as 8 weeks. The athlete should not return to full activity until there is clear evidence of radiographic union and there is no residual palpatory tenderness. This usually occurs between 3 and 4 months.

When the fracture site is displaced or is demonstrating delayed union or nonunion, surgical intervention may be indicated. Internal fixation with a screw or pin through the styloid and possible bone grafting may expedite an early return to activity. Such surgical intervention should take into consideration the athletic level and activity. A dancer or basketball player is unlikely to be able to return to activity without a fully united fracture, whereas a rower or cyclist may be able to participate comfortably with nonunion (23, 42).

Fractures of the Metatarsals

In athletes, metatarsal fractures usually occur secondary to compressive forces, such as when someone steps on another's foot. This may be common in football, rugby, basketball, and volleyball. Stress fractures are a common occurrence in the second and third metatarsals. With progression these may become complete.

Inversion and plantarflexion injuries may fracture the dorsal base of the metatarsals (Fig. 16.46).

Fractures of the Phalanges

Toe fractures are a common occurrence and generally result from one of three mechanisms: avulsion, crush, or longitudinal blow. Fractures of the hallux, particularly those involving the metatarsal phalangeal joint, may result in secondary hallux rigidus or limitus. Chip fractures may result from hyperextension or hyperflexion of a toe. Crush injuries, in athletes, generally result from the phalanges being stepped on, whereas direct blows result from the athlete kicking an object. Unless comminuted, these fractures can be treated conservatively and frequently require no direct treatment other than the application of ice and a shoe with ample forefoot room. Those fractures involving a joint space need to have proper rehabilitation, after the fracture has healed, to restore normal joint mechanics and prevent degenerative changes within the articular structures. Toe injuries will often create compensatory sites of stress and hence injuries to other parts of the body due to mechanical compensation. Therefore, care should be taken to ensure that the athlete is not preforming antalgically on return to activity and competition.

AVASCULAR NECROSIS (OSTEOCHONDROSES) OF THE FOOT

Diaz' Disease (Avascular Necrosis of the Talus)

Diaz' disease is an avascular necrosis of the talus. It is likely that it occurs secondary to trauma to the talar body, particularly fracture. Signs of necrosis generally appear within 1 to 3 months after injury. Radiographic signs demonstrate a collapse of the articular surface and increased density of the talar body.

Köhler's Disease (Avascular Necrosis of the Navicular)

Köhler's disease is an avascular necrosis of the tarsal navicular. This condition frequently occurs in boys and predominates at age 5. The condition is characterized by local swelling and pain. Mild edema and pes planus may be present. Gait is generally antalgic on the affected side. Radiographs demonstrate a narrowed diameter of the navicular in an anterior to posterior direction. Radiographically, this appears as flattening and sclerosis of the navicular with irregular fragmentation.

Treatment will vary depending on the severity

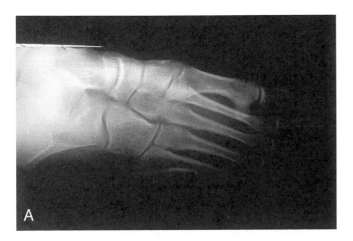
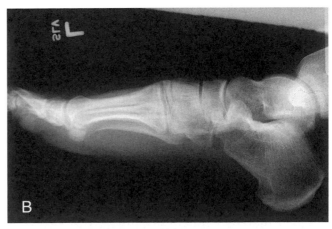

Figure 16.46. A. Fracture at the base of the first through fourth metatarsals, with good alignment. **B.** At the first metatarsal the fracture extends into the articular margin with the first cuneiform. (Courtesy of T.L. Forcum.)

of the condition. Treatment may consist of limited activity with the use of low dye strapping and arch strapping supported by arch supports. In more severe cases, non–weight-bearing short leg casting for 6 to 8 weeks is necessary. Generally this condition resolves without deformity or disability, and complete resumption of activity is possible.

Sever's Disease (Calcaneal Apophysitis)

The crescent-shaped calcaneal apophysis begins ossifying in females at 4 to 6 years of age, fusing at approximately age 16. In males, ossification occurs between the ages of 5 and 9, fusing at approximately age 20. During the normal course of ossification and fusion, the apophysis may appear sclerotic, irregular, and fragmented. Thus, some debate the existence of Sever's as a disease. This situation also demonstrates that the diagnosis of this condition should not be based on radiographic findings.

Patients will generally present with palpatory tenderness over the posterior aspect of the calcaneus. There may be mild edema and painful weight bearing. The athlete may present with antalgic gait on the affected side. This condition has a high incidence in those demonstrating overpronation and equinus syndrome. It is possible that a traction apophysitis is secondary to tension from the plantar fascia or the Achilles tendon.

This condition is self-limiting and should be treated symptomatically by decreasing offending activities. The use of heel lifts and orthotics will decrease biomechanical stress at the os calcis. General stretching of the calf and plantar fascia is recommended, along with moist heat before activity and stretching and ice after activity.

Freiberg's Disease (Avascular Necrosis of the Metatarsal Heads)

Freiberg's disease represents avascular necrosis of the metatarsal heads, most commonly the second metatarsal. This condition presents radiographically with a crushed appearance, irregularity, sclerosis, and marginal osteophytes. This condition predominates in girls (75%) after the age of 13. The cause of this condition is unclear, and may be associated with trauma or overuse. The patient generally presents with pain and swelling at the site of the involved metatarsal. This swelling decreases metatarsal phalangeal range of motion, and crepitus may be present.

Freiberg's disease can be classified into Types I through IV. This classification system depicts progressive severity, articular involvement, and the number of metatarsals involved.

Type I demonstrates no articular degeneration and is treated with reduction of weight bearing, accommodative padding or orthotics, and a reduction of shoe heel height. Steroid injection should be avoided because this may interfere with the normal repair process. Generally this condition is considered self-limiting.

Type II demonstrates periarticular spurring and metatarsal head flattening, but the articular cartilage remains intact. Treatment for Type II metatarsal head avascular necrosis consists of the use of non–weight-bearing casting and the same measures as described in Type I.

Type III demonstrates severe degenerative joint disease with loss of articular cartilage. Frequently, there will be an associated phalangeal subluxation. This level of progression is best treated surgically.

Type IV involves multiple metatarsal heads. This is rare, but when it does occur, treatment depends on level of severity and follows that described for Types I, II, and III.

ADDENDUM: BIOMECHANICAL PRESCRIPTION OF ATHLETIC FOOTWEAR

Athletic footwear is designed for four functions.

1. *Protection of the foot from the environment.* Protection of the foot from the environment can come in many forms. For example, the use of thermal insulation in golf and hiking shoes can protect the foot from environmental temperatures and assist in keeping the foot dry. Toe guards can help protect the distal toes from compression or abrasion. Proper midsole thickness and rigidity protect the foot from sharp, uneven surfaces such as rocks, glass, or other hazards to the plantar foot.

2. *Fit.* Fit and comfort of the shoe are important for the prevention of pressure sores, blisters, corns, and calluses. If the shoe does not fit properly, the athlete may encounter other biomechanical faults in compensation. Improper fit of the shoe, such as being too long or too short, may also produce biomechanical compromise to several joints, particularly the metatarsal phalangeal joints. Generally, there should be an index finger width from the longest toe to the end of the shoe for adequate space. A shoe that is too narrow can cause interdigital nerve compression, which may result in an interdigital neuroma. A shoe that is too

wide may cause blistering from friction created when the foot slides from side to side. Shoe lacing must be accessed to prevent neural or vascular encroachment of the ankle and dorsal foot. In such cases, skipping an eyelet, heel lock lacing, Lydiard lacing, or variable width lacing may be necessary.

3. *Shock absorption.* Shoe shock absorption is generally adequate if the shoe is worn for its intended function. Frequently, however, athletes will cross-train, using a basketball or court shoe (which may not provide adequate cushioning for a prolonged period) for running. Most shoes are designed to be worn for approximately 500 miles. At this point, 70% of shock absorption has been lost. This seems to be the critical point at which shock absorption injuries occur.

4. *Control of functional biomechanics.* Biomechanical control or motion control is critical for those who have biomechanical faults. The shoe with strong biomechanical control can often cause injury to an individual with no faults by overcorrecting a biomechanical pattern. An example is a neutral gait athlete who wears a shoe that is highly controlled for pronation. In such a situation, the athlete may underpronate.

SHOE FEATURE DESIGNS FOR BIOMECHANICAL CONTROL

Neutral Gait

A. Semicurve lasted.
B. A nonposted midsole with a combination lasted upper, or a medial posted shoe with a slip lasted upper.

Underpronation

A. Curved or banana lasted shoe.
B. Slip lasted shoe.
C. Soft, flexible midsole.
D. In rare instances, a lateral post or kinetic wedge can be found to assist in encouraging inward rotation of the forefoot.

Overpronation

A. Straight or semicurve last.
B. Full or combination board last, Kevlar or other rigid material in the hindfoot.
C. Medial posted midsole, foot bridge, or plastic plug in the medial midsole.
D. Firm heel counter.
E. Appropriately placed arch support.

When orthotics are combined with footwear, the shoe's biomechanical features must be considered. A patient's condition may be worsened by the use of an orthotic with an inappropriate shoe. The author recommends that an athlete rotate or alternate the use of shoes with at least two pairs. Each shoe is slightly different biomechanically and will work the musculature to different degrees. Rotating shoes will reduce repeated stress and aid in the prevention of overuse injury. In addition, allowing ample recovery between use allows for complete reexpansion of the midsole materials. Allowing the shoes to dry and decompress will add life to the shoe and increase its shock-absorbing capacities. The use of a second shoe brought into play midway through the life of the first shoe prevents a cyclical lull as the patient goes through new shoes with proper shock absorption and downgrades to shoes with improper shock absorption.

References

1. Agur AR. Grant's atlas of anatomy. Baltimore: Williams & Wilkins, 1991.
2. Moore KL. Clinically oriented anatomy. Baltimore: Williams & Wilkins, 1980.
3. Draves DJ. Anatomy of the lower extremity. Baltimore: Williams & Wilkins, 1986.
4. Chusid JG. Correlative neuroanatomy and functional neurology. Los Altos, CA: Lange Medical Publications, 1985.
5. Wiley JP, Short WB, Wiseman DA, et al. Ultrasound catheter placement for deep posterior compartment pressure measurements in chronic compartment syndrome. Am J Sports Med 1990;18:74–79.
6. Egan TD, Joyce SM. Acute compartment syndrome following a minor athletic injury. J Emerg Med 1989;7:353–357.
7. Beadnell SW, Saunderson JR, Sorenson DC. Compartment syndrome following oral and maxillofacial surgery. J Oral Maxillofac Surg 1988;46:232–234.
8. Bergquist D, Bohe M, Ekelund G, et al. Compartment syndromes after prolonged surgery with leg supports. Int J Colorectal Dis 1990;5:1–5.
9. Williams TM, Knopp R, Ellyson JH. Compartment syndrome after antishock trouser use without lower-extremity trauma. J Trauma 1982;22:595–597.
10. Templeman D, Lange R, Harms B. Lower-extremity compartment syndromes associated with use of pneumatic antishock garments. J Trauma 1987;27:79–81.
11. Kikta MJ, Meyer JP, Bishara RA, et al. Crush syndrome due to limb compression. Arch Surg 1987;122:1078–1081.
12. McKee MD, Jupiter JB. Acute exercise-induced bilateral anterolateral leg compartment syndrome in a healthy young man. Am J Orthop 1995;24:862–864.
13. Lutz LJ, Goodenough GK, Detmer DE. Chronic compartment syndrome. Am Fam Physician 1989;39:191–196.
14. Pedowitz RA, Hargens AR, Mubarak SJ, et al. Modified criteria for the objective diagnosis of chronic compartment syndrome of the leg. Am J Sports Med 1990;18:35–40.
15. Melberg PE, Styf J. Posteromedial pain in the lower leg. Am J Sports Med 1989;17:747–750.
16. Hoffmeyer P, Cox JN, Fritschy D. Ultrastructural modification of muscle in three types of compartment syndrome. Int Orthop 1987;11:53–59.
17. Reid DC. Sports injury assessment and rehabilitation. New York: Churchill Livingstone, 1992.

18. Styf J. Chronic exercise-induced pain in the anterior aspect of the lower leg: an overview of diagnosis. Sports Med 1989;7:331–339.

19. Styf JR, Korner LM. Diagnosis of chronic anterior compartment syndrome in the lower leg. Acta Orthop Scand 1987;58:139–144.

20. Bourne RB, Roraback CH. Compartment syndromes of the lower leg. Clin Orthop 1989;240:97–104.

21. Roy S, Irvin R. Sports medicine. Englewood Cliffs, NJ: Prentice-Hall, 1993.

22. Evans RC. Illustrated essentials in orthopedic physical assessments. St. Louis: Mosby Year Book, 1994.

23. Oloff LM. Musculoskeletal disorders of the lower extremities. Philadelphia: WB Saunders, 1994.

24. Baxter DE. Functional nerve disorders in the athlete's foot, ankle and leg. Instr Course Lect 1993;42:185–194.

25. Turnipseed WD, Pozniak M. Popliteal entrapment as a result of neurovascular compression by the soleus and plantaris muscles. J Vasc Surg 1992;15:285–293. Discussion.

26. Schon LC, Baxter DE. Neuropathies of the foot and ankle in athletes. Clin Sports Med 1990;9:489–509.

27. Edwards MS, Hirigoyen M, Burge PD. Compression of the common peroneal nerve by a cyst of the lateral meniscus. Clin Orthop 1995;316:131–133.

28. Michaud TC, Fowler SM. Superficial peroneal nerve entrapment resulting from a congenital plantar flexed first ray. J Neuromusculoskeletal System 1995;3:27.

29. Stoica E, Voiculescu V. Transient peripheral ischemia may restore quickly the motility in patients with compression neuropathy. Rom J Neurol Psychiatry 1993;31:139–150.

30. Michaud TC. Foot orthoses and other forms of conservative foot care. Baltimore: Williams & Wilkins, 1993.

31. Uncini A, Di Muzio A, Gambi D. Compressive bilateral peroneal neuropathy: serial electrophysiologic studies and pathophysical remarks. Acta Neurol Scand 1992;85:66–70.

32. Perlman MD. Os peroneum fracture with sural nerve entrapment neuritis. Foot Surg 1990;29:119–121.

33. Shaffrey ME, Jane JA, Persing JA, et al. Surgeon's foot: a report of sural nerve palsy. Neurosurgery 1992;30:927–930.

34. Peri G. The critical zones of entrapment of the nerves of the lower limb. Surg Radiol Anat 1991;13:139–142.

35. DiRisio D, Lazaro R, Popp AJ. Nerve entrapment and calf atrophy caused by a Baker's cyst: case report. Neurosurgery 1994;35:333–334.

36. Ekelund AL. Bilateral nerve entrapment in the popliteal space. Am J Sports Med 1990;18:108.

37. Meisterling RC, Boyum GP, Lane-Larsen CI. Posterior tibial nerve impingement from a tibial spine fixation screw: a case report. Am J Sports Med 1993;21:326–328.

38. Logigian EL, Berger AR, Shahani BT. Injury to the tibial and peroneal nerves due to hemorrhage in the popliteal fossa. Two case reports. J Bone Joint Surg 1989;71:768–770.

39. Subotnick SI. Podiatric sports medicine. Mount Kisco, NY: Futura Publishing Company, 1975.

40. Schon LC. Nerve entrapment, neuropathy, and nerve dysfunction in athletes. Orthop Clin North Am 1994;25:47–59.

41. Boc SF, Kushner S. Plantar fibromatosis causing entrapment syndrome of the medial plantar nerve. J Am Podiatr Med Assoc 1994;84:420–422.

42. McGlamry ED. Fundamentals of foot surgery. Baltimore: Williams & Wilkins, 1987.

43. Taylor P, Taylor D. Conquering athletic injuries. Champaign, Il: Leisure Press, 1988.

44. Johnston MR. Nerve entrapment causing heel pain. Clin Podiatr Med Surg 1994;11:617–624.

45. Johnson ER, Kirby K, Lieberman JS. Lateral plantar nerve entrapment: foot pain in a power lifter. Am J Sports Med 1992;20:619–620.

46. Cheung Y, Rosenberg ZS, Magee T, et al. Normal anatomy and pathologic conditions of the ankle tendons: current imaging techniques. Radiographics 1992.

47. Plattner PF. Tendon problems of the foot and ankle: the spectrum from peritendinitis to rupture. Postgrad Med 1989;86:155–162, 167–170.

48. Sobel M, Pavlov H, Geppert MJ, et al. Painful os peroneum syndrome: a spectrum of conditions responsible for plantar lateral foot pain. Foot Ankle Int 1994;15:122–143.

49. Johnson KA, Strom DE. Tibialis posterior tendon dysfunction. Clin Orthop 1989;239:196.

50. Anouchi YS, Parker RD, Seitz WH Jr. Posterior compartment syndrome of the calf resulting from misdiagnosis of a rupture of the medial head of the gastrocnemius. J Trauma 1987;15:678–680.

51. Scioli MW. Achilles tendinitis. Orthop Clin North Am 1994;25:177–182.

52. Nichols AW. Achilles tendinitis in running athletes. J Am Board Fam Pract 1989;2:196–203.

53. O'Reilly MA, Massouh H. Pictorial review: the sonographic diagnosis of pathology in the Achilles tendon. Clin Radiol 1993;48:202–206.

54. Soma CA, Mandelbaum DR. Achilles tendon disorders. Clin Sports Med 1994;13:811–823.

55. Smart GW, Taunton JE, Clement DB. Achilles tendon disorders in runners: a review. Med Sci Sports Exerc 1980;12;231–243.

56. Lehtinen A, Peltokallio P, Taavitsainen M. Sonography of Achilles tendon correlated to operative findings. Ann Chir Gynaecol 1994;8:322–327.

57. Leppilahti J, Orava S, Karpakka J, et al. Overuse injuries of the Achilles tendon. Ann Chir Gynaecol 1991;80:202–207.

58. Schafer RC. Chiropractic management of sports and recreational injuries. Baltimore: Williams & Wilkins, 1982.

59. Wall JR, Harkness MA, Crawford A. Ultrasound diagnosis of plantar fasciitis. Foot Ankle 1993;14:465–470.

60. Ryan J. Use of posterior night splints in the treatment of plantar fasciitis. Am Fam Physician 1995;52:891–898:901–902.

61. Karlsson J, Lansinger O. Chronic lateral instability of the ankle in athletes. Sports Med 1993;16:355–365.

62. Verhagen RA, De Keizer G, van Dijk CN. Long-term follow-up of inversion trauma of the ankle. Arch Orthop Trauma Surg 1995;114:92–96.

63. Bennett WF. Lateral ankle sprains. part 2: acute and chronic treatment. Orthop Rev 1994;23:504–510.

64. Seto JL, Brewster CE. Treatment approaches following foot and ankle injury. Clin Sports Med 1994;13:695–718.

65. Stiell IG, Greenberg GH, McKnight D, et al. Decision rules for the use of radiography in acute ankle injuries. JAMA 1993;269:1127–1132.

66. Mazion JM. Illustrated manual of neurological reflexes/signs/tests and orthopedic signs/tests/maneuvers. Arizona City, AZ: Dr. J.M. Mazion, 1980.

67. Ward DW. Syndesmotic ankle sprain in a recreational hockey player. J Manipulative Physiol Ther 1994;17:385–394.

68. Wilers GB, Horn-Kingery HM. Treatment of the inversion ankle sprain: comparison of different modes of compression and cryotherapy. J Orthop Sports Phys Ther 1993;17:240–246.

69. Myerson MS, Henderson MR. Clinical applications of a pneumatic intermittent impulse compression device after trauma and major surgery to the foot and ankle. Foot Ankle 1993;14:198–203.

70. Johannes EJ, Sukul DM, Spruit PJ, et al. Controlled trial of a semi-rigid bandage ("scotchrap") in patients with ankle ligament lesions. Curr Med Res Opin 1993;13:154–162.

71. Karlsson J, Andreasson GO. The afield of external ankle support in chronic lateral ankle joint instability: an electromyographic study. Am J Sports Med 1992;20:257–261.

72. Justin KA, Gwynn-Brett KA, Marshall SC. Illustrated guide to taping techniques. Baltimore: Mosby-Wolfe, 1994.

73. Eiff MP, Smith AT, Smith GE. Early mobilization versus immobilization in the treatment of lateral ankle sprains. Am J Sports Med 1994;22:83–88.

74. Hedrick MR, McBryde AM. Posterior ankle impingement. Foot Ankle Int 1994;15:2–8.

75. Sandmeirer RH, Renstrom PA. Ankle arthroscopy. Scand J Med Sci Sports 1995;5:64–70.

76. Meyer SA, Callaghan JJ, Albright JP, et al. Midfoot sprains in collegiate football players. Am J Sports Med 1994;22:392–401.

77. Shapiro MS, Wascher DC, Finerman G. Rupture of Lisfranc's ligament in athletes. Am J Sports Med 1994;22:687–691.

78. Richardson EG. Injuries to the hallucal sesamoids in the athlete. Foot Ankle 1987;7:229–244.

79. McBryde AM Jr, Anderson RB. Sesamoid foot problems in the athlete. Clin Sports Med 1988;7:51–60.

80. Yochum TR, Rowe LJ. Essentials of skeletal radiology. Baltimore: Williams & Wilkins, 1987.

81. Lomer R, Fisher C, Lloyd-Smith R, et al. Osteochondral lesion of the talus. Am J Sports Med 1993;21:13–19.

82. Hough DO, Ray R. Stress Fractures. Sports Science Exchange 1994;7:48.

83. Hulkko A, Orava S. Diagnosis and treatment of delayed and non-union stress fractures in athletes. Ann Chir Gynaecol 1991;80:177–184.

84. Ryaby J, Fitzsimmons R, Magee F, et al. Biophysical stimulation of tissue healing mediated by IGF-II. Am Acad Orthop Surg New Orleans, Louisiana 1994. Scientific Exhibit.

85. Brown MA, George CR, Dunstan R, et al. Aluminum-related bone disease presenting with calcaneal stress fractures. Br J Rheumatol 1993;32:260–262.

86. Orava S, Karpakka J, Hulkko A, et al. Stress avulsion fractures of the tarsal navicular, an uncommon sports-related overuse injury. Am J Sports Med 1991;19:392–395.

87. Dietzen CJ. Great toe sesamoid injuries in the athlete. Orthop Rev 1990;19:966–972.

88. Mallik AR, Chase MD, Lee PC, et al. Calcaneal fracture-dislocation with entrapment of the medial neurovascular bundle: a case report. Foot Ankle 1993;14:411–413.

Section III

SPECIAL CONSIDERATIONS

The Female Athlete

Abigail A. Irwin

AN HISTORICAL PERSPECTIVE

No women took part in the first Olympic Games in 4 A.D. Females were forbidden even to watch the Games—under penalty of death. As we rapidly approach the 21st century, it is astounding to reflect on the events that have allowed the female athlete to gain the respect, admiration, and freedom that, until the past few decades, had been reserved for her male counterparts.

This long quest for equality of women in sports has been a struggle. Many talented and determined athletes were instrumental in this rise to athletic freedom. The dedication and hard work of a number of famous women such as Babe Didrickson Zaharias, Wilma Rudolph, Billie Jean King, Jackie Joyner-Kersee, Martina Navratilova, and Joan Benoit, to name a few, have made possible the growing acceptance in sports participation that female athletes enjoy today (Figs. 17.1 to 17.3).

The passage of Title IX of the United States Education Amendment in 1972 was a major catalyst in permitting the U.S. female athlete to excel in sports, as she does today. Title IX states that educational institutions must not discriminate on the basis of gender. Federally funded schools are required to provide equal facilities and opportunities for girls and women. As a result of this amendment, athletic scholarships were made available to women. These changes facilitated a new era of competitiveness for the female athlete that precipitated changes in traditional social attitudes surrounding women in sports. With these changes came a growing acceptance of women and girls in sports participation.

More than 20 years after the passage of Title IX, most collegiate sports programs have failed to comply adequately with this amendment. The bulk of programs and scholarships continue to go to revenue-producing men's sports. The NCAA is attempting to rectify this long-standing problem by enforcing "gender equity" in NCAA-governed colleges. Gender equity is designed to provide an equal percentage of funding to either the percentage of female athletes participating in intercollegiate sports or the number of female students enrolled. The NCAA has formed a Gender Equity Task Force that, by 1998, must assure that these schools have at least 40% female athletes receiving 40% of available funding (1).

Now girls are beginning their initiation into organized athletics at ages comparable to those for boys. In addition, they are intensifying their training and conditioning programs. These new trends are creating changes in the traditional or common injuries that female athletes typically encounter. Many studies have concluded that the most common injuries sustained by women are overuse injuries, usually secondary to lack of training and muscular strength. Initially, with the surge of participation, there was an overall increase in the number of injuries suffered by women when compared with men in the same sport. Today there is virtually no difference in the overall injury rate between the sexes (2).

For many years it was thought that women should not participate in endurance competitions. It was believed that women were physically incapable of withstanding the gruelling demands of an endurance sport—it might be too stressful and too dangerous! In 1896 a Greek woman, Melpomene, secretly ran in the Olympic marathon. That event marks the first attempt of a woman to gain acceptance as an Olympian endurance athlete. It was not until 88 years later that Joan Benoit won the first official women's Olympic marathon. Her time in that race was 2:24:52. That time would have won 11 of the 20 previous men's Olympic marathons (3).

What does the future hold for the female athlete and sports competition? Whipp and Ward (4) examined the world records of men and women for running events from the 200 meter to the marathon over the past century. During this period, women's records improved nearly twice as fast as men's. Using this information, the au-

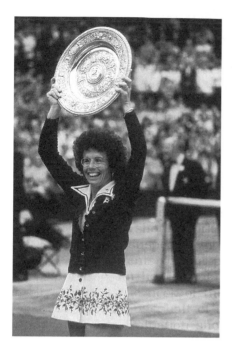

Figure 17.1. Billie Jean King, Wimbledon champion 1975. (Courtesy of Allsport.)

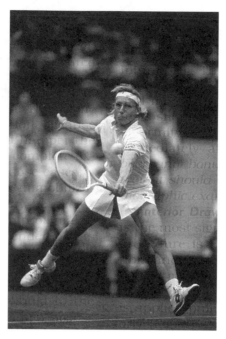

Figure 17.2. Martina Navratilova, U.S. Open 1993. (Courtesy of Chris Cole/Allsport.)

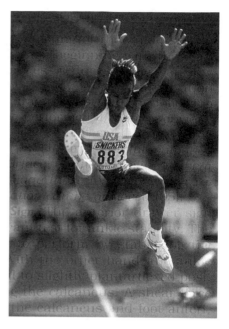

Figure 17.3. Jackie Joyner-Kersee, Heptathlon World Championships 1993. (Courtesy of Tony Duffy/Allsport.)

thors extrapolated the record progressions into the future and suggested that women's records are closing in on the men's records. They predicted that women may outrun or equal men's records in the marathon as early as 1998 (4). In reviewing these data, it would appear unlikely that this prediction will come true. The inaccuracies of this study can be attributed to the unequal length of time that the genders have had the opportunity to compete. Given the overall strength difference between men and women, it is doubtful that women will achieve the predictions of this study, yet it is likely that they will continue to narrow the gap.

Will women experience the same trends in sports as men? In his writing on athletic performance, Patrick Murphy investigated athletic potential in sports. Men have continued to improve their athletic performances over the years but they may be closer to reaching their limits of performance than women are because men have been competing for a longer period. Murphy cites eight reasons for improved performances by athletes.

1. The greater number of persons participating in sports.
2. The improved health status of the general population.
3. Better facilities and equipment.
4. Improved medical care.
5. Increased external rewards.
6. Improved competitive strategy.
7. Improved diet and ergogenic aids.
8. Better training methods that result in an improved physiologic state (5).

Women are in their infancy as far as sports performance is concerned. By virtue of the continued advances being made in sports science, it seems safe to predict that women are only beginning to approach the limits of their athletic potential and will continue to excel.

ANATOMICAL AND PHYSIOLOGIC CONSIDERATIONS

The boom in women's participation in sports and exercise along with the rising number of well-conditioned women have stimulated research on the physiologic differences and similarities between the genders. How do these gender differences affect women's performance and training in sports? Whereas structural and anatomical differences are of considerable interest, it is typically the physiologic or functional differences that are more important in terms of physical performance (6).

There are distinct differences between the male and female skeleton, as summarized in Table 17.1. Female bone is less dense; therefore, a woman will weigh less than a man of comparable size. Women are generally shorter and have a lower center of gravity, which can be helpful in sports that require strength and balance, such as in gymnastics. Women have proportionately shorter limbs and a greater carrying angle at the elbow, which has an effect on the arm as a lever (see Chapter 12). Arms that do not hang vertically and an increased shoulder slope create different arm mechanics when throwing, making it easier to throw sidearm rather than the typical male overhand delivery (3, 6).

The female pelvis is wider, and the femurs tend to slant more toward the knee. This can change gait biomechanics in running. For example, a woman with excessive genu valgum (knock-knees) greater than 15° will appear to swing her lower leg in a slight circle as she runs. The shape of the pelvis causes a greater quadriceps (Q) angle (Fig. 17.4), which some claim predisposes women to an increased incidence of knee injuries (3). However, this increased Q angle results in a wider articular surface between the femur and the tibia, and may actually provide greater knee stability than in the male (3, 6). Athletic women do not demonstrate the same Q angle variance as the general female population.

There are also physiologic differences between men and women. A woman has a smaller heart (heart volume) than does a man of the same stature. The smaller heart means she will have a smaller stroke volume; even with a higher heart rate than men, women have 30% less maximal cardiac output. Also because of smaller body size, a woman has a smaller thorax than a man. Hence, women have a higher respiratory rate and less total lung capacity than men (6). These differences are significant when comparing overall endurance.

It is well documented that at sexual maturity, the average male will be 10% taller and 25 pounds heavier than the average female (3, 7, 8). In addition, males will have 8 to 10% less body

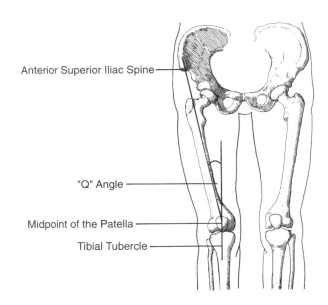

Figure 17.4. Measuring the Q angle.

fat and a larger proportion of muscle, resulting in a greater lean body weight and a larger total muscle mass. Muscle mass affects strength, power, muscular endurance, and speed, which in turn influence many types of sports performance. Thus, in the many sports requiring force and power, women are often at a disadvantage.

There are apparently no gender differences in muscle fiber composition; however, there are differences in muscle fiber size. Men tend to have larger fast twitch and slow twitch fibers than women. The slow twitch fibers have a high capacity for aerobic metabolism and are thus better suited for prolonged endurance exercise. Fast twitch fibers generally have a higher capacity for anaerobic metabolism and are designed for larger force production associated with short-term, high-intensity exercise. It has been shown that the fast twitch and slow twitch muscle fibers can be hypertrophied and strengthened with increases in physical activity. Women athletes appear to have muscle fiber compositions similar to those of men in the same sport, but the size (cross-sectional area) of the fibers remains smaller (3, 8).

The strength differences between the sexes have been well documented (3, 6–9). Understanding these differences can be instrumental in designing a proper weight training program for the female athlete. Currently, there is an enormous difference between the upper body strength of the adult female compared with the adult male (43 to 63% weaker in the female); however, this difference is much less when comparing lower body strength (27% weaker). The discrepancy between the upper and lower body strength is believed to be a result of lack of use of the upper

Table 17.1. Skeletal Characteristics in Women Compared with Men*

Item	Result
Size: usually smaller, shorter	Lower center of gravity
Pelvis: wider	Lighter body frame
	Different running mechanics
Thighs: slant inward toward knees	Injury may be more likely
Lower leg bones: less "bowed"	because of knee instability
Limbs (relative to body length): shorter	Shorter lever arm for movement—important for use of implements
Shoulder: narrower, greater sloping	Different mechanics of upper limb motion
Upper arms: do not hang vertically	
Elbows: marked "carrying angle"	Important in throwing pattern

From Wells CL. Women, sport & performance: a physiological perspective. Champaign, IL: Human Kinetics Publishers, 1991:17. Reprinted by permission.
*Information courtesy of C. Wells, Arizona State University.

body by most women. With adequate weight training, the relative differences between upper and lower body strength can be diminished. It appears that the weakness of the upper extremities in the female is more socially than genetically determined (6, 7).

Women and men respond to strength training in very similar ways from their individual pretraining baselines. In general, women have smaller bodies, have less absolute muscle mass and smaller individual muscle fibers, and display approximately two thirds of the absolute overall strength and power of men. However, unit for unit, female muscle tissue is similar to male muscle mass in force output, and there is some evidence to support similar, proportional increases for men and women in strength performance and hypertrophy of muscle fibers relative to pretraining status. There is no evidence that women should weight-train differently than men, but training programs should be individually tailored (9).

Current recommendations for cardiovascular exercise in men and women are similar. A recent study looked at the serum lipoprotein (SLP) levels of women after a single period of submaximal exercise of 45 minutes or less on a treadmill. In this study, no significant positive changes of the SLP levels were produced after a single bout of submaximal exercise. However, positively affected SLP levels have been observed in men under the same circumstances. One might conclude from this research that longer sessions of submaximal cardiovascular exercise may be necessary for women to produce positive changes in SLP levels (10).

There are also various metabolic differences between men and women. Women tend to have a slower metabolism than do men; metabolic rate represents the conversion of food to energy for use by the body. Basal metabolic rate (BMR) is believed to be lower in women because of the greater lean-body mass of the male and the greater proportion of relatively inactive adipose tissue in the female (3). Maximal oxygen uptake ($\dot{V}O_2max$) is widely accepted as the best single measure of cardiovascular fitness and maximal aerobic power. Absolute values of $\dot{V}O_2max$ are typically 40 to 60% higher in men than in women. When adjusted for the differences in size and weight of the women, the relative expression of $\dot{V}O_2max$ reduces this difference to 20 to 30%. Values of $\dot{V}O_2max$ vary among athletes in different sports. Generally, the higher the aerobic demand of the sport, the greater the $\dot{V}O_2max$. For example, female long-distance skiers and run-

ners have a much higher maximal aerobic capacity than men who excel in tennis, baseball, football, and ice hockey.

It has been observed that the response to heat and exercise differs between men and women. Women tend to begin sweating at a higher body temperature and sweat less than men. In addition, the heart rate and the core (rectal) temperature increase more rapidly in women, especially in humid conditions (7). Hence, an improved sweating efficiency in humid heat has been reported in women, perhaps resulting from a larger surface area-to-mass ratio than in men (11). Men, however, appear to have an advantage in more severe dry heat, having a larger absolute fluid reserve with which to increase sweating. Although women tend to lose less fluid through sweating, the loss represents a larger fraction of body fluid (11).

Do women have an advantage exercising in cold temperature due to their layer of subcutaneous fat? Witnessing Lynne Cox (33% body fat), the world's top endurance swimmer, swim across the Bering Strait in 38° temperature might lead one to agree. Currently, there is no evidence that gender alone limits exercise of humans in a cold environment. This has more to do with surface area-to-mass ratio; because this ratio is greater in women, exercising in the cold would appear to be disadvantageous (11).

Developmental Variances

During the prepubertal period, the difference in height and weight between boys and girls is minimal. Mixing of sexes in athletic activities is no longer the exception but is fast becoming the rule. Social and cultural influences still somewhat dictate a girl's athleticism or acceptance in competitive sports participation (6). Studies have demonstrated equality in the motor skills of prepubertal children between the ages of 5 and 12, except for certain "masculine" activities such as throwing. However, when the nondominant arm of boys was tested, these differences were negated (7). Questions of safety may arise as organized sports allow co-recreational activity among prepubertal boys and girls. Most studies concur that as long as participation in contact sports is controlled according to equal size, weight, and maturity, the risk of injury to girls will be very low (7).

It has been shown that preadolescent athletes have a later onset of menses than nonathletes (3, 6, 12). Does vigorous exercise cause this delay, or are girls with delayed menses better athletes? A study by Stager and Hatler addressed this question. They compared the age of onset of menses

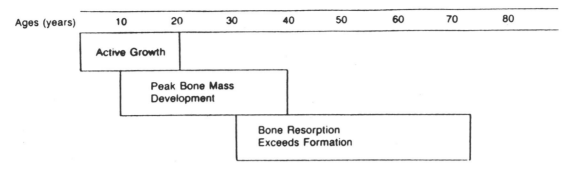

Figure 17.5. Phases of bone growth. (Reprinted with permission from Sanborn CF, Tietz CC, eds. Menstrual dysfunction in the female athlete. In: Scientific foundations of sports medicine. St. Louis: Mosby-Year Book, 1989:138.)

with preadolescent swimmers and their sisters. Findings confirmed other researchers' observations that early athletic training does delay age of menarche in girls, but they did not rule out the possibility of a genetic predisposition. They concluded that swimmers are older at menarche than their sisters and that athletes' sisters are older at menarche than all nonathletic controls (13). Late-onset menses may be a sport-specific phenomenon. For example, in one study, runners had a later onset than gymnasts, and both had a later onset than swimmers (7).

It has been theorized that low body weight and body fat less than 17% are factors that may delay menarche in young athletes. A recent study of premenarcheal athletes and nonathletes refuted this hypothesis, concluding that sexual maturation is not related to a low percentage body fat in either premenarcheal athletes or nonathletes (14). When an amenorrheic young girl reduces her physical activity, menses will usually occur in 3 to 6 months. If not, further investigation is indicated. Until recently, it was believed that delayed-onset menstrual function had no significant health ramifications. Drinkwater et al. found that athletes with a history of amenorrhea or oligomenorrhea may have a lower vertebral bone mineral density (12). Peak bone mass is laid down between the ages of 10 and 30 (Fig. 17.5). If girls are hypoestrogenic during adolescence, their ability to develop peak bone mass may be decreased. Even if they begin menstruating regularly, the bone mineral density loss may be irreversible. These athletes may be vulnerable to stress (and early osteoporotic fractures) later in life (12).

For the most part, proper training can be an important adjunct to normal growth and maturation for children. In sports such as female gymnastics, for which the average age of participants is in the prepubescent and pubescent range, strenuous and prolonged training may predispose these young athletes to increased risk of overuse injuries to growing bone (15). This risk is increased during the growth spurt, which may cause increased muscle-tendon tightness around the joints with accompanying loss of flexibility. Problems do not ordinarily arise at normal levels of activity; however, the more frequent and intense training of young female athletes today merits close scrutiny. Signs of overuse injuries should be monitored, and the training regimen of the young athlete adjusted accordingly (16).

Girls tend to reach puberty approximately 2 years earlier than boys. Puberty in girls occurs as a result of the secretion of pituitary hormones (estrogen) to stimulate the development of the ovaries. Along with the eventual onset of menses, puberty brings developmental changes in the skeleton, breasts, hair follicles, fat, and lean tissue. Sexual maturation stimulates tremendous increases in the rates of growth of various body parts (3). At age 11, a girl is taller and heavier than a boy. At 12 to 15 years of age, a girl may be more mature and physically stronger than a boy; however, during this period the girl may bow to social pressure to do more "feminine" activities and thus may not compete as actively with adolescent boys (7). In puberty, the increasing amount of estrogen accelerates the closing of the growth plates in the bones of girls. Generally, girls complete their growth in height 2 years earlier than boys. When the long bones stop growing at approximately age 18, the average U.S. woman is 5 feet 4.5 inches tall and weighs 123 pounds. Men end up approximately 10% taller because they have approximately 2 years longer to grow (3).

GYNECOLOGIC ISSUES

Menstruation

There has been a great deal of ongoing research in the area of menstrual function and exercise. Just how does menstrual function affect exercise? Conversely, what are the effects of exercise on

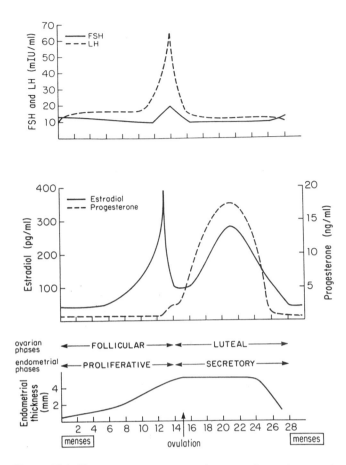

Figure 17.6. Hormone concentrations and patterns during the normal menstrual cycle.

menstrual function? It might be expected that fluctuations in sex hormone levels during the normal menstrual cycle (Fig. 17.6) would influence exercise performance because estrogens and progesterone are known to affect a variety of physiologic factors. In addition, the exercise performance of women who experience premenstrual syndrome and dysmenorrhea might be affected (17). To date, studies investigating these questions are somewhat contradictory. A recent study by Lamont (18) was conducted to determine if energy metabolism varied across the menstrual cycle by examining the response of blood lactate to 60 minutes of exercise at the different phases of the cycle. The author found that blood lactate concentration was not significantly different among the phases of the menstrual cycle when 1 hour of moderate-intensity, steady-state exercise was performed (cycle ergometer), thus indicating that the menstrual cycle has no effect on this index of anaerobic glycolysis during prolonged steady-state exercise (18).

The effects of periodic variation of the menstrual cycle on swimming performance were studied in 20 female team swimmers aged 18 to 22 years. This study found that female swimmers' times for sprint swimming can be affected by their menstrual cycle. The times were usually best on cycle day 8 and worst at the onset of menstruation. Eighteen subjects reported menstrual problems of some type. Fatigue or weakness was most frequent, followed by backache and stomachache. Approximately 50% of subjects reported breast soreness, especially premenstrual. The subjects' views of the effect of menstruation on performance were unrelated to actual performance. Swimming performance was best in the postmenstrual period in this study (19). It is not understood whether the effects are the result of psychological or physiologic factors.

A study by Dibrezzo et al. (20) investigated the effects of three different phases of the menstrual cycle on dynamic strength and work performance of the knee flexors and extensors. Of 21 women aged 18 to 36 tested, no significant differences among the strength variables during the three phases of the menstrual cycle were noted. These data would indicate that the physical capabilities of women are far greater than previously believed. Active women with a normal menstrual cycle should experience no discernible change in strength and work performance as a result of cycle changes (20–22). Many women still have preconceived notions of the negative effect of menstruation on exercise performance. Wells cites several studies in which some athletes had their best performances during menstruation, some had worst performances, and the majority of women had no change in performance (3). World records and Olympic gold medals have been won during menstruation and during all other phases of the menstrual cycle (7).

Consequently, research has presented conflicting views of the effects of menstrual function on exercise performance. It is evident that the performance of some women is affected by their menstrual cycle, and coaches should be aware of this and adjust their competitive schedules accordingly.

Premenstrual Syndrome and Dysmenorrhea

Premenstrual syndrome (PMS) is a symptom complex that includes a variety of physiologic and psychological symptoms occurring 4 to 10 days (mid to late luteal phase) before the onset of the menstrual cycle. As many as 150 physical and psychological symptoms have been attributed to PMS. The most common symptoms are fatigue, headache, abdominal bloating, breast tenderness and swelling, and acne. Anxiety, hostility or anger, and depression occur in more than

94% of women with the syndrome. Many have psychological reactions such as guilt, decreased self-esteem, and shame; many also report notably disturbed family and work lives (23). To confirm a diagnosis of PMS, cycle symptoms must repeat for at least 3 months and only be present 4 to 10 days before menses.

Although many women suffer from PMS, its cause is still unknown. Researchers suspect PMS to be a condition resulting from a disturbance of the neuroendocrinologic system but greatly influenced by psychosocial factors (23–26). PMS is most likely due to the sequential hormonal changes that take place during the menstrual cycle. There may be a link to the ratio of progesterone to estrogen; increased levels of progesterone have been observed in some cases (25). Because the manifestations can vary in severity and because PMS has a tremendous placebo response, it is difficult to evaluate the effectiveness of many types of therapy. Few pharmacologic interventions have been found to be more effective (14) than placebo (26). Nutritional intervention and exercise have been reported to have positive effects on the symptoms of PMS (24–27). Several conservative treatment suggestions for PMS are listed in Table 17.2.

Primary dysmenorrhea refers to the pain associated with uterine contractions or ischemia during menstruation. This problem, commonly referred to as cramps, can manifest as painful cramps causing a dull ache or pressure low in the abdomen. The pain can come and go, remain constant, or be severe enough to cause nausea, vomiting, diarrhea, backache, sweating, and achiness spreading to the hips, lower back, and thighs (28). Almost half of all women suffer from primary dysmenorrhea (29). In 1 in 10 women, dysmenorrhea is painful enough to impair normal function unless medication is taken (28). Primary dysmenorrhea is believed to be caused by prostaglandins (F-series) released by the endometrium (17). These prostaglandins act by causing uterine contractions that may be strong enough to temporarily cut off the blood supply of the uterine muscles,

thus causing pain (28). Secondary dysmenorrhea is pain caused by some type of disease. Endometriosis (major cause of secondary dysmenorrhea), uterine fibroids, adenomyosis, pelvic inflammation or infection, and cervical stenosis are examples of causative disorders (28).

Pharmacologic management of dysmenorrhea uses various antiprostaglandin medications. Oral contraceptive administration is occasionally recommended for the treatment of dysmenorrhea; however, relieving dysmenorrhea should not be the reason for taking birth control pills (28). A recent study by Kokjohn et al. looked at the effects of spinal manipulation on primary dysmenorrhea (29). Perceived pain and blood levels of prostaglandins were monitored in 38 women with dysmenorrhea 15 minutes before treatment and 60 minutes after treatment. Either a sacral manipulation or a "sham" adjustment was administered to the patients. The women who received chiropractic spinal manipulation reported significant reductions in back pain and menstrual distress; blood levels of prostaglandins decreased in both groups (29). This is encouraging information for women who prefer a nonpharmacologic approach to treating their dysmenorrhea.

Many clinicians recommend exercise to alleviate the symptoms of both PMS and dysmenorrhea, although there is limited evidence to support these recommendations. A study by Prior et al. investigated the theory that premenstrual symptoms can be decreased with exercise. Results showed that moderate exercise significantly decreased premenstrual symptoms without significant changes in weight, hormonal, or menstrual cycle (27). Golub et al. prescribed a program of calisthenic exercises for 302 junior high school students and questioned them twice yearly for 3 years about premenstrual and menstrual symptoms and regularity in exercise performance. By the end of the third year, dysmenorrhea had developed in 61% of girls who did not perform the exercises regularly and in 39% of girls who continued to exercise (30).

To summarize, regular exercise may improve the symptoms of PMS and dysmenorrhea in some women. This phenomenon may be related to exercise-induced secretion of endorphins or vasodilating prostaglandins, although more research is needed to determine the mechanism.

Less common uterine bleeding abnormalities such as polymenorrhea (bleeding too frequently), menorrhagia (heavy bleeding at the appropriate time for menstruation), intermenstrual bleeding (bleeding between periods), and premenstrual spotting (spotting on the days immediately pre-

Table 17.2. Conservative Treatment of Premenstrual Syndrome

Nutritional supplements	Eating adequate complex
B6	carbohydrates
Magnesium	Whole grains and polyunsaturated fats
Multivitamin and mineral supplements	Acupuncture and/or homeopathy
Lowering salt intake	Exercise
Moderating caffeine and alcohol intake	

ceding the onset of menstruation) can all adversely affect athletic performance. Demonstration of any of these abnormal bleeding patterns by the female athlete should be evaluated, diagnosed, and treated accordingly (31).

Exercise-Induced Menstrual Dysfunction

As women began to enjoy their new-found exercise freedom, their intensity of exercise and training steadily increased. Soon researchers discovered a direct correlation between women who train heavily and menstrual dysfunction; however, there is inadequate information regarding why some athletes, and not others, become reproductively dysfunctional. Most studies indicated that exercise training does not appear to be the major factor associated with athletic amenorrhea (32). Factors such as stress, poor nutrition, low body fat, weight loss, delayed menarche, and training itself were implicated (Table 17.3) (33).

Myburgh et al. (34) examined prevalence of risk factors and menstrual dysfunction in 618 ultramarathoners. The results of their study indicated that no one risk factor, such as low body fat or training intensity, can accurately predict a runner's predisposition to menstrual dysfunction. This study did reveal that runners with current menstrual dysfunction had more risk factors than their matched control subject counterparts (34). A study by Myerson et al. (35) compared resting metabolic rate and energy balance in amenorrheic and eumenorrheic runners. It is common for endurance athletes to take in too few calories to compensate for their high level of activity. Lower resting metabolic rate (RMR) is associated with caloric deprivation. Cessation of reproductive function may also be an energy-conserving adaptation to inadequate diet. The findings of this study demonstrated a significantly lower RMR in amenorrheic runners compared with eumenorrheic runners and sedentary control subjects. This suggests that reduced resting metabolic rate

Table 17.3.   Proposed Causes of Athletic Amenorrhea

Low body weight or fat	Immature reproductive axis
Absolute weight loss	Young athlete
Critical level, set point	Nulliparity
Late menarche	Prior menstrual irregularities
Training before menarche	Psychological stress
Diet	Multiple factors
Energy drain—caloric deficit	Others?
Hormonal alterations	
Acute hormonal response	
Chronic hormonal response	

From Menstrual dysfunction in the female athlete. In: Sanborn SF, Tietz CC, eds. Scientific foundations of sports medicine. St. Louis: Mosby–Year Book, 1989:122. Reprinted by permission.

and amenorrhea in runners are part of an adaptive syndrome to conserve energy and maintain stable weight in response to the caloric demands of a high-level training program with a low caloric intake (35).

Abnormalities in menstrual function may not be apparent to all athletes. Among normally menstruating athletes, up to one third can be anovulatory whereas another third may have shortened luteal phases (Fig. 17.6). The adverse conditions associated with a shortened luteal phase are infertility, loss of bone density, and increased risk of breast cancer. As the dysfunction increases and less progesterone is produced, the athlete may acquire anovulatory oligomenorrhea. The chronic, unopposed estrogen production can lead to unpredictable and at times heavy bleeding. There is an increased risk of endometrial hyperplasia and possible adenocarcinoma, although this has never been reported in athletic women (36, 37).

Oligomenorrhea and Amenorrhea

Oligomenorrhea (infrequent menses) and amenorrhea (absent menses) are more prevalent in athletic women than in the general population. In athletes, these types of menstrual disorders are found in 10 to 20% of women compared with up to 5% in nonexercising women (36). The prevalence can be as high as 50% in elite runners and professional ballet dancers (37). An athlete with oligomenorrhea usually has 3 to 6 menstrual cycles per year. These women demonstrate lower levels of reproductive hormones. Until recently, oligomenorrhea was considered harmless. Drink-water et al. determined that women with extended periods of oligomenorrhea and/or amenorrhea may suffer from an irreversible decrease of vertebral bone mineral density resulting in an increased risk of stress fractures (12).

Primary amenorrhea refers to women who have never had menstrual bleeding. Secondary amenorrhea occurs in women who have had at least one episode of menstrual bleeding before the absence of their menses (37). The criteria for defining secondary amenorrhea have not been standardized, but a generally accepted definition is anywhere from 3 to 12 months without menses (37). The most common cause of amenorrhea is pregnancy. Other causes could include ovarian failure (menopause), pituitary tumors or abnormalities, or hypothalamic dysfunction (36). Hypothalamic amenorrhea can be caused by excessive weight loss, increased levels of stress, and overexercising. Gonadotropin-releasing hormone (Gn-RH) is produced by the hypothalamus. In hypothalamic amenorrhea, secretion of Gn-RH by the hypothalamus is diminished. GnRH directly affects the luteinizing hormone (LH) and follicle stimulating hormone (FSH) producing cells in the pituitary. Decreased levels of LH and FSH retard follicular growth, resulting in lower levels of estrogen production by the ovaries. Hypothalamic amenorrhea may ensue (6, 37). Exercise-induced amenorrhea is a type of hypothalamic amenorrhea. The cause of this affliction appears to be multifactorial. A profile of a woman with exercise-induced amenorrhea is shown in Table 17.4.

Initially, exercise-induced amenorrhea was thought to be benign and probably reversible. Later, researchers reported findings of low bone density in amenorrheic athletes (38–40). This discovery eventually led to findings of a predisposition to stress fractures in these athletes (41–43). In 1986, Drinkwater et al. (44) investigated the vertebral bone mineral density of amenorrheic athletes after 1 year to determine whether resumption of normal menstrual cycles after an extended period of amenorrhea was sufficient to affect bone mass. The results of this study demonstrated that the athletes who regained menses showed a significant increase in bone density.

Until recently, it was thought that the effects of this secondary amenorrhea were not permanent. In 1990, Drinkwater et al. (12) investigated the long-term effects of athletic amenorrhea on female runners. The results showed that although the bone density did begin to increase after the athletes resumed normal menses, these increases in bone density ceased after approximately 2 years. Other findings from this study demonstrated that athletic women who had never had regular menses showed 17% less vertebral bone density than athletic women whose cycles were regular. These amenorrheic runners had estrogen

Table 17.4. Profile of a Woman with Exercise-Induced Amenorrhea

Adolescent female with primary amenorrhea or adult female with secondary amenorrhea

Competitive long-distance runner, gymnast, and professional ballet dancer at highest risk

Low weight plus loss of weight after training initiates

Low body fat for weight

Decreased % of protein in diet—vegetarian

High incidence of menstrual abnormalities before vigorous training

Associates higher level of stress with training than do athletes with normal menses

May have return of menses during intervals of rest, even without weight gain or change

"Anorectic reaction" is common

More likely to have begun training at an early age

Table 17.5. Diagnostic Evaluation of Amenorrhea

History, including dietary intake

Physical examination, including pelvic examination

Laboratory examination

Pregnancy test—order liberally

TSH—hypothyroidism an infrequent cause

FSH—if greater than 40, repeat once more before the diagnosis of ovarian failure is made

Prolactin—pregnancy, pituitary adenoma, or microadenoma can all elevate prolactin levels

Estrogen level—if consistently less than 50 pg/ml, ERT may be beneficial

Progestin challenge test—useful to assess the amount of endogenous estrogens and the normalcy of the genital outflow tract

levels equivalent to those of postmenopausal women, with the main difference being that the runners showed bone loss in only the vertebrae, whereas women with postmenopausal osteoporosis also have bone loss in the distal radius. Although it is premature to state that this bone density loss is irreversible, it is clear that this is a topic of concern. Further research is ongoing.

These findings pose a dilemma for women. They are told to exercise to prevent osteoporosis; yet they are also told if they exercise too much, they may become amenorrheic and thus hypoestrogenic, predisposing themselves to osteoporosis (45). It seems that the simple solution to this perplexing problem is to exercise in moderation. It is up to the practitioner to monitor carefully those athletes who are having menstrual irregularities secondary to exercise. Women with an increased number of stress fractures should be questioned about their training habits and menstrual function and educated about methods of preventing further problems in this area.

It is common for women to welcome cessation of their menses. To ignore the long-term effects of oligomenorrhea and amenorrhea could be damaging to the athlete and lead to increased risk of injury. Athletic amenorrhea is a diagnosis of exclusion and should only be diagnosed after a full history, physical examination, and laboratory tests (Table 17.5) have eliminated other common causes (Table 17.3) (33). The following management protocol is recommended.

1. Review the goals of the patient.
2. Review diet and exercise pattern.
3. Evaluate for other causes of amenorrhea.
4. Evaluate bone density by bone density measurement if athlete has been amenorrheic for at least 6 months.
5. Counsel, based on the above. If the athlete has had a skeletal injury and her bone density falls 1 standard deviation below normal, then hormone intervention should be

Table 17.6. Contraindications to Estrogen Replacement Therapy

Absolute	Relative
Abnormal liver function	Hypertension
History of thromboembolic or vascular disease	Diabetes mellitus
	Fibrocystic disease of the breast
Breast or endometrial carcinoma	Uterine leiomyomata
Undiagnosed vaginal bleeding	Familial hyperlipidemia
	Migraine headaches
	Gallbladder disease

seriously considered (estrogen therapy or oral contraceptives).

6. Ensure a minimum total calcium intake of 1500 mg daily.
7. Encourage a moderate exercise regimen addressing all components of fitness: cardiovascular endurance, muscular strength, flexibility, and body composition.
8. Follow-up every 6 months or more with repeat evaluations as needed (46).

Treatment of menstrual dysfunction in athletes may vary depending on the needs of the athlete. Many women shy away from estrogen replacement therapy (ERT) because it has been shown to cause endometrial cancer in some women (36). ERT now includes concurrent administration of conjugated estrogen and medroxyprogesterone. This combination is thought to eliminate the risk of endometrial cancer. There are, however, various absolute and relative contraindications to ERT (Table 17.6). If the woman with athletic amenorrhea is sexually active, oral contraceptives are recommended. Many women choose to treat this menstrual disorder conservatively by decreasing their exercise intensity and optimizing their nutritional intake (including 1500 mg of calcium/day).

Iron Loss in the Female Athlete

Iron deficiency is the most common nutritional deficiency in the United States today. Because of menstrual iron loss, women are especially at risk. This deficiency may be accompanied by anemia. The athlete may complain of lassitude, fatigue, and listlessness; however, the onset is typically insidious and often only discovered by a routine blood test. Many female athletes have been shown to have lower serum hemoglobin and iron levels than sedentary individuals (47–52). Proposed theories for the low levels of the iron variables are (1) inadequate dietary intake, (2) low bioavailability of iron, and/or (3) high rates of iron loss (50). As many as 80% of female long-distance runners show iron deficiency (52, 53).

Several explanations have been offered for iron deficiency, including inadequate iron in the diet, low gastrointestinal tract absorption, excessive blood loss from the bowel during exercise, accelerated iron loss through the skin (sweating), red blood cell (RBC) losses through the urine, and RBC fragmentation or trauma-induced hemolysis with hemoglobinuria, particularly in athletes with abnormal RBC membranes (52, 54, 55). Urinary losses and loss via sweating are considered negligible by most authorities (50, 51, 53).

Steenkamp et al. (52) investigated the theory of traumatic RBC fragmentation in marathon runners. They did not find severe mechanical damage in the blood of these runners and concluded that mechanical trauma to the blood is not a likely cause of iron deficiency in most female marathon runners. They suggest that a more likely cause is the nutritional status of women athletes. Other studies confirm this theory (50, 51, 54, 55). Many female athletes have been reported to ingest only 1600 to 2000 kcal/day, which provides approximately 12 mg of iron, well below the Recommended Daily Allowance (RDA) of 18 mg/day (50). In addition, many female athletes are vegetarians or modified vegetarians (no red meat). Meats contain heme iron, which is highly bioavailable and therefore an excellent source of iron. Heme iron also increases the bioavailability of iron from nonheme sources, such as deep green leafy vegetables, whole grain or enriched breads, and legumes (50). Thus, even if vegetarian female athletes consume enough calories (3000 kcal/day recommended), they may not be getting enough iron in their diets to avoid becoming iron deficient. A recent investigation of iron status and diet in athletes by Telford et al. (53) found that the dietary factor that most closely correlated with iron status was the percentage of protein consumed. These data suggest that the proportion, rather than the total amount of protein, in the athlete's diet may be more important in facilitating the absorption of iron. Daily iron supplementation is an effective means for treating female athletes with iron loss, whether or not anemia is present. Without proper nutritional counseling, however, supplementation alone is not sufficient (56).

It is well documented that iron deficiency, when manifested as anemia, generally impairs work capacity, decreases endurance, decreases oxygen delivery, and enhances lactic acid production, hence, adversely affecting performance (57). Yet the effects of nonanemic iron deficiency on athletic performance continue to be controversial. Because the female athlete is often on the

Table 17.7. Prevention of Iron Deficiency Anemia

Increase dietary intake of iron
   Lean red meat, dark meat of poultry
   Leafy green vegetables, grains, nuts
   Iron-fortified cereals
   Cook in iron skillets
   Enhance absorption: vitamin C, animal proteins
   Avoid inhibitors of absorption: tea, coffee, milk, eggs
Iron supplementation (RDA = 18 mg Fe per day)
   Multiple vitamin with iron

brink of anemia, her hemoglobin should be monitored carefully and iron supplements should be prescribed accordingly. Ferrous gluconate taken orally may cause less gastrointestinal distress than ferrous sulfate (36). The athlete should also avoid certain foods (such as tea, cereal grains, and coffee) and drugs (such as antacids, tetracycline, and H2-blockers) because they are often detrimental to iron absorption (54). Table 17.7 lists suggestions for prevention of iron deficiency.

EXERCISE DURING PREGNANCY AND POSTPARTUM

There have been concerns expressed by pregnant women that exercise during pregnancy can lead to miscarriage, premature delivery, or poor fetal outcome. Is it safe to exercise while pregnant? The consensus is that exercise is beneficial to the pregnant woman (58–65). Theoretical benefits of exercise are listed in Table 17.8. Whether it is safe to exercise and how much the pregnant woman should exercise can only be answered on an individual basis. In 1985, the American College of Obstetricians and Gynecologists (ACOG) introduced guidelines for exercise during pregnancy. These guidelines were designed more for the "average" woman, not necessarily for the more active one. Much controversy has surrounded the ACOG recommendations and their conservative nature. A metaanalytic review of the effects of physical exercise on pregnancy outcomes was recently conducted by Lokey et al. (61). They compared groups that complied with the 1985 ACOG guidelines and those that exceeded the guidelines. Results indicated no difference in pregnancy outcomes between the groups, although women performed bouncy, jerky types of movements and exercise heart rates exceeded 140 bpm (61).

Recognizing that these guidelines were not based on any hard clinical data, in 1994 the ACOG issued new guidelines (Table 17.9). These revised guidelines contain recommendations based on extrapolations of the most recent data

regarding exercise and pregnancy. No limit is placed on training heart rate for pregnant women. It is suggested that the rate of perceived exertion be used as the best guide for optimal heart rate level. Ultimately, prescribing an exercise program for a pregnant woman should be done on a individual basis. Encourage these women to listen to their bodies while exercising. During the advanced stages of pregnancy, the ability to exercise will be limited and women will diminish levels of activity accordingly. Professionals should use the ACOG recommendations as a guide to assist them in providing exercise prescriptions to pregnant women. As more research is conducted in this area, the ACOG guidelines will be adjusted accordingly (63). Table 17.10 presents recommendations for and contraindications to exercise during pregnancy.

Postural changes occur during pregnancy because of weight gain distributed primarily in the breasts and abdomen, and laxity in ligamentous and connective tissue caused by hormonal changes. These changes are not necessarily pathologic, yet they may lead to loss of balance and acute or chronic lower back and sacroiliac

Table 17.8. Benefits of Exercise during Pregnancy

To the fetus
   Shorter/easier labor
   Decreased body fat
To the mother
   Avoidance of excessive weight
   Maintenance of fitness and muscle tone
   Improvement of self-image and sense of well-being
   Improved appearance and posture
   Less backache, less water retention
   Increased energy
   Better labor outcome
   Shorter postpartum recovery

Table 17.9. Recommendations for Exercise During Pregnancy and Postpartum: ACOG Guidelines (Revised February 1994)

Regular exercise 3 times a week
Avoid supine exercise after first trimester
Modify exercise intensity according to maternal symptoms (RPE)
Non–weight-bearing exercise recommended to minimize injury
Avoid balancing-type exercises or contact sports
Increase caloric consumption, additional 300 kcal/d
Hydrate adequately
Resume postpartum exercise 4–6 weeks after birth or as soon as woman is physically capable
No exercise if any contraindications are present or consult physician

From American College of Obstetricians and Gynecologists. Exercise during pregnancy and the postpartum period. Washington, DC: ACOG Technical Bulletin no. 189, 1994. Reprinted by permission.

Table 17.10. Contraindications to Exercise in Pregnancy

Absolute contraindications
- Active myocardial disease
- Congestive heart failure
- Rheumatic heart disease (class II and above)
- Thrombophlebitis
- Recent pulmonary embolism
- Acute infectious disease
- At risk for premature labor, incompetent cervix, multiple gestations
- Uterine bleeding, ruptured membranes
- Intrauterine growth retardation or macrosomia
- Severe isoimmunization
- Severe hypertensive disease
- No prenatal care
- Suspected fetal distress

Relative contraindications*
- Essential hypertension
- Anemia or other blood disorders
- Thyroid disease
- Diabetes mellitus
- Breech presentations in the last trimester
- Excessive obesity or extreme underweight
- History of sedentary lifestyle

From Exercise during pregnancy. In: Strauss R, ed. Sports medicine. Philadelphia: WB Saunders, 1991:513. Reprinted by permission.
*Patients may be engaged in medically supervised exercise programs.

pain syndromes. The three most common postural changes that occur with pregnancy that may lead to chronic pain are (1) increased lordosis in the cervical and lumbar region, (2) protraction of the shoulder girdle, and (3) hyperextension of the knees (58). By understanding the biomechanical abnormalities that are common in pregnancy, the practitioner can design an exercise program to strengthen these vulnerable areas (especially trunk, abdomen, and back), with the ultimate goal of preventing some of the common musculoskeletal problems of pregnancy.

Pregnant women need a safe, efficient, and productive means of improving or maintaining muscular and cardiovascular strength and endurance throughout gestation. This will allow their bodies to meet the progressive physical demands of pregnancy in a more comfortable manner. Not only will exercise during pregnancy provide the mother with a feeling of well-being psychologically and physiologically, it has been found to minimize the discomfort of labor and delivery without risk to the fetus (59). It is recommended that each woman check with her obstetrician to be sure that she does not have a high-risk pregnancy. If she has been exercising at a particular level before pregnancy and is not at risk for problems during pregnancy, she should be able to continue that activity throughout the pregnancy.

After the birth of a child, many women are eager to return to their previous activity level and regain their prepregnancy condition. Weight loss typically is the prime motivation for an early return to exercise. It is thought that many different types of stress, including excessive activity, can disrupt a woman's ability to breast feed successfully, especially in the first 4 to 6 weeks. The results of studies indicate that moderate aerobic exercise has little effect on the quantity of mothers' milk or on infant growth (66). Recent research indicates that the quality of milk is adversely affected by exercise (65). Postexercise breast milk contains more lactic acid, a by-product of exercise. Even after less strenuous workouts, lactic acid in some women's breast milk increases by 200%. Babies rejected this milk although they had not been fed for 2 to 3 hours (65). It is recommended that women who breast feed either nurse before exercising or collect milk for later feedings before exercising. Women should also be sure to maintain adequate caloric and fluid intake to meet the higher energy demands needed for breast feeding while exercising.

Some physicians recommend a recovery period of at least 2 weeks after childbirth, whereas others say it is safe to resume exercise as soon as the mother feels ready. After cesarean section, 6 to 10 weeks are recommended before return to exercise (67). Walking is probably the best early exercise choice; however, other exercises from aerobic dance to long-distance running are acceptable, provided the mother feels up to it and is careful to avoid excessive fatigue. Not only can moderate exercise boost energy levels and reduce fatigue in nursing mothers, it can also help many women to avoid postpartum depression. The absence of physical activity can contribute to depressed moods, hence accentuating depression. Overall, one can conclude that the sooner a woman can return to exercise after delivery, the better she is going to feel (67).

Exercise in Postmenopausal Women

Regular physical exercise for postmenopausal women can reduce their risk of developing several medical illnesses, including osteoporosis, cardiovascular disease, obesity, and depression. Regular exercise can also benefit flexibility, coordination, mood, and alertness. A carefully structured, physician-guided program can offset structural and functional losses that accompany aging (68). Table 17.11 shows the functional adaptations to exercise from which elderly women benefit (69).

Menopause usually occurs around age 51, but can happen between ages 38 and 55. At this time, the ovaries gradually stop producing estrogen. In the early stages of menopause, a woman may begin to experience changes in her menstrual cycle (longer, shorter, heavier, or lighter). She may have such symptoms as hot flashes, night sweats, vaginal dryness, menstrual spotting, urine leakage, insomnia, headaches, depression, and irritability (70). Menopause officially begins when a woman goes for 1 year without a period. At menopause ovarian function ceases, and women are at a greater risk of becoming osteoporotic. Osteoporosis is characterized by a decreased bone mineral content, increased porosity of bone, and decreased resistance to fracture. Various risk factors (Table 17.12) are helpful in identifying women who are more vulnerable to osteoporosis (70). Osteoporosis affects 15 to 20 million persons per year in the United States, producing 1.3 billion fractures per year (45). One third of U.S. women older than 65 will have a spinal fracture, and approximately 15% will fracture a hip. Most fractures in the elderly occur as result of falls. At a cost of approximately $10 billion annually, osteoporosis can have a devastating effect on the public health system. Although the case for treatment seems straightforward, researchers are still exploring how best to combine the following therapies to prevent osteoporosis.

ERT is the most effective means of preventing osteoporosis today (45, 56, 69–71). Studies have shown that ERT combined with exercise helped women gain bone mass, outperforming the effects of calcium supplementation and exercise (71). ERT has also been proven to decrease the risk of coronary artery disease, congestive heart failure, arterosclerotic cardiovascular disease, and hypertension (70). Before the current practice of estrogen administration with progesterone, there was an increased risk of endometrial cancer with ERT. With this worry eliminated, there is new focus on the increased risk of breast cancer with long-term ERT (58, 70). This is a controversial topic, and more research is needed to either confirm or dispel these fears. Consequently, a physician may instruct a menopausal women to undergo ERT to prevent osteoporosis, yet she may shy away from this therapy for fear of cancer. In addition, many women do not like the idea of returning to monthly menstruation and the necessity of obtaining a yearly endometrial biopsy, which are other possible aspects of ERT (45). Most experts agree that ERT begun early in menopause retards the process of osteoporosis, although estrogen alone is not the answer. Dietary intake of calcium and a regular exercise program are also recommended.

Conservative preventive measures for osteoporosis in postmenopausal women currently consist of 1000 to 1500 mg/day intake of dietary calcium along with individualized exercise programs. A recent study compared bone mineral content (BMC) of weight-lifting resistance exercise (body builders) and nonresistance endurance exercise (runners and swimmers) and inactive nonathletes. They found that the BMC of the body builders was greater than the runners, swimmers, and nonathletes. The swimmers had greater bone mineral density than runners and controls, although the differences were not significant (72).

Weight-bearing exercise is the most common type of exercise recommended for postmenopausal women. Exercise not only increases bone mineral density, but also enhances strength and balance, thus reducing the risk of falls and fracture (69). Until more research is conducted in this area, it is suggested that a combination of weight-bearing exercise and weight-lifting resistance exercise (preferably free weights) should be encouraged in the postmenopausal woman. The optimal type, intensity, frequency, and duration of exercise have not been established (45). It is suggested that women obtain bone density measurements beginning at age 40 as a baseline, and then 1 year after menopause and at 2-year intervals thereafter (70).

Table 17.11. Functional Adaptations to Exercise in Elderly Women*

Cardiovascular	Miscellaneous
↑ Work capacity	↑ Mental outlook (mood, self-esteem)
↓ Resting heart rate	
↓ Total cholesterol	↑ Socialization, reduced loneliness
↑ HDL cholesterol	↓ Idle time
↓ Blood pressure	↓ Anxiety
↑ Maximum oxygen consumption	↓ Symptoms of depression
Respiratory	↑ Fat and carbohydrate metabolism
↑ Minute ventilation	
↑ Vital capacity	↑ Insulin receptor sensitivity
Musculoskeletal	↑ Fibrinolysis
↑ Bone density	↑ Plasma volume
↑ Flexibility	↑ Weight control
↑ Range of motion	↑ Metabolic rate
↑ Muscle tone and strength	↓ Appetite
↑ Coordination	Maintenance of lean body mass

From Barry HC, Rich BSE, Carlson RT. How exercise can benefit older patients. Phys Sportsmed 1993;21:124–140. Reprinted by permission of McGraw-Hill.
*These effects are not unique to the frail elderly. Some are seen only with vigorous exercise.

Table 17.12. Risk Factors for Osteoporosis

Calcium intake	Bilateral oophorectomy (before age 50)
Caffeine consumption	
Dietary phosphorus (sodas, pop)	Heavy alcohol use
Smoking	Corticosteroid use
Age of natural menopause	Sedentary lifestyle
Postmenopausal estrogen use	Family history

DRUG USE AMONG FEMALE ATHLETES

Steroid Use

With increasing pressure to "go for the gold," women are falling into the same kind of win-at-all-cost traps that bedevil men's sports. It is common to see the side effects of anabolic steroid use in women in such sports as body building, weight lifting, track and field, cycling, and swimming. The use of anabolic steroids is not so common with women as it is with men; however, not much research has been done on the prevalence of steroid use in female athletes. A study of adolescent high school students found that 3% (27 of 901) used anabolic steroids—5% (23 of 462) of all males and 1.4% (6 of 439) of all females admitted to steroid use (73). In the few other studies that have looked at anabolic steroid use by women, incidence ranged from 0.005 to 1% in high schools (male usage is 6.6%), to 1% in college, to 3 to 5% in elite and professional women athletes (74).

Underreporting by athletes is often a problem in assessing the accuracy of the prevalence of steroid use. Yesalis et al. (75) conducted a study of NCAA division I athletes asked to estimate the level of their competitors' steroid use. The mean overall projected rate of use of anabolic steroids across all sports surveyed was 14.7% for male and 5.9% for female athletes. In women's sports, the greatest projected use was among track and field athletes (16.3%). These results may be overestimates of actual steroid use among athletes. True percentages probably lie somewhere between these percentages and self-reported figures.

Athletes use steroids because they expect to increase their muscle mass and strength and enhance their overall performance. The performance-enhancing effects of steroids are somewhat controversial (see Chapter 24). In humans, increases in muscular strength while using steroids have been demonstrated in approximately half of controlled investigations (76–79). The level of testosterone seems to be most responsible for increases in strength. There is probably a greater opportunity for women than for men to increase muscle mass while using steroids because of their lower levels of natural circulating testosterone.

Steroids often have an extreme virilizing effect on women who take them. Women may have hair growth on the upper lip, chin, and cheeks; baldness; deepening of the voice; shrinkage of breast size; enlargement of the clitoris; uterine atrophy; and irregularity or cessation of the menstrual cycle. In addition, some of these side effects may be irreversible, even after cessation of use, in-

Table 17.13.   Side Effects of Steroids

Facial hair	Decreased sexual drive
Baldness	Irreversible
Deepening of voice	Facial hair growth and baldness
Shrinkage of breast size	Enlargement of clitoris
Enlargement of clitoris	Deepening of voice
Irregular menstrual cycle	Long-term effects (possible)
Amenorrhea	Abnormal liver and heart
Acne/skin rash	function
Irritability/aggressiveness	Hepatocellular carcinoma
Depression	Peliosis hepatitis

cluding baldness, growth of facial hair, enlargement of the clitoris, and deepening of the voice (Table 17.13). Many other findings concerning long-term effects of steroid use are inconclusive at this time, but it has been found that prolonged use in high doses can lead to decreases in high-density lipoprotein (HDL) cholesterol, hepatocellular carcinoma, and peliosis hepatitis (77). It has been suggested that they also have adverse effects on reproductive function (73, 76–79).

It is clear that women have been ill-informed about the risks of anabolic steroid use. Individual response to these drugs varies greatly, and the androgenic-anabolic effects are different with each compound. Women can be misled by other users who experience no or few masculinizing side effects (74).

The best way to stop steroid use is through education and drug testing (76). However, detection through drug testing is becoming more difficult as new methods are being discovered to mask the use of steroids. This is especially true in women because they get good results by using shorter courses and lower doses of steroids than men. These abbreviated and lower dosing schedule during training may make detection harder and masking easier during precompetition testing (74).

Oral Contraceptive Use

Oral contraceptives are a common form of birth control for many female athletes. It is thought that the pill hampers peak athletic performance, although findings are inconclusive at this time. In the past, side effects of the pill included weight gain, nausea, fatigue, and headaches. The increased risks of thromboembolic disease, hypertension, and altered glucose and lipid metabolism associated with oral contraceptive use were more significant concerns. These side effects were associated with the original, higher dose oral contraceptive formulations rather than with today's biphasic or triphasic pills. Today's oral contraceptives can reduce the amount of bleeding, risk of iron deficiency, and frequency of cramps, thus possibly helping to improve athletic performance (66). The pill also allows elite athletes to manipulate their menstrual cycles around competitive events. For many women, oral contraceptives also offer protection against the risks of endometrial hyperplasia and bone loss associated with oligomenorrhea and amenorrhea, which may result from intense exercise, weight loss, or both.

The effect of oral contraceptives on athletic performance is not yet clear (7). However, the added weight gain has been found to affect performance adversely in some athletes. A recent study on whether the use of oral contraceptives influenced the rate of injury during any part of the menstrual cycle found that women taking the pill seemed to have a lower injury rate than women not taking the pill (80). Until more studies have been done in this area, caution is advised in prescribing the contraceptive pill for prevention of injuries. Today's oral contraceptives are not only a convenient form of birth control; they are also safer than earlier forms of the pill and do offer some relief for those women who are vulnerable to the dangers of menstrual dysfunction (81).

ATHLETIC INJURIES SPECIFIC TO WOMEN

Pelvic Injuries

In the early stages of women's sports participation, fear arose that more strenuous activity, as in contact sports, might predispose women to injure their reproductive organs. Contrary to these misconceptions, pelvic injuries are rare. Pelvic contusions occur only occasionally and are usually just surface bruises not affecting the internal structures of the ovaries, vagina, or uterus. The reproductive organs of women are extremely well protected by bony, ligamentous, and muscular structures, especially compared with those of men (3). As a result of some reports in the literature of laceration injuries to the vagina by "forceful vaginal douches" in waterskiing and jet skiing, it is recommended that women participating in these sports wear reinforced neoprene rubber pants or a pant girdle (7, 82). A rare case of perforation of a uterus by an intrauterine device (IUD) after a blow to the pelvis was cited by Haycock and Gillette (1976) (83). Based on present research, one can conclude that injuries to the reproductive organs of female athletes are unlikely.

Exercise-related incontinence is an inconvenience suffered by some female athletes. In a study performed at the University of Michigan Medical Center, 108 of 326 women surveyed reported some bladder leakage during exercise. Running and high-impact aerobics are the two forms of exercise most likely to cause people to leak. Many women use sanitary napkins or participate in less jarring exercise to remedy the problem of incontinence. This problem can be treated by strengthening the muscles of the pelvic floor. Two methods are commonly recommended to build up those muscles: Kegel exercises and new devices called vaginal weights. Kegel exercises strengthen the perivaginal muscles through repetitions of contractions and relaxations. Vaginal weights are inserted like tampons, and women wear them between 20 and 30 minutes a day. As gravity pulls out the weight, the muscles contract and push the weight back in (84). Many women with this problem are embarrassed to consult a physician, so it is recommended that health-care providers routinely question their patients about urinary control problems.

Breast Injuries

Injuries to the breast are very rare in sports today. Problems of the breast secondary to excessive motion or improper protective wear, particularly sports bras, are more common. Jogger's nipple results from prolonged rubbing of the nipple against the bra or shirt. This problem is most common in running sports and is not unique to women. To protect nipples from becoming raw or from bleeding, most athletes can wear a well-designed sports bra or cover the nipple with an adhesive bandage before sporting activity (36, 85). Bicyclist's nipple is an unusual condition caused not by friction, but by exposure to cold. Cold weather and perspiration result in the combination of evaporation and wind chill to lower the temperature, causing cold and painful nipples. To prevent this problem, the cyclist should wear layers of clothing and wind-breaking jackets. Haycock (85) states that significant injuries to the breasts can occur among female athletes who participate in contact and racket sports. Trauma to the breasts usually results in contusions, lacerations, and hematomas, most of which are not serious (85). Applying ice and direct pressure to the injured area if bleeding is present can minimize damage to the tissue. There is no evidence that trauma to the breast causes cancer (36).

Breast soreness secondary to excessive movement can usually be prevented by wearing the proper sports bra. Studies of breast motion while running show that the breasts not only move up and down but also move in a circular motion. This causes excessive strain on the supportive ligaments of the breasts (Cooper's ligaments), resulting in discomfort during and/or after exercise. A study of selected sports bras was performed by Lorentzen and Lawson (86). They concluded that the woman who is large breasted should use a more rigidly constructed bra, whereas the small-breasted woman may use a more elastic bra. Other important factors when selecting a sports bra include the type of sport, fabric preferences and sensitivities, protection needs, and quality of design and construction (86). A supportive sports bra may provide relief in exercising women who experience discomfort from premenstrual breast tenderness and fibrocystic changes (36).

It is recommended that all women practice monthly breast self-examination. In addition, mammography is useful in early detection of breast cancer. Baseline mammography is suggested between ages 35 and 40, every 1 to 2 years between ages 40 and 49, and annually thereafter.

The Question of Knee Injury Predisposition in Women

The knee is one of the most frequently injured body parts in athletics, especially in contact sports. This has been found to be true in both men and women, although the injury rate for knees appears to be greater for women (36). Initially, it was believed that women were more predisposed to knee injuries because of biomechanical variances created by a wider pelvis. It is now evident that the injuries noted in earlier studies that showed a higher prevalence of injuries in women were due to the lack of adequate conditioning (36). As a result

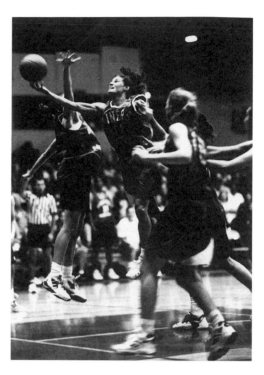

Figure 17.8. Jennifer Azzi, Member of the 1996 Olympic basketball team. (Courtesy of Kim Larson.)

of their wider pelvis, women have a greater Q angle (12°–15° versus 8°–12° in men), causing the kneecap to slide laterally when the leg is flexed.

The Q angle measures the relationship between a line drawn down the femur following the quadriceps pull and another line drawn up the tibia from the tibial tuberosity. The two lines intersect at the midpatellar region (Fig. 17.4) (6). Because the patella serves as a fulcrum for increasing the leverage of the quadriceps on the tibia, the patellofemoral joint is subjected to enormous pressure approaching several times the body weight. The vastus medialis obliquus (VMO) muscle acts to evenly distribute the loads across the patella (Fig. 17.7). Some theorize that in women the VMO is inherently weaker, which again leads to lateral tracking of the patella and hence a higher prevalence of patellofemoral tracking problems, chondromalacia patella, and patellar subluxation (87–89).

Messier et al. (90) studied etiologic factors associated with patellofemoral pain in runners. Q angle was found to be a strong discriminator between the injured and noninjured groups. Based on their results, it is suggested that Q angles in excess of 16° may be significantly associated with patellofemoral pain in male or female runners (90). Some common methods used in the prevention and treatment of patellofemoral injuries include strengthening of the quadriceps muscula-

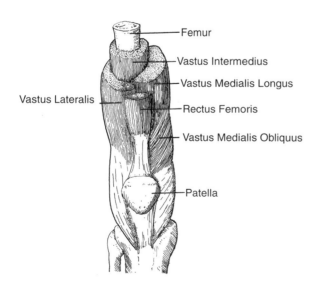

Femur

Vastus Intermedius

Vastus Medialis Longus

Vastus Lateralis

Rectus Femoris

Vastus Medialis Obliquus

Patella

Figure 17.7. The quadriceps muscles (note course of the VMO).

ture, especially the VMO; fitting the patient with orthotics if there is subtalar instability and pronation; and correcting biomechanical joint dysfunction at the knee, ankle, and hip (91).

Recent data collected by the NCAA Injury Surveillance System (ISS) has shown an increased rate of injury to the anterior cruciate ligament (ACL) in women compared with men, especially in basketball (Fig. 17.8). Theories of why this type of injury is more prevalent point toward both intrinsic (ligament size, ligament laxity, limb alignment) and extrinsic (level of skill, experience, shoe/floor interface) factors (92). Because of the serious nature of ACL injuries, further research in this area is indicated. Prevention is generally the best treatment of the majority of knee injuries suffered by female athletes. Adequate preseason conditioning and maintenance programs that continue throughout the season need to be implemented and followed.

Foot Injuries in Women

Woman inherently seem to have a greater risk for bunions than men based on the anatomy of their feet and on genetics (87). Bunions have plagued women for years; some relate their cause to heredity; others claim that wearing high-heeled or "pump" shoes is the causative factor. Hyperpronation creates altered joint biomechanics resulting in excessive medial weight-bearing and hence increased stress at the great toe, possibly causing the bunion. A bunion (hallux valgus abductus) is described as instability of the first metatarsophalangeal joint with concurrent deviation of the great toe. It is characterized by pain over the first metatarsal head, and there may be some pain with range of motion of the first toe (2).

Conservative treatment of bunions begins with correcting the altered biomechanics of the foot, usually by the use of an orthotic device. Strengthening the intrinsic foot musculature, wearing wider shoes, and using protective pads to reduce pressure on the painful toe are often helpful in diminishing bunion symptoms (36, 87). Surgery is a common procedure for treatment of painful bunions (2).

COMMON TYPES OF INJURIES IN THE EXERCISING FEMALE

Overuse Syndromes

Overuse syndromes are described as repetitive forces on a structure beyond the abilities of that specific structure to withstand such a force. These types of injuries usually take the form of stress fractures or inflammatory processes such as tendinitis or bursitis (3). Overuse injuries are usually caused by doing "too much, too soon," and the "culprits" in most cases are training errors. Stress fractures appear to be more common in the female athlete, predominantly in the lower extremity. A study by the U.S. Army of women in the military found this to be true. In the 1980 basic training class, 10 men and 9 women had 19 stress fractures, representing an incidence of 1% for men and 10% for women (93). Training changes were made that resulted in fewer stress fractures in the class of 1990. In the past 3 years, these researchers found that 5.1% of the men and 10.5% of the women sustained a stress injury of the lower leg during the first summer of training (93). They, along with others, concluded that women were more prone to stress injuries because of their lower level of previous athletic activity and lack of appropriate conditioning, along with their competitive nature when competing with more fit counterparts (7, 93).

The amenorrheic athlete has also been shown to have an increased incidence of stress fractures. Osteoporosis with decreased bone mineral density can ensue in these athletes, making it difficult for the bones to withstand the stress of training. Dietary and training changes need to be recommended for these high-risk athletes (94).

Tendinitis is another common overuse problem. It is characterized as an inflammation to the musculotendinous unit as a result of overuse. As in stress fractures, inadequate training plus muscle weakness can cause tendinitis. This problem can be an early precursor to a stress fracture, as illustrated in the medial tibial stress syndrome. Posterior tibialis tendinitis can lead to periostitis (medial shin splint), which over time may result in a tibial stress fracture. An appropriate strength and flexibility program along with a slower progression into activity can help to reduce the incidence of this type of injury.

Sport-Specific Injuries

CONTACT SPORTS

"The Committee on the Medical Aspects of Sports maintains that it is very unlikely that girls competing in contact sports will sustain more injuries than boys engaged in similar activities. It is even conceivable that girls may suffer fewer injuries because of their lesser muscle mass in relation to body size which means that they cannot generate the same momentum and potential trauma forces on body contact" (3).

A recent study by Havkins (95) on head, neck, face, and shoulder injuries in female and male

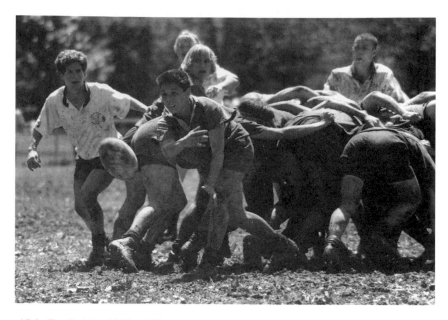

Figure 17.9. The Berkeley All Blues, Women's National Rugby Champions 1994. (Courtesy of Debra Dennis.)

rugby players found that the numbers of injuries among women and men did not differ significantly (Fig. 17.9). Men had more face and shoulder injuries than women, but women had more head and neck injuries. There was a significant difference in the severity of injuries between men and women; 83% of women's injuries were minor and 7.8% were major, whereas 55% of men's injuries were minor and 13.7% were major. The remaining percentages were moderate injuries. The greater incidence of neck injuries in women may be related to inadequate upper body strength and inexperience with collision sports (95). This study confirms the preceding prediction by the Committee on the Medical Aspects of Sports. It also illustrates that gender differences in injuries can be expected in women as they begin to participate in contact sports. This margin of difference is expected to narrow as women become more skilled.

There is much concern about the safety of coed competition in contact sports such as football. Title IX has made it possible for girls and women to take part in male-dominated sports that are not offered to them by federally funded schools. Are women therefore at an increased risk for injury because of differences in strength, size, and speed? H.B. Falls, a professor of biomedical sciences at Southwest Missouri State University, has discussed the hazards and implications of women's participation in coed football. He holds that women and girls are at a greater risk for injury owing to anatomical, strength, and conditioning differences (88). It seems clear that more studies should investigate this topic to substantiate or refute Falls' assumptions.

NONCONTACT SPORTS

Running

The majority of injuries that occur in running are caused by repetitive trauma. Training errors appear to be the major cause of these overuse injuries. Excessive mileage, intense workouts, rapid changes in training routines, or running on hills or on hard surfaces is responsible in most cases, although other extrinsic and some anatomical factors are often implicated (2, 3, 7). Some of the more common overuse injuries are illustrated in Table 17.14. Injuries are common in both sexes, although it appears that women may have an overall greater incidence of injury. Injury patterns are similar, but women appear to have a higher incidence of stress fractures and shin splints and a lower incidence of certain types of tendinitis. Studies have found knee injuries to be the most common, followed by those of the lower leg (3).

Aerobic Dance

Participation in aerobic dance as a form of cardiovascular fitness has grown in popularity since the 1970s. Although both men and women are active in the various types of aerobic dance (e.g., high-impact, low-impact, step, boxing), female participation is greater. As in running, most aerobic dance injuries are the result of overuse. The lower leg and foot are the most common injury sites. A recent study by Mutoh et al. found instructors to be injured at a rate of 72.4% (of 161 instructors) compared with students at 22.8% (of 800 students) during a 5-year period (96). In the past, many of the lower extremity injuries in aerobic dance were attributed to improper footwear. Recent technology in the development of improved aerobic shoes has helped to diminish this as a major problem. Moderating the frequency and duration of participation, along with a more individualized strengthening program, will help reduce the number of injuries that occur in aerobics.

Ballet Dance Injuries

Ballet is probably one of the most physically demanding of all sports. Most dancers begin participation at a very young age, and they practice for several hours a day, 6 to 7 days a week. Ballet requires very high levels of strength, flexibility, speed, coordination, agility, and balance (3). It is not surprising that most injuries are due to overuse, primarily of the ankle, foot, and knee. Back injuries are also common (97). Scoliotic curvature of the spine is more common in ballet dancers than in the general population. A study by Hamilton et al. on musculoskeletal characteristics of elite professional ballet dancers found an incidence of scoliosis in 50% of the study group compared with 3.9% in the general population (98). Ballet shoes have no cushioning, no shock-absorbing material, and no room for orthotics. Dance floors are often wood overlying concrete, which offers little cushioning for the frequent jumps and leaps required. The most common complaint of ballet dancers is plantar fascial strain (3). This is not surprising considering the forces absorbed by the foot during this activity. Along with inadequate floor surfaces and shoes, faulty technique is also a common cause of dance injuries (85).

Turnout or external hip rotation is necessary for all dance positions. Excessive turnout that maximally stresses the hip joint can often lead to injuries, not only of the hip, but also to the knee and foot. The plié is often implicated in knee injuries. This is performed by the dancer planting her feet in the turnout position with the knees bent and then straightening the legs by using the floor as a lever (Fig. 17.10). The plié has a rotational effect on the knee and places great strain

Table 17.14.   Incidence of the 10 Most Common Overuse Injuries in Runners

Injury	Men		Women		Total	
	%	No.	%	No.	%	No.
Patellofemoral pain syndrome	24.3	262	27.9	206	25.8	468
Tibial stress syndrome	10.7	115	16.8	124	13.2	239
Achilles peritendinitis	7.9	85	3.2	24	6.0	109
Plantar fasciitis	5.3	57	3.9	28	4.7	85
Patellar tendinitis	5.6	60	2.8	21	4.5	81
Iliotibial band friction syndrome	4.6	50	3.8	28	4.3	78
Metatarsal stress syndrome	3.3	36	3.0	22	3.2	58
Tibial stress fracture	2.4	26	2.8	21	2.6	47
Tibialis posterior tendinitis	1.9	21	3.2	24	2.5	45
Peroneal tendinitis	2.0	22	1.6	12	1.9	34
Total	68.0	734	69.0	510	68.7	1244

Clement DB, Taunton JE, Smart GW, et al. A survey of overuse running injuries. Phys Sportsmed 1981;9:50. Reprinted with permission of *The Physician and Sportsmedicine*, a McGraw-Hill publication.

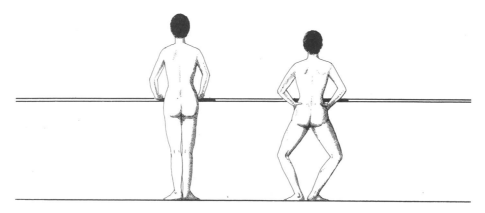

Figure 17.10. Plié.

on the supportive ligaments and muscles of the knee (97). In Hamilton's study, total injuries and overuse syndromes were more common in women with less turnout and less plié (98).

Most dancers are obsessive about weight and often have eating disorders. Decreased body fat and increased levels of activity may lead to cessation of the menstrual cycle with resultant loss of bone density. Stress fractures are common in ballet dancers not only because of athletic amenorrhea, but because of decreased shock absorption of the performing surface. If athletic amenorrhea is suspected, it is recommended that instructors, coaches, athletic trainers, and physicians educate at-risk athletes on proper nutrition and weight control techniques (99).

It has been suggested that ballet dancers should participate in strengthening programs to help prevent injuries. Most ballet dancers do not engage in training activities outside daily technique class and rehearsal. Many dancers believe that strength and conditioning programs may cause them to develop bulky muscles resulting in loss of range of motion and flexibility, which are essential in ballet. Stalder et al. (100) investigated the effects of supplemental weight training for ballet dancers. Seven female dancers participated in progressive weight training and stretching for 9 weeks. Results of this study showed that the dancers had increased functional leg strength, endurance, and anaerobic power with no detriment to the artistic or physical requirements of ballet. Therefore, specific weight training exercises for ballet dancers will improve, not harm, a dancer's performance and prevent injury.

Gymnastic Injuries

Most studies comparing injury rates in men and women have demonstrated few gender-related difference in rates of injury (2). Doctors at Ohio State University prospectively studied eight matched men's and women's intercollegiate varsity sports teams for 1 academic year to determine the incidence of athletic injury and disability (101). Men and women were injured at comparable rates, 42% versus 39%, except for gymnastics. Women gymnasts incurred 0.82 injury per 100 person-hours of exposure, compared with 0.21 injury for men (99). The authors suggest that the increased injury rate among women gymnasts is a consequence of the different types of events and apparatus, rather than of gender. Male gymnasts use predominately upper body musculature, whereas women use primarily lower body musculature (102). In a study by Lowry and Leveau, it was concluded that the level of competition seems to be the most important factor related to the rate of injury in women's gymnastics, meaning that the higher the level of competition, the greater the chance of injury (103).

As in ballet dance, female gymnasts begin training at young ages (5 to 6 years) and training is vigorous (5 to 6 hours/day, 5 to 6 days/week) (102). Injury rate and the severity of injury for gymnasts are nearly as high as those with football players and wrestlers (104). According to Garrick and Requa, sprains and strains are the most common types of injuries in women's gymnastics. They found that ankle sprains were the most common of all traumatic or overuse injuries, and the floor exercise was the event that had the highest incidence of injuries (105). Other studies have found that the highest incidence of injuries occurs in the lower extremity, followed by those in the upper extremity and trunk (102, 104).

Chronic overuse injuries of the spine have been a significant problem in gymnastics. Typically it is the chronic, repetitive flexion, rotation, and extension of the spine that causes spinal injury (106). Common problems include damage to the pars interarticularis with resultant spondylolysis and spondylolisthesis, discogenic pathology, and vertebral end plate abnormalities (106).

Gymnastics is somewhat unique because the most competitive age for girls is usually younger than 20 years. Growth plate injuries are common, especially to the wrist (104). In addition, because strong value is placed on a thin and lean appearance, eating disorders are prevalent. Many of these athletes experience menstrual dysfunction (oligomenorrhea and amenorrhea) with resultant decreased bone mineral density and increased risk for stress fractures (7). Injury prevention in women's gymnastics begins with an appropriate preseason conditioning program. Coaches can be instrumental in decreasing the high incidence of injury in this sport by implementing the following.

1. Avoid premature attempts at new skills.
2. Avoid overloading the wrists at an early age.
3. Use cyclical progressive training.
4. Alternate swinging and support events in workout.
5. Use supportive bracing and/or taping of wrists and ankles.
6. Have athletes undergo a preparticipation physical to determine vulnerable areas for injury (102).

PREVENTION OF ATHLETIC INJURIES IN FEMALES

Stretching

Stretching has been advocated as one of the most important tools in the prevention of athletic injury. Part of every complete training program should include a well-rounded stretching program. Levine et al. (107) analyzed the individual stretching programs of intercollegiate athletes and found that overall, women stretched significantly more than men, although men have tighter muscles than women. Nearly all athletes sampled participated in some kind of stretching program. Only 39% of athletes stretched daily, and only 33% stretched both before and after exercise. Men tend to stretch only before activity. The authors concluded that women athletes tended to be more attentive and balanced in their programs than men, suggesting the probability of decreased injury risk (107). Further studies would be helpful to determine the incidence of injury in relation to increased flexibility via stretching.

Proper Equipment

Use of proper equipment can be helpful in preventing sports injuries. Protective gear such as chest protectors in ice hockey, neoprene wetsuits in waterskiing, and specialized sports bras are important in the avoidance of specific injuries to women (108). Women can be injured by using equipment designed for men. Only recently have

manufacturers started producing bicycles designed to accommodate women. In 1985, a new line of high-quality bicycles was designed for women, who have proportionately shorter torsos than men of the same height (109)). This bike has a smaller, 24-inch front wheel paired with the standard 27-inch wheel in the rear. As a result, it has a shorter top tube, so that riders with shorter torsos can reach the handlebars without straining their backs. Nautilus has its own line of isotonic exercise equipment for women. Although many of its general machines are adjustable, some women are just too small to fit properly and may risk injury working out on these machines (36). As technology in the area of equipment design grows, the injury rate related to equipment should begin to decrease.

Currently, girls and women do not seem to have a higher prevalence of sports-related injuries than do boys or men. It appears that types of injuries do vary with the sexes (Fig. 17.11) (101). With improved conditioning and coaching techniques, one can surmise that the incidence of athletic injuries in the female athlete will decrease even more. With increasing social acceptance, girls are beginning sports participation at an earlier age. This will be helpful in developing enhanced skill and technique in their sport and, one hopes, in preventing injuries. Research is providing us with more accurate information concerning types of injury, prevalence of injury, and areas vulnerable to injury. This information will provide coaches and trainers with the tools

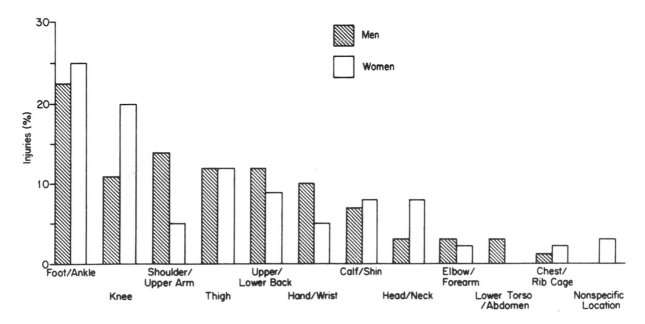

Figure 17.11. Percentage of injuries by site among male and female athletes. (Reprinted with permission from Lanese RR, et al. Injury and disability in matched men's and women's intercollegiate sports. Am J Public Health 1990;80:1461.)

they need in devising sport- and gender-specific preseason and maintenance conditioning programs, with the ultimate goal of preventing injuries before they occur.

PSYCHOLOGICAL CONSIDERATIONS IN THE FEMALE ATHLETE

Many of the existing barriers that need to be broken in women's sports are not so much physiologic or anatomic as they are psychological. There has been tremendous resistance to change in both the attitudes of society and of the women athletes themselves. As women have become participants at all levels and in all types of sports, there has been a diminishing of these psychosocial barriers (5). Being a tomboy does not have the same negative connotation it did years ago. U.S. culture has traditionally stressed that girls and women be nonaggressive, passive, and dependent rather than achievement-oriented. This gender-role stereotype is certainly considered passé by today's standards, yet these beliefs still strongly influence women's participation or lack of participation in sports (2). A study on role conflict and the high school female athlete found overall role conflict in this group to be low. Women appear to adjust to their role and self-image as athletes, but the external conflict remains prominent. Usually, forces outside the domain of sports cause the most conflict. The old stereotype still has some power in influencing female attitudes toward the appropriateness of sports involvement (110).

Sports provide not only feelings of physical well-being but also feelings of mental health. Involvement in sports may serve different purposes for men and women. Studies have indicated that men are more concerned with the competitive aspect of winning, whereas women participate more to enjoy interacting and socializing with other players (2). According to Mariah Burton Nelson, author of "Are We Winning Yet," the female approach to sports (1) rejects the military sports model consisting of a "battle with the enemy"; (2) states that humiliating a player is not how to get the best out of her; (3) emphasizes nonviolence and discourages play when athletes are injured; (4) empowers, encourages, and supports players; and (5) includes athletes of all levels, adjusting the rules as necessary to accommodate different skill levels (111).

With the ongoing success of professional women's sports, however, women are becoming more and more competitive. Some women can set their sights on becoming a professional athlete and even make a decent living that way. However, examining the existing professional sports for

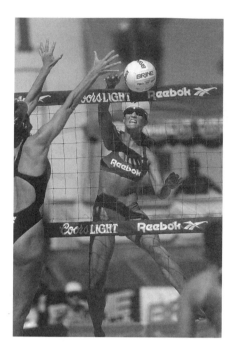

Figure 17.12. Liz Masakayan, Women's Pro Beach Volleyball Tour 1995. (Courtesy of F.E. Goroszko.)

women, such as tennis, golf, and bowling, leads one to return to the old stereotypes of "lady-like" sports. During the past few years, attempts have been made to professionalize the sports that are considered more masculine in nature, such as basketball, softball, and volleyball. Currently, only volleyball survives in the ranks of professional sports (Fig. 17.12). Women's professional basketball is slated to begin again in the fall of 1996. Previous attempts at professionalizing women's basketball have failed. The problem is not the lack of excellent athletes in these sports but the lack of media, financial, and spectator support.

As traditional views and values about women in sports continue to change, so will the quality of performance. Men will learn to accept that women are not far behind them in some of the traditionally male-dominated sports. Events such as Billie Jean King defeating Bobby Riggs at tennis, Susan Butcher winning Iditarod dogsled races, or Janet Gutherie winning major race car events are signals that women athletes can and do compete successfully with men and will continue to narrow the gap of sports performance between the genders.

Eating Disorders: Anorexia and Bulimia Nervosa

With the increased opportunities in sports and the correspondingly greater pressures to win,

Table 17.15. DSM-IV Criteria for Anorexia and Bulimia Nervosa

Diagnostic Criteria for 307.1 Anorexia Nervosa

A. Refusal to maintain body weight at or above a minimally normal weight for age and height.

B. Intense fear of gaining weight or becoming fat, even though underweight.

C. Disturbance in the way in which one's body weight or shape is experienced, undue influence of body weight or shape on self-evaluation, or denial of the seriousness of the current low body weight.

D. In postmenarchal females, amenorrhea, i.e., the absence of at least three consecutive menstrual cycles.

Specify type:

Restricting Type: during the current episode of anorexia nervosa, the person has not regularly engaged in binge-eating or purging behavior.

Binge-Eating/Purging Type: during the current episode of anerexia nervosa, the person has regularly engaged in binge-eating or purging behavior.

Diagnostic Criteria for 307.51 Anorexia Nervosa

A. Recurrent episodes of binge eating. An episode of binge eating is characterized by both of the following:

  (1) eating, in a discrete period of time (e.g., within any 2-hour period), an amount of food that is definitely larger than most people would eat during a similar period of time and under similar circumstances.

  (2) a sense of lack of control over eating during the episode (e.g., a feeling that one cannot stop eating or control what or how much one is eating)

B. Recurrent inappropriate compensatory behavior in order to prevent weight gain, such as self-induced vomiting; misuse of laxatives, diuretics, enemas, or other medications; fasting; or excessive exercise.

C. The binge eating and inappropriate compensatory behaviors both occur, on average, at least twice a week for 3 months.

D. Self-evaluation is unduly influenced by body shape and weight.

E. The disturbance does not occur exclusively during episodes of anorexia nervosa.

Specify type:

Purging type: during the current episode of bulimia nervosa, the person has regularly engaged in self-induced vomiting or the misuse of laxatives, diuretics, or enemas.

Nonpurging type: during the current episode of bulimia nervosa, the person has used other inappropriate compensatory behaviors, such as fasting or excessive exercise, but has not regularly engaged in self-induced vomiting or the misuse of laxatives, diuretics, or enemas.

From American Psychiatric Association. Diagnostic and statistical manual of mental disorders. 4th ed. Washington, DC: American Psychiatric Association, 1994. Reprinted by permission of American Psychiatric Association.

some women have found themselves vulnerable to drug use and eating disorders. It is well documented that eating disorders such as anorexia nervosa and bulimia are common among female athletes (112–116). Increasing demands—not only made by themselves but also by their coaches—are placed on these athletes to improve their techniques and physical states. A study of 182 varsity-level female athletes found that self-induced vomiting and laxative abuse occurred with almost equal frequency—14% and 16%. Diet pills were used by 25% of subjects. Thirty-two percent of athletes practiced at least one of the pathogenic weight control behaviors. The highest incidence was seen in gymnasts and distance runners, although they have the lowest body fat percentage. According to this study, swimmers, golfers, and basketball players did not seem at high risk for this type of behavior (112).

Anorexia nervosa is characterized by a preoccupation with food and body weight, behavior directed toward losing weight, peculiar patterns of handling food, weight loss, intense fear of gaining weight, body image distortions, and amenorrhea (113). Bulimia is characterized by an episodic pattern of binge-eating that is sometimes followed by vomiting, a fear of not being able to stop eating voluntarily, great concern about weight, self-criticism, depressive mood after episodes of binge-eating, and rapid weight fluctuations within a normal weight range (113). The diagnos-

Table 17.16. Physical Effects of Starvation and Purging

Starvation	Purging
Amenorrhea	Swollen parotid glands
Fat and muscle loss	Chest pain
Dry hair and skin	Sore throat
Cold extremities	Abdominal pain
Decreased body temperature	Esophageal tears
Light-headedness	Erosion of tooth enamel
Decreased ability to concentrate	Face and extremity edema
Bradycardia, other cardiac effects	Diarrhea and/or constipation
Menstrual irregularities	
Cardiac effects	

tic criteria for anorexia and bulimia according to the Diagnostic and Statistical Manual of Mental Disorders (DSM-IV) are listed in Table 17.15 (117). An athlete is classified as having "disordered eating" if she does not meet the DSM-IV criteria for either anorexia or bulimia. Long-term practice of anorexia and/or bulimia can cause malnutrition, dehydration, loss of vital electrolytes, hypoglycemia, or excessive adrenergic stimulation resulting in impaired strength, speed, endurance, and reflexes. Eventual serious injury and potentially life-threatening physiologic malfunctioning can ensue (114). Some physical effects of starvation and purging are listed in Table 17.16 (36).

Studies have shown a strong correlation between female athletic activity and pathologic eating disorders. Athletes involved in sports that em-

Table 17.17. Signs of Disordered Eating

Repeatedly expressed concerns about being or feeling fat, even when weight is average or below average

Refusal to maintain a minimal normal weight

Preoccupation with food, calories, and weight

Increasing criticism of one's body

Consumption of huge amounts of food not consistent with athlete's weight

Secretly eating or stealing food

Eating large meals, then making trips to the bathroom

Bloodshot eyes, especially after bathroom, swollen parotid glands

Vomitus, or odor of vomit in toilet, sink, shower, or wastebasket

Foul breath, poor dental hygiene

Wide fluctuations of weight over short time span

Periods of severe calorie restriction or repeated days of fasting

Excessive laxative use, or packages lying around

Relentless, excessive physical activity

Depressed mood and self-deprecating thoughts following eating

Avoiding eating with others

Use of diet pills

Mood swings

Wearing baggy or layered clothing

Complaints of bloating or light-headedness that cannot be attributed to other medical causes

phasize leanness are especially at risk. Women involved in weight lifting and particularly competitive body building fall into this category. In a recent study, the majority of competitive body builders questioned had excessive concern about body weight and overeating, but did not display the full complement of psychological abnormalities indicative of eating disorders. It appears that these athletes may be restricting energy intake to satisfy their desire for weight loss (115). Most authorities conclude that teachers, coaches, and parents of female athletes should not overemphasize leanness, especially for athletes in activities that already focus on the need for leanness (113). Telling an athlete that she is too fat or giving her undue praise for losing weight beyond original goals may be an iatrogenic cause of anorexia nervosa or the binge-purge syndrome (116).

Recognition of eating disorders in athletes can often be difficult. Most athletes are very secretive and usually deny having a problem. Table 17.17 lists various signs and symptoms of disordered eating (111–118). Intervention in eating disorders should be gentle. It is recommended that the physician present evidence of the athlete's abnormal behavior and express concern about the athlete's health and the effect of this problem on athletic performance. The physician should never criticize and should avoid direct confrontation. It should be suggested to the athlete that a consultation with an eating disorder specialist, rather than treatment, should be the first step (119).

Treatment of eating disorders involves a multidisciplinary team including the physician, nutritionist, therapist or psychologist, coach, and athlete. Prevention begins with educating the athlete not specifically about eating disorders but about sports nutrition, body weight and composition, and performance. Coaches should be educated by recommending that they deemphasize the importance of weight, eliminate group weigh-ins, discourage unhealthy practices, and treat each athlete individually (118, 119). Ultimately, until society in general—and sports in particular—eliminates the pressures that encourage disordered eating, this problem will continue. The physician must play a key role in recognizing, treating, and preventing eating disorders (118).

CONCLUSION

There is a strong correlation between being physically fit and having high self-esteem (120, 121). This is true in both men and women. Balogun (121) found that relative strength of the upper back, chest, and arms was significantly related to overall self-concept in women. Strong women are more satisfied with themselves in general (121).

As the year 2000 approaches, many myths regarding the female athlete are being discarded. Notions that women are genetically inferior, are more likely to be injured, are not strong enough, or lack endurance are no longer acceptable; research has shown many of these conceptions to be unfounded. There are undeniably physiologic and anatomic differences between the sexes. Women may not be able to compete against men in sports in which strength is the determining factor, but some women may be able to compete against men in events in which endurance prevails.

Will professional female athletes ever approach the salaries that male athletes enjoy? Multimillion dollar salaries for women athletes seem utterly unimaginable, but women have not yet come close to their potential in sports performance; they have only been participating on a competitive level for the past century. Only since the advent of Title IX in 1972 have they had equal opportunities in schools and colleges. Records continue to be broken, records that would have bettered those of the male athlete 20 years ago. The changing of women's traditional ideas about participating in sports and the loosening of social attitudes are enabling female athletes to surge forward. In a world in which it is no longer "un–lady-like" for a woman to be competitive, aggressive, independent, and strong in her sport, the cultural reinforcements and rewards that men receive from athletic participation should also become a reality for women.

Acknowledgments

The author thanks the following for their assistance, cooperation, and understanding in the completion of this chapter: Andrea Sullivan, D.C., Jennifer Caldwell, Zane Irwin Brown, Beth Davidson, D.C., and the staff of the library at Life Chiropractic College West.

References

1. Anonymous. The implications of gender equity in college sports. Phys Ed J Sports Med 1993;2:2.
2. Haycock CE, ed. Sports medicine for the athletic female. Oradell, NJ: Medical Economics Company, 1980.
3. Wells CL. Women, sport & performance: a physiological perspective. Champaign, IL: Human Kinetics Publishers, 1985.
4. Whipp D, Ward S. Will women soon outrun men? Nature 1992;355:25.
5. Murphy P. Longer, higher, faster: athletes continue to reach new heights. Phys Sportsmed 1986;14:140–149.
6. Hale RW. Factors important to women engaged in vigorous physical activity. In: Strauss RH, ed. Sports medicine. 2nd ed. Philadelphia: WB Saunders, 1991:487–502.
7. Roy S, Irvin R. Sports medicine: prevention, evaluation, management, and rehabilitation. Englewood Cliffs, NJ: Prentice-Hall, 1983:457–467.
8. Holloway JB, Baechel TR. Strength training for female athletes. Sports Med 1990;9:216–228.
9. Cureton KJ, Collins MA, Hill DW, et al. Muscle hypertrophy in men and women. Med Sci Sports Med 1988;20:338–344.
10. Hughes RA, Housh TJ, Hughes RJ, et al. The effect of exercise duration on serum cholesterol and triglycerides in women. Res Q Exerc Sport 1991;62:98–104.
11. Mitchell JH, Tate J, Raven P, et al. Acute response and chronic adaptation to exercise in women. Med Sci Sports Exerc 1992;24:258–265.
12. Drinkwater BL, Bruemner B, Chestnut CH. Menstrual history as a determinant of current bone density in young athletes. JAMA 1990;263:545–548.
13. Stager JM, Hatler LK. Menarche in athletes: the influence of genetics and prepubertal training. Med Sci Sports Exerc 1987; 15:219–222.
14. Plowman SA, Liu NY, Wells CL. Body composition and sexual maturation in premenarcheal athletes and nonathletes. Med Sci Sports Exerc 1991;23:23–29.
15. Nattiv A, Mandelbaum BR. Injuries and special concerns in female gymnasts. Phys Sportsmed 1993;21:66–82.
16. Caine DJ, Koenroad JL. Overuse injuries of growing bones: the young female gymnast at risk? Phys Sportsmed 1985;13:51–64.
17. Carlberg K, Peake GT, Buckman MT. Exercise and the menstrual cycle. In: Appenzeller O, ed. Sports medicine, fitness, training, injuries. 3rd ed. Munich: Urban and Schwarzenberg, 1988:246–250.
18. Lamont LS. Lack of influence of menstrual cycle on blood lactate. Phys Sportsmed 1986;14:159–163.
19. Bale P, Nelson G. The effects of menstruation on performance of swimmers. Aust J Sci Med Sport 1985;17:19–20.
20. Dibrezzo R, Fort IL, Brown B. Dynamic strength and work variations during three stages of the menstrual cycle. J Orthop Sports Phys Ther 1988;10:113–116.
21. Quadagno D, Faquin L, Lim G, et al. The menstrual: does it affect athletic performance. Phys Sportsmed 1991;19:121–124.
22. De Souza MJ, Maguire MS, Rubin KR, et al. Effects of menstrual phase and amenorrhea on exercise performance in runners. Med Sci Sports Exerc 1990:22:575–580.
23. Keye WR. Premenstrual syndrome. West J Med 1988;149:765.
24. Miller-Jones J. PMS. The Melpomene Report March 1986;12–17.
25. Shangold MM. Premenstrual syndrome. Sports Med Dig 1992;14:5.
26. Shangold MM. Treatment for premenstrual syndrome: what works and what doesn't. Sports Med Dig 1993;15:7.
27. Prior JC, Vigna Y, Alojada N. Conditioning exercise decreases premenstrual symptoms: a prospective controlled three month trial. Eur J Appl Physiol 1986;55:349–355.
28. Anonymous. Fight dysmenorrhea with exercise. Phys Ed J Sports Med 1992;2:2.
29. Kokjohn K, Schmid DM, Triano JJ, et al. The effect of spinal manipulation on pain and prostaglandin levels in women with primary dysmenorrhea. J Manipulative Physiol Ther 1992;15:279–285.
30. Golub LJ, Menduke H, Lange WR, et al. Exercise and dysmenorrhea in younger teenagers: a 3-year study. Obstet Gynecol 1968;32:508–511.
31. Shangold MM. Women in sports, abnormal uterine bleeding and the athlete. Sport Med Dig 1991;13:5.
32. Kaiserauer S, Snyder AC, Sleeper M, et al. Nutritional, physiological, and menstrual status of distance runners. Med Sci Sports Exerc 1989;21:120–125.
33. Sanborn CF. Menstrual dysfunction in the female athlete. In: Tietz CC, ed. Scientific foundations of sports medicine. Philadelphia: B.C. Decker, 1989.
34. Myburgh KH, Watkin VA, Noakes TD. Are risk factors for menstrual dysfunction cumulative? Phys Sportsmed 1992;20:114–125.
35. Myerson M, Gutin B, Warren MP, et al. Resting metabolic rate and energy balance in amenorrheic and eumenorrheic runners. Med Sci Sports Exerc 1991;23:15–21.
36. Shangold M, Mirkin G, eds. Women and exercise: physiology and sports medicine. 2nd ed. Philadelphia: FA Davis, 1994.
37. Lynch JM, Waters DU. The female athlete. In: Grana WA, Kalinak A, eds. Clinical sports medicine. Philadelphia: WB Saunders, 1991:197–208.
38. Caldwell F. Light-boned and lean athletes: does the penalty outweigh the reward? Phys Sportsmed 1984;12:139–149.
39. Cook SD, Harding AF, Thomas KA, et al. Trabecular bone density and menstrual function in women runners. Am J Sport Med 1987;15:503–506.
40. Baker E, Demers L. Menstrual status in female athletes: correlation with reproductive hormones and bone density. Obstet Gynecol 1988;72:683–687.
41. Sutton JR, Nilson KL. Repeated stress fractures in an amenorrheic marathoner. Phys Sportsmed 1989;17:65–71.
42. Otis CL, Puffer JC, Mandelbaum BR. Tibial pain in an amenorrheic runner. Phys Sportsmed 1988;16:115–119.
43. Barrow GW, Saha S. Menstrual irregularity and stress fractures in collegiate female distance runners. Am J Sports Med 1988;16:209–215.
44. Drinkwater BL, Nilson K, Ott S, et al. Bone mineral density after resumption of menses in amenorrheic athletes. JAMA 1986;256:380–382.
45. Munnings F. Exercise and estrogen in women's health: getting a clearer picture. Phys Sportsmed 1988;16:152–161.
46. Highet R. Athletic amenorrhea: an update on aetiology, complications and management. Sport Med 1989;7:82–108.
47. Prior JC, Vigna YM, Schechter MT, et al. Spinal bone loss and ovulatory disturbances. N Engl J Med 1990;323:1221–1227.
48. Debrezzo R, Fort IL, Brown B. Relationships among strength, endurance, weight and body fat during three phases of the menstrual cycle. J Sports Med Phy Fitness 1991;31:89–94.

49. Grimston SK, Sanborn CF, Miller PD, Huffer WE. The application of historical data for evaluation of osteopenia in female runners: the menstrual index. Clin Sports Med 1990;2:108–118.

50. Snyder AC, Drorak LL, Roepke JB. Influences of dietary iron source on measures of iron status among female runners. Med Sci Sports Exerc 1989;21:7–10.

51. Risser WL, Lee EJ, Poindexter HBW, et al. Iron deficiency in female athletes: its prevalence and impact on performance. Med Sci Sports Exerc 1988;20:116–121.

52. Steenkamp I, Fuller C, Graves J, et al. Marathon running fails to influence RBC survival rates in iron-depleted women. Phys Sportsmed 1986;14:89–95.

53. Telford RD, Cunningham RB, Deakin V, et al. Iron status and diet in athletes. Med Sci Sports Exerc 1993;25:796–800.

54. Selby GB. When does an athlete need iron? Phys Sportsmed 1991;19:96–102.

55. Risser WL, Risser JMH. Iron deficiency in adolescents and young adults. In: Goldberg B, ed. Pediatrics series. Phys Sportsmed 1990;18:87–101.

56. Magazanik A, Weinstein Y, Abarbanel J, et al. Effect of an iron supplement on body iron status and aerobic capacity of young training women. Eur J Appl Physiol 1991;62:317–323.

57. Blum SM, Sherman AR, Boileau RA. The effects of fitness-type exercise on the iron status in adult women. Am J Clin Nutr 1986;43:456–463.

58. Gleeson PB, Pauls JA. Obstetrical physical therapy, review of the literature. Phys Therapy 1988;68:1699–1702.

59. Hall DC, Kaufmann DA. Effects of aerobic and strength conditioning on prepregnancy outcomes. Am J Obstet Gynecol 1987;157:1199–1203.

60. Artral R. Exercise during pregnancy. In: Strauss RH, ed. Sports medicine. Philadelphia: WB Saunders, 1991:503–514.

61. Lokey EA, Tran ZV, Wells CL, et al. Effects of physical exercise on pregnancy outcomes: a meta-analytic review. Med Sci Sports Exerc 1991;23:1234–1239.

62. Clapp JF, Rokey R, Treadway JL, et al. Exercise in pregnancy. Med Sci Sports Exerc 1992;24(Suppl):294–299.

63. American College of Obstetricians and Gynecologists. Exercise during pregnancy and the postpartum period. Washington, DC: ACOG Technical Bulletin no. 189, 1994.

64. Anonymous. Prenatal care for the active woman. Phys Ed J Sports Med 1992;1:4–5.

65. Wallace J. Babies prefer pre-exercise breast milk. Pediatrics 1993;89:1245–1247.

66. Schelkun PH. Exercise and breast-feeding mothers. Phys Sportsmed 1991;19:109–116.

67. Warren MP. Exercise in women. effects on reproductive system and pregnancy. In: DiNubile NA, ed. Clinics in sports medicine. Philadelphia: WB Saunders, 1991:131–139.

68. Buchmann GA, Grill J. Exercise in the postmenopausal woman. Geriatrics 1987;42:75–85.

69. Barry HC, Rich BSE, Carlson RT. How exercise can benefit older patients. Phys Sportsmed 1993;21:124–140.

70. Anonymous. Menopause does not stop active women. Phys Ed J Sports Med 1992;1:2.

71. Marcus R, Drinkwater BL, Dalsky G, et al. Osteoporosis and exercise in women. Med Sci Sports Exerc 1992;24(Suppl):301–307.

72. Heinrich CH, Going SB, Pamenter RW, et al. Bone mineral content of cyclically menstruating female resistance and endurance trained athletes. Med Sci Sports Exerc 1990;22:558–563.

73. Windsor R, Dumitru D. Prevalence of anabolic steroid use by male and female adolescents. Med Sci Sports Exerc 1989;21:494–497.

74. Otis CL. Women and sports. women and anabolic steroids. Sports Med Dig 1990;12:4.

75. Yesalis CE, et al. Athlete's projections of anabolic steroid use. Clin Sports Med 1990;2:155–171.

76. Duda M. Female athletes: targets for drug abuse. Phys Sportsmed 1986;14:142–146.

77. Nevole GJ, Prentice WE. The effect of anabolic steroids on female athletes. Athletic Training 1987;22:297–299.

78. Haupt HA, Rovere GD. Anabolic steroids: a review of the literature. Med Sci Sports Exerc 1984;12:469–483.

79. Lamb DR. Anabolic steroids in athletics: how well do they work and how dangerous are they? Med Sci Sports Exerc 1984;12:31–37.

80. Moller-Nielsen J, Hammar M. Women's soccer injuries in relation to the menstrual cycle and oral contraceptive use. Med Sci Sports Exerc 1989;21:126–129.

81. Schelkun PH. Exercise and the pill. Phys Sportsmed 1991;19:143–152.

82. Wein P, Thompson DJ. Vaginal perforation due to jet ski accident. Aust N Z J Obstet Gynaecol 1990;30:384–385.

83. Haycock CE, Gillette JV. Susceptibility of women athletes to injury: myths and reality. JAMA 1976;236:163–165.

84. Nygaard IE, DeLancey JOL, Arnsdorf L, et al. Exercise and incontinence. Obstet Gynecol 1990;75:848–851.

85. Haycock CE. How I manage breast problems in athletes. Phys Sportsmed 1987;15:89–95.

86. Lorentzen D, Lawson L. Selected sports bras: a biomechanical analysis of breast motion while jogging. Phys Sportsmed 1987;15:128–140.

87. Potera C. Women in sports: the price of participation. Phys Sportsmed 1986;14:149–153.

88. Falls HB. Coed football: hazards, implications, and alternatives. Phys Sportsmed 1986;14:207–222.

89. Giel D. Women's weight lifting: elevating a sport to world-class status. Phys Sportsmed 1988;16:163–168.

90. Messier SP, Davis SE, Curl WW, et al. Etiologic factors associated with patellofemoral pain in runners. Med Sci Sports Exerc 1991;23:1008–1015.

91. Eng JJ, Pierrynowski MR. Evaluation of soft foot orthotics in the treatment of patellofemoral pain syndrome. Phys Ther 1993;73:62.

92. NCAA Injury Surveillance System. Men's and women's basketball 1993-94. Overland Park, KS: NCAA, 1994:49.

93. Welch MJ. Women in the military academies US Army. Phys Sportsmed 1989;17:89–96.

94. Sutton JR, Nilson KL. Repeated stress fractures in an amenorrheic marathoner. Phys Sportsmed 1989;17:65–71.

95. Havkins SB. Head, neck, face, and shoulder injuries in female and male rugby players. Phys Sportsmed 1986;14:111–118.

96. Mutoh Y, Sawai S, Takanashe Y, et al. Aerobic dance injuries among instructors and students. Phys Sportsmed 1988;16:81–96.

97. Wheeler LP. Common musculoskeletal dance injuries. Chiro Sport Med 1987;1:17–23.

98. Hamilton WG, Hamilton LH, Marshall P, et al. A profile of the musculoskeletal characteristics of elite professional ballet dancers. Am J Sports Med 1992;20:267–272.

99. Rosen LW, McKeag DB, Hough DO, et al. Pathogenic weight-control behavior in female athletes. Phys Sportsmed 1986;14:79–86.

100. Stalder MA, Noble BJ, Wilkinson JG. The effects of supplemental weight training for ballet dancers. J Appl Sport Sci Res 1990;4:95–102.

101. Lanese RR, Strauss RH. Leizman DJ, et al. Injury and disability in matched men's and women's intercollegiate sports. Am J Pub Health 1990;80:1459–1462.

102. Snook GA. Injuries in women's gymnastics. Am J Sports Med 1979;7:242–244.

103. Lowry CB, Leveau BF. A retrospective study of gymnastics injuries to competitors and noncompetitors in private clubs. Am J Sports Med 1982;10:237–239.

104. Wadley G, Albright JP. Women's intercollegiate gymnastics. Am J Sports Med 1993;21:314–320.

105. Garrick JG, Requa RK. Epidemiology of women's gymnastic injuries. Am J Sports Med 1980;8:261–264.

106. Weber MD, Woodall WR. Spondylogenic disorders in gymnastics. J Orthop Sports Phys Ther 1991;14:6–13.

107. Levine M, Lombardo J, McNeeley J, et al. An analysis of individual stretching programs of intercollegiate athletes. Phys Sportsmed 1987;15:130–136.
108. Shangold M, Mirkin G. The complete sports medicine book for women. New York: Simon and Schuster, 1985:166.
109. Weaver S. So you want to buy a bike. Women Sports 1987;12:23.
110. Anthrop J, Allison MT. Role conflict and the high school female athlete. Res Q Exerc Sport 1983;54:104–111.
111. Anonymous. Women are changing the nature of sports. Phys Ed J Sports Med 1993;2:2.
112. Rosen LW, McKeag DB, Hough DO, et al. Pathogenic weight-control behavior in female athletes. Phys Sportsmed 1986;14:79–86.
113. Borgen JS, Corbin CB. Eating disorders among female athletes. Phys Sportsmed 1987;15:89–95.
114. Rosen LW, Hough DO. Pathogenic weight-control behaviors of female college gymnasts. Phys Sportsmed 1988;16:141–144.

115. Walberg JL, Johnston CS. Menstrual function and eating behavior in female recreational weight lifters and competitive body builders. Med Sci Sports Exerc 1991;23:30–36.
116. Zucker P, Avener J, Bayder S, et al. Eating disorders in young athletes. Phys Sportsmed 1985;13:89–106.
117. American Psychiatric Association. Diagnostic and statistical manual of mental disorders. 4th ed. Washington, DC: American Psychiatric Association, 1994.
118. Wichman S, Martin DR. Eating disorders in athletes. Phys Sportsmed 1993;21:126–135.
119. Anonymous. Athletes with eating disorders. Phys Ed J Sports Med 1993;2:1–2.
120. Young ML. Estimation of fitness and physical ability, physical performance and self-concept among adolescent females. J Sports Med 1985;25:144–150.
121. Balogun JA. Muscular strength as a predictor of personality in adult females. J Sports Med 1986;26:377–383.

The Young Athlete: Special Considerations

Marianne S. Gengenbach and Robin A. Hunter

No text on athletic injuries would be complete without a discussion of pediatric and adolescent athletes. In these age-groups, one finds uniquely vulnerable and impressionable athletes. Not only physicians, but also coaches, parents, and teachers may all influence these individuals, in both a positive and negative manner. For the physician to be able to provide adequate guidance and injury management, it is imperative to understand the unique physical and psychological characteristics that affect the child involved in athletic activity. Such understanding must encompass a knowledge not only of those sports-induced injuries or conditions most commonly seen in this age-group, but also of their special musculoskeletal characteristics. Similar injury mechanisms produce far different tissue responses in children than in adults. Other concepts of particular importance include the interaction that sports and exercise may have with growth and development, nutritional needs of the exercising child, and relationship between sports-induced competition and psychological well-being of the child/adolescent. This chapter provides an overview of these topics and information on the involvement of both healthy children and those with special health problems in appropriate physical activity.

HISTORICAL PERSPECTIVES AND CURRENT ISSUES

The History of Youth Sports

The use of highly organized competitive sports programs for adolescents is a phenomenon that arose during the first half of the 20th century (1). With the inclusion of sports in the school curriculum in the 1900s, there was a direct influence on the promotion and acceptance of youth involvement in athletic programs.

In the 1930s, sports emerged as an after-school recreational activity developing into a highly win-at-all-cost competition. Consequently, public school educators condemned having youths in organized sports. As athletic competition was eliminated from elementary school programs, physical education and intramural programs were introduced in their place. The withdrawal of support for competitive athletics by health education leaders and public school educators in the 1930s has had a lasting influence on youth sport programs (2). Organized athletic activity became more a primary function of family-oriented agencies and youth-related groups such as the YMCA, YWCA, and Police Athletic League. Because these groups had no educationally imposed restrictions on them, children's sports programs began to flourish. By the 1960s, millions of preadolescents were involved in sports competition such as Little League Baseball, Pop Warner Football, Pee Wee Hockey, and National Junior Tennis League. By 1970, the opportunities for regional and national competition in children's athletics had expanded to include virtually every sport in which competition was available at the adult level (2).

Today, approximately 40 million children and adolescents participate in sports programs. Virtually all children up to the age of 10 participate in some form of organized play or sports (3). There are important issues to consider such as children competing at ages as young as 4 and 5, the elite young athlete becoming more common, and more young athletes getting injured. When is the appropriate time to begin competition? How is healthy competition best fostered? When does exercise become too demanding and stressful for the young athlete?

The Role of Athletic Activity

Sports competition is particularly important to children. It is an arena in which individuals can compare their motor and athletic abilities, which are highly valued attributes, with other children of elementary and secondary school age (4, 5). Thus, success in athletics becomes a significant form of positive social reinforcement.

Research suggests that the early elementary school years are when most children are first able to compete and seek out competitive situations for their social comparison value (6). Not until the age of 5 or 6 do children begin to compare their performance with that of other children spontaneously to evaluate their own competence. This social comparison continues to strengthen in the early school years and becomes an independent social motive around the age of 7 or 8 (6–8). However, if younger children are to compete, there is no need to formalize and structure physical activity into highly organized and competitive games. The emphasis on athletic activity before the age of 7 or 8 should be on the development of skills, fitness, and fun. It is important for parents to keep athletic activity in proper perspective, particularly when children are young. Free play and unstructured periods of exercise are vital for the youngster in exploring newly acquired or developing skills and in developing self-esteem.

Maturation, Motivation, and Sport Readiness

Is a given child ready for the demands of competitive sports? Readiness is closely related to the notion of maturation. Maturation is most often viewed in the context of genetic regulation of developmental changes and in combination with learning (6, 9). Therefore, maturation refers to the potential or limitations of a given child. Readiness should be decided in terms of a match between a child's level of growth and development and the tasks and demands presented by competitive sport. All too often the physical size (biologic maturity) and motor components (skill) are emphasized in selecting youngsters for sports. Normal growth and development for the child-to-adolescent transformation is a physiologic continuum. Between the ages of 8 and 16, changes take place that convert the child to a young adult. Specifically, between 8 and 14 years of age the highest number of participating athletes are found (10). During these critical growth years, increases in size and strength occur, as well as maturation of the nervous system producing quick reflexes, good balance, and improved muscular control. Coordination of larger muscle groups is extremely variable and must be accounted for when matching children to play any competitive sport.

Size and age alone do not suffice; any two children of the same age may vary greatly in levels of coordination. Children undergoing major changes in height and weight may be exceedingly clumsy, because muscular and skeletal growth have surpassed neurologic maturation. Time will improve this situation for the young athlete, and this is when coach and parental understanding, proper guidance, and placement become crucial. In addition, the maturity factor must be considered. The Tanner rating (Fig. 18.1) classifies development of children on a scale from 1 (very little pubertal change) to 5 (fully developed). Because many athletic skills (muscular power, coordination, oxygen consumption) develop rapidly with hormonal changes of puberty (especially in boys), equal height and weight alone are not enough in matching capabilities. A boy or girl with a Tanner rating of 1 or 2 should not compete against a youth with a rating of 4 or 5. For young male athletes, the evidence indicates that early maturing boys of mesomorphic type (approximately 10 to 13 years) have a distinct advantage over the late maturing boys (9). With advanced skeletal maturity, larger size and strength are noted. Owing to this, the early maturers are more likely to participate in and be selected for sports such as football, baseball, swimming, cycling, and track and field. However, as adolescence approaches its termination, the size and maturity status is of less significance; the late maturing boys catch up with the early maturers.

Among young female athletes, delayed biologic maturity has been noted compared with nonathletes (9). The late maturing girl characteristically has long legs for her stature, relatively narrow hips, a linear physique, less height, and less fatness than peers who matured at an earlier age (9). Because of this, the late maturing girl is more apt to participate in sports such as gymnastics, figure skating, swimming, tennis, and dance.

There are other important factors to consider that also influence the selection process. Parental encouragement and support are the primary influence on the young child and the beginning of involvement in sports. Economic factors are a significant consideration, particularly in sports such as gymnastics, figure skating, swimming, and tennis.

Those most suited to the demands of a sport, which usually means those most capable of adapting physically, psychologically, and emotionally, are presumably more successful and may eventually comprise the elite competitors. As a child gets older, self-selection is a critical factor, as is the influence of parents and coaches (11). Ultimately, it is the child who must train, perform, and compete. Therefore, the motivation of the child to train and be receptive to coaching is important for success in sports as well.

The Fitness of Our Youth

Recent studies have shown that U.S. youth are at low levels of physical fitness compared with 25 years ago (12–14). Researchers, school adminis-

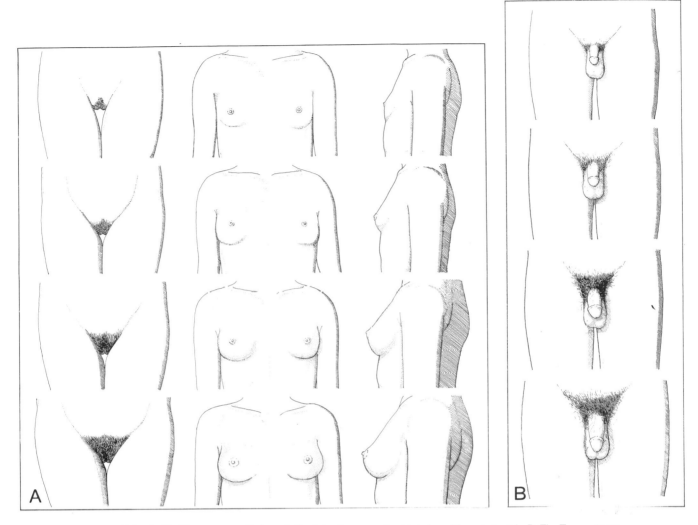

Figure 18.1. A. The Tanner stages (2 through 5) of development of pubic hair and breasts in girls. **B.** The Tanner stages (2 through 5) of development of pubic hair and genitalia in boys.

trators, and medical experts have hypothesized many different reasons for this dilemma. Foremost considerations have been the affluence of the U.S. lifestyle, television viewing, adopting of sedentary lifestyles, and lack of support from schools in educating students in the importance of healthful eating habits and proper physical fitness (13–17). An increasing concern of pediatricians today is the evidence of poor physical fitness and its correlation to increased risk of health problems such as cardiovascular disease, hypertension, obesity, and associated elevated serum lipids (12). Adolescents are not immune to these health problems. Obesity is directly related to elevated blood pressure and increased risk of coronary problems (12). Childhood obesity has become a definite problem; however, the recent upsurges in sports involvement and physical fitness may be changing these health problems in a few years. It has been estimated that 5 to 25% of

children and adolescents are obese (18). Approximately 11 million school-age children are obese, and obesity of younger children (aged 6 to 11) rose 54% from 1963 to 1980 (17).

PROPOSED SOLUTIONS

The Heart Healthy program begun in 1981 was developed to address the issues of poor physical fitness. The project, developed for elementary school students, was designed to increase students' consumption of complex carbohydrates; decrease consumption of saturated fat, cholesterol, sodium, and sugar; and increase the level of habitual physical activity. Although notable improvements were seen in children's eating habits, there was a failure to observe positive changes in fitness activity levels (15). The problem of improving the fitness of youth is believed by many experts to be the prime responsibility of the educational system (16). Virtually all children

(97%) are enrolled in physical education classes; however, only 36.5% of these children take those classes daily (14). It has been found that the less time schools allow for physical education, the more time they allow for recess. A recent study has shown that only four states require students in all grades to take physical education courses. And only one state, Illinois, requires students to take physical education every day (14).

There is also a growing concern that there is too much emphasis being put on competitive sports and not enough time dedicated to developing habits for long-term fitness. Duncan et al. (12) suggested straightforward alternatives and a possible solution to this national dilemma. Their study was performed with fifth grade students for the purpose of comparing the relative effectiveness of a structured physical fitness program stressing conditioning, strength, and flexibility against the customary skill and team sports emphasis. The standard physical fitness tests of the American Alliance for Health, Physical Education, and Recreation (AAHPER) were used to measure fitness. The findings revealed a significant improvement in percentile score in seven of nine fitness tests performed by the children in the experimental program.

An innovative program called Fit Youth Today, developed by William G. Squires, Ph.D., was introduced in some Texas school districts. The 8-week fitness program was designed to improve cardiovascular fitness through regular structured exercise activity such as running and calisthenics (12). The emphasis was on fitness versus athletic prowess.

Programs that provide the opportunity for adolescents to develop and maintain physical fitness should be emphasized. Relatively few high school students and even fewer elementary school children participate in conditioning programs. Healthcare professionals have urged schools to provide regular programs in circulatory enhancing and endurance activities for children in grades K through 12. The general consensus is that cardiovascular conditioning activities should be emphasized, consisting of 30 minutes a day of vigorous activities (although even 10 minutes, 3 times a week, will provide some improvement) (12).

Fostering Healthy Competition

Children's sporting environments should reflect the youths' priorities and not those of adults. Children believe the most important aspects of their sports are opportunities to play, to play as well as they are able, and to have fun, whereas the least important factor is to beat their opponent (19). Adults, coaches, and parents all seem to place too much emphasis on winning. However, the relationship between the players and coach, in particular, is a primary determinant of the ways in which children are ultimately affected by their participation. Coaches become the vital element in establishing a psychologically healthy environment for children in their sport. A possible solution is to have coaches' training courses. Less than 50% of coaches (and probably closer to 30%) have received any formal training. Surveys in Canada, the United States, and southern Australia revealed that few coaches would be willing to take lengthy courses of training; however, most would consider attending workshops (20). Because many coaches are aware of their inadequate training and want some education, workshops may be a step to fill the void.

The committees of Sports Medicine and School Health of the American Academy of Pediatrics (AAP) have set forth policies and statements regarding fostering healthy youth sports competition (21).

The goals of a program and the adults' (parents and coaches) behavior should focus on assisting the child to develop the following seven key objectives.

1. Enjoyment of sports and fitness.
2. Physical fitness.
3. Basic motor skills.
4. Positive self-image.
5. Balanced perspective on sports in relation to the child's scholastics and life.
6. Commitment to values of teamwork, fair play, and sportsmanship.
7. Safe sport.

In addition, the following guidelines were recommended for implementation for any youth sporting activity.

1. The game or sporting event should allow each child equal playing time.
2. The game rules and equipment should be modified to accommodate age appropriateness.
3. Participants should be grouped according to size, skill, and maturation level rather than age. This becomes particularly important with the growth spurts between 11 and 14 years of age.
4. There must be unconditional approval for participating and having fun.

Attrition, Overtraining, and Burnout

It is estimated that 35% of U.S. children who become involved in sports annually will withdraw

(22). Researchers have found that children cite multiple motives for sports involvement, focusing primarily on such reasons as having fun, improving skills, being with friends, enjoying the excitement, experiencing success, and becoming fit. Similarly, children who dropped out cited multiple motives for sports withdrawal, including conflict of interest, lack of play time, lack of success or skill improvement, competitive stress, lack of fun, dislike of the coach, boredom, and injury (23).

The major risk of intensive training, aside from injury, is the eventual loss of interest that can occur when children and adolescent athletes train too hard and compete too often (24, 25). Until recently, this syndrome has been more common in U.S. sports systems characterized by short seasons and by inadequate training time in school sports programs. Continued interest usually does not occur when the young athletes are pushed to the limit every season. The club sport approach, which is prevalent in Europe, allows a longer view of participation that helps to reduce the tendency for overtraining and overcompetition in the early years. Club systems are now making a comeback in the United States.

ATHLETIC INVOLVEMENT

The Preparticipation Evaluation

PURPOSE AND GOALS

Most children will undergo a preparticipation evaluation of some sort during their school years. Surveys by Feinstein et al. (26) show that at least 35 states require a yearly preparticipation physical examination (PPE) of school children; other states have varying requirements of lesser stringency. It is also well known that these preparticipation examinations are considered a child's annual health assessment in a majority (80%) of cases (27, 28). Schichor and Beck (28) reported that 43% of children and adolescents use the preparticipation physical in the school setting as their only form of health assessment.

This has led to some controversy centering around the cost-effectiveness and yield of such examinations, as well as the purported goals of such an examination. Risser et al., for example, report an unfavorable cost–benefit ratio for standard PPE (29) based on yield of significant negative information. However, Goldberg et al. and others have argued that the use of these PPEs as a means of primary health assessment points to a continued need for such evaluations (27, 30). The PPE also provides one of the few occasions during which a physician can actively prevent sports injuries from occurring (31). Therefore,

more recent literature has focused on how to construct a valid and reliable PPE and what components should be included to increase the yield of useful information.

What emerges is that current information on the PPE must be viewed as a set of guidelines, rather than a cookbook of what to do (32), and must be combined with clinical judgment specific to the presenting situation. Examples of modifying factors for any set of PPE guidelines include the age of the individuals being examined, intended sport or activity, and anticipated level of competition (32). The findings of Goldberg et al. (27) and McKeag (32) would indicate that although the cost-effectiveness of PPE may be controversial, they can be justified if they are adapted to the characteristics of the potential athlete. Although McKeag describes as many as 11 potential goals for such an examination, Goldberg et al. narrow the various goals to two. These authors and others also agree that the highest yield from such evaluations comes from the history and neuromusculoskeletal portions of the evaluation (27, 32, 33). Goldberg et al. even suggest that a routine physical examination need not be part of a preparticipation screening assessment for athletic competition, but should be a prerequisite responsibility of a primary care physician (27). Such a preassessment requirement might eliminate the substitution of the PPE for a primary care assessment and allow the screening to focus on more realistic goals. The simplest yet most thorough delineation of these goals is provided by Kibler (34):

1. Provide an objective, sport-specific musculoskeletal profile of fitness.
2. Determine negative information that prohibits, modifies, or delays participation.
3. Determine positive information that can decrease injury risk and/or increase performance.
4. Provide a reproducible baseline for subsequent examinations.
5. Provide a base for sport-specific conditioning.

An ideal situation is one in which the baseline medical evaluation is required before the PPE. This would allow the PPE to focus on those activities with the highest yield of information pertinent to the goals quoted above (i.e., a primarily musculoskeletal assessment). However, current experience indicates that this ideal is not yet an accepted norm. Therefore, armed with the knowledge that this assessment may be the only evaluation received by the athlete, one should strive to create evaluations sensitive enough to at least identify any underlying abnormalities.

TIMING AND CONTENT

Faced with the reality that the PPE can be a viable and reliable vehicle when properly administered, the questions of timing, content, and format of these examinations must be addressed. With respect to timing, the current practice seems to coincide more or less with the thinking of McKeag (32), who recommends that any such evaluation be carried out 4 to 6 weeks before the beginning of a particular sports season. This time frame presumably allows for sufficient time to follow up on required consultations, rehabilitate injuries, identify predisposing factors to injury, and begin to correct deficiencies in conditioning. This timing should also achieve the objective of not giving too much time for new problems to develop between the time of examination and the actual beginning of participatory activity. With respect to format, the two most common forms of evaluation are the individual in-office evaluation and the station evaluation (32). Whereas one might assume that the in-office examination has the best chance of being the most thorough, there is some evidence to indicate that a team of multiple examiners will actually bring a higher yield of clinically significant information (35). Regardless of format, however, it is ideal if any examination (beyond the general medical evaluation) can be modified toward a more sports-specific approach (34). Although there are many possible ways to establish a station-type screening examination, Table 18.1 is an example. The content of this table also illustrates the minimum information that should be elicited in a screening evaluation of this type. Many modifications in this setup are possible, but one requirement is that each station be administered by personnel competent to perform a particular task. This not only provides accurate infor-

mational yield, but also helps to provide legal defensibility of the process.

The initial registration station is designed to check for proper execution of any paperwork required before the examination itself. This would be especially important if, as mentioned previously, the baseline medical evaluation had been done before the PPE.

The history station should be staffed by personnel who are competent in eliciting proper histories. Goldberg et al. (27) have stated that when performed for the purpose of restricting participation or referring for additional evaluation, the history and musculoskeletal examination have the highest yield of significant information. Yet the history in station examinations is often elicited from a form that the athlete's parents are required to fill out in advance. Anyone who has ever performed these physical examinations is well aware that these forms are often not filled out adequately (especially when a student has chosen to bypass the parents). Therefore, it is crucial that the history station include an actual questioning of the athlete.

Time constraints usually prohibit the history from being reviewed, so it is suggested that the personnel at this station be trained to spot-check the histories. It is often a good idea, for example, to ask a question in a different way than asked on the form itself. In addition, it is wise to focus on questions that may have particular relevance to a given sport (e.g., questions about previous head trauma would be considered crucial in contact/collision sports). In Table 18.2, sports are listed by classification that is used in the establishment of clearances for athletes. It should also be noted that current guidelines for items to incorporate into a PPE history form include the following: personal and family medical history, orthopedic history, exercise-induced bronchospasm history (34), and questions about any current medications, allergies, last tetanus vaccination, and use of any orthotic appliances such as temporomandibular joint (TMJ) splints, retainers, contact lenses, or other items (31).

If the baseline medical evaluation has not been performed previously, stations 3 through 7 will provide this evaluation. In addition to standard vital signs, height and weight will provide useful baseline information for competition in various sports and will establish potential dehydration status in the athlete. The need for a minimal testing for visual acuity is self-explanatory. The visual instrumentation of ears, eyes, nose, and throat are performed in a standard manner; in many a dental examination should be included. Kibler

Table 18.1.   Example of Possible Organization of Stations for Preparticipation Physical Examination

Station	Required Tasks
1	Registration
2	History taking, questioning on all positive responses, spot-checking negative responses
3	Vital signs (pulse, respiration, blood pressure, height, weight)
4	Visual acuity (Snellen chart)
5	Ears, eyes, nose, throat (visual instrumentation)
6	Heart and lung auscultation
7	Abdomen and hernia (palpatory examination), Tanner staging
8–?	Musculoskeletal examination (dependent activity or degree of screening)
Final	Summary station (qualified personnel to check correlation among areas of information)

Table 18.2.   Classification of Sports

Contact/Collision	Limited Contact/Impact	Strenuous Noncontact	Moderately Strenuous Noncontact	Nonstrenuous Noncontact
Boxing	Baseball	Aerobic dancing	Badminton	Archery
Field hockey	Basketball	Crew	Curling	Golf
Football	Bicycling	Fencing	Table tennis	Riflery
Ice hockey	Diving	Field		
Lacrosse	Field	Discus		
Martial arts	High jump	Javelin		
Rodeo	Pole vault	Shot put		
Soccer	Gymnastics	Running		
Wrestling	Horseback riding	Swimming		
	Skating	Tennis		
	Ice	Track		
	Roller	Weight lifting		
	Skiing			
	Cross-country			
	Downhill			
	Water			
	Softball			
	Squash, handball			
	Volleyball			

Reprinted with permission from Pediatrics May 1988;81(5). Copyright 1988, American Academy of Pediatrics.

(34) recommends that one even use a dentist with an interest in sports medicine. Heart and lung auscultation should focus on the possibility of heart murmurs, extra heart sounds, and obstructive respiratory conditions such as asthma.

The abdominal examination should focus on finding organomegaly, as well as any other masses, and should include a hernia check. To yield more accurate results, care should be taken to ensure the proper modification of the examination environment. For example, a quiet area is essential for auscultation, privacy is imperative for abdominal and hernia examinations, and a darkened area aids in eye instrumentation.

The abdominal and hernia examination station is an ideal time at which to note and record the Tanner rating of the athlete. Although still notably absent on many PPE forms (26), this item provides useful data. It also provides valuable information for counseling an athlete about choosing an appropriate sport or even deferring entry into a particular competition level until further development is achieved. At least one state has proposed guidelines for restricting children below a Tanner 3 rating from participating in collision sports (36). Also, recently published recommendations about strength training by children and adolescents have warned against power lifting and repetitive use of maximal amounts of weight in anyone below a Tanner rating of 5 (37). It is, therefore, recommended that the physician make a note of the Tanner rating, even if paperwork in a particular situation does not require it.

LABORATORY WORK

Many schools and competitive organizations also require the PPE to include some form of laboratory analysis. Most common is the inclusion of the dipstick urinalysis, although complete blood counts (CBC), hemoglobin, and/or hematocrit values may also be required. Although several authors (32, 38) have stated that there is little benefit from performing blood tests and urinalysis in a PPE performed on children and adolescents, many groups continue to maintain that certain inexpensive and easily performed laboratory tests such as the dipstick urinalysis may be of some help (34). It may also be a good idea to screen young female athletes in sports that emphasize thinness for the presence of iron deficiency anemia.

THE MUSCULOSKELETAL EXAMINATION

If the only goal of a PPE was to elicit negative information that prohibits, modifies, or delays participation in a sport, then the usual yield of information hovers around 1.5% (27). However, if one adds the goal of delineation of positive information to decrease injury risk and increase performance, at least one study has estimated that the yield of significant information rises to 55 to 80% (30, 32). It is the musculoskeletal portion of the examination that provides the most significant proportion of findings of this type and therefore dictates that particular attention should be paid to this portion of the examination. Although there are many different interpretations for what should be included in the general musculoskeletal examination, most authors agree on the following items: range of motion of the major paired joints, strength of major muscle groups, spinal posture (scoliosis check), alignment of all major extremity joints, stability of shoulders and knees, and cursory evaluation of gait.

Whereas the above scenario has been used for many years, a greater emphasis has recently been placed on the development of a sports-specific musculoskeletal evaluation. Such an evaluation can help to increase the yield of significant information obtained during a PPE. In addition, the development of such an examination will allow the physician to identify predisposing factors to injury and possibly "prehabilitate" them. Kibler (34) has created a system of construction of sports-specific evaluations that can ultimately identify those parameters that need to be developed for optimal sports performance for the athlete.

Table 18.3. Parameter Rating Scale, Based on the Relative Importance of a Parameter to a Specific Sport

Rating	Need
4	Maximally required for optimum performance (e.g., aerobic endurance in running, strength in football)
3	Synergistic for optimum performance (e.g., flexibility in basketball, power in tennis)
2	Necessary for injury reduction (e.g., strength in tennis, aerobic endurance in football)
1	Minimally needed (e.g., aerobic endurance in golf)

Reprinted with permission from Kibler WB. The sports preparticipation fitness examination. Champaign, IL: Human Kinetics, 1990.

Table 18.4. Sports Profiles, Based on Application of the Parameter Rating Scale (Table 18.3) to Some Common Sports

Sport	Flexibility	Strength	Power	Anaerobic Endurance	Aerobic Endurance
Football	3	4	4	3	2
Halfbacks	3	4	4	4	3
Basketball	3	3	4	4	4
Baseball	3	3	4	4	2
Tennis	4	2	3	4	3
Swimming	4	4	2	2	4
Sprinting	4	4	2	4	2
Long-distance running	3	2	2	2	4
Sprinting	3	3	3	4	2
Golf	3	4	4	2	1
Soccer	3	2	3	4	4
Bicycling	3	3	4	3	4
Ice skating	3	2	4	3	4
Skiing	3	3	4	3	2
Volleyball	3	2	4	4	2
Cheerleading	3	3	4	2	2

Reprinted with permission from Kibler WB. The sports preparticipation fitness examination. Champaign, IL: Human Kinetics, 1990.

Table 18.5. Tests Often Used to Evaluate the Five Basic Sports Parameters

Parameter	Test
Flexibility	Sit-and-reach exam of lower back
	Goniometric exam of the following:
	Shoulder internal/external rotation
	Shoulder flexion/extension
	Elbow flexion/extension
	Wrist flexion/extension
	Hip flexion/extension
	Hip internal/external rotation
	Knee flexion (quadriceps flexibility)
	Knee extension (hamstring flexibility)
	Iliotibial band flexibility
	Gastrocnemius flexibility
Strength	Sit-ups
	Push-ups
	Handgrip dynamometer
	One repetition squat
	Dips
	Cybex exam peak torque
Power	Cybex exam time to peak torque
	Vertical jump
	Medicine ball throw
Anaerobic endurance	Jumping jacks in 1 minute
	40- or 20-yard dash
	Shuttle run
	Hexagon drill
	Sit-ups in 1 minute
Aerobic endurance	Step test
	Timed mile run
	Submaximal treadmill or bicycle stress test

Reprinted with permission from Kibler WB. The sports preparticipation fitness examination. Champaign, IL: Human Kinetics, 1990.

This type of sports-specific examination will allow, in some measure, the separation of extrinsic factors that affect injury potential (such as rules of a sport, equipment, and environmental conditions) from intrinsic factors (39), which are potentially modifiable. Kibler (34) uses characteristics of muscles to develop five parameters that can serve as the basic intrinsic factors to evaluate in a sports-specific examination. These five parameters are flexibility, strength, power, anaerobic endurance, and aerobic endurance.

He then establishes a rating scale for these parameters that ranks a parameter's relative importance to either performance or injury reduction (Table 18.3). He then creates a profile for each sport that ranks the importance of each of the five parameters for that particular activity (Table 18.4). Finally, he lists various tests that are generally used to evaluate each parameter (Table 18.5). This elegant system allows an examiner to design a musculoskeletal PPE that is specific to a given sport. For example, in football, which carries a profile from the listed tables of 3, 4, 4, 3, and 2 for the five parameters (34), only a few flexibility tests will be used and they will concentrate on the risk areas of shoulder, back, knees, and ankles. Strength and power assessments will incorporate all listed tests because of their relative importance. Aerobic endurance, because it is less important in football, will be evaluated with only one test. Some of the tests described in the Kibler system are pictured in this text (Figs. 18.2 and 18.3). However, the reader who desires more detailed information about this excellent evaluation system, as well as a listing of normal values for many of the assessments, is referred to the original text that outlines this system (34). Ultimately, the physician has the opportunity (perhaps especially by relegating the baseline medical evaluation to a prior physician–patient encounter as mentioned previously) to obtain an evaluation that truly considers the interaction between an athlete's capability and the demands of a sport.

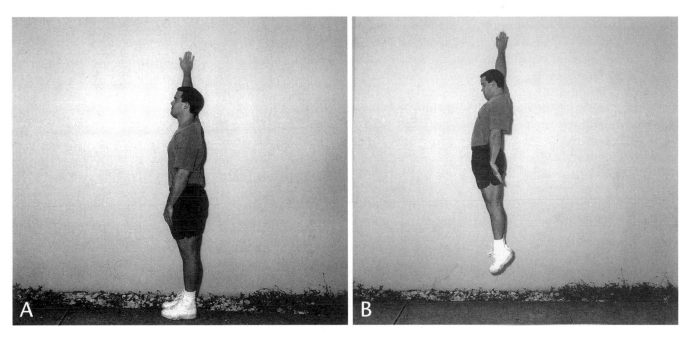

Figure 18.2. A. Vertical jump, starting position. **B.** Vertical jump measurement. The athlete may touch a tape attached to a wall, or use a piece of chalk to mark the starting position and highest position reached.

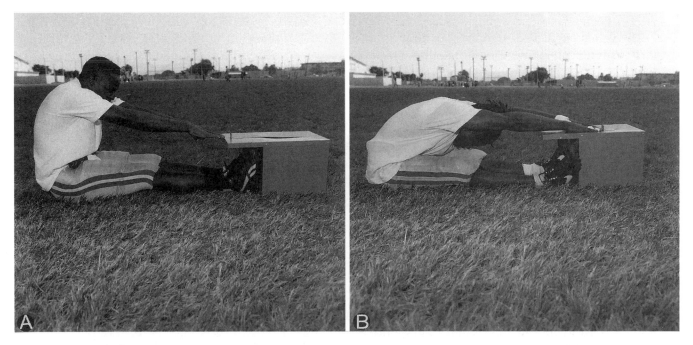

Figure 18.3. The sit-and-reach test for lower back flexibility. **A.** The feet are against the box, and the knees are straight. **B.** The athlete flexes forward as far as possible.

THE SUMMARY STATION

The final station of a good PPE will provide more than just a place to drop off paperwork and make sure that the young athlete visited all the stations. This station should be staffed by one or several physicians, whose job it is to peruse the findings from the individual stations and attempt to correlate any significant findings. This physician should then render an assessment of the findings and record this, along with specific recommendations for items such as additional consultations, stretching, strengthening, weight reduction or increase, or alternate activities should a blanket clearance be inappropriate. Failure to correlate the sometimes fragmented information from the various stations into identifiable problems and—it is hoped—some identifiable solutions, can not only lead to missed diagnoses, but also help to perpetuate the somewhat antagonistic view that young athletes often develop toward the whole PPE system. The physicians who engage in these examinations are, after all, a potential obstacle between the athlete and participation; any physician who becomes involved in planning and executing PPE would do well to remain mindful of this fact.

CLEARANCES FOR ACTIVITY

McKeag (31) has identified four basic categories of clearance that are available to the physician at the conclusion of a PPE.

1. Clearance without limitation for sports and level desired.
2. Clearance deferred pending consultation, treatment, equipment, fitting, or rehabilitation.
3. Clearance with limitation to include medical recommendation for an alternative sport.
4. Disqualification from any sport.

The physician is limited by standards for exclusion from participation that are revised by the Academy of Pediatrics approximately every 10 years (Table 18.6). However, great care should be taken not to create a situation in which an athlete is needlessly excluded from any athletic activity. Every attempt to allow young athletes to find something that they can participate in safely should be made, and level 4 clearances should be a rare exception. Clearances that include limitations should be discussed with parents and coaches whenever possible, and all appropriate personnel should be advised of recommendations made even in those cases in which no significant limitation is imposed. Such personnel might again include parents, coaches, primary care physicians, school nurses, and team physicians (27, 30, 32).

LEGAL CONSIDERATIONS

Kibler has suggested the following protection for a physician involved in organizing and performing PPE (34).

1. A letter sent to parents/guardians that explains the attached medical history form and the screening nature of the examination to be performed.
2. A parental or personal consent form giving the testers the authority to perform all aspects of all examinations and stating the minimal risk associated with the examinations themselves. This form should also attest to the confidentiality of discovered information and have a space for authorization of release of such information to appropriate personnel such as coaches or school representatives.
3. A contract with the institution or group for which the physician is performing these examinations, which spells out the relationship among the sponsoring organization, athletes, and testing organization.

Following these basic guidelines and carefully documenting all examinations should minimize the risk of litigation in the preparticipation examination environment. Although the screening nature of such examinations is well known, the sensitivity should always be high enough to discover underlying medical abnormalities.

THE SPECIAL OLYMPICS

In the past several years, more physicians have been involved in the preparticipation screenings of competitors in the Special Olympics (Fig. 18.4). Although the yield of negative information from PPE performed in nondisabled school-aged populations has been shown to be low, the yield of sports-significant abnormalities in Special Olympics participants has been documented as high as 39% (40). The most common problems involve atlantoaxial instability (especially in individuals with Down syndrome), orthopedic disorders, and cardiac lesions.

Orthopedic disorders seen in this group include a higher than average incidence of patellar instability, metatarsus primus varus, hallux varus or valgus, scoliosis, pes planus, and slipped capital femoral epiphysis. Cardiac problems include ventricular septal defect (VSD) and endocardial cush-

Table 18.6.   Recommendations for Participation in Competitive Sports

	Contact/ Collision	Limited Contact/ Impact	Strenuous Noncontact	Moderately Strenuous Noncontact	Nonstrenuous Noncontact
Atlantoaxial instability	No	No	Yes*	Yes	Yes
*Swimming: no butterfly, breaststroke, or diving starts					
Acute illnesses	*	*	*	*	*
*Needs individual assessment, eg, contagiousness to others, risk of worsening illness					
Cardiovascular					
Carditis	No	No	No	No	No
Hypertension					
Mild	Yes	Yes	Yes	Yes	Yes
Moderate		*	*	*	*
Severe	*	*	*	*	*
Congenital heart disease	†	†	†	†	†
*Needs individual assessment					
†Patients with mild forms can be allowed a full range of physical activities; patients with moderate or severe forms, or who are postoperative, should be evaluated by a cardiologist before athletic participation					
Eyes					
Absence or loss of function in one eye	*	*	*	*	*
Detached retina	†	†	†	†	†
*Availability of eye guards approved by the American Society for Testing and Materials may allow competitor to participate in most sports, but this must be judged on an individual basis					
†Consult ophthalmologist					
Inguinal hernia	Yes	Yes	Yes	Yes	Yes
Kidney: Absence of one	No	Yes	Yes	Yes	Yes
Liver: Enlarged	No	No	Yes	Yes	Yes
Musculoskeletal disorders	*	*	*	*	*
*Needs individual assessment.					
Neurologic					
History of serious head or spine trauma, repeated concussions, or craniotomy	*	*	Yes	Yes	Yes
Convulsive disorder					
Well controlled	Yes	Yes	Yes	Yes	Yes
Poorly controlled	No	No	Yes†	Yes	Yes‡
*Needs individual assessment					
†No swimming or weight lifting					
‡No archery or riflery					
Ovary: Absence of one	Yes	Yes	Yes	Yes	Yes
Respiratory					
Pulmonary insufficiency	*	*	*	*	Yes
Asthma	Yes	Yes	Yes	Yes	Yes
*May be allowed to compete if oxygenation remains satisfactory during a graded stress test					
Sickle cell trait	Yes	Yes	Yes	Yes	Yes
Skin: Boils, herpes, impetigo, scabies	*	*	Yes	Yes	Yes
*No gymnastics with mats, martial arts, wrestling, or contact sports until not contagious					
Spleen: Enlarged	No	No	No	Yes	Yes
Testicle: Absent or undescended	Yes*	Yes*	Yes	Yes	Yes
*Certain sports may require protective cup					

Reprinted with permission from Pediatrics May 1988;81(5). Copyright 1988, American Adacemy of Pediatrics.

ion defects. Therefore, a very careful orthopedic examination, preferably by a single examiner, and a careful auscultation for heart murmurs are essential (40).

In addition, radiographic screening of all children who have Down syndrome, beginning at age 5 to 6, is currently recommended by the AAP (41). This screening involves neutral lateral, flexion, and extension views of the cervical spine. A fixed transition gap (between the odontoid process and anterior arch of the atlas) greater than 4.5 mm is considered to warrant a diagnosis of atlantoaxial

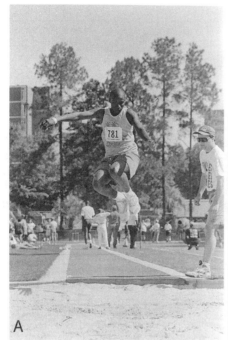
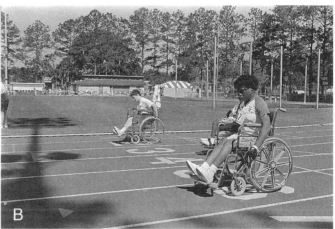

Figure 18.4. A and B. The Special Olympics bring the joy and gratification of athletic activity to a variety of physically and mentally challenged athletes. A preparticipation examination for these athletes brings special challenges.

instability (42). Current Special Olympics policies do permit an athlete with subluxation of the atlantoaxial joint to participate in noncontact sports, if the abnormality is documented and the parents or guardians are made aware of the condition (43). These important considerations dictate an especially cautious and thorough approach to this population of special athletes.

Physical Conditioning of the Young Athlete

Physical conditioning has been related to both sports performance and injury prevention in much of the literature regarding the adult athlete. General consensus in the literature reflects the emerging belief that physical conditioning of the young athlete is just as important as it is in the adult, both from the standpoint of fitness and in terms of improved performance and lessened chance of injury. It has been speculated, for example, that the increased injury rate sometimes seen in adolescent girls when they begin involvement in competitive sports is related to a lack of conditioning relative to that seen in most adolescent boys (44). This speculation centers around the socialized gender differences and the emphasis put on exercise for younger children (45). However, lessening of gender differences in injury rates has been noted when elite male and female athletes are compared (46).

If one is to make recommendations for conditioning in pediatric and adolescent athletes, one must first take a closer look at several issues raised by the inherent physical and developmental differences in this age-group. It must be determined whether conditioning can have a positive effect, and whether exercises used for conditioning have a potential deleterious effect.

Pate and Fox (47) have identified three key variables in children's responses to conditioning principles, the first of which is initial fitness level. Children tend to be closer to their physiologically attainable values for aerobic endurance and therefore can be expected to be less responsive in an absolute sense to endurance training. It is unknown whether this is also true for strength and flexibility parameters.

The second variable is that of growth and developmental stage of the child. Ongoing processes of growth and development can alter training responses. For example, prepubescent children are less responsive to strength training than postpubescent children. In addition, heavy training may pose some risk of injury for the growing child. Stanitski (48) has found that during the time when an adolescent is at a Tanner 3 maturational rating, strength at the epiphyses is decreased, causing significant increase in the risk of injury. The growth spurts characteristic of this developmental stage lead to decreased flexibility and relative strength, both of which add potential factors for injury. In general, conditioning and fitness parameters such as strength and flexibility seem to be better correlated with maturational age (Tanner rating) than with chronologic age (49).

The third variable mentioned by Pate and Fox (47) is the psychological immaturity of the typical child when compared with the average adult. This may make the young athlete less capable of tolerating the stress that accompanies high-level conditioning programs for elite sports performance.

The aforementioned variables notwithstanding, it has been shown that physical conditioning of youths positively affects physical fitness, aerobic endurance and strength capacity, and even auditory and visual reaction times (50–52). Therefore, it becomes important to have an understanding of the effects and guidelines for the implementation of the various parameters involved in physical conditioning. Although numerous authors have established general guidelines for conditioning and exercise (47, 53–56), a separate discussion of each major parameter will help to define better the appropriate conditioning goals.

ENDURANCE

Several authors have established that, despite the high relative initial fitness levels found in youths, aerobic endurance training can achieve increases in both absolute and relative maximal oxygen uptake ($\dot{V}o_2$max) values (57, 58). Ventilatory threshold (or anaerobic threshold) has also been shown to increase with training (58, 59). In addition, this improvement seems to be somewhat independent of whether continuous or interval training is used as the primary stimulus (60). Unfortunately, the types of exercise often recommended for endurance conditioning, coupled with the ability of the child to respond positively to such training, sometimes lead to increased risk of injury, particularly if the training is excessive. Overuse injuries have been cited as a significant problem in endurance training to excess (61) and include epiphyseal injuries, stress fractures, patellofemoral pain syndromes, and chronic tendinitis. The AAP has also cited thermal injuries as risks in this type of training (56). This is due to the child's decreased efficiency at maintaining thermal homeostasis, particularly at extremes of temperature. In addition, Stager et al. and others (56, 62) have associated delayed menarche in adolescent girls with excessive endurance training.

Given the potential positive effects of endurance training, it becomes necessary to prescribe training that will avoid the obvious risks of excessive stress on the growing body. Pate and Fox (47) have made the following recommendations.

1. Endurance training programs for children should begin at low levels of frequency, duration, and intensity and should emphasize the enjoyable aspects of the activity.
2. Very gradual incremental increases in training are the rule; abrupt increases and large exercise doses should be avoided.
3. Total dose of exercise should be kept well below the level that might be applied to mature persons. This is to protect against adverse psychological and physiologic effects.

An example of the third point above can be seen in the recommendations of Micheli (63) and others with regard to distance running. Micheli states that prepubescent children should be limited to distances of 5 km in competition and training, whereas pubescent children should be limited to 10-km distances. McKeag (54) has added the recommendation that frequency be kept to between 3 and 5 times a week for training, and that training should be carried out between 70% and 90% of maximum heart rate.

FLEXIBILITY

The relationship of flexibility to sports performance and injury prevention has been documented in the literature. The best means of attaining such flexibility have been the subject of significant controversy. However, the relationship of flexibility to sports performance and injury has recently been explored in the specific realm of the youthful athlete. Klemp and Chalton (64) have shown that flexibility is at least partly acquired through training in this age group. This acquired flexibility is often sports specific, as in the study of junior elite tennis players by Chandler et al. (65). Their findings suggested a need for sports-specific flexibility programs to promote maximum performance and to help prevent flexibility-related injuries. In addition, Smith et al. (66) found that flexibility in adolescent elite figure skaters was actually related to the incidence of reported knee pain. In their study, improved flexibility through training lowered the incidence of knee pain; the participants in the study who lost flexibility showed an increase in reported knee complaints.

Micheli (63) has stated that early incorporation of flexibility training for children will assist in the ability to remain flexible. This is particularly important because the altered bone to muscle strength growth ratios will often render the body least flexible during a growth spurt (67, 68). Inflexibility has been implicated in the causation of overuse injuries and the more traditionally recognized musculotendinous injuries (63).

Although a significant controversy exists about the types of stretching that work best to create maximum flexibility, agreement seems to have been reached on the following recommended criteria (63).

1. Muscle stretching should be specific. The child should know where the stretch is supposed to be felt and what is being stretched.
2. The stretch should be performed slowly and gradually with attempts to allow the muscle to relax. Ballistic movements are to be avoided.
3. There should be no pain during the stretch. Children must be taught to distinguish between pain and the sensation of stretching.
4. The low back should always be protected from hyperextension during stretching exercises. (This may not be the case when the exercise is specifically for the low back.)
5. Only warm muscles should be stretched, both to avoid injury and to render stretching more effective. Muscles can be warmed up by intervals of low-intensity continuous activity.

Strength

Because of the automatic association that is made between strength training and terms such as weight lifting, power lifting, and body building, there has been much confusion and controversy surrounding the issue of strength training for children and adolescents. For a long time, strength training in this age group was generally discouraged, due to the perceived risk of injury from weight lifting and also due to the belief that children (especially prepubescent) could not achieve significant strength gains because of their lack of androgenic hormones (69). More recently, the consensus on this issue has been modified significantly, especially in light of the recent data on lack of fitness and conditioning in our youth. Numerous authors have now reported the finding that resistance training for strength has consistently resulted in significant increases in muscle strength in the prepubescent and adolescent age group (31, 53, 55, 69, 70). Supervised strength training programs have been shown to have a low incidence of injury (53, 71) and have positive effects on flexibility and motor performance.

Fripp and Hodgson (72) have also reported favorable alterations in high-density lipoprotein/low-density lipoprotein (HDL/LDL) ratios with resistance training in adolescents. This is not to say that the risk of injury does not exist for children participating in such training programs. Both overuse and acute injuries have been re-

ported to occur, with axial loading being by far the most common mechanism of injury (52). However, both the AAP and the National Strength and Conditioning Association have issued guidelines for involving youths in strength training, which should help to eliminate any inordinate risk of such injury. A summary of these guidelines is as follows.

1. All issued guidelines have in common the requirement for adequate supervision and training of the supervising personnel.
2. Starting age for training seems to be less important than the correlation of training program construction to the maturational age of the participant and the emotional maturity required for participating in such a program under supervision.
3. Strength training is defined as progressive resistance training using weight training principles, such as weights, the person's own body weight, machines, elastic tubing, or other devices. It is specifically not defined as using weight lifting or power lifting techniques, which imply the use of maximum lifting ability of specific weights in specific exercises (55).
4. The AAP has specifically stated that children and adolescents should avoid the practice of weight lifting or power lifting and body building, as well as the repetitive use of maximal weights in strength training programs, until they have reached Tanner stage 5 of developmental maturity (37). (This level is reached at a mean age of 15 in both genders, but significant variation does occur.)
5. Children should not participate in any strength training program without a preparticipation examination, which focuses on identifying those body areas that may need rehabilitation (52). Areas to especially consider for such evaluation, owing to their lag in development, are the shoulder, abdominal wall, and trunk muscles (73).
6. For optimum injury prevention with optimum gains, resistance training should be submaximal and composed of combined strength and muscular endurance exercises with a strong emphasis on form over quantity (52).

INJURIES IN YOUNG ATHLETES

Incidence

Sports are an integral part of life for U.S. children. By participating in recreational activities, organized youth leagues, and interscholastic sports, children obtain both enjoyment and the health benefits of regular exercise. Currently, more than 40 million children and adolescents participate in community-based athletic programs and more than 6 million are involved in high school sports (10, 74, 75).

Unfortunately, participation in athletics entails risk of injury. The National Electronic Injury Surveillance System (NEISS) has shown annually that 1 of every 14 teenagers requires hospital treatment of a sports-related injury (76). Of the millions of children participating in sports programs each year, 3 to 11% will be injured (26). Goldberg (74) found that injury rates by grade level in school were 3% for elementary school, 7% for junior high school, and 11% for high school. Boys sustained 67% of the injuries. However, other studies have shown that injuries to girls are on the rise, particularly with involvement in gymnastics and coed sports such as soccer (77). For both sexes, the most common areas injured were the knee and ankle, with sprains/strains and contusions being the most common injuries (77–79).

The highest injury rates in organized sports were seen in football, basketball, baseball, soccer, and wrestling. Injuries were also seen in soccer, field hockey, gymnastics, baseball, and track and running sports (74, 77, 78, 80–82). High injury rates sustained on playground equipment and activities cannot be ignored either (83). The factors that contributed most frequently to injury were recklessness on the part of the injured party, falling down in particular, and foul or illegal play by another player (82, 84).

SPORT-SPECIFIC PATTERNS

Epidemiologic studies show that different sports pose different types and degrees of risk and injury (74, 77, 78, 80, 84).

Football Injuries

These injuries occur primarily because football is a collision sport. Injuries arise primarily from forces generated at the time of contact. The injury experience among preadolescent players is significantly different from that of high school players. Whereas the overall injury rate with youths is approximately 15%, it ranges from 25 to 65% with high school players (74). The body parts most commonly injured are the knee, ankle, thigh, neck, and shoulder (74, 81). Sprains, strains, and contusions are the most common types of injury, with epiphyseal fractures accounting for 3% of youth football injuries (74).

Baseball Injuries

Baseball exposes players to the risk of traumatic collision injuries and microtraumatic overuse problems. Overuse problems caused by repetitive throwing most often result in the condition known as Little League elbow (85, 86). Because of the nature of throwing a baseball hard, especially by pitchers, the arm is put through unusual repetitive strain at the shoulder, wrist, and elbow. The throwing mechanism puts tremendous compression forces across the lateral side of the elbow joint and tension forces across the medial side of the joint (87–89). Damage to the medial joint produces chronic apophyseal injury presenting as aching pain, tenderness, and swelling. Radiographically, fragmentation or separation of the apophysis may be seen. On the lateral side, osteochondritic lesions of the capitellum and/or radial head occur. Treatment consists of rest and cessation of pitching, followed by gradual resumption of activity. Due to the potential of chronic pathologic conditions of the baseball player, the National Little League Administration has put an emphasis on controlling the types of pitches thrown and on restricting the number of innings pitched per week (85).

Basketball Injuries

Basketball, both interscholastic and recreational, is one of the most popular sports among children. It is also one of the top four injury-causing sports (83). A 10% injury rate among children on organized school teams has been reported. The areas most frequently injured are in the lower extremity at the ankle, knee, and leg, with ankle sprains being the most common. Boys sustained a greater number of shoulder injuries, and girls sustained a greater number of knee injuries (74).

Soccer Injuries

Soccer is the most popular sport in the world, with more than 22 million individuals participating annually (90). Soccer has emerged in the United States as the fastest growing team sport. Approximately 1.6 million children and adolescents participate in leagues and 220,000 participate in high school programs (Fig. 18.5) (74). Most injuries are caused by direct contact with a player, the ball, or the ground. Several studies have reported that the younger soccer player has a lower incidence of injury compared with the older youth (90, 91). Contusions are the most frequent injury with the ankle, knee, and shin being the most common sites. Among older players,

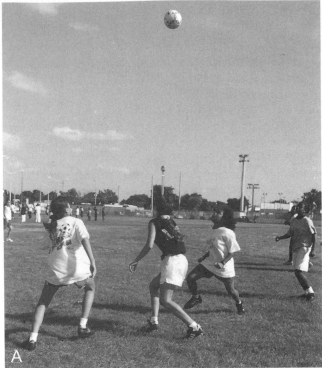

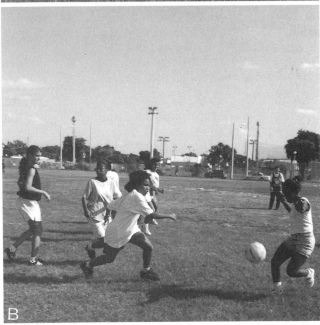

Figure 18.5. A and B. Soccer represents one of the premier recreational sports available to young athletes.

overuse injuries and internal knee derangement syndromes are prevalent (74, 90). With younger players, head and upper extremity injuries are more common (90).

Gymnastics Injuries

Gymnastics has experienced a tremendous growth in participation. In the past decade, women's gymnastics has become the fastest growing individual sport in the United States (92). This sport has experienced an increase of almost 500% in interscholastic participants between 1974 and 1980 (93, 94). Since 1980, the number of clubs has increased and thus the number of young participants. The trend of earlier participation has been accompanied by increased levels of training. Increased involvement at an early age with the extreme training intensity required has led to a concomitant increase in the risk of injury. There is also a growing body of evidence that has suggested that the process of growth through puberty renders the female gymnast more susceptible to injury than the postpubescent athlete, who characterized the elite level of this sport in the past (93). It has been found that gymnastic injury rates are consistently approaching those of football and wrestling (74, 92). The risk of injury has also appeared to be proportional to the athlete's level of skill (92).

Floor exercise/tumbling has been reported as the event with the greatest number of injuries, with the balance beam and uneven parallel bars second in frequency of injury. There is a broad distribution of injuries that involve the lower extremity most frequently, as well as upper extremity, spine, and head. Sprains, strains, contusions, and fractures occur most commonly. Approximately half of these injuries are acute and half are overuse syndromes (74). Certain injuries appear to be unique to gymnastics. The evidence of spondylolysis of the lumbar region is 4 times greater than would be expected in the general population (74). The stress placed on the spine in hyperextension maneuvers appears to be the mechanism of injury. Fractures and dislocations of the elbow, stress fractures of the distal radial epiphysis, and wrist sprain syndromes occur frequently because of the upper extremity being used for weight bearing (74, 94, 95). The sprained/strained ankle is the most frequent injury (93). The most common knee injury is inflammation of the patellofemoral articulation (74). There has been much concern expressed in the gymnastics arena because of unusually high reinjury rates, which may point to a need for complete rehabilitation before return to full participation (93).

Wrestling Injuries

Injury rates of 23 to 75% have been reported among high school wrestlers (74). Injuries are most commonly caused by the direct blows of an opponent, friction from hitting the mat, falls, and twisting and leverage forces during maneuvers (96). Sprains and strains are the most common injuries. Injuries appear to be equally distributed among the upper extremity, lower extremity, spine, and trunk (74). Spinal strains, acromioclavicular sprains, shoulder dislocations, and knee sprains are common injuries (96). In one study, wrestling was second only to football as a cause of knee injuries requiring surgery (97). With the requirements of headgear, rules prohibiting slams, and new mat surfaces, the incidence of mat abrasions, cauliflower ears, and severe neck injuries has decreased in frequency (97).

Mechanical/Traumatic Back Pain in Children

Complaints of back pain are relatively uncommon but highly significant in the pediatric age group (98, 99). In many cases of pediatric back pain, subtle clinical signs and symptoms may be due to major pathology. A complete history and physical examination are the initial steps in evaluating a child with back pain. Several characteristics of pain must be specifically sought. The mode of onset is important. An acute, posttraumatic pain episode must be distinguished from pain gradually increasing in severity. Pain that occurs suddenly after trauma suggests strain/sprain, dislocation, fracture, and/or mechanical injury. Overuse injuries that occur secondary to repetitive unrepaired microtrauma are also common in children and may affect the back. Mild soft tissue and ligamentous injuries may lead to acute episodes of back pain that can be self-limiting, may resolve in 2 to 3 weeks, and must be differentiated from more serious injury.

NATURE, DURATION, AND SEVERITY OF PAIN

The nature, duration, and severity of pain are the next important part of history taking. Is it constant or intermittent? Is it localized or does it radiate into the legs? A cough or sneeze may aggravate the pain of intraspinal pathology. Any associated systemic symptoms should be sought. Any specific neurologic changes should be noted. A change in bowel or bladder habits suggests intraspinal pathology. A change in gait pattern, muscle use, or foot deformity and/or foot weakness should all elevate the doctor's level of suspicion regarding the possibility of a progressive neurologic process involving the spine. Most children are extremely active and rarely suffer the postexercise muscle strain seen so frequently in adults. However, occasionally a child who has recently started a very active and high-level competitive sport will present with pain of muscular origin. The widespread participation in athletics by young people may result in pain more charac-

teristic and secondary to overuse syndromes owing to repeated unrepaired microtrauma. This frequently results from incorrect technique or excessively rapid advances in activity without proper conditioning. The diagnosis is usually made based on history and examination; however, if pain does not resolve or if it recurs, other causes must be pursued carefully (100).

Mechanical or spondylogenic causes of back pain are most common and regularly treated by the chiropractic physician. The adolescent athlete with mechanical low back pain (for treatment of low back pain, see Chapter 9) will be managed similar to the adult athlete. Potentially more serious infective, metabolic, and neoplastic conditions must be considered as well (101).

Discitis presumably has an infectious cause. It most commonly occurs in children younger than 10 years of age; the average age is 6 (102). Symptoms include nonradiating back pain, refusal to walk or crawl, anorexia, irritability, and malaise. Blood cultures are usually normal; erythrocyte sedimentation rate may be elevated, but white blood count may be normal. Cultures of biopsy material from the involved disc are positive in only approximately 25% of cases. The most commonly demonstrated growth is *Staphylococcus aureus.* A complete imaging evaluation of these children, including radionuclide bone scanning and magnetic resonance imaging (MRI), is often necessary to make the diagnosis because plain film radiographs are negative early in the disease (103).

Vertebral osteomyelitis presents clinically in a manner that is similar to discitis although it is usually seen in children older than 10 years of age (98,99). As with discitis, bone scan and MRI are extremely helpful in making a diagnosis long before radiographs become positive. Tumors of the spinal cord are usually slow-growing lesions with often subtle and slowly progressive clinical manifestations. Diagnosis of these neoplasms, therefore, often occurs late in the course of the disease (104). Weakness is the most common presenting complaint, with 25 to 30% of these children having pain as their initial presentation (99).

An aggressive diagnostic approach should be taken when evaluating a child with back pain. Familiarity with the differential diagnosis in back pain in children is essential for proper evaluation.

SPONDYLOLYSIS AND SPONDYLOLISTHESIS

Spondylolysis is a defect in the pars interarticularis of the vertebrae. The defect is most commonly caused by recurrent mechanical stress (repetitive hyperextension) with resultant fracture (105).

Defects in the pars interarticularis are uncommon in children younger than 5 years of age. However, they increase significantly after age 5 and are most often seen between ages 10 and 15 (105). Discerning the mechanism of injury during history taking is extremely important in these cases. Patients generally present with low back pain that is aggravated by activity and relieved by rest. It has been identified that up to 40% of the complaints of low back pain that persist over 3 months in young athletes are due to stress reaction at the lumbar pars interarticularis area. Stress reactions can eventually progress to a defect in the pars interarticularis, leading to stress fracture (106, 107).

Repetitive hyperextension activity—such as with blocking in football, military press in weight training, pole vaulting, diving, pitching in baseball, gymnastics maneuvers, and serving in tennis—have all been cited as common activities that aggravate or precipitate this condition.

Spondylolisthesis traditionally has been described as an anterior slipping of one vertebral segment over another. According to Yochum and Rowe (105), a more precise term for this anatomical disrelationship should be an anterolisthesis with or without the presence of spondylolysis. Spondylolisthesis (anterolisthesis) may occur without a defect in the vertebral arch (nonspondylolytic spondylolisthesis). Approximately 90% of all spondylolisthesis involves the fifth lumbar vertebra. In children, it is almost always the result of bilateral pars defects (105).

Clinical Manifestations

Children with spondylolisthesis will often have distinct postural changes. Buttocks are prominent with the increased lumbar lordosis, and spondylolytic spondylolisthesis reveals a prominence of the spinous process at the affected level. Tightness of the hamstring muscles with a decrease in straight leg raising ability is present and usually symmetrical. A peculiar gait may be present due to tightness of the hamstrings that limits flexion of the hips and shortens the stride length.

Spondylolysis/spondylolisthesis may be found in asymptomatic patients, and in most cases a lesion has been present since the age of 5 or 6 (105).

It is thought by many that by the age of 10, the greatest degree of displacement has already been reached and that progression of displacement seldom occurs after the age of 18. Approximately one half of patients with radiologic signs never have symptoms. Experts believe that a spondylolysis/spondylolisthesis is not the cause of pain but may be related to biomechanical stresses originating from the posterior joints, as in facet syndromes (108).

A child older than 10 years of age with a spondylolysis/spondylolisthesis should be permitted to enjoy normal activity during childhood and adolescence without fear of progressive displacement or disabling pain, unless there is the possibility of a traumatically induced new fracture. Bone scan can rule this out. When spondylolisthesis has been detected in a child younger than 10 years of age, recommendation is limitation of gymnastics and sports activities until a series of flexion/extension upright lumbar views are taken 6 months apart to demonstrate that there is no evidence of progressive displacement or instability in the involved segment. Traction/compression radiography may be substituted for flexion/extension views and is currently thought to be more sensitive (109). Therefore, the existence of these conditions does not justify creating a "spondylo invalid" (105). These adolescents do not need to be restricted from activity in any way and can be allowed to fully participate in sports. Recent studies do not support discouraging these individuals from participation even in rigorous sports. However, those patients who demonstrate biomechanical instability with persistent symptoms warrant further clinical consideration.

SCHEUERMANN'S DISEASE

More than a dozen theories have been proposed to explain Scheuermann's disease. In 1920, Scheuermann postulated that the vertebral wedging seen in this condition was secondary to avascular necrosis of the cartilage ring apophysis. A more recent hypothesis states that it is a stress spondylodystrophy secondary to minor repeated traumas, which results in traumatic growth arrest and end-plate fractures (110). This typically occurs during the heightened vulnerability phase of the adolescent growth spurt.

This condition is exacerbated by excessive load bearing in youth owing either to overvigorous attempts at mobilization, i.e., gymnastics training, or to the too early acceptance of a heavy weight training program. Generally, it is advisable that loads exceeding the body weight not be accepted as part of a weight training program until after skeletal maturity. The subsequent distortion of the vertebral bodies may predispose these children to degenerative joint disease later in life.

Clinical Manifestations

The adolescent will present with a prominent fixed kyphosis most commonly involving the thoracic spine, with the chief complaint usually being poor posture. Back pain is a dull, nonradiating fatigue type of pain aggravated by periods of activity and promptly relieved by rest or changes in position; it is located primarily at the apex of the kyphosis.

Treatment of a Scheuermann's kyphosis depends on the existence of back pain, neurologic compromise, or cosmetic concerns. Thoracic kyphosis of less than 50° is rarely symptomatic or of cosmetic concern. When the kyphosis exceeds 50°, however, young patients may complain of back pain and may have compensatory hyperlordosis of the lumbar spine and cervical spine (111). Adolescent athletes with Scheuermann's disease may participate in many sports activities including contact sports, so long as they are not symptomatic or currently being treated through the use of bracing.

DISCOGENIC LOW BACK PAIN

Discogenic low back pain is rare in prepubescent children, but its prevalence in athletic adolescents appears to be increasing (112). There is often a preceding history of trauma. Herniated discs in adolescents have also shown a high prevalence (19%) of an associated fracture with the vertebral end-plate. This occurs because the ring apophysis does not fuse to its adjacent vertebrae until 18 years of age, and an associated avulsion fracture of the vertebral end-plate may occur if disc herniation occurs before this fusion (113).

Repetitive unrepaired microtrauma to the spine—as in compressive forces during activities such as running, jumping, and playing contact sports—may lead to an overuse and abuse injury to the immature nucleus pulposus and vertebral bodies of young athletes.

Clinical Manifestations

Almost two thirds of adolescents with a disc herniation will present with a chief complaint of back pain, and one third will present with a chief complaint of sciatica. Back stiffness and hamstring tightness with gait disturbance are common. Significant limitation of straight leg raising is common and often more dramatic in children than adults (112).

SCOLIOSIS

Idiopathic scoliosis is seen in females to males in a ratio of 9:1, with the most rapid changes occurring between the ages of 12 and 16. Scoliosis is a condition that is regularly treated by the chiropractic physician. It is also usually painless.

However, children with scoliosis in whom pain is a prominent presenting complaint should be considered to have another primary condition until diagnosed otherwise. Painful scoliosis may result from persistent muscle spasm caused by an osseous lesion located on one side of a vertebra, neural arch, or posterior end of a rib. The most common causes are osteoid osteoma, benign osteoblastoma, infection, eosinophilic granuloma, and aneurysmal bone cyst.

LOWER AND UPPER EXTREMITY INJURIES

Mechanical Injury

SLIPPED CAPITAL FEMORAL EPIPHYSIS

Slipped capital femoral epiphysis (SCFE) refers to the displacement of the epiphysis of the femoral head and can be considered a special form of the Type I Salter-Harris epiphyseal fracture (114). It most commonly occurs during the adolescent rapid growth period (10 to 15 years of age). Boys are more commonly affected than girls, with the peak incidence in boys occurring at age 13 and in girls at age 12. Blacks are more commonly affected than whites (114, 115).

Initial examination reveals bilateral involvement in approximately one third of patients, but patients with unilateral involvement have little risk of a subsequent slip on the contralateral side. The cause is unclear although various traumatic, inflammatory, and endocrine factors have been proposed (113).

A mechanical onset has been hypothesized. The position of the growth plate of the approximate femur normally changes from horizontal to oblique during preadolescence and adolescence. Weight increase occurring during the adolescent growth spurt puts extra strain on the growth plate. This condition is also characterized by obesity and deficient gonadal development (115). These findings suggest an endocrine basis for the skeletal problem. The major complications are avascular necrosis, chondrolysis, and later degenerative osteoarthritis. With chondrolysis, the articular cartilage degenerates and erodes, and the capsule and synovial membrane become inflamed and fibrotic. This usually develops during or after treatment and may progress to the point that the joint space is nearly obliterated.

Clinical Manifestations

Most children with SCFE present with hip, knee, or thigh pain and a limp. Pain in the thigh and knee is a more common initial presentation than pain in the hip; therefore, a proper orthopedic examination of the hip should be performed in all children with thigh/knee pain (114). Tenderness around the hip will be present. When the slippage is extreme, the gluteus medius is rendered inadequate, and the Trendelenburg test is positive. Severity and onset of symptoms reflect three types of slips.

The most common type is the chronic slip (60% of cases), which can cause persistent pain that refers to the hip or distal knee. In some cases, patients present only with pain in the area of the vastus medialis, and the slip itself is overlooked. Limping pain and loss of hip motion are the usual presenting symptoms. Restricted abduction becomes more pronounced as the slip increases. The most important diagnostic finding is the loss of internal rotation. This is easily detected on examination because, if the hip is flexed, it automatically rolls into external rotation and abduction.

The acute slip (11% of cases) occurs after significant trauma, with a sudden onset of pain severe enough to prevent weight bearing. The young patient usually reports minimal or no previous symptoms.

The acute-on-chronic-slip patient will first experience persistent aching in the hip, thigh, or knee. Sometimes a limp that is a result of a chronic slip will develop. Subsequent trauma, even a minor accident, causes an acute slip superimposed on the chronic. The acute slip is heralded by sudden, severe pain. Treatment of SCFE requires immediate medical attention. Primary goals of treatment are to keep displacement to a minimum, while maintaining a close general range of hip motion and delay the onset of osteoarthritis.

Treatment

In the patient with a chronic slip, bedrest and traction are prescribed before definitive treatment to stabilize the femoral head and maintain hip motion. These measures help reduce the risk of cartilage necrosis. If surgery is indicated, two pins are placed in the femoral neck and head.

For the acute slip, gentle repositioning under anesthesia is attempted to reduce the deformity. Gradual reduction is attempted, and it appears to be safer than the acute manipulative reduction. The most serious complication during reduction is the danger of disrupting blood supply to the femoral head leading to avascular necrosis. Two or three threaded pins are then inserted through the epiphyseal line to secure the reduction. Pinning is the initial treatment of choice for all grades of slip.

Avascular Necrosis

LEGG-CALVÉ-PERTHES DISEASE

Legg-Calvé-Perthes (LCP) disease is an idiopathic avascular necrosis of the epiphysis of the femoral head in the growing child. The disease is more often found in boys than in girls (incidence 5:1) and can occur between the ages of 2 and 12 years, with the average age being 7 (116). The disorder represents a true avascular necrosis of bone; it is self-limited, resolving within 2 to 8 years, and results in a variable degree of deformity (117).

When involvement is bilateral, changes usually appear in one hip at least 1 year earlier than in the other. LCP may be a manifestation of unknown systematic disorder, rather than an isolated abnormality of the hip joint.

Bone age of affected children is typically 1 to 3 years lower than their chronologic age (116). As a consequence, affected children are usually shorter than their peers, with disproportionate growth abnormalities in skeletal growth maturation, and elevated serum levels of somatomedin have also been demonstrated (116).

Clinical Manifestations

Early findings include an antalgic gait, muscle spasm, restricted hip range of motion, atrophy of the proximal thigh, and short stature. Antalgic gait is noticed when the young patient shortens the time of weight bearing on the involved limb during walking to reduce pain or discomfort. Pain from the irritable hip can also cause a reflex inhibition of the hip abductors that results in a positive Trendelenburg test (a common early sign). Previous trauma to the hip is often associated with this condition (117). Initial symptoms are mild and intermittent and consist of pain in the anterior thigh, a limp, or both. Although many children do not complain of pain, on close questioning most admit to mild pain in either the anterior thigh or knee. The onset of pain can be acute or insidious. Because a child's initial symptoms are typically mild, parents frequently do not seek medical attention for several weeks or more after clinical onset.

Treatment

The only justification for treatment is for the prevention of femoral head deformity and secondary osteoarthritis. Until the 1960s, treatment of LCP was complete and prolonged bedrest with or without traction or abduction of the involved limb (116). Currently, management ranges from observation to surgery. If there is no limitation of hip motion and no subluxation of the hip, observation is appropriate for children 6 years or younger. Temporary or periodic bedrest and abduction stretching exercises are then used in conjunction with observation. Bedrest may be necessary during these times, as hip irritability with a temporary decrease in motion occurs during the subchondral fracture and resorption phases. If two or three recurrent episodes of irritability occur, this may indicate the need for 2 to 3 months of nonsurgical containment to reduce the risk of extrusion.

Soft Tissue Injuries

More than 50% of all injuries to young athletes are from contusions, sprains, and strains. Causative factors for soft tissue injuries are muscle tightness, muscle imbalance across an involved joint, previous injury, lack of warm-up, and reckless and illegal play (84, 89). During the adolescent growth spurt, children are particularly predisposed to injury owing to the musculotendinous unit elongating in response to the growth of the long bones (75). Clinical manifestations and treatment of soft tissue injuries are similar to presentation in the adult athlete. Treatment typically includes rest, ice, compression, and elevation (RICE) followed by passive range-of-motion exercises and soft tissue treatment.

Fractures

Although the incidence of soft tissue injuries is high in the young athlete, the doctor must be constantly aware of the tendencies for epiphyseal and apophyseal injuries in individuals with open growth plates. Injury that results in a sprain or strain frequently results in a musculotendinous rupture causing an avulsion of the apophysis in athletes with unfused apophyses. Most commonly, this is seen around the pelvis where ischial tuberosity avulsion may occur at the site of the hamstrings.

APOPHYSEAL INJURIES

Traction epiphyses or apophyses act as an insertion for major muscles but do not contribute to bone growth. The mechanism of injury is either a sudden, violent muscular contraction or an excessive amount of muscle stretch across an open apophysis (sudden deceleration, as in coming to a quick stop or landing from a jump). Injury occurs most often in adolescent athletes between the ages of 14 and 17 and is seen in boys more often than girls (116). Common sites are the anterior/superior iliac spine (origin of sartorius), anterior/inferior iliac spine (rectus femoris), is-

chial tuberosity (hamstrings and adductor magnus), lesser trochanter (iliopsoas), and iliac crest (abdominal oblique muscles) (Fig. 18.6). These injuries are seen particularly in sprinters, runners, and soccer and football players.

Clinical Manifestations

Apophyseal injuries exhibit localized swelling, tenderness, and limitation of motion around the site of the avulsion fracture. The pain may be extreme, and radiographs confirm the diagnosis.

Treatment is primarily conservative and includes the following.

1. Bedrest with appropriate positioning, ice application.
2. The athlete is allowed to increase gradually the exertion on injured musculotendinous unit when pain has subsided.
3. The athlete institutes resistive exercise program when full active range of motion is obtained.
4. When 50% of anticipated strength is achieved, the athlete integrates use of the injured unit with other muscles of the pelvis and lower extremity. At this stage, there is a high risk of reinjury.
5. Only when the athlete has achieved normal strength and function is return to full competitive sports approved. The majority of athletes can be treated successfully and nonoperatively with a guided rehabilitation program.

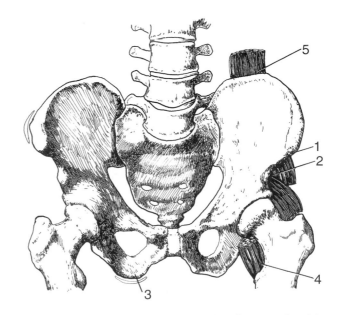

Figure 18.6. The most common sites of apophyseal injury in the adolescent athlete. 1: Anterior/superior iliac spine; 2: anterior/inferior iliac spine; 3: ischial tuberosity; 4: lesser trochanter; 5: iliac crest.

6. Surgical repair with open reduction and internal fixation is advocated only when there is significant displacement of the fragment.

EPIPHYSEAL INJURIES

The young athlete is musculoskeletally unique. The bones of children are in a dynamic state of constant growth and remodeling. Differences in biomechanical properties make fracture less common in children overall, generally occurring after much greater trauma, with the mode of bone failure differing. However, mechanisms of injury that lead almost exclusively to soft tissue injuries in adults may elicit bony deformation in children, due to the altered bone to muscle strength ratios seen during and after growth spurts (63). Torus fractures, greenstick fractures, epiphyseal fracture, and plastic deformation (bowing fractures) of bones are seen in children and adolescents (118). Also, because their bones have not yet matured, young athletes are subject to unique types of injuries to the growth centers of bones consisting of the epiphysis, physis or growth plate, and metaphysis.

From 6 to 18% of sports-related injuries in children are reported to involve the physis (119, 120). Physeal injuries of young athletes can occur from violent forces or through chronic stress. The most frequent occurrence is cited in football and hockey, particularly with a shear-type force from a violent, sudden blow. In noncombative skilled sports such as gymnastics, physeal injury is due to mechanical stresses and recurrent microtrauma.

In skeletally immature children, ligaments have been determined to be 2 to 5 times as strong as the physeal plate (75, 121, 122). Therefore, the physis has been identified as the weakest link in the musculoskeletal system of adolescents. Thus,

a force that causes sprain/strain in the adult may cause epiphyseal damage in the youngster. Due to the possibility of permanent damage to maturing bones, early diagnosis and treatment are essential. If a sprain/strain has not been incurred, one should always assume epiphyseal damage, unless proven otherwise, due to the dire consequences. Patients with epiphyseal fractures usually have a history of a falling injury (seen more often in recreational activities), a sudden onset from a violent muscular contraction at the injury site, or a blow from an opponent. In gymnastics, injuries have been seen in the distal radial epiphysis, in part due to the conversion of the upper extremity to a weight-bearing support (123). The incidence of physeal injury is not escalating, and most injuries are not severe. However, so much emphasis has been put on this area because growth disturbances can occur.

Epiphyseal fractures are typically categorized using the Salter-Harris classification system (124). The most common epiphyseal fractures are Type I or II. Distal tibial epiphyseal separation is one of the more common epiphyseal injuries seen in athletes due to the high incidence of ankle injuries, as well as phalangeal epiphyseal injury due to their exposed position (125, 126) (Fig. 18.7).

Clinical Manifestations

Taking an accurate history and obtaining a good description of the mechanism of injury are essential. The patient will frequently present with deformity around the joint as well as swelling and pain at the area of the epiphyseal plate.

If the injury is not severe enough to produce deformity, the physician must make careful note of the exact site of pain. Pain will be present over the growth plate area, rather than nearby structures (ligaments, tendons). Physical examination

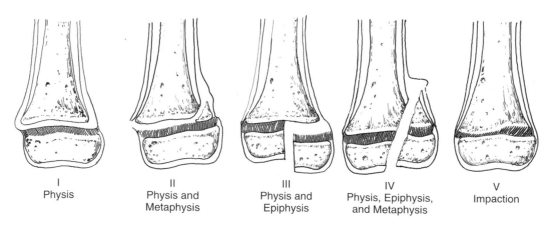

I	II	III	IV	V
Physis	Physis and Metaphysis	Physis and Epiphysis	Physis, Epiphysis, and Metaphysis	Impaction

Figure 18.7. The Salter-Harris classification of growth plate injury (Types I–V).

should also include isometric contraction of the muscles attached to the joint; pain will be reproduced at the epiphyseal plate or apophyseal growth center.

Age is a key factor in making the proper diagnosis. Epiphyseal injuries often occur during the periods of rapid growth, i.e., 11 to 12 years of age in girls and 13 to 14 years of age in boys, but can continue up to age 15 in girls and age 16 in boys. Boys are injured more frequently than girls (125, 126).

Diagnostic Imaging

When ruling out epiphyseal damage, it is important to take bilateral views. Although an epiphysis may have been injured, there may be little or no displacement. Therefore, comparison studies are necessary to detect any slight alterations in anatomical positioning. Slight widening or irregularity of the growth plate may be noted. However, stress radiographs (often under anesthesia) may be needed to prove that an epiphyseal fracture (Type I) has occurred. Applying a stressed application to the injury site shows, a gapping at the damaged growth plate.

Classification of Epiphyseal Fractures

The injuries are divided into five types: Type I producing the least damage and Type V producing the most damage to the epiphysis.

- Type I fractures separate through the epiphyseal plate.
- Type II fractures separate through the epiphyseal plate and also take a small triangular fragment of metaphyseal bone with them. Frequently, radiographs will show only the chip fracture if it is displaced.
- Type III fractures violate the joint space, fracture the epiphysis, and vertically traverse the epiphyseal plate.
- Type IV fractures traverse the epiphysis, epiphyseal plate, and also into the metaphysis.
- Type V fractures are crushing injuries to the epiphyseal plate.

Treatment and Prognosis

The determinants of prognosis for the young athlete with growth plate fractures are the age of the child at time of injury, nature of the fracture (whether closed or open), degree of displacement, region of injury (knee location carries poorest prognosis), type of Salter-Harris fracture, integrity of blood supply to the physis, and management of the injury. Generally, it is important that Types I and II fractures are not overtreated

and that Types III and IV are not undertreated (120).

Type I and II injuries are the most common and the most benign (120, 125). They usually heal quickly, and long bone growth will continue. If minimal separation is present, approximately 3 weeks of cast immobilization are necessary, followed by rehabilitation. If there are slightly more separation, approximately 6 weeks of cast immobilization are necessary, followed by rehabilitation before returning to participation. Overall, the prognosis is good and the young athlete can eventually return to full participation.

Type III and IV fractures are more serious. Because the fractures extend into the joint space, the fractures must be reduced perfectly and usually require surgery. The adolescent should avoid contact and collision sports for at least 1 year after such an injury. If a weight-bearing joint is involved, there should be no running activities for at least 1 year. Non–weight-bearing activities such as swimming provide a good alternative. The prognosis for these injuries is poor, because these fractures have the potential to cause bony growth disturbance.

Type V fractures, although rare, are the most drastic injury because these occur from an impact or crushing injury to the growth plate. The compressive forces damage the germinal cells of the plate, and total growth arrest can occur, causing angulation and deformity. Complete cessation of activity and immobilization are required, similar to the treatment for Types III and IV. Usually, the athlete is not permitted to resume any vigorous athletic participation.

Overuse Syndromes

To excel in sports today, the young athlete is forced to train longer, harder, and earlier in life. However, there is a price to pay for intense training. Hours of practicing the same movements produce gradual wear on specific parts of the body, eventually leading to an overuse injury. The overuse injury is characterized by pain, tenderness, swelling, and disability. Bursae, tendons, muscles, ligaments, joints, and bones are all subject to overuse. Repetitive microtraumas, as in one structure rubbing against another (patellofemoral pain syndrome), repetitive traction on a ligament or tendon (plantar fasciitis, Osgood-Schlatter's disease), or impact and shear forces (stress fractures) are the commonly seen factors in overuse injuries (127, 129). In 80% of cases of overuse injuries, the young athlete has only recently taken up the sport or significantly increased training intensity (128–130). Overuse injuries of the lower extremity are the most common, because most sports and training involve running.

STRESS FRACTURES

Stress fractures are generally considered to be an exercise-related condition that characteristically occurs in normal bone subjected to repeated cyclic loading (130). According to Rettig and Beltz (131), the young athlete may be more susceptible to stress injuries than the adult athlete, particularly when undergoing the adolescent growth spurt. During the growth spurt the musculotendinous unit may be insufficient to protect the bone from the repetitive demands made on it, and stress fractures occur (131, 132). Tibial stress fractures are the most frequent and are considered to be common in children (128). Complications of stress fractures can lead to delayed unions and complete fracture (133).

Clinical Manifestations

The patient presents with a (limping) pain of insidious onset. Symptoms may have been present for weeks or months. The pain is typically relieved with rest and aggravated by repetitive activity. Examination reveals normal ranges of motion of all joints with normal muscle bulk.

Localized tenderness and a visible, palpable swelling are frequently present. Films and bone scans are used to confirm the diagnosis (128, 130). However, early stress fractures are not always apparent on radiographs; bone scans will be positive long before the characteristic changes on plain films are seen (127).

Treatment

Treatment of the adolescent athlete is similar to the management for the adult athlete. The important principle of successful therapy is reduction, if not cessation, of the offending activity, restraint from activity being at least 4 to 12 weeks (127). Alternative exercises can be used, such as swimming, pool running, or a stationary bicycling program. An important key to proper rehabilitation may lie in a thorough evaluation of the patient's training techniques to eliminate the training error responsible for the stress fracture. This may involve a change in running, distance, frequency or duration, a modification of footwear, or an alteration of training location (127, 129, 130).

OSGOOD-SCHLATTER'S DISEASE

The current thinking on Osgood-Schlatter's disease holds that it is an overuse syndrome that results in partial avulsion of the tibial tuberosity (134, 135). The process occurs in late childhood or early adolescence and is more common in boys than in girls. Major or repetitive tensile stress on the tuberosity may cause the developing bone and the overlying cartilage or both to fail (136). The involved fragment or fragments and the intact portion of the tuberosity continue to grow and fill in, resulting in the typical overgrowth and bony prominence of the tuberosity seen in this condition.

Clinical Manifestations

Localized swelling and tenderness are present at the tibial tuberosity. Pain is aggravated by direct pressure as in kneeling, or by traction as in running and jumping in forced flexion. On examination, extension of the knee against resistance and palpation of the prominence are also painful. Sports participation exacerbates the symptoms, and rest tends to alleviate the pain.

Treatment

This condition is often self-limiting, and avoidance of strenuous exercise involving the knee is often the only treatment necessary. Activities that produce pain are avoided until symptoms completely resolve. Ice can be used to reduce swelling and ease discomfort. When the acute pain decreases, the athlete should start on a quadriceps stretching program, with the goal of treatment directed at relieving the tensile force on the tibial tuberosity exerted by the quadriceps. Stretching of the quadriceps should be instituted twice daily and followed by 20-minute applications of ice to the affected area. When the athlete can easily touch the buttock with the heel of the affected leg while lying prone, quadriceps strengthening is added. At this point, resumption of athletic participation may be allowed. Some patients may require some bracing or a neoprene tracking sleeve, and surgery should only be considered in rare cases when conservative treatment has failed (127).

OSTEOCHONDROSES

The osteochondroses are developmental disorders of unknown etiology and self-limited progression. They are usually diagnosed in growing children and are associated with anatomic sites undergoing transition from cartilage to bone (136).

Some investigators have viewed the osteochondroses as overuse syndromes; however, Pappas (136) considers them overdemand syndromes. As a growing athlete enters developmental stages that change skeletal maturation patterns, complaints of discomfort may be reported that were not previously present. Factors determining outcome include skeletal maturation of the patient, stage and extent of involvement, biomechanical effects on skeletal and articular development, functional demands on the involved area, and recommendations and compliance with treatment (136).

The course of osteochondroses is mostly influenced by factors such as repetitive microtrauma. Clinical complaints and subsequent deformity are directly related to the frequency and intensity of physical stress. The most common location to be affected is the knee, followed by the ankle, elbow, and hip (137).

OSTEOCHONDRITIS DISSECANS

Current knowledge now suggests that osteochondritis dissecans may be more appropriately referred to as osteochondrosis dissecans, because no evidence of inflammation has been found (137). It is a condition of unknown cause that occurs in children and adolescents. It is characterized by a small necrotic segment of subchondral bone. The lesion may heal spontaneously, or it may separate and become displaced into the joint cavity forming an intra-articular loose body. The most frequent age of onset is between 11 and 20 years, and this condition is seen more predominantly in boys than in girls (137). The most common location affected is the lateral aspect of the medial condyle of the knee. Mechanical injury has been proposed as the mechanism of injury. Shearing, rotatory, and tangentially applied forces to the cartilage and subchondral bone appear instrumental in initiating the segmental area of avascular necrosis or separation of fragment (137).

Clinical Manifestations

Onset may be insidious, from an acute traumatic event, or it may be caused by a group of factors. The young patient may have vague complaints of intermittent, poorly localized aching. Pain intensifies with exercise but may persist even at rest. The knee may feel stiff with catching or locking due to a loose fragment. If the fragment is sufficiently large, it may become entrapped in the joint, with the patient feeling sudden pain and the knee giving way. Episodes of entrapment can produce synovial effusions. On physical examination, forceful compression of the affected side of the knee joint elicits crepitation during knee flexion and extension. There may also be tenderness on the affected femoral condyle with palpation.

Similar manifestations exist when other joints, such as the elbow, are affected.

Treatment

Conservative measures can suffice in the early stages, particularly if the fragment has not separated from the underlying bone and cartilage. The lesion is considered to be more of a healing fracture. Walking with crutches to avoid placing weight on the affected limb is the most important treatment while symptoms persist. Immobilization is rarely needed and should be avoided whenever possible, because motion is beneficial to the health of the articular cartilage. If the condition is diagnosed after skeletal maturation, it is more likely to require surgical intervention and carries a greater likelihood of functional impairment, with the possible development of osteoarthritis later in life (136).

LITTLE LEAGUE ELBOW

The articular surfaces in Little League elbow (LLE) demonstrate the ill effects of overuse with excessive, repeated compression and tensile forces. During the acceleration phase of pitching, compressive forces on the lateral aspect of the elbow occur between the capitulum and the radial head, and osteochondritis dissecans is a common sequela. At the same time, tensile forces occur at the medial aspect of the elbow, causing possible avulsion of the medial epicondyle or chronic medial epicondylitis (127). Lack of rest, too many innings pitched, repetitive valgus overload, and an attempt to throw curve balls contribute to this condition (85).

Clinical Manifestations

The most common finding in young athletes with LLE is medial elbow pain. It can also be accompanied by locking or catching in the elbow, and occasionally lateral elbow pain or aching is noted (127). If symptoms have been occurring for some time, a flexion contracture of the elbow may be present. Tenderness is found over the medial epicondyle and/or ligaments, and pain can often be elicited at the medial epicondyle with wrist or finger flexion against resistance.

Treatment

With treatment of LLE, temporary cessation of the offending activity is mandatory. Depending on the extent of the injury, a slow return to throwing may be permitted if the patient is pain-free and range of motion has improved. If osteochondral fracturing, loose bodies, or extensive osteochondritis is present, surgery may be required (86). In pitching injuries in which no anatomical change has occurred but symptoms persist, alterations in pitching style may be advocated to take emphasis away from the offended infrastructures. As mentioned previously, restricting the number of innings pitched, including the time spent practicing and the number of pitches thrown per week, is also important (85). Because this injury can also occur in catchers and outfielders, the general amount of throwing may need to be reduced until appropriate rehabilitation has been completed.

DRUG ABUSE IN YOUNG ATHLETES

It is unfortunate that this section of an athletic injuries text must, by necessity, be included. However, it is impossible to escape the fact that drug use and abuse have become part of any discussion involving health issues in the pediatric and adolescent populations. A practitioner dealing with this population must be mindful of the use of recreational drugs and those that can be related to sports activity. For the sake of brevity, this section will focus only on those drugs that have a direct link to sports activity and performance. For the most part, such drugs have come into use because of their purported or actual effects on sports performance. Whereas these ergogenic substances pose important ethical questions about unfair performance enhancement, they also have important health effects that often create unique problems for the younger population.

Drugs used as potential ergogenic aids in the younger athletic community fall primarily into two groups: anabolic steroids (and other hormones such as growth hormone) and stimulants. In addition, the use of miscellaneous products and practices such as smokeless tobacco and blood doping have also become more common. Each grouping and its effect on young athletes are examined in the following sections.

Anabolic Steroids and Growth Hormone

ANABOLIC STEROIDS

The derivation and use of anabolic steroids are discussed in Chapter 24. Whereas the use of anabolic steroids is well known in many adult sports, and their use in college sports is documented in approximately 5% of all athletes (138), recent attention has focused on the increasing use of these drugs by young students in high schools. Various reported estimates of high school students' use of steroids range from 4.4 to 11% (139), and the more recent and well-documented work of Buckley and Yesalis (140) shows that 6.6% of all high school male seniors have tried anabolics by age 18. This may represent as many as 500,000 adolescents. What is even more astounding and also disturbing is that 27% of the individuals in this study reported using these drugs not for athletic performance and enhancement, but for improvement of appearance.

Despite much published information about the side effects of steroids, the true extent of damage that can potentially be caused by these substances is difficult to determine because the illegal nature of their use for athletic performance enhancement makes it difficult to obtain populations who are totally honest about their intake of steroids. What is known is that many athletes use dosages that are 10 to 40 times higher than are prescribed medically (141). In addition, most athletes who use steroids use them in "stacking" regimens (more than one steroid at a time) in cycles lasting 7 to 14 weeks (142). Most commonly, two or three oral agents are taken in conjunction with one or more injectable forms.

Anabolic steroids have been shown to be effective in increasing size and strength of musculature (143, 144). Athletes also experience psychological effects including increased aggressiveness and diminished fatigue, which can contribute to enhanced training programs (145). However, numerous side effects can help in detecting steroid use. These include increased acne, changes in sex drive, decreased endogenous testosterone production, testicular atrophy, decreased fertility, gynecomastia in males, breast atrophy in females, water retention, and abnormal liver function. Most of these side effects are considered reversible when steroid use is discontinued. There are, however, several side effects that are considered permanent. These include male pattern baldness, hirsutism, and female genital enlargement and deepened voice (146).

By far, the most significant immediate side effect in children and adolescents is acceleration of epiphyseal closure, which can result in permanent short stature (145, 147). It is this particular effect that makes the higher rate of use in younger athletes particularly disturbing.

Long-term effects of steroids are less well understood and documented. Reports of increased rates of peliosis hepatitis and liver tumors exist, but rely heavily on data from patients taking steroids for the purpose of medical treatment. Dosages were continuous over a longer period than traditionally seen in athletic use. Another long-term effect that warrants mention is extreme alterations of lipoprotein ratios in favor of LDL (143). Although this alteration is transient, its long-term effect in cardiovascular risk has not been determined. Several recent reports of stroke in athletes taking steroids raises the question of whether today's generation of steroid users will be tomorrow's victims of cardiovascular disease.

Steroid use can lead to a degree of both psychological and physical addiction (148). This may be somewhat related to the psychological compulsion regarding distorted body image that often accompanies a young athlete's entry into the realm of building the dream body. For competitive athletes, the understanding that they may well be in a minority if they remain drug free, and the effect that this may have on competitive status, provides additional pressure for use.

Two other dangers have been linked to steroid use in the recent literature. One is that athletes who are well educated about the side effects of steroids are now taking other drugs to counter these side effects. Examples are the use of furosemide to counteract water retention, human chorionic gonadotropin to maintain endogenous testosterone production, and tamoxifen to block the development of steroid-induced gynecomastia (149).

In dealing with the child or adolescent who is using steroids, each physician must make a personal decision as to what role to play in the education of the patient. Goldberg et al. (150) have published results that indicate that the use of scare tactics is less effective in warning youth away from ergogenic drugs than balanced education about positive and negative effects. Strauss (144) has also warned against the adoption of moralistic or judgmental attitudes with youngsters who take these drugs, and even reminds us that body language and facial expressions should be guarded carefully against displaying judgment. A young athlete needs to be able to trust the physician, and if the athlete knows that matter-of-fact, balanced information can be gained from the physician, the athlete may be more likely to return if problems do ensue.

Questions are often asked by physicians about monitoring the potentially damaging effects of steroids on their patients. Haupt has developed a screening procedure, which he has made available to his young athletic patients on an anonymous basis. These laboratory tests consist of ALT, AST, GGT, the liver-specific isoenzymes of LDH, alkaline phosphatase, and HDL/LDL ratios (143).

GROWTH HORMONE

Growth hormone is used by some athletes to mimic the effects of anabolic steroids. In addition, some parents occasionally ask that their children be injected with human growth hormone to induce greater height before epiphyseal closure. Preliminary evidence does indicate that muscle hypertrophy may be possible with growth hormone (151). However, long-term studies are not yet conclusive. The potential side effects include the development of giantism in children and adolescents and acromegalic changes in adults. The development of myopathy in acromegaly patients has led to the speculation that HGH use by athletes may lead to hypertrophy overshadowed by pathology. Growth hormone has not been studied extensively enough to substantiate high degrees of any of these side effects. It is, however, banned by both the NCAA and the USOC (143).

Stimulants

The most common stimulants used by athletes are amphetamines, cocaine, caffeine, and phenylpropanolamine. Most of these substances stimulate the sympathetic nervous system and can increase alertness, elevate mood, and potentially enhance performance (152). Adolescents also use amphetamines and phenylpropanolamine to help with weight loss before competitive events owing to their appetite-suppressing properties. Common side effects of the more powerful stimulants include restlessness, insomnia, anxiety, tremors, heart palpitations, psychosis, hypertension, dehydration, and addiction. Stimulants vary in which side effects are the most prominent. All of these have been declared illegal ergogenic aids, and their use should be discouraged and avoided.

Miscellaneous Drugs and Doping Practices

Whereas any ergogenic drug taken by adult athletes can eventually find its way into the hands of youths, the use of smokeless tobacco and the practice of blood doping seem to have found their way into adolescent ranks more quickly. Both are discussed briefly next.

SMOKELESS TOBACCO

The practice of using smokeless tobacco is prevalent among teenagers in general (153). Young athletes in particular seem to turn to this drug, not only because it is purported to act as a stimulant, but because the use of smokeless tobacco has been popularized by professional

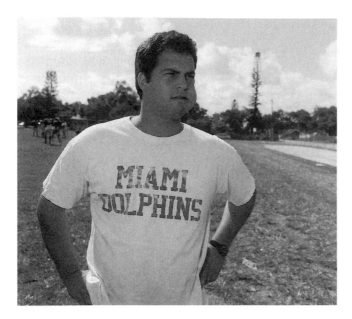

Figure 18.8. Smokeless tobacco use by college and professional athletes has been one of the promoting factors of its use by younger athletes.

sports figures, particularly in baseball (Fig 18.8). Although estimates of snuff use vary, a large proportion of male adolescents (40 to 50%) and a smaller proportion of females (7%) have reported the use of the substance (153–155). Common terminology for the use of smokeless tobacco includes chewing, dipping, and the use of plugs.

Studies of smokeless tobacco in nonathletes and athletes have shown that heart rate does increase from the use of smokeless tobacco, most probably from its nicotine content. However, studies have not been able to show any enhancement of athletic performance in terms of reaction time, movement time, or total response time (154, 156). There are, however, severe side effects from the use of these substances, the most dramatic of which is a 50-fold increase in the rate of gum and buccal mucosa cancers and a 4-fold increase in the rate of oral and pharyngeal cancers (154, 157). Additional side effects include an increase in dental caries, gingival and periodontal inflammation, hyperkeratotic lesions, and leukoplakia. The overall 5-year survival rate for oral cancers is 40% (154). The nicotine component of smokeless tobacco makes it an addictive substance. Use often becomes chronic, and the individual in unable to quit.

In an effort to curb the burgeoning use of smokeless tobacco products in athletics, the NCAA and the National Association of Professional Baseball Leagues have taken steps to prohibit the use of such products in competitions, although at least in one case the prohibition is extended to championship games and practices only (158). It is hoped that such tactics, and educational efforts by other agencies that publicize the health problems that have been experienced by athletes who use snuff, will help to stop its use.

Blood Doping and Erythropoietin

The practice of blood doping is relatively new in athletics and is a practice used primarily by endurance athletes. It involves the withdrawal and storage of a volume of blood from an athlete, with retransfusion 24 to 48 hours before an event in an attempt to increase red blood cell volume. A small increase in endurance capacity is subsequently experienced by the athlete (143). Increases in $\dot{V}o_2$max of 3.9 to 12.8% have been documented (159). Donor transfusion may also be used but carries obviously higher risks. Although declared illegal by both the NCAA and the USOC, this practice cannot be detected by testing.

In an effort to bypass the complicated procedures of phlebotomy, blood storage, and transfusion, some athletes have begun to experiment with the use of erythropoietin as a way of inducing endogenous red blood cell production increases. Erythropoietin is a substance normally found in the body that stimulates stem cells in bone marrow to differentiate into red blood cells. The athlete uses concentrated amounts of a synthetic form of this chemical into his or her system to gain an edge similar to that seen with standard blood doping. Although this system is thought to be effective, recent reports indicate that there may be an increased death rate among athletes who practice this ergogenic technique due to thrombosis or myocardial infarction (160). This seems to be a result of the dramatically increased blood viscosity seen with erythropoietin.

NUTRITIONAL CONSIDERATIONS FOR YOUNG ATHLETES

Although the nutritional needs of young athletes are not remarkably different from those of adult athletes, there are several significant variables that should be explained. In addition, several special issues related to nutrition in this age group warrant mention in the context of how they relate to exercise and athletic performance.

Growth and development require nutrition, both in the form of additional calories and in terms of specific nutrients (161). In childhood, especially during adolescence, additional calories are needed to maintain weight compared with the adult. For example, a child between the ages of 11 and 14 needs an average of 25 kcal/lb of body weight compared with an average 16.5 kcal/lb of body weight for the adult between 23 and 50 years of age (162). This calculation includes basal metabolic rate needs and moderate activities of daily living. It does not include the extra needs that arise from vigorous exercise, and such energy costs must be taken into account if malnutrition is to be avoided. Healthy children and adolescents have somewhat higher fat needs than those currently recommended for adults (between 30 and 50% of total calories, compared with 30% or below in adults) (161). However, even with this increased need, children's diets often exceed necessary fat percentages.

Thermal Regulation

A similar caution must be expressed regarding hydration of young athletes. The presence of decreased thermoregulation ability in children when compared with adults has been well documented (163). Studies have repeatedly found that young adolescents, compared with adults, are physiologically less able to regulate their body temperatures. Three factors contribute to this.

1. Children generate more metabolic heat per unit body size than adults.
2. Children demonstrate reduced sweat rates.
3. Children do not initiate sweating until they reach a higher core temperature than an adult.

Susceptibility for thermal injury is a risk in this population; therefore, a special emphasis is placed on adequate hydration because it is a significant component of thermoregulation. Children should be taught early that regular drinking of fluids is essential during exercise, and that thirst is not an adequate indicator of fluid need (164).

Cold water is still the hydration method of choice, and if exercise is being carried out within appropriate guidelines for this age group, electrolyte and carbohydrate replacement during exercise are probably unnecessary. Smith and Wroble (165, 166) have made the following recommendations concerning fluid replacement.

1. Fluid should be cold (preferably water).
2. Small volumes should be consumed.
3. During exercise, fluids should be consumed every 15 to 20 minutes.
4. Good taste may be a factor in compliance, but if commercial drinks are used, they should be diluted to half strength.

Chen et al. (167) have observed that rational, balanced nutrition is the basis of an athlete's good health, conditioning, and performance. Taken as a whole, athletic populations often have somewhat better nutritional practices than less active populations (168).

Emphasis on nutrient balance should be relatively similar to recommendations made for adults. The diet should be high in carbohydrates, particularly complex carbohydrates, with care being taken not to overload either fat or protein. Excessive fat or protein intake increases the metabolic load on hepatic and renal systems (167), whereas proper emphasis on carbohydrates will optimize energy stores for activity.

Because athletes will often heed supplement advertising's call for large protein intakes, it is worth mentioning that although most athletes do require more protein than their sedentary counterparts, this requirement is usually already present in the average diet (162, 169). Tarnopolsky has also shown that body builders, who are often noted for their excessive protein intake, may actually require less protein for lean body mass maintenance than do endurance athletes (169).

Pre-Event Eating

One should always remind young athletes that their performance during an event is less dependent on the pre-game meal than it is on the cumulative energy storage from food that has been eaten over the past several days. However, the pre-event meal is often an important ritual for athletes and should certainly be constructed in such a way as to optimize energy stores and prevent impairment. Smith (165) and Wroble (166) have made several recommendations regarding pre-event nutrition.

1. The meal should be high in carbohydrates and low in fat.
2. The meal should take place at least 3 to 4 hours before competition.
3. The meal should avoid excessive protein, high salt content, extremely spicy foods, or gas-producing foods.
4. Within these broad guidelines, the athlete should be allowed to consume those foods and those amounts that are believed to help performance.
5. Adequate fluids should be taken with the meal.

Special Issues

Although the athletic population as a whole may have generally good nutritional practices, there are several sports that seem to cause nutritional concerns. These are primarily sports in which weight control is an issue, e.g., wrestling, gymnastics, figure skating, and ballet dancing. On the other end of this spectrum, it is also important to examine childhood obesity and its relationship to both exercise and nutritional practices. The subsequent sections will address these issues.

CHILDHOOD AND ADOLESCENT OBESITY

Childhood obesity has been mentioned elsewhere in this chapter as affecting a significant number of individuals in the United States. Development of obesity in childhood and adolescence has been shown to correlate very strongly with obesity in adulthood (170), which carries with it not only psychological and emotional burdens, but also increased risk of cardiovascular diseases, gallbladder disorders, certain types of cancer, and other disorders (170, 171). Rocchini et al. (172) have noted that obese adolescents already have structural changes present in blood vessels that contribute to the higher incidence of hypertension in this group of young people.

It is important to establish the most effective treatment of childhood and adolescent obesity. At least one author has stated that obesity in children is not a reliable indicator of fitness (173). However, numerous authors have implicated lack of exercise and nutrition as significant factors in childhood obesity, along with genetic predisposition (170). Therefore, management must focus on both increasing activity levels and establishing proper nutritional practices.

Reduction of obesity has been shown to be most effective when nutritional restriction, nutritional education, and exercise are combined (174–177). Rocchini et al. (178) and Epstein et al. (179) have shown that some of the physiologic characteristics associated with obesity, such as adverse lipoprotein ratios and increased blood pressures, are actually reversible with successful treatment of obesity. Weight loss coupled with increases in lean muscle mass has also been shown to improve self-esteem and psychological well-being (176, 180).

Diet and physical activity patterns seem to be learned at an early age (181), suggesting the need for early intervention, especially based in the school systems. Indeed, follow-up studies of several multicomponent, multidisciplinary school programs aimed at behavior modification, increased aerobic exercise, and nutritional education have yielded promising results. Results have included a 25% increase in physical activity in one study coupled with a 30% reduction in sodium and 28 to 42% reduction in fat in selected foods served at school lunches. Another study yielded

an 11% reduction of weight while maintaining lean body mass coupled with improved exercise and eating behaviors. Almost all reviewed studies indicated that the best compliance and most favorable results were achieved when exercise was combined with nutritional education/behavior modification—neither technique alone proved to be as effective (175, 176, 178, 180). School support was also found to be an integral factor (173, 182, 183).

In summary, childhood and adolescent obesity is related to both activity levels and nutritional practices. Therefore, intervention must be aimed at both components to be effective.

WEIGHT LOSS AND WRESTLING

Although wrestling is not the only sport in which potentially pathogenic means of weight control are used, it has become, by far, the most publicized. Recent studies indicate that wrestlers at the high school and college level use numerous means to "make weight" in a particular weight class, often attempting to achieve weights that are unhealthy for their particular stage of growth and development. The means used include dietary restriction, bingeing and purging (vomiting), induced vomiting without bingeing, sweating, fluid restriction, thermal dehydration, diuretics, laxatives, and enemas (184, 185).

Such methods of weight control potentially impair adolescent growth and development in the long run (185) and have been estimated to cause months of growth arrest during the wrestling season (165). They have been shown to decrease serum testosterone levels as well (186).

In addition, Steen et al. (187) have shown that repetitive cycles of weight loss and gain in wrestlers lead to a lowering of the mean resting metabolic rate, which could have significant predisposing effects on obesity later in life. However, on the more immediate front, such practices almost uniformly lead to dehydration, temporary undernourishment, and nutritional deficiencies; in addition, they have been shown to decrease blood plasma volume, muscle strength, muscular endurance capacity, and performance as well as detrimentally altering electrolyte imbalance (164, 165, 184, 188). These results have been documented at losses of greater than 2% body weight dehydration. One author has stated that losses up to 5% of body weight can be tolerated and the effects reversed within the customary 5 hours between weigh-in and competition (189). However, most other authors agree that 5 hours is not sufficient time to restore electrolyte imbalance, replace glycogen stores, or rehydrate adequately. In addition, the above mentioned means of weight loss are often achieved at the expense of lean body mass, which is essential to performance.

In establishing an appropriate weight for a wrestler, the most proper goal is to be able to enter competition with the maximum amount of strength, endurance, and speed for each pound of body weight taken into competition (190). This calls for optimization of lean body mass, because body fat is a relatively inert component of performance. Although there are several equations that can be used to calculate optimum weight for a wrestler (191), a relatively simple estimation of appropriate weight class can be performed by using 5 to 7% as the optimum amount of body fat desired for the wrestler (166, 190).

Smith (190) has outlined the following steps, which are easy to follow. One must know the athlete's current weight and estimated body fat percentage to perform this calculation.

1. Multiply the wrestler's total weight by estimated body fat to determine fat weight.
2. Subtract the fat weight from the total weight to obtain the total lean body weight.
3. Divide the lean body weight by the desired percentage of lean body weight (for 5% desired fat this number would be 95%). This calculates the best competing weight for the wrestler.

Such measurements should be done well in advance of the wrestling season, so that an appropriate weight loss and training program can be designed. This program should aim at a reduction in fat weight of not more than 2 lb/wk (166, 190) and should be achieved at an energy deficit of no greater than 1000 kcal/day. This will still allow an intake of approximately 1800 to 2000 cal/day by the athlete, allowing him to have enough energy intake to meet growth and development demands and activities of daily living. Resistive strength training during this time is also a good idea, because this will help to maintain or even increase the lean body mass. Increasing lean body mass will be especially desired if the new calculated optimum weight for the wrestler is slightly below the desired weight class; increased strength and lean body mass have positive correlations with performance.

Unfortunately, there are still too many instances in which coaching and training personnel, especially in high schools, adhere to the traditional means of "making weight." As an informed physician, it becomes just as important to educate the individual coaching and training the team as it is to make sound recommendations for the individual athlete.

EATING DISORDERS

Although the nutritional practices of wrestlers include those identified with eating disorders, these pathologic means of weight control are seen in other sports as well.

Although wrestlers are usually not defined as having a clinical eating disorder per se, such disorders have been identified in other sports, primarily those in which losing or maintaining weight are important and monitored at a high frequency, for example, dance and gymnastics.

Swimming and diving have also been implicated. Recent studies indicate that athletes may have a higher incidence of eating disorders than the regular population, in some cases reaching as high as 25% (192–194). Bulimia and mixed eating disorders seem to be somewhat more common than anorexia nervosa in the athletic population (195). This compounds the issue of diagnosis because mixed eating disorders and bulimia are harder to spot. These disorders often do not involve the high degree of weight loss that we see in anorexia nervosa, yet they are associated with many serious medical problems, including menstrual irregularities, esophageal inflammation, tooth erosion, hormone imbalances, osteoporosis, impaired renal function, electrolyte imbalances, and associated mood disorders (195).

Furthermore, once an eating disorder pattern is established, it is addictive and therefore extremely difficult to break. The prevalence of such disorders is higher in females, particularly in adolescence, possibly due to a higher psychological burden associated with body image than for males (196). Also, if someone already has a tendency toward this type of disorder, it is possible that pressures of athletic performance may exacerbate such a tendency. Although no one has ever stated that coaches cause eating disorders, coaching methodology that overemphasizes weight and its monitoring, when coupled with the compulsive personalities of many athletes, may well be a contributory factor. This means that physicians and coaches must be aware of and responsible for their actions and recommendations.

Recognition of the signs of eating disorders is also important, but will be compounded by the fact that these conditions are particularly difficult to diagnose in athletes. This is because athletes can often continue to perform adequately even under severe dietary deprivation (195). Signs to watch for include the following (197).

1. Changes in eating behavior such as recurrent episodes of binge eating, obsession

with dieting, starvation periods, loss of control during bingeing periods.

2. Frequent weighing, inappropriate concern with weight, overexercising, excessive use of laxatives or diuretics.
3. Constipation, dry skin and hair, skin rashes, especially when coupled with depressed behavior, sluggishness.
4. Distortion of perception of body size.
5. In women, absence of three consecutive menstrual cycles (must rule out other causes).

If an eating disorder is suspected, it is extremely important that an appropriate psychological referral be arranged. Care must be taken to do this in a personal, nonthreatening way, with the intent of maintaining a supportive relationship with the athlete. As with other addictive disorders, denial may be a significant factor, so these situations should be handled carefully.

A WORD ABOUT ANEMIA

Although anemias are generally not a problem unique to children, the common finding of nonanemic iron deficiency in the athletic population warrants mention. This is particularly true because those sports that lead to nutritional deficiency because of caloric undernourishment (in the face of increased activity) can also lead to iron deficiency and deficiencies of other micronutrients. In some sports, such as running, increased incidence of iron deficiency seems to be related to training; in others, such as swimming, iron-deficient states seem to be more related to dietary intake (198). As with adults, it must be remembered that girls and women are more vulnerable owing to the additional variable of menstrual blood loss. Iron deficiency can be treated adequately with full therapeutic doses of iron supplementation (199). However, it should be noted that many physicians do not treat iron deficiency until it leads to frank anemia.

Recent literature suggests that nonanemic or preanemic iron deficiency may also lead to a subjective perception of decreased performance on the part of the athlete (200). Therefore, more studies are being undertaken to assess what may well be a high prevalence of nonanemic iron deficiency in young athletes, which may impair performance (201).

YOUNG ATHLETES WITH SPECIAL HEALTH PROBLEMS

Much of this chapter has dealt with the benefits of exercise for the pediatric and adolescent age group. However, there is a significant portion of this population that is affected by various chronic health problems.

Goldberg (202) has estimated that more than 1 million children in the United States have chronic disease. These children are estimated to have 2 to 3 times the incidence of psychosocial problems when compared to the healthy population. This may be due to a combination of self-esteem issues related to having a chronic disease and the immediate issues involved in medical management of such states. Sports and exercise involvement can help such children obtain a greater sense of accomplishment and independence. In most cases, this fact can be coupled with the intrinsic benefits of exercise to promote both psychological and physical health.

A text of this nature cannot address all existing types of chronic disease in this population. However, the most common conditions and their special considerations are discussed below.

Diabetes

Insulin-dependent diabetes mellitus is the most common metabolic endocrine disorder affecting children and adolescents, having an incidence of 1.4 in 1000 children (203). This disease brings with it the management challenges involved in maintaining adequate metabolic control of serum glucose levels. This can be particularly challenging in early adolescence, when there is often a significant change in glucose regulation, concomitant with deteriorating metabolic control (204).

Exercise has been noted to be an effective way of increasing fitness in children with diabetes mellitus and, more importantly, has been shown to improve glycemic control and sometimes decrease the need for exogenous insulin (205–207). Therefore, the involvement of children and adolescents in exercise should be encouraged strongly and is not contraindicated (203). However, the physiologic response to exercise in the diabetic child must be understood and appropriately compensated for.

In nondiabetic athletes, exercise brings about a 10-fold increase in the use of circulating glucose. Glucose needs are supplied by both calories from the diet and liver glycogenolysis; in later stages, gluconeogenesis is also a contributor. These changes are accompanied by a decrease in insulin secretion. Diabetics are unable to modulate their insulin levels, and since their insulin is from an injected exogenous source, insulin may actually be absorbed more quickly during exercise. This suppresses glucose production and, coupled with the increased glucose use in muscle during exercise, can cause exercise-induced hypoglycemia (203). The diabetic athlete will automatically have an increased need for calories and will often require reduction in insulin dosage. It is very important to help athletes to exercise a degree of control over their glycemic state. Anderson et al. (204) have shown that teaching athletes to monitor their blood glucose and to use the informational yield appropriately can improve metabolic control in those individuals, even during exercise.

Exercise hypoglycemia can have from mild to severe manifestations, depending on the degree of glucose depletion. Mild versions are accompanied by inattentiveness, mood changes, pallor, shakiness, fatigue, headache, nausea, abdominal pain, and poor motor performance. As the condition worsens, confusion, loss of coordination, and staggering occur, followed by loss of consciousness and convulsions in the most severe instances (203). It is important for the physician, coach, and trainer to recognize these symptoms and take appropriate action, which involves immediate administration of exogenous glucose. Appropriate sources of glucose include fruit juices, raisins, and even granola bars. Other sources that have been suggested such as jelly beans, Lifesavers, and sugar packets will certainly do in an emergency, but are obviously less healthful alternatives.

When athletes are so severely affected that they are unable to ingest solids or liquids, glucagon should be available for subcutaneous injection. The need for such availability dictates another important tenet in management of diabetic athletes. Coaches, trainers, and on-the-field physicians must be aware of athletes who are diabetic, so that appropriate management is undertaken rapidly in an emergency. The behavioral changes associated with exercise hypoglycemia might otherwise be mistaken for drug- or alcohol-induced behaviors.

Asthma

Children and adolescents with asthma have an 80 to 90% incidence of exercise-induced bronchospasm (EIB), whereas nonasthmatic individuals have a 35 to 50% incidence of EIB (208). This condition is characterized by varying airway obstruction after 3 to 8 minutes of vigorous continuous exercise, followed by a moderate to severe obstruction 5 to 15 minutes after exercise (209). Symptoms include coughing, wheezing, and chest tightness, usually of sufficient intensity to affect or even cause cessation of the activity. Children with asthma have also been shown to be less fit, which seems to be related not only to

decreased activity levels in these children, but also to the increased body fat that often accompanies the administration of systemic corticosteroids (a common management tool in more severe cases of asthma) (210).

Children with asthma and EIB can safely participate in exercise programs (211). Exercise program participation in this population has been shown to increase work capacity and aerobic endurance (209, 211). The AAP (212) has stated that children with asthma should be encouraged to participate in sports activity. However, a few pointers about how to minimize asthmatic attacks in the athlete with EIB will assist in managing this problem. EIB is usually managed with a combination of pharmacologic and nonpharmacologic measures. Pharmacologic management most commonly involves the use of various forms of inhalant therapy immediately preceding exercise. These can include albuterol and cromolyn sodium, sometimes in combination. If control cannot be achieved, other medications such as theophylline or corticosteroids are added to the regimen.

Nonpharmacologic management tools include the following (209).

1. Aerobic training. The highly trained athlete will be less affected by EIB. This is because training increases vital capacity and airway function.
2. Vigorous warm-up. If warm-up exercise is pursued vigorously enough to induce maximum symptoms of EIB, the athlete will experience a refractory period devoid of attacks for 2 to 3 hours after recovery. Timing of warm-ups is crucial in this instance.
3. Warm, humid air. Breathing of such air causes less bronchoconstriction than dry and especially cold air. The athlete can be encouraged to participate in sports activities that optimize such conditions, or at least avoid cold, dry air.
4. Face masks. The use of face masks can promote the rebreathing of warm, moister air. The degree of EIB can be somewhat controlled with this practice.
5. Avoidance of food within 2 hours before exercise. Food ingestion within 2 hours of onset of exercise seems to promote EIB.

It is important for the physician to remember that there are extrinsic factors that can exacerbate EIB. These include exercising in polluted air, exposure to pollens and other allergens in a sensitive individual, some medications such as beta blockers, and the presence of upper respiratory infections such as colds or sinusitis.

Epilepsy

Epilepsy has unfortunately been defined as a condition in which two or more unprovoked seizures have occurred in an individual. This definition does not consider the time between occurrences or the severity of seizures (213). Therefore, the "diagnosis" of epilepsy can actually encompass a startlingly broad range of conditions. Each child with epilepsy must be evaluated separately, and individual recommendations regarding sports participation must be made.

In general it can be stated that so long as seizures are well-controlled, or only occur at night, physical activity is not precluded. In fact, current recommendations allow for participation in contact sports, if the above criteria are met. There is no evidence that contact sports induce more seizures than any other type of activity. There is even some evidence that participation in exercise can make seizures less likely to occur (213). It is important that children with seizure disorders be supervised in their activities and that they do not exercise alone. In addition, it is important that those children taking medication continue to take it while exercising. This is particularly important because some individuals will skip medication if they feel that it impairs their performance. If a young athlete wants to alter the medication because of interference with performance, this should be done only with the aid of a physician experienced in dealing with seizure disorders. Some studies have shown that if a child's seizures have been controlled for 2 years or longer and the EEG looks good, then the child can discontinue medication with a 90 to 95% chance of remaining seizure free (213).

Overprotection of children with seizure disorders is to be avoided. However, if training for a particular activity does seem to provoke seizures, then an alternate activity or a change in medication might be in order.

Congenital Heart Problems and Cystic Fibrosis

The importance of differentiating potentially dangerous heart murmurs in children has been discussed in the section on preparticipation examination. However, even for children in whom a significant congenital abnormality is found to exist, participation in exercise programs has been found to be beneficial. Children who have had correction of tetralogy of Fallot and those with transportation of the great vessels have been studied (209). In both cases, children were able to increase their $\dot{V}O_2$max and decrease their body fat in response to aerobic exercise programs. These children must undergo a complete preprogram assessment including echocardiogram, stress testing, and Holter monitor use before beginning to exercise. Vaccaro et al. (214) have recommended that exercise consist of 10 to 20 minutes of exercise conducted at 60% to 75% of the maximum heart rate performed 3 times a week. In addition, recommendations also exist for use of flexibility and muscle strengthening programs along with aerobic exercise recommendations.

Cystic fibrosis also causes cardiovascular compromise, usually in the form of chronic obstructive pulmonary disease (COPD). Children with cystic fibrosis have altered exercise responses when compared with healthy children. However, mild exercise carried out over time (3 months in one study) has been shown to improve exercise tolerance, increase $\dot{V}O_2$max, and improve response of respiratory muscle and heart rate without adverse effects.

Goldberg (202) and Strauss et al. (215) have also reported that the addition of high-repetition, low-weight training for strength to an aerobic exercise program has led to increased weight, muscle strength, and muscle size as well as decreased residual lung volume in the subjects studied. All of this translated into an increased tolerance of activities of daily living for children who were normally impaired by this disease.

In summary, all children and adolescents seem to be able to glean positive benefits from involvement in exercise and sports. This seems to be the case regardless of infirmity, so long as rational thought is put into an exercise prescription. In making recommendations for children with impairment or chronic disease, one should keep in mind the principle outlined by John Freeman, M.D. (212): "We should not paternalistically impose disability on the handicapped!"

Acknowledgments

The authors thank Rebecca Corson, D.C., Jeffrey Hunter, D.C., and Joseph Tangaro, D.C. for their invaluable encouragement as well as research and editing contributions. In addition, we thank Ms. Terri Tillman for her untiring assistance in manuscript preparation.

References

1. Berryman JW. The rise of highly organized sports for preadolescent boys. In: Magill RA, Ash MJ, Smoll FL, eds. Children in sport. 3rd ed. Champaign, IL: Human Kinetics, 1988:3–10.
2. Seefeldt V. The future of youth sport in America. In: Smoll FL, Magill RA, Ash MJ, eds. Children in sport. Champaign, IL: Human Kinetics, 1988:335–348.

3. Pappas AM. Children and sports. In: Southmayd W, Hoffman M, eds. Sports health: the complete book of athletic injuries. New York: Pataman, 1981:424–445.
4. Scanlan TK. Social evaluation: a key developmental element in the competition process. In: Magill RA, Ash MJ, Smoll FL, eds. Children in sport. Champaign IL: Human Kinetics, 1986:138–152.
5. Malina RM. Readiness for competitive youth sport. In: Broekhoff JB, Ellis MJ, Tripps DG, eds. Sport for children and youths. Champaign IL: Human Kinetics, 1986.
6. Passer MW. When should children begin competing? a psychological perspective. In: Broekhoff JB, Ellis MF, Tripps DG, eds. Sport for children and youths. Champaign IL: Human Kinetics, 1986:55–58.
7. Toda M, Shinotsuka H, McClintock GG, et al. Development of competitive behavior as a function of culture, age and social comparison. J Pers Soc Psychol 1978;36:825–839.
8. Coakley J. When should children begin competing? A sociological perspective. In: Broekhoff JB, Ellis MJ, Tripps DG, eds. Sport for children and youths. Champaign IL: Human Kinetics, 1986:59–63.
9. Malina RM. Growth and maturation of young athletes: biological and social considerations. In: Smoll FL, Magill RA, Ash MJ, eds. Children in sport. Champaign IL: Human Kinetics, 1988:83–101.
10. Murray JJ. Pediatric sports medicine. In: Vinger PF, Hoerner EF, eds. Sports injuries: the unthwarted epidemic. Littleton, MA: PSG Publishing Co., 1986:325–343.
11. Halbert JA. When should children begin competing? a coach's perspective. In: Broekhoff JB, Ellis MJ, Tripps DG, eds. Sport for children and youths. Champaign IL: Human Kinetics, 1986:65–69.
12. Duncan B, Boyce WT, Itami R, et al. A controlled trial of a physical fitness program for fifth grade students. J Sch Health 1983;53:467–471.
13. President's Council on Physical Fitness and Sports. 1985 National School Population Survey. Washington, D.C.: U.S. Government Publishing Office, 1986.
14. Raithel K. Are American children really unfit? Phys Sports Med 1988;16:146–154.
15. Coates TJ, Jeffrey RW, Slinkard LA. Heart healthy eating and exercise: introducing and maintaining changes in health behaviors. Am J Public Health 1981;71:15–23.
16. DeMarco T, Sidney K. Enhancing children's participation in physical activity. J Sch Health 1989;59:337–340.
17. Hunter RA, Marsh MT. American youth and physical fitness. J Chiro 1988;12:39–42.
18. Price JH, Desmond SM, Ruppert ES, et al. School nurses' perceptions of childhood obesity. J Sch Health 1987;57:332–336.
19. Orlick T. Evolution in children's sport. In: Weiss MR, Gould D, eds. Sport for children and youths. Champaign IL: Human Kinetics, 1986.
20. Smoll FL, Smith R. Improving self-awareness of youth sport coaches. J Phys Educ Recreation 1980;51:46–49.
21. American Academy of Pediatrics: Committees on Sports Medicine and School Health. Organized athletics for preadolescent children. Pediatrics. 1989;84;583–584.
22. Gould D. Understanding attrition in children's sport. In: Gould D, Weiss M, eds. Advances in pediatric sport sciences: behavioral issues. Champaign IL: Human Kinetics, 1987:61–85.
23. Gould D, Petlichkoff L. Participation, motivation, and attrition in young athletes. In: Smoll FL, Magill RA, Ash MJ, eds. Children in sport. Champaign IL: Human Kinetics, 1988:161–178.
24. Sharkey BJ. When should children begin competing? a physiological perspective. In: Broekhoff JB, Ellis MF, Tripps DG, eds. Sport for children and youths. Champaign IL: Human Kinetics, 1986:51–54.
25. Feigley DA. Psychological burnout in high level athletes. Phys Sport Med 1984;12:109–119.
26. Feinstein RA, Soileau EJ, Daniel WA. A national survey of preparticipation physical examination requirements. Phys Sportsmed 1988;16:5;51–59.
27. Goldberg B, Saraniti A, Witman P, et al. Pre-participation sports assessment: an objective evaluation. Pediatrics 1980;66:736–745.
28. Schichor A, Beck A. School-based follow-up care for sports physicals. J Sch Health 1988;58:200–202.
29. Risser WL, Hoffman HM, Bellah GG, et al. A cost-benefit analysis of preparticipation sports examinations of adolescent athletes. J Sch Health 1985;55:270–273.
30. Kibler WB, Chandler TJ, Uhl T, et al. A musculoskeletal approach to the preparticipation physical examination. Am J Sports Med 1989;17:525–531.
31. McKeag DB. Preseason physical examination for the prevention of sports injuries. Sportsmedicine 1985;2:413–431.
32. McKeag DB. Preparticipation screening of the potential athlete. Clin Sports Med 1989;8:373–397.
33. Linder CW, DuRant RH, Seklecki RM, et al. Preparticipation health screening of young athletes. Am J Sports Med 1981;9:187–193.
34. Kibler WB. The sport preparticipation fitness examination. Champaign, IL: Human Kinetics, 1990.
35. DuRant RH, Seymore C, Linde CW, et al. The preparticipation examination of athletes: comparison of single and multiple examiners. Am J Dis Child 1985;139:657–661.
36. Caine DJ, Broekhoff J. Maturity assessment: a viable preventive measure against physical and psychological insult to the young athlete? Phys Sports Med 1987;15:67–80.
37. Anonymous. Strength training by children and adolescents: report of the AAP committee on sportsmedicine. Sports Med Dig 1991;13:7.
38. Runyan DK. The preparticipation examination of the young athlete. Clin Pediatr 1983;22:674–679.
39. Rooks DS, Micheli LJ. Musculoskeletal assessment and training: the young athlete. Clin Sports Med 1988;7:641–677.
40. Tanji JL. The preparticipation exam: special concerns for the Special Olympics. Phys Sports Med 1991;19:61–68.
41. Anonymous. American Academy of Pediatrics committee on sports medicine: atlantoaxial instability in Down syndrome. Pediatrics 1984;74:152–154.
42. Pueschel SM, Scola FH, Perry CD, et al. Atlanto-axial instability in children with Down syndrome. Pediatr Radiol 1981;10:129–132.
43. Anonymous. 1986–1987 Program guide (revised 1985). Austin, TX: Texas Special Olympics, 1987:54.
44. Potera C. Women in sports: the price of participation. Phys Sports Med 1986;14:149.
45. Raithel KS. Are girls less fit than boys? Phys Sports Med 1987;15:157–163.
46. Haycock CE, Gillette JR. Susceptibility of women athletes to injury: myth vs. reality. JAMA 1976;236:163–165.
47. Pate RR, Fox EL. Training of youth for sport. In: Kelly VC, ed. Practice of pediatrics. Hagerstown, MD: Harper & Row, 1987.
48. Stanitski CL. Management of sports injuries in children and adolescents. Orthop Clin North Am 1988;19:689–698.
49. Pratt M. Strength, flexibility, and maturity in adolescent athletes. Am J Dis Child 1989;1:560–563.
50. Hascelik Z, Basgoze O, Turker K, et al. The effects of physical training on physical fitness tests in auditory and visual reaction times of volleyball players. J Sports Med Phys Fit 1989;29:234–239.
51. Mero A, Kauhanen H, Peltola E, et al. Physiological performance capacity in different prepubescent athletic groups. J Sports Med Phys Fit 1990;30:57–66.
52. Hakkinen K, Mero A, Kauhanen H. Specificity of endurance, spring and strength training on physical performance capacity in young athletes. J Sports Med Phys Fit 1989;29:27–35.
53. Webb DR. Strength training in children and adolescents. Pediatr Clin North Am 1990;30:1187–1210.
54. McKeag DB. The role of exercise in children and adolescents. Clin Sports Med 1991;10:117–130.
55. National Strength and Conditioning Association. Position paper on prepubescent strength training. National Strength and Conditioning Association Journal 1985;7:27–31.

56. Anonymous. Risks in distance running for children. Sports Med Dig 1991;13:3.
57. Docherty D, Wenger HA, Collis ML. The effects of resistance training on aerobic and anaerobic power of young boys. Med Sci Sports Exerc 1987;19:389–392.
58. Mahon AD, Vaccaro P. Ventilatory threshold and $\dot{V}O_2max$ changes in children following endurance training. Med Sci Sports Exerc 1989;21:425–431.
59. Haffor AA, Harrison AC, Catledge-Kirk PA. Anaerobic threshold alterations caused by interval training in 11-year-olds. J Sports Med Phys Fit 1990;30:53–56.
60. Adeniran SA, Torioloa AL. Effects of continuous and interval running programs on aerobic and anaerobic capacities in school girls age 13 to 17 years. J Sports Med Phys Fit 1988;28:260–266.
61. Leard JS. Flexibility and conditioning in the young athlete. In: Micheli LJ, ed. Pediatric and adolescent sports medicine. Boston: Little, Brown & Co., 1984.
62. Stager JM, Wigglesworth JK, Hatler LK. Interpreting the relationship between age of menarche and prepubertal training. Med Sci Sports Exerc 1990;22:54–58.
63. Micheli LJ. Risks in distance running for children. Sports Med Dig 1991;13:3. Commentary.
64. Klemp P, Chalton D. Articular mobility in ballet dancers: a follow-up study after four years. Am J Sports Med 1989;17:72–75.
65. Chandler TJ, Kibler WB, Uhl TL, et al. Flexibility comparisons of junior elite tennis players to other athletes. Am J Sports Med 1990;18:134–136.
66. Smith AD, Stroud L, McQueen C. Flexibility and anterior knee pain in adolescent elite figure skaters. J Pediatr Orthop 1991;11:77–82.
67. Kendall H, Kendall F. Normal flexibility according to age-groups. J Bone Joint Surg 1948;39:424.
68. Leighton J. Flexibility characteristics of males ten to eighteen years of age. J Assoc Phys Ment Rehabil 1956;10:494.
69. Jacobson BH, Kulling FA. Effect of resistive weight training in prepubescents. J Orthop Sports Phys Ther 1989;11:96–98.
70. Pfeiffer RD, Francis RS. Effects of strength training on muscle development in prepubescent, pubescent, and postpubescent males. Phys Sports Med 1986;14:134–143.
71. Rians CB, Weltman A, Cahill BR, et al. Strength training for prepubescent males: is it safe? Am J Sports Med 1987;15:483–489.
72. Fripp RR, Hodgson JL. Effect of resistive training on plasma lipid and lipoprotein levels in male adolescents. J Pediatr 1987;111:926–931.
73. Yessis MP. Pre-Post-pubescent weight training. Proceedings of the California Strength and Conditioning clinic, Los Angeles. 1987.
74. Goldberg B. Injury patterns in youth sports. Phys Sports Med 1989;17:175–186.
75. Zito M. Musculoskeletal injuries of young athletes: the new trends. In: Gould JA, ed. Orthopedic and sports physical therapy. Baltimore: CV Mosby, 1990:627–650.
76. Wetterhall SF, Waxweiler RJ. Injury surveillance at the 1985 national boy scout jamboree. Am J Sports Med 1988;16:534–538.
77. DeHaven KE, Litner DM. Athletic injuries: comparison by age, sport and gender. Am J Sports Med 1986;14:218–224.
78. Backx FJ, Erich WB, Kemper AB, et al. Sports injuries in school-aged children: an epidemiologic study. Am J Sports Med 1989;17:234–240.
79. Martin RK, Yesalis CE, Foster D, et al. Sports injuries at the 1985 Junior Olympics. Am J Sports Med 1987;15:603–608.
80. McClain LG, Reynolds S. Sports injuries in a high school. Pediatrics. 1989;84:446–450.
81. Prager BI, Fitton WL, Cahill BR, et al. High school football injuries: a prospective study and pitfalls of data collection. Am J Sports Med 1989;17:681–685.
82. Shephard RJ. Physical activity and wellness of the child. In: Boileau RA ed. Advances in pediatric sport sciences. Champaign, IL: Human Kinetics, 1984:1–27.
83. U.S. Consumer Product Safety Commission. National Electronic Injury Surveillance System. Washington, D.C.: U.S. Government Printing Office, 1989.
84. Tursz A, Crost M. Sports-related injuries in children. Am J Sports Med 1986;14:294–299.
85. Pappas AM. Elbow problems associated with baseball during childhood and adolescence. Clin Orthop 1984;184:30–41.
86. Tullos HS, King JW. Lesions of the pitching arm in adolescents. JAMA 1972;220:264–271.
87. Adams JE. Osteochondrosis of the proximal humeral epiphysis in boy baseball pitchers. California Med 1966;105:22–25.
88. Adams JE. Injury to the throwing arm. California Med 1964;102:127–132.
89. Herndon WA. Acute and chronic injury: its effect on growth in the young athlete. In: Gana WA, Lombardo JA, Sharkey BJ, et al., eds. Advances in sports medicine and fitness. Chicago: Year Book Medical Publishers, 1990:127–146.
90. Keller CS, Noyes FR, Buncher CR. The medical aspects of soccer injury epidemiology. Am J Sports Med 1987;15:230–237.
91. Nielson AB, Yde J. Epidemiology and traumatology of injuries in soccer. Am J Sports Med 1989;17:803–807.
92. McAuley E, Hadash G, Shields K, et al. Injuries in women's gymnastics. Am J Sports Med 1987;15:124–131.
93. Caine D, Cochrane B, Caine C, et al. An epidemiologic investigation of injuries affecting young female gymnasts. Am J Sports Med 1989;17:811–820.
94. Mandelbaum BR, Bartolozzi AR, Davis CA, et al. Wrist pain syndrome in the gymnast. Am J Sports Med 1989;17:305–317.
95. Priest JD. Elbow injuries in gymnastics. Clin Sports Med 1985;4:73–83.
96. Snook GA. The injury problem in wrestling. Am J Sports Med. 1976;4:184–188.
97. Requa R, Garrick JG. Injuries in interscholastic wrestling. Phys Sport Medicine. 1981;9:44–51.
98. Bunnell WP. Back pain in children. Orthop Clin North Am 1982;13:587–604.
99. King HA. Back pain in children. Pediatr Clin North Am 1984;31:1083–1095.
100. Boston HC. Branch AJ. Jr., Rhodes KH. Disc space infections in children. Orthop Clin North Am 1975;6:953–964.
101. Clark A. Standish WD. An unusual case of back pain in a young athlete. Am J Sports Med 1985;13:51–54.
102. Spiegl PG, Kengla KW, Isaacson AS, et al. Intervertebral disc space inflammation in children. J Bone Joint Surg Am 1972;54:284–296.
103. Heller RM, Szalay EA, Green NE, et al. Disc space infection in children: magnetic resonance imaging. Radiol Clin North Am 1988;26:207–209.
104. Epstein F, Epstein N. Intramedullary tumors of the spinal cord. In: Shilito J, Matson DD, eds. Pediatric neurosurgery of the developing nervous system. New York: Grune & Stratton, 1982:529–540.
105. Yochum TR, Rowe LJ. The natural history of spondylolysis and spondylolisthesis. In: Yochum TR, Rowe LJ, eds. Essentials of skeletal radiology. Baltimore: Williams & Wilkins, 1987:243–272.
106. Commandre FA, Gagnerie G, Zakarian M, et al. The child, the spine and sport. Am J Sports Med 1988;28:11–19.
107. Commandre FA, Taillan B, Gagnerie F, et al. Spondylolysis and spondylolisthesis in young athletes: 28 cases. Am J Sports Med 1988;28:104–107.
108. Banks SD. Athletic low back pain originating from the neural arch. Chiro Sports Med J 1988;2:51–54.
109. Gengenbach MS. The symptomatic lumbar spine. DC Tracts 1990;2:74–79.

110. Alexander C. Scheuermann's disease: a traumatic spondylodystrophy. Skeletal Radiol 1977;128:5.

111. Pizzutillo PD. Osteochondroses. In: Sullivan JA, Grana WA, eds. The pediatric athlete. Park Ridge, IL: American Association of Orthopedic Surgeons, 1990:227–230.

112. Afshani E, Kuhn J. Common causes of low back pain in children. Radiographics 1991;11:269.

113. Kent C. Pediatric back pain: imaging considerations. ICA Intl Review Chiro 1991;47:59–63.

114. Rowe LJ, Yochum TR. Trauma: slipped capital femoral epiphysis. In: Yochum TR, Rowe LJ, eds. Essentials of skeletal radiology. Baltimore: Williams & Wilkins, 1987: 465–468.

115. Anonymous. Slipped capital femoral epiphysis. In: Dingle RV, ed. The CIBA collection of medical illustrations: the musculoskeletal system. Summitt, NJ: CIBA-Geigy, 1990:69–71.

116. Anonymous. Legg-Calvé-Perthes disease. In: Dingle RV, ed. The CIBA collection of medical illustrations: the musculoskeletal system. Summitt, NJ: CIBA-Geigy, 1990:59–69.

117. Rowe LJ, Yochum TR. Hematological and vascular disorders. In: Yochum TR, Rowe LJ, eds. Essentials of skeletal radiology. Baltimore: Williams & Wilkins, 1987: 995–998.

118. Kettner N. Acute plastic bowing fractures: a review. CSMJ 1987;4:141–143.

119. Salter RB, Harris WR. Injuries involving the epiphyseal plate. J Bone Joint Surg 1963;45:587–622.

120. Connelly JF. Fractures in children: when the growth plate is damaged. J Musculoskeletal Med 1991;8:82–97.

121. Roy S, Irvin R. Sports medicine: prevention, evaluation, management, and rehabilitation. Englewood Cliffs, NJ: Prentice-Hall, 1983:133–140.

122. Singer K. Injuries and disorders of the epiphysis in young athletes. In: Broekhoff JB, Ellis MJ, Tripps DG, eds. Sport for children and youths. Champaign IL: Human Kinetics, 1986:141–150.

123. Roy S, Caine D, Singer KM. Stress changes of the distal radial epiphysis in young gymnasts. Am J Sports Med 1985;13:301–307.

124. Salter RB. Specific fractures and joint injuries in children. In: Salter RB, ed. Textbook of disorders and injuries of the musculoskeletal system. Baltimore: Williams & Wilkins, 1983:434–436.

125. Larson RL. Epiphyseal injuries in the adolescent athlete. Orthop Clin North Am 1973;4:839–850.

126. Larson RL, McMahan RO. The epiphyses and the childhood athlete. JAMA. 1966;196:99–104.

127. Clain MR, Hershman EB. Overuse injuries in children and adolescents. Phys Sport Med 1989;17;111–123.

128. Donati RB, Echo BS, Powell CE. Bilateral tibial stress fractures in a six-year old male. Am J Sports Med 1990;18:323–325.

129. Harvey JS. Overuse syndromes in young athletes. In: Broekhoff JB, Ellis MF, Tripps DG, eds. Sport for children and youths. Champaign IL: Human Kinetics, 1986:151–163.

130. Aspergen DA, Cox JM, Benak DR. Detection of stress fractures in athletes and non-athletes. J Manipulative Physiol Ther 1989;12:298–303.

131. Rettig AC, Beltz HF. Stress fracture in the humerus in an adolescent tennis tournament player. Am J Sports Med 1985;13:55–58.

132. Caine DJ, Lindner KJ. Overuse injuries of growing bones:the young female gymnast at risk? Phys Sports Med. 1985;13:51–64.

133. Pecina M, Bojanic I, Dubravcic S. Stress fractures in figure skaters. Am J Sports Med. 1990;18:277–279.

134. Mirbey J, Besancenot J, Chambers RT, et al. Avulsion fractures of the tibial tuberosity in the adolescent athlete. Am J Sports Med 1988;16:336–340.

135. Bowers KD. Patellar tendon avulsion as a complication of Osgood-Schlatter's disease. Am J Sports Med 1976;4: 253–263.

136. Pappas AM. Osteochondroses: diseases of growth centers. Phys Sports Med 1989;17:51–62.

137. Rowe LJ, Yochum TR. Hematological and vascular disorders. In: Yochum TR, Rowe LJ, eds. Essentials of skeletal radiology. Baltimore: Williams & Wilkins, 1987:1009–1013.

138. Anderson WA, McKeag DB, McGrew CA. A national survey of alcohol on drug use by college athletes. Phys Sportsmed 1991;19:91–104.

139. Cowart VS, Wright JE. Anabolic steroids: altered states. Carmel: Benchmark, 1990.

140. Buckley WE, Yesalis CE, Friedl KE. et al. Estimated prevalence of anabolic steroid use among male high school seniors. JAMA 1988;260:3441–3445.

141. Rich SE, Hough DO. Performance enhancing drugs. Sports Med Dig 1992;14:1–2.

142. Perry PJ, Anderson KH, Yates WR. Illicit anabolic steroid use in athletes: a case series analysis. Am J Sports Med 1990;18:422–428.

143. Haupt HA. Ergogenic aids. In: Reider B, ed. Sports medicine: the school age athlete. Philadelphia: WB Saunders 1991:52–56.

144. Strauss RH. Anabolic steroid use by young athletes. In: Smith NJ, ed. Common problems in pediatric sports medicine. Chicago: Year Book Medical Publishers 1989:131–135.

145. Haupt HA, Rover GD. Anabolic steroids: a review of the literature. Am J Sports Med 1984;12;469–484.

146. Strauss RH, Liggett MT, Lanese RR. Anabolic steroid use and perceived effects in ten weight trained women athletes. JAMA 1985;253:2871–2874.

147. Lamb DR. Anabolic steroids in athletics: how well do they work and how dangerous are they? Am J Sports Med 1984;12;31–38.

148. Tennant FS, Black DL, Voy RO. Anabolic steroid dependence with opioid features. N Engl J Med 1988;7:578.

149. Anonymous. Medication risks in patients taking steroids. Sports Med Dig 1992;14:2–3.

150. Goldberg L, Bents R, Bosworth E, et al. Anabolic steroid education and adolescents: do scare tactics work? Pediatrics 1991;87:283–286.

151. Macintyre JG. Growth hormone and athletes. Sports Med 1987;4;129–142.

152. Laties VG, Weiss B. The amphetamine margin in sports. Fed Prog 1981;40:2689–2692.

153. Murray DM, Roche LM, Goldman AI, et al. Smokeless tobacco use among ninth graders in a north-central metropolitan population: cross sectional and prospective associations with age, gender, race, family structure and other drug use. Preventive Med 1988;17:449–460.

154. Glover ED, Edmundson EW, Edwards SW, et al. Implications of smokeless tobacco use among athletes. Phys Sportsmed 1986;14:94–105.

155. Gerber RW, Newman IM, Martin GL. Applying the theory of reasoned action to early adolescent tobacco chewing. J Sch Health 1988;58:410–413.

156. Edwards SW, Glover ED, Schroeder KL. The effect of smokeless tobacco on heart rate and neuromuscular reactivity in athletes and non-athletes. Phys Sportsmed 1987;15:141–147.

157. Duda M. Snuffing out the use of smokeless tobacco. Phys Sportsmed 1985;13:171–175.

158. Strauss RH. Spittin' image: breaking the sports-tobacco connection. Phys Sportsmed 1991;19:46–48. Editorial.

159. American College of Sportsmedicine. Position and stand on blood doping as an ergogenic aid. Med Sci Sports Exerc 1987;19:540–543.

160. Anonymous. Cyclists' deaths linked to erythropoietin? Phys Sportsmed 1990;18:48–50.

161. Colon AR. Nutrition. In: Ziai M, ed. Pediatrics. 4th ed. Boston: Little, Brown & Co., 1990:117–124.

162. Williams MH. Nutrition for fitness and sport. Dubuque, IA: WC Brown, 1983:160.

163. Rowland TW. Exercise and children's health. Champaign, IL: Human Kinetics, 1990:252–253.

164. Oded Bar-Or. Children and performance in warm and cold climates. In: Boileau R, ed. Advances in pediatric sport sciences. Champaign, IL: Human Kinetics, 1984: 117–129.

165. Smith NJ. Nutrition in children's sports. In: Micheli LJ, ed. Pediatric and adolescent sports medicine. Boston: Little, Brown & Co., 1984:134–143.

166. Wroble RR, Hoegh JT, Albright JP. Wrestling. In: Reider B, ed. Sports medicine: the school age athlete. Philadelphia: WB Saunders, 1991:550.

167. Chen JD, Wang JF, Lee KJ, et al. Nutritional problems and measures in elite and amateur athletes. Am J Clin Nutr 1989;49:1084–1089.

168. Hickson JF, Duke MA, Risser WL. et al. Nutritional intake from food sources of high school football athletes. J Am Diet Assoc 1987;87:1656–1659.

169. Tarnopolsky MA, MacDougall JD, Atkinson SA. Influence of protein intake and training status on nitrogen balance and lean body mass. J Appl Phys 1988;64: 187–193.

170. Leung AK, Robson WL. Childhood obesity. Postgrad Med 1990;87:123–133.

171. Becque MD, Katch VL, Rocchinin AP, et al. Coronary risk incidence of obese adolescents: reduction by exercise plus diet intervention. Pediatrics 1988;81:605–612.

172. Rocchini AP, Katch V, Anderson J, et al. Blood pressure in obese adolescents: effect of weight loss. Pediatrics 1988;82:16–23.

173. Cooper DM, Poage J, Barstow TJ, et al. Are obese children truly unfit? minimizing the confounding effect of body size on the exercise response. J Pediatr 1990;116: 223–230.

174. Hill J, Schlunt DG, Sbrocco T, et al. Evaluation of an alternating calorie diet with and without exercise in the treatment of obesity. Am J Clin Nutr 1989;50:248–254.

175. Reybrouck T, Vinckx J, Vandenberghe G, et al. Exercise therapy and hypocaloric diet in the treatment of obese children and adolescents. Acta Poediatr Scan 1990;79: 84–89.

176. Marshall Hoerr SL, Nelson RA, Essex-Sorlie D. Treatment and followup of obesity in adolescent girls. J Adolesc Health Care 1988;9:28–37.

177. Katch V, Becque MD, Marks C, et al. Basal metabolism of obese adolescents: inconsistent diet and exercise effects. Am J Clin Nutr 1988;48:565–569.

178. Rocchini AP, Katch V, Schork A, et al. Insulin and blood pressure during weight loss in obese adolescents. Hypertension 1987;10:267–273.

179. Epstein LH, Kuller LH, Wing RR, et al. The effect of weight control on lipid changes in obese children. Am J Dis Child 1989;143:454–457.

180. Segal KR, Pi-Sunyer FX. Exercise and obesity. Med Clin North Am 1989;73:217–236.

181. Simmons Morton BG, Parcell GS. O'Hara NM. Implementing organizational changes to promote healthful diet and physical activity at school. Health Educ Q 1988;15:115–130.

182. Price JH, Desmond SM, Ruppert ES, et al. School nurses' perceptions of childhood obesity. J Sch Health 1987;57:332–336.

183. Perry CL, Mullis RM. Maile MC. Modifying the eating behavior of young children. J Sch Health 1985;55:399–402.

184. Tipton CM. Commentary: physicians should advise wrestlers about weight loss. Phys Sportsmed 1987;15: 160–165.

185. Woods ER, Wilson CD, Masland JR. Weight control methods in high school wrestlers. J Adolesc Health Care 1988;9:394–397.

186. Strauss RH, Lanese RR, Malarkey WB. Weight loss in amateur wrestlers and its effect on serum testosterone. JAMA 1985;254:3337–3338.

187. Steen SN, Opplinger RA, Brownell KD. Metabolic effects of repeated weight loss and regain in adolescent wrestlers. JAMA 1988;260:47–50.

188. American College of Sports Medicine. Position stand on weight loss in wrestlers. Med Sci Sports Exerc 1976;8: 11–13.

189. Klinzing JE, Karpowics W. The effects of rapid weight loss and rehydration on a wrestling performance test. J Sports Med 1986;26:149–156.

190. Smith NJ. Weight control in a high school wrestling program. In: Smith NJ, ed. Common problems in pediatric sports medicine. Chicago: Year Book, 1989: 176–180.

191. Opplinger RA, Tipton CM. Iowa wrestling study: cross validation of the Tcheng-Tipton minimal weight prediction formulas for high school wrestlers. Med Sci Sports Exerc 1988;20:310–316.

192. Brownell K, Forey JP. Handbook of eating disorders. New York: Basic Books, 1986.

193. Rosen LW, McKeag DB, Hough DO, et al. Pathogenic weight control behavior in female athletes. Phys Sportsmed 1986;14:79–86.

194. Rosen LW, Hough DO. Pathogenic weight control behaviors of female college gymnasts. Phys Sportsmed 1988;16:141–146.

195. Thornton JS. Feast or famine: eating disorders in athletes. Phys Sportsmed 1990;18:4:116–122.

196. Thompson RA. Management of the athlete with an eating disorder: implication for the sports management team. Sports Psychol 1987;1:114–126.

197. Gerschoff S. The Tufts university guide to total nutrition. New York: Harper & Row, 1990:185–186.

198. Rowland TW, Kelleher JF. Iron deficiency in athletes: insights from high school swimmers. Am J Dis Child 1989;143:197–200.

199. Nickerson JH, Holubets MC, Wheiler BR, et al. Causes of iron deficiency in adolescent athletes. J Pediatr 1989;114:657–663.

200. Risser WL, Lee EJ, Poindexter HB, et al. Iron deficiency in female athletes: its prevalence and impact on performance. Med Sci Sports Exerc 1988;20:116–121.

201. Nichols BL. Pediatric nutrition and nutritional disorders. In: Behrman RE, Kliegman R, eds. Nelson essentials of pediatrics. Philadelphia: WB Saunders, 1990:669.

202. Goldberg B. Children, sports, and chronic disease. Phys Sportsmed 1990;18:45–56.

203. Lefebvre JF. The young athlete with diabetes mellitus. In: Smith NJ, ed. Common problems in pediatric sports medicine. Chicago: Year Book, 1989:81–90.

204. Anderson BJ, Wolf FM, Burhart MT, et al. Effects of peer-group intervention on metabolic control of adolescents with IDDM: randomized outpatient study. Diabetes Care 1989;12:179–183.

205. Merrero DG, Fremeion AS, Golden MP. Improving compliance with exercise in adolescents with insulin-dependent diabetes mellitus: results of a self-motivated home exercise program. Pediatrics 1988;81:519–525.

206. Stratton R, Wilson DP, Endres RK, et al. Improved glycemic control after 8-wk exercise program in insulin-dependent diabetic adolescents. Diabetes Care 1987;10: 589–593.

207. Huttunen NP, Lankela SL, Knip M, et al. Effect of once-a-week training program on physical fitness and metabolic control in children with IDDM. Diabetes Care 1989;12:737–740.

208. Pierson WE. Exercise-induced bronchospasm in children and adolescents. Pediatr Clin North Am 1988;35: 1031–1040.

209. Pierson WE. The young athlete with exercise induced respiratory distress. In: Smith NJ, ed. Common problems in pediatric sports medicine. Chicago: Year Book, 1989;115–121.

210. Strunk RC, Rubin D, Kelley L, et al. Determination of fitness in children with asthma: use of standardized tests for functional endurance, body fat composition, flexibility, and abdominal strength. Am J Dis Child 1988;142: 940–944.

211. Orenstein DM. Exercise tolerance and exercise conditioning in children with chronic lung disease. J Pediatr 1988;112:1043–1047.
212. American Academy of Pediatrics. Exercise in the asthmatic child. Pediatrics 1989;84:392–393.
213. Freeman JM. The young athlete with epilepsy. In: Smith NJ, et al. Common problems in pediatric sports medicine. Chicago: Year Book, 1989:91–95.
214. Vaccaro P, Galioto FM, Bradley LM, et al. Effects of physical training on tolerance of children following surgical repair of D-transposition of the great arteries. J Sports Med 1987;27:443–448.
215. Strauss GD, Osher A, Wang CI, et al. Variable weight training in cystic fibrosis. Chest 1987:92:273–276.

19

The Senior Athlete

D. A. Lawson

For the past decade, older adults have been encouraged to become more physically active by such organizations as the American Heart Association, the President's Council on Fitness, and the American Association of Retired Persons. Exercise programs for seniors and opportunities for athletic competition, such as the Senior Olympics, are thriving. This truly is the coming of age for the senior athlete.

There are two distinctly different groups of older athletes: the well-seasoned athlete who is continuing a program of sports participation into the senior years and the relative newcomer who has taken up an interest in exercise later in life.

This chapter primarily addresses the physiologic changes and sports injuries in the currently participating athlete, with a brief discussion of exercise evaluation and prescription in the older athlete and an introduction to the Senior Olympics.

BIOLOGIC CHANGES WITH AGING

Support of the older athlete in performance or exercise necessitates an awareness of the physiologic changes associated with aging. In the past, the hallmark of aging was considered to be a reduction in function of most of the major organ systems. However, what was once regarded as the physiology of "aging" is now being redefined as the physiology of "disuse." It is becoming clearer that much of the reduction in organ function associated with aging is the result of disuse in an increasingly sedentary population (1). This is emphasized by the fact that the maintenance of chronically high levels of physical activity over the course of a lifetime, as in the case of master athletes, often leads to an apparent separation of chronologic and physiologic aging (2–6). Similarly, resuming activity, even after many years of sedentariness, can reverse certain deficits in physiologic structure and function at one time thought to be irreversible. This includes muscle weakness, limitation of joint motion, loss of aerobic capacity, and metabolic potential of skeletal muscle (7–11). Table 19.1 outlines the important interactions of aging, disuse, and exercise.

There are changes that occur with aging, and it is important to keep in mind the differences between aging and disuse. From the limited research available, it appears that much of the age-related loss of function is due to a combination of aging and decreased physical activity. Losses resulting from the combination of these factors may not have the capacity for complete recovery. Losses caused by disuse alone may be able to be regained through exercise rehabilitation (12). This section discusses the alterations in exercise capacity secondary to aging itself, with a focus on how this might apply to the older athlete. The commonly held view is that age-related changes may predispose the older athlete to injury or affect the rehabilitation time associated with recovery from injury. This has yet to be confirmed, and evidence to the contrary is increasing.

Cardiovascular System

The most consistently described change in the aging cardiovascular system is a decrease in maximal heart rate (HR_{max}) (13–16). This phenomenon has been observed in all populations studied to date, including well-trained master athletes (2). It is thought to be the result of an age-related decrease in myocardial sensitivity to sympathetic stimulation. This limitation in HR_{max} appears to be the underlying cause for the decline in maximal oxygen consumption ($\dot{V}O_2max$) often observed with aging (1).

Rodeheffer et al. (17) showed that despite the lower peak heart rate, submaximal exercise cardiac output was maintained in healthy elderly subjects by augmentation of end-diastolic and stroke volumes. In these subjects, exercise cardiac output was maintained by reliance on the Frank-Starling mechanism to compensate for the

Table 19.1.   Comparison of Aging, Disuse, and Exercise

Physiologic Characteristic (Reference)	Aging	Disuse	Exercise
Body composition (2,8,13,16,23,26,28)			
Fat mass	I	I	D
Lean mass	D	D	I
Bone mass	D	D	I
Cardiovascular function (6,7,13,14,15,16,17)			
V̇o₂max	D	D	I
Cardiac output	D, NC	NC	NC
Heart rate			
Resting	I, NC	I	D
Maximal	D	NC	NC
Stroke volume			
Resting	D, NC	D	I, NC
Maximal	D, NC	D	I
Skeletal muscle (5,8,12,19,21,22,24,25,26,27,29,30,34,35)			
Fiber number	D	NC	NC
Mean fiber area	D	D	I, NC
Type II fiber area	D	D	I, NC
Muscle strength	D	D	I
Enzyme capacity	D	D	I
Glycogen storage	D	D	I
Capillary density	D, NC	I	I, NC, D
Fat and connective tissue content	I	I	D
Nervous system (36,37,38,39,40,41,42)			
Nerve conduction velocity	D	NC	NC
Reaction time	D	D, NC	NC
Cognitive processing	D	D, NC	NC

I, increased; D, decreased; NC, no change.

inability to raise the heart rate adequately. However, a negative age-related trend was observed in the ejection fraction, suggesting that contractility was impaired. This may be the result of the decreasing sympathetic responsiveness of the myocardium described earlier. It should be noted that when relying on the Frank-Starling mechanism, the heart must function at a larger volume, which implies more wall tension stress and produces a greater myocardial oxygen demand.

Muscle Function

Age-related changes in muscle appear to be present even in the absence of disease and despite the maintenance of contractile demands on the muscle fibers (12, 16, 18–22). The most obvious change is the loss of muscle mass, beginning in approximately the fourth decade (18, 23–25). For those who have been particularly sedentary, this may result in a 40% reduction in peak muscle mass by age 70 or 80.

Morphologic studies of aging muscle demonstrate loss of motor fibers with predominant atrophy of Type II (fast twitch) fibers and lean tissue replacement by connective tissue and fat (26–31). The functional implications of this age-related atrophy is the loss of strength. Muscle strength is directly related to the cross-sectional area of the fibers (24, 25). The lower extremities in particular appear to be affected preferentially by this age-related weakness (32, 33).

Other changes investigated in skeletal muscle include reductions in mitochondrial density (34), oxidative enzyme activity (27), and capillary density (35). These changes limit the supply of substrate available to skeletal muscle for aerobic and anaerobic work, as well as the tissue capacity for oxygen consumption. This reduced oxidative capacity of skeletal muscle may also contribute to the decline in V̇o₂max described earlier.

Neurologic System

Changes that occur in the central and peripheral nervous systems include lengthening of reaction times, slowing of conduction velocities, and altering of cognitive function (13). Nerve conduction velocity declines approximately 10 to 15% over the life span (13). Physically active older adults have been shown to have faster reaction times and improved cognitive abilities when compared with their sedentary peers, suggesting that these functions may be modulated by disuse (36–38).

Short-term exercise studies have not been effective in detecting changes in neurologic function (39–41). Rikli and Edwards, however, showed significant improvement in simple and choice reaction times as well as balance during a 3-year study using previously sedentary women, aged 57 to 85 (42). These findings suggest the effectiveness of exercise in reversing or at least slowing certain age-related declines in motor performance and cognitive processing speed when sustained over longer periods.

Skeletal System

Bone density is known to decrease with age and proceeds at different rates among persons and in different parts of the skeleton. Cortical bone is found primarily in the long bones of the appendicular skeleton, and trabecular bone is found in the axial skeleton. The skeleton as a whole is composed of approximately 80% cortical bone and 20% trabecular bone (43).

Women lose bone at a greater rate than men and have an accelerated period of bone loss after menopause at some skeletal sites (21). This accelerated loss, particularly of cortical bone, has been linked to declining estrogen levels (44). The spine especially appears to be sensitive to estrogen withdrawal (21). Over a lifetime, women may lose 30 to 35% of their cortical bone compared with 20% in men (16).

In men, the average rate of loss of cortical bone is 0.3% of adult peak bone mass per year; the rate of loss of trabecular bone is slightly higher and has an earlier onset of loss (12). Cortical bone is less metabolically active than trabecular bone, which may explain its maintenance until later in life (21). In women, the average rate of loss is approximately 1% of adult peak bone mass per year for both cortical and trabecular bone (43). This rate is accelerated for approximately 5 years after menopause. By age 80, a woman has lost approximately 50% of her axial bone.

Bone density is affected by three categories of factors: genetic (heavy-boned persons lose less bone mass than do small-boned persons), endocrine/nutritional (this includes calcium-regulating and systemic hormones as well as calcium and vitamin D and its metabolites), and mechanical stress (exercise) (43). Cross-sectional studies of athletes have demonstrated that those who are most active have a higher bone mass or density compared with age-matched control subjects (12). Exercise in combination with estrogen appears to be the most effective means to improve bone mineral density (44).

EXERCISE EVALUATION AND PRESCRIPTION IN THE OLDER ATHLETE

Although this chapter focuses on the currently participating athlete, a few comments are in order regarding preexercise evaluation and exercise prescription in the older athlete.

Exercise evaluation should include the following: identification of risk factors for heart disease and diabetes, a stress test to determine aerobic capacity and to evaluate the heart under demand conditions, tests for flexibility and strength, sensory testing, and screening for deformities and joint pain. This information is used to formulate the individual exercise prescription. Accommodations for physical limitations are defined, and the appropriate mode and intensity of exercise are selected (45).

Risk Factors and Stress Testing

Two or more risk factors for heart disease and diabetes place an individual at higher risk for exercise. According to the guidelines published by the American College of Sports Medicine, an examination and diagnostic exercise testing are desirable for the higher risk individual before beginning a vigorous exercise program (46). Target exercise heart rates can be established using the stress test data.

Muscle Strength

Assessment of ankle and knee strength is beneficial for exercise prescription. Isometric quadriceps data can be used as an index of general body strength; those with an output of 50% or less body weight should participate in a remedial strengthening program before any cycling or track work. Major strength deficits predispose to muscle strain, and exercise more strenuous than moderate walking may be detrimental. Individuals with quadriceps capability of less than 50% of body weight also tend to have a positive Trendelenburg test while walking or even standing on one leg (47). Weakness in the gluteus medius may result in hip pain during jogging and vigorous walking.

Flexibility

An evaluation of lower extremity flexibility may assist in identifying those at risk for injury due to a lack of mobility. Hip and ankle excursion are particularly important. The straight leg test for hamstring contractures and the modified Thomas test for hip flexion contractures, rectus femoris tightness, and iliotibial band tightness are generally sufficient for hip evaluation. Tight hip flexors may result in hip, knee, or back pain (47). Fast walking, for example, requires a 60° arc of hip motion. Reduced ranges of motion will impose undue stress on the lumbar spine to recruit the additional needed movement.

A minimum of 0° of ankle dorsiflexion is required for walking or jogging programs; 10° is preferred. A short stride or calf pain will result with less than 0°. A good pair of walking or running shoes may sufficiently accommodate for a reduction in motion. However, women who for many years have worn moderate to high heels may be unable to walk comfortably in low shoes; the heelcords may need to be stretched in these cases.

Sensory Testing

Sensitivity on the dorsum and plantar surfaces of the foot is important. Impaired sensation necessitates particular attention to proper-fitting footwear with excellent shock absorption, the use of double-thickness socks, and conscientious care of the nails.

Deformities and Joint Pain

Inspection of the feet and lower extremities may reveal overt arthritic changes. Joint pain or degeneration is rarely considered a contraindica-

Table 19.2. Location of Injury in Older and Younger Groups

Location	Older No.	Older %	Younger No.	Younger %
Knee	202	29.5	294	40.7
Foot	135	19.7	98	13.6
Lower leg	73	10.7	90	12.5
Ankle	54	7.9	52	7.2
Shoulder	50	7.3	45	6.2
Lumbosacral spine	42	6.1	47	6.5
Elbow	26	3.8	18	2.5
Hip/pelvis	25	3.6	22	3.0
Upper leg	20	2.9	30	4.2
Neck	9	1.3	5	0.7
Wrist/hand	6	0.9	6	0.8
Multiple sites	43	6.3	15	2.1
Total	685	100.0	722	100.0

From Matheson GO, MacIntyre JE, Taunton DB, et al. Musculoskeletal injuries associated with physical activity in older adults. Med Sci Sports Exerc 1989;21:379–385.

tion for exercise. Selecting weight-supported exercises such as swimming, bicycling, Nordic track, or chair exercises may be more appropriate than walking, jogging, or stair climbing (48).

Other Considerations

If balance is poor, it is advisable to avoid such activities as cycling or skiing. Also, adverse environmental conditions may not be tolerated well by the older athlete. Thermoregulation can be affected by such common medications as beta-blocking agents, and exercise during hot spells should be performed in air-conditioned facilities or in the water. Exercise in severely cold temperatures can cause reflexive increases in blood pressure and coronary vasoconstriction and may provoke myocardial ischemia. Finally, swimming or pool exercises may be followed by hypotension, particularly if an individual is receiving antihypertensive medication. It is important to ensure that pools have adequate handrails and nonslip decks (48).

SPORTS INJURIES IN THE OLDER ATHLETE

Despite the increase in sporting activities in the aging population, there are relatively few studies that have addressed the frequency, profile, and specific features of sports injuries occurring among older athletes (49–53). Matheson et al. (53) documented the clinical pattern of sports injuries in older individuals (50 years of age and older) who had been referred by a physician to an outpatient sports medicine clinic over a 5-year period. These findings were compared with a younger group from the same population. The anatomical locations of injury and the diag-

noses in each group are presented in Tables 19.2 and 19.3.

Matheson et al., in agreement with other studies (49, 50, 52–54), found that 85% of the diagnoses in the older athlete were associated with overuse syndromes. The knee was the most common site of injury.

Running appears to be the most common physical activity associated with injury; this may explain the high proportion of injuries to the knee, lower leg, and foot (49, 52, 54). Several studies agree, however, that the long-term runner does not develop injuries or greater degenerative changes compared with any other individual (49, 54, 55). An important study found that older runners had less physical disability and sought medical services less often than age-matched control subjects (49). The age-related development of musculoskeletal disability appears to occur at a lower rate in runners, thus prolonging the functional capacity of this system with age.

Specific sports injuries in the older athlete will be discussed relative to the most common modes of exercise in this group. These include running, tennis, golf, swimming, and cycling (Table 19.4).

Running and the Older Athlete

The popularity of running has increased considerably since the early 1970s. The older athlete has become more prevalent in the sport; some have been running since the 1970s, and others have recently started a program. Almost without exception, running injuries are due to overuse;

Table 19.3. Diagnoses in Older and Younger Age Groups

Diagnosis	Older No.	Older %	Younger No.	Younger %
Tendinitis	173	25.3	189	26.2
PFPS	75	10.9	163	22.6
Ligament sprain	54	7.9	91	12.6
Muscle strain	48	7.0	65	9.0
Metatarsalgia	47	6.9	20	2.8
Osteoarthritis	45	6.6	12	1.7
Plantar fasciitis	45	6.6	18	2.5
Meniscal injury	37	5.4	10	1.4
DDD	33	4.8	11	1.5
Stress fracture/periostitis	29	4.2	81	11.2
Morton's neuroma	22	3.2	4	0.5
Inflammatory arthritis	18	2.6	8	1.1
Vascular/compartment	10	1.5	2	0.3
Bursitis	7	1.0	16	2.2
Multiple diagnoses	16	2.3	10	1.3
Unknown	26	3.8	22	3.1
Total	685	100.0	722	100.0

From Matheson GO, MacIntyre JE, Taunton DB, et al. Musculoskeletal injuries associated with physical activity in older adults. Med Sci Sports Exerc 1989;21:379–385.
PFPS, patellofemoral pain syndrome; DDD, degenerative disc disease.

Table 19.4. Injuries in Senior Athletes by Sport

Sport	Location	Overuse Syndrome
Running	Knee	Patellofemoral pain syndrome
		Iliotibial band friction syndrome
Tennis	Shoulder/arm	Acute injury
		Rotator cuff rupture
		Chronic injuries
		Tennis elbow
		Rotator cuff tendinitis
	Knee/leg	Acute injuries
		Meniscal tears
		Medial gastrocnemius tears
		Achilles tendon rupture
		Chronic injury
		Degenerative knee joint
	Lumbar spine	Chronic pain syndrome
Golf	Cervical spine	Chronic pain syndrome
	Lumbar spine	Chronic pain syndrome
	Shoulder	Rotator cuff impingement
	Elbow	Golfer's elbow
		Lateral epicondylitis
	Wrist	Chronic pain syndrome
		Tendinitis
Swimming	Shoulder	Swimmer's shoulder
		Injuries of the rotator cuff and
		long biceps tendon
		Degenerative joint changes
	Knee	Patellofemoral pain syndrome
Cycling	Wrist	Compression syndromes
		Carpal tunnel
		Ulnar nerve (Guyon's canal)
	Shoulder/arm	Inflammatory syndromes
		Lateral epicondylitis
		Subacromial bursitis

the cause is multifactorial (54, 55). Factors leading to overuse injuries can be divided into intrinsic and extrinsic categories. Intrinsic factors, such as alignment abnormalities, leg length discrepancies, muscle weakness or imbalance, and poor flexibility, can lead to abnormal stress and load on articular and soft tissue structures (56). Extrinsic factors include training errors such as poor technique; excess mileage or intensity; too-rapid changes in routines; running on surfaces that are too hard, uneven, or sloping; and inadequate running shoes.

Identifying the underlying causes of injury is important in the treatment and prevention of overuse syndromes. However, the realization that the incidence of running injuries is directly related to the weekly mileage of the runner is particularly important. Increases in mileage appear to be the most important factor in the development of overuse injuries (54, 56).

The most common injuries affecting the older runner involve the knee, lower leg, and foot (53–58). These injuries share a common cause—repetitive trauma that overwhelms the tissue's ability to repair itself.

KNEE

Knee injuries in runners are different from those of athletes in collision or twisting and cutting sports. Distance running involves straight-line motion rather than torsional forces on the knee (57). Meniscal and ligamentous injuries are uncommon but may be present because of previous injury, and musculotendinous disorders tend to predominate (56).

Treatment modalities applicable to most overuse syndromes of the knee include attenuation of activity; management of pain and inflammation; stretching and strengthening exercises, particularly of the abdominal and quadriceps muscles; proper shoe selection; and the use of orthoses when indicated.

Regarding reduced activity levels, most injured runners are not willing to totally discontinue physical activity. The goal is usually gentle progression to full running after a period of complete cessation of running. The use of relative rest may be necessary to ensure compliance to treatment. The runner is encouraged to engage in activities that do not aggravate the injury, such as cycling, cross-country skiing, walking, swimming, or running in a swimming pool. Water walkers are foam flotation devices that can be attached around the waist, allowing total immersion in the water up to the shoulder level. Buoyancy is maintained without effort, and full ranges of motion against the resistance of the water are achieved with minimal joint strain (59).

Patellofemoral Pain Syndrome

Patellofemoral pain syndrome, also termed chondromalacia patella, runner's knee, or capsular pain, is the most common disorder in runners (60). Retropatellar pain, variable in its presentation, is the primary feature. The pain tends to be aggravated by going up and down hills, but may vary throughout the period of the run or from day to day. Prolonged sitting in one position, such as in an automobile or movie theater, may also cause pain. Other symptoms include joint effusion and a sensation of "instability" in the knee.

Treatment, in addition to the modalities already mentioned, may include the use of a knee sleeve while running and control of hyperpronation if present. Careful shoe selection or an orthosis that provides medial longitudinal support may be helpful.

Iliotibial Band Friction Syndrome

Lateral knee pain may be due to the iliotibial band friction syndrome or less defined causes.

Friction caused by the iliotibial band rubbing the lateral femoral condyle may induce an inflammatory response. There is usually point tenderness over the lateral femoral excrescence, or at Gerdy's tubercle, and a positive iliotibial band test (55). Conservative measures such as replacement of worn running shoes and exercises to stretch the iliotibial tract are usually sufficient to treat most cases (60).

Some patients will present with lateral knee pain but lack the specific findings of the previously mentioned condition. Point tenderness may be present in the lateral knee structures, and fullness may occasionally be observed over the popliteal area. The symptoms are related to a change in the training program or overuse. Treatment is the same as that for iliotibial band friction syndrome.

A note should be made regarding the older runner with varying amounts of degenerative changes involving the knee. Runners, in particular, are athletes that are known to persist in their sport regardless of the pain or potential impairment it may produce. Maintaining muscular strength around an affected joint will give support to the area. Proximal and distal musculature is prone to weakness (53). Sport-specific muscle imbalances, occurring in athletes participating in only one sport, are also likely sources of problems in the aging distance runner.

LOWER LEG AND FOOT

Achilles Tendinitis

Achilles tendinitis is the most common injury in sports, and the chronic incidence of this disorder in the senior runner is high (55, 56). Some of the causes include faulty biomechanics, poor cushioning or stiff-soled shoes, or excessive downhill running. Most symptoms tend to occur 2 to 5 cm proximal to the insertion, an area of the tendon that has a relatively poor blood supply. The runner often experiences a burning pain early in the run, which becomes less severe during the run and then worsens afterward (60). The pain may also appear when the patient gets out of bed in the morning but gradually subsides during the day.

Acute exacerbations may respond to rest, ice massage, and antiinflammatory measures. When the symptoms subside, gentle stretching of the tendon (along with exercises to strengthen the anterior compartment muscles) are indicated. The running shoe must have a flexible sole, a well-molded Achilles pad, a heel wedge at least ⅔ inch high, and a rigid heel counter. Bilateral heel lifts

worn in everyday shoes helps relax the Achilles tendon. Hyperpronation should be corrected, and in the case of the cavus foot, a Schuster heel wedge may help (60).

Plantar Fasciitis

Plantar fasciitis is the most common cause of heel pain in runners. It is an inflammatory reaction due to chronic traction on the plantar aponeurosis at its insertion into the calcaneus. Although a bone spur may develop, it is the inflammation and not the heel spur that causes the painful symptoms. Similar to other overuse syndromes, the pain occurs at the beginning of a workout, diminishes during running, then recurs later. Pain with the first few steps in the morning is often present. Point tenderness may be elicited at the attachment of the plantar aponeurosis to the heel.

Conservative procedures include the use of heel pads, plastic heel cups, rest, and ice. Management should also include the bent-knee exercise, which gently stretches the plantar aponeurosis. Correction of underlying biomechanical imbalances is necessary for permanent relief. This may require specific orthoses to stabilize the foot (60).

Tennis and the Older Athlete

Tennis is a sport that relies on quickness, strength, and flexibility. Quickness is reflected in the ability of the tennis player to move from point to point, bringing the racquet rapidly into position. Muscular strength influences performance by its effect on the player's power and endurance on the court and may also be important in the avoidance of injury. Decreases in forearm strength, for example, can lead to tendinitis of the elbow and rotator cuff (61).

Flexibility also affects both performance and injury; for example, loss of shoulder extension will directly affect serving motion. Additional areas of importance to the tennis player are the adductor muscles, hamstrings, lower back muscles, and posterior calf muscles. Running with the quickness of stride needed on the court places special demands on the calf muscles. Loss of flexibility in these muscles can result in acute rupture of the Achilles tendon or chronic Achilles tendinitis. Slow, sustained stretching for 12 to 18 seconds before play appears to be effective in maintaining tendon length and muscle flexibility (62).

ACUTE INJURIES

Although the majority of injuries in the senior tennis player are chronic, several acute injuries have been reported (56). These include tears of the meniscus and medial head of the gastrocnemius tendon, and acute rupture of the Achilles tendon and rotator cuff.

Meniscal Tears

The most common meniscal tear is a cleavage lesion of the posterior horn of the medial meniscus. The clinical presentation in the older patient tends to be somewhat different than that in the younger patient. Pain with activity is more likely the presenting complaint than acute swelling, locking, or giving way of the joint. The most consistent physical finding is posterior joint line tenderness. This, with pain on extension and a positive history, supports the diagnosis of posterior horn tear. Débridement of the tear with arthroscopic surgery may be necessary. Some patients may play within several weeks; however, it is more effective to keep the patient off the court for approximately 6 weeks while working in a rehabilitation program (61).

Tears of the Gastrocnemius

Partial tears of the medial head of the gastrocnemius tendon were formerly called plantaris tendon tears. The major episode of pain is acute and almost always follows impact of the forefoot as the person starts toe-off when running. Occasionally, a tearing sensation is felt in the calf. Swelling occurs during the first 24 hours. Treatment consists of rest, compression, ice, and partial weight bearing with crutches. Flexibility of the posterior structures should be regained before a full return to tennis, usually between 21 and 42 days after the injury.

Achilles Tendon Rupture

Ruptures of the Achilles tendon are common in players of racquet sports, particularly in those older than the age of 35 (61). Injury occurs during running with the knee extended; as the foot is forced into dorsiflexion, the tendon is stretched and may rupture. The rupture may produce an audible snap, but pain may not be a major feature (63). The patient may not seek care for 24 to 72 hours after injury. A positive Thompson's test, plus the inability to stand on tip toes on the injured side, will confirm the diagnosis. Evidence of bleeding into the pseudosheath of the Achilles tendon will also be present.

Although controversy exists as to the appropriate method of treatment, surgical repair is probably best for the individual intending to return to tennis (61, 63). Early rehabilitation, di-

rected toward regaining muscle strength and flexibility, should be encouraged. Cast immobilization for approximately 6 weeks should be followed by strengthening exercises at 8 weeks or 1 to 2 weeks after cast removal (61). A patient that has regained a strong Achilles tendon and good muscle power should be able to return to tennis within 6 months.

Rotator Cuff Rupture

An acute rupture of the rotator cuff will present with the inability to abduct or externally rotate the arm against resistance. Partial ruptures may be more subtle, as function tends to improve somewhat after the acute episode. The supraspinatus tendon is most commonly involved; however, the infraspinatus and the tendon of the long head of the biceps may also be included.

Large tears require surgery. Partial tears may be treated nonoperatively, but surgical repair tends to result in a better functioning shoulder in the long run. Rehabilitation is particularly important to regain the strength and mobility necessary to return to play safely. The major determinants of long-term outcome are dependent on the size of the tear and the condition of the local tissues.

CHRONIC INJURIES

Chronic or overuse injuries occur more commonly than acute injuries. Although the majority are not disabling, the player's performance or endurance can be affected. The areas most often involved are the knee, elbow, shoulder, and back.

Degenerative Changes of the Knee

Knee pain in the senior player may stem from earlier injuries to the joint, ligaments, or patella. Degenerative changes may subsequently develop that lead to chronic pain. Degeneration of the meniscus or the articular cartilage surface are likely sites of involvement, and arthroscopic débridement may be necessary in some cases. Many players can continue to play tennis, but may need to decrease the amount of play and seek out clay courts rather than asphalt. Ongoing rehabilitation may be useful to increase quadriceps strength and maintain mobility in extension.

Tennis Elbow

Chronic tendinitis of the wrist extensors is more common in the 40- to 55-year-old age group than in younger players, especially in those hitting a lot of tennis balls. Involvement of the lateral epicondyle tends to be more common and appears to be the result of overuse and muscle imbalances in the experienced player (63). Many players will have treated themselves for a number of months before seeking the care of a physician. The chronic inflammation and pain must be addressed, but rehabilitation is the critical factor in treatment. Increasing the strength of the forearm muscles and restoring normal flexibility are the primary goals (64). The use of counterforce braces and decreased playing time may also be helpful.

Rotator Cuff Tendinitis

This disorder is less common than tendinitis of the wrist extensors, but more devastating because it frequently prevents play. The actions of abduction and external rotation, needed for serving or hitting overhead shots, produce pain. Players will tend to have weakness of the supraspinatus muscle plus local tenderness. The arm placed in position for a high backhand volley against resistance will reproduce pain in the anterior shoulder. Chronic tendinitis and small rotator cuff tears may be difficult to distinguish (61).

Treatment involves pendulum exercise or overhead pulleys to regain ranges of motion, followed by strengthening of the rotator cuff in internal and external rotation. Elastic bands of varying resistance are useful aids for the strengthening exercises.

Back Pain

Back pain is a significant cause of disability in tennis players. Certain movements of the sport, such as the serve or overhead shot, require extension of the back and can stress the facets and soft tissues of the spine. Strong abdominal muscles are critical, as most strokes are performed in a semiflexed position or going from extension into flexion (61). Rehabilitation the tennis player should include strengthening the abdominal and extensor muscles and increasing the flexibility in flexion and extension.

Golf and the Older Athlete

Golf is an activity that is often sustained over a lifetime. It is one of the few sports in which the playing frequency may actually increase with age. Skill is of greater importance to performance than is the aerobic or anaerobic capacity of the athlete. Skill is obtained through repetitive, sustained practice; this practice is often the cause of the overuse injuries associated with the sport.

Adequate strength and flexibility will help support the older athlete during the repetitive movements demanded by the game. Areas of importance in stretching include the rotator cuff muscles, particularly the posterior portion of the shoulder capsule; the anterior chest muscles, such as the pectoralis major; the muscles associated with trunk flexibility, such as the back flexors, back extensors, and lateral flexors; and the calf muscles, particularly if walking the course.

Strengthening exercises specific to golf include rotator cuff muscles; abdominal muscles and trunk extensors for stabilizing the upper extremities; hip extensors to control forward lean; neck musculature; and especially forearm and wrist muscles. Pronation and supination exercises for the forearm can be performed using light hand weights. Strengthening of the wrist must include radial and ulnar deviation as well as flexion and extension.

Overuse syndromes affecting the senior golfer tend to involve the cervical and lumbar spine, shoulder, elbow, and wrist (65).

CERVICAL PATHOLOGY

Many mature golfers suffer from cervical pathology, whether discal or osteoarthritic. The reason for cervical pain is often misunderstood. It does not result from the golfer rotating the neck and "taking the eye off the ball." It occurs as a result of the position inherent in the swing: the head is held steady, forward flexed, and the body rotates around and under the stationary head. Improved swing mechanics, using a more upright stance and lessening the forward head thrust, may assist in reducing the discomfort (65).

Additional measures may include decreasing the frequency of play, especially during the acute phase; limiting the absolute number of practice swings, either during the game or on the driving range; and isometric neck strengthening exercises.

LOW BACK PAIN

Low back pain is the most frequent complaint among golfers of any age (66). The position used to address the ball and the posture throughout the swing, in particular planting the feet and rotating through the lumbar spine, are motions that may produce problems. Weakness of the trunk muscles combined with repetitive swinging actions will eventually produce back pain (65). Strengthening the abdominals, long trunk extensors, and shorter paraspinal muscles will support the torso and improve the player's endurance against the repetitive demands of the game.

In addition, the high torque placed on the lumbar vertebra and discs during a golf swing contributes to the high incidence of low back injuries. This can be reduced; a swing that requires less torque is the "classic" swing. The hip and shoulder turn almost equally, with the player rising up on the lead toe. The swing is shortened by keeping the elbow close to the body to prevent collapse of the wrist. The back swing of the club is reduced, which results in less stress for the golfer with low back pain (67).

Chronic injuries may require some changes in equipment and technique to assist the golfer in resuming play. Use of one of the newer extralong putters, for example, demands less flexion in the stance when addressing the ball. Static stresses on the lumbosacral spine and back musculature are significantly reduced by this postural alteration (67).

Prevention remains the most effective treatment. Attention to strengthening and stretching exercises, careful warm-up routines before participation, and the development of proper technique, perhaps through lessons by a teaching professional, will help improve performance and decrease the risk of injury.

SHOULDER PAIN

Rotator Cuff Impingement

Rotator cuff impingement is a common finding in the older golfer. Specific programs of stretching and strengthening the rotator cuff muscles and other supportive musculature of the shoulder girdle are important components in managing the disorder. Specific programs for shoulder rehabilitation have been outlined in other texts (63, 65, 68, 69).

Instability in the nondominant shoulder (i.e., left shoulder in a right-handed golfer) may also pose problems for the senior golfer. Pain is often felt posteriorly. Strengthening of the rotator cuff, scapular rotators, and glenohumeral stabilizers is indicated. Stretching, especially of the posterior capsular region, should be performed only if tightness is demonstrated.

ELBOW PAIN

Golfer's Elbow

Golfer's elbow, or medial epicondylitis, is the traditional diagnosis associated with elbow pain. However, it appears that there are an equal number of problems involving the lateral epicondyle,

which has been characteristically associated with racquet sports (65). Elbow pain is probably most often caused, or exacerbated, by the sudden impact loading that occurs when the golfer creates a divot.

Treatment includes ice or heat as required, stretching if needed, and antiinflammatory measures if warranted (64). Rest from the offending activity is important, but may not mean complete cessation of play. Switching to the driving range or the putting green until the acute pain subsides may suffice. Additional support of the forearm and wrist with muscle strengthening exercises may help avoid exacerbation or reduce the susceptibility to injury during the game. If not playing competitively, a player may lessen the pain by teeing the ball up on all shots. This maneuver avoids the elbow and wrist trauma when a divot is taken.

WRIST PAIN

Many overuse syndromes associated with the wrist can be prevented with strengthening exercises. Wrist pain almost always occurs on the nondominant side and is related to repeated extension and radial deviation during the swing. Strengthening the area and improving the swing mechanics usually resolve the problem (65). Tendinitis is often involved but will usually respond to conservative therapy, particularly if an eccentric exercise program is included (70). Players with chronic wrist syndromes or arthritis involving the hands and wrists may benefit from the use of a golf club with a curved shaft-grip design. The BioCurve club (Chicago Golf and Sport, Clearwater, FL) uses a handle with a 19° bend. This design reduces the amount of ulnar deviation of the lead wrist at impact. Golfers with normal and pathologic conditions of the hand, wrist, and elbow have reported greater comfort and less sensation of shock transmission to the hands when using the BioCurve grip (71).

Swimming and the Older Athlete

The non–weight-bearing status of swimming is considered noninjurious to almost all degenerative problems of the major joints and is an excellent mode of exercise for the older athlete (72). However, preexisting injuries or degenerative disorders with loss of strength and flexibility may result in overuse or chronic pain syndromes.

Flexibility is a high priority in swimming. Stretching, on a regular basis, is recommended as a means to maintain the necessary ranges of motion and muscle elasticity necessary in the prevention of injury (62, 72).

SHOULDER

Swimmer's Shoulder

Swimmer's shoulder is an overuse syndrome that classically refers to impingement of the supraspinatus and biceps tendons under the coracoacromial arch. It is influenced by intensity or duration of activity (long distances or sprint swimming), the primary stroke used (freestyle, butterfly, or backstroke), and swimming biomechanics (i.e., limited body roll during the stroke leads to a greater incidence of pain) (73). Pain is the primary feature and may be anterior, anterolateral, or diffuse. Radiation to the side or "root" of the deltoid is common. This pattern is due to the embryologic relationship of the shoulder to the C5 somatotome (74). Symptoms occur during the recovery or pull-through phases of the stroke, especially at or just after hand entry, when the shoulder is fully abducted.

Treatment may include the use of an upper-arm strap for swimming; this is believed to prevent some of the excursion of the biceps and deltoid muscles (59). Prevention is attained through slow static stretching before and after the workout, a warm-up period of easy swimming before more vigorous activity, and the altering use of different strokes (63, 74).

A note of caution is advised in the use of hand paddles. Hand paddles are often used by younger swimmers to increase the resistance of pulling the hand through the water, thereby increasing the strength and endurance of the shoulder muscles. This considerably increases the incidence of impingement syndromes and may affect senior swimmers to an even greater extent (72). The use of hand paddles should be avoided in the older swimmer.

Rotator Cuff Injuries

Rupture or tearing of the rotator cuff, especially the supraspinatus tendon, is more common in the older swimmer. Pain around the acromion that is more pronounced at night and with overhead activities is characteristic. Recommendations for management of this condition have been addressed earlier.

Long Biceps Tendon

The bicipital tendon is subject to the same stresses as the rotator cuff. Rupture is common in the older swimmer and can be especially debilitating as forceful elbow flexion is essential to forward propulsion in all swimming strokes (72). Surgical intervention is indicated for this condition.

Degenerative Changes of the Shoulder

Degenerative changes of the joints of the upper extremity are not as common as those of the lower extremity and are often the result of previous injury. Arthritis involving the glenohumeral joint, and to a lesser degree the acromioclavicular joint, most likely to affect the activities of a swimmer.

Degenerative changes of the acromioclavicular joint will produce pain with the overhead activities of swimming, but rarely lead to restricted ranges of shoulder motion. Combined with other appropriate treatment procedures, swimming may be beneficial in the ongoing management of the condition. Modifications of stroke style, frequency of workout, and intensity of the workout need to be determined on an individual basis.

Degenerative arthritis of the glenohumeral joint is more difficult and debilitating to the swimmer. Pain and restricted ranges of motion are common in this condition. Conservative treatment and continued swimming during the nonacute phases may help sustain the older athlete for prolonged periods. Worsening conditions, however, may require the use of antiinflammatory measures and surgical intervention (72).

LOWER EXTREMITY

Patellofemoral Pain Syndrome

Degenerative changes in the knee and patellofemoral joint may produce painful symptoms with kicking using any of the major swimming strokes. Pain is most commonly associated with the breaststroke (75). Whereas the flutter or dolphin kick require an average of 90° of flexion, the whip kick used in the breaststroke demands approximately 130° (73). Forward propulsion in swimming is achieved by forced extension of the knee against the resistance of the water. This maneuver may be aggravating for swimmers with patellofemoral pain syndromes (72).

Treatment may include the use of neoprene patellar stabilizing knee supports, minimum-flex quadriceps strengthening exercises, ice packs, anti-inflammatory measures, and the use of relative rest procedures such as pulling only routines or using a pull-buoy. The breaststroke, other aggravating strokes, and swimming fins should be avoided. Swimming fins increase the resistance to knee extension and are contraindicated for athletes with patellofemoral disorders.

Cycling and the Older Athlete

Injuries in cycling result from accidents or overuse. Accidents most frequently result in injuries to the upper extremities and generally involve soft tissues. There appears to be no difference in the incidence of injury from accidents between younger and older cyclists; the overall prevalence ranges from 3.2% to 4.6% (76). Although cycling accidents can rarely be avoided, experience of the rider, rather than age, is the more important factor. The neophyte rider is much more likely to sustain an injury from an accident (77).

Overuse injuries tend to result from training errors, malposition, and excessive stress. Injuries are composed of compressive syndromes, inflammatory syndromes, and muscle strains. Injury patterns in the older cyclist tend to involve compression and inflammatory syndromes of the upper extremity. There is a predominance of subacromial bursitis, lateral epicondylitis, and conduction problems of the median and ulnar nerves (Guyon's canal and carpal tunnel syndromes) (77).

Upper extremity overuse syndromes can be prevented by careful attention to the size and fit of the bicycle, good positioning, appropriate saddle height, use of padded gloves, frequent change of hand positions, not resting on the hands, and strengthening the abdominal muscles.

The older athlete may be able to cycle indefinitely. Patients with debilitating arthritis, degenerative disc disease, or even total hip replacement have managed to continue this sport by modifying their intensity and altering their technique and position (77).

COMPRESSION SYNDROMES

Nerve tissue is subject to overuse injury. Repetitive motion and loading, muscular hypertrophy, direct trauma, decreased flexibility, and pathomechanics have all been implicated in the nerve entrapments of sports participants (56). Injury is clinically characterized by sensory and/or motor changes specific to the involved nerve distribution.

Carpal Tunnel Syndrome

Carpal tunnel syndrome is the most common entrapment neuropathy of the wrist in athletes (56). The cause is usually a thickening of the flexor synovialis in the carpal tunnel, resulting from inflammation due to repetitive wrist movements. Compression of the median nerve causes neural symptomatology in the hand and upper extremity. Pain is described as burning or aching, usually in the hand, but may extend proximally to the shoulder or neck areas (78).

Tingling and numbness in the hand or fingers and a loss of sensibility to light touch and pain may occur.

Treatment procedures for this condition have been widely documented (68, 78). The avoidance of factors that initiate and aggravate compression—such as proper positioning, use of padded gloves, frequent changes of hand position, padded handlebars, and maintenance of wrist and forearm flexibility—is of particular importance in the cyclist (56).

Ulnar Nerve Compression

Direct compression of the ulnar nerve at Guyon's canal produces a syndrome called handlebar palsy. The cyclist will present with motor weakness involving the ulnar innervated muscles of the hand. Minimal sensory findings are present. Prevention consists of applying sufficient padding to the handlebars and changing the position of the hand at frequent intervals while cycling (63).

INFLAMMATORY SYNDROMES

In overuse injuries, the additive effects of repetitive forces lead to microtrauma, which triggers the inflammatory process. Inflammation of the musculotendinous unit or tendinitis is frequently seen with overuse injuries. Repetitive submaximal loading of even a strong tendon can produce fatigue. The relatively poor blood supply, particularly at the bone-tendon interface, may contribute to injury production and delayed healing.

Lateral Epicondylitis

Lateral epicondylitis in the cyclist is a result of tendinitis of the forearm extensors (64). Prolonged positioning of the hands on the handlebars and infrequent changes of hand position are thought to contribute to the development of this condition. Management includes the avoidance of aggravating factors.

Subacromial Bursitis

Overuse injuries involving the bursa are caused by friction of the overlying tendon or external pressure. Inflammation results in effusion and thickening of the bursal wall. Although subacromial bursitis may be secondary to other disorders such as calcific supraspinatus tendinitis, prolonged and improper loading forces can initiate the disorder in the cyclist. Proper riding technique and flexibility exercises may assist in the management of this disorder.

THE SENIOR OLYMPICS

In 1969, the first organized, local, multisport competition for seniors took place in Los Angeles. This marked the first time that senior athletes could participate in competitions that consisted solely of seniors. Over the next 20 years, multisport competitions for older adults came into being all over the United States. In 1987, more than 2500 athletes competed in the first U.S. National Senior Olympics, held in St. Louis. A major result of this event was the establishment of the U.S. National Senior Sports Organization (USNSO). Its primary purposes were to ensure the continuation of the national games and to promote physical fitness among older adults.

To participate in the biennial National Games, an athlete must be at least age 55 and meet USNSO qualifying requirements. Qualifying for most USNSO events requires an athlete to place first, second, or third in that event at a local senior game, which has been designated by the USNSO.

There are 18 sport categories in the National Games competition, including archery, badminton, basketball, bowling, cycling, golf, horseshoes, shuffleboard, softball, swimming, table tennis, tennis, track and field, triathlon, race walk, racquetball, road race, and volleyball. With the exception of the team sports of basketball, softball, and volleyball, all competitions are classified in 5-year increments from age 55 to age 100+ for both men and women. At the 1991 national event, the most popular categories were swimming and track and field, and the largest age group was 60 to 64 (79). More information can be obtained from the resources at the end of this chapter.

SUMMARY

Sport injuries in the older athlete are almost exclusively due to overuse syndromes. Improper technique is an important contributor; unless corrected, the athlete is destined to recurrence (80). Maintaining muscle strength and balance and flexibility is necessary in the rehabilitation of the athlete and in prevention of injury and unnecessary painful conditions (47). The goals of rehabilitation of overuse syndromes are pain-free ranges of motion, strength and endurance, and continued athletic participation.

Resources (From Lindeman [81])

U.S. National Senior Sports Organization
14323 S. Outer Forty Road
Suite N300
Chesterfield, MO 63017
Phone: 314-878-4900

U.S. Tennis Association-League Tennis
707 Alexander Road
Princeton, NJ 08540-6399
Phone: toll-free 800-223-0456
In New Jersey: 609-452-2580

Bruce Douglass
Athletics Congress of the U.S.A.
Race Walking Committee
36 Canterbury Lane
Mystic, CT 06355

Barbara Kousky
Masters Track and Field Committee
5319 Donald Street
Eugene, OR 97405

Charles DesJardins
Masters Long Distance Running Committee
5428 Southport Lane
Fairfax, VA 22032

Dorothy Donnelly
U.S. Masters Swimming, Inc.
2 Peter Avenue
Rutland, MA 01543
Phone: 508-886-6631
Fax: 508-886-6265

Al Sheahen
National Masters News
PO Box 2372
Van Nuys, CA 91404
Phone: 818-785-1895
(monthly newsletter: $22 a year)

References

1. Bortz W. Disuse and aging. JAMA 1982;248:1203–1208.
2. Heath GW, Hagberg JM, Ehsani AA, et al. A physiological comparison of young and older endurance athletes. J Appl Physiol 1981;51:634–640.
3. Nakamura E, Moritani T, Kanetaka A. Biological age versus physical fitness age in women. Eur J Appl Physiol 1990;61:202–208.
4. Nakamura E, Moritani T, Kanetaka A. Biological age versus physical fitness age. Eur J Appl Physiol 1989;58:778–785.
5. Seals DL, Hagberg JM, Allen WF, et al. Glucose tolerance in young and older athletes and sedentary men. J Appl Physiol 1984;56:1521–1525.
6. Steinhaus LA, Dustman RE, Ruhling RO, et al. Cardiorespiratory fitness of young and older active and sedentary men. Br J Sports Med 1988;22:163–166.
7. Frontera WR, Meredith CN, O'Reilly KP, et al. Strength training and determinants of $\dot{V}O_2$max in older men. J Appl Physiol 1990;68:329–333.
8. Frontera WR, Meredith CN, O'Reilly KP, et al. Strength conditioning in older men: skeletal muscle hypertrophy and improved function. J Appl Physiol 1988;64:1038–1044.
9. Hamdorf PA, Withers RT, Penhall RD, et al. Physical training effects on the fitness and habitual activity patterns of elderly women. Arch Phys Med Rehabil 1992;73:603–608.
10. Naso F, Carner E, Blankfort-Doyle W, et al. Endurance training in the elderly nursing home patient. Arch Phys Med Rehabil 1990;71:241–243.
11. Posner JD, Gorman KM, Windsor-Landsberg L, et al. Low to moderate intensity endurance training in healthy older adults: physiological response after four months. J Am Geriatr Soc 1992;40:1–7.
12. Wilmore JH. The aging of bone and muscle. Clin Sports Med 1991;10:231–244.
13. Elia EA. Exercise and the elderly. Clin Sports Med 1991;10:141–155.
14. Fuchi T, Iwaoka K, Higuchi M, et al. Cardiovascular changes associated with decreased aerobic capacity and

aging in long-distance runners. Eur J Appl Physiol 1989;
58:884–889.

15. Seals DR, Hagberg JM, Hurley BF, et al. Endurance training in older men and women. part 1. cardiovascular response to exercise. J Appl Physiol 1984;57:1024–1029.

16. Stamford BA. Exercise and the elderly. Exerc Sports Sci Rev 1988;16:341–379.

17. Rodeheffer RJ, Gerstenblith G, Becker LC, et al. Exercise and cardiac output are maintained with advancing age in healthy human subjects: cardiac dilatation and increased stroke volume compensate for a diminished heart rate. Circulation 1984;69:203–212.

18. Gersten JW. Effect of exercise on muscle function decline with aging. West J Med 1991;154:579–582.

19. Klitgaard H, Ausoni S, Damiani E. Sarcoplasmic reticulum of human skeletal muscle: age-related changes and effect of training. Acta Physiol Scand 1989;137:23–31.

20. LaForest S, St-Pierre DMM, Cyr J, et al. Effects of age and regular exercise on muscle strength and endurance. Eur J Appl Physiol 1990;60:104–111.

21. Rutherford OM, Jones DA. The relationship of muscle and bone loss and activity levels with age in women. Age Ageing 1992;21:286–293.

22. Sarianna S, Suominen H. Ultrasound imaging of the quadriceps muscle in elderly athletes and untrained men. Muscle Nerve 1991;14:527–533.

23. Steen B. Body composition in aging. Nutr Rev 1988;46:45–51.

24. Young A, Stokes M, Crowe M. Size and strength of the quadriceps muscles of old and young women. Eur J Clin Invest 1984;14:282–287.

25. Young A, Stokes M, Crowe M. Size and strength of the quadriceps muscles of old and young men. Clin Physiol 1985;5:145–154.

26. Alnaqeeb MA, Al Zaid NS, Goldspink G. Connective tissue changes and physical properties of developing and ageing skeletal muscle. J Anat 1984;139:677–689.

27. Aniansson A, Hedberg M, Henning GB, et al. Muscle morphology, enzymatic activity and muscle strength in elderly men: a follow-up study. Muscle Nerve 1986;9:585–591.

28. Borkan G, Hults D, Gerzof S, et al. Age changes in body composition revealed by computer tomography. J Gerontol 1983;38:673–677.

29. Lexell J, Henriksson-Larsen K. Distribution of different fiber types in human skeletal muscles: effects of aging studied in whole muscle cross section. Muscle Nerve 1983;6:588–595.

30. Maclennan W, Hall M, Timothy J, et al. Is weakness in old age due to muscle wasting? Age Ageing 1980;9:188–192.

31. Menard D, Stanish WD. The aging athlete. Am J Sports Med 1989;17:187–196.

32. Aniansson A, Sperling L, Rundgren A, et al. Muscle function in 75 year old men and women: a longitudinal study. Scand J Rehabil Med Suppl 1983;9:92–102.

33. Aniansson A, Grimley G, Rundgren A. Isometric and isokinetic quadriceps muscle strength in 70 year old men and women. Scand J Rehabil Med 1980;12:161–168.

34. Orlander J, Kiessling KH, Larsson L, et al. Skeletal muscle metabolism and ultrastructure in relation to age in sedentary men. Acta Physiol Scand 1978;104:249–261.

35. Pariskova JE, Eisett E, Sprynarova S, et al. Body composition, aerobic capacity, and density of muscle capillaries in young and old men. J Appl Physiol 1971;31:323–325.

36. Clarkson-Smith L, Hartley AA. Relationships between physical exercise and cognitive abilities in older adults. Psychol Aging 1989;4:183–189.

37. Dustman RE, Emmerson RY, Ruhling RO, et al. Age and fitness effects of EEG, ERPs, visual sensitivity, and cognition. Neurobiol Aging 1990;11:193–200.

38. Stones MM, Kozma A. Age, exercise, and coding performance. Psychol Aging 1989;4:190–194.

39. Blumenthal JS, Emery DF, Madden DJ, et al. Long-term effects of exercise on psychological functioning in older men and women. J Gerontol 1991;46:352–361.

40. Panton LB, Graves JE, Pollock ML, et al. Effect of aerobic and resistance training on fractionated reaction time and speed of movement. J Gerontol 1990;45:26–31.

41. Whitehurst M. Reaction time unchanged in older women following aerobic training. Percept Mot Skills 1991;72:251–256.

42. Rikli RE, Edwards DJ. Effects of a three-year exercise program on motor function and cognitive processing speed in older women. Res Q Exerc Sport 1991;62:61–67.

43. Sinaki M. The role of exercise in preventing osteoporosis. J Musculoskel Med 1992;9:67–83.

44. Oyster N, Morton M, Linnell S. Physical activity and osteoporosis in post-menopausal women. Med Sci Sports Exerc 1984;16:44–50.

45. Topp R. Development of an exercise program for older adults: pre-exercise testing, exercise prescription and program maintenance. Nurse Pract 1991;16:16–26.

46. American College of Sports Medicine. Guidelines for exercise testing and prescription. 4th ed. Philadelphia: Lea & Febiger, 1991.

47. Brown M. Special considerations during rehabilitation of the aged athlete. Clin Sports Med 1989;8:893–901.

48. Shephard RJ. The scientific basis of exercise prescribing for the very old. J Am Geriatr Soc 1990;38:62–70.

49. Kirk S, Sharp CF, Elbaum N, et al. Effect of long-distance running on bone mass of women. J Bone Miner Res 1989;4:515–522.

50. DeHaven KE, Lintner DM. Athletic injuries: comparison by age, sport, and gender. Am J Sports Med 1986;14:218–224.

51. Kannus P, Niittymaki S, Jarvinen M, et al. Sports injuries in elderly athletes: a three-year prospective, controlled study. Age Ageing 1989;18:263–270.

52. Lane N, Block DA, Wood PD, et al. Aging, long-distance running, and the development of musculoskeletal disability. Am J Med 1987;82:772–780.

53. Matheson GO, MacIntyre JG, Taunton JE, et al. Musculoskeletal injuries associated with physical activity in older adults. Med Sci Sports Exerc 1989;21:379–385.

54. Marti B, Vader JP, Minder CE, et al. On the epidemiology of running injuries: the 1984 Bern Grand-Prix study. Am J Sports Med 1988;16:285–294.

55. Lutter LD. The knee and running. Clin Sports Med 1985;4:685–698.

56. Herring SA, Nilson KL. Introduction to overuse injuries. Clin Sports Med 1987;6:225–239.

57. Cox JS. Patellofemoral problems in runners. Clin Sports Med 1985;4:699–715.

58. Ting AJ. Running and the older athlete. Clin Sports Med 1991;10:319–325.

59. Heyneman CA, Premo DE. A water walkers exercise program for the elderly. Public Health Rep 1992;107:213–217.

60. Brody DM. Running injuries. Clin Symp 1987;39.

61. Leach RE, Abramowitz A. The senior tennis player. Clin Sports Med 1991;10:283–290.

62. Taylor DC, Dalton JD, Seaber AV, et al. Viscoelastic properties of muscle tendon units: the biomechanical effects of stretching. Am J Sports Med 1990;18:300–309.

63. Roy S, Irvin R. Sports medicine: prevention, evaluation, management, and rehabilitation. Englewood Cliffs, NJ: Prentice-Hall, 1983.

64. Leach RE, Miller JK. Lateral and medial epicondylitis of the elbow. Clin Sports Med 1987;6:259–273.

65. Jobe FW, Schwab DM. Golf for the mature athlete. Clin Sports Med 1991;10:269–282.

66. Stanish WD. Low back pain in athletes: an overuse syndrome. Clin Sports Med 1987;6:321–344.

67. Stover CN, Mallon WJ. Golf injuries: treating the play to treat the player. J Musculoskel Med 1992;9:55–72.

68. Gatterman MI, Goe DR. Muscle and myofascial pain syndromes. In: Gatterman MI, ed. Chiropractic management of spine related disorders. Baltimore: Williams & Wilkins, 1990:285–329.

69. Kisner C, Colby LA. Therapeutic exercise: foundations and techniques. 2nd ed. Philadelphia: FA Davis, 1990.

70. Fyfe I, Stanish WD. The use of eccentric training and stretching in the treatment and prevention of tendon injuries. Clin Sports Med 1992;11:601–624.

71. Cahalan TD, Cooney WP, Tamai K, et al. Biomechanics of the golf swing in players with pathologic conditions of the forearm, wrist, and hand. Am J Sports Med 1991;19: 288–293.

72. Richardson AD, Miller JW. Swimming and the older athlete. Clin Sports Med 1991;10:301–316.

73. Richardson AR. The biomechanics of swimming: the shoulder and knee. Clin Sports Med 1986;5:103–113.

74. Ciullo JV. Swimmer's shoulder. Clin Sports Med 1986;5: 115–137.

75. Fowler PJ, Regan WD. Swimming injuries of the knee, foot and ankle, elbow, and back. Clin Sports Med 1986;5:139–148.

76. Kiburz D, Jacobs R, Reckling F, et al. Bicycling accidents and injuries among adult cyclists. Am J Sports Med 1986;14:416–419.

77. McLennan JG, McLennan JC. Cycling and the older athlete. Clin Sports Med 1991;10:291–299.

78. Gerow G, Matthews B, Jahn W. Musculoskeletal system: extremities. In: Lawrence DJ, ed. Fundamentals of chiropractic diagnosis and management. Baltimore: Williams & Wilkins, 1991:365–497.

79. U.S. National Senior Olympics Organization. USNSO and the U.S. national senior sports classic: the senior Olympics. Chesterfield, MO: USNSO, 1993.

80. Gieck JH, Saliba EN. Application of modalities in overuse syndromes. Clin Sports Med 1987;6:427–465.

81. Lindeman L. Beating time. Mod Maturity 1991;34:26–33.

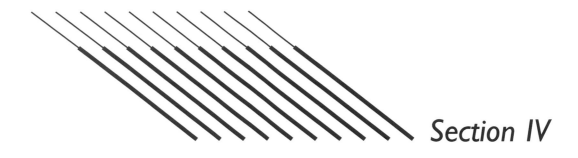

Section IV

SIGNIFICANT ISSUES
IN SPORTS MEDICINE

Diagnostic Imaging of Athletic Injury

Norman W. Kettner and Michael S. Barry

Athletic injury may result from a number of pathomechanical interactions ranging from chronic overuse to acute high-velocity impacts. Imaging these abnormalities presents a frequent challenge for the chiropractic sports physician. Information about appropriate imaging modalities, indications, advantages, and contraindications is presented in this chapter. In addition, an overview of the common plain film manifestations of athletic injuries is presented. Acute fractures, joint instability, and overuse syndromes will be emphasized. Technical aspects of optimal film production, positioning, and use of a directed plain film search pattern will be provided. This chapter is designed to highlight the role of diagnostic imaging as it applies to sports medicine. A definitional overview of the role of nuclear bone scan, computed tomography (CT), and magnetic resonance imaging (MRI) will be included.

The increased awareness of the benefits of participation in a diverse number of sports has resulted in greater numbers of athletic injuries. Young and old, amateur and professional, athletes place great demand on their bodies and, in particular, the musculoskeletal system. Injury to the musculoskeletal system constitutes a frequent indication for diagnostic imaging. This chapter is designed to review the broad spectrum of techniques and applications of the most useful modalities. The indications and limitations of these modalities will be emphasized.

Athletic injuries vary from minor to life-threatening and from acute to chronic. Selection of the appropriate imaging techniques requires a complete understanding of the pathomechanics of injury. A reasonable differential diagnosis and a clear understanding of the role of the diagnostic imaging technology will ensure a cost-effective approach in the management of athletic injury.

The evaluation of the symptomatic athlete requires careful attention to differential diagnosis (1). There is an inherent bias to attribute the athlete's pain to the particular endeavor. A delayed diagnosis could be life-threatening or, at the least, frustrate the athlete's return to optimal function. There must be a balance struck between a cost-effective evaluation and the need for a timely diagnosis. An approach that is logical and concise is cost-effective and should provide the clinical solution necessary for appropriate management and follow-up.

A STRATEGY FOR DIFFERENTIAL DIAGNOSIS

The sequence in obtaining a differential diagnosis begins with the patient history. This will be followed by the physical examination, selection of systems, differential diagnostic categories, and differential diagnosis. The testing strategy may include diagnostic imaging, laboratory tests, and/or electrophysiologic examination. The results of these examinations help establish the provisional diagnosis. The differential diagnosis is iterative and dynamic, allowing the clinician to reformulate or provide additional diagnoses as necessary.

History

The chief complaint obtained from the athlete typically revolves around a pain complex. As with patients in general, the onset, provocative and palliative features (including treatment), quality of pain, radiation, anatomical location, and timing are mandatory historical inquiries. The assessment of athletic pain also requires an understanding of the athlete's level of motivation and personal desire. Additional athletic history is important. This should include the specifics of conditioning, training surfaces, previous history of injury, and underlying biomechanical complications that could predispose to injury. The time of day at which the injury occurred and the athlete's stretching program may provide additional differential value.

Physical Examination

Evaluation of the athlete presenting with a pain complex generally revolves around a biomechanical assessment. The specific region under evaluation requires assessment of muscle strength and a search for obvious defects such as swelling or erythema. Fever, weight loss, and other constitutional signs or symptoms should alert the clinician to obtain a more extensive and multisystem examination.

System Association and Analysis of Findings

Disturbances of a biomechanical nature generally arise from the musculoskeletal system. It is important for the clinician to remember that the causes of pain may arise outside this system and obscure the correct diagnosis. Other systems should be given consideration, such as respiratory, cardiovascular, neurologic, genitourinary, gastrointestinal, dermatologic, and endocrine. For example, compression of the brachial plexus by cervical ribs or cervical spondylosis has been reported to cause angina-like pain (2). This may be provoked by exercise. Pelvic pain in the female athlete with a fever is suggestive of infectious disease, such as urinary tract infection or pelvic inflammatory disease. The latter, however, may occur without fever.

Differential Diagnostic Categories

The differential diagnostic categories that should be considered include vascular, infection, congenital, trauma, arthritide, neoplasm, and endocrine. The acronym VIC TANE serves as a useful reference for these categories. In most cases, the athlete presents with a history of injury, prompting the consideration of the trauma category. Acute or chronic joint injury is also common, making arthritide a frequent consideration. Vascular and neurologic injury often poses a greater diagnostic challenge. Metabolic disorders frequently manifest constitutional signs that assist in the diagnosis. Congenital disorders, if unknown to the patient, are usually diagnosed on the basis of incidental radiographic findings. The selection of one or more differential diagnostic categories then permits the individual diagnoses to be considered.

Differential Diagnosis

The selection of a differential diagnostic category is followed by the construction of the differential diagnosis. The individual diagnostic considerations may be numerous or in some cases solitary. More than one category may be under consideration. Athletic injury usually traumatizes the musculoskeletal system, resulting in a diagnosis of an acute or chronic nature. The differential diagnosis serves as the focus for the testing strategy.

Testing Strategy

The testing strategy consists of the subcategories of diagnostic imaging, laboratory testing, and electrophysiologic testing. The category of diagnostic imaging includes plain film radiography and advanced imaging. The proper selection of a diagnostic test requires at least superficial understanding of the principles of sensitivity and specificity. Sensitivity refers to the rate of positivity in a population with a given disorder. Specificity refers to the rate of negative tests in a patient population without the disorder. These two factors should always be given consideration to maintain cost-effective test selection. Highly sensitive tests, when negative, allow the presence of disorders to be excluded confidently. Highly specific tests, when abnormal, serve to confirm confidently the presence of a given disorder. Once the goal of a diagnostic study is clear, the clinician can select and perform the accurate, rapid, and cost-effective tests to delineate the differential diagnosis. This saves time and conserves financial resources, while minimizing patient discomfort and risk. When the results of a study are negative, but the clinical findings compel further investigation, the next diagnostic examination should then be performed. A shotgun approach to diagnostic testing should be avoided because of expense and results that are often confusing. In addition, such an approach may delay a diagnosis. As a rule, multiple tests are most helpful if the results are all positive, thus confirming the diagnosis; or if the results are all normal, thus adding confidence that a disorder has been excluded.

Treatment

The treatment of athletic injury includes a prognosis and rehabilitation program. The objective of treatment, whether it be operative or conservative, is pain reduction and a restoration of maximal function. The response of the athlete under management may provide additional diagnostic information. Treatment itself can be viewed in the light of a testing modality. The failure of adequate healing raises the suspicion of an underlying complication and, if necessary, a new testing strategy may be devised.

PLAIN FILM RADIOGRAPHY

The mainstay of diagnostic imaging in the evaluation of injured athletes is plain film radiography. These examinations are usually performed to detect the presence of soft tissue, bone, or joint injury. Several radiographic tenets should be considered axiomatic. Radiographic examination should always consist of a series including at least two views at right angles to each other. The entire osseous structure, as well as the joint above and below the injury, should be visualized. Injuries involving a joint or the vertebral column will require angulated, oblique, or special views.

Stress, weight bearing, or traction views may provide additional information not found on routine plain film examinations. They may document the presence and extent of joint instability, which in turn is a measure of ligamentous or capsular compromise. These views are frequently used in the evaluation of ankle, knee, wrist, shoulder, and spinal instability (3).

Fluoroscopic examination is often used in the evaluation of ligamentous instability. In addition, occult fractures may be better visualized. Fluoroscopic examination should be conducted with strict indications, optimal technology, and great care taken to reduce the radiation exposure.

SEARCH PATTERN

A complete radiographic series should demonstrate optimal technical quality. Factors including collimation, radiographic contrast, and the inclusion of the appropriate anatomy should be assessed. Patient motion can degrade the anatomical detail, rendering the examination suboptimal. The use of patient restraining devices should be considered, and cautious implementation should be used. The use of a table bucky is mandatory for trauma evaluation because stability is easily provided. Patients in pain are more likely to require retake films; the physician must resist the tendency to accept lower film quality in a high-risk population.

A directed search pattern permits a thorough and comprehensive analysis of the radiographic series. The musculoskeletal search pattern consists of evaluation of the soft tissues, bone, and joint structures.

The radiographic assessment of soft tissue in the injured athletic patient will often reveal the presence of soft tissue swelling (4). This nonspecific sign should direct one's attention to the underlying osseous or joint structures. Posttraumatic hemorrhage with heterotopic ossification and dystrophic calcification following overuse are frequent sources of increased density in the soft tissues. Foreign bodies such as gravel are occasionally encountered. Soft tissue swelling distorting the normal fascial planes and arising within a few days of a closed, although more often, open injury should alert the clinician to the possibility of osteomyelitis or septic arthritis. Subcutaneous air can be seen after a laceration. Infection is another source of air within soft tissues, most likely arising within the foot of a diabetic patient.

The directed search pattern of the osseous structure is subdivided into evaluation of the periosteum, cortex, and medullary cavity. A periosteal reaction always constitutes an important radiographic finding. Trauma, as well as ischemia and invasive processes, may stimulate an osteoblastic response within the periosteal layers. A periostitis stimulated by an overuse mechanism generates a thick, uninterrupted pattern that eventually is incorporated into the cortex of a long bone. Patterns of periostitis associated with aggressive processes, such as infection or neoplasm, are likely to stimulate multiple layers of periosteal reaction that are thin, interrupted, and on occasion radial or spiculated (sunburst). A periosteal response should always prompt the clinician to obtain further diagnostic imaging.

Cortical interruption, whether complete or incomplete, constitutes the definition of a fracture. Incomplete fractures (greenstick) are often encountered in the pediatric population (Fig. 20.1). The subtle bowing fracture is another fracture seen only in the pediatric population. Contralateral views for comparison are often necessary to

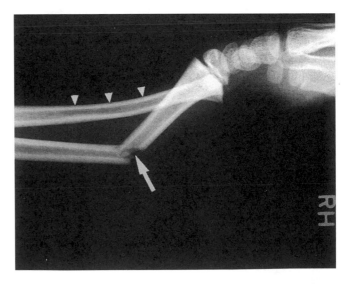

Figure 20.1. Distal radial (Galeazzi's) fracture. There is an anteriorly angulated fracture of the distal radius (arrow) with dislocation of the distal radioulnar joint. Also note the post-traumatic bowing deformity of the ulna (arrowheads). (Courtesy of Michael J. Silberstein, M.D.)

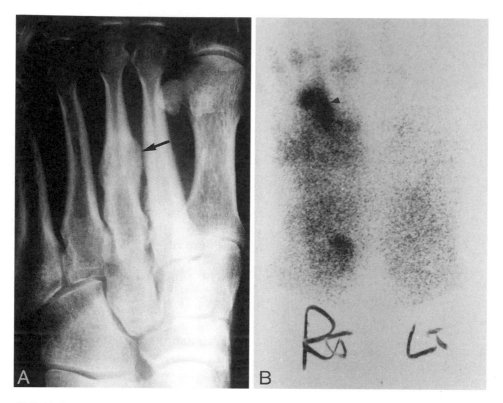

Figure 20.2. Healing stress fracture. **A.** Radiographs show callus surrounding a stress injury to the third metatarsal (arrow). **B.** Nuclear scintigraphy reveals increased radionuclide uptake in this area (arrowheads).

obtain the diagnosis. Occult fractures should be considered when soft tissue swelling or joint effusion is encountered in the absence of a fracture.

Stress fractures result when stress is applied to the skeleton and bone resorption exceeds osteoblastic repair. These injuries are termed fatigue fractures and are frequently seen in runners and other athletes whose training generates unusually large stresses on their skeleton. A stress fracture can occur abruptly or, as is typically the case with athletes, in a slowly progressive fashion. Pathomechanical disturbances of the walking or running gait, improper training, poor equipment, and postural stress are important factors. The radiologic findings of a stress fracture depend on the stage of presentation.

Stress fractures seen in chronic overuse syndromes also fail to generate radiographic findings for at least 10 days to 2 weeks. A horizontal, linear pattern of sclerosis becomes evident as the pain pattern persists. Radionuclide bone imaging and MRI permit early detection. Chronic mechanical stress applied to the cortex produces an acceleration of bone remodeling followed by localized appositional bone growth. If stress patterns persist, the formation of a cortical stress fracture will ensue (Fig. 20.2).

Avulsion injuries are often seen in the adolescent athlete at the time of epiphyseal or apophyseal closure. Avulsion injury mechanisms usu-

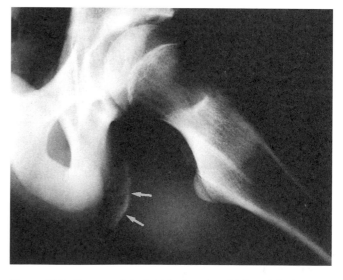

Figure 20.3. Fracture of the ischial tuberosity with lateral displacement of the avulsed fragment (arrows).

ally revolve around a violent contraction of a musculotendinous unit or repetitive loading. The most common sites of avulsion injury are the ischial tuberosity (Fig. 20.3), anterior superior and anterior inferior iliac spine, symphysis pubis, and iliac crest. At times, the presence of an ununited epiphysis or supernumerary bone (ossicle) may pose difficulty in radiologic interpretation. Avulsion fracture should display an irregular fracture margin just opposite its host site. An ossicle will demonstrate a sclerotic bony margin around the entire circumference. In addition, no defect site will be noted.

The cancellous or medullary component of bone can demonstrate the presence of a stress fracture. Osteoblastic activity (sclerosis) is noted after the collapse and repair of bony trabeculae. Ischemic necrosis of the medullary cavity may present as a serpentine pattern of increased density due to osteonecrosis. Osteonecrosis is also a complication of a scaphoid fracture. The finding of a permeative pattern of destruction in the metaphysis of a long bone is strongly suggestive of a destructive process, such as osteomyelitis or osteosarcoma. Generalized radiolucency subsequent to trauma raises the consideration of reflex sympathetic dystrophy syndrome (RSDS). Disuse or immobilization may also result in rapid bone loss and osteopenia. Generalized demineralization raises the consideration of endocrinopathy or long-standing use of medications (corticosteroids, methotrexate) that demineralize the skeleton.

The radiographic evaluation of an articulation is the third step in this search pattern. The thickness of the articular cartilage should be focused on first. Focal joint space narrowing surrounded by sclerosis, subchondral cysts, and marginal osteophytes is consistent with osteoarthrosis. Generalized joint space reduction, accompanied by para-articular osteopenia and soft tissue swelling, raises the suspicion of an inflammatory or infectious arthropathy. Septic arthritis should be considered whenever an articulation displays the cardinal signs of inflammation. The failure of a traumatic arthralgia to respond to several days of management warrants consideration of a septic cause. Irreversible chondrolysis may be initiated within days of an acute septic arthritis. The long-term sequelae of septic arthritis are devastating and can include osteoarthrosis, osteonecrosis, subluxation, and bony ankylosis (5).

Traumatic disruption of the articular surface can produce osteocartilaginous fragmentation such as that seen in osteochondritis dissecans (Fig. 20.4). Observed most frequently in the knee joint, it can also be seen in the ankle and elbow joints. Fractures that extend to the articular surface may disrupt hyaline or fibrocartilage, leading to premature osteoarthrosis.

The alignment of an articulation is the second phase of the joint assessment. It is largely dependent on the stabilizing structures, including cartilage, subchondral bone, surrounding capsule, and ligaments. The musculotendinous unit provides minimal stability relative to the aforementioned structures. Chronic degenerative and acute traumatic etiologies are the most common causes of a disturbance in alignment across an articulation.

During the assessment of alignment in the cervical spine, attention should be directed to the spinolaminar junction. A line formed by visually connecting these vertically oriented opaque landmarks should be curved or straight, depending on the patient's posture. Anterolisthesis or retrolisthesis is established when alignment is disturbed at the spinolaminar reference. In addition, the cervical canal diameter should be evaluated carefully to exclude congenital stenosis. The diameter of the sagittal canal divided by the width of the vertebra should not be less than 80%. Athletes with cervical spinal stenosis are at risk for spinal cord neurapraxia and should avoid contact sports.

Intracapsular hematoma and abscess, as well as inflammatory or traumatic disruption of the periarticular tendon and/or ligaments, can also result in acute traumatic subluxation. Displacement of fat pads or fat planes are reliable signs of hemarthrosis (6).

The analysis of function constitutes the third feature in the assessment of the joint search pattern. The use of weight bearing, traction, or stress views permits the radiographic assessment of the active or passive joint range of motion. The judicious introduction of passive forces across an injured articulation is warranted. Stressing an acute ligamentous injury or

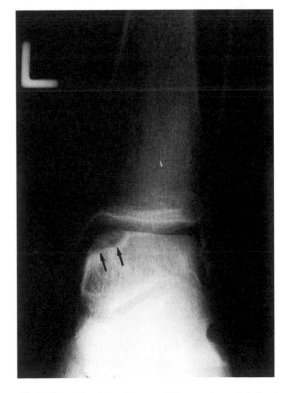

Figure 20.4. Osteochondritis dissecans. Observe the well-defined subarticular lucency at the superomedial aspect of the talus (arrows).

fracture of the vertebral column is strictly contraindicated. Flexion and extension, traction, compression, and lateral bending views have been used in the plain film examination of the minimally unstable vertebral articulation.

The high incidence of spondylolisthesis in competitive athletes often raises the diagnostic consideration of segmental instability. The use of traction-compression radiography for the detection of segmental instability has been demonstrated to be more accurate than the use of flexion-extension radiography (7). Traction-compression radiography can be used to demonstrate translatory motion in an unstable segment with little expense and only minimal patient discomfort.

In the extremities, evaluation of unstable joints in the hand, wrist, shoulder, knee, and ankle can provide valuable information leading to diagnostic and appropriate therapy.

The presence of an epiphysis within a traumatized articulation warrants cautious evaluation for the presence of cartilaginous injury. Physeal or epiphyseal injury is more frequently encountered than soft tissue injury in the adolescent population (8). Epiphyseal alignment may be normal in the presence of a nondisplaced physeal fracture. Stress views may be helpful in this setting. Particular caution is urged in the assessment of weight-bearing joints, in which an incorrect diagnosis can lead to lifelong sequelae, pain, and premature osteoarthrosis. This is particularly important in the hip joint where the slipped capital femoral epiphysis is encountered. Ischemic necrosis of an epiphysis may be encountered in the pediatric or adolescent athlete with an asymptomatic or minor history of trauma. A gait analysis revealing the presence of a limp should raise the suspicion of epiphyseal injury.

SKELETAL SCINTIGRAPHY

Nuclear medicine has played an important role in the diagnosis of a wide variety of musculoskeletal injuries. It is a highly accurate and useful modality for evaluating athletic injuries when radiographs are equivocal or negative. Radionuclide scintigraphy allows for a physiologic evaluation of the athlete's soft tissues, bones, and joints. This is in contrast to the relatively static and anatomical perspective of plain film radiography. Detection of abnormalities by bone scanning may precede clinical or radiographic changes by days, weeks, or months (9).

The bone scan is performed by the intravenous administration of a bolus of Tc99m- labeled phosphate compound. The technetium isotope has a short half-life of 6 hours and results in total body

radiation exposure similar to that of a radiographic examination of the lumbar spine. The isotope emits photons of 140 Kev, which are detected by a gamma camera and a series of collimators (10, 11). The camera detects the tracer flow and distribution as it moves from the vascular to extravascular space over a period of minutes. Several hours later, the isotope is taken up in the skeleton. Areas of increased uptake (hot spots) identify increased blood flow and metabolic activity.

The detection of photon activity is generally the highest in areas of trabecular bone because they are subject to considerable stress. A normal bone scan is symmetrical around the midline in the sagittal plane; that is, the right and left halves of the body should be mirror images. Uniform uptake of the radiopharmaceutical agent will be seen throughout most of the skeleton and kidneys.

Thus, physiologic and pathophysiologic information is provided, but without the resolution of CT or MRI. Recent advances in nuclear medicine technology with single photon emission computed tomography (SPECT) have provided greater anatomical resolution. The SPECT technique involves the use of a scintillation detector that is rotated around the area of interest in a circular orbit. Images are then obtained at multiple positions surrounding the body. Reconstruction of these tomographic images in the transverse, sagittal, and coronal planes provides greater information on tracer localization than can be obtained on planar camera images. When infection or inflammatory conditions are suspected in association with skeletal trauma, the radiopharmaceuticals used are gallium (Ga67) citrate or indium-labeled (In111) white blood cells. Intravenous injection is followed by delayed images obtained at 24 or 48 hours. The white cells of a patient are labeled and reinjected, followed by scanning in 18 to 24 hours.

Soft Tissues

Contact sports frequently involve trauma to large muscle groups such as the thigh and upper arm. Traumatic myositis ossificans results when calcium is deposited in the muscle and fascial soft tissues (Fig. 20.5). It is typically a self-resolving process. If pain persists, mechanical irritation or increased compartment pressure may be the causative factor. Surgical excision should be performed only after several negative bone scans demonstrate maturation of the calcification (12). Reflex sympathetic dystrophy syndrome was described more than 100 years ago but its pathophysiology is still controversial. Soft tissue injury that is often trivial may be followed by the onset of diffuse, exquisite pain, joint stiff-

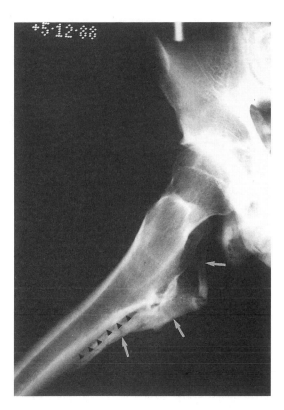

Figure 20.5. Post-traumatic myositis ossificans. There is ossification of the medial soft tissues adjacent to the right femur (arrows). Note the cleavage plane separating the intact bony cortex from the abnormal ossification (arrowheads).

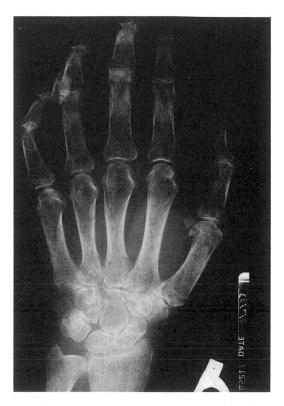

Figure 20.6. Reflex sympathetic dystrophy syndrome. Plain radiographs demonstrate spotty osteopenia of the left hand. (Courtesy of National College of Chiropractic, Department of Radiology, Lombard, IL.)

ness, swelling, and soft tissue trophic changes. The hand or foot is often involved after blunt trauma. Radionuclide bone scanning is the most sensitive examination for diagnosis (13). The delayed bone scanning phase demonstrates diffuse increased periarticular uptake. Radiographic changes in reflex sympathetic dystrophy syndrome are nonspecific, revealing generalized soft tissue swelling and osteopenia (Fig. 20.6).

The medial tibial stress syndrome, or shin splints, is a traumatic periostitis of the soleus muscle with tearing of the Sharpey's fibers from their bony insertion. Although this diagnosis can be established clinically, the bone scan appearance is characteristic (Fig. 20.7). It demonstrates linear increased uptake along the superficial aspect of the long bone cortex (14). This contrasts with the more focal increase seen in a stress fracture.

Injury to muscles in marathon and ultramarathon runners can be detected by bone-seeking radiopharmaceuticals that localize in the area of damage. Detection with scintigraphy shows abnormal uptake within a few hours of the injury, most intense activity by 48 hours, and a gradual decline to normal levels of activity by approximately 1 week. This information may be useful in an athlete when rhabdomyolysis is associated

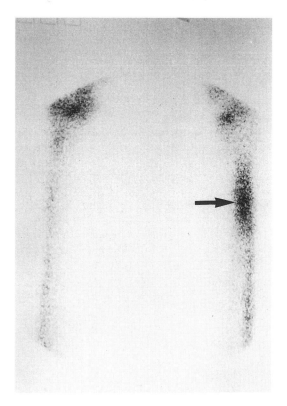

Figure 20.7. Shin splints. Delayed images of the triple phase bone scan display the typical vertically oriented linear photon activity along the tibial cortex (arrow).

with overuse syndromes seen in hurdlers, football players, or weight lifters.

Bone

Stress fractures are often associated with normal radiographs (15). The bone scan appearance of a stress fracture is a dense focal or fusiform site of uptake. All three phases of the bone scan are usually positive during the acute stage. The stress fracture is the most frequent athletic injury associated with a normal radiograph and persistent skeletal pain (16). This injury is the result of persistent abnormal activity that results in accelerated bone resorption and ultimately bone fatigue (Fig. 20.8). It is a result of numerous resorption cavities. Radionuclide bone scanning permits earlier detection than plain film. Stress fractures display a spectrum of abnormality from minimal periosteal reaction to full-thickness stress fracture. Five stages have been described (17).

In Stages I and II, periosteal reactions result in the deposition of the radiopharmaceutical at the site of injury. This produces a faint linear band along the periphery of the bone. Radiographs at this stage of abnormality are usually normal. The advanced stages of stress fracture demonstrate radiopharmaceutical concentration in a fusiform fashion extending throughout the entire cortex of the bone (Fig. 20.9). Stress fractures at Stages I and II demonstrate scintigraphic reversion to normal by 2 to 3 months. A Stage V abnormality may require 6 months or more. Early detection of

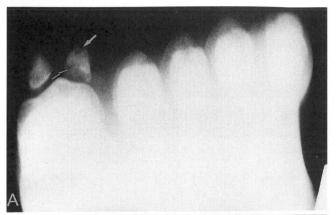
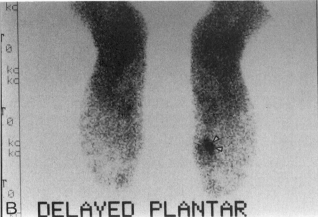

Figure 20.8. Osteonecrosis in a sesamoid bone. This long-distance runner had pain on the plantar aspect of her foot. **A.** The radiograph shows ill-defined cystic areas within the fibular sesamoid (arrows). **B.** Nuclear scintigraphy reveals increased uptake at this area (arrowheads). (Courtesy of Canadian Memorial Chiropractic College, Radiology Department, Toronto, Ontario,

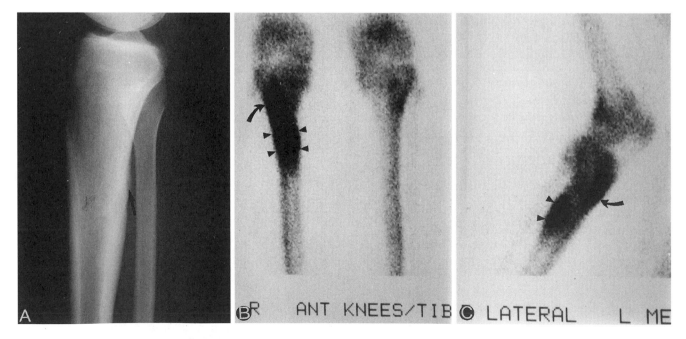

Figure 20.9. Stress fracture. **A.** The radiograph shows focal periosteal new bone formation along the posterior aspect of the proximal tibia (arrow). **B** and **C.** Nuclear scintigraphy reveals significant uptake of the bone-seeking radioisotope posteriorly (arrowheads) and more proximally in an anterior location (curved arrows), due to chronic stress at the insertion of the patellar tendon.

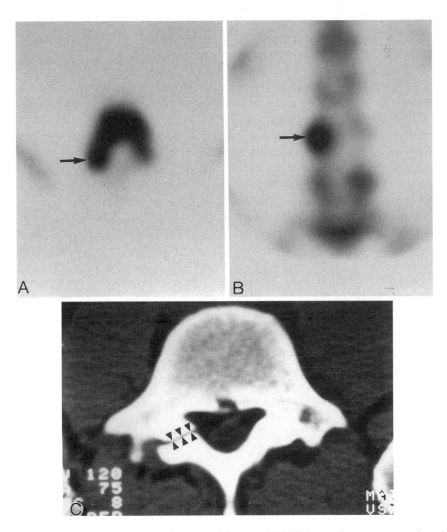

Figure 20.10. Spondylolytic spondylolisthesis. **A.** Axial and **B.** coronal SPECT images demonstrate a unilateral increase in radioisotope uptake at the L4 level (arrows). This corresponds to a unilateral pars defect (arrowheads) seen on CT **(C).** (Courtesy of David Volarich, D.O.)

a stress fracture can prevent fracture progression to cortical interruption. The sites of stress fractures are determined by the type of athletic activity and the presence of other predisposing factors including pathomechanics, substandard athletic equipment, and inappropriate training techniques. The most common sites of stress fractures are in the lower extremity involving the tibia, metatarsals, and femur.

Another valuable role for bone scanning is in the detection of occult fractures. A substantially large percentage of fractures may be detected within 24 hours of injury when compelling physical findings are coupled with negative plain films. An example of a common occult fracture involves the hamate. Fractures of the hook of the hamate can result from falls or the use of bats, clubs, or racquets in which the butt of the handle impacts the hook and fractures it. Occult fractures can also be seen in the scaphoid, femoral neck, tibial plateau, and ribs.

Differential diagnosis between soft tissue trauma and a fracture may be assisted by skeletal scintigraphy if images are obtained within a few days of injury. The fracture will demonstrate discrete and intense uptake relative to the soft tissue injury. A delayed bone scan from 8 to 24 hours may be helpful because soft tissue radioisotope is decreased. SPECT imaging may also be helpful.

Low back pain in a young athlete, especially pain that is aggravated by hyperextension and twisting, is often mechanical. Spondylolysis is often occult on the plain film examination. Radionuclide bone scanning should be performed even if the radiograph is abnormal, because the injury can be dated and the level of activity substantiates further supportive treatment. These injuries are particularly common in weight lifters and gymnasts. One or more levels may be involved. Recently, SPECT imaging has been advocated in the evaluation of suspected spondylolysis (Fig. 20.10) (16, 18).

Dual photon absorptiometry (DPA) is a nuclear medicine procedure capable of monitoring skeletal mass. The differential attenuation of two different energy peaks by bone and soft tissues allows the calculation of bone density. A typical examination delivers a total dose of 100 to 200 mrem.

The capability of quantifying bone density in athletes has proven to be beneficial. Decreases in bone density secondary to amenorrhea have been reported in runners (19). This translated into more running-related fractures. A reduced level of lumbar bone density has also been reported in male long-distance runners (20). Both of these studies suggest that endurance training may promote hormonal changes leading to osteoporosis.

Joints

Athletes who are injured in areas surrounding an articulation may experience pain and diminished range of motion. Plain films obtained in the setting of persistent pain are often negative. Radionuclide bone scanning is helpful in excluding an occult fracture. If delayed images demonstrate focal intense uptake around an articulation, post-traumatic arthritis is present. Runners may be prone to osteoarthrosis in the weight-bearing articulations of the hip, knee, and ankle, although recent evidence refutes this association (21).

MUSCULOSKELETAL ULTRASOUND

Diagnostic ultrasound has gained an increasingly greater role as an imaging modality in the diagnosis of musculoskeletal injury. It is particularly useful in the evaluation of soft tissues. During the past decade, technical advances have improved the contrast and spatial resolution of this modality. Published data offer a variety of opinions as to the sensitivity, specificity, and overall accuracy of musculoskeletal sonography. Ultrasound is highly dependent on the operator's skill and experience. This creates difficulty in establishing ultrasound as a reliable means for evaluation of injury. The radiologist's experience with the musculoskeletal application of ultrasound, type of injury, body part, and type of examination equipment are additional variables for consideration.

Ultrasound operates according to the piezoelectric principle. Electrical energy is used to create mechanical energy (sound). Sound waves pass from the transducer, through a conducting medium, and into the tissues to be examined. Tissues demonstrate varying acoustic properties based on their composition. Thus, varying frequencies of sound are reflected and returned to the transducer. These echoes are compared with the differential transmission of the remaining sound, and an image is produced. High-frequency transducers (7.5 to 10 MHz) allow for increased contrast and spatial resolution, but are somewhat limited in their depth of view. Using a lower frequency transducer (3.5 MHz) increases depth of view while sacrificing detail. The selection of the type and frequency of transducer head used is a decision based primarily on the sonographer's preference and the body part being examined.

Ultrasound provides several advantages over other imaging modalities. Examinations are painless, relatively inexpensive, readily available at most imaging centers or hospitals, and are performed in a timely fashion (usually less than 30 minutes). Dynamic evaluation of tendons and muscles during contraction and relaxation may provide additional information that is useful in the differential reasoning process (22). Additionally, ultrasound is noninvasive and uses no radiation, so that comparison studies with the opposite normal side and post-treatment follow-up are easily performed.

Limitations of ultrasound revolve primarily around the fact that it images only soft tissues, particularly of the appendicular skeleton. Because the image is composed of echoes returning to the transducer, sound that is completely transmitted or completely absorbed by a tissue contributes nothing to the image.

Normal skeletal muscle, when examined longitudinally, demonstrates multiple fine parallel echoes (23). This is contrasted by the increased echogenicity of the surrounding connective tissue and subcutaneous fat. Tendons are moderately echogenic (increased when compared with skeletal muscle) with fine parallel internal echoes (23). The tendon is surrounded on either side by a hyperechoic line representing the peritendon (23). Normal synovial sheaths are anechoic (22–24). Fibrocartilaginous structures (e.g., knee meniscus) are homogeneously hypoechoic (22).

Rotator cuff tears are frequently observed in competitive sports. These injuries are the result of stress placed on the glenohumeral joint. Stabilization of this joint is primarily the responsibility of the surrounding soft tissues, leaving it extremely vulnerable to athletic trauma. Middleton et al. (25) have defined three sonographic criteria indicative of a rotator cuff tear: (1) discontinuity of the normal echogenicity of the tendon, (2) replacement of the normal homogeneous echogenicity by a central hyperechoic band, and (3) nonvisualization of the cuff (Fig. 20.11). Kaplan et al. (23) consider focal thinning of the rotator cuff

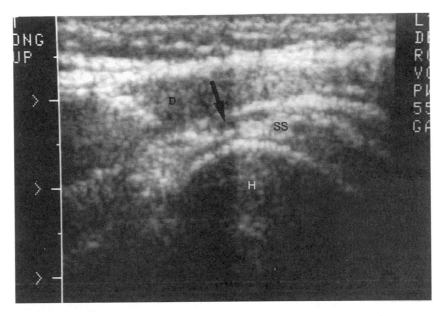

Figure 20.11. Rotator cuff tear. Ultrasonography demonstrates discontinuity (arrow) of the supraspinatus tendon. D: deltoid muscle; H: humerus; SS: supraspinatus tendon.

tendon also to be highly suggestive of a tear. Focal areas of echogenicity representing calcification within the cuff may be misinterpreted as a partial tear (22). Plain film radiography will help avoid this misdiagnosis. By far, most tears occur in the distal portion of the supraspinatus tendon or "critical zone." At this location the tendinous fibers are obliquely oriented, and the inexperienced sonographer may misinterpret this finding as a tear.

Ultrasonography of the knee has been reported to be reliable for examination of the patellar tendon and menisci. Evaluation of the cruciate ligaments has been reported (26). Tears of the patellar tendon usually occur proximally at the junction of the patella and the tendon (23, 27). These can be demonstrated as focal hypoechoic areas. Local hematomas within the tendon are also hypoechoic (28). Early evidence of osteoarthritis can be demonstrated with high-resolution ultrasound before plain film manifestations exist. Diminished thickness and surface irregularity of the meniscal fibrocartilage have been reported by Aisen et al. (29) as a reliable sign of degeneration. Suprapatellar effusions represent an echo-free area interposed between the quadriceps tendon and the femur (27).

Ultrasound provides an accurate method with which to image injuries of the Achilles tendon. It is most helpful in differentiating tears requiring surgery from those that can be treated conservatively (23). Complete tears appear as an echo-free zone within a retracted muscle (27). Partial tendon rupture is sonographically similar, but some areas of the tendon have a normal appearance

and there is preservation of tendon continuity (30). Hematoma formation within the tendon may produce a variable echo pattern (23). Ruptures of the Achilles tendon most commonly occur 2 to 6 cm cephalad to the calcaneal insertion site. This site is where the tendon is thinnest and its vascular supply is most deficient (27).

Injuries to muscles may be sonographically detected. During the acute phase, hematoma and surrounding edema appear relatively echolucent. Subsequent fibrosis and organized hematoma most commonly demonstrate an echogenic pattern. Normal relaxed muscle produces a relatively echogenic pattern compared with the contracted state. With injury, resting muscular tonicity tends to flatten and smooth an area of discontinuity, potentially masking the abnormality. In cases of rupture, muscular contraction causes the lesion to appear larger, especially when imaged longitudinally (30).

Diagnostic ultrasound has emerged as a primary imaging technology. The clinical applications of musculoskeletal sonography, however, are limited. High-resolution, functional capability and the absence of ionizing radiation are its key advantages. Its role is likely to complement that of CT or MRI in the assessment of athletic injury.

ARTHROGRAPHY

Arthrography is an imaging modality that evaluates the cartilage and soft tissues of an articulation. This technique, which began in the early 1900s, was originally coupled with plain film radiography. Technological advances have since used arthrography with fluoroscopy, tomography (both computed axial images and conventional methods), and digital radiography. Preliminary work using MRI coupled with arthrography has demonstrated favorable results in the shoulder joint (31).

The first intra-articular contrast agent used was air (pneumoarthrography). Since then both iodinated and, more recently, noniodinated positive contrast materials have been used. Currently, examinations may be performed with either radiopaque contrast alone (single-contrast technique) or with both air and positive contrast matrial injection (double-contrast technique).Indications for a single-contrast exaination versus a double-contrast examination vary, depending on the arthrographer's training and experience.

The past 10 years have seen an overall decline of approximately 20% in the number of arthrograms performed (32). Reasons for this decline include the increased use of arthroscopy and MRI. Despite the decreasing number of examinations performed today, arthrography remains a popular imaging tool because of its relatively low cost and comparatively accurate diagnostic information.

Shoulder

Arthrography is a commonly used technique in evaluating athletic injuries to the shoulder joint. Rotator cuff tears, recurrent dislocations of the glenohumeral joint, glenoid labrum injuries, and abnormalities of the long head of the biceps tendon are some of the common shoulder injuries adequately evaluated with arthrography (33). Many of these lesions are directly related to the throwing mechanism.

Most abnormalities can be demonstrated sufficiently using double-contrast techniques. Single-contrast examinations are, however, the procedure of choice for evaluating adhesive capsulitis of the glenohumeral joint (32). Additionally, small partial-thickness tears located on the deep surface of the rotator cuff tendon are best demonstrated with the single-contrast technique (34).

Double-contrast techniques allow adequate evaluation of rotator cuff tendon abnormalities. Specific information may be obtained concerning the defect size, quality of the torn tendon edges, amount of retraction, and size of the remaining intact tendon (34). Because of the overlying air and contrast-filled subscapularis bursa and bicipital tendon sheath, anterior labral abnormalities may be difficult to evaluate with conventional arthrography (35).

Postarthrography CT offers exquisite detail of both osseous and soft tissue structures of the shoulder joint in the axial plane. The accuracy and overall sensitivity in detecting labral abnormalities, capsular lesions, and osseous defects surpass those of plain film arthrography (35, 36). If clinical evidence of recurrent dislocation or joint instability exists, double-contrast arthrography followed by CT is the procedure of choice (33). Capsular evaluation is particularly important, as it is capsular pathology that is most commonly implicated as the causative lesion in glenohumeral instability. The determination of the exact site and extent of capsular and labral abnormalities may assist in determining the appropriate surgical or nonsurgical treatment (37). Additional advantages of computed arthrotomography include the potential for image reformatting in coronal and sagittal planes, reduced patient radiation, and less patient repositioning during the examination (a significant consideration in patients experiencing extreme pain) (36).

Digital arthrography of the glenohumeral joint is a less often used technique. Stiles et al. (38) suggest that it may offer significant advantages over standard single- and double-contrast techniques. It is, however, a costly procedure. The widespread use of computed arthrotomography has reduced the need for advances in digital techniques.

Lesions of the rotator cuff are present as either complete or incomplete tears. Complete tears are diagnosed by the visualization of air or contrast in the subacromial subdeltoid bursa located superior or lateral to the greater tuberosity and adjacent to the inferior aspect of the acromion (33, 39–41). Using double-contrast techniques, the width of the tear and the degree of degeneration within the disrupted tendon can be assessed (41). Incomplete tears may involve the superior surface or inferior surface or they may exist as an entirely intrasubstance lesion. Visualization of incomplete tears with conventional arthrographic techniques is considered difficult and unreliable (42). Tears of the superior surface and intrasubstance tears routinely escape arthrographic detection (41). Only those tears involving the inferior surface of the tendon can be assessed accurately (33, 41). These abnormalities are demonstrated as an irregular or linear collection of contrast material superior to the opacified joint cavity near the anatomical neck of the humerus (33).

Glenoid labrum abnormalities are commonly seen with shoulder instability. Disruption of the integrity of the labrum (usually anterior and inferior) is the most frequent form of internal derangement in recurrent shoulder dislocations (41). These lesions may be purely fibrocartilaginous or may involve portions of the bony glenoid

(Bankart lesions). Hill-Sachs deformity (impaction fracture) may also be associated and is demonstrated as a bony defect along the posterolateral aspect of the humeral head. Although commonly associated with glenohumeral instability, labral tears are rarely the primary cause (39). Tears of the superior labrum have been specifically attributed to the throwing mechanism in stable shoulders (36). CT arthrography offers comprehensive evaluation of labral pathology. The normal anterior labrum appears longer and thinner than the posterior with its sharper margins (41). Singson et al. (43) defined the following labrum abnormalities: tears, truncation, attrition (diminished cartilage thickness), thickening, and detachment with or without fragmentation.

As mentioned previously, capsular lesions are usually the causative factor in shoulder instability. Anatomical variations of the capsule insertion may produce large recesses that may be a predisposing or major contributing factor to the instability of the joint (37). The posterior capsule always inserts on the posterior labrum; the anterior capsular insertion is variable (39). These have been divided into three types: type 1 inserts on or near the anterior labrum, and types 2 and 3 insert in a progressively medial direction along the scapular neck (43). Arthrographic evidence of capsular pathology includes significant medial scapular insertion of the anterior capsule (type 3), marginal stripping or detachment of the glenoid, and tears or loss of intervening scapular marginal soft tissues (43).

Double-contrast arthrography is a reliable means with which to evaluate bicipital tendon pathology (35). Acute ruptures can be evaluated more accurately than subacute ruptures, as shrinking of adjacent tissues may obscure the abnormal findings (41). Incomplete tears of the tendon produce distortion of the synovial sheath accompanied by increased width of the tendon (41). Arthrography is also suited for evaluation of the osseous anatomy of the intertubercular groove and the diagnosis of medial dislocation of the tendon (35).

A patient with a clinical history suggesting adhesive capsulitis should be evaluated using single-contrast arthrographic techniques. Findings of adhesive capsulitis include diminished joint volume, irregularity of the capsular insertion, and decreased size of the axillary recess and subscapular bursa (33). "Brisement" is a form of treatment using arthrography to progressively distend the joint capsule (44). This technique has achieved limited success, and its full description is beyond the scope of this text.

Elbow

Single- or double-contrast arthrography of the elbow with plain film radiography or conventional tomography enhances the diagnosis of post-traumatic intra-articular abnormalities. The addition of CT provides imaging in the transaxial plane with superior soft tissue resolution. In addition, computer manipulation of the image and the ability for reconstruction allow for multiplanar visualization of the joint (45). This eliminates most of the painful joint repositioning with other techniques and diminishes total examination time (reducing image degradation from air and contrast resorption) (46).

Indications for elbow arthrography include demonstration of osteochondral loose bodies, articular surface irregularity, and capsular abnormalities (e.g., rupture, post-traumatic synovitis, adhesive capsulitis). In post-traumatic situations, the double-contrast technique is preferred. The coated articular surfaces and synovial lining are highlighted against the intra-articular air (47).

Although useful in adult athletes, arthrography is even more valuable in younger athletes. The immature developing elbow is complex, and injuries to the physeal cartilage may escape detection with plain film radiography (41). Contrast opacification of the articulation is especially helpful in delineating physeal (Salter-Harris) injuries and osteochondritis dissecans. Much of the same information may be gained from alternatively using MRI; however, because the joint is not distended with air, precise localization of fragments relative to the joint space may not always be possible.

Wrist

Arthrography of the posttraumatic wrist should be performed only when there is suspicion of ligamentous injury coupled with negative plain films and fluoroscopy. Traditionally, contrast was injected into the radiocarpal joint. The extension of contrast into either the midcarpal or distal radioulnar joint was then observed fluoroscopically (47). Recent advances in wrist arthrography include tricompartmental injection of contrast and the use of digital subtraction techniques. These newer techniques allow greater diagnostic capabilities for identifying subtle ligamentous abnormalities. The normal radiocarpal, midcarpal, and distal radioulnar joints do not communicate. The significance of intracompartmental communications is greater in the young athlete due to "normal" communications with advancing age (presumed to be degenerative) (33, 41). Other post-traumatic soft tissue abnormalities demonstrated by arthrography include triangular fibrocartilage complex (TFCC) injury, traumatic synovitis, capsular disruption, adhesive capsulitis, and transchondral fractures.

Sequential injection of contrast into the radiocarpal compartment, distal radioulnar joint, and midcarpal compartment with fluoroscopic assistance may offer superior diagnostic accuracy in identification and localization of intracompartmental ligament abnormalities. Levinsohn et al. (48) found that 17% of TFCC perforations were diagnosed with radiocarpal joint injection (negative when injected only into the distal radioulnar joint); 33% of detached TFCC were demonstrated only with distal radioulnar joint injection (negative when injected only with the radiocarpal joint; and 28% of scapho-lunate or lunatotriquetral ligament perforations were identified with midcarpal injection (negative when injected only into the radiocarpal joint). Occasionally, synovial reflections of the radiocarpal compartment will retain a large amount of contrast, thereby obscuring fine detail at the scapholunate and lunatotriquetral ligaments (49).

Digital subtraction radiography has been used widely to image vascular abnormalities. Its limited use in the diagnosis of soft tissue joint injuries has emerged in the past decade. Its greatest contribution is in demonstrating interosseous ligament abnormalities of the wrist.

Initially a precontrast image is acquired. Contrast is then injected into the radiocarpal joint while multiple sequential images are obtained at a rapid rate (1 to 2/sec for approximately 20 to 30 sec). The osseous structures are then subtracted from subsequent contrast images using the initial noncontrast images as a "mask." This allows for real-time monitoring and continuous frame-by-frame evaluation of flow dynamics of the contrast injection. The examination can then be reviewed in a closed-loop movie format (41).

Sequential opacification of the joint spaces allows for precise determination of interosseous ligament or TFCC injury. This technique is superior to conventional arthrography and possibly MRI at demonstrating small perforations. Pittman et al. (50) reported the use of a double-contrast subtraction protocol following a negative single-contrast subtraction examination. The addition of air into a distended joint containing contrast allows air to pass through small ligament perforations (50). Postarthrography CT of the wrist offers excellent anatomical detail. However, significant diagnostic information is not acquired when compared with multiple compartment arthrography, and clinical management decisions are not significantly influenced by this costly procedure (51).

Knee

Single- and double-contrast arthrography provides information in evaluation of the ligaments, menisci, and articular surfaces of the knee. The use of regular and high-resolution CT has increased diagnostic accuracy, especially when investigating the cruciate ligaments and articular surfaces of the patella.

Meniscal pathology is observed most frequently to involve the medial meniscus, more specifically the posterior horn. Lateral meniscus involvement is less common. This is partially due to poor visualization of the more complex anatomy of the posterior horn of the lateral meniscus. Improved anatomical detail may be obtained with the addition of postarthrographic analysis using high-resolution CT.

The normal menisci are triangular when viewed tangentially and semilunar, wedge-shaped when viewed axially. The anterior and posterior horns of the lateral meniscus are of approximately equal size, whereas the anterior horn of the medial meniscus is noticeably smaller than the posterior horn. After intra-articular contrast injection, the menisci may be observed as radiolucent structures outlined by radiopaque contrast. Any contrast material demonstrated within the meniscus proper is abnormal. Many different arthrographic classifications of meniscal tears have been proposed. These systems of classification are often inaccurate, and their effect on clinical management is suspect. It is of greater importance to localize and estimate the severity of the meniscal abnormality (41, 52). It is with the previous statement in mind that common arthrographic patterns of meniscal tears are described.

Any tear of the meniscus that extends from one surface to the other can be considered a bucket-handle tear (52). Contrast will be observed in an intrameniscal location either vertically or in oblique orientation. Displacement of the inner fragment may be evident arthrographically. Horizontal tears are usually observed in older individuals and are presumed to be degenerative. A single specific injury usually cannot be implicated as a causative factor. Horizontally oriented intrameniscal contrast is demonstrated extending to either the superior or inferior meniscal surface. The third major category of meniscal tear is the radial tear. These vertical tears occur along the inner contour of the meniscus (33). Arthrographic evidence of this type of tear appears as blunting of the meniscal border.

Ligamentous abnormalities are somewhat more difficult to assess with arthrography. Normal cruciate ligaments are seen as water density structures coated by a layer of positive contrast material and surrounded by air (52). The arthrographic examination is performed in the stressed anterior drawer position. This causes the ligaments to be taut and appear well marginated. Cruciate ligament tears can be diagnosed when the ligament is not in its anticipated location. It presents with an angulated, wavy, or bowed contour or demonstrates an irregular inferior ligamentous attachment (53).

The collateral ligaments are usually adequately evaluated with clinical examination and supplemental plain film radiography performed in varus and valgus stressed positions (52). The lateral collateral ligament (LCL) is separate from the joint capsule. Therefore, tears will infrequently disrupt the capsular integrity. The capsular integrity must be violated before contrast extravasation into the surrounding soft tissues is exhibited. The medial collateral ligament (MCL), however, represents a blending of fibers from the medial joint capsule and the more superficial tibial collateral ligament. Only a complete tear through both the superficial and deep portions of the ligament will be arthrographically demonstrable. A tear involving the deep ligament fibers (capsule) without superficial fiber disruption allows contrast to outline the vertically oriented superficial fibers (33). Tears involving only the superficial portion of the ligament demonstrate a normal arthrogram.

According to Hughston et al. (54), it is damage to the posterior aspect of the medial capsule that produces knee instability. They report damage to this structure to be of even greater importance than anterior cruciate ligament (ACL) injury. The two abnormalities often occur together and frequently include a tear of the medial meniscus producing "O'Donaghue's unhappy triad."

Injuries to the articular surfaces of the knee include transchondral fractures and chondromalacia patella. Conventional arthrography and, more recently, computed arthrotomography and MRI can aid in the diagnosis of these abnormalities.

Transchondral fractures may consist entirely of articular cartilage or may involve a portion of the subchondral bone. Those fragments with an osseous component are usually visible without the use of contrast, particularly if a defect of the host bone is demonstrated. The addition of contrast will, however, allow a more accurate assessment of the size of the fragment.

Arthrography may be helpful in the patient who presents clinically with persistent knee pain or joint locking following shearing, rotatory, or tangentially directed forces to the knee. The cutting maneuver in football is a common mechanism. The majority of these transchondral fractures are produced by the relocation of a dislocated patella (52). Most dislocations occur laterally when the knee is flexed and in a valgus position. The knee is then extended and the patella is driven into the surface of the lateral femoral condyle. A cartilage fragment is then produced from either the medial facet of the patella or the lateral femoral articular surface. Arthrography may demonstrate a normal, swollen, or depressed cartilage surface. Dissection beneath the chondral (osteochondral) fragment is also considered abnormal (41).

The patellar cartilage fissuring, fibrillation, and ulceration seen with chondromalacia patella cannot be seen with conventional arthrography, but is well demonstrated with the addition of CT.

Ankle

Ankle arthrography may be performed as either a single- or double-contrast examination, with or without the use of CT. A single-contrast examination is recommended for acute injuries, whereas double-contrast examinations better demonstrate articular cartilage abnormalities (e.g., intra-articular loose bodies) and synovial lesions (e.g., adhesive capsulitis) (55). The normal arthrogram demonstrates filling of the articular capsule without extravasation of contrast medium outside the confines of the capsule. Three normal recesses are observed: (1) anteriorly, (2) posteriorly, and (3) at the distal tibiofibular syndesmosis (contrast normally extends 1 to 2.5 cm proximally from the joint) (41).

Indications for ankle arthrography in the athlete include acute ligamentous injury, ligamentous instability (chronic ligamentous injury), transchondral fracture, and adhesive capsulitis.

The anterior talofibular ligament is the most commonly injured ligament of the ankle, occurring with inversion trauma. Because it maintains an intimate relationship with the capsule, tearing of this ligament results in capsular disruption (56). Arthrography exhibits extravasation of contrast inferior, anterior, and lateral to the distal fibula (41, 55, 56). The amount of contrast that leaks from the torn capsule, however, is not indicative of the extent of injury (56). These findings can be observed only when the examination is performed within 24 to 36 hours of injury (55). After this period healing of the capsule occurs, eliminating extra-articular extravasation of contrast. Therefore, a delay in performing the arthrographic examination may lead to a false-negative result, inadequate treatment, and subsequent long-term chronic ankle instability.

Tearing of the calcaneal fibular ligament also results in rupture of the inner aspect of the proximal peroneal tendon sheath (41, 55). This results in communication between the capsule and tendon sheath (55, 56). It is demonstrated arthrographically as extravasation of contrast along with the laterally located peroneal tendon. These injuries are often associated with tears of the anterior talofibular ligament (41). Another injury associated with inversion trauma is rupture of the tibiofibular syndesmosis. Diagnosis of this entity is often inferred from separation of the tibia and fibula or fracture of the fibula demonstrated on plain film radiography. Proximal leaking of contrast beyond the normal tibiofibular recess indicates a rupture of this ligament (55).

Eversion injuries may produce a tear of the deltoid ligament. Because this ligament is extremely strong and offers a tremendous amount of support to the medial ankle, complete rupture is unusual. Tears of the deltoid ligament are usually confined to only the anterior segment (54). When injury exists, contrast is present in the medial soft tissues, beyond the confines of the articular capsule (41).

Adhesive capsulitis of the ankle is best demonstrated with single-contrast arthrography. As in other articulations, this abnormality is observed as diminished joint volume and synovial irregularity.

Although immediate arthrographic assessment of the injured ankle is beneficial in demonstrating acute tears, abnormalities of the chronically unstable ankle can also be demonstrated adequately. Previous ligamentous disruptions that have undergone healing with fibrotic tissue appear as small, well-defined recesses extending beyond the normal lateral capsular margins (56).

Evaluation of a clinically suspected transchondral fracture is best achieved with the double-contrast technique (55). The addition of CT may improve diagnostic accuracy. Fragments may be entirely cartilaginous or contain both cartilage and bone. They may lie free within the joint cavity or be attached to the synovium.

The role of CT arthrography, as applied to the evaluation of joint trauma, is likely to give way to MRI. This prediction, however, may not see fulfillment for many years. Until then, CT arthrography remains well established in diagnostic imaging algorithms for joint trauma.

COMPUTED TOMOGRAPHY

The use of CT in the workup of athletic injury has gained wide use, especially in imaging cranio-cerebral, facial, chest, abdominal, spinal, and pelvic trauma. Through axial and reconstructed coronal and sagittal images, CT can "unravel" complex osseous and soft tissue anatomy (Fig. 20.12). CT has eliminated more invasive diagnostic studies for examination of blunt trauma to the abdomen and head injuries.

CT combines a finely collimated x-ray beam with high-efficiency detectors. The detectors transmit their data to a computer, where it is processed using a series of mathematical formulas. This information is then manipulated into tiny two-dimensional squares (pixels) that represent a three-dimensional volume of tissue (voxel). The pixels are arranged in a matrix (e.g., 256×256 or 512×512) to produce an axial image. Additionally, the density of a pixel is assigned a number (Hounsfield unit) according to the attenuation coefficient of the tissue being examined. These assigned numbers can be accentuated by targeting select tissues. Because this information is stored as numerical data within the computer, it can display axial images or be manipulated to construct sagittal, coronal, and oblique reformatted images.

Head

Most head injuries in the athlete result from unintentional trauma. The sport of boxing is one notable exception. In no other sport is victory determined by the opponent's physical demise; thus victories can be obtained by decision or by knockout. The possibility of serious head injuries also exists with other sports such as football, baseball, ice hockey, rugby, skiing, and cycling.

Sports-related brain injuries may be either diffuse or focal. The diffuse lesion results from external force inducing rotational acceleration of the brain as it collides with the osseous calvarium (57). Cerebral concussion (Grades I–III) and diffuse brain swelling are included in this category of injury (57). Concussions are the most common sports-related head injury (58). This injury demonstrates varying levels of consciousness and temporary disorientation. Generally, these injuries produce no structural brain lesions and resolve within 24 hours. Diffuse brain swelling is a poorly understood entity. Whether this represents a primary form of brain injury or traumatic sequela is yet to be resolved (59). It occurs in both mild and severe types of head injury, and its CT appearance may present a diagnostic challenge for the inexperienced clinician.

Focal lesions constitute a more severe form of brain injury and include cerebral contusion as well as intracerebral, epidural, and subdural

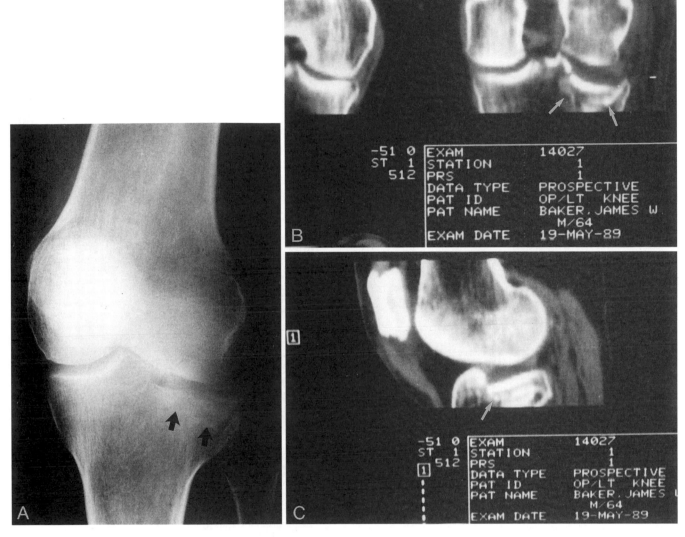

Figure 20.12. Lateral tibial plateau fracture. **A.** The radiograph demonstrates a depressed fracture of the lateral tibial plateau (arrows). CT reconstruction images in the **(B)** coronal and **(C)** sagittal planes better define the plateau fracture. (Courtesy of Mahmoud Ziaee, M.D.)

hematomas. Cerebral contusions and intracerebral hematomas occur in the athlete suffering a blow to the head. Persistent headache and post-traumatic amnesia without loss of consciousness or neurologic deficit closely follow the traumatic event (60). The mechanisms producing such a lesion have been categorized into coup and contrecoup (59). Coup injury occurs when the stationary calvarium is impacted by an object (e.g., hockey puck, baseball). The overlying calvarium produces a lesion within the ipsilateral cerebral parenchyma. Contrecoup injuries are produced when the brain and calvarium are in motion and suddenly undergo a dramatic reduction in velocity, leaving the brain in relative motion. Lesions occurring with this form of injury occur opposite the side of impaction. Both contusions and in-

tracerebral hematomas are well demonstrated on CT. Initially there is an area of increased density. The subsequent repair usually occurs within 2 to 3 weeks, producing varying degrees of diminished attenuation of the lesion. This is secondary to edema and necrotic tissue.

Acute subdural and epidural hematomas are the most severe brain injuries. Because athletic head injuries generally result from lower inertial loading than other forms of head trauma (i.e., motor vehicle accidents and falling from heights), acute subdural hematomas are 3 times more common than epidural hematomas (57). This injury generally yields an unconscious patient with neurologic deterioration. These lesions characteristically present without skull fractures. Initially, CT examination demonstrates crescentic density paralleling the calvarium with or without demonstrable mass effect.

Epidural hematomas result from disruption of the meningeal arteries on the surface of the dural covering of the brain. Calvarial fractures are present in almost all situations (59). The classic patient demonstrates immediate loss of consciousness with lucid recovery and subsequent increasing headache, diminishing levels of consciousness, pupillary changes, and decerebrate posturing and weakness (57). Signs and symptoms generally develop 1 to 4 days after injury. Although classic, this presentation only represents one third of cases (56). Initially, CT demonstrates a biconvex density, most commonly in the temporoparietal region. With resolution, both acute subdural and epidural hematomas exhibit varying degrees of hypodense/isodense regions relative to adjacent brain parenchyma.

The use of CT has reduced the need for more invasive procedures such as angiography and surgical intervention. Although not a replacement for skull radiography, CT provides a valuable adjunctive imaging modality that, in certain instances, may preempt plain radiography. Although MRI use exceeds CT in a number of centers, CT remains the primary technique for evaluation of acute trauma to the head (61).

The facial skeleton and associated soft tissues pose a complex diagnostic challenge. CT has replaced plain film radiography for the athlete sustaining facial injury. The physical examination concentrates on facial asymmetry and contour. Deformity should prompt the plain film examination. CT should then be used. Although often less serious than head injuries, facial injuries may result in impaired function and permanent disfigurement if not correctly diagnosed and treated. The development of software capable of supplying three-dimensional reconstruction has allowed better definition of complex facial fractures. This aids the surgeon in planning the reconstruction necessary to restore facial symmetry.

Injury to the paranasal sinuses may occur as an isolated finding or as part of a more complex injury (Fig. 20.13). These injuries may be diagnosed adequately with plain film radiography; however, CT often provides additional information regarding the extent of injury (e.g., intracranial extension) (Fig. 20.14).

Orbital fractures, like paranasal sinus injuries, may present as an isolated entity or in combination with more extensive injuries (i.e., tripod and LeFort fractures). Perhaps the most well-known and clinically significant orbital fracture is the blowout fracture. Classically, this

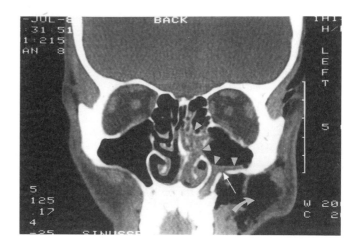

Figure 20.13. Maxillary sinus fracture. CT shows a depressed anterior wall of the left maxillary sinus (arrow). Note the hemorrhage and edema within the maxillary sinus cavity, nasal cavity, and ethmoid sinus (arrowheads). There is also subcutaneous emphysema (curved arrow) reflecting the escape of maxillary sinus air dissecting through the soft tissues. (Courtesy of Claude Pierre-Jerome, M.D., D.C.)

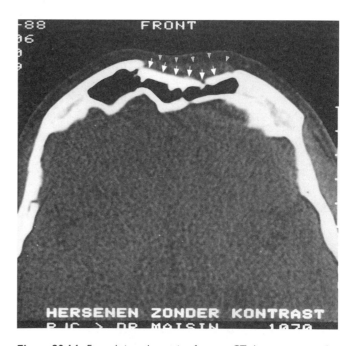

Figure 20.14. Frontal sinus depression fracture. CT shows posterior displacement of the comminuted fracture involving the anterior wall of the frontal sinus (arrows). Also note the swelling of the anterior soft tissues (arrowheads). (Courtesy of Claude Pierre-Jerome, M.D., D.C.)

fracture involves only the orbital walls (most commonly the posteromedial wall or lamina papyracea of the ethmoid bone). An "impure" type has also been described in which the contour of the orbital rim has been disrupted. These injuries are produced by a sudden increase in intraorbital pressure such as that generated by an impacting fist or ball. A major complication of this type of injury is diplopia from inferior displacement of periorbital fat or entrapment of the inferior rectus muscle within the maxillary sinus (Fig. 20.15). Large fractures may also cause inferior displacement of the globe.

Fractures of the zygoma include the zygomatic arch and the tripod. The tripod fracture separates the malar eminence of the zygoma from its normal frontal, temporal, and maxillary attachments (62). The usual components of this injury are diastasis of the zygomaticofrontal suture, zygomatic arch fracture, and fracture of the medial portion of the inferior orbital rim.

Spine

The primary indication for the use of CT in sports-related spinal injury is the identification and evaluation of fractures. Although the spinal cord, intervertebral disc, and other soft tissues are more accurately evaluated with MRI, the ability of CT to depict bone fragments and foreign

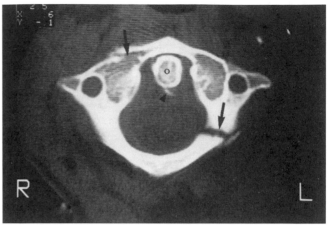

Figure 20.16. Jefferson's fracture. CT shows the fractures through the anterior and posterior arches of C1 (arrows). The osseous fragment (arrowhead) posterior to the odontoid (o) represents volume averaging from an associated fracture of C2. (Reprinted from Yochum and Rowe: Essentials of Skeletal Radiology, Second Edition. 1996. Baltimore: Williams & Wilkins. Used with permission.)

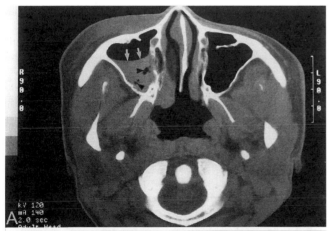

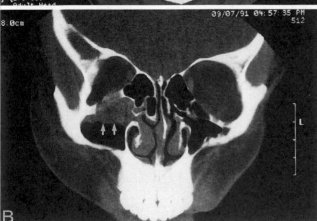

Figure 20.15. Orbital blowout fracture. **(A)** Axial and **(B)** coronal CT show hemorrhage into the right maxillary sinus (arrows). The low attenuation areas (arrowheads) within the blood represent orbital fat displaced into the sinus cavity. The fracture is not demonstrated on these images.

bodies within the spinal canal is unmatched (62). Postmyelography CT is often beneficial in visualizing the spinal canal when the neurologic picture does not correlate with the noncontrast examination findings. Athletes particularly prone to spinal injuries include those that participate in football, rugby, wrestling, diving, and gymnastics. The most serious spinal injuries incurred by the athlete usually involve the cervical spine. Most investigated injuries consist of the sprain/strain complex, but unstable dislocation and/or fractures carry the most serious complications.

Burst fractures of the bony ring of the atlas occur as a result of axial compression between the occiput and the atlas (Fig. 20.16). CT demonstrates fractures through both the anterior and posterior portions of the osseous ring. Fractures of the odontoid process occur as a result of forced hyperextension. These injuries have been classified into three categories: Type 1—an avulsion fracture from excessive tension placed on the apical and/or alar ligaments; Type 2—fracture at the junction of the odontoid process and the C2 body (most common type and most likely to demonstrate nonunion and/or subsequent instability); and Type 3—fracture through the body of C2 (odontoid remains contiguous with the superior aspect of the C2 body) (Fig. 20.17).

Fractures that parallel an axial CT slice are often missed. Coronal or sagittal reconstruction images greatly diminish this oversight (Fig. 20.18). Rotatory fixation of C1/C2 is actually a rotational dislocation and is well demonstrated by CT. Clinical suspicion of this entity should be suggested when the athlete complains of persistent torticollis following a traumatic incident to the head and

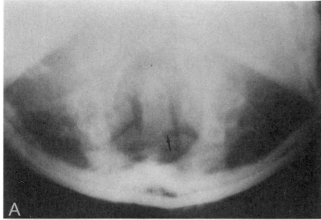

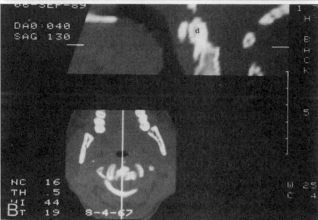

Figure 20.17. Type II dens fracture. **A.** The submentovertex view shows tilting of the odontoid and a faint lucency through the base (arrow). **B.** The sagittal reconstruction CT reveals anterior displacement of the dens (d). (Reprinted from Yochum and Rowe: Essentials of Skeletal Radiology, Second Edition. 1996. Baltimore: Williams and Wilkins. Used with permission.)

neck. Traumatic bilateral neural arch disruption of C2 (hangman's fracture) results from cervical hyperextension. Although the diagnosis in most instances should be obtained from the plain film examination, CT is helpful in excluding osseous fragments in the neural canal (Fig. 20.19).

Another common injury resulting from forced hyperextension is the teardrop fracture. This avulsion fracture occurs at the anterior inferior aspect of the vertebral body as a result of excessive stress placed on the anterior longitudinal ligament. The articular pillars are commonly fractured as a result of the cervical spine undergoing forced hyperextension and rotation. These may be detected with CT as a compression deformity; however, coronal reconstruction images are almost always necessary to appreciate the abnormality (Fig. 20.20).

Flexion injuries produce compression fractures of the vertebral body and unilateral or bilateral facet subluxation/dislocation. Compression fractures, although not always depicted on axial images, can be evaluated accurately with sagittal reformatting.

The thoracic spine is stabilized by the surrounding bony thorax, and the lumbar spine by powerful paraspinal musculature; therefore, the thoracic spine and lumbar spine are not as sus-

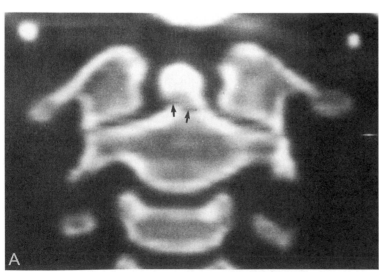

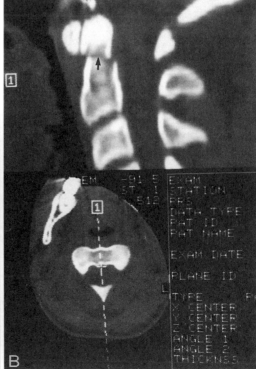

Figure 20.18. Type II dens fracture. CT reconstruction in the **(A)** coronal and **(B)** sagittal planes shows the fracture (arrows) with anterior and lateral displacement. (Courtesy of Mahmoud Ziaee, M.D.)

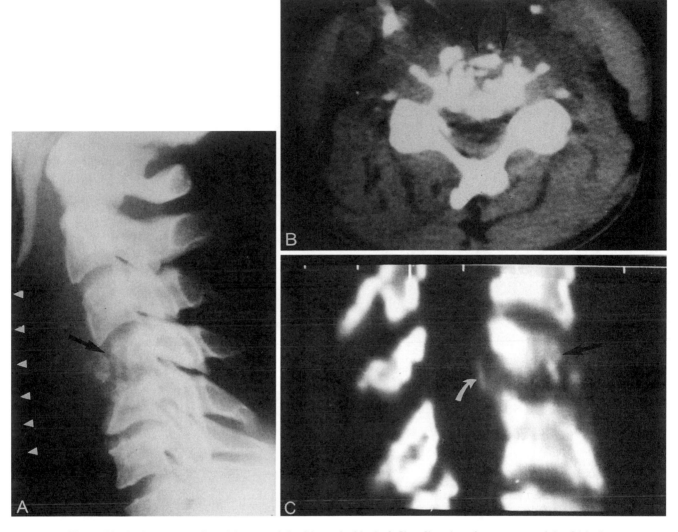

Figure 20.19. Comminuted (burst) fracture of the C4 vertebral body. **A.** Plain films show fragmentation of the C4 body (arrow) and a large hematoma within the prevertebral soft tissues (arrowheads). Also note the acute cervical kyphosis. **B** and **C.** Axial and sagittally reconstructed CT images reveal retropulsion of the posterior vertebral body margin into the neural canal (curved arrow). (Courtesy of Mark Roesler, D.C.)

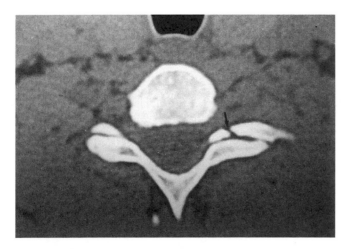

Figure 20.20. Articular pillar fracture. CT reveals a fracture of the superior articular process of C6 (arrow). (Courtesy of Brian Batenchuk, D.C.)

ceptible to osseous injury as the cervical spine. Axial and hyperflexion trauma may produce simple compression fractures of the vertebral body, burst fractures (comminuted compression fracture often displacing a fracture fragment into the neural canal), and nonosseous seat-belt–type injuries (Figs. 20.21 and 20.22). The latter form of injury is similar to the bilateral facet dislocation accompanying flexion injuries to the cervical spine. This injury may also be associated with anterior compression deformity of the vertebral body.

Spondylolisthesis and its many etiologic factors can be demonstrated accurately with CT. Combining the high sensitivity of bone scans (see previous section) with the high specificity of CT results in an overall increase in diagnostic accu-

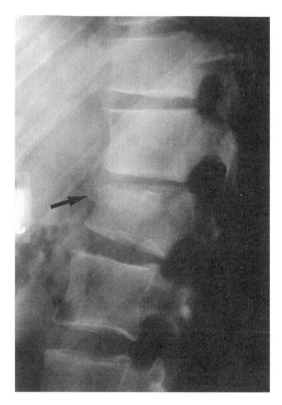

Figure 20.21. Spinal compression fracture. There is a simple anterior compression deformity of the L1 vertebral body. Note the step defect at the anterosuperior portion of the vertebrae (arrow).

racy (Fig. 20.23). Persistent lumbar pain in a young athlete should trigger the suspicion of a stress reaction involving the pars interarticularis (63). Active participation in sports such as diving, football, wrestling, gymnastics, and weight lifting should increase clinical suspicion.

Pelvis

Athletic injuries that disrupt the complex osseous and soft tissue structures of the pelvis can be demonstrated magnificently by CT. Injuries to the pelvis have been described and are categorized by many different classifications. The most accepted method is described by Key and Conwell (64). This method divides all pelvic fractures into four categories.

- Type 1—single bone involvement without disruption of the pelvic ring.
- Type 2—single fractures to the pelvic ring.
- Type 3—double fractures of the pelvic ring.
- Type 4—acetabular fractures.

Type 1 fractures are stable and include avulsion fractures. They usually occur in young athletes as a result of forced muscle contraction of the lower extremity. Fractures of a single ramus, isolated sacral fractures, and iliac wing fractures

(Duverney's fracture) are included. Type 2 fractures are also stable and include fractures through two ipsilateral rami and fractures near or subluxation of the symphysis pubis or sacroiliac joint. The more serious Type 3 fractures include bilateral superior and inferior rami fractures (straddle fractures), simultaneous diastatic fractures of the symphysis pubis and sacroiliac joints (sprung pelvis), and fractures of the anterior and ipsilateral posterior (Malgaigne) or contralateral posterior (bucket-handle) portions of the bony pelvis. These injuries are unstable and result in the most severe visceral damage (i.e., bladder contusion, ureteral laceration). Type 4 fractures are

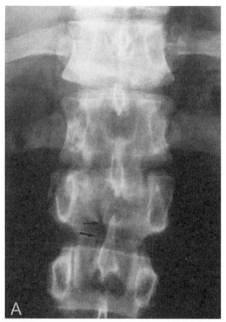

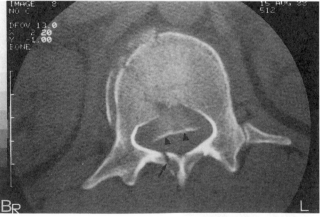

Figure 20.22. L1 burst fracture. **A.** The AP radiograph demonstrates an asymmetrical decrease in vertebral body height and an increase in the interpediculate distance. Note the lucency extending through the neural arch on the right (arrows). **B.** CT reveals fracture fragments displaced anteriorly and posteriorly (arrowheads) into the neural canal. (Reprinted from Yochum and Rowe: Essentials of Skeletal Radiology, Second Edition. 1996. Baltimore: Williams & Wilkins. Used with permission.)

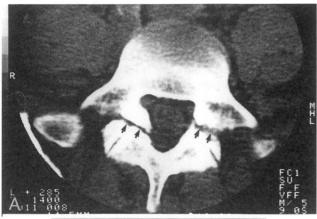

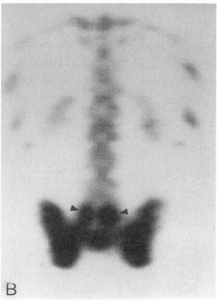

Figure 20.23. Spondylolytic spondylolisthesis. **A.** CT demonstrates bilateral pars interarticularis disruption (arrows). **B.** Nuclear scintigraphy shows increased uptake at the L5 vertebral level in the region of the pars, bilaterally (arrowheads). (Courtesy of Thomas E. Hyde, D.C.)

Abdomen

Blunt abdominal trauma in the athlete is far less common than injury to the musculoskeletal system. These injuries, however, can present serious and life-threatening complications. Contact sports such as football and rugby, as well as high-velocity noncontact sports such as bicycling and skiing, have been implicated in the production of abdominal injury. The wide use of CT in evaluation of blunt abdominal trauma has virtually replaced other imaging methods, including radionuclide scanning, angiography, exploratory laparotomies, and diagnostic peritoneal lavage in the stable patient (66). CT examinations have demonstrated both superb sensitivity and specificity in evaluation of the abdominal viscera. Prompt evaluation can reveal both intraperitoneal and retroperitoneal blood (Fig. 20.24) and the status of the liver, spleen, pancreas, and genitourinary system (67). Oral contrast medium should be used, when possible, to identify the gastrointestinal tract and to avoid confusion with abnormal fluid collections. Intravenous contrast is extremely helpful in the identification of hemorrhage from the visceral organs.

Patients with blunt abdominal injuries usually present with pain, but the frequently subtle nature of presenting signs and symptoms may preclude a correct diagnosis. Peritoneal irritation from visceral laceration may produce abdominal rigidity, pain (mild to severe), and decreased or absent bowel sounds. Before seeking CT examination, the injured patient must first be determined to be in stable condition. The spleen is the most commonly injured organ in the abdomen (68, 69). These injuries result from trauma to the left upper

acetabular fractures. These injuries are important because of their high association with vascular and genitourinary tract injury.

Complications of pelvic fractures include urethral tears (almost exclusively male), bladder rupture/contusion, diaphragm rupture, vascular injury, and neurologic damage. The most common organ to sustain injury from pelvic fractures is the urinary bladder. Bladder contusion (incomplete tearing of the bladder mucosa) is the most common form of bladder injury (65). Rupture of the bladder can be demonstrated on CT following intravenous injection of contrast material by the presence of contrast material within the peritoneal cavity or in a retroperitoneal location. Although bladder rupture is present in only 10% of pelvic fractures, 83% of patients with bladder rupture secondary to blunt trauma have pelvic fractures (65).

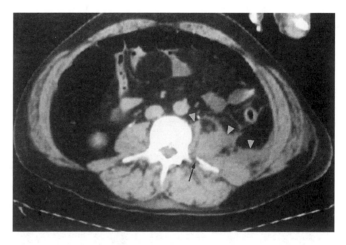

Figure 20.24. Transverse process fracture with hematoma. CT shows a minimally displaced fracture of the L3 transverse process (arrow). Additionally, hematoma is seen within the retroperitoneum and surrounds the ipsilateral psoas muscle (arrowheads).

quadrant, commonly associated with fracture of the lower rib cage. Injuries include splenic laceration (with subcapsular or perisplenic hematoma) and transection. Differentiation between splenic hematoma and laceration is possible with CT (Fig. 20.25). This is a clinically important differentiation because hematoma formation is not necessarily an indication for surgical intervention.

CT findings in hepatic injury include the demonstration of laceration, subcapsular fluid (blood bile), and fragmentation. The predominant site of injury is the right lobe (70, 71). Hepatic injury should also be considered in the athlete with an acute abdomen following right upper quadrant injury (with or without rib fracture).

The pancreas is an uncommon site of injury in sports-related trauma. Fracture of the body of the gland is the most common major injury of the pancreas due to its prevertebral location (72). Suspicion of pancreatic injury follows a history of a direct blow to the upper abdomen with resultant epigastric pain. Elevated serum amylase, when present, may assist in proper diagnosis. Complications can include pseudocyst formation and posttraumatic pancreatitis. The kidney is a commonly injured organ in many sports (66). Renal injury should be suspected in the athlete sustaining a blow to the flank, lower ribs, or upper abdomen. Clinical manifestations include hematuria, ecchymosis at the flank, and an enlarging flank mass following injury (73). Renal injuries have been classified into three categories based on severity (74).

- Minor—small cortical laceration or contusion.
- Intermediate—deep laceration with or without involvement of the collecting system.
- Major—renal pedicle injury or renal transection/fragmentation.

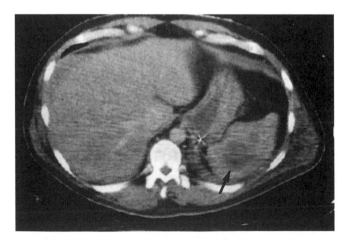

Figure 20.25. Splenic hematoma. CT demonstrates a central lucency within the substance of the spleen (arrow).

Intravenous urography is adequate in the diagnosis of most renal injuries, but CT following bolus injection of contrast material can be used in the stable patient to provide information about localization of injury, extent of injury, and renal function. Sports commonly implicated in the production of renal injury include karate, boxing, football, and rugby.

Chest

CT plays a limited, yet important role in evaluating chest injuries. Whereas injury to the thorax from sports-related trauma is often uncomplicated and adequately diagnosed with plain-film radiography, CT offers better delineation of the sometimes confusing plain-film findings. CT is better at demonstrating chest wall fracture complications and parenchymal injury sustained from chest wall fractures than it is at identifying the osseous lesion itself. Pulmonary contusions are the most common sequelae of blunt trauma to the chest (75). These appear as a nonspecific focal area of parenchymal consolidation occurring shortly after a traumatic event. Although CT identifies contusions more accurately than plain radiographs, those demonstrating clinical significance are seen on both plain film and CT examination (76).

Rib injuries in the athlete can be classified as "bruised ribs" and uncomplicated or complicated rib fractures. Uncomplicated rib fractures are an isolated injury and are clinically insignificant. However, these fractures may signify a more complex injury than is readily apparent on clinical examination. Complicated rib fractures resulting in hemothorax or pneumothorax must be excluded cautiously (Fig. 20.26). The sensitivity of CT for differences in density permits the discrimination of blood from other pleural fluids. The most common location for rib fractures is the 4th through 10th ribs. When the upper three ribs sustain enough force to fracture, the suspicion of a life-threatening major vessel or bronchial injury must be entertained (77). As previously mentioned, fractures of the lower ribs may produce splenic, hepatic, or renal injury.

CT has the capacity to discern subtle attenuation differences between adjacent soft tissue densities and is the modality of choice for imaging mediastinal injury. Hemomediastinum or pneumomediastinum, hemopericardium or pneumopericardium, rupture of the great vessels, bronchial fracture, and esophageal rupture will usually demonstrate a mediastinal abnormality on plain-film examination. Although diagnostically nonspecific, mediastinal widening or the presence of air is sensitively detected by plain-film radiography. CT following abnormal

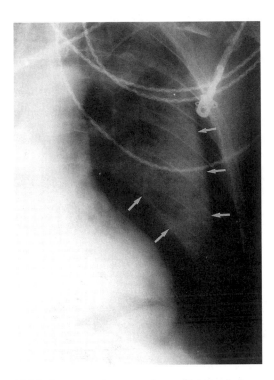

Figure 20.26. Posttraumatic pneumothorax. Multiple rib fractures (not shown) of the lower ribs resulted in this pneumothorax. The peripheral margins of the left lung are retracted away from the chest wall (arrows), indicating a partial collapse. (Courtesy of Claude Pierre-Jerome, M.D., D.C.)

plain-film examination will usually delineate the precise cause of the abnormality.

CT provides the sports physician with the means to detect subtle traumatic conditions and monitor complications arising from complex injury. Convenient access, ease of examinations, clinical use, and high-resolution imaging are factors that will ensure CT a lasting position in the diagnostic imaging strategy of the athlete.

MAGNETIC RESONANCE IMAGING

The most recent and likely the most significant advance in imaging since the discovery of x-rays is MRI. Magnetic resonance technology has been used for several decades by chemists in the laboratory. The past decade has seen this technology evolve from chemical analysis to anatomical imaging. MRI shares with CT an ability to provide sectional images from data gathered and stored by a computer; however, MRI produces an image with far greater contrast resolution while maintaining comparable spatial resolution (41). An in-depth discussion of MRI physics is beyond the scope of this text. The following brief discussion will provide an introduction to the essentials of magnetic resonance image production.

MRI is dependent on both the hydrogen ion concentration and its physicochemical environ-ment (78). Hydrogen nuclei are normally rotating around their axis in a random orientation. When a strong external magnetic field is applied to the tissue, these nuclei act like tiny bar magnets and align themselves in one of two possible positions—parallel or antiparallel. The nuclei aligned in a parallel orientation with the magnetic field are slightly more in number than those in the antiparallel orientation. This produces a net magnetization parallel to the external magnetic field. While in their respective alignments, the nuclei are in constant motion. In addition to rotating around their axes, they also "wobble" or process in a manner similar to that of a slowly spinning top. A radio frequency (RF) pulse is then applied to the nuclei. This RF pulse, which is matched to the frequency of the processing nuclei (Larmor frequency), results in a 90° deflection of the hydrogen proton from the longitudinal plane to the transverse plane (41).

In their new alignment, nuclei maintain their coherent spinning motion, but have absorbed energy from the RF pulse (78, 79). With the termination of this pulse, the protons regress to their original lower energy state (80). This occurs by a mechanism known as relaxation (79). During this process, energy is reemitted in the form of a radio signal. It is this loss of energy by the nuclei that produces the magnetic resonance signal. The rate at which relaxation occurs depends on the local environment of the protons in the sample; that environment reflects chemical structure and ultimately human anatomy (81).

Relaxation is governed by two sample-related time constants: spin-lattice (T1) relaxation and spin-spin (T2) relaxation (80). Both T1 and T2 relaxation times are determined by the mobility of the nuclei in their molecular environment (79). T1 is the rate at which energy is transferred from the hydrogen protons to its surrounding environment (lattice). The time required for coherently spinning nuclei to lose their cohesiveness by interactions with adjacent nuclei is known as T2 relaxation. Every magnetic resonance image contains both T1 and T2 information; by the appropriate choice of the timing and length of the RF pulses, the image can be weighted to represent primarily T1, T2, or proton density (the number of spinning nuclei per unit volume) (78).

Magnetic resonance signal intensity can be manipulated by controlling the timing of the RF pulses—repetition time (TR) and echo time (TE) (81). A short TR and short TE results in a T1-weighted image, whereas a long TR and a long TE produces a T2-weighted image. Proton density images are the result of a long TR with a short TE.

Spin echo imaging is the most commonly used method of magnetic resonance image formation (80). This uses an RF pulse to tip the hydrogen nuclei 90°, then an additional 180° pulse that refocuses the protons and subsequently produces the spin echo image. Other more advanced pulse sequences include low flip angle techniques (such as gradient echo, FLASH, and FLIP sequences), fat suppression techniques, and three-dimensional images.

Initially, MRI demonstrated excellent images of the brain, spine, and spinal cord. More recent technological advances using surface coil magnets and new software packages have become available. This newer technology combined with high field strength magnets enables the production of excellent signal-to-noise ratios. This, in turn, allows for a comprehensive and accurate evaluation of musculoskeletal injury. Additionally, MRI offers multiplanar imaging capabilities without the adverse effects of ionizing radiation or other harmful biologic effects.

Shoulder

Disorders of the shoulder joint are common in the athlete. MRI allows accurate evaluation of both osseous and soft tissue structures frequently implicated in the production of shoulder pain. Common lesions of the glenohumeral articulation include rotator cuff tears (complete and partial), tendinitis, bursitis, labral and capsular pathology, and osseous abnormalities. MRI can provide the clinician with useful information, assisting in the facilitation of an accurate diagnosis. A spectrum of clinical disorders ranging from impingement syndrome to glenohumeral instability, as well as their associated pathomechanical abnormalities, can be evaluated.

Impingement syndrome is a relatively common condition characterized by chronic entrapment of the soft tissues of the subacromial space (supraspinatus tendon, biceps tendon, and subacromial bursa) between the humeral head and the acromion (35, 82). Participation in sports requiring repetitive overhead motion such as throwing and swimming places an increased stress on this region. Hypertrophy of the acromioclavicular joint capsule, osteophytes extending from the acromioclavicular joint margins, or an anterior inferiorly placed acromion may further predispose to shoulder impingement (Fig. 20.27) (83–85).

The impingement syndrome is a pathophysiologic process, with variability of clinical symptomatology and MRI findings. These range from mild tendinitis to complete tendon rupture (82). Neer (86) has categorized impingement lesions

into three progressive stages. Stage I is represented by edema and hemorrhage within the rotator cuff tendon (Fig. 20.28). This reversible process usually occurs in the younger athlete. With repeated injury, fibrosis and tendinitis occur. This represents the Stage II category. At this level, a more aggressive regimen of treatment must be pursued. These lesions occur most frequently

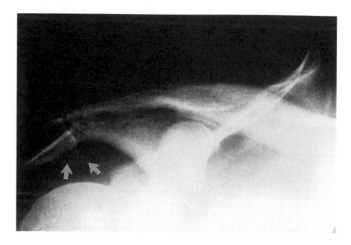

Figure 20.27. Impingement syndrome. This 45-year-old weight lifter complained of shoulder pain exacerbated by abduction and flexion of the right arm. There is a large subacromial spur at the inferior aspect of the acromion (arrows).

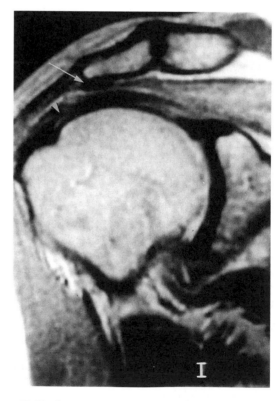

Figure 20.28. Grade I impingement syndrome. Proton density (TR 2000/TE 35 msec) MRI shows subacromial bony proliferation (arrow) and diffuse hyperintense area within the supraspinatus tendon (arrowheads). (Courtesy of Joseph S. James, D.C.)

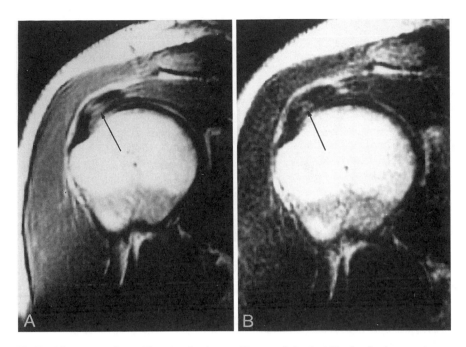

Figure 20.29. Partial rotator cuff tear. There is a focal area of increased signal within the distal supraspinatus tendon (arrows) seen on these proton density **(A)** and T2-weighted **(B)** images (TR 2000/TE 20/80 msec). (Courtesy of Metropolitan MRI Center, St. Louis, MO.)

in the third to fourth decades of life. Stage III lesions are the most severe and include rotator cuff tears, biceps ruptures, and osseous degenerative changes (Fig. 20.29). Early diagnosis and conservative management of impingement syndrome can impede the progression to rotator cuff tears. MRI is the only noninvasive modality that accurately assesses Stage I and Stage II lesions (87).

According to Neer (86), 95% of all rotator cuff tears are initiated by subacromial impingement. Rotator cuff injury is considered to be a chronic process occurring only in tendons that have been significantly degenerated (87, 88). The most common location for rotator cuff tears is at the insertion of the tendon on the greater tuberosity (zone of relative avascularity). As mentioned previously, the anatomy of this "critical zone" often eludes correct diagnosis by diagnostic ultrasound. Oblique coronal and oblique sagittal magnetic resonance images optimally display the structures in this important anatomical region.

Clinical distinction between severe tendinitis and partial rotator cuff tear or partial tears and small complete tears can be extremely challenging (82). Several studies (88–91) have demonstrated MRI to be as accurate or more accurate than CT arthrography in identifying the presence or absence of rotator cuff tears. MRI also demonstrates secondary bone changes of chronic impingement and allows direct visualization of osseous impingement on the rotator cuff tendons and mus-

cles (90). Surgical correlation has consistently shown that MRI can accurately define the size and severity of a cuff tear (87). MRI is particularly helpful in the diagnosis of intrasubstance tears and partial tears occurring on the superior surface of the tendon. Both of these lesions would be overlooked routinely with CT and arthroscopy.

Glenohumeral instability is a common cause of chronic pain and disability (84). History and physical examination may be unrewarding. Although there is often a history of trauma preceding the development of the shoulder complaint, many patients cannot recall a specific event (82, 92). The most common clinical complaint is anterior shoulder pain, particularly during abduction and external rotation. Subclinical instability, however, may present with vague symptoms such as nonspecific pain, decreased range of motion, and arm numbness (92).

Posttraumatic anterior glenohumeral dislocation producing unidirectional instability is by far the most common scenario (83, 93). This occurs after an abduction and external rotation injury mechanism. Posterior instability and multidirectional instability are much less common, but may occur in contact sports such as football and rugby. Abnormalities associated with an unstable shoulder include labral injury (such as tearing, detachment, and attenuation from recurrent subluxation), stripping of the capsule from the scapula, Hill-Sachs lesion (osseous impaction

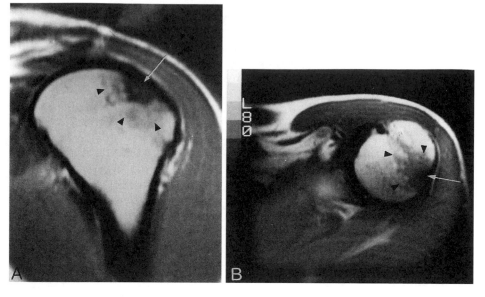

Figure 20.30. Humeral impaction (Hill-Sachs) fracture. T1-weighted (TR 800/TE 25 msec). **(A)** Parasagittal and **(B)** axial MRI show a relatively well-defined hypointense area within the proximal humerus (arrows). The diffuse low signal represents associated bone marrow edema (arrowheads).

fracture), and Bankart fracture (fracture of the anterior glenoid rim; may be purely cartilaginous, osseous, or both) (Fig. 20.30) (84, 87).

MRI provides a noninvasive method for accurate evaluation of glenohumeral instability and its associated abnormalities (89, 93–96). Axial images provide the best visualization for evaluation of the humeral head, labrum, anterior capsule, and glenoid (97, 98). With intraarticular effusion, these structures are even better appreciated as tissue plane delineation is better defined (93).

Elbow

Injuries to the elbow are frequently encountered in noncontact sports such as baseball and tennis, as well as in contact sports like football and rugby. Plain film radiography is the most frequently used imaging modality. Radiographs (and CT) are relatively effective for the identification of osseous lesions but lack the sensitivity to assess soft tissue injury and occult bony lesions. When clinical suspicion of elbow injury exists and plain radiographs are negative or demonstrate nonspecific findings, MRI should be used. MRI can provide a relatively accurate and comprehensive evaluation of the musculotendinous, ligamentous, neural, and osseous components of the elbow.

MRI can disclose information related to soft tissue injury only inferred from clinical and radiographic examination. The medial and LCL are common sites of acute and chronic trauma sustained during athletic activities (96). Discontinuity or thickening of fibers and increased internal signal intensity on T2-weighted images signify rupture or partial tearing (99). Evaluation of musculotendinous injuries such as tendonitis, tenosynovitis, and intramuscular hematoma is possible with MRI. Tunnel syndromes (e.g., radial tunnel syndrome and sulcus ulnaris syndrome) can also be appreciated on MRI.

Direct assessment of the articular cartilage may yield thinning, irregularity, or inhomogeneous signal as evidence of chondral abnormality (99). Osteochondritis dissecans is one such abnormality. The cause of this entity is poorly understood; however, trauma is consistently implicated by most investigators as the causative factor. Patients are usually within the first or second decade and participate in sports requiring the throwing motion. Clinical findings include dull pain, joint effusion, and a lack of full extension. Negative plain films should raise the suspicion of osteochondritis dissecans, and MRI should be used as the next imaging modality. Other occult lesions that can be detected by MRI include early cartilage degeneration (osteoarthritis), transchondral and osteochondral fractures, and small intraarticular fragments.

Subtle growth plate injuries in the elbow (particularly Salter-Harris Types III and IV) are commonly missed radiographically (97). In addition to these injuries, subtle impaction fractures and bone contusions can be demonstrated with MRI when plain radiographs yield negative results.

Wrist

Injuries to the wrist are responsible for a significant number of athletic injuries. A large percentage of these injuries involve only soft tissue structures. The initial lack of radiographic evidence of injury often results in misdiagnosis and delayed treatment. Progression may lead to chronic wrist instability, possibly endangering the athlete's participation in that sport. Early diagnosis, therefore, is imperative for proper clinical management of the injured wrist. MRI provides exquisite detail of soft tissue and occult osseous injuries in the wrist. This information is useful in arriving at a correct diagnosis and may ultimately affect the prognosis.

Fractures of the carpal bones are frequently observed. The most commonly fractured bone in the wrist is the scaphoid (39, 79, 100, 101). The usual mechanism of injury is a fall on an outstretched hand (39, 79, 102). Other, less common carpal fractures involve the triquetrum, pisiform, and hamate hook. These injuries are often correctly diagnosed with plain film radiography. Occasionally, signs of osseous injury may be absent or overlooked due to the complex anatomy of this region. MRI can demonstrate subtle cortical disruptions and nondisplaced fractures (103). Identification of these lesions is of great importance, as delay in diagnosis and inadequate treatment are cited as the primary causes of scaphoid nonunion (Fig. 20.31) (97, 100). Radiographically occult microfractures and medullary bone contusions are also accurately detected with MRI (103).

Traumatic osteonecrosis may occur after disruption of the vascular supply to the carpal bones. This occurs most often after fracture of the scaphoid (104). Radiographs are capable of demonstrating end-stage manifestations of osteonecrosis. Comparatively, MRI can depict early marrow changes before plain film evidence of injury (39, 47, 97, 103–105).

Wrist stability is provided by the intercarpal and radiocarpal ligaments and the TFCC (102, 104). Injuries to these structures may be as common as scaphoid fractures but are frequently undiagnosed and untreated, being passed off as simple sprains (106). MRI is effective in evaluating tears involving both the intercarpal ligaments (particularly the scapholunate ligament) and radiocarpal ligaments (107). The TFCC is composed of the articular disc, meniscus homolog, dorsal and volar radioulnar ligaments, ulnar collateral ligament, and sheath of the extensor carpi ulnaris (97, 104). These structures act as a cushion between the ulna and the carpus, in addition to providing stability to the distal radioulnar joint (108). Injuries to the TFCC joint produce weakness of grip (107). MRI provides accurate and comprehensive evaluation of the TFCC (Fig. 20.32). Future advances in imaging techniques, such as stress images and cine-MRI examinations, should

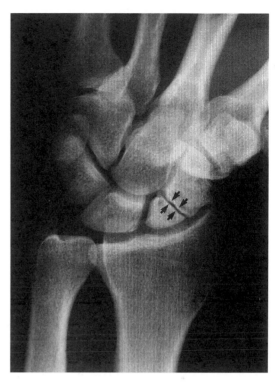

Figure 20.31. Scaphoid fracture with nonunion. The radiograph reveals two smoothly marginated fragments at the site of a previous fracture (arrows).

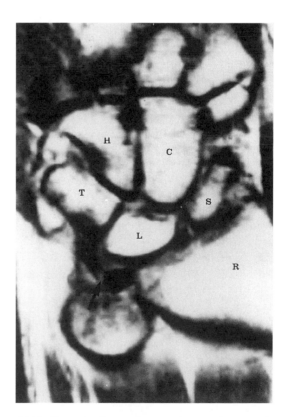

Figure 20.32. Triangular fibrocartilage tear. An area of high signal (arrow) is seen within the TFCC on these coronal proton density (TR 2400/TE 26) images (R: radius; S: scaphoid; L: lunate; T: triquetrum; H: hamate and; C: capitate). (Courtesy of Claude Pierre-Jerome, M.D., D.C.)

enhance the ability of this modality to evaluate carpal instability patterns.

Overuse and repetitive athletic activities with considerable recruitment of the wrist flexors and extensors may result in tenosynovitis. The most common site is the first extensor compartment involving the abductor pollicis longus and brevis tendons at the level of the radial styloid (de Quervain's synovitis) (105). The edema surrounding the signal void of the tendon is easily depicted with MRI (97, 103). Tenosynovitis is a common cause of carpal tunnel syndrome (CTS) in the athlete (104). Clinical findings and nerve conduction studies have been the mainstay of diagnosing CTS (109).

Until recently, imaging CTS was rarely a productive venture. With axial magnetic resonance images, objective signs of median nerve encroachment within the carpal tunnel can be demonstrated (109). Direct visualization of nerve flattening and edema flattening, as well as bowing of the flexor retinaculum, can be identified with MRI (Fig. 20.33) (104, 110). CTS occurs as a result of athletic activities, such as gymnastics,

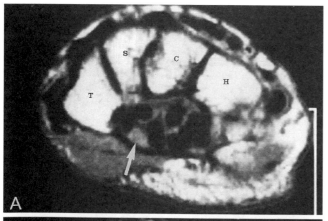

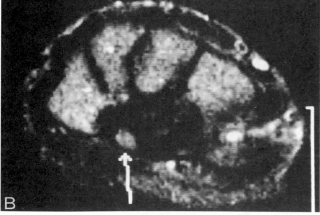

Figure 20.33. Carpal tunnel syndrome. **(A)** Axial proton density and **(B)** T2-weighted spin echo sequences (TR 2800/TE 22/80) show increased signal and slight enlargement of the median nerve (arrow). Note the high signal (edema) surrounding the flexor tendons (T: trapezium; S: scaphoid; C: capitate and; H: hamate). (Courtesy of Claude Pierre-Jerome, M.D., D.C.)

body building, tennis, and golf, which use repetitive powerful flexion maneuvers (79). Another nerve compression syndrome may occur by entrapment of the ulnar nerve within Guyon's canal. This follows fracture of the pisiform and hamate or occurs when chronic stress is placed on that region, such as the hand position on the handlebars of a touring cyclist (101).

Moderate and large articular cartilage defects can be characterized by MRI (97, 107). These lesions are most commonly identified at the proximal lunate, triquetrum, and distal ulna in athletes with TFCC tears (107).

Hip

Athletic injuries of the hip may present a confusing clinical picture. Most significant injuries can eventually be diagnosed from plain film examination. Early detection of occult injury, however, may be the difference between short-term and long-term disability. MRI has proven to be an accurate method for evaluating the soft tissue, chondral, and osteochondral lesions that escape early plain film diagnosis.

Osteonecrosis occurs after disruption of the vascular supply, producing ischemia and eventual necrosis of the subchondral bone. Trauma to the hip or acetabulum is the most common cause in sports. Nontraumatic osteonecrosis may also occur in scuba divers when they ascend to the water surface too quickly (Caisson's disease). Signs and symptoms vary from mild symptomatic complaints to severe pain with functional impairment (111).

Early diagnosis is crucial to prevent undesirable complications (112). When negative plain films and a high index of clinical suspicion are maintained, MRI should be used. MRI is the most accurate diagnostic imaging tool for the early detection of ischemic necrosis of the femoral head (112–115). Although plain films are specific, they lack the sensitivity for early diagnosis. Nuclear bone scans provide the necessary sensitivity for early detection but lack diagnostic specificity. MRI provides both superb sensitivity and specificity, outperforming both plain films and nuclear scans (Fig. 20.34) (111, 115, 116).

MRI demonstrates local areas of signal abnormality that extend from the subchondral portions of the femoral head into the distal marrow cavity (114). These changes reflect cellular and chemical alterations that precede disruption of the trabecular architecture (116). This provides MRI with the capacity to identify epiphyses at risk for subsequent articular surface collapse by depicting the volume and location of necrotic tissue

(117). When subchondral collapse occurs, osteonecrosis is irreversible. With early diagnosis, subchondral fracture can be avoided and a more conservative course of therapy may be pursued (111). Ficat (118) has described a staging classification for the evaluation of osteonecrosis with plain radiography.

- Stage I—hip pain (negative radiographs).
- Stage II—increase density of the femoral head.
- Stage III—contour changes of the femoral head (subchondral fracture and subsequent collapse).
- Stage IV—progressive joint space narrowing (mixed cystic and sclerotic changes of the femoral head, often mimicking osteoarthritis) Hauzeur et al. (119) demonstrated 100% correlation between MRI and the histologic findings of osteonecrosis.

Stress fractures in athletes occur when abnormal stress is applied to bone with normal elastic resistance (98, 120). These injuries commonly occur in the young athlete engaged in sports such as jogging, gymnastics, and ballet. Clinically, patients present with pain and tenderness exacerbated with activity and relieved by rest. Plain films initially may be negative, often lagging 2 to 6 weeks behind the onset of symptoms (120). MRI provides evidence of stress fractures much earlier than radiographs (Fig. 20.35) (111).

The ability of MRI to detect subtle marrow abnormality has also proved useful in the identifi-

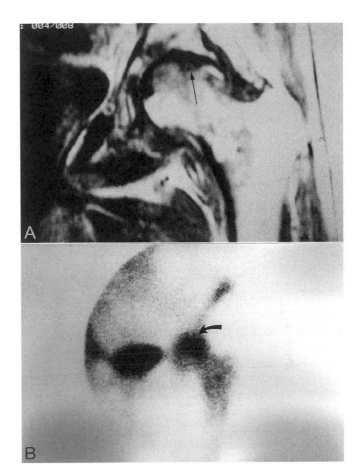

Figure 20.34. Ischemic necrosis. **A.** T1-weighted (TR 600/TE 20 msec) MRI shows a hypointense band (arrow encompassing a central area of mixed signal intensity). **B.** This corresponds to an area of increased radionuclide uptake (curved arrow) with nuclear scintigraphy. (Courtesy of Dennis Adams, D.C.)

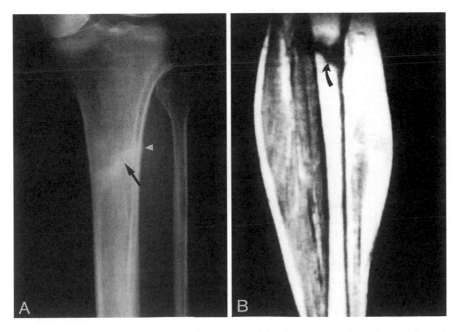

Figure 20.35. Stress fractures. **A.** Radiographs show an area of ill-defined sclerosis (arrow) and slight periosteal elevation (arrowhead) within the proximal tibia. **B.** Proton density (TR 1000/TE 40 msec) coronal MRI demonstrates mixed signal (curved arrow) at the fracture site. (Courtesy of Mahmoud Ziaee, M.D.)

cation of occult fractures (115). The fracture line, hemorrhage, and surrounding edema within the marrow space can be visualized (114). Often, occult fractures can be differentiated from stress fractures with MRI based on location (occult fractures are usually located in the epiphysis, whereas stress fractures generally occur in the metaphysis or diaphysis) (114).

Nuclear bone scans are highly sensitive at demonstrating occult fractures; however, they lack specificity. Synovitis and arthritis (degenerative or inflammatory) can mimic fractures in certain patients, necessitating the use of additional examinations for confirmation and further characterization (121). Once again, the exceptional sensitivity and specificity of MRI may eliminate the need for additional imaging.

Bone bruises and chondral and osteochondral lesions of the hip are also well demonstrated with MRI. These lesions present with identical MRI features regardless of their anatomical location.

Knee

Almost all sports rely on proper functioning of the knee. It provides both agility and stability during the variety of complex motions required in sports. Consequently, knee injuries are the leading cause of long-term disability from athletics (122). MRI provides an excellent noninvasive method of directly visualizing injuries to the knee. It is particularly valuable in the acutely injured patient, for whom it serves as a painless extension of the physical examination (123). For internal knee derangements and most other clinical questions concerning the knee, MRI has replaced arthrography and CT (124–126).

The most frequent clinical indication for MRI of the knee is for evaluation of the menisci (123, 125). MRI not only allows screening of suspected meniscal injury, but can also distinguish surgically significant meniscal lesions from those that are adequately managed with conservative therapy (127).

The most common lesions of the menisci are tears (126, 128). Tears can be detected with MRI when there are morphologic changes of the contours of the meniscus or by an abnormal high signal within the meniscus (Fig. 20.36) (123, 126, 129). Crues et al. (128) have described a grading system for meniscal tears. Grades I and II represent progressive stages of degeneration, ultimately resulting in frank (Stage III) tears. This is of prognostic importance, as Grade II lesions (especially those occurring in the posterior horn of the medial meniscus) would be expected to progress to Stage III tears (130). MRI may accurately depict

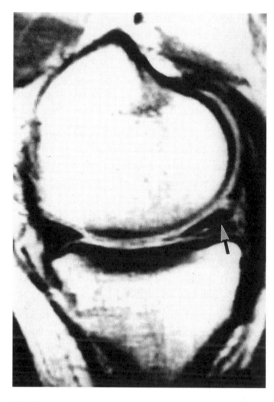

Figure 20.36. Meniscal tear. Proton density (TR 2900/TE 22 msec) MRI. Note the linear high-signal area within the posterior horn of the medial meniscus (arrow). (Courtesy of Claude Pierre-Jerome, M.D., D.C.)

meniscal lesions of all three stages, whereas arthrography and arthroscopy routinely provide information regarding only frank tears (125, 130).

Clinically, tears are found in athletes complaining of pain, locking, popping, or "slipping out of joint" (122, 131). Asymptomatic athletes, however, also frequently display increased meniscal signal (129). Recently, two studies (132, 133) have examined the menisci of both recreational and trained runners after repetitive impulse loading (jogging/running). It was found that after activity, the recreational joggers demonstrated increased signal within their menisci. The authors suggest this may represent the earliest demonstrable changes secondary to chronic biomechanical stress. The trained marathoners, however, demonstrated no increased signal within their menisci. This suggests these athletes adapted to the chronic stress of their activity. Reinig et al. (134) have reported an increased signal in the menisci of asymptomatic college football players over a single season. They contend that with each season of football, a slightly greater chance of further meniscal degeneration and eventual tear exists in young athletes.

Most vertical longitudinal tears of the menisci occur in knees in which there is an accompanying tear of the ACL (122, 126, 129). Of the knee ligaments, the ACL is the most common to be injured (97, 123, 125). The ACL serves to provide stability and limit hyperextension of the knee. Injury occurs after sudden deceleration that produces a valgus twisting (135). Clinically, this lesion may go undetected if only minimal instability is appreciated. The athlete will frequently complain of the knee "giving way" during pivoting motions (122).

Generally, acute ACL injury can be depicted with MRI as increased signal within the substance of the ligament. Nonvisualization of the ACL and/or acute angulation of the posterior cruciate ligament (PCL) are additional signs of acute ACL injury (Fig. 20.37) (125, 129, 136). Chronic ACL injury may preclude MRI diagnosis secondary to replacement of the normally low-signal intensity ligament with low-signal intensity scar tissue.

Posterior cruciate ligament injuries are less common than ACL injuries (125, 129, 137). Considerable force is required to injure the PCL and often leads to significant instability (126). These injuries are usually associated with other serious intra-articular injuries, particularly detachment of the posterior horn of the medial meniscus, tears of the MCL and LCL, disruption of the posterior medial and lateral capsular ligaments, and avulsion of the tibial insertion of the PCL (126). Mechanisms for injury include forceful posterior translation of the tibia in the flexed knee, forced hyperextension, and continued valgus angulation following rupture of the ACL and MCL (137).

Clinically, the patient with a complete tear of the PCL may be asymptomatic (122, 129). The patient will often exhibit discomfort and a feeling of unsteadiness and insecurity when the knee is in a semiflexion position (as when descending stairs) (137). Early detection of acute rupture is important in avoiding chronic instability and early osteoarthritis. MRI is effective at demonstrating PCL injury and associated complications.

The MCL and LCL provide stability and limit the amount of varus and valgus stress placed on the joint. The MCL is more commonly injured than the LCL (97, 123, 125). Injury to the MCL occurs after excessive valgus stress. MCL sprain is a frequently overlooked lesion and may be the only positive finding in a patient with a history of minor knee trauma (136). If injury to the MCL is present, close inspection of the contralateral distal femur and proximal tibia with MRI may reveal the presence of trabecular microfractures (see later discussion) (125, 136).

Coronal MRI accurately display both the superficial and deep fibers of the MCL. Mink and Deutsch (123) have described a clinical grading system for MCL injury using MRI. Grade I demonstrates edema and hemorrhage around the tendon with no visible morphologic changes. Grade III is characterized by thickening, discontinuity, and serpiginous contours of the ligament. Lesions that demonstrate some features of both Grade I and Grade III injury are classified as Grade II lesions. The edema and pain of Grade III lesions make arthrography and comprehensive clinical examination difficult (123).

Lateral collateral ligament injuries occur after excessive varus stress across the knee joint. Injuries to this complex structure demonstrate the same features as MCL injury. Because the LCL complex is under maximum tension when the leg is extended while walking, these lesions may be more disabling than MCL injuries (97).

The extensor mechanism of the knee is composed of the quadriceps muscle and tendon, the patella and its tendon, the tibial tubercle, and retinaculum (123). This complex is often the site of chronic tendinitis from overuse (Fig. 20.38). In the adult athlete, this condition is associated with jumper's knee and in the adolescent athlete it is known as Osgood-Schlatter's disease (138). Conventional radiographs may demonstrate small osseous fragments at the inferior pole of the patella or at the tibial tubercle, with blurring of the normally well-marginated patellar tendon (136). MRI is helpful because it establishes the diagnosis, detects associated chronic microtears of the musculotendinous and ligamentous structures, and may help determine appropriate clinical management (138). Detection of the soft tissue abnormalities is an exclusive advantage of MRI.

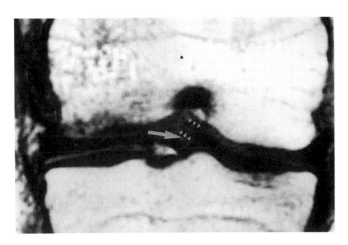

Figure 20.37. ACL tear. On this T1-weighted (TR 810/TE 15 msec) MRI, there is significant replacement of the ACL by intermediate-signal intensity hemorrhage (arrow). A few remnant ACL fibers remain (arrowheads).

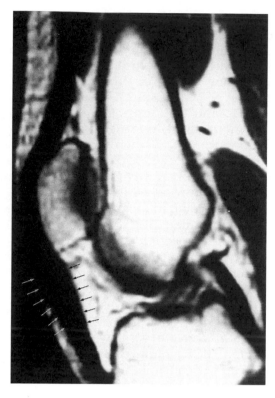

Figure 20.38. Chronic patellar tendinitis. Proton density (TR 2700/TE 22 msec) sagittal MRI shows thickening of the patellar tendon (arrows). (Courtesy of Claude Pierre-Jerome, M.D., D.C.)

Clinically, the athlete may present with exquisite anterior knee pain and swelling. This condition often eludes correct clinical diagnosis and management. Delayed or improper treatment may lead to worsening of the pain and possible rupture of the tendon (138).

Chondral and osteochondral abnormalities may be directly visualized with MRI. This capability is further enhanced when an effusion is present because of the "arthrogram" effect (139, 140). With T2-weighted sequences, the high-signal edema is contrasted against the low-signal cartilage.

Osteochondritis dissecans occurs most frequently in adolescent or young adult athletes. As mentioned previously, trauma is the most likely cause. The mechanism of injury is thought to result from rotatory motion when the tibial spine impacts the femur, usually the lateral aspect of the medial femoral condyle (97). Clinically, patients may present with pain or be asymptomatic with no history of trauma. MRI not only allows identification of the osteochondral fragment, but is also useful in evaluating whether the lesion is stable (129, 141). The most common injury to the osteochondral structures in the knee is dislocation-relocation of the patella (96). This usually occurs laterally, resulting in a chondral or osteochondral fragment arising from the medial facet of the patella or lateral femoral condyle.

Impaction forces may injure the cartilage and subchondral bone. These lesions typically occur directly over the anterior horn of the lateral meniscus and are often associated with ACL tears (142). MRI is superior to other modalities in the detection of subtle osteocartilaginous abnormalities. Symptoms of chondral injuries include catching, locking, and giving way of the knee (139). These findings mimic those of a meniscal lesion and are, therefore, commonly misdiagnosed.

Chondromalacia patella is another frequent cause of knee pain in young individuals (143). The etiologic factors responsible for producing these lesions are currently under debate. Trauma and mechanical tracking abnormalities are most frequently cited (144). Pathologically, this lesion is characterized by various degrees of chondral softening and irregularity. Conway et al. (144) have described a grading system to further classify this abnormality.

- Grade 1—superficial cartilage softening.
- Grade 2—blister-like lesion that may extend to the cartilage surface.
- Grade 3—cartilage fibrillation.

MRI offers the only means of direct visualization of these various grades of chondromalacia patella. Accurate assessment of these lesions, particularly Grades 2–4, is possible with MRI (144).

MRI has been useful in demonstrating a previously undescribed entity, the bone bruise. These lesions occur after an impact force and are self-limiting, healing with no subsequent evidence of injury. Bone bruises are characterized by trabecular microfractures without disruption of the cortex or osteochondral surface. MRI is useful for the identification of these lesions because of its high sensitivity in the detection of secondary fluid changes (edema, hyperemia, and hemorrhage) in the bone marrow (126, 145). MRI reveals low-signal intensity on T1-weighted sequences and high-signal intensity on proton density and T2-weighted images (Fig. 20.39).

The bone bruise should be suspected after significant knee trauma when radiographs are normal (136). They are most commonly encountered in the knee after significant collateral ligament tear (Grades II and III), acute ACL disruption, or both (97). In a study by Vellet et al. (146), 81% of occult trabecular microfractures visible on MRI were demonstrated in the lateral joint compartment (distal femur or proximal tibia). This occurs as a result of compressive forces on the osseous structures opposite the applied stress. Common mechanisms of injury include significant relative rotation of the tibia and femur, sudden deceleration, and valgus stress injuries (146). It is difficult to ascertain whether bone bruise, as an isolated entity, will produce pain because these lesions are usually associated with ligamentous damage (97).

Occult stress fractures are also demonstrated with MRI. These lesions may appear similar to bone bruises; however, clinical history should provide the differentiating factor.

Spontaneous osteonecrosis has been postulated to occur in conjunction with tears of the menisci, most commonly medial (125). MRI demonstrates marrow signal abnormality before radiographs and may even reveal evidence of osteonecrosis before radionuclide scans (126). Clinically, the athlete will complain of sudden nonspecific knee pain. The symptoms may mimic that of a stress fracture. MRI can differentiate the linear appearance of a stress fracture from the diffuse amorphous appearance of osteonecrosis (136).

Visualization of the intramedullary abnormalities also includes replacement of normal marrow

fat by hematopoietic tissue. Shellock et al. (147) have described this phenomenon in the distal femora of asymptomatic marathon runners. It has been attributed to sports anemia commonly found in aerobically trained athletes. The MRI appearance is characterized by intermediate or low signal on T1-weighted sequences, contrasting with the high signal of normal marrow fat.

Ankle

The ankle allows the athlete both agility and flexibility by providing complex motions like supination, pronation, dorsiflexion, and plantarflexion. Unfortunately, with complex motion comes the potential for injury and subsequent instability. Timely diagnosis and proper management are necessary to avoid unwanted complications. Clinical and radiographic examinations permit the identification of many general types of injury. The exact site and extent of damage, particularly in the soft tissues, often cannot be assessed completely (148). MRI is useful in evaluation of the ligaments, tendons, cartilage, and osseous structures of the ankle.

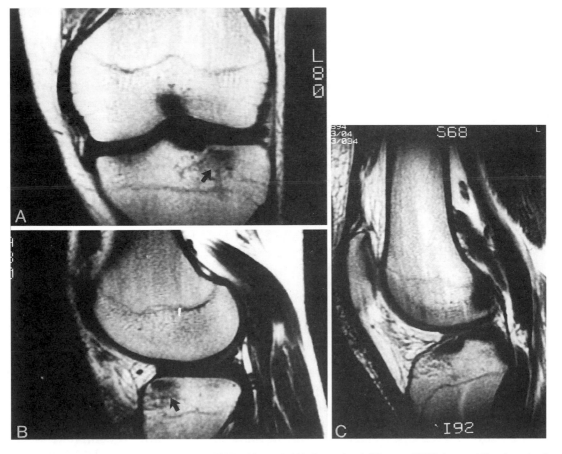

Figure 20.39. Bone bruise. T1-weighted (TR 700/TE 20 msec). **(A)** Coronal and **(B)** sagittal MRI show a diffuse low-signal area within the medial tibial plateau (arrows). **C.** The signal increases on proton density (TR 2000/TE 20 msec) images. (Courtesy of Metropolitan MRI Center, St. Louis, MO)

Localized soft tissue swelling after a twisting injury without evidence of fracture suggests tendon or ligament damage. Ankle ligament injuries most commonly result from inversion trauma and involve the LCL (anterior talofibular ligament, calcaneofibular ligament, and posterior talofibular ligament). Of these, the anterior talofibular ligament (ATFL) is injured most frequently (97, 120). Grade I injury consists of partial tearing of the ATFL. Partial tearing of the calcaneofibular ligament (CFL) combined with ATFL injury constitutes a Grade II injury. Complete tears of the ATFL and CFL ligaments result in a Grade III injury (120).

Posterior talofibular ligament (PTFL) and CFL injuries occur much less commonly and are almost always associated with injury to the ATFL (97, 149). Traumatic eversion injuries usually involve the medially located deltoid ligament. MRI can be used to demonstrate isolated ligament injuries or those that accompany other ankle injuries (150). Identification and characterization of ligamentous damage with MRI can aid in management decisions.

Tendon injuries typically result from overuse or direct trauma. They are a common source of acute and chronic pain and often lead to disability of the ankle (148). Injuries include inflammation of the tendon sheath (tenosynovitis), the tendon itself (tendinitis), and complete and partial tears. Clinical evaluation may prove unrewarding, as many of these entities produce nonspecific symptoms (150). Some of the more common tendon injuries of the ankle will be discussed briefly.

Achilles tendinitis occurs in sports with frequent running and jumping (151). Ignored or misdiagnosed tendinitis may progress to a partial tear and possibly result in a complete tearing of the tendon. Tears usually occur 2 to 6 cm proximal to the calcaneal insertion (150, 151). The posterior tibial tendon (PTT) is one of the principal stabilizers of the hindfoot and functions to support the medial longitudinal arch and invert the foot (97). This tendon is placed under increased stress by sports that require quick changes in direction such as basketball, football, and tennis (151).

The primary cause of PTT rupture occurs secondary to chronic stress placed on an already inflamed and degenerated tendon (150). Other less commonly injured tendons in athletics include the anterior tibial tendon and flexor hallucis longus tendon. Anterior tibial tendon inflammation occurs in runners training on hilly terrain (150, 151). Flexor hallucis longus tendinitis occurs in dancers of whom repetitive flexion and extension of the forefoot are required (152).

Acute tendinitis is visualized on MRI as a focal area of increased signal within the tendon. This appearance is often characteristic of both tendinitis and partial tendon tears; however, clinical history should provide the differentiating information. Complete tears are diagnosed by loss of continuity of the tendinous structure, retraction of the two tendon fragments, and the demonstration of high or intermediate signal areas between the separated tendon margins. The intrasubstance signal represents edema, hemorrhage, or reparative granulation tissue.

Mechanical tenosynovitis results from overuse, chronic stretching, and bone and shoe friction (152). The clinical presentation is identical to overuse tendinitis. Edema is demonstrated within the synovial sheath surrounding an intact tendon in acute situations. Chronic changes can lead to the formation of fibrous or scar tissue around the tendon, as noted with stenosing tenosynovitis (152). This appears as a low-signal area surrounding the tendon.

Retrocalcaneal bursitis may produce symptoms similar to those of Achilles tendinitis (151). Demonstration of a swollen high-signal bursa positioned between the Achilles tendon and calcaneus is characteristic (150).

A common cause of heel pain in runners is plantar fasciitis. Its cause has been attributed to mechanical stress on the plantar fascia, resulting in microtears and fascial and perifascial inflammation (153). MRI demonstrates thickening of the fascia with increased intrasubstance signal (153).

Muscle injury is usually assessed clinically. For the professional athlete, however, further evaluation may be beneficial in determining the extent and nature of injury. Additionally, injuries requiring surgical intervention must be differentiated from those likely to respond to conservative therapy (154). MRI readily differentiates muscle strains and tears from delayed-onset muscle soreness and confirms the absence of focal hematomas and fascial herniations (Fig. 20.40) (121, 155). Fat suppression techniques are more effective than standard spin echo sequences at demonstrating these abnormalities (135, 155).

Osteochondral fractures may accompany ligamentous injury and represent a commonly overlooked cause of persistent ankle pain (150). The possibility of an osteochondral fracture of the talus must be considered in those patients with previous ligamentous injury and no signs of instability who continue to complain of pain and disability despite apparently normal radiographs (156). Most osteochondral fractures of the ankle involve the talar dome, either the posterior one

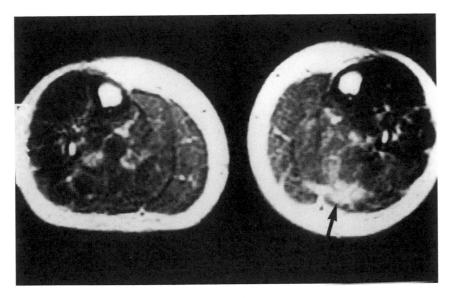

Figure 20.40. Acute muscle injury. There is an area of increased signal intensity within the gastrocnemius and soleus muscles of the left leg (arrow), as seen on these T2-weighted (TR 1500/TE 70 msec) magnetic resonance images. This finding is consistent with hemorrhage and/or edema. (Reprinted from Yochum and Rowe: Essentials of Skeletal Radiology, Second Edition. 1996. Baltimore: Williams & Wilkins. Used with permission.)

third of the medial aspect or the middle one third of the lateral portion of the talus (97). The mechanism of injury is variable. With ankle eversion, the posteroinferior lip of the tibia compresses and fractures the medial talar dome; inversion compresses the talus against the medial border of the fibula, resulting in an osteochondral fracture of the lateral aspect of the talus (149, 151, 156, 157).

Anderson et al. (156) have described a method useful for staging osteochondral fractures with MRI.

- Stage I—subchondral trabecular compression (negative plain film radiographs; MRI demonstrates edema/hemorrhage).
- Stage II—incomplete separation of the fragment.
- Stage IIA—formation of subchondral cyst (Stage I fractures may progress to an attached or unattached fragment or to formation of the subchondral cyst).
- Stage III—unattached, undisplaced fragment.
- Stage IV—displaced fragment.

MRI can accurately assess stability of the fragment, aiding in patient management. Additionally, progression from a stable lesion to an unstable lesion may be appreciated (158). If the fragment remains attached, revascularization and healing are more likely. Complete detachment results in nonhealing and subsequently a loose body within the articulation (159).

Clinical differentiation between stress fractures and tendinitis can be difficult, as identical activities can initiate both conditions. As previously mentioned, MRI is useful in identification and evaluation of stress fractures before their recognition on plain film. The navicular and calcaneus are the two tarsal bones most vulnerable to stress fractures in athletes (150). Clinically, these lesions present with focal pain that is exacerbated with activity and somewhat relieved by rest.

Osteonecrosis involves the talus more than any other bone in the ankle. This frequently follows displaced fracture of the talar neck (150).

MRI is the earliest and most accurate method of detecting avascular necrosis in the ankle (147).

Spine

Spinal injuries account for only 5% to 15% of all sports-related trauma, but they represent a higher proportion of the most devastating injuries in sports medicine (79). The extent of injury ranges from simple mechanical pain to fracture to spinal cord injury. Plain films remain the first line in detection of injury. CT is unmatched in detection of suspected and occult osseous injury. These two modalities, however, have only been able to provide substandard information regarding soft tissue injury. MRI accurately displays extraspinal soft tissue, osseous vertebral abnormality, and spinal cord injury without injection of myelographic contrast material or the poor resolution of CT reconstruction images (160–162).

The imaging sequence parameters commonly used in imaging spinal abnormalities are discussed here. T1-weighted sequences (low TR/low TE) provide good anatomical detail combined with a short examination time. T2-weighted sequences (high TR/high TE) are more time-consuming but are sensitive to increased quantities of water (edema). Proton density images (long TR/short TE) deemphasize the importance of T1 and T2 effects and rely on the hydrogen ion concentration. Consequently, these images tend to reinforce the findings of T2-weighted sequences, but with better anatomical detail. Low flip angle and intermediate flip angle techniques are often referred to by various acronyms such as FISP, FLASH, and GRASS. These pulse sequences are obtained with very short examination times (rapid acquisition). Their primary advantage stems from the myelogram-like image, producing enhanced spinal cord and thecal sac visualization. Fat suppression techniques are not widely used. By suppressing the normal signal of fat, subtle areas of edema can be depicted.

The most serious of all injuries to the spine are those that involve the spinal cord. These injuries are not common in sports; however, they can occur in high-velocity activities such as automobile, motorcycle, and marine racing events. Additionally, football, skiing, and diving injuries may be severe enough to include embarrassment to the spinal cord. MRI provides both the extent and pattern of cord injury. Kulkarni et al. (162) described three patterns of MRI signal intensities in cord injury. Type I is the most severe injury pattern and is associated with either complete spinal cord transection or incomplete transection without significant neurologic improvement. This pattern represents hemorrhage within the substance of the cord. The second pattern most likely represents cord edema and often appears with no demonstrable skeletal injury. Patients may present with or without neurologic signs. When clinical evidence of neurologic injury is present, rapid improvement should be expected. The third pattern is a mixed pattern representing a combination of cord hemorrhage and edema. These patients should also be expected to experience neurologic improvement.

The capability of MRI to examine the condition of the spinal cord enhances treatment planning and permits a more accurate prognosis (163–165). MRI can aid in the differentiation between irreversible (hemorrhage) and potentially reversible damage (edema) (164). Acute intramedullary hematoma exhibits diminished signal intensity on both T1- and T2-weighted sequences, whereas acute extradural hemorrhage usually demonstrates increased signal intensity on T1-weighted images and isointense signal on T2-weighted sequences (160, 163, 166–168). Cord edema is isointense on

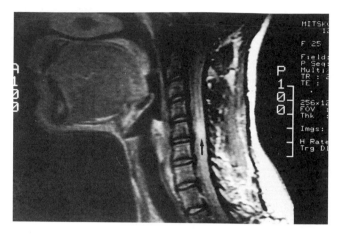

Figure 20.41. Spinal cord edema. Observe the focal hyperintense area (arrow) seen on these proton density (TR 2069/TE 30 msec) MRI. These findings are consistent with a Type II cord injury. (Courtesy of Alisa Mitskog, D.C.)

T1-weighted and increased on T2-weighted sequences (Fig. 20.41) (167, 168).

Spinal MRI is indicated in all athletes with a neurologic deficit and no obvious osseous or discoligamentous injury on plain films and CT. If obvious fractures are present, MRI can provide additional information regarding cord injury. In the acutely injured patient with incomplete neurologic deficit, MRI offers the most benefit by allowing identification and commencement of aggressive therapy directed at limiting further cord deterioration (160).

The sequelae of spinal cord trauma include atrophy, tethering, myelomalacia, and syringohydromyelia (160). Included in this spectrum of chronic injury is a syndrome known as posttraumatic progressive myelopathy. This consists of delayed onset of motor and sensory dysfunction after cord injury (169).

Before MRI, direct visualization of ligamentous injury was impossible. MRI can accurately assess the continuity of the anterior and posterior longitudinal ligaments, as well as the interspinous ligaments and surrounding large muscle groups. Ligamentous injury is suggested when the normally low-signal ligament is discontinuous or replaced by a focal high-signal intensity area, representing edema or hematoma (166). Indirect osseous abnormalities such as increased posterior disc angulation and splaying of the spinous processes are also apparent. Intramuscular hematoma may also be present and evidenced by increased signal intensity within the injured muscle. This information may impact clinical management and alert the treating physician to the risk of chronic instability and delayed spinal cord compression (160).

Assessment of the osseous integrity may be accomplished with T1-weighted sequences (167). Acute fractures can be demonstrated when T2-weighted and gradient echo sequences are used (166). Use of the latter pulse sequences demonstrating increased signal, combined with decreased signal on T1-weighted sequences, is a reliable sign of marrow edema indicating acute osseous fracture. Spondylolysis is more difficult to assess with MRI because it represents chronic microtrauma and separation of the pars interarticularis. If anterolisthesis is present, however, these lesions may be readily identified.

Normal intervertebral discs appear with a high signal of T2-weighted images. Many sports requiring repeated axial loading or torquing of the lumbar spine (weight lifting, gymnastics, tennis) result in tearing of the intradiscal connective tissue and subsequent loss of disc hydration. This is detectable with T2-weighted images as diminished intradiscal signal intensity. MRI is currently the only modality capable of directly assessing intervertebral disc degeneration.

MRI is more accurate than noncontrast CT and equivocal to CT myelogram examinations in identification of disc herniations. Posttraumatic disc herniations may be the cause of neurologic injury in unstable spinal injuries (especially cervical spine) (161). Increased signal on T2-weighted sequences differentiates acute disc herniations from those occurring secondary to chronic injury (166). CT myelography does not provide such information.

MRI offers a noninvasive, accurate, and convenient method for the evaluation of soft tissue, bone, and joint injuries in the athlete. It is the initial procedure of choice in some clinical settings and may be the only one necessary in many instances. MRI has revolutionized the examination of musculoskeletal injury (170, 171). In light of its continuing technical evolution, it is likely that MRI will sustain its imaging dominance.

References

1. Kettner N. Differential diagnosis: a strategic approach. DC Tracts 1989;1:3.
2. Jacobs B. Cervical angina. NY State J Med 1990;90:8–11.
3. Kettner N, Guebert G. The radiology of cervical spine injury. J Manipulative Physiol Ther 1991;14:518–526.
4. Williams A, Evans R, Schirley P. Imaging of sports injuries. London: Bailliere-Tindall, 1989.
5. Yochum T, Rowe L. Essentials of skeletal radiology. Baltimore: Williams & Wilkins, 1996.
6. Murphy WA, Siegel MJ. Elbow fat-pads with new signs and extended differential diagnosis. Radiology 1977;124:659–665.
7. Friberg O. Lumbar instability: a dynamic approach by traction-compression radiography. Spine 1987;12:119–129.
8. Ogden J. Skeletal injury in the child. Philadelphia: Lea & Febiger, 1982.
9. Rupani H, Holder L, Espinola D, et al. Three-phase radionuclide bone imaging in sports medicine. Radiology 1985;156:187–196.
10. Fogelman I, Maisley M. An atlas of clinical nuclear medicine. St. Louis: CV Mosby, 1988.
11. Martire J. The role of nuclear medicine bone scans in evaluating pain in athletic injuries. Clin Sports Med 1987;6:713–737.
12. Freed JH, Hahn H, Menter R, et al. The use of the three-phase bone scan in the early diagnosis of heterotopic ossification (HO) and in the evaluation of Didronel therapy. Paraplegia 1982;20:208–216.
13. MacKinnon S, Holder L. The use of three-phase radionuclide bone scanning in the diagnosis of reflex sympathetic dystrophy. J Hand Surg Am 1984;9:556–563.
14. Mubarak SJ, Gould RN, Lee YF, et al. The medial tibial stress syndrome: a cause of shin splints. Am J Sports Med 1982;10:201–205.
15. Daffner RH. Stress fractures: current concepts. Skeletal Radiol 1979;2:221–229.
16. Belkin RC. Stress fractures in athletes. Orthop Clin North Am 1980;11:735–742.
17. Matin P. Basic principles of nuclear medicine techniques for detection and evaluation of trauma and sports medicine injuries. Semin Nucl Med 1988;18:90–112.
18. Collier BD, Johnson RP, Carrera GP, et al. Painful spondylosis or spondylolisthesis studies by radiography and single-photon emission computed tomography. Radiology 1985;154:207–211.
19. Marcus R, Cann C, Madvig P, et al. Menstrual function and bone mass in elite women distance runners. endocrine and metabolic features. Ann Intern Med 1985;102:158–163.
20. Bilanin JE, Blanchard MS, Russek-Cohen E. Lower vertebral bone density in male long distance runners. Med Sci Sports Exerc 1989;21:66–70.
21. Lane NE, Block DA, Jones HH, et al. Long distance running, bone density and osteoarthritis. JAMA 1986;255:1147–1151.
22. Kaplan PA, Anderson JC, Norris MA. Ultrasonography of post-traumatic soft tissue lesions. Radiol Clin North Am 1989;27:973–982.
23. Kaplan PA, Matamoros A, Anderson JC. Sonography of the musculoskeletal system. AJR 1990;155:237–245.
24. Fornage BD, Rifkin MD. Ultrasound examination of tendons. Radiol Clin North Am 1988;26:87–107.
25. Middleton WD, Edelstein G, Reinus WR. Sonographic detection of rotator cuff tears. AJR 1985;144:349–353.
26. Lane NE, Bloch DA, Jones HH, et al. Long-distance running, bone density, and osteoarthritis. JAMA 1986;255:1147–1151.
27. Pathria MN, Zlatkin M, Sartoris DJ. Ultrasonography of the popliteal fossa and lower extremities. Radiol Clin North Am 1988;26:77–85.
28. Richardson ML, Selby B, Montana MA. Ultrasonography of the knee. Radiol Clin North Am 1988;26:63–75.
29. Aisen AM, McCune WJ, MacGuire A, et al. Sonographic evaluation of the cartilage of the knee. Radiology 1984;153:781–784.
30. Laine HR, Harjula A, Peltokallio P. Ultrasonography as a differential diagnostic aid in achillodynia. J Ultrasound Med 1987;6:351–362.
31. Flannigan B, Kursunoglu-Brahme S, Snyders S, et al. Magnetic resonance arthrography of the shoulder: comparison with conventional magnetic resonance imaging. AJR 1990;155:829–832.
32. Hall FM. Arthrography: past, present and future. AJR 1987;149:561–563.
33. Gundry CR, Schils JP, Resnick D, et al. Arthrography of the post-traumatic knee, shoulder and wrist, current status and future trends. Radiol Clin North Am 1989;27:957–971.

34. Bernageau J. Roentgenographic assessment of the rotator cuff. Clin Orthop 1990;254:87–91.

35. Deutsch AL, Resnick D, Mink JH, et al. Computed and conventional arthrotomography of the glenohumeral joint: normal anatomy and clinical experience. Radiology 1984;153:603–609.

36. Rafii M, Firooznia H, Bonamo JJ, et al. Athlete shoulder injuries: CT arthrographic findings. Radiology 1987;162:559–564.

37. Rafii M, Firooznia H, Golimbu C, et al. CT arthrography of capsular structures of the shoulder. AJR 1986;46:361–367.

38. Stiles RG, Resnick D, Sartoris DJ, et al. Rotator cuff disruption: diagnosis with digital arthrography. Radiology 1988;168:705–707.

39. Kerr R. Diagnostic imaging of the upper extremity trauma. Radiol Clin North Am 1989;27:891–908.

40. Wilson AJ, Totty WG, Murphy WA, et al. Shoulder joint: arthrographic CT and long-term follow-up, with surgical correlation. Radiology 1989;173:329–333.

41. Resnick D, Niwayana G. Diagnosis of bone and joint disorders. 2nd ed. Philadelphia: WB Saunders, 1988.

42. Ellman H. Diagnosis and treatment of incomplete rotator cuff tears. Clin Orthop 1990;254:64–74.

43. Singson RD, Feldman F, Bigliani L. CT arthrographic patterns in recurrent glenohumeral instability. AJR 1987;149:749–753.

44. Zlatkin MB, Bjorkengren AG, Gylys-Morin V, et al. Cross-sectional imaging of the capsular mechanism of the glenohumeral joint. AJR 1988;150:151–158.

45. Sauser DD, Thordarson S, Fahr LM. Imaging of the elbow. Radiol Clin North Am 1990;28:923–940.

46. Singson RD, Feldman F, Rosenberg ZSR. Elbow joint: assessment with double-contrast CT arthrography. Radiology 1986;160:167–173.

47. Levinsohn EM. Imaging of the wrist. Radiol Clin North Am 1990;28:905–921.

48. Levinsohn EM, Palmer AK, Coren AB, et al. Wrist arthrography: the value of the three compartment injection technique. Skeletal Radiol 1987;16:539–544.

49. Tirman RM, Weber ER, Snyder LL, et al. Midcarpal wrist arthrography for detection of tears of the scapholunate and lunotriquetral ligaments. AJR 1985;144:107–108.

50. Pittman CC, Quinn SF, Belsole R, et al. Digital subtraction wrist arthrography: use of double contrast technique as a supplement to single contrast arthrography. Skeletal Radiol 1988;17:119–122.

51. Quinn SF, Belsole RS, Greene TL, et al. Work in progress: postarthrography computed tomography of the wrist: evaluation of the triangular fibrocartilage complex. Skeletal Radiol 1989;17:565–569.

52. Wolfe RD. Knee arthrography: a practical approach. Philadelphia: WB Saunders, 1984.

53. Langer JE, Meyer SJ, Dalinka MK. Imaging of the knee. Radiol Clin North Am 1990;28:975–990.

54. Hughston JC, Andrews JR, Cross MJ. Classification of knee ligament instabilities: part I. the medial compartment and cruciate ligaments. J Bone Joint Surg Am 1976;58:159–172.

55. Pavlov H. Imaging of the foot and ankle. Radiol Clin North Am 1990;28:991–1018.

56. Dory MA. Arthrography of the ankle joint in chronic instability. Skeletal Radiol 1986;15:291–294.

57. Bruno LA, Gennarelli TA, Torg JS. Management guidelines for head injuries in athletics. Clin Sports Med 1987;6:17–29.

58. Wilberger JE, Maroon JC. Head injuries in athletes. Clin Sports Med 1989;8:1–9.

59. Zimmerman RA. Evaluation of head injury: supratentorial. In: Tavaras JM, Ferrucci JT, eds. Radiology: diagnosis-imaging-intervention. Philadelphia: JB Lippincott, 1987;3:1–18.

60. Bleichrodt RP, Kingma LM, Binnendijk B, et al. Injuries of the lateral ankle ligaments: classification with tenography and arthrography. Radiology 1989;173:347–349.

61. Hackney DB. Skull radiology in the evaluation of acute head trauma: a survey of current practice. Radiology 1991;181:711–714.

62. Pathria MN, Blaser SI. Diagnostic imaging of craniofacial fractures. Radiol Clin North Am 1989;27:839–853.

63. Kraus DR, Shapiro D. The symptomatic lumbar spine in the athlete. Clin Sports Med 1989;8:59–69.

64. Key JA, Conwell HE. Management of fractures, dislocations and sprains. St. Louis: CV Mosby, 1951.

65. Sandler CM, Hall JT, Rodriguez MB, et al. Bladder injury in blunt pelvic trauma. Radiology 1986;158:633–638.

66. Wing VM, Federle MP, Morris JA Jr, et al. The clinical impact of CT for blunt abdominal trauma. AJR 1985;145:1191–1194.

67. McCort JJ. Caring for the major trauma victim: the role for radiology. Radiology 1987;163:1–9.

68. Diamond DL. Sports related abdominal trauma. Clin Sports Med 1989;8:91–99.

69. Jeffrey RB, Laing FC, Federle MP, et al. Computed tomography of splenic trauma. Radiology 1981;141:729–732.

70. Foley WD, Cates JS, Kellman GM. Treatment of blunt hepatic injuries: role of CT. Radiology 1987;164:635–638.

71. Moon KL Jr, Federle MP. Computed tomography in hepatic trauma. AJR 1983;141:309–314.

72. Van Steenbergen W, Samain H, Pouillon M. Transection of the pancreas demonstrated by ultrasound and computed tomography. Gastrointest Radiol 1987;12:128–130.

73. Lang EK. Trauma of the urinary tract. In: Tavaras JM, Ferrucci JT, eds. Radiology: diagnosis-imaging-intervention. Philadelphia: JB Lippincott, 1987;4:1–24.

74. Toombs BD, Lester RG, Ben-Menachem Y, et al. Computed tomography in blunt trauma. Radiol Clin North Am 1981;19:17–35.

75. Schild HH, Strunk H, Weber, et al. Pulmonary contusion: CT versus plain radiograms. J Comput Assist Tomogr 1989;13:417–420.

76. Smejkal R, O'Malley KF, David E, et al. Routine initial computed tomography of the chest and blunt torso trauma. Chest 1991;100:667–669.

77. Heare MM, Heare TC, Gillespy T III. Diagnostic imaging of pelvic and chest wall trauma. Radiol Clin North Am 1989;27:873–889.

78. Armstrong P, Keevil SF. Magnetic resonance imaging: part 1. basic principles of image production. BMJ 1991;303:35–40.

79. Osteaux M, Demeirleir K, Shahabpour M. Magnetic resonance imaging and spectroscopy in sport medicine. Berlin: Springer-Verlag, 1991.

80. Seeger LL. Physical principles of magnetic resonance imaging. Clin Orthop 1989;244:7–16.

81. Huang HK, Aberle DR, Lufkin R, et al. Advances in medical imaging. Ann Intern Med 1990;112:203–220.

82. Kursunoglu-Brahme S, Resnick D. Magnetic resonance imaging of the shoulder. Radiol Clin North Am 1990;28:941–954.

83. Meyer SJ, Dalinka MK. Magnetic resonance imaging of the shoulder. Semin Ultrasound CT MR. 1990;11:253–266.

84. Seeger LL, Gambhir S, Bassett LW. Magnetic resonance imaging of the shoulder. Rheum Dis Clin North Am 1991;17:693–703.

85. Vellet AD, Muak PL, Marks P. Imaging techniques of the shoulder: present perspectives. Clin Sports Med 1991;10:721–756.

86. Neer CS. Impingement lesions. Clin Orthop 1983;173:70–77.

87. Tsai JC, Zlatkin MB. Magnetic resonance imaging of the shoulder. Radiol Clin North Am 1990;28:279–291.

88. Rafii M, Firooznia H, Sherman O, et al. Rotator cuff lesions: signal patterns at magnetic resonance imaging. Radiology 1990;177:817–823.

89. Iannotti JP, Zlatkin MB, Esterhai JL, et al. Magnetic resonance imaging of the shoulder. Sensitivity, specificity and predictive value. J Bone Joint Surg Am 1991;73:17–29.

90. Zlatkin MB, Iannotti JP, Roberts MC, et al. Rotator cuff tears: diagnostic performance of magnetic resonance imaging. Radiology 1989;172:223–229.
91. Burk DL, Karasick D, Mitchell DG, et al. Magnetic resonance imaging of the shoulder: correlation with plain radiography. AJR 1990;154:549–553.
92. Seeger LL. Magnetic resonance imaging of the shoulder. Clin Orthop 1989;244:48–59.
93. Silliman JF, Hawkins RJ. Current concepts and recent advances in the athlete's shoulder. Clin Sports Med 1991;10:693–705.
94. Seeger LL, Gold RH, Bassett LW. Shoulder instability evaluation with MR imaging. Radiology 1988;168:695–697.
95. Legal JM, Burchard TO, Off WB, et al. Tears of the glenoid labrum: magnetic resonance imaging of 88 arthroscopically confirmed cases. Radiology 1991;179:241–246.
96. Gross ML, Seeger LL, Smith JB, et al. Magnetic resonance imaging of the glenoid labrum. Am J Sports Med 1990;18:229–234.
97. Deutsch AL, Mink JH. Magnetic resonance imaging of musculoskeletal injuries. Radiol Clin North Am 1989;27:983–1002.
98. Pykett IL, Newhouse JH, Buonanno FS, et al. Principles of nuclear magnetic resonance imaging. Radiology 1982;143:157–168.
99. Ho CP, Sartoris DJ. Magnetic resonance imaging of the elbow. Rheum Dis Clin North Am 1991;17:705–720.
100. Posner MA. Injuries to the hand and wrist in athletes. Orthop Clin North Am 1977;8:593–618.
101. McCue FC, Baugher WH, Kulund DN, et al. Hand and wrist injuries in the athlete. Am J Sports Med 1979;7:275–286.
102. Barry MS, Kettner NW, Pierre-Jerome C. Carpal instability: pathomechanics and contemporary imaging. Clin Sports Med 1991;5:38–44.
103. Linn MR, Mann FA, Gilula LA. Imaging the symptomatic wrist. Orthop Clin North Am 1990;21:515–543.
104. Kursunoglu-Brahme S, Resnick D. Magnetic resonance imaging of the wrist. Rheum Dis Clin North Am 1991;17:721–739.
105. Kursunoglu-Brahme S, Gundry CR, Resnick D. Advanced imaging of the wrist. Radiol Clin North Am 1990;28:307–320.
106. Jones WA. Beware the sprained wrist. J Bone Joint Surg Br 1988;70:293–297.
107. Zlatkin MB, Chao PC, Osterman AL, et al. Chronic wrist pain: evaluation with high-resolution magnetic resonance imaging. Radiology 1989;173:723–729.
108. Mandelbaum BR, Bartolozzi AR, Davis CA, et al. Wrist pain syndrome in the gymnast. Pathogenetic, diagnostic, and therapeutic considerations. Am J Sports Med 1989;17:305–317.
109. Mesgarzadeh M, Schneck CD, Bonakdarpour A. Carpal tunnel: magnetic resonance imaging. Part II: carpal tunnel syndromes. Radiology 1989;171:749–754.
110. Mesgarzadeh M, Schneck CD, Bonakdarpour A. Carpal tunnel: magnetic resonance imaging. Part I: normal anatomy. Radiology 1989;171:743–748.
111. Hiehle JF, Kneeland JB, Dalinka MK. Magnetic resonance imaging of the hip with emphasis on avascular necrosis. Rheum Dis Clin North Am 1991;17:669–692.
112. Meyer SJ, Vahey TN. Imaging algorithm for avascular necrosis of the hip. Rheum Dis Clin North Am 1991;17:799–802.
113. Bassett LW, Gold RH. Magnetic resonance imaging of the musculoskeletal system: an overview. Clin Orthop 1989;244:17–28.
114. Lang P, Genant HK, Jergesen HE, et al. Imaging of the hip joint. Computed tomography versus magnetic resonance imaging. Clin Orthop 1992;274:135–153.
115. Brower AC, Kransdorf MJ. Imaging of hip disorders. Radiol Clin North Am 1990;28:955–974.
116. Jergensen HE, Heller M, Genant HK. Signal variability in magnetic resonance imaging of femoral head osteonecrosis. Clin Orthop 1990;253:137–149.
117. Vande Berg B, Malghem J, Labaisse MA, et al. Avascular necrosis of the hip: comparison of contrast-enhanced and nonenhanced magnetic resonance imaging with histologic correlation. Radiology 1992;182:445–450.
118. Ficat RP. Idiopathic bone necrosis of the femoral head: early diagnosis and treatment. J Bone Joint Surg Br 1985;67:3–9.
119. Hauzeur JP, Pasteels JL, Schoutens A, et al. The diagnostic value of magnetic resonance imaging in non-traumatic osteonecrosis of the femoral head. J Bone Joint Surg Am 1989;71:641–649.
120. Mitchell MJ, Ho C, Resnick D, et al. Diagnostic imaging of lower extremity trauma. Radiol Clin North Am 1989;27:909–928.
121. Fleckenstein JL, Weatherall PT, Parkey RW, et al. Sports-related muscle injuries: evaluation with magnetic resonance imaging. Radiology 1989;172:793–798.
122. Zarins B, Adams M. Knee injuries in sports. N Engl J Med 1988;318:950–961.
123. Mink JH, Deutsch AL. Magnetic resonance imaging of the knee. Clin Orthop 1989;244:29–47.
124. Stoller DW, Genant HK. Magnetic resonance imaging of the knee and hip. Arthritis Rheum 1990;33:441–449.
125. Kursunoglu-Brahme S, Resnick D. Magnetic resonance imaging of the knee. Orthop Clin North Am 1990;21:561–572.
126. Langer JE, Meyer SJ, Dalinka MK. Imaging of the knee. Radiol Clin North Am 1990;28:975–990.
127. Stull MA, Nelson MC. The role of magnetic resonance imaging in diagnostic imaging of the injured knee. Am Fam Physician 1990;41:489–500.
128. Crues JV, Mink J, Levy TL, et al. Meniscal tears of the knee: accuracy of magnetic resonance imaging. Radiology 1987;164:445–448.
129. Weissman BN, Hussain S. Magnetic resonance imaging of the knee. Rheum Dis Clin North Am 1991;17:637–638.
130. Stoller DW, Martin C, Crues JV, et al. Meniscal tears: pathologic correlation with magnetic resonance imaging. Radiology 1987;163:731–735.
131. Singson RD, Feldman F, Staron R, et al. Magnetic resonance imaging of displaced bucket-handle tear of the medial meniscus. AJR 1991;156:121–124.
132. Kursunoglu Brahme S, Schwaighofer B, Gundry C, et al. Jogging causes acute changes in the knee joint: a magnetic resonance study in normal volunteers. AJR 1990;154:1233–1235.
133. Shellock FG, Mink JH. Knees of trained long-distance runners: MR imaging before and after competition. Radiology 1991;179:635–637.
134. Reinig JW, McDevitt ER, Ove PN. Progression of meniscal degenerative changes in college football players: evaluation with MR imaging. Radiology 1991;181:255–257.
135. Hernandez RJ, Keim DR, Chenevert TL, et al. Fat-suppressed magnetic resonance imaging of myositis. Radiology 1992;182:217–219.
136. Burk DL, Mitchell DG, Rifkin MD, et al. Recent advances in magnetic resonance imaging of the knee. Radiol Clin North Am 1990;28:379–393.
137. Grover JS, Bassett LW, Gross ML, et al. Posterior cruciate ligament: magnetic resonance imaging. Radiology 1990;174:527–530.
138. Bodne D, Quinn SF, Murray WT, et al. Magnetic resonance images of chronic patellar tendinitis. Skeletal Radiol 1988;17:24–28.
139. Speer KP, Spritzer CE, Goldner JL, et al. Magnetic resonance imaging of traumatic knee articular cartilage injuries. Am J Sports Med 1991;19:396–402.
140. Hayes CW, Conway WF. Evaluation of articular cartilage: radiographic and cross-sectional imaging techniques. Radiographics 1992;12:409–428.
141. DeSmet AA, Fisher DR, Graf BK, et al. Osteochondritis dissecans of the knee: value of magnetic resonance

imaging in determining lesion stability and the presence of articular cartilage defects. AJR 1990;155:549–553.

142. Mink JH, Deutsch AL. Occult cartilage and bone injuries of the knee: detection, classification, and assessment with MR imaging. Radiology 1989;170:823–829.

143. McCauley TR, Kier R, Lynch KJ, et al. Chondromalacia patellae: diagnosis with magnetic resonance imaging. AJR 1992;158:101–105.

144. Conway WF, Hayes CW, Loughran T, et al. Cross-sectional imaging of the patellofemoral joint and surrounding structures. Radiographics 1991;11:195–217.

145. Lynch TC, Crues JV, Morgan FW, et al. Bone abnormalities of the knee: prevalence and significance at magnetic resonance imaging. Radiology 1989;171:761–766.

146. Vallet AD, Marks PH, Fowler PJ, et al. Occult posttraumatic osteochondral lesions of the knee: prevalence, classification, and short-term sequelae evaluated with magnetic resonance imaging. Radiology 1991;178:271–276.

147. Shellock FG, Morris E, Deutsch AL, et al. Hematopoietic bone marrow hyperplasia: high prevalence on magnetic resonance images of the knee in asymptomatic marathon runners. AJR 1992;158:335–338.

148. Feldman F, Staron RB, Haramati N. Magnetic resonance imaging of the foot and ankle. Rheum Dis Clin North Am 1991;17:617–636.

149. Pavlov H. Imaging of the foot and ankle. Radiol Clin North Am 1990;28:991–1018.

150. Kerr R, Forrester DM, Kingston S. Magnetic resonance imaging of foot and ankle trauma. Orthop Clin North Am 1990;21:591–601.

151. Forrester DM, Kerr R. Trauma to the foot. Radiol Clin North Am 1990;28:423–433.

152. Cheung Y, Rosenberg ZS, Magee T, et al. Normal anatomy and pathologic conditions of ankle tendons: current imaging techniques. Radiographics 1992;12:429–444.

153. Berkowitz JF, Kier R, Rudicel S. Plantar fasciitis: magnetic resonance imaging. Radiology 1991;179:665–667.

154. Deutsch AL, Mink JH, Waxman AD. Occult fractures of the proximal femur: MR imaging. Radiology 1989;170:113–116.

155. Greco A, McNamara MT, Escher RM, et al. Spin-echo and STIR magnetic resonance imaging of sports-related muscle injuries at 1.5T. J Comput Assist Tomogr 1991;15:994–999.

156. Anderson IF, Crichton KJ, Grattan-Smith T, et al. Osteochondral fractures of the dome of the talus. J Bone Joint Surg Am 1989;71:1143–1152.

157. Deutsch AL, Mink JH, Shellock FG. Magnetic resonance imaging of injuries to bone and articular cartilage: emphasis on radiographically occult abnormalities. Orthop Rev 1990;19:66–75.

158. De Smet AA, Fisher DR, Burnstein MI, et al. Value of magnetic resonance imaging in staging osteochondral lesions of the talus (osteochondritis dissecans): results in 14 patients. AJR 1990;154:555–558.

159. Nelson DW, DiPaola J, Colville M, et al. Osteochondritis dissecans of the talus and knee: prospective comparison of magnetic resonance and arthroscopic classifications. J Comput Assist Tomogr 1990;14:804–808.

160. Kerslake RW, Jaspan T, Worthington BS. Magnetic resonance imaging of spinal trauma. Br J Radiol 1991;64:386–402.

161. Pratt ES, Green DA, Spengler DM. Herniated intervertebral discs associated with unstable spinal injuries. Spine 1990;15:662–666.

162. Kulkarni MV, McArdle CB, Kopanicky D, et al. Acute spinal cord injury: magnetic resonance imaging at 1.5T. Radiology 1987;164:837–843.

163. Yamashita Y, Takahashi M, Matsuno Y, et al. Acute spinal cord injury: magnetic resonance imaging correlated with myelopathy. Br J Radiol 1991;64:201–209.

164. Bondurant FJ, Cotler HB, Kulkarni MV, et al. Acute spinal cord injury: a study using physical examination and magnetic resonance imaging. Spine 1990;15:161–168.

165. Mirvis SE. Applications of magnetic resonance imaging and three-dimensional computed tomography in emergency medicine. Ann Emerg Med 1989;18:1315–1321.

166. Flanders AE, Schaefer DM, Doan HT, et al. Acute cervical spine trauma: correlation of magnetic resonance imaging findings with degree of neurologic deficit. Radiology 1990;177:25–33.

167. Pathria MN, Petersilge CA. Spinal trauma. Radiol Clin North Am 1991;29:847–865.

168. Schaefer DM, Flanders A, Northrup BE, et al. Magnetic resonance imaging of acute cervical spine trauma: correlation with severity of neurologic injury. Spine 1989;14:1090–1095.

169. Wittenberg RH, Boetel U, Beyer HK. Magnetic resonance imaging and computer tomography of acute spinal cord trauma. Clin Orthop 1990;260:176–185.

170. Kettner NW, Pierre-Jerome C. Magnetic resonance imaging of the wrist: occult osseous lesions. J Manip Physiol Ther 1992;15:599–603.

171. Levinsohn EM. Imaging of the wrist. Radiol Clin North Am 1990;28:905–921.

Thermal Imaging of Sports Injuries

David J. BenEliyahu

The use of infrared thermography (IRT) as a clinical tool for the diagnosis and management of sports injuries has been documented in the world scientific literature. IRT has been used as a diagnostic, prognostic, risk assessment, and treatment assessment tool. Thermographic equipment basically consists of two different types of technologies: liquid crystal equipment and electronic infrared telethermography.

NEUROPHYSIOLOGY

Thermography measures surface skin temperature, which is reflective of the underlying sympathetic autonomic function or dysfunction. Cutaneous temperature is governed by hypothalamic control, local nervous system control, and the effects of any local chemical mediators (e.g., histamine, substance P). In normal situations, surface skin temperature from right to left sides of the body varies only within tenths of a degree. Several studies have been performed to document small interside temperature differences and to demonstrate their short- and long-term stability. Uematsu et al. found that the small interside temperature differences were reliable and reproducible at 2- and 5-year follow-up study (Table 21.1) (1). Generally, temperature differentials rarely exceed a quarter of a degree centigrade. Goodman et al., So et al., and Feldman and Nickoloff published similar findings (2–4). The Feldman and Nickoloff study documented that temperature differentials in excess of 0.65°C were consistent with underlying pathology.

Thermal imaging can detect either decreased or increased temperature in response to an injury (Table 21.2). If there is sympathetic or unmyelinated nerve irritation, there will be an increase in circulating catecholamines that will have a vasospastic effect on the local dermal microcirculation. This will be observed as a hypothermic (decreased thermal cutaneous emission) response. The neural modulation for this phenomenon may occur centrally due to increased preganglionic and postganglionic sympathetic function. Preganglionic fibers synapse with postganglionic cell bodies and have acetylcholine as the neurotransmitter. The postganglionic fibers influence the dermal microcirculation via the local alpha receptors and catecholamines (adrenaline/noradrenaline).

Hypersensitization of the alpha receptors can also cause hypothermia. Conversely, hyperthermia may be seen in situations in which decreased postganglionic function (such as in denervation or blockade of the alpha receptors) is due to increased levels of local vasodilatory substances such as histamines, bradykinin, and substance P. This may typically be seen in an acute injury (Table 21.2) (5).

In sports injuries an athlete may injure ligament, nerve, muscle, tendon, or periosteal bone. It has been shown that temperature changes deeper than 0.5°C cannot be detected at the surface. Therefore, thermographic equipment detects cutaneous thermal changes controlled by local autonomic reflex. In a study by Hobbins, athletes exercising on a treadmill displayed cutaneous vasoconstriction and cooling (6). It is evident that injured tissue will cause referred pain to a somatocutaneous referral pain zone. This work has been documented by Kellgren for muscle and scleratogenous structures (7). Similar work has been documented by many others (8–13). Travell and Simons have published much work on the referred pain patterns of myofascial trigger points and their pain reference zones (12). Jinkins and Whittemore recently documented autonomic lumbosacral head zones in the lower extremity for patients with disc protrusions (13). The pain reference zones of trigger points have been documented by Kruse et al. to be thermologically active and detectable (14). BenEliyahu has documented that the lumbosacral head zones and autonomic pain reference zones are thermologically active as well (15).

Table 21.1. Thermal Symmetry of the Skin

Confidence Factor Body Segment	50% X	sd	84% +1sd	98% +2sd
Forehead	0.12	0.093	0.22	0.30
Cheek	0.18	0.186	0.37	0.56
Chest	0.14	0.151	0.19	0.34
Abdomen	0.18	0.131	0.31	0.44
Cervical spine	0.15	0.091	0.24	0.33
Thoracic spine	0.15	0.092	0.24	0.33
Lumbar spine	0.25	0.201	0.45	0.65
Scapula	0.13	0.108	0.24	0.35
Arm—biceps	0.13	0.119	0.35	0.37
Arm—triceps	0.22	0.155	0.38	0.54
Forearm—lateral	0.23	0.198	0.43	0.63
Forearm—medial	0.32	0.158	0.48	0.64
Palm—lateral	0.25	0.166	0.42	0.59
Palm—medial	0.23	0.197	0.43	0.63
Fingers—average	0.38	0.064	0.44	0.50
Thigh—anterior	0.11	0.085	0.20	0.29
Thigh—posterior	0.15	0.116	0.27	0.39
Knee—anterior	0.23	0.174	0.40	0.57
Knee—posterior	0.12	0.101	0.22	0.32
Leg—anterior	0.31	0.277	0.59	0.87
Leg—posterior	0.13	0.108	0.24	0.35
Foot—dorsum	0.30	0.201	0.50	0.70
Foot—heel	0.20	0.220	0.42	0.64
Toes—average	0.50	0.143	0.64	0.78
Trunk—average	0.17	0.042	0.21	0.25
Extremities—average	0.20	0.073	0.27	0.34

Table 21.2. Summary of Mechanisms Observed in Thermography

Hyperthermia
  Loss of postganglionic fiber function (denervation, sympathetic block, peripheral neuropathy)
  Alpha receptor blockade (chemical mediators, substance P, histamine PG, skin trauma, drugs)
Hypothermia
  Increased postganglionic fiber function (nerve dysfunction, reflex sympathetic dysfunctions)
  Increased alpha receptor sensitivity (noradrenaline, denervation)

These somatocutaneous referral pain zones are thermally active via the neurophysiologic mechanisms previously described. For example, when a joint is injured, there will be capsular and ligamentous activation of nociceptors, mechanoreceptors, and chemoreceptors. This will cause an afferent barrage and a reflex efferent response. The autonomic component of the efferent response causes the cutaneous thermal asymmetry detected by IRT. In an acute injury, one would normally expect to see a hyperthermic response. This is usually due to local release of vasodilatory substances such as substance P. The substance P theory has been postulated by Christiansen and Gerow (16). According to this theory, thermal symmetry will return in a typical injury as the substance P stores are depleted and the patient is healing. A hypothermic finding will appear later if the injury does not heal properly and there remains some degree of pathophysiology. Sometimes for reasons poorly understood, an acute injury may yield a global hypothermic appearance of the extremity of approximately 2.0°C or more. This is usually synonymous with a poorer prognosis and longer recovery time. This type of injury is termed posttraumatic reflex sympathetic dysfunction (RSD), which displays characteristics of sympathetic hypertonia. Sometimes there is no thermal difference from right to left parts (isothermia), and these injuries are usually mild with good prognosis and recovery.

CLINICAL APPLICATIONS OF INFRARED THERMAL IMAGING

Lower Extremity: Knee Pain

IRT can be helpful in the differential diagnosis of knee pain. There are many causes of knee pain, which can include injury to the menisci, ligaments, patellofemoral joint, plica, arthritis, and epiphysitis. IRT will generally have a consistent pattern for some of the more common disorders.

Patellofemoral pain syndrome (PFPS), which presents with anterior knee pain, is usually made worse by descending or ascending stairs, prolonged sitting (positive cinema/movie sign), or running. This condition is often mislabeled as chondromalacia patella and is actually representative of patellar malalignment, vastus medialis weakness, and dyskinetic tracking. IRT scans of this condition will typically display a global hypothermia around the local patellar region (Fig. 21.1). There have been many studies to support this finding (17–20).

In a study by the author, IRT was found to have a 97% sensitivity and 90% specificity in the detection of PFPS when compared with clinical and radiographic findings (20). Similar studies have documented good sensitivity for IRT and PFPS (17–19). Perelman and Adler's study (18) found 82% sensitivity and 90% specificity for detection of patellar thermal asymmetry and hypothermia.

There have been attempts to use magnetic resonance imaging (MRI) and bone scintigraphy for the diagnosis of PFPS, but they have not been very helpful. IRT is a noninvasive, risk-free, cost-effective, and sensitive diagnostic tool. IRT is also helpful as a treatment outcome assessment tool because IRT scans may be repeated throughout the course of patient care.

PFPS has many contributing biomechanical and kinesiologic etiologies that must be taken into consideration for successful treatment; e.g., Q angle, hyperpronation, genu valgum, patella alta, vastus medialis obliquus (VMO) weakness. The IRT scan will continue to display patellar hypothermia if there is still an offending biomechanical or muscular dysfunction. In several cases seen by the author, the simple addition of foot orthotics allowed full clinical relief and patellar thermal symmetry. IRT has also displayed the efficacy of conservative chiropractic management for PFPS with pretreatment and post-treatment thermograms (21). Chiropractic care included knee and spinal manipulation, knee ultrasound, knee rehabilitative exercises, and orthotics when indicated.

IRT scans of patients with osteoarthritis, meniscal lesions, ligament lesions, and synovial plica syndromes typically display hyperthermia of the affected knee. In meniscal or ligament le-

sions of the knee, there will typically be a 1.5°–2.5°C rise in temperature around the patellar region (Fig. 21.2). This pattern is contrasted with that of PFPS, which shows hypothermia. IRT is the test of choice when one suspects RSD of the knee (Fig. 21.3) (22–27). RSD may occur after casting, surgery, or minor trauma for reasons poorly understood. The patient will complain of some or all the following: persistent, unrelenting pain; tingling; burning; hyperhydrosis; muscle wasting; allodynia; and hyperalgesia. These signs and symptoms represent sudomotor and vasomotor disturbances secondary to sympathetic hyperreflexia. IRT scans are the diagnostic test of choice when one suspects RSD, because no other

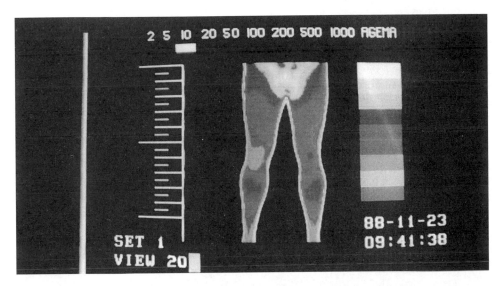

Figure 21.1. An anterior-patellar IRT scan showing patellar hypothermia compatible with PFPS.

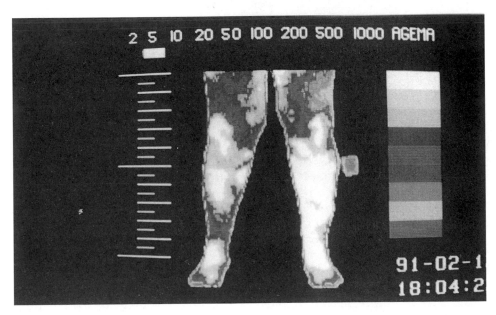

Figure 21.2. An anterior knee IRT scan depicting diffuse hyperthermia compatible with meniscal lesion and internal derangement.

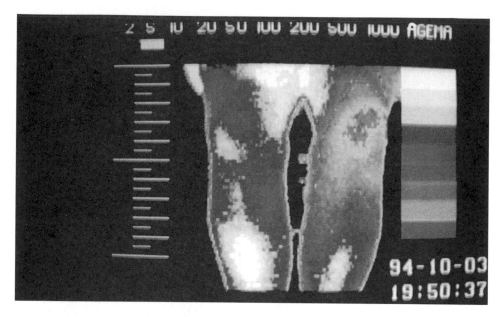

Figure 21.3. A knee IRT scan showing extensive hypothermia extending into the knee, calf, and thigh compatible with postsurgical RSD.

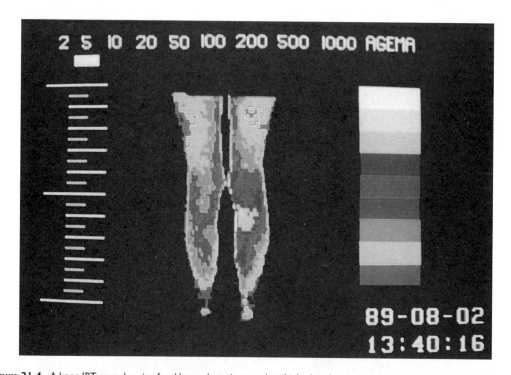

Figure 21.4. A knee IRT scan showing focal hyperthermia over the tibial tubercle consistent with Osgood-Schlatter's disease.

readily tests for sympathetic dysfunction. It is extremely important to diagnose this condition early because successful treatment depends on it. IRT findings include not only patellar hypothermia, but a spreading effect of hypothermia to the thigh and calf as well.

IRT is also useful in Osgood-Schlatter's disease, which is a tibial epiphysitis of the tibial tubercle. The patient, typically an athlete who does much jumping with running, will present with anterior knee pain typically over the tibial tubercle and patellar tendon. IRT scans will detect a focal hyperthermia over the tibial tubercle on the order of 2.0°C. As the patient is treated, IRT scans may be repeated to determine a return to thermal symmetry and a cessation of underlying pathoneurophysiology (28). This is useful because IRT may be used to determine when the athlete can safely return to competition without the great risk of relapse (Fig. 21.4).

LOWER EXTREMITY: ANKLE SPRAIN

The most common ankle sprain is an inversion sprain that will most typically affect the anterior talofibular ligament and, to a lesser degree, the calcaneofibular ligament. Thermographically, increased thermal emission over the lateral ankle and dorsal foot is most commonly seen. The hyperthermia response is most likely due to a release of local chemical mediators such as substance P, histamines, and bradykinin. Isothermia (thermal symmetry) and hypothermia (decreased thermal emission) may also be seen, but not as frequently.

A study done by Schmitt and Guillot in France on 200 patients with ankle sprains revealed three basic findings: isothermia (symmetry), hyperthermia, and hypothermia (29). The cases of isothermia indicated a minor injury, and recovery time was 1 to 2 weeks. Hyperthermia, which is the usual finding, varied from 1.0°–4.0°C, with an average right to left asymmetry of 1.5°–2.0°C. They found hyperthermia resolved in 4 weeks, which is when they allowed their athletes to resume full competition. Some patients displayed decreased thermal emission of the ankle and foot on the IRT scan. This category was broken up into two groups. One group of hypothermic ankles had thermal asymmetry less than 1.0°C compared with the good ankle. This subgroup also had a prognosis of 6-week healing time. In the second group, a regional global hypothermia was ob-

served both proximal and distal to the area of the sprain. This has been termed posttraumatic reflex sympathetic dysfunction (RSD) or posttraumatic pain syndrome by Pochachevsky (30). It is most probably a reflex efferent vasoconstriction due to afferent C-nociception from severe damage to synovium ligaments and muscle.

The finding of hypothermia in RSD will generally display a right to left temperature differential of approximately 3.0°–4.0°C (normal difference, 0.20°C) (Fig. 21.5). This finding of RSD and vast cooling carries with it a protracted recovery and rehabilitation time varying from 3 to 6 months. Clinical recovery (pain) seems to happen before thermal and neurophysiologic recovery, as seen on thermographic images, but full thermal symmetry does return with continued conservative care. Thermal symmetry and a return to normal biomechanics and neurophysiology are desired to inhibit the risk of relapse and reinjury.

LOWER EXTREMITY: MEDIAL TIBIA STRESS SYNDROME

Stress Fractures

Goodman et al. studied 17 athletes with exertional leg pain who were scanned by IRT, bone scan, and x-ray to assess their legs for stress fracture (31). They found that IRT had a 90% positive predictive value, an 82% sensitivity, an 83% specificity, and a 71% negative predictive

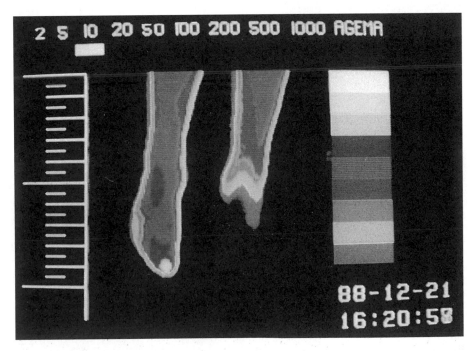

Figure 21.5. An ankle/foot IRT scan showing hypothermia with a temperature differential of 4°C compatible with posttraumatic pain syndrome or RSD.

value for stress fractures of the tibia. These values were based on a blind comparison to radiographs and bone scans. The athletes with hyperthermic patterns had a poorer prognosis when compared with the hypothermic group and were unable to resume their original activity. The authors also found IRT to be a useful marker for bone healing in observing the thermal transition from hot to cold.

Another study by Devereaux et al. produced similar findings with stress fractures in athletes (32). The thermographic findings of a stress fracture generally will be that of a focal hyperthermic hot spot (Fig. 21.6). Medial tibial stress syndrome, or shin splints, are thermographically hyperthermic but are generally nonfocal. The hyperthermia is diffuse along the tibia margin (Fig. 21.7). These patterns are similar to those seen in bone scan or nuclear medicine images.

LOWER EXTREMITY: TARSAL TUNNEL SYNDROME

Tarsal tunnel syndrome is a rare condition that involves entrapment of the medial plantar nerve at the medial malleolus. IRT is a sensitive test for this condition and will show thermal asymmetry and hyperthermia at the heel and big toe (33). Hyperthermia will be a typical finding in an entrapment syndrome because of denervation and loss of sympathetic tone. Thermographic findings are generally limited to the foot.

METATARSALGIA/MORTON'S NEUROMA

The patient will complain of pain at the plantar aspect of the foot at the metatarsal heads, most commonly at the third/fourth metatarsal heads. A neuroma develops due to postural stresses of the foot at the interdigital nerve. Hyperpronation has been suggested as one cause. IRT scans will reveal a focal hyperthermia at the metatarsal head of the level involved and often at the toe of involvement (Fig. 21.8) (34).

ACHILLES TENDINITIS

Santilli has documented the clinical use of IRT for the detection of Achilles tendionopathies. Thermographic imaging will display hyperthermia at the inner precalcaneal region and the lateral Achilles region (35).

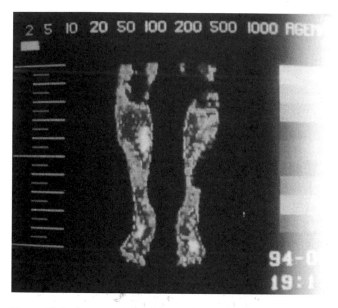

Figure 21.6. An IRT scan of the anterior calf showing focal hot spot compatible with stress fracture.

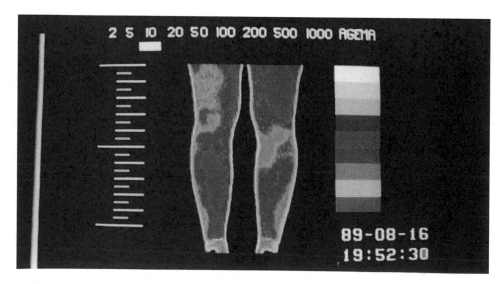

Figure 21.7. A tibial IRT scan with diffuse hyperthermia compatible with medial tibial stress syndrome (shin splints).

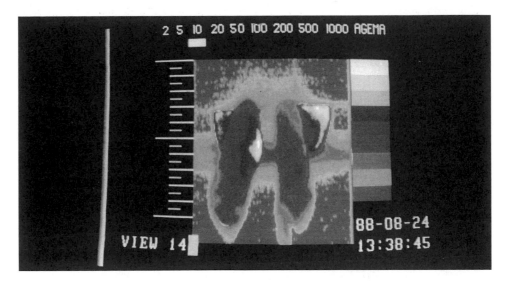

Figure 21.8. A foot IRT scan consistent with Morton's neuroma.

TENNIS LEG

The patient will experience a sudden sharp pain in the posterior aspect of the calf. There will be a palpable defect in the gastrocnemius muscle representing a tear. The calf will be swollen, hot, and palpably hard. The differential diagnosis must include thrombophlebitis, posterior compartment syndrome, and tennis leg. The thermogram will not show a diffuse calf hyperthermia compatible with thrombophlebitis, but will show a focal hot spot over the region of the tear. Thus, IRT is helpful in the differential diagnosis of posterior calf pain in conjunction with clinical findings and history.

GASTROCNEMIUS TRIGGER POINT

The gastrocnemius can develop myofascial trigger points as a result of overload. Calf pain that can be quite painful will develop. The thermography scan will reveal a focal hot spot approximately 2° warmer than the surrounding areas. The focal hot spot is representative of the trigger point, and this area is sensitive to palpation. On successful treatment of the trigger point (i.e., ischemic compression massage, ultrasound), the trigger point will resolve and the thermogram will return to normal.

UPPER EXTREMITY: SHOULDER

Thermography is useful as an adjunctive aid in the diagnosis of shoulder impingement syndrome (28, 36). The patient will typically complain of shoulder pain exacerbated by upper extremity hyperabduction and hyperflexion. There will be weakness on manual testing of some or all of the rotator cuff muscles and positive impingement sign with Hawkins test. The patient will also have pinpoint tenderness over the rotator cuff. Most commonly, the impingement will be subacromial and involve the supraspinatus tendon. MRI is very useful for anatomic diagnosis. However, it has been documented that healthy populations will have a positive MRI for structural abnormalities, despite having no symptoms.

IRT is useful, in that when there is clinical evidence of a condition, it offers supportive physiologic data reflective of underlying somatic dysfunction. IRT will display a somatocutaneous reflex hyperthermia of the involved shoulder (Fig. 21.9). Maultsby has found a common area of diffuse hyperthermia over the shoulder in documented cases of impingement syndrome (36). Rotator cuff tears show a more focal hot spot over the area of the tear. Thermography can be useful in the differentiation of impingement syndrome and rotator cuff tears, in that a tear will show a more focal spot of hyperthermia and an impingement syndrome will show a more diffuse area of hyperthermia.

Biceps tendinitis will show an area of hyperthermia over the biceps tendon on thermography scan. This will support the clinical findings of palpation and physical orthopedic tests (i.e., Yergason's, Abbot Saunders').

UPPER EXTREMITY: ELBOW

Thermography has been shown to be useful in the diagnosis and management of epicondylitis. Several authors have documented that epicondylitis will appear as a focal hyperthermia over the lateral epicondyle (Fig. 21.10) (28, 37–39). In

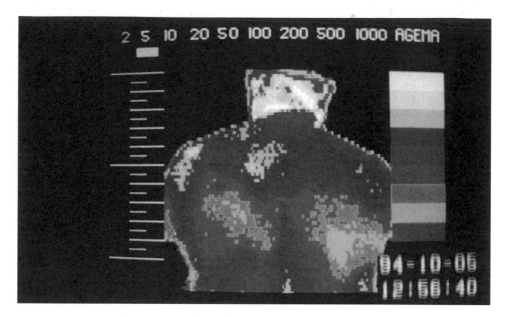

Figure 21.9. An IRT scan of the shoulder revealing shoulder impingement syndrome.

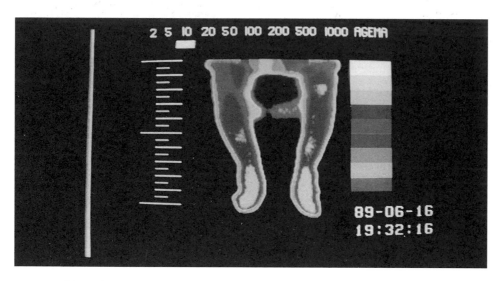

Figure 21.10. An IRT scan of the elbow compatible with tennis elbow/epicondylitis.

a study by Binder and Parr (39) of patients with epicondylitis, a high sensitivity was found for IRT. IRT is useful in the differential diagnosis of forearm pain because the IRT scan will show classic focal hyperthermic findings over the epicondyle. There are times when the patient will have forearm pain due to more proximal osseous or myofascial dysfunction, which will show a different thermal pattern. Patients with a "loose body" or joint mouse in the elbow will have pain and restricted range of motion with joint locking. IRT scan will display a diffuse blush hyperthermia at the elbow unlike that of epicondylitis.

UPPER EXTREMITY: NERVE ENTRAPMENT

Median Nerve

Carpal tunnel syndrome is an entrapment of the median nerve at the wrist. When nerve entrapment occurs, there will be some degree of denervation. Because it is documented by neurophysiologists that 8% to 30% of all peripheral nerves carry sympathetic fibers, there will be loss of sympathetic tone (1, 5, 6). With a loss of sympathetic tone, the IRT scan will show reflex hyperthermia at the hand and median nerve distribution (Fig. 21.11).

UPPER EXTREMITY: ULNAR NERVE ENTRAPMENT

Cyclists are prone to ulnar nerve entrapments due to their upper extremity posture while on the bicycle for prolonged periods. Ulnar nerve entrapment will result in hyperthermia of the hand along the ulnar nerve distribution.

UPPER EXTREMITY: MYOFASCIAL TRIGGER POINTS

Myofascial trigger points are a common finding in a sports practice. Travell et al. have extensively documented the referred pain patterns of trigger points (40). IRT is an objective tool to document myofascial trigger points. The use of IRT to document trigger points has been well established in the scientific literature (28, 40–44). Trigger points of the levator scapula will reveal a focal hyperthermia at the superior angle of the scapula (Fig. 21.12). Trapezius trigger points will reveal cutaneous focal hyperthermia overlying the area of the trigger point. Trigger points can cause vasomotor changes into the referred pain zone, which is often very distal to the offending trigger point (i.e., infraspinatus trigger point can cause thermal asymmetry into the upper extremity). This has been documented by Christiansen and Kruse (41). Pectoralis minor trigger points can be detected by IRT and can often cause a thoracic

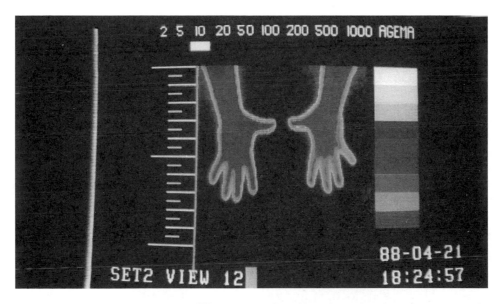

Figure 21.11. A hand IRT scan compatible with carpal tunnel syndrome.

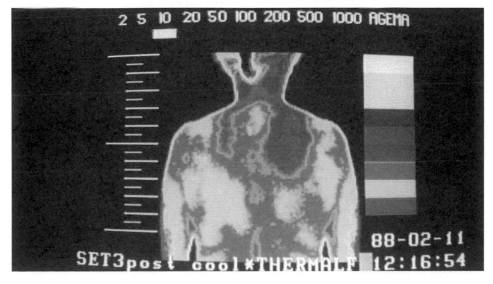

Figure 21.12. An IRT scan showing focal hot spots consistent with myofascial trigger points.

outlet syndrome due to neurovascular compression under the pectoralis minor tendon (45). Thermal asymmetry will be observed in the lower cervical neurologic levels of C8/T1 due to irritation of the medial cord of the brachial plexus.

UPPER EXTREMITY: THORACIC OUTLET SYNDROME

Thoracic outlet syndrome, which is a common syndrome in swimmers, can be due to several factors including the presence of a cervical rib, anterior scalene spasm, costoclavicular compression, and pectoralis minor tendon/spasm and trigger points. Compression of the neurovascular bundle can cause pain and numbness into the extremity in a C8/T1 distribution (Fig. 21.13). IRT can add to the clinical examination and radiographs in helping the treating physician to make an accurate diagnosis. Pavot and Ignacio documented good sensitivity and reliability for thermographic imaging in their study of patients with thoracic outlet syndrome (45). IRT may be used in stress views by raising the patient's arms overhead in hyperabduction stress and studying thermal changes in real time. If thoracic outlet syndrome is present, the hyperabduction stress will reveal a thermal change in the forearm and hand due to compression in the stress position.

FACIAL/CEPHALIC STUDIES

Temporomandibular Joint Syndrome

Temporomandibular joint syndrome (TMJ) is common in athletes and has been documented to affect athletic performance. Numerous studies have been performed on the sensitivity and specificity of IRT for the diagnosis and management of TMJ (46–49). Weinstein published a thermographic protocol that has become the standard in TMJ thermography (46, 47). All TMJ studies should be performed at a 0.5° sensitivity and must include the anterior face and right/left lateral face. It should also include anterior cervical, posterior cervical, and interscapular trigger point studies. A positive finding should encompass a 1.0°C temperature differential from right to left homologous parts. Weinstein has stated that IRT has high sensitivity and reliability in the diagnosis of TMJ syndrome.

Steed has stated that liquid crystal thermography is invaluable in the diagnosis and management of TMJ syndrome (48).

IRT will reveal focal hyperthermia over the involved TMJ and focal hyperthermia over any existing trigger points in the masseter and temporalis muscles (Fig 21.14) (46–49).

Cephalgia

Headaches can be due to cervical spine disorders, muscle tension, vascular disorders, trigger points, TMJ syndrome, hypertension, brain tumors, metabolic disorders, and other causes. Thermography can be useful in the differential diagnosis of headaches because there are different patterns for TMJ, migraine, cluster, and tension headaches as well as carotid stenosis.

Migraine headaches yield a pattern of focal hyperthermia over the inner canthus of the eye and a "cold patch" over the supraorbital region (50). Cluster headaches reveal a "Chai pattern" of ipsilateral hyperthermia on the IRT scan (51). TMJ

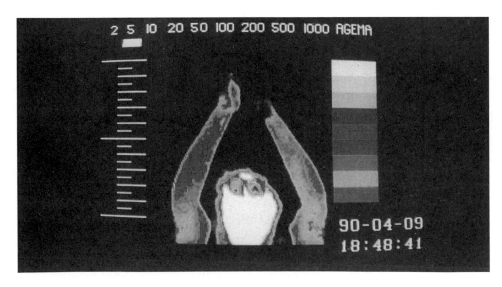

Figure 21.13. An IRT scan of the upper extremity in the overhead stress position revealing C8 nerve irritation secondary to thoracic outlet syndrome.

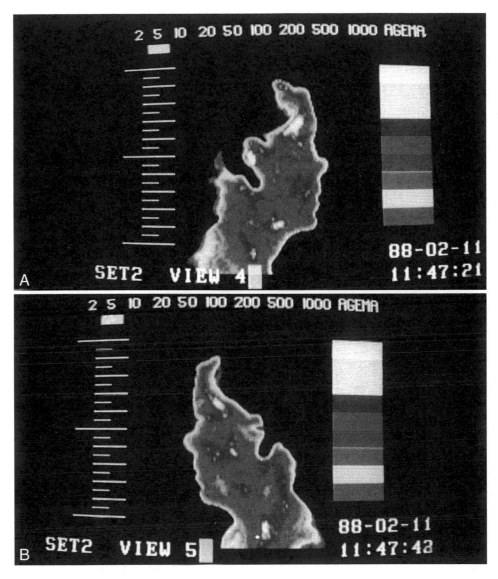

Figure 21.14. A. and B. Facial IRT scan compatible with TMJ syndrome. Note focal hyperthermia over the TMJ and blush hyperthermia over the temporalis muscle.

syndrome reveals a focal hyperthermia over the involved TMJ and a blush hyperthermia over the temporalis region (46–49). Cervicogenic headache will typically reveal focal hyperthermia over the facet joint of the offending segmental motor unit with no facial asymmetry. Myofascial trigger point headaches from trigger points of muscles, including the trapezius, levator scapulae, and sternocleidomastoid (SCM), will reveal focal hyperthermia over the cutaneous region of the involved trigger point. In cases of carotid stenosis (i.e., internal carotid), there will be a characteristic thermal asymmetry over the forehead often called the Flame of Capistrand (11, 16, 52). In terms of clinical management, the IRT scan will be useful to the treating physician by helping with the differential diagnosis.

SPINE IMAGING

Athletes will be prone to cervical, thoracic, and lumbar spinal injuries. In contact sports such as football, cervical spine injuries will be common and will include sprains/strains, facet syndrome, myofascial syndromes, and disc injuries. IRT is helpful in the differential diagnosis of these disorders.

Facet syndrome will reveal a focal hyperthermia over the region and level of the involved facet joint (Fig. 21.15) (53–55). Typically, there are no asymmetric findings in the lower extremity. However, if these findings are present, they are patchy and inconsistent. This may be reflective of thermal instability due to c-nociception from mechanoreceptors and proprioceptors in the joint capsule. In a study by the author, IRT was shown to provide consistent findings in the diagnosis of lumbar facet syndrome (53).

The thermal findings in facet syndrome cases will be unlike those in radiculopathy or disc syndrome cases. Disc protrusions, whether by direct nerve root compression or irritation of the sinuvertebral nerve in the anulus, will cause thermal asymmetry in the lower extremity dermatome/thermatomes (15). In direct nerve root compression, a dermatomal pattern will typically be seen (i.e., an L5/S1 disc herniation causing a purely S1 pattern). In cases of vertebrogenic disc herniation with no direct root compression, there will be c-nociception from mechanical distention of the anulus and c-nociception from chemoreceptors due to the release of proinflammatory enzymes (VIP PLA 2, etc.) (56, 57). As opposed to showing a dermatomal pattern with thermal asymmetry in only one dermatomal region, the thermal asymmetry will appear across two to three dermatomes in an autonomic pattern (Fig. 21.16). In studies published by the author, IRT was shown to be useful in the diagnosis of nerve dysfunction in both cervical and lumbar disc herniations (58, 59). IRT has also been shown to be a useful diagnostic tool in measuring the efficacy of chiropractic treatment for cervical and lumbar disc herniations (58–60).

Disc and facet conditions are problems that can be encountered in clinical sports practice. They can be seen in all sports, including running. IRT will display a different pattern for facet syndrome cases and disc/radiculopathy cases (Figs. 21.15 and 21.16).

Myofascial trigger points syndromes of the lower extremity can often present symptomati-

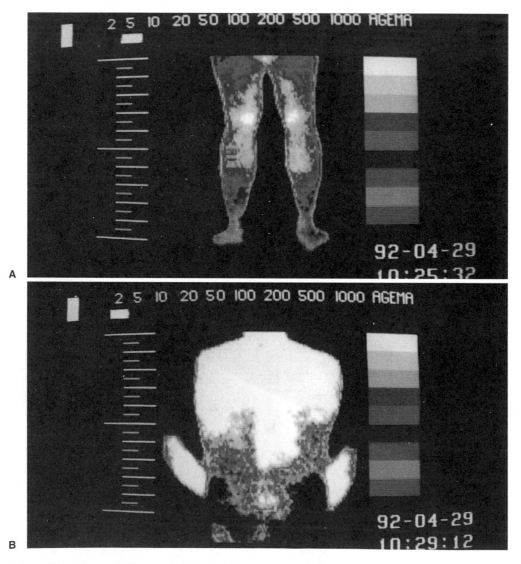

Figure 21.15. A and B. IRT scan displaying focal hot spots over the facet joint in a case of lumbar facet syndrome.

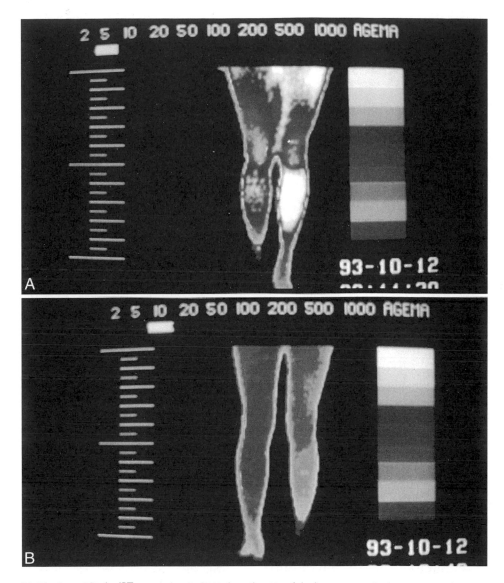

Figure 21.16. A and B. An IRT composite displaying hypothermia of the lower extremity in an autonomic pattern crossing multiple dermatomes secondary to lumbar disc herniation.

cally and clinically like a facet syndrome or chronic disc syndrome. IRT will clearly show trigger points at the involved muscle. Typical trigger points seen can include the quadratus lumborum, gluteus minimus/medius, piriformis, psoas, and gluteus maximus. These trigger points can be involved alone or in conjunction with a facet syndrome, sacroiliac syndrome, or disc syndrome. Therefore, IRT is helpful in identifying all involved causes for the patient's pain and discomfort so the clinician can address each one.

Sacroiliac syndrome has been documented by Diakow as an area of hyperthermia over the involved sacroiliac (61). Diakow documented that IRT was dynamic; after a trial of chiropractic sacroiliac adjustments, the hyperthermic finding reverted to normal.

THERMOGRAPHY AS A PROGNOSTIC TOOL

Thermal imaging can be useful as a prognostic tool. In most cases of acute sprain, swelling and inflammation are routinely seen clinically on observation and palpation. Occasionally a great deal of pain at the sprained joint is not proportional to the observed swelling or injury. If no thermal asymmetry (isothermia) is seen on IRT, the patient will generally heal quickly and return to competition within 1 to 2 weeks. However, if a diffuse global hypothermia is evident at the joint, as well as above and below the joint involved, one can expect a prolonged recovery. For reasons poorly understood at this time, the sympathetic nervous system at the region involved is hypersensitized and causes a violent cutaneous vasoconstriction in the area. This seems to impair healing and is reflective of RSD or sympathetically maintained pain.

THERMOGRAPHY AS A TREATMENT ASSESSMENT TOOL

As a treatment assessment tool, thermography can be useful to assure that the care given for a sports injury is helping the patient (58–61). It can also help the physician detect secondary problems that may develop during the evolution of the injury, such as compensatory reactions with respect to biomechanics and myofascial disorders. IRT is also useful because the athlete's pain will often diminish, but the underlying pathologic condition has not completely healed. A premature cessation of therapy and rehabilitation with a return to full competition and participation may result in reinjury or worse injury of the afflicted area. IRT is thus an objective tool to help the patient understand why continuing care is necessary. The author and others have documented IRT to be an effective treatment assessment tool in sports injuries, including chiropractic management of facet joint and disc disorders (58–62).

THERMOGRAPHY AS A RISK ASSESSMENT TOOL

Thermography may be used as a screening tool for preseason testing. The author has used IRT to detect subclinical problems or problems the athletes have become accustomed to over time and pay little or no attention to. These small or subclinical problems during the course of a vigorous season and/or practices can often become full-blown clinical sports injuries. For example, a high school football team with 24 players was screened with IRT. The knee region overlying the patella was found to be asymmetrical in 75% of players. This IRT finding has been shown to be characteristic of patellofemoral dysfunction. It is postulated that these players are predisposed to future clinical patellofemoral dysfunction. On examination, 65% had crepitus and positive orthopedic testing. By having this type of information, strengthening programs, exercises, and supportive devices may be used to prevent injury and lost time during the season. It will also allow the athlete to compete at optimal levels of performance. We have also screened baseball teams and were able to identify clinical and subclinical problems with the shoulder, elbow, and lumbar and cervical spine and then help institute corrective measures and strengthening before a full-blown in-

jury occurred during the season, causing the athlete to have "down time."

CONCLUSION

Infrared thermal imaging is an invaluable aid for the diagnosis and clinical management of sports injuries. It adds an important dimension to sports practice with noninvasive, neurophysiologic information about the athlete's condition. Although thermography equipment is costly and not within the budgets of all physicians, thermography laboratories and certified thermographers are available in all major suburban and urban areas. The sports-oriented practice and practitioner should incorporate the use of thermography in the referral network and make use of this invaluable diagnostic tool. Thermography's largest and most valuable contribution is in the identification of RSD.

References

1. Uematsu S, Edwin DH, Jankin WR, et al. Quantification of thermal asymmetry: part I. normal values and reproducibility. J Neurosurg 1988;69:552–555.
2. Goodman PH, Murphy MG, Siltanese G. Normal temperature asymmetry of the back and extremities by computer assisted infra-red imaging. Thermology 1986;1:195–202.
3. So YT, Arminoff MJ, Olney RK. Thermography in the evaluation of lumbosacral radiculopathy. Neurology 1989;39:1154–1158.
4. Feldman F, Nickoloff E. Normal thermographic standard in the cervical spine and upper extremities. Skeletal Radiol 1984;12:235–249.
5. Hobbins WB. Basic concepts of thermology and its application in the study of the sympathetic nervous system. Second Albert Memorial symposium, Washington, DC. 1986.
6. Hobbins WB. Thermography and pain. In: Gauthrie M, ed. Biomedical thermology. New York: Alan R. Liss, 1982:361–375.
7. Kellgren JH. On the distribution of pain arising from deep somatic structures with charts of segmental pain. Clin Sci 1939;4:35–36.
8. Head S. Brain 1893;4:1–158.
9. Richter CP. Nervous control of electrical resistance of the skin. Bulletin of John Hopkins University 1929;45:56–74.
10. McCall J. Induced pain referral from posterior lumbar elements in normal subjects. Spine 1979;4:441–446.
11. Mooney W, Robertson J. The facet syndrome. Clin Orthop 1976;115:149–156.
12. Travell JG, Simons DG. Myofascial pain dysfunction. In: The trigger point manual. Baltimore: Williams & Wilkins, 1980.
13. Jinkins JR, Whittemore AR. The anatomic basis of vertebrogenic pain and the autonomic syndrome associated with lumbar disc extrusion. AJR 1989;512:1277–1289.
14. Kruse R, Silber J. Thermographic imaging of myofascial trigger points. Am J Chiropractic Med 1990;3:67–70.
15. BenEliyahu DJ. Infrared thermography in the diagnosis and management of sports injuries. Chiro Sports Med 1990;4:46–53.
16. Christiansen J, Gerow G. Thermography. Baltimore: Williams & Wilkins, 1990.
17. Davidson JW, Bass AL. Thermography and patellofemoral pain. Acta Thermograph 1979;4:98–103.
18. Perelman RB, Adler D. Electronic thermography of the knee. J Acad Neuromusc Thermogr 1989;1:89–92.

19. Devereaux MD, Parr GR. Thermographic diagnosis in athletes with patellofemoral arthralgia. J Bone Joint Surg 1986;688:42–44.
20. BenEliyahu DJ. Infra-red thermographic imaging in the detection of sympathetic dysfunction in patients with patellofemoral syndrome. J Manipulative Physiol Ther 1992;15:57–63.
21. BenEliyahu DJ. Conservative chiropractic management of patellofemoral pain syndrome: clinical case study. Chiro Sports Med 1992;6:57–63.
22. Uematsu S, Hendler N, Hungerford D. Thermography and electromyography in the differential diagnosis of chronic pain syndrome and reflex sympathetic dystrophy. Elect Clin Neurophys 1981;21:165–182.
23. Lewis R, Racz G, Fabian G. Therapeutic approaches to reflex sympathetic dystrophy of the upper extremity. Clin Issues in Regional Anesthesia 1984;19:12–14.
24. Hobbins WB. Thermography and sports medicine. In: Appenzeller O, ed. Sports medicine. 3rd ed. Urban & Schwarzenberg, 1988:395.
25. AMA Council on Scientific Affairs Report. Thermography in neurological and musculo-skeletal conditions. Chicago: AMA Council on Scientific Affairs Report, 1987.
26. Policy Statement on Thermography. American Academy of Physical Medicine and Rehabilitation, 1991.
27. ACA Council on Diagnostic Imaging. Policy Statement. Arlington, VA, 1988.
28. BenEliyahu DJ. Infra-red thermography in the diagnosis and management of sports injuries: a clinical study and literature review. Chiro Sports Med 1990;4:46–53.
29. Schmitt M, Guillot Y. Thermography and muscular injuries in sports medicine. In: Ring EFJ, Phillips B, eds. Recent advances in medical thermology. New York: Plenum Press, 439–455.
30. Pochachevsky R. Thermography in post-traumatic pain. Am J Sports Med 1987;15:243–249.
31. Goodman PH, Heasley MW, Pagliano JW. Stress fractures: diagnosis by computer assisted thermography. Phys Sports Med 1985;13:114–131.
32. Devereaux MD, Graham RP, Lachman SM. The diagnosis of stress fractures in athletes. Phys Sports Med 1987;52:531–533.
33. Dudley WN. Thermography: tracking nerve traps. J Chiro 1987;21:63–65.
34. Chapman G. Clinical thermography, diagnostic manual. Chula Vista, CA: CTA Publishers, 1984;3.
35. Santilli G. Achilles tendinopathy and paratendinopathy. J Sports Med 1979;19:245–259.
36. Maultsby JA. Thermography and the shoulder impingement syndrome. J Acad Neuromusc Thermogr 1989;1:52–53.
37. Lelik F, Kezy G. Contact thermography in sports medicine. Acta Thermograph 1984;27;14–17.
38. Shilo R, Engel J. Thermography as a diagnostic aid in tennis elbow. Hand Surgery 1976;8:101.
39. Binder AL, Parr G. A clinical and thermographic study of lateral epicondylitis. Br J Rheum 1983;22:77–81.
40. Travell, Simons JG, Simons DG. Myofascial pain and dysfunction. Postgrad Med 1983;73:81–108.
41. Christiansen J, Kruse R. Thermographic evaluation of a chronic rotator cuff. Myofasc Trigger Point Chiro 1990;6:34–36.
42. BenEliyahu DJ. Thermography in clinical practice. JACA 1989;26:59–71.
43. Diakow P. Thermographic imaging of myofascial trigger points. J Manipulative Physiol Ther 1988;11:114–117.
44. Fischers AA. Documentation of myofascial trigger points. Arch Phys Med Rehabil 1988;69:286–291.
45. Pavot AP, Ignacio DR. Infra-red imaging in the diagnosis of thoracic outlet syndrome. Thermology 1986;1:142–145.
46. Weinstein SA. Facial thermography, basis, protocol and clinical value. Cranio 1991;9:201–209.
47. Weinstein SA, Gelb M. Thermophysiologic anthropometry of the face in Homo sapiens. Cranio 1990;8:252–257.
48. Steed PA. Utilization of contact liquid crystal thermography in the evaluation of temporomandibular dysfunction. J Craniomandib Pract 1991;9:120–129.
49. Chapman G. TMJ imaging and thermal imaging. J Chiro Products 1988:98–101.
50. Swerdlow B, Dieter JN. Validity of the vascular cold patch in the diagnosis of headache. Headache 1986;26:22–26.
51. Kudrow L. A distinctive facial thermographic pattern in cluster headache: the chai sign. Headache 1985;25:33–36.
52. BenEliyahu DJ. Clinical utility of thermography. Chiropractic 1989;1:9–16.
53. BenEliyahu DJ, Duke SG. Pathoneurophysiology assessed by infra-red thermography in patients with lumbar facet syndrome. J Chiro Res Clin Invest 1991;8:3–9.
54. McFadden J. Thermography used to diagnose facet syndrome. J Neurol Orthop Surg 1983;4:354–355.
55. Leary PC, Christian CR. Diagnostic thermography in low back pain syndromes. Clin J Pain 1985;1:4–13.
56. Weinstein JN. Recent advances in the neurophysiology of pain. Phys Med Rehabil 1990;4:201–212.
57. Saal JS. The role of inflammation in lumbar pain. Phys Med Rehabil 1989;4:191–196.
58. BenEliyahu DJ. Infra-red thermographic assessment of chiropractic treatment in patients with lumbar disc herniations: an observational study. Chiro Tech 1991;3:123–133.
59. BenEliyahu DJ. Infra-red thermographic assessment on the efficacy of chiropractic treatment for MRI documented cervical disc herniations: a clinical study. J Manipulative Physiol Ther 1991;14:337.
60. BenEliyahu DJ. Chiropractic management and manipulative therapy for MRI documented of cervical disc herniation. J Manipulative Physiol Ther 1994;17:177–185.
61. Diakow PR. Thermographic assessment of sacroiliac syndrome. J Can Chiro Assoc 1990;34:131–134.
62. Giani E, Rochi L, Tavoni A. Telethermographic evaluation of NSAID's in the treatment of sports injuries. Med Sci Sport Exerc 1989;21:1–10.

Strength and Conditioning

Michael Leahy

Strength and conditioning should be an integral part of an athlete's training. When properly implemented, such programs can improve performance and enable the athlete to tolerate the stresses of training and competition in a better manner. This chapter reviews the rationale behind such programs and provides guidelines for their design and use. Many of the programs described are being used at the United States Air Force Academy. All terms are defined in Table 22.1.

Goals of a conditioning program include improved strength, flexibility, cardiovascular and cardiorespiratory capability, and improved performance. Conditioning can also be a goal in itself.

When designing a conditioning program, limitations (or "weak links") must be considered. When problems in biomechanics or the mechanics of sports performance are identified, the individual muscle or muscle groups that lack sufficient strength or function can be isolated. These should be trained first. The muscles that support the joints during activity should be tested and specifically strengthened to improve stability. The training of these two groups will provide the base on which to build overall strength and to prevent injury.

PROGRAM TYPES

Competitive Weight Lifting

There are two forms of competitive weight lifting: Olympic lifting and power lifting. An Olympic-style lifter will perform the snatch and the clean and jerk. The power lifter will perform the bench press, dead lift, and squat. Olympic lifts require a greater development of speed, flexibility, and agility. Elite athletes in this category produce some of the highest power outputs of any athletes (2).

The snatch (Fig. 22.1) is performed in a single, uninterrupted motion. Using a wide grip with the arms straight, the athlete lifts the barbell from a position in front of the legs to one above the head. The clean and jerk (Fig. 22.2) involves two movements. In the first, the athlete lifts the bar from the floor to the shoulders; in the second, the athlete lifts the barbell overhead to extended arms.

Injuries in Olympic lifting include fractures, dislocation at the elbow, tendinitis, meniscal tears, lumbar sprain/strain, and quadriceps or patellar tendon rupture (3). Rotator cuff problems will quickly become evident in these overhead lifts, especially those involving the subscapularis, as this inhibits complete external rotation of the humerus required in the final position. As evident in Figure 22.3, the "split snatch" results in less extension and external rotation of the shoulder and consequently causes fewer shoulder disorders. It should be recommended to lifters with shoulder problems. Young lifters may also avulse the distal radial epiphysis as the weight is caught with the arms and chest (3).

The power lifter performs the deadlift (Fig. 22.4) by rising to a standing position, holding the barbell with a one overhand/one underhand grip. This grip prevents the barbell from rolling out off the fingers. Weights have exceeded 900 pounds. Biceps tendon rupture is common, as are patellar tracking disorders from knee wraps. The bench press (Fig. 22.5) is a popular exercise, but one that often leads to shoulder injury when weight is added too abruptly. The subscapularis and pectoralis major are the commonly injured muscles in this exercise. In the squat (Fig. 22.6), the bar is held on the shoulders and the knees bent to more than 90°. Care must be taken to avoid extension of the lumbar spine, as this can cause facet jamming.

WEIGHT LIFTER'S BLACKOUT

Many lifters will hyperventilate before a lift. This can cause reduced cerebral oxygen supply. Intrathoracic pressure has been shown to increase during a lift. Increases in intratruncal pressure aid in support of the spine during a lift, but this pressure reduces venous return to the heart, which reduces stroke volume. During the lifting phase, the heart size becomes greatly reduced; at the end of the clean phase of the clean and jerk, the lifter will catch his breath, causing intrathoracic pressure to drop. Arterial pressure falls to as low as 50 mm Hg, the splanchnic vessels and great veins fill, and stroke volume decreases for up to four beats (4). The lifter then faints from cerebral ischemia. To avoid this sequence, the lifter should not hyperventilate, should be brief in the squat position, lift quickly, and resume normal breathing.

Body Building

Body building is popular as a fitness regimen and as a sport. Much is written in the lay literature about

Table 22.1. Definitions of Terms Used in This Chapter

Term	Definition
Absolute strength	The maximum force an athlete can produce regardless of body weight (1).
Relative strength	The maximum force an athlete can produce relative to body weight, expressed as "strength per kilo of body weight" (1).
Optimal strength	Strength needed to benefit performance above which there is no gain in performance (1).
Power	The amount of force produced per unit of time (1).
Aerobic training	Exercise in which the oxygen transport mechanisms are trained.
Anaerobic threshold	Minimum exercise intensity at which oxygen debt begins to occur. Also known as lactate threshold.
Cross training	Training in more than one discipline when designed to support overall fitness or athletic fitness synergistically.

special techniques for set/repetition schemes. Evidence shows that the number of muscle fibers does not seem to change with exercise, but increases in power and force attainable do vary with set/rep schemes (5). Muscle size (or hypertrophy), symmetry, and definition are the goals of the body builder and these are less quantifiable (6). Consistency of effort, completeness, and variability of program design aid in achieving these goals. Injuries can occur when one exercise is given a disproportionate share of attention, causing imbalances. It is common to see chest and internal rotators of the shoulders developed before the back and external rotators, thus causing posture and shoulder disorders.

Exercises in body building are numerous, and these athletes become adept at isolating muscles. Speed and agility are usually exceptional with these athletes. Cardiorespiratory fitness is usually limited, and the effects of severe diet changes before competition are negative aspects of the sport. The adverse effects of anabolic steroid use should be made known to all body builders because the pressure to use them is common (6).

Circuit Training

Weight training can be adapted to provide an increased cardiovascular component. In traditional circuit training programs, a series of weight exercises are organized under a timed format. Typically, 2 minutes are allotted for the completion of an exercise station, and a 20-second rest is allowed as the athlete changes stations. This pro-

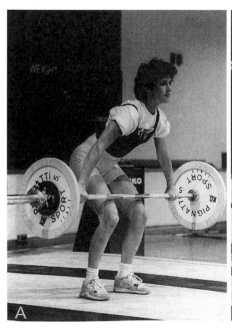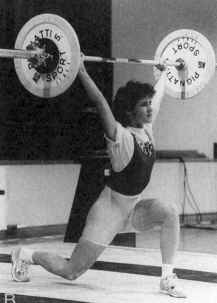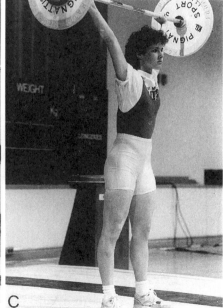

Figure 22.1. The snatch.

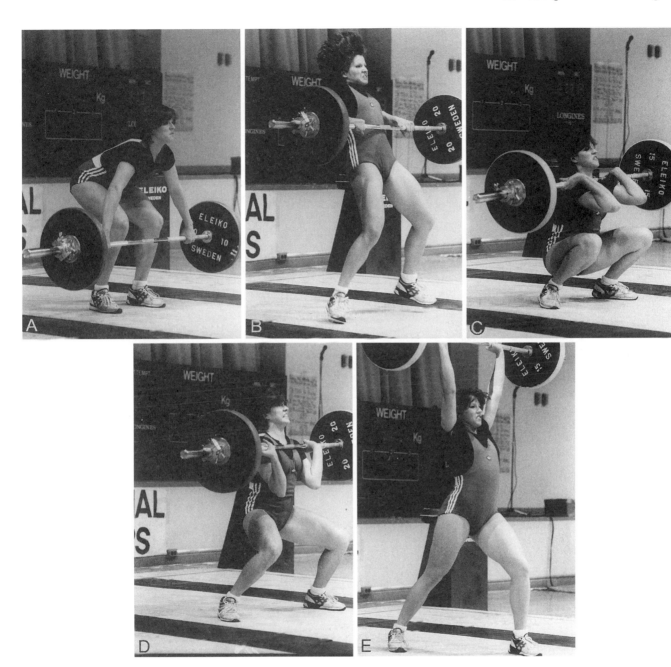

Figure 22.2. The clean and jerk.

tocol keeps the heart rate near the level dictated by the exercises. It also allows for maximum use of equipment during the session.

Plyometrics

Plyometrics is a form of exercise that links strength with speed to produce dynamic movement. When properly administered, plyometric training enables athletes to run faster, jump higher, react more quickly, and produce greater muscular power (7). Because of the many misunderstandings concerning this form of training and the high potential for injury with improper

program design and execution, a more in-depth description of this type of training is offered.

A plyometric contraction is characterized by a rapid stretching of muscles immediately followed by a dynamic shortening of those muscles. Chu offers the following explanation of how plyometrics work:

A plyometric exercise is an exercise in which the athlete utilizes the force of gravity to store energy within the muscular framework of the body. The storing of energy is then immediately followed by an equal and opposite reaction, using the natural elastic tendencies of the muscle to produce a kinetic energy system (8).

A plyometric contraction can be compared with the action of a spring. A spring reacts to compression (eccentric work) by producing a dynamic response (concentric work) on the release of that compression. Although often associated with jumping exercises, any movement that involves this dynamic "stretch/shortening cycle" can be classified as plyometric. A push-up can be considered a plyometric activity. Most techniques in sports involve some form of plyometric activity.

PRECAUTIONS

An athlete can become injured performing plyometrics by underestimating the intensity of the exercises, thus exceeding standard recommendations of work. Many plyometric drills seem so easy that the athlete does not feel that the work performed is significant. However, plyometrics can place considerable stress on the musculoskeletal system, so training must be carefully planned and monitored.

Poor technique, inappropriate landing surfaces, and shoes with inadequate support (most lower body plyometrics should never be performed in bare feet) are several factors that increase the likelihood of becoming injured from plyometrics. Because of the complexity of many plyometric exercises, personal instruction or use of video tapes demonstrating this form of training is recommended over printed material.

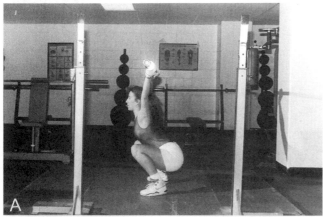

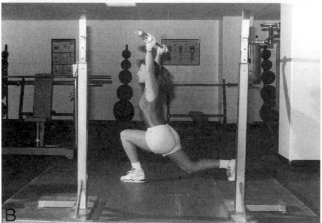

Figure 22.3. A. Regular snatch. **B.** Split snatch.

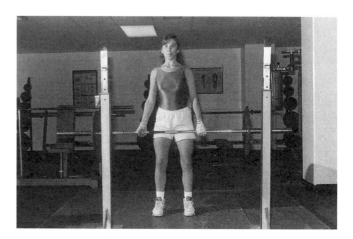

Figure 22.4. Dead lift finishing position.

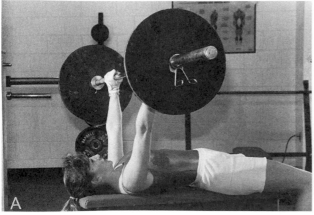 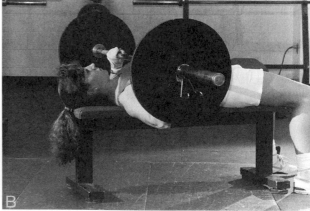

Figure 22.5. Bench press.

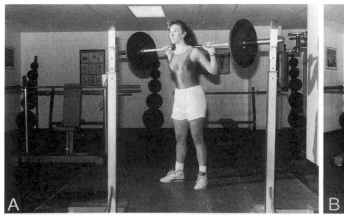

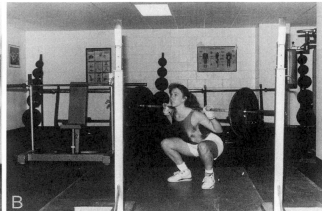

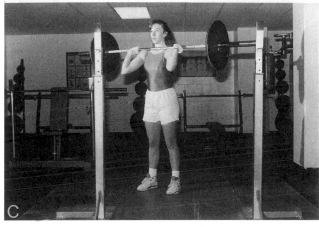

Figure 22.6. Squat and front squat.

Because it increases the stress tolerance of the connective tissues, weight training should be an integral part of a plyometric program. Some coaches from Eastern Bloc countries believe that athletes should be able to squat one and a half times their body weight before performing high-stress plyometrics, such as the intense in-depth jumps that require the athlete to step off platforms from various heights (7).

Another popular test to determine whether athletes are ready for advanced plyometric training is to have them attempt to perform five squats with 60% of body weight within 5 seconds. This protocol measures an athlete's eccentric strength. Regardless of the method used, it is important to realize that a strength base is a necessary component of plyometric training.

An athlete's body type must also be taken into consideration when designing plyometric workouts. Heavier athletes should avoid higher intensity plyometrics because these athletes must overcome greater stress levels associated with their higher body mass during these types of exercises.

The nature of the sport an athlete is training for should also be taken into consideration when designing plyometric programs. For example, a basketball player may need to discontinue all lower body plyometrics during the season. That person may not be able to handle the added stress of playing on hardwood court surfaces without developing overuse injuries.

An athlete's medical history should also be reviewed when designing a plyometric program. An athlete with a history of knee and ankle injuries may need to avoid many plyometric exercises for the lower extremities until the condition improves.

METHODS

Many plyometric exercises require no equipment, and equipment for special exercises is usually simple to make or inexpensive (such as medicine balls and jumping boxes). When building plyometric boxes, the landing surfaces should be large enough to provide stability. Padding to help minimize the shock of landing, prevent slipping, and reduce the risk of bruises is also desirable.

Medicine balls, which can be used for upper body plyometrics, are traditionally made of soft leather and are available in a variety of weights and shapes. An alternative is a soft, loosely packed ball that bounces only slightly. Because these balls are soft, they are easier to catch and will not jam the fingers. Rubber medicine balls that rebound on impact are also available to increase variety of exercises. Athletes and coaches on a tight budget should consider making their own medicine balls with sturdy tape, a used soccer or volleyball, and some loose material for filling.

EXERCISE SELECTION

Lower body plyometrics are commonly classified into three major categories: jumps, bounds, and hops (7). Jumps are vertical leaps for height, whereas bounds are horizontal leaps for distance. Hops are a specific type of bound with an emphasis on maximum foot speed.

Upper body plyometrics performed with medicine balls are commonly classified as either swings or throws (7). Throws involve releasing the ball, whereas swings do not. As with jumps, hops, and bounds, explosiveness is the key to achieving the desired results.

When selecting plyometric exercises, the concept of "specificity of training" must be addressed. In other words, to attain the most benefit from training, the exercises performed must closely approximate the speed and technique of the movements that occur in the activity that one is trying to master.

TECHNIQUE

Plyometrics can improve basic athletic skills, but best results occur only if each repetition of every exercise is performed with explosiveness. Plyometric workouts must therefore be brief, with seldom more than 15 minutes devoted to lower extremity exercises. Longer training sessions will reduce the quality of the workout and increase the risk of injury. Also, plyometrics should be performed at the start of the workout when the athlete is fresh, or at least immediately after sports-specific training.

PROGRESSION

One popular method for planning lower body plyometric training is to regulate the number of foot contacts during each workout. A young or novice athlete may be able to tolerate only 50 foot contacts per workout in certain exercises, whereas an advanced athlete may perform 200 or more in those exercises.

The intensity of a lower body workout can be increased with weighted vests, higher boxes, more difficult exercises, and more repetitions. An off-season plyometric program might start with jumps on low boxes and double-leg bounds and progress to taller boxes and single-leg bounds.

With medicine ball workouts, training can be regulated by the number of throws or swings. Intensity can be increased with heavier balls, more difficult exercises, more repetitions, greater distances, or faster swings. As a general rule, athletes can tolerate more repetitions in upper body plyometric exercises than in lower body exercises.

The exercise textbook by Stone and O'Bryant (6) offers an excellent review of the types of plyometric exercises. Also included is a rating system that accesses the intensity level of these movements.

The intensity of exercise must be taken into consideration when determining the number of repetitions for each exercise. Higher intensity exercises are performed for less repetitions.

REST

Adequate rest is required between sets. For quality training, more rest is necessary between bouts of higher intensity exercises. When performing depth jumps, an exercise technique that can require rest intervals as high as 10 minutes between sets, the athelete can perform an upper body plyometric exercise during the rest periods.

FREQUENCY

Seldom are more than 2 days a week of plyometric training recommended during the offseason. However, many of the lower intensity exercises could be performed daily as part of a warm-up for sports training; many upper body plyometrics can also be performed daily.

SAMPLE PROGRAM

Table 22.2 presents an 8-week program designed to improve vertical jumping ability for basketball and volleyball. Note how the volume (total repetitions) decreases during the program while the intensity (type of exercises used) increases. The height of the jumps must be appropriate for the ability of the athlete.

Table 22.2. Vertical Jump Plyometric Program

	Exercise	Repetitions	Sets
Weeks 1 and 2	Static box jumps	10	6
Weeks 3 and 4	Static box jumps	10	1
	Box jumps	8	5
Weeks 5 and 6	Static box jumps	10	1
	Box jumps	8	1
	Box jumps with step	6	4
Weeks 7 and 8	Static box jumps	10	1
	Box jumps	8	1
	Box jumps with step	6	1
	In-depth jumps	5	3

Running as Conditioning

The type of running training an athlete should perform (aerobic versus anaerobic) depends on the distance for which the athlete is training. Longer races involve more aerobic components, whereas shorter races require a higher contribution of anaerobic work. For example, an 800-meter run requires 33% aerobic contribution and 67% anaerobic. A marathon is 98% aerobic and 2% anaerobic, and a mile is virtually an even split (9).

Although many types of training methods are availiable for running, most can be classified as continuous, interrupted, or competition.

CONTINUOUS RUNNING

This type of training can involve both steady- and uneven-paced workouts. Steady-paced running is primarily aerobic training, with common regimens consisting of either medium-paced runs (2 to 6 miles in anaerobic threshold) or long slow distance runs in the aerobic zone below anaerobic threshold.

INTERRUPTED RUNNING

This type of running consists of repeated runs with periods of rest between each run. This type of training is most often used on tracks. The elements that are varied include the following:

1. Distance
2. Speed
3. Repetition (number of intervals)
4. Rest
5. Recovery methods (complete rest, jog, stride)

There are three types of interrupted running:

1. Interval training
2. Speed-endurance
3. Tempo
   A. Tempo-endurance
   B. Competitive pace running

FARTLEK

Fartlek training, also known as speed play or mixed paced running, is a type of interrupted training involving efforts of long duration in which low-intensity work is interspersed with bouts of high-intensity work or uses varying terrains (hills). Fartlek training is used to improve endurance and increase the athlete's ability to handle the effects of running at faster speeds. For beginners, it is better to have planned workouts because they find it difficult to evaluate their training levels. Conversely, elite athletes find that the less-stringent structure of fartlek running is a welcome break from the more structured intervals.

At the easiest level, the starting pace will be slow (100 to 160 bpm), but the faster speeds will force an oxygen debt by anaerobic workout. This debt will be repaid during the lower intensity phase. This method educates the body to improve its oxygen uptake and speed of recovery.

A sample schedule is as follows: Jog 5 minutes, run fast for 3 minutes, do easy runs interspersed with sprints of 50 meters, do easy running with bouts of runs, jog 5 minutes.

COMPETITION

Competition running includes races or situations with training partners that simulate races. The pace is high to maximum intensity. Opponents are involved to stimulate effort.

Cycling

Training for cycling varies by distance and type of event. On the track, a cyclist will depend more on power than when on the road, where a series of stages may last more than 2 weeks and distances are in excess of 130 miles. Strength training is integral to the track cyclist's program and will include lower extremity exercises to develop maximum absolute strength and power. Workouts on the track are usually of the interval nature and are performed at high percentages of maximum effort. Cadence or revolutions of the pedals per minute are also high in both training and competition. Because of the increased flexion at the hip caused by the low handlebars, the hamstring musculature becomes more important and must be included in a training program.

Weight training is used to a lesser degree in road cycling. Primary training is done on the bike, and there is no substitute for "putting in the miles." Training is often performed by heart rate, with long-distance training done in the neighborhood of 130 to 170 bpm. For hill work, cadence is kept high (85 to 105) and the heart rate will approach or exceed anaerobic threshold. For long climbs, lower back strength is important and should be addressed in a training program.

Cycling programs frequently involve the following techniques.

1. Spinning: riding at higher than normal cadence in an attempt to raise efficiency. Sometimes a fixed gear will be used instead of a freewheel to force a higher cadence.
2. Motor pacing: the rider will follow a vehicle very closely to draft and use a high cadence.

Power output can be much lower than that normally required to maintain speed.

A common muscle imbalance is that the medial quadriceps are comparatively weaker than the lateral, but this can be corrected with strength training. When this imbalance is present, the cyclist will attempt to set the cleats with excessive toe-in position.

Cross Training

With the advent of multisport events such as triathlon and biathlon, the concept of cross training has gained more acceptance. There are distinct advantages to this concept.

1. More complete fitness and conditioning of musculature.
2. Ability to train despite injury (as in swimming with leg strain)
3. Avoidance of psychological overtraining with variety in the type and intensity of workouts.
4. Flexibility of schedules, which allows workouts to fit into crowded schedules.

Examples are weight training for football and cycling for running. The most common form of cross training is the use of weight training for another sport.

EQUIPMENT

Free Weights: Types

The category of free weights includes barbells, dumbbells, kettlebells, swingbells, and accessory equipment such as benches, squat racks, and plate stands. In addition to being less expensive than most machines, free weight equipment allows the athlete to perform a greater variety of exercises and provides more effective work for stabilizing muscles. The primary disadvantage is that spotting is often necessary because weights can fall on the athlete. Because free weights require more balance and skill, it is necessary to begin these programs with lighter weights and more direct supervision than for similar exercises with machines.

All free weight equipment should be sturdy, have a minimum of sharp corners, and where appropriate contain a sufficient amount of firm padding (for benches, approximately 1 inch). A flat bench usually stands approximately 18 inches high and 12 inches wide. For the bench press exercise, the height should be such that the athlete can place the feet flat on the floor without arching the back and wide enough so that the bench does not dig into the athlete's

shoulders. Squat racks should be adjustable or set at a height 2 to 4 inches below shoulder level. Platforms should be at least 8×8 feet, with a smooth surface such as wood. The surface should not be waxed or finished because this can cause improper traction.

Space provided for any equipment must allow the exercise to be performed, mistakes to be made, and room left for safe traffic flow. Several manufacturers have equipment templates that make exercise room layout simpler and safer.

Weight bars should have an efficient device for securing the plates to the bar. An exercise should not be performed without first securing the plates. For standing lifts, "bumper" plates made of rubber will increase safety when the bar is dropped or released.

A weight belt helps the torso muscles compress the gases and fluids in the abdominal cavity to relieve compressive forces on the spine. Most belts are 10 cm wide in back (competition width), and some new designs are also wider in the abdominal area. For better fit, instead of leather belts some use Velcro-type material.

Machines: Types

Guided resistance machines encourage proper form, and their ability to isolate specific muscle groups makes them valuable for specific training and injury rehabilitation. An important advantage that machines have over free weights is safety—the weights cannot drop or fall. Beginners will find this feature especially reassuring because they are learning the techniques of the exercises.

Among the first multistationed machines marketed for mass appeal was the jungle gym, so named because its single cage bases are surrounded by a safari of cables, pulleys, and levers. Jungle gyms are especially popular in high schools and colleges; they are difficult to steal, easy to maintain, and usually contain no loose parts. Additionally, the units are compact, making them ideal for circuit training. Circuit training involves moving from one exercise to another with minimal rest, thus reducing workout time and effectively conditioning the heart and lungs (see Circuit Training).

In 1970, inventor Arthur Jones introduced his Nautilus machines to the fitness community. These single-stationed machines were among the first to use the now popular shell-shaped cams to vary the resistance during the exercise, instead of the circular cams that keep resistance constant. Jones stated that his "variable resistance" machines matched a person's natural strength curves, thereby working the muscles harder and more completely (11).

The first single-stationed exercise machines (Nautilus included) were primarily suited for professional and college-level male athletes, especially football players. Consequently, many women and smaller stature men had trouble adjusting to these machines and handling the large weight increases. But today many equipment companies manufacture adjustable, scaled-down machines that possess smaller weight increments. Other manufacturers of single-stationed machines include Cybex, David, Hydra-Gym, Mini-Gym, Polaris, Paramount, and Universal.

As with all forms of exercise, proper instruction is necessary with machines to decrease the likelihood of injuries and to ensure maximum effectiveness. The natural safety advantages of machines can give the athelete a false sense of security.

A few performance guidelines apply to almost every exercise machine. One should always be positioned in a straight, aligned manner. On machines with adjustable seats and backrests, one will usually need to align the center of the body part being worked with the center of the pulley apparatus.

Regardless of the exercise, twisting or shifting the body during the exercise should be avoided. If a machine has handgrips, they should not be squeezed during the exercise; instead, they should be grasped with a loose, comfortable grip. Any sudden or jerky movements should be avoided. A good rule to remember is that it should take twice as long to lower the weight (eccentric work) as it does to raise it (concentric work). For example, one should lift to the count of three, pause, and lower to the count of six. The reason for this method of training is that momentum may develop in the linkage of the machine and cause the resistance to move the limbs beyond their normal range of motion or at a speed that cannot be controlled safely (12). One-on-one instruction is necessary for the first-time user. Figures 22.7 through 22.10 show proper use of equipment for specific exercises.

The following are some tips and precautions for using specific types of exercise machines.

LOWER BODY MACHINES

Leg Extension

One of the most popular exercise machines, leg (knee) extension machines provide direct resistance to the quadriceps. During the exercise one should sit upright and pause momentarily at the peak contraction. Lowering the bar too fast and "bouncing" out of the starting position reduce the effectiveness of the exercise and subject the knee joint to excessive stress. The feet may be rotated laterally or medially to accentuate the vastus medialis and lateralis, respectively.

Leg Press

Leg press machines take the leg extension exercise one step farther by also involving the muscles of the hip. When using this machine, the weight should be lowered slowly to avoid stretching knee ligaments. Using excessive upper body effort should be avoided because this can increase the stress on the lower back.

Leg Curl

The leg curl strengthens the hamstrings. Hips should be kept flat against the bench throughout the movement. Raising the hips in an effort to lift more weight reduces the range of motion of the hamstrings and places potentially harmful stress on the lower back.

Inner and Outer Thigh

The adductors and abductors are problem muscles for many athletes, and these machines are excellent for developing these areas. To avoid muscle pulls in the groin area, these exercises should be performed in a smooth, controlled manner.

UPPER BODY MACHINES

Seated Press and Other Shoulder Machines

Whether these machines require raising the elbows to the sides or lifting the arms overhead, during this movement there is a tendency to arch the low back, placing great strain on the lumbar spine. A weight-lifting belt will help ensure a proper, stable position.

Pullover

The pullover machine primarily affects the latissimus dorsi muscles. Pullover machines usually come with a seat belt to keep the back flat against the backrest and to hold the hips down during the exercise. Allowing the lower back to arch during the upward portion of this exercise is improper and suggests that the weight is excessive.

Pect Deck

The pectoralis major and minor are trained with this machine. To avoid shoulder injury, it is important not to allow the elbows to move too far posteriorly or at too high a rate.

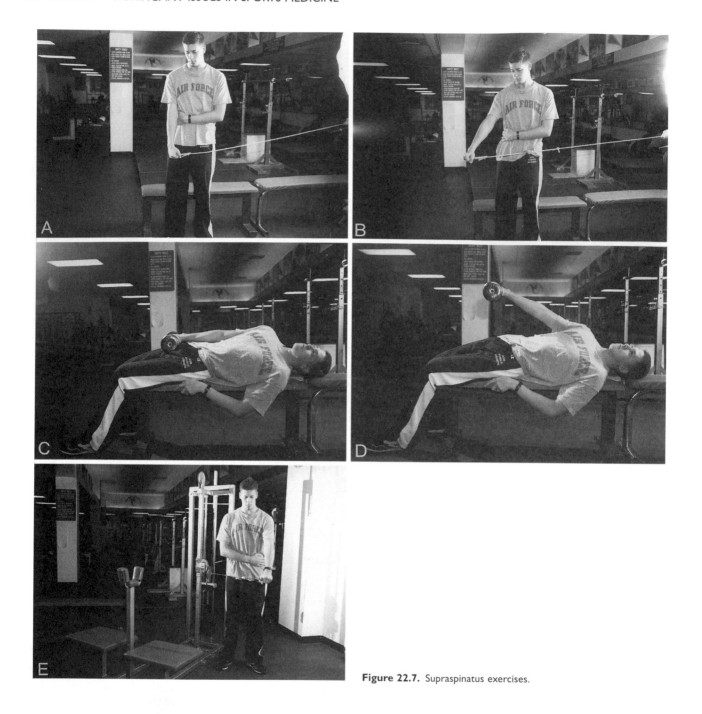

Figure 22.7. Supraspinatus exercises.

Arm Curl and Triceps Extension

The major problem with exercise machines for the arms is that it is difficult to accommodate all statures. Varying the sitting height and hand position and using seat pads are often all that is necessary. Hyperextension of the elbow is a common mistake that the athlete must avoid.

Trunk Curl (Abdominal)

The first abdominal machines required pulling against handles aligned alongside the neck, a design that often limited the amount of weight us-

able in this exercise. The newer machines have bypassed this problem—they are designed so that the force is directed against a large pad that rests across the chest. If lumbar facet problems exist, the feet should not be held in place by any pad or other apparatus. By keeping the feet free, the psoas will not be able to draw the lumbar spine anteriorly.

Common Factors

Weight training exercises can be classified as isolation (single-joint) or compound (multijoint) movements. Both types of exercises can be performed with free weights or machines. By arranging isolation machines in a circuit, it is possible to handle large groups of people efficiently and safely with less space, assets especially popular with physical education and corporate fitness directors. With free weights it takes more time to arrange the equipment and change resistance.

Because they permit proper technique, some exercises should be performed only with free weights. If the joints are allowed to move through their natural range of motion during a weight training exercise, tolerance to stress can be increased. For example, during a bench press the barbell leaves the chest and travels anteriorly and superiorly. During a bench press on a Smith machine, an apparatus that consists of a bar on guided rails, the barbell cannot travel through this natural arc. The machine movement can place an unnatural stress on the shoulder, increasing the risk of injury.

Power, which is expressed mathematically as force (strength) × velocity (speed), may determine what type of muscle fibers are recruited during an exercise (6). With most machines, it is not possible to perform high-power movements to recruit the maximum amount of fast-twitch fibers

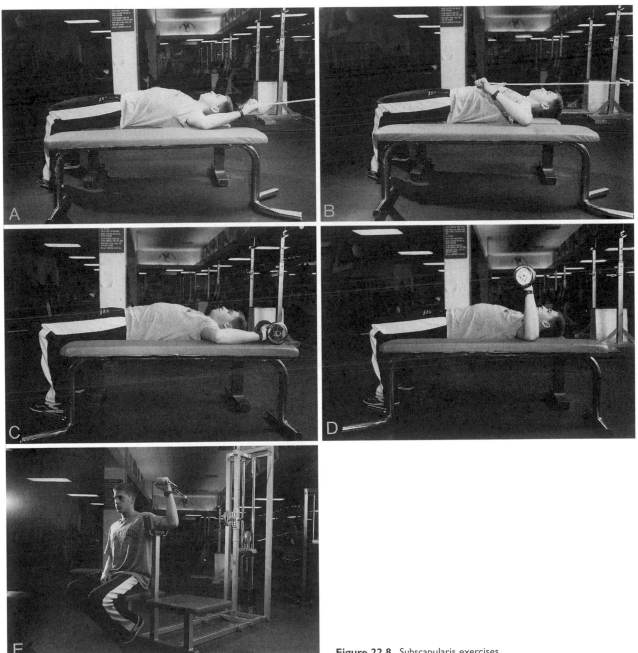

Figure 22.8. Subscapularis exercises.

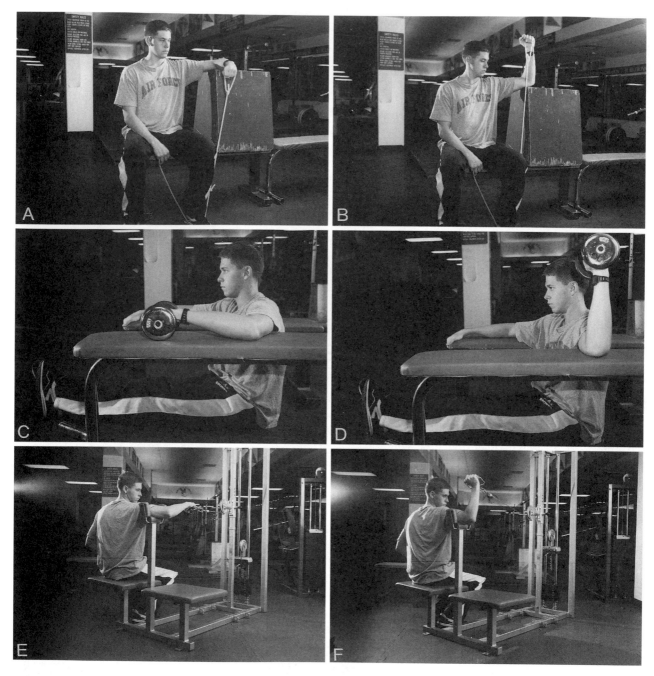

Figure 22.9. Infraspinatus exercises.

because momentum builds up in the linkage mechanism of the machine. This buildup is especially true for machines with variable resistance cams; momentum can become so great that the machine literally moves by itself.

Some machine manufacturers recommend that the first few repetitions of a set be performed slowly to fatigue the muscle to avoid producing momentum. Only then should the weight be moved as fast as possible—a speed that will be relatively slow because the muscles are fatigued— to stress the fast-twitch muscle fibers. A problem

with this method is that the fast-twitch fibers may only be stimulated during the last few repetitions of the set, whereas with free weights every repetition can stimulate the fast-twitch fibers (e.g., clean and jerk) (12). Some also believe that the best method of training muscle fibers of both types is to perform repetitions slowly throughout the exercise session.

Isometric machines have not been popular in recent years, but this is changing due to new evidence of good results in spinal strengthening. The best results in this area are obtained by using several positions along the available range of motion and performing maximum effort isometric contractions at each of these positions. The individual also performs a work capacity activity that requires movement through that range of motion with a variable resistance. True isolation of the spine is the key to success in this case.

Despite much effort to place isokinetic machinery into the strength and conditioning arena, to date most programs do not use them. Some reasons include cost, technical operating characteristics, and injury. There are some hydraulic isokinetic machines that solve the cost and technical

aspects. When the exercise involves the spine, technique becomes important to get good results without injury (squats, leg press).

Other Equipment

TRAMPOLINE

Mini-trampolines can help teach balance and develop strength in muscles that help stabilize the lower extremities (peronei, tibialis, popliteus, gluteus medius, and gluteus minimus). Simple standing, jogging, squatting, and jumping exercises are much more difficult when performed

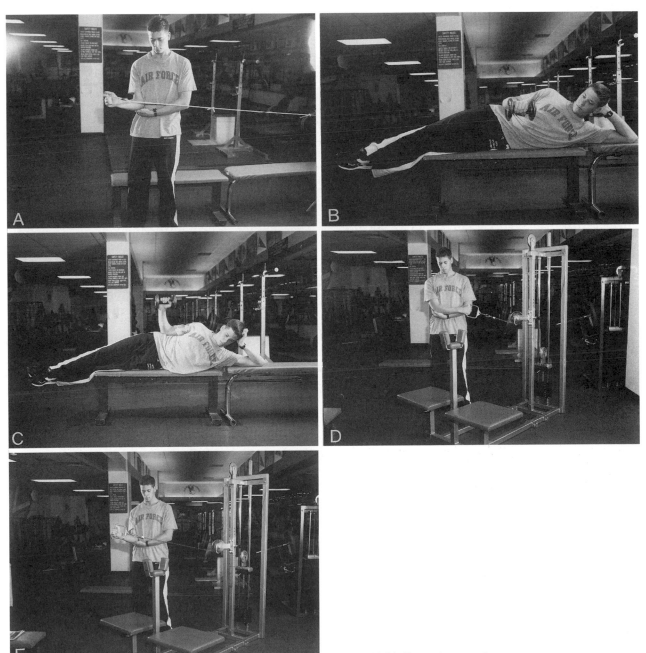

Figure 22.10. Teres minor exercises.

in this manner, but abrupt impact forces are avoided.

Large trampolines are valuable for teaching maintenance of stability in awkward positions. However, in 1976 the American Academy of Pediatrics recommended that this type of equipment be banned in schools because of the number of neck injuries attributed to this type of training (12).

BALANCE BOARDS

Balance boards have been primarily used in elementary schools to teach movement skills and more recently they have also been used in rehabilitation programs. They are made with a platform and a smaller board across an inferior surface so that it tilts when standing alone. Balancing on these boards develops balance and the musculature needed for control.

HEAVY BALLS

Medicine ball training was covered in the plyometric section of this chapter, but it is worth noting that medicine balls can also be used for general strengthening exercises. See Table 22.2 for a sample workout.

TUBING

Surgical tubing is an excellent device for providing resistance in the exact plane of motion of athletic movements. Surgical tubing is made of natural rubber or synthetic substances that offer increased resistance as the tubing stretches. When proper wall thickness and cord length are chosen, the modulus of elasticity will allow proper resistance to be applied to the musculature throughout the range of motion. Advantages include low cost, convenience, portability, and specificity. Exercises can also be performed at maximum speed, a feature often not possible with other equipment. Minimum length should be 4 feet.

PROGRAM DESIGN AND MANAGEMENT

Principles of Training

The first published description of progressive resistance exercise is credited to DeLorme (13). Much has been written concerning the ideal method of training, but no one method provides all the answers. Muscles grow stronger only if they are continually exposed to a variety of exercises, sets, and repetition schemes. Most athletes instill this variety into workouts by following their instincts, but sometimes their instincts fail and much time is lost with poor results.

Designing effective weight training programs for athletes must involve properly manipulating the following variables of training: specificity, volume, intensity, variety, and continuity. The popularity of strength and conditioning programs has often confused many physical educators and coaches, and the demand for more complex individualized programs often leaves them overwhelmed.

Programs are now available that record and analyze data and print sports-specific workouts that are adjusted to an athlete's strength level. Other programs help in body composition and fitness reports.

SPECIFICITY

The "law of specificity" in weight training states that to acquire the most benefit from training, the exercises performed must closely approximate the movements that occur in the sport. This principle also requires that the movement be performed at the same velocity required of the sporting activity. Most training programs can improve athletic ability, but to achieve the highest levels of performance athletes must continually strive to increase the specificity of their workouts (14). This is especially true with more advanced athletes (see Periodization).

Because it is biomechanically similar to a vertical jump, the power clean would be an excellent exercise for volleyball or basketball. Despite being relatively short for their body weight, weight lifters are among the best jumpers of any athletes. Even the Russian weight lifting champion Vasily Alexeev, weighing in excess of 330 pounds, could high jump over 6 feet and was ranked as a Class 1 volleyball player.

In another example, running distances of 4000 meters can improve performance for an athlete specializing in the 5000-meter run because the distance is similar, the pace is nearly the same, and the energy system is primarily aerobic. In contrast, running distances of 100 meters would not be as effective in training this athlete because the pace is much faster and the energy system is primarily anaerobic (without oxygen).

At the Air Force Academy, cadets are continually tested on the 600-yard run and sit-ups, and at one time the 600-yard run was performed within 3 minutes after the sit-ups test. This protocol causes fatigue in the hip flexor (front hip) muscles that help lift the legs during running. Applying the principle of specificity in training, these cadets should perform some running immediately after hip flexor exercises (such as sit-ups or leg raises) to become accustomed to running with fatigue in the hip flexor muscles. This is why triathletes often run immediately after a bike workout.

To select the appropriate weight training exercises for athletes, it is important to understand that lifting affects not only the muscles, but also the nervous system. If athletes perform all the training exercises slowly, they may not develop the speed necessary for their sport.

Olympic-style weight lifting exercises, such as the clean and jerk, are especially valuable in training athletes because more weight can be lifted only with good technique. In many body building exercises, such as the biceps curl, more weight can be lifted with poor technique by swinging the weight up with the back muscles. Unfortunately, this technique reduces the training effect on the biceps and places adverse stress on the spine.

Another important aspect of the specificity principle is that the complex (multijoint) exercises are superior to simple (single-joint) exercises. Performing a few complex exercises (such as the power clean) that will work all the major muscles used in an athlete's event will produce far better results than performing numerous simple exercises for those same muscle groups. This approach also reduces the time that athletes need to spend in the weight room because only a few exercises are needed to work all the major muscle groups.

It is often necessary, however, to isolate a muscle group with simple exercises. Simple exercises can help rehabilitate an injury, correct a muscle imbalance, and strengthen a specific area of the body that endures extreme stress during the sport. For these reasons, many strength coaches often have their swimmers, baseball players, and volleyball players perform rotator cuff (shoulder) exercises; gymnasts perform back extension exercises for the lower back.

VOLUME

Volume is the measure of the amount of work that athletes perform during training. Runners measure training volume by how far they run, javelin throwers by how many times they throw. In the weight room, volume can be measured by the number of repetitions performed. If an athlete can bench press 100 pounds for 3 sets of 10 repetitions, the total volume would be 30 repetitions ($3 \times 10 = 30$); the amount of weight lifted is irrelevant in this formula.

Because the human body is an especially adaptive organism, training volume must be increased gradually at the beginning level to guarantee continual progress. Also, a higher volume of training increases the recovery ability of the athlete. This effect is dramatically illustrated with elite distance runners, who often find it necessary to run in excess of 80 miles per week to progress.

In weight training, the beginner may improve on a program of 200 total repetitions per week. But an advanced athlete may need 2000 or more repetitions per week to see results. One reason why Bulgarian athletes were so competitive in the sport of Olympic-style weight lifting after the 1984 Olympics is that the athletes have been known to train 4 or 5 times a day to achieve the necessary volume of training (15).

Although training volume must be steadily increased throughout an athlete's career, for most sports a maintenance program is recommended during the season. This program is necessary so that the athlete can devote more time and energy to the sport. Two 30-minute workouts per week are usually sufficient during this period to minimize any strength loss (16). However, athletes involved in sports that require a high degree of strength, such as the shot put, must actually train considerably harder with weights during the season.

One of the major problems with weight training programs in the United States is the relatively low training volume used compared with training programs in other countries. Because high-volume training strengthens connective tissues, U.S. athletes tend to suffer more injuries to these areas than athletes from Eastern Bloc countries. In this regard, quantity (volume) is just as important as quality (intensity).

INTENSITY

To ensure continual progress, athletes need to increase steadily both the number of high-intensity lifts in each training cycle and the average amount of weight lifted. If an athlete can lift 100 pounds once in a specific exercise, to get stronger that athlete would have to train with weights approaching 100 pounds (when using low repetitions). If this athlete has never performed workouts that required lifting higher intensity weights, the strength level will stay the same or even decrease.

An exception to this principle of increasing training intensity occurs during in-season training. For most athletes, workout intensity must be decreased dramatically during the season so that more energy can be devoted to the sport. Also, young children and adolescents should not perform high-intensity lifts because of the high risk of developing chronic injury to the skeletal system (17).

VARIETY

A monotonous training program will lead to boredom and create physiologic adaptations that

Table 22.3. Variations in Training

Variation	Sport
Hand paddles	Swimming
Motor pacing	Cycling
Jumps with heavy ball	Basketball, volleyball

will prevent progress (i.e., overtraining) (16). One way to get better at push-ups is simply to perform more push-ups every day. Perhaps a highly motivated athlete can make good progress with this system, but the lack of variety makes it difficult to stick with. A better method would be to perform not just the standard push-ups, but push-ups with different hand spacings and push-ups with the feet or hands elevated.

Variety can also provide improved training results. Altering resistance to a specific sport motion should be considered. Just as a baseball player uses weights on the bat for warm-up swings, this technique can be applied to almost any sport. Runners will use a slightly downhill grade to develop a faster turnover in stride, or an uphill grade to develop strength. Other examples are presented in Table 22.3.

CONTINUITY OF TRAINING

Strength training must be performed on a continual basis or the body will eventually return to its pretraining strength levels. This means that an athlete should perform strength training year-round. If an athlete takes extended layoffs from strength training during the year, it is unlikely that this person will be able to fulfill individual physical potential. This is especially true with elite athletes (18).

Practical Guidelines For Strength Training

REPS AND SETS

Intensity is defined as the difficulty of an athletic activity; it is one of the key variables to consider when designing weight training programs. Runners measure intensity by how fast they run, javelin throwers by how far they throw. In the weight room, intensity is measured by how much weight is lifted because this determines the degree of tension generated by the muscle. It is muscular tension that stimulates the strength training response (16).

The way to measure intensity is to calculate how close a specific resistance is to the maximum amount of weight an individual can lift for one repetition. Using 100 pounds as a 1-repetition maximum (1RM), lifting 95 pounds would be an intensity of 95%.

Intensity is often confused with degree of effort. Lifting 75% of a 1RM for 10 repetitions may seem much harder than lifting 80% of a 1RM for one repetition, but the intensity is lower because the muscular tension is not as great. The reason why less muscular tension occurs with high repetitions sets is because the motor units are fired in sequence, rather than simultaneously (16).

The development of maximum strength is best achieved by using weights that fall between 70% and 100% of an individual's 1RM. For optimal results, an advanced athlete should emphasize higher intensity lifts because the nervous system is more efficient at recruiting motor units. Thus, an advanced athlete can lift higher intensity weights with less muscular tension than an athlete with less training experience (16).

Because it is not possible to perform a great number of repetitions with higher intensity weights, specific guidelines must be followed when planning strength training programs. One formula to determine the relationship between intensity and repetitions (when performed to exhaustion) is as follows: 100% allows one more repetition, 95% allows two repetitions, and each subsequent 2.5% allows one repetition (19). Some muscle groups fatigue at different rates, so the intensity/repetition pattern would be different from the above model (16). For example, because the calves have greater muscular endurance than the biceps, the calves respond better to higher repetitions. Nevertheless, for practical reasons, the above formula provides an excellent model for planning workouts. This formula also allows for the prediction of 1RM after testing for maximum number of repetitions with less than 1 RM weight.

Just as there is a relationship between intensity and repetitions, there is also a relationship between repetitions and sets. In general, the more repetitions performed, the fewer sets are needed to achieve the training effect because with higher repetitions the muscle generates tension for longer periods. See Table 22.4 for one way of determining how many sets to use based on repetitions performed (16).

The above formula does not include warm-up sets. In this regard, more warm-up sets are needed for higher intensity weights. If 8 to 10 repetitions

Table 22.4. Determining Number of Sets

Percentages	Repetitions	Sets Required
100–95	1–2	4 or more
95–90	2–4	3–4
90–85	4–6	3
85–80	6–8	2–3
80–75	8–10	2

Table 22.5. Sample Set/Repetition Schemes

Goal	Method	Repetitions/Sets
Hypertrophy	1	75% × 10r × 5s
(high repetitions)	2	70% × 12r
		80% × 8r × 3s
	3	70% × 12r
		75% × 10r
		80% × 8r
		75% × 10r
		70% × 12r
	4	70% × 12r
		80% × 8r × 2s
		70% × 12r × 2s
Strength	1	70% × 10r
(medium repetitions)		75% × 8r
		80% × 6r × 2s
	2	75% × 8r
		80% × 6r
		85% × 4r × 3s
	3	00% × 8r × 2s
		85% × 6r × 4s
	4	85% × 6r
		90% × 4r × 4s
		85% × 6r
Strength without	1	90% × 3r
hypertrophy		95% × 2r
(low repetitions)		100% × 1r × 3s
	2	85% × 5r
		90% × 3r
		95% × 2r × 3s
	3	85% × 5r
		90% × 3r
		95% × 2r
		100% × 1r × 2s
		90% × 3r
		100% × 1r
		95% × 2r
	4	85% × 3r
		90% × 2r
		95% × 2r
		90% × 2r
		95% × 1r
		100% × 1r
		85% × 4r × 2s

r, repetitions; s, sets.

are performed with lighter weights, only 1 warm-up set will probably be necessary; if 1 to 2 repetitions are performed with heavier weights, additional sets are needed. The goal of warm-up sets is to get ready for the primary weights as quickly as possible with as little fatigue as possible (17).

Although poorly documented, current thought in weight training lay literature indicates broad principles. Determining which set/rep schemes are appropriate for an athlete's training program, involves the following.

Low repetitions (1 to 3) will develop maximum strength with little increase in muscle size. It is ideal for athletes such as wrestlers and weight lifters who benefit from a high level of relative strength. This type of training is considered advanced and should be performed only by athletes with 2 years of weight training experience in lower intensity programs.

Medium reps (4 to 7) will develop strength and hypertrophy, but not to absolute levels of both. This type of training requires at least 1 year of weight training experience in a program that emphasizes hypertrophy.

High reps (8 to 12) will develop maximum hypertrophy, but is not as effective at building strength as medium- and low-repetition programs. High repetitions are recommended for introductory programs; such training will help an athlete reach top competitive body weight at an earlier age without the increased injury potential of the higher intensity lifts.

Table 22.5 presents several examples of training programs that emphasize the three major set/rep combinations. Because the body adapts quickly to a specific workout, use of several of these methods throughout the training year is desirable (20, 21).

SUPERSETS

Supersets commonly combine exercises for opposing muscle groups, such as performing a set of curls for the biceps followed by a set of French presses for the triceps. Because fewer rest periods are taken when performing supersets, this method of training reduces the time it takes to complete a workout. This stepped-up pace is also traditionally considered to condition the cardiovascular system more effectively.

Exercise physiologists at Louisiana State University in Baton Rouge conducted a 16-week study on supersets. Subjects were divided into two groups: one that was required to perform an arm routine with the exercises arranged in superset fashion, and another that performed the same exercises and set-rep schemes arranged in the conventional manner. Arm measurements were taken throughout the experiment. After 16 weeks, the researchers found no significant difference in strength gains between the two groups (22).

Supersets should not be used for exercises that involve a considerable amount of technique or that can be performed with relatively heavy weights. The shortened rest periods fatigue the athlete faster, and moving quickly to the second exercise diminishes concentration. These factors can increase the risk of injury.

CIRCUIT TRAINING

Because most traditional weight training programs produce only minor cardiorespiratory im-

Table 22.6. Circuit Programs

Circuit 1	Circuit 2
Squat	Squat
Bench press	Shoulder shrug
Leg press	Push press
Rowing	Leg curl
Leg curl	Leg extension
Incline press	Rowing
Leg extension	Bench press
Shoulder press	Pulldowns

Table 22.7. Small Circuit Design

Mini-circuit 1	Mini-circuit 2
Squat	Leg curl
Bench press	Incline press
Leg press	Leg extension
Rowing	Shoulder press

provements (Vo₂max), many lifters occasionally experiment with circuit training. This type of training has produced significant improvements in all cardiovascular risk factors that are improved by aerobic exercise (23).

Instead of performing multiple sets of one exercise in succession, with circuit training only one set is performed followed by another exercise. A circuit is completed when each exercise is performed once.

Table 22.6 lists typical circuit programs. Circuit 1 alternates upper body exercises with lower body exercises, whereas circuit 2 matches pulling exercises with pushing exercises.

Because they are self-contained and offer convenient methods of changing resistance, multistationed exercise machines are ideal for circuit training. Many gyms have complete lines of single-station exercise machines, such as the Polaris and Nautilus machines, and arrange this equipment in circuits.

Different muscle groups are used in each circuit station, so one can move through a circuit with short rests between stations. For maximum cardiovascular stimulation, the recovery time between rest periods is justified only after exhaustive exercise, such as the squat and the power clean, or during use of a heavy resistance.

When high equipment usage or crowds are a problem, a circuit can be divided into smaller circuits (Table 22.7). These circuits are called mini-circuits.

Mini-circuits allow for greater specialization than traditional circuits. For example, when concentrating on weak areas, exercises that work those body parts should be chosen for the first circuit while energy levels are higher. Table 22.8

presents a mini-circuit program designed to emphasize areas of the body.

Many will try to achieve better aerobic results from circuit training by adding 15 to 30 seconds of aerobic work, such as jogging in place, between each station. This type of circuit is referred to as a super circuit.

Variety is one of the most important principles in designing a weight training workout. Intelligent use of supersets and circuit training are additional techniques that help prevent overtraining.

PERIODIZATION

The effects of training are specific to the type of training. Therefore, training schedules are designed to accomplish given objectives such as strength, power or endurance, and performance in competition. These objectives can be met individually with a scheduling method termed periodization.

Periodization is the process of organizing all the components of training (running, weight training, etc.) so that athletes can achieve best performance in their major competitions. A periodization plan, or model, consists of six components: macrocycle, period, phase, microcycle, training sessions, and training unit (24).

A macrocycle is a complete program of training, from early preparation to a major competition. A calendar year consists of several macrocycles.

Each macrocycle is divided into smaller categories called periods, with each period emphasizing different training components. A typical macrocycle will consist of a preparation period, followed by a competition period and a transition period. The preparation period develops the primary athletic requirements of training, the competition period refines these requirements to reach peak condition, and the transition period is devoted to recovering from the stress developed during the first two periods.

Training periods are divided into smaller categories called phases. The preparation period, for example, could be broken down into a general conditioning phase and a specific conditioning phase. For a sprinter, the general conditioning

Table 22.8. Focused Mini-circuit

Mini-circuit 1	Mini-circuit 2	Mini-circuit 3
Squat	Bench press	Incline press
Prone leg curl	Rowing	Lat pulldown
Leg press	Shoulder press	French press
Standing leg	Pulldown	Arm curl

phase might emphasize heavy weight training for the legs to build a strength base; the specific conditioning phase could emphasize more dynamic strength training such as downhill running to increase speed.

Phases are divided into smaller categories called microcycles. Most microcycles last 1 week or less.

Microcycles are divided into smaller categories called training sessions, and the number of training sessions in a day should increase with the level of ability. For example, a beginning weight lifter may make optimal progress on one training session per day, three times per week, whereas international-caliber weight lifters often train several times per day.

Training sessions are divided into training units, which are the single components of a training session. Warm-up exercises could be considered a training unit.

CONDITIONING

Endurance sports are gaining in popularity and number of participants. Conditioning programs apply to all sports, but their necessity is never more obvious than in these cases.

The question of quality versus quantity always comes up, but there are no black and white answers. In a conditioning program, just as in strengthening, many of the same elements must be stressed. The term conditioning has the connotation of including more than strength alone.

Consistency

Infrequent workouts for conditioning the cardiovascular and respiratory systems seem to offer poor results. Three to six times per week schedules are better.

Intensity

The systems must be stressed to make progress—this is the quality side of the equation. There is a point of diminishing return, but training at high intensity is advisable for the healthy athlete. This means using "pace of effort" levels just below, at, or above the lactate threshold.

Volume

This quantity measure is important also. To prepare for a 12-hour endurance event successfully, one must consider exercise sessions in the 4- to 9-hour range. No amount of intensity-driven workouts can prepare the athlete for the physiologic needs of the longer events.

The longer the event, the longer the workouts must be. Workouts for shorter events should stress intensity, but in all events both intensity and volume should be addressed. When determining how much of each to use, certain measures are helpful. Heart rate monitors can help in performing workouts, as well as in gauging the athlete's condition. Triathletes have noted that maximum heart rate during workouts is lower when poor diet and fatigue are prominent. Some use resting heart rate on waking as a gauge of overtraining; a sharp rise in heart rate signifies the need for more rest.

Ultraendurance

When training for events longer than 5 hours, new factors come into play. The athlete's ability to provide glucose to the muscles, maintain electrolyte balance, and maintain fluid levels becomes critical. For example, the Ironman triathlon consists of a 2.4-mile swim, a 112-mile bike, and a 26.2-mile run. It is common for low blood sugar and altered sodium and ferritin levels to occur. It is therefore necessary to incorporate food and fluid ingestion into the training regimen to find the proper quantities and rates of ingestion. Mistakes in this area can easily lead to a failure to finish.

Overtraining

Exhausting the recovery systems leads to overtraining. The chronic fatigue associated with this condition can make the athlete irritable and depressed, and can eventually cause a loss in body weight. There is also an increased susceptibility to injury, particularly overuse injuries (6).

Although high-intensity training is essential to stimulate the muscles to develop, efforts will be wasted if the body cannot recover from such training. Some argue that the best way to identify excessive training may be through evaluation of the athlete's mental attitude. Blood chemistry and other methods of direct measurement have produced possible indicators, but have not produced effective and practical means of identifying the overtrained situation (16).

The best method of preventing overtraining is rest. If training is yielding poor results, simply taking a few days off can correct the situation. To prevent loss of strength or conditioning, an athlete needs to keep the muscles active during a layoff. Instead of complete rest, the mind and muscles should be given a change of pace by participating in another sport. Basketball, volleyball, and racquetball are excellent cross-training activities for this purpose.

Rest is also a key concept to consider when planning training cycles. Research and experience tell us that the larger muscle groups require more rest after high-intensity workouts. Although a body builder may be able to train calves and forearms everyday and still make gains, this athlete will probably be able to max out on a heavy bench press only once a week and a heavy squat only once every 2 weeks.

STARTING OUT

Before starting a strength or conditioning program, it is advisable to do a biomechanical analysis. This can be accomplished in many ways. A video or observation is made with the athlete performing the sport or motion involved; then a series of manual muscle tests are performed. In this way, weak links are discovered. In addition to traditional methods such as manipulation used to correct imbalance, these weak links must be given special attention in the first phase of training. Exercises that isolate these weak areas are begun immediately, and only when the joints are sufficiently stable will the main program be initiated.

SAMPLE EXERCISE COMBINATIONS FOR INDIVIDUAL SPORTS AND SPECIFIC INJURIES

During extended or intense workout, an adequate water supply and/or carbohydrate solution should be available. When used throughout the workout, the symptoms of faintness, nausea, and excessive fatigue can often be minimized or eliminated. The following is a list of exercises, by sport, that is currently being used for intercollegiate athletics at the U.S. Air Force Academy. The 11 categories that follow do not include trunk and ankle exercises also performed by these athletes.

1. Baseball. Back squat, bent-arm pullover and press, chin-up, French press, hyperextension, rotator cuff exercises, side lunge, wrist curl.
2. Basketball. Bench press (narrow), dumbbell row, power clean and push press, side lunge, step-up, wrist curl.
3. Cycling. Bench press (narrow), dumbbell row hyperextension, incline dumbbell press, lat pulldown to throat, leg curl, leg extension, step-up.
4. Football. Bench press (narrow), incline press (narrow), dumbbell row, power clean and push press, side lunge, step-up.
5. Golf. Bent-arm pullover and press, chin-up, dumbbell row, hyperextension, step-up, side lunge, wrist roller.
6. Racquet sports. Bent-arm pullover and press, dumbbell row, hyperextension, incline press, leg curl, lunge, rotator cuff exercises.
7. Running. Bench press (narrow), dumbbell curl, dumbbell row, leg curl, lunge, calf raise. (For sprint events, add the power clean and push press.)
8. Soccer. Incline press (narrow), leg curl, lunge, neck exercises, power clean, running curl, side lunge.
9. Swimming. Bench press (narrow), dumbbell row, hyperextension, incline press, leg extension, lat pulldown (front), leg extension, rotator cuff exercises.
10. Volleyball. Same as basketball.
11. Wrestling. Curls, power clean and jerk, hyperextension, incline press (narrow), neck exercises, pullover and press, pull-up, wrist roller.

RECURRENT ANKLE SPRAIN

Ankle table: tibialis anterior and posterior, peroneus longus, brevis, and tertius.

Patella Femoral Arthralgia

This condition is usually present with clicking of patella and vastus medialis weakness. Leg extensions with three foot positions and hamstring curls should be performed.

Post Surgical Knee

Leg extensions with three foot positions, hamstring curls, popliteus exercise with tubing, leg press, and calf raises should be performed.

Recurrent Shoulder Pain

Dumbbell and tubing rotator cuff exercises, dumbbell flies, lat pulldowns, cable or dumbbell rows with elbow flexion, then elbow fixed in extension should be performed.

Acknowledgments. The author acknowledges Mr. Kim Goss, assistant strength coach at the U.S. Air Force Academy, for his assistance in the preparation of most of the material presented here.

References

1. Poliquin C, Patterson P. Classification of strength qualities. National Strength and Conditioning Association 1989;6:48–50.
2. Garhammer J. Power outputs by Olympic lifters. Med Sci Sports Exerc 1980;12:54–60.
3. Kulund DN, Dewey JB, Brubaker CE, et al. Olympic weight-lifting injuries. Phys Sportsmed 1978;6:111–119.
4. Compton D, et al. Weight-lifter's blackout. Lancet 1973;2:1234–1237.

5. Weiss L. Differential effects of repetition number on strength and power development. Proceedings of the First IOC Congress on Sport Sciences. 1989;49–50.
6. Stone M, O'Bryant H. Weight training: a scientific approach. Minneapolis: Burgess, 1984.
7. National Strength and Conditioning Association. Practical considerations for utilizing plyometrics: part 1. round-table. National Strength and Conditioning Association 1986;3:14–22.
8. Chu D. Plyometrics. Proceedings of the National Conference on Strength Training and Conditioning, June, 1990.
9. Freeman W. Peak when it counts. Los Altos: Tafnews Press, 1989;55.
10. Jones A. Nautilus training principles. Deland: Nautilus Sports/Medical Industries, 1971;87–90.
11. Stone M. Considerations in gaining a strength: power training effect (machines vs. free weights). National Strength and Conditioning Association 1982;2:22–24, 54.
12. Dominquez RH. The complete book of sports medicine. New York: Warner Books, 1979:47.
13. DeLorme T, Watkins A. Techniques of progressive resistance exercise. Arch Phys Med 1948;29:263–273.
14. Bompa T. Theory and methodology of training. Dubuque, IA: Kendall/Hunt Publishing, 1983:17–33.
15. Abadjiev I. The preparation of international class weightlifters. Proceedings of the IWF Coaching-Medical seminar, Budapest. 1984:57–63.
16. Poliquin C. Practical methods in developing strength: absolute, explosive, speed and endurance. Proceedings of the National Strength and Conditioning Association, June, 1990.
17. Weight training and weight lifting: information for the pediatrician. Pediatrics 1987;15:483–489.
18. Laputin N, Oleshko G. Managing the training of weight-lifters: optimization of training loads as a factor of managing the training process. Livonia: Sportivny Press, 1982.
19. Landers J. Maximum based on reps. National Strength and Conditioning Association 1985;6:60–61.
20. Medvedyev A. A system of multi-year training in weightlifting: the methods of weightlifters speed-strength training. Livonia: Sportivny Press, 1989;83.
21. Ajan T, Baroga L. Weightlifting fitness for all sports: strength training methods. Budapest: Medicina Publishing House, 1988;161–171.
22. Goss K. Supersets for super shape. Strength Training for Beauty 1985;6:56–60.
23. Stone M, Wilson G, et al. Cardiovascular responses to short-term Olympic style weight training in young men. Can J Appl Sports Sci 1983;8:134–139.
24. Freeman W. Peak when it counts: the language of periodization. Los Altos: Tafnews Press, 1989;4–8.
25. Garhammer J. US weightlifting federation safety manual. Colorado Springs: USWF, 1990:60.
26. Stone M. Physical and physiological preparation for weightlifting. In: US weightlifting federation safety manual. Colorado Springs: USWF, 1990:82.
27. Kristensen J. The problematic effects of overtraining. International Olympic Lifter 1977;2:8–9, 26.
28. Costill D. Carbohydrate: fuel for optimal training and performance. Proceedings of the first IOC Congress on Sport Sciences 1989:12–16.
29. Budgett R, et al. Overtraining syndrome/staleness. Proceedings of the first IOC Congress on Sport Sciences 1989:118–119.

Sports Nutrition

James M. Gerber

It is well understood that nutrition is important for optimum performance in sports (1). The specific rules for applying this fact, however, are subject to a great deal of uncertainty, debate, and individual experimentation by athletes, coaches, trainers, and health professionals (2). This chapter attempts to shed some light on the extent and limitations of present knowledge regarding nutrition and athletic performance. Guidelines intended to form a practical basis for advising athletes are provided.

Athletes are not a homogeneous group. Not only do they vary in their aptitude for certain sports and in their mastery of specific skills; they also come in a wide range of sizes, shapes, ages, and levels of fitness. Thus, their nutritional needs cannot be stated simply, but must be ascertained on a somewhat individual basis (3). Athletes are subject to a variety of human shortcomings with respect to their eating habits. They may have just as poor an understanding of food, may be as limited in food budget, or may be as careless about eating regularly and properly as any other person (2).

DIETARY NEEDS OF THE ATHLETE

When helping the athlete design the best training diet, several factors should be considered.

1. The diet should be consistent with what is generally known about basic human nutritional requirements for optimum health. Many athletes will learn dietary habits during training that will stay with them for years. It would not be advisable, therefore, to consume a diet that is either excessive or inadequate in any of the myriad nutrients or other components found in today's food supply.
2. The individual nutritional needs of the athlete as a unique person must be considered. There may be preexisting health conditions

or other acquired or even genetic dissimilarities compared with the average person. These differences may impose additional needs or limitations on the athlete's diet.
3. There may be special dietary requirements dictated by the athletic endeavors themselves. The demands for various blends of power and endurance required for superior performance in a particular sport may suggest training and competition strategies that include nutritional considerations.

The Healthful Diet

The athlete's diet must begin with enough of the right nutrients to sustain a normal, healthy individual. If the diet is to be ongoing, it should also not be an unhealthy diet with respect to long-term disease risk (1, 4).

An athlete's current diet may not be adequate by the above definition (2). The typical U.S. diet is often criticized for being excessive in certain components such as fat, sugar, sodium, and chemical additives while being inadequate in some nutrients and dietary fiber (5). These are some of the most important nutritional concerns to be addressed by sports health professionals.

Various national authorities, including the U.S. Department of Health and Human Services, the American Heart Association, and most recently the Surgeon General, have attempted to develop guidelines for Americans to use in adopting more healthful eating habits in line with the maintenance of health and prevention of disease. These various guidelines can be summarized as follows (6).

1. Maintain desirable body weight through appropriate caloric intake and appropriate physical activity.
2. Eat a variety of foods.
3. Increase consumption of fruits, vegetables, and whole grains to ensure adequate starch and fiber.

4. Decrease consumption of refined and other processed sugars and foods high in such sugars.
5. Decrease consumption of food high in total fat and partially replace saturated fats, whether obtained from animal or vegetable sources, with unsaturated fats.
6. Decrease consumption of animal fat, and choose meat, poultry, and fish that will reduce saturated fat intake.
7. Except for young children, substitute low-fat and nonfat milk for whole milk, and low-fat dairy products for high-fat dairy products.
8. Decrease consumption of butterfat, eggs, and other high-cholesterol sources.
9. Decrease consumption of salt and foods high in salt content.
10. Use alcoholic beverages in moderation, if at all.

The above recommendations were primarily designed to prevent atherosclerotic disease, which is the most common cause of death in older adults. More recently, in response to a growing awareness of the role of nutrition in the development of cancer, several national authorities have produced guidelines for cancer prevention that include the following additional recommendations (6).

• The daily diet should include fruits and vegetables high in vitamin C and beta-carotene, as well as cruciferous (cabbage family) vegetables.
• The consumption of smoked and nitrite-cured foods should be minimized.
• Foods containing extraneous chemicals and additives should be minimized in the diet.

Following the above guidelines in the design of the athlete's diet will address most, if not all, of the issues of nutritional excesses that may be hazardous to health. Whether the above recommendations will prevent deficiencies of the many known essential vitamins and minerals is not at all clear. This must be addressed before assuming that no further guidelines are needed.

Although the typical U.S. diet appears to be adequate for many vitamins and minerals, recent national nutrition surveys have identified several examples of problem nutrients (7). These micronutrients include vitamin B_6, folic acid, magnesium, iron, and zinc. In some cases, the prevalence of deficiencies in these nutrients has been only recently appreciated.

For some time, the standard for teaching the public how to achieve a balanced (i.e., adequate

in nutrients) diet has been the Basic Four Food Group Guide. This guide is often used for evaluating the adequacy of nutritional intake as well. Reliance on the Basic Four Food Group Guide, a product of nutrition knowledge of the late 1950s, as a basis for designing an adequate diet is questionable in light of the progress made in understanding nutritional needs and availabilities since its development. Recent reevaluations of the Guide have pointed out numerous inadequacies in menus resulting from its use (8). Improved guidelines will appear to require more variety and selectivity in food choices, including the daily use of wholesome foods from each of the following groups (8, 9).

• Milk and milk products.
• Meat, poultry, fish, and eggs.
• Legumes and nuts.
• Whole grain cereal products.
• Fruits and vegetables rich in vitamin C.
• Dark green vegetables.
• Additional fruits and vegetables.
• Polyunsaturated fats and oils.

Special Needs of the Athlete

CALORIES

Adequate calorie intake, regardless of source, will guarantee adequate energy for normal body processes, training effort, and muscle tissue synthesis when this is a goal of the conditioning program. Inadequate intake has been associated with various problems including early fatigue, reduced muscle growth or muscle tissue loss, and amenorrhea in women. Intake levels below 1800 kcal/day may result in vitamin and mineral deficiencies if replacement supplements are not used (10).

Calorie requirements for an athlete will depend primarily on training and performance intensity. The athlete who trains to exhaustion on a daily basis will require more fuel than one who performs a milder regimen two or three times per week. Factors such as metabolic rate and other physiologic factors may have minor effects on energy needs (11).

It is common for a lean athlete undergoing intense training to require in excess of 5000 kcal per day to sustain such activity (11, 12). However, each individual must find the proper caloric intake, using appetite as a general guide, but ultimately by trial and error.

Weight for height is the most commonly used measure for assessing the adequacy of caloric intake. In athletes it may be more appropriate to measure body composition using procedures such as skinfold thickness, underwater weighing, and bioelectric impedance (13). In the final analysis, however, the athlete's performance and general health are the best indicators of the adequacy of caloric intake (1).

Athletes who are at special risk for calorie deficiency include those who want to compete in lower weight categories (wrestlers, boxers), those whose sport favors small body size (gymnasts, swimmers, jockeys), and those who must display the socially accepted aesthetic body shape (dancers, figure skaters) (10). These individuals may feel pressured to restrict their energy intakes to extreme degrees to gain a competitive edge (14) (see Nutrition-Related Problems in Athletes).

CARBOHYDRATE

Carbohydrate is the most efficient fuel the body can use for energy production (15, 16). It can also be stored as glycogen in significant amounts in muscle and liver, functioning as a readily available energy source for athletic effort under strenuous conditions. Carbohydrate intake, therefore, may be the most important aspect of the nutritional enhancement of sports performance.

Carbohydrate may be provided through such dietary sources as grain products, starchy vegetables, legumes, fruit, and refined sugars. It can also be produced as glucose in the liver by the process of gluconeogenesis. This process uses many types of precursors: other dietary sugars such as fructose, certain amino acids, lactic acid from glycolytic processes in muscle tissues, and glycerol from mobilization of triglycerides in adipose tissue.

Dietary complex carbohydrates, or starches, are an inexpensive source of energy compared with fats and proteins. In addition, these carbohydrates appear to be one of the least hazardous dietary components, according to studies and recommendations by leading nutrition authorities. Diets containing up to 70% complex carbohydrates do not seem to pose any danger to overall health or health risk (4).

Refined sugars are of questionable value in the athlete's diet. Although providing a dense source of calories, other nutrients such as vitamins and minerals are lacking. Furthermore, refined sugar consumption may increase certain health risks, such as dental caries and glucose intolerance. During athletic competitions, however, dilute solutions of sugar may help maintain glucose levels in the blood and muscle tissues and may help replenish depleted glycogen stores (see nutrition and the endurance athlete). This will result in greater exercise endurance in most cases and

may possibly improve precision in certain sports such as tennis (17).

Because athletic events differ in the type of energy demands made on the body, carbohydrate requirements may not be the same for all athletes (15, 18). Short-term, high-intensity efforts rely on anaerobic use of stored muscle glycogen. Training regimens for these events will encourage muscle cell hypertrophy, which will increase the capacity for storing glycogen. Consumption of a high complex carbohydrate diet will assure that maximum glycogen deposition occurs (see Nutrition and the Power Athlete).

Aerobic endurance and other heavily training athletes do not depend totally on muscle glycogen for energy needs. However, their endurance capacity will depend on maintenance of blood glucose levels, using liver glycogen stores as a major source (16, 18). This represents a much greater demand for carbohydrate reserves than do short-term efforts. The importance of a high complex carbohydrate diet is essential for heavy training regimens. Moreover, special diet techniques such as carbohydrate-loading may be able to increase carbohydrate reserves beyond ordinary levels (see Nutrition and the Endurance Athlete).

FAT

Fat as derived from the diet functions primarily as an energy source for the body. A small amount provides essential fatty acids for cell membrane structure and prostaglandin synthesis. It contains the most calories per gram of all the macronutrients, which makes fat the most efficient form for the storage of energy.

Dietary fats are abundant in the U.S. diet, largely owing to its ample presence in many snack and convenience foods as well as the rich fare preferred by many people. The use of frying oils in the production of much of our meals and snacks has greatly contributed to an excessive intake of fat by most Americans in the past few decades (4).

The presence of fat in the athlete's diet can serve at least two purposes (10). First, it lends palatability to the diet. Diets containing less than 20% fat are often considered unappetizing and unsatisfying. Second, it allows an intake of concentrated calories in those athletes who require large amounts to sustain intense training on a regular basis. These benefits, however, must always be weighed against the hazards of excessive fat consumption.

Dietary fat should represent 30% or less of the athlete's diet. Within this amount, choices among various types of fat are important. As saturated fat is associated with many health risks, one third or less of daily fat intake should be saturated. The remainder may be distributed among the various unsaturated fats (4).

PROTEIN

Protein has many functions in the human body. In addition to its primary role in the structure of muscle and other tissues, protein contributes to energy needs and provides precursors for specialized molecules such as hormones and neurotransmitters. Because it cannot be stored, excesses must be catabolized actively, primarily in the liver. The calories represented by the carbon skeleton of the amino acids must then be used or stored, and the nitrogen component excreted by the kidneys (19). The protein needs of the athlete must take into account all these issues.

Protein occurs in the diet in a wide variety of foods, although foods of animal origin are often much higher in protein concentration. Vegetable proteins may also suffer from a relative lack of one or more essential amino acids, necessitating some attention to variety in diets low in animal protein. Former beliefs in the need for optimum protein-combining at every meal have been discredited, however, since the discovery that a 50- to 100-g pool of surplus amino acids stored in the liver, blood, and muscle tissue is constantly available to augment dietary intake (20).

The typical U.S. diet is considered abundant in protein, the average intake being well over the Recommended Daily Allowance, which itself contains a margin for safety (21). As calorie consumption goes up with heavy athletic training, the natural presence of protein in many foods results in even greater protein intake above the norm. Additionally, athletes and body builders frequently emphasize high-protein foods in their diet and often use supplemental protein powders. This practice of high-protein intake, although it appears to be unnecessary, has been popular since the days of the ancient Greek Olympians (22).

High-protein diets are often discouraged because they are frequently high in fat content as well. The potential health risks of excess lean protein intake, on the other hand, are poorly understood (4). There does not seem to be any significant risk of heart disease, hypertension, or stroke if the diet is not also high in fat. Population studies on cancer cannot show a definite correlation, although animal studies suggest that a 20% to 25% protein diet is tumorigenic (23). Protein supplements, but not food proteins, have been shown to increase urinary calcium loss, which increases the risk of osteoporosis (24).

High protein intake may increase age-related deterioration of kidney function (25). Finally, unabsorbed proteins and amino acids may be used by certain intestinal bacteria, which excrete toxic nitrogenous waste products having deleterious local or systemic effects (26, 27).

The adult U.S. RDA for protein is given as 0.8 g/kg ideal body weight (i.e., not actual weight in underweight or overweight individuals). The requirement is increased to 0.9 to 1.0 g/kg for older children and adolescents due to growth requirements (21). Whether the metabolic cost of athletic training increases the need for dietary protein beyond the RDA has been controversial for the past few decades. It would seem logical that increased muscle energy consumption, stresses and strains on muscle fiber integrity, and requirements for muscle growth would combine to cause a significant additional need for protein intake.

There is growing agreement that absolute protein requirements are higher for many types of athletes (see Nutrition and the Power Athlete). However, it does not appear that any special emphasis on dietary protein is called for, owing to the natural abundance of protein in the typical U.S. diet. The safe and adequate range for protein intake for athletes has been given as 12 to 20% of daily calorie intake, with an ideal level of 15% (20). This amount should be attainable through a normal diet.

VITAMINS

Many vitamins play direct roles in exercise metabolism by virtue of their coenzyme functions in many basic body processes. Deficiencies of certain vitamins have been shown to impair work performance, and other research has proven that exercise increases vitamin metabolism (28). Furthermore, theories have been proposed that suggest that by maximizing enzyme function, larger doses of vitamins may produce sufficient improvements in performance to warrant regular supplementation by athletes (29).

Nevertheless, no special requirements for athletes have been proposed other than those for vitamins B_1, B_2, and B_3, which are tied to calorie intake. There may be several reasons for this (18). The Recommended Dietary Allowances for each micronutrient are set with a margin for safety that is assumed to allow for increased needs in some individuals, such as athletes (21). If a true deficiency cannot be demonstrated, the RDA is considered to be adequate. Moreover, the dietary intake of many heavily training athletes is so large that sufficient micronutrient intake is easily achieved. Finally, the evidence for benefits of individual or multiple vitamin supplements is generally lacking (21, 30). Issues pertaining to individual micronutrients will be discussed below.

Thiamine (vitamin B_1) plays a pivotal role in carbohydrate metabolism and is also necessary for normal neurophysiologic functioning. It is not a common deficiency in the United States. Few controlled studies have investigated the need for thiamine in athletes, and the results of these are conflicting (31–33). It is not possible at this time to recommend a specific thiamine intake for athletes. The RDA for this vitamin is 0.5 mg/day for every 1000 kcal consumed (34).

Riboflavin (vitamin B_2) is important in energy production and in one antioxidant enzyme system used in the body to protect against tissue-damaging free radicals. Deficiency in healthy persons is unusual in the United States. Exercise, at least in untrained individuals, appears to increase riboflavin requirements, possibly due to increased activities in one or both of the above processes (35, 36). At least 1.0 mg/day for every 1000 kcal consumed may be required (34). However, supplemental riboflavin has not been shown to enhance performance in trained athletes (37).

Niacin (vitamin B_3) functions in the human body in two coenzymes that are essential for many oxidation-reduction processes, including energy production and protein metabolism. Deficiency in the U.S. population is rare. Strenuous physical activity may somewhat increase the requirements for this vitamin, the current RDA being 6.6 mg/1000 kcal (34). No specific recommendations can be made for athletes, but supplemental doses in the form of nicotinic acid (as opposed to niacinamide) should be avoided, as this form appears to impair fatty acid mobilization and increases glycogen depletion during endurance exercise (38, 39).

Pantothenic acid (vitamin B_5) has been known for some time to be the essential component of coenzyme A. As such, it participates in energy production from all fuel sources and is necessary for steroid hormone synthesis as well. Animal studies have suggested an ergogenic effect of pantothenic acid above nutritional requirement levels. Both animal and human research have reported that blood and tissue pantothenate levels are decreased by exercise (29, 34). One human study found no effect at 1000 mg/day (40), but another study showed positive effects on exercise performance at 2000 mg/day (41). This appears to be a safe level, although it is much higher than the 4 to 7 mg/day estimated requirement set by the RDA Committee (21).

Pyridoxine (vitamin B_6) is closely associated with protein synthesis and amino acid metabolism in humans. Requirements are proportional to protein intake at 0.02 mg B_6/g protein/day. Significant deficiencies of this vitamin may exist in some athlete populations (42). Exercise has been shown to influence pyridoxine status in animals and humans, but the significance (if any) of these findings is unclear. It has been suggested that pyridoxine supplementation may increase glycogen use, which could lead to earlier depletion during endurance exercise (42, 43). Most studies on the effects of vitamin B_6 supplementation on exercise performance have shown no positive results (29, 34).

Biotin plays an important role in the metabolism of the branched-chain amino acids used as fuel by muscle tissue, as well as other reactions in energy and amino acid metabolism. The quality of the U.S. diet for adequate biotin is not well understood, although outright deficiency is rare. Excessive consumption of raw egg white (not an unknown practice among certain athletes) may seriously reduce biotin absorption. Additionally, because biotin is synthesized by intestinal bacteria, an important source may be lacking in those individuals taking antibiotic medications for prolonged periods. No studies on biotin and physical performance have been reported (21, 34).

Folic acid is a required cofactor for many aspects of nucleotide and amino acid metabolism. It plays a crucial role in the production of red blood cells and other rapidly dividing tissues. Once considered the most common vitamin deficiency in humans, recent revisions of the Recommended Dietary Allowances have reduced the requirement by 50% to 180 to 200 mcg/day as a result of improved understanding of the bioavailability of the vitamin (21). Whereas anemia resulting from folic acid deficiency is likely to increase fatigue, no research has been done to determine any special relationships between exercise and folic acid (34).

Cobalamin (vitamin B_{12}) is also vital for DNA synthesis and cell division, as well as for normal nerve function. Its deficiency will produce an anemia similar to that of folic acid. However, B_{12} is well conserved by the body and is required at merely 2.0 mcg/day. Nevertheless, it is widely used by athletes and other individuals in the belief that it boosts energy. No studies have shown positive effects of vitamin B_{12} supplementation on athletic performance, although specific research on trained athletes is lacking (21, 34).

Ascorbic acid (vitamin C) is a water-soluble antioxidant and is an important cofactor in many processes, including iron absorption and synthesis of collagen, neurotransmitters, steroid hormones, and carnitine. Whereas the RDA is set at 60 mg/day, up to 200 mg/day saturate body tissues (21). Many studies, although not all, have suggested that vitamin C intake of at least 80 mg/day is required for optimum physical performance and/or prevention of deficiency during heavy exercise (29, 34). Up to 1000 mg/day has been associated with positive results on performance in some studies (44, 45), but others using these or higher levels have shown no benefit (29, 46). One study revealed a detrimental effect of chronic supplementation (47). Recent controlled research on vitamin C and exercise has demonstrated both beneficial and detrimental effects as well as no effect at all (29, 34). Thus, no definite recommendations for increased ascorbic acid intake can be made. The role of vitamin C in muscle soreness and tissue healing is discussed later (see Nutrition and Sports Injuries).

Retinol (vitamin A) does not play a direct role in energy metabolism, although it is essential for normal vision as well as growth and repair of many tissues (see Nutrition and Sports Injuries). Very few human or animal studies involving vitamin A and physical performance have been performed, and none has suggested any relationship between them. Similarly, vitamin D (cholecalciferol) and vitamin K (phylloquinone) have neither a theoretical nor research basis suggesting any interaction with exercise (34).

Tocopherol (vitamin E) is a fat-soluble antioxidant and may have other, as yet poorly understood, functions related to energy production. Overt deficiency appears to be rare; therefore, the RDA has been set at typical dietary levels, i.e., 8 to 10 mg/day (12 to 15 IU/day) (21). Research has suggested a stabilizing effect of vitamin E on muscle cell membranes, which may be important in minimizing the damaging effects of intense muscular effort. In this regard, actual requirements may increase 50 to 100% (48). Performance studies have not demonstrated consistent results from the use of large supplemental doses of vitamin E. Improved physical endurance at high altitudes has been shown, but most of the well-controlled research on vitamin E at lower altitudes has found no clear effect on athletic performance (29, 34).

MINERALS

Minerals play a wide variety of structural, metabolic, and enzyme-cofactor roles in human physiology. Some of these roles may influence athletic performance as discussed below. However, as with vitamins, no special recommendations have been made for increasing mineral intake by athletes, except in special situations such as bone loss, anemia, and electrolyte depletion, which are discussed elsewhere.

Calcium is the predominant mineral in the human body due to its major contribution to the structure of bone. It also performs crucial roles in nerve conduction, muscle contraction, cardiac function, and many other physiologic processes. Current recommendations range from 800 to 1200 mg/day, depending on age and gender (21). Although the effects of calcium deficiency on risk of bone loss are well accepted (see Nutrition-Related Problems in Athletes), the effect of calcium deficiency on muscle cramps and spasms has not been adequately studied (see Nutrition and Sports Injuries). No effects on exercise performance have been attributed to calcium (29).

Most athletes appear to consume the Recommended Daily Allowance of calcium (49). Nonetheless, the effects of high-protein diets on calcium balance suggest that certain athletes may need even more than the RDA (24). However, low–body-weight athletes, especially women, are very likely to be eating calcium-deficient diets (50). This is a potentially serious problem in athletes who are at increased risk for bone loss (see Nutrition-Related Problems in Athletes).

Phosphorus is a major structural mineral in bone, a component of cell membrane phospholipids and adenosine triphosphate (ATP), and participates in more metabolic functions than any other mineral. Dietary requirements are equivalent to those for calcium; thus a 1:1 ratio is ideal (21). Although deficiency is rare, phosphate ion has been investigated as a possible ergogenic aid (see Ergogenic Aids).

Magnesium is an important cofactor in energy metabolism and protein synthesis. It also interacts in a complex manner with calcium in neuromuscular activity. Magnesium requirements, normally 300 to 400 mg/day, may be increased in athletes undergoing strenuous training (21, 51). Recent reports have suggested potential gains in endurance capacity (52, 53) and muscle strength (54) with magnesium supplementation, but more studies are needed. For a discussion of the role of magnesium in the cause of muscle cramps, see Nutrition and Sports Injuries.

Iron is a crucial element in many energy-yielding processes in the human body. Not only is its presence in hemoglobin essential for oxygen transport, but it is a critical component of the mitochondrial cytochromes that function directly in ATP synthesis. Although requirements have been recently lowered to 10 to 15 mg/day (21), iron deficiency remains one of the most common mineral deficiencies in the U.S. and has been found in substantial numbers of athletes (55). Athletic performance may be impaired significantly by iron deficiency, especially if it results in clinical anemia (see Nutrition-Related Problems in Athletes).

Sodium, potassium, and chloride are the major electrolytes in the human body and a major part of the U.S. diet. Their importance in sports nutrition is discussed later (see Water and Electrolytes).

Zinc is a cofactor for more than 200 enzymes, including some with important roles in protein and bone synthesis as well as cell membrane function and energy metabolism. Requirements have been set at 12 to 15 mg/day. Exercise appears to increase zinc losses from the body, and athletes often show subnormal zinc levels in their blood (56). Marginal zinc deficiency does not appear to affect performance (55). However, in cases of athletic injury, such a deficiency may slow the healing process (see Nutrition and Sports Injuries).

Copper is also a ubiquitous enzyme cofactor in human metabolism. It is essential for iron transport, mitochondrial energy production, and catecholamine synthesis, functions that are relevant to athletic performance. It also plays a role in collagen synthesis, an important factor in tissue healing (see Nutrition and Sports Injuries). Exercise appears to influence copper levels in the blood and various tissues, but the significance of this is unclear. No studies have been reported on the effects of copper status on performance (55).

Chromium has been associated with optimal insulin function and control of blood sugar. Because insulin is necessary for uptake of glucose and amino acids into muscle cells, this mineral would seem to be important for athletic performance. Moreover, not only is dietary chromium intake marginal in the United States, but strenuous exercise is known to increase urinary excretion of chromium (55). Of four studies testing the anabolic effect of chromium during weight training, two reported positive results (57), one found significant effects in women only (58), and the fourth demonstrated no changes in either body composition or strength (59).

Most of the remaining trace elements have no obvious theoretical or research basis suggesting any interaction with exercise (29). Manganese, which participates in certain aspects of connective tissue synthesis, may be important in recovery from injuries (see Nutrition and Sports Injuries).

WATER AND ELECTROLYTES

Water is the most abundant substance in the human body and is essential for normal physiologic function. In it are dissolved various amounts of sodium, potassium, chloride, and magnesium—the electrolytes, which perform many basic body functions such as nerve transmission, muscle contraction, and fluid balance (60).

During exercise, sweating causes the greatest depletion of body fluids, with other losses occurring through urine formation and expired air. The purpose of sweating is to help control the buildup of heat in the exercising body. Blood that is brought near the skin surface by subcutaneous capillaries carries heat from the body's muscles and other core tissues. The evaporation of sweat allows increased skin cooling, thus more effective heat removal (60).

Exercise intensity, exercise duration, and climate all contribute to the loss of fluids and electrolytes through sweat during sports activities. Thus, heavy training or highly competitive contests lasting several hours present great demands for maintaining adequate intake of fluids and electrolytes. Higher air temperatures, ground temperatures, and relative humidity will also contribute to additional losses, with humidity having the greatest effect. Fluid depletion during intense exercise can exceed 2 liters (68 oz) per hour (60, 61).

Water intake is the most important nutritional activity during the act of exercising. It allows the maintenance of normal plasma volume and helps prevent serious elevation of core body temperature. The athlete must not depend on thirst to signal the need for water but should instead use it preventively before the need is felt. Fluids should be ingested before exercise and during exercise as well, if indicated by current conditions of intensity, duration, and climate (60).

Electrolyte replacement appears to be of only limited importance in most athletic endeavors. Although water losses in sweat can be costly in terms of fatigue after a moderate aerobic effort, electrolytes such as sodium and potassium are actually conserved and concentrated in the plasma during perspiration (60). Several hours of exercise is usually necessary before sodium depletion becomes significant, longer for potassium, chloride, and magnesium (see Dehydration and Water Intoxication). However, the presence of sodium in drinking fluids will often increase total voluntary water intake and facilitate absorption (see Nutrition and the Endurance Athlete).

The role of water and electrolytes in the cause of muscle cramps, is discussed later (see Nutrition and Sports Injuries).

NUTRITION AND ATHLETIC TRAINING

Nutrition and the Overfat Athlete

Excessive weight in most sports, although not all, is thought to hamper performance, especially when the additional mass is fat. Ideal body compositions have not been determined for different sports or team positions, yet each variety of athletic activity appears to favor specific body types or certain ranges of body composition (13). Thus, an athlete may desire to make changes in weight and/or body composition to satisfy the perceived demands of the chosen sport.

ASSESSMENT AND MONITORING TOOLS

Although it is the most commonly used measure for monitoring the effects of overall caloric intake, weight for height is not suitable for assessing body composition changes in athletes. Measurement of body lean/fat ratios requires one of several possible procedures such as skinfold thickness, underwater weighing, or bioelectric impedance (13).

Underwater weighing remains the most accepted commercial method for precise determinations and is available at many large collegiate athletic departments. Bioelectric impedance, infrared, and ultrasonic devices have the advantage of lower cost and portability. Of these however, only bioelectric impedance has a significant body of research. Limitations of bioelectric impedance include: (1) it measures body water, which may be affected by hydration status; and (2) it may not accurately measure trunk fat (62, 63). Skinfold caliper measurements assess subcutaneous fat in a limited number of sites (as do infrared and ultrasonic methods) and are usually valid only in the hands of trained, practiced individuals (62–64). Periodic muscle girth measurements may be useful in monitoring changes in lean body mass (64). In the final analysis, however, the athlete's performance is the best indicator of success in achieving best weight and body composition (1).

GOAL-SETTING

Weight loss during athletic training should be accomplished in such a way that performance is not impaired and lean body mass is preserved if not enhanced. Body fat should be measured, and a safe, suitable goal should be targeted within the normal ranges of 12 to 18% for men and 15 to 25% for women. Depending on the sport, elite athletes often have body fat percentages below these ranges (as low as 5% for men and 8% for women), but these extremes may be neither achievable nor desirable for all aspirants (1, 13).

The target weight or body composition goal should be achieved gradually at no more than 2 or 3 lb per week to preserve lean body mass. A young athlete's growth and maturation stage must be considered; weight loss may be inappropriate during periods of rapid growth (10, 65).

WEIGHT-LOSS STRATEGIES

Moderate calorie restriction and/or suitable aerobic exercise to achieve gradual changes should form the basis for a weight-loss plan. Replacing higher calorie items with similar but lower calorie foods will allow comparable quantities to be eaten, which may improve compliance. For example, lower fat meat, dairy, and grain products will permit the consumption of full meals without excessive calorie intake.

Nutritional adequacy must be guaranteed if training capacity is not to be compromised. Careful food choices will maximize the nutritional value of a restricted-calorie diet and prevent deficiencies (see Designing the Athlete's Diet). If the athlete is not likely to eat a sufficiently nutritious diet, supplementation should be considered (65).

If athletes appear to maintain weight on very low calorie intake, they may be attempting to achieve a level of body weight or body fat that is below their natural potential (18). In these individuals, it may be very difficult to accomplish weight loss without severely compromising health or performance.

Nutrition and the Endurance Athlete

Endurance considerations apply not only to athletes who compete in this type of sport, but also to all athletes who train intensively for long periods.

PHYSIOLOGIC CONSIDERATIONS

As exercise duration lengthens beyond 1 minute, whether continuous or in short bursts with little available recovery time, ATP production will depend more and more on aerobic oxidative processes to keep up with energy demands. Muscle glycogen will yield much more energy under these conditions compared with glycolysis. In addition, along with the required oxygen, the blood will deliver other fuels, principally glucose and fatty acids, that will increase the sustainability of long-term exercise activities (66).

At the same time, the muscle tissue can release amino acids into the blood, where they can be converted to glucose by the liver, thereby contributing to the maintenance of blood sugar, a process that may be very important during long-term exercise. As much as 10 to 15% of the energy needs during endurance exercise may be provided by the muscle tissue pool of amino acids. The actual amount of protein and amino acid degradation that occurs appears to depend on the intensity and duration of the exercise and the magnitude of muscle glycogen reserves (20).

Endurance training accomplishes many aspects of physiologic conditioning that benefits the optimal use of fuels during exercise. Enhancement of cardiovascular and respiratory function will ensure efficient delivery of oxygen and fuels to the muscle tissue. The muscle cells will respond to conditioning with increased glycogen deposition (assuming adequate dietary intake), increased use of oxygen for aerobic energy production, and greater use of free fatty acids as fuel for ATP production. Faster mobilization of free fatty acids from adipose tissue and faster production of glucose in the liver from other substrates may also result from endurance training (12, 66).

CALORIES

Athletes who train daily must consume enough calories to sustain their training intensity, body composition goals, and growth needs in the case of adolescents and strength-training athletes. The type of sport will also influence energy expenditure. For example, distance runners commonly use approximately 100 kcal/mile, and cyclists expend 1000 to 1200 kcal/hour at training speeds. Combined with normal metabolic requirements, athletes in heavy training may require 50 to 85 kcal/kg body weight/day (see Designing the Athlete's Diet). Insufficient caloric intake may result in easy fatigue or loss of lean body mass (16).

The complexity of and individual variation in energy requirements make it difficult to calculate the proper caloric intake for a given athlete at that person's training level (see Designing the Athlete's Diet). If the athlete is neither overweight nor motivated to overrestrict calories, then appetite will be a convenient starting point. Monitoring of weight or body composition during training will provide additional insight into the appropriateness of the athlete's calorie intake. Performance, as usual, will be the final outcome measure to determine if the athlete has achieved proper calorie balance (1).

CARBOHYDRATES

A high-carbohydrate diet is necessary to replace daily losses of liver and muscle glycogen, which may reach 500 to 700 g on days of heavy training. If this is not done, training will become increasingly more difficult as glycogen depletion approaches critical levels. Depending on training intensity and duration, athletes require 7 to 10 g carbohydrate/kg body weight or 60 to 70% of total calories as carbohydrate, whichever is greater (15, 16) (see Designing the Athlete's Diet).

Postexercise Glycogen Repletion

The activity of the enzyme responsible for glycogen synthesis is significantly increased immediately after a long bout of exercise. If the blood sugar is kept elevated during the hours after exercise, maximum glycogen synthesis will occur. Therefore, repletion with carbohydrate should begin immediately after exercise (67, 68).

Optimum postexercise intake appears to be approximately 40 to 60 g carbohydrate/hr. This may be accomplished using 1.5 g carbohydrate/kg of body weight, taken as soon as possible after exercise and repeated every 2 hours for the 4 to 6 hours after exercise. Simple sugars appear to be more effective than complex carbohydrates during this period, but foods with a high glycemic index may be acceptable substitutes. Sucrose, glucose, and glucose polymer produce greater increases in muscle glycogen, whereas fructose is best for liver glycogen repletion. A liquid carbohydrate source providing fluid replacement as well may be the most acceptable and efficient method for immediate postexercise supplementation (15, 67, 68).

After the initial hours postexercise, high-complex carbohydrate meals will allow further glycogen repletion to occur as discussed above (Table 23.1) (15, 16).

Carbohydrate Supercompensation (Loading)

Carbohydrate loading or supercompensation regimens are chosen to increase the storage of glycogen in muscle and liver to levels beyond normal values. Two methods of carbohydrate supercompensation have been investigated (16).

Originally, it was proposed that the athlete begin supercompensation by first exercising to exhaustion 1 week before an event. This was followed by 2 successive days of low (10%) dietary carbohydrate intake. On the third day, another

Table 23.1. Examples of Low-Fat, High-Carbohydrate, Moderate Protein Diets

Breakfast: oatmeal, whole grain cold cereals, pancakes, muffins, low or nonfat milk and yogurt, fresh fruit, juices

Lunch or dinner: turkey or tuna sandwiches, bean and pea soups, pasta with tomato sauce, thick-crust vegetarian pizza, broiled fish or poultry, baked potatoes, winter squash, cornbread, corn tortillas, cooked rice or other grains, raw vegetables and salads with low-calorie dressings, corn on the cob, low or nonfat milk and yogurt, fresh fruit, juices

Snacks: fruit and fruit juices, vegetables, crackers, pretzels, bagels, air-popped corn, low or nonfat yogurt, low-calorie desserts

bout of exhaustive exercise was undertaken; after that, the diet was changed to one of very high (90%) carbohydrate intake. This diet was continued up to the day of competition. Studies demonstrated that glycogen content more than doubled with this procedure (69).

Problems with the extreme nature of exercise and diet required by the original supercompensation method led to the development of a modified procedure that has been shown to yield comparable results (70). Instead of exhaustive exercise close to the day of competition, training effort is gradually reduced day by day during the prior week, ending with at least one day of rest. The diet is maintained at a typical 50% carbohydrate level for the first half of the week, then boosted to 70% carbohydrate or 10 g/kg body weight for the second half (16, 70) (see Designing the Athlete's Diet).

Recently, it has been suggested that simply 2 to 3 days of rest along with a carbohydrate intake of 8 to 10 g/kg body weight is sufficient to achieve supercompensation in endurance-trained athletes (16). Success may be detected by a 1- to 2-kg increase in body weight measured in the morning before breakfast and after emptying the bladder. Some athletes will gain more benefit in performance than others from carbohydrate loading, but it appears that the modified procedures are at least harmless (16).

Precompetition Carbohydrate Intake

Carbohydrate intake before competition has been shown to benefit endurance athletes, although the precise timing and quantity for optimal performance are unclear (16). Various methods may be considered, as discussed below.

The precompetition meal should be eaten 3 to 6 hours before the event. It should be individualized to the athlete by testing various regimens during training. Carbohydrate content should be at least 100 g, and as much as 4.5 g/kg body weight may be beneficial (16, 71). Fat and protein content should be low. Table 23.1 presents examples of appropriate meal items (see Designing the Athlete's Diet).

Consumption of carbohydrate 30 to 45 minutes before exercise should be avoided in some cases. Performance may be impaired due to a rise in insulin and a fall in blood sugar during the first few minutes of exertion. However, all athletes are not equally susceptible to this phenomenon. In those who are found to be sensitive, using fructose-based sources may prevent this side effect, but it should be kept in mind that fructose in amounts over 75 g may cause gastric distress (16, 71).

Within 30 minutes or less of the starting time, an additional 50 to 100 g of carbohydrate without added fat or protein may be taken. Solid or liquid supplements may be ideal for this purpose as long as they are fairly rapidly digested and absorbed. Again, fructose products should be limited to less than 75 g to avoid gastric distress (71).

Carbohydrate Supplementation During Exercise

Carbohydrate must be available to muscle and other tissues throughout exercise. Even in later stages when fatty acid use is high, some glucose must be present to allow maximum energy production to proceed. Sources of glucose during exercise include muscle and liver glycogen stores and ingested carbohydrate (16, 72).

Prolonged exercise for more than 1 hour can significantly deplete muscle glycogen, even in supercompensated tissues. When this occurs, exogenous glucose from the blood becomes a critical factor in sustaining maximum performance. Because liver glycogen stores are also likely to be depleted late in endurance exercise, other sources of blood glucose are needed (16, 72).

Maintaining blood sugar levels and supplying muscles with exogenous glucose appear to be the benefits of consuming carbohydrate during exercise lasting more than 1 hour. Fatigue is delayed and performance is improved by consuming at least 20 to 30 g of carbohydrate per half hour. A liquid supplement used for this purpose would have the advantage of more rapid absorption and of providing needed fluids. However, solid forms have also been shown to be effective (16, 72).

Commercial sports drinks, several examples of which can be seen in Table 23.2, usually contain 6 to 8% carbohydrate in the form of glucose, sucrose, fructose, and/or glucose polymer. Fructose content is not as useful for supplying quick energy sources and may cause gastric distress in high concentrations. Glucose polymer solutions are effective in concentrations up to 25% or more and may be useful in supporting intense exercise when maximum fluid replacement is not an issue. The nutritional and electrolyte content of several beverages are presented in Table 23.2. Up to 16 oz or more of carbohydrate-containing beverages per half hour may be optimal. Small, frequent doses may be less likely to cause gastric upset, but large (1 to 2 cups) portions appear to enhance gastric emptying. Each athlete will have to determine best intake (73).

PROTEIN

Endurance exercise initially appears to have a catabolic effect on body proteins. This is probably

Table 23.2. Sports Drink and Beverage Comparison (8 oz portions)

Product	CHO source	% CHO	Na (mg)	K (mg)	Other nutrients	
Fluid/energy replacement products						
Gatorade (Quaker Oats)	SUC, GLU	6	110	25	Chloride Phosphate	
Exceed Fluid Replacement (Ross Labs)	GP, FRU	7.2	50	45	Chloride Calcium	Magnesium Phosphate
Recharge (Knudsen)	FRU, GLU	7.6	15	25	Chloride Phosphate	Magnesium Calcium
PowerBurst (PowerBurst)	FRU	5.9	25	50	Chloride Magnesium	Vitamin C B vitamins
Breakthrough (Weider)	MD, FRU	8.9	56	48	Chloride Calcium	Magnesium
Hydra Fuel (Twinlab)	GP, GLU, FRU	7	25	50	Phosphate Chloride Magnesium	Chromium Vitamin C
Powerade (Coca-Cola)	FRU, GLU MD	7.9	55	30	Chloride Phosphate	
Revive (Purepower)	FRU	4.2	100	100	Chloride Phosphate L-carnitine	Calcium Magnesium Vitamin C
Sqwincher (Universal Prods.)	GLU, FRU	6.8	60	36	Chloride Phosphate Calcium	Magnesium Vitamin C
Quickick (Cramer)	FRU, SUC	4.7	116	23	Calcium Chloride	Phosphate
10-K (Beverage Prods.)	SUC, GLU, FRU	6.3	52	26	Vitamin C Chloride	Phosphate
Coca-Cola (Coca-Cola)	FRU, GLU, SUC	11	9.2	0	Phosphate	
Orange Juice	FRU, SUC, GLU	11.8	2.7	474	Vitamin C Phosphate Calcium	Magnesium B vitamins
Homemade recipe[a]	Depends on sugar source	6.5–10	72–112	55–65	Chloride Vitamin C	Phosphate Magnesium
Human sweat	None		54–540[b]	28–74	Chloride Magnesium	Iron
Recovery drink products						
GatorLode (Quaker Oats)	MD, GLU	20	63	0	Vitamin C B vitamins	
Exceed High Carbohydrate Replacement (Ross Labs)	GP, FRU	25	117	42–84[c]	Magnesium Potassium Phosphate	Calcium B vitamins
Ultra Fuel (Twinlab)	GP, FRU FRU	21	0	50	Vitamin C Phosphate Magnesium	Chromium B vitamins

CHO, carbohydrate; Na, sodium; K, potassium; SUC, sucrose; GLU, glucose; GP, glucose polymer; FRU, fructose; MD, maltodextrin.
[a] 1 quart water + ½ cup orange juice + ⅛ tsp salt + ¼ cup sugar, honey or sugar syrup
[b] Depending upon heat acclimatization
[c] Estimated

due to use of amino acids for energy production in the muscle and for glucose production in the liver (74). Thus, athletes beginning a training regimen will usually lose more protein nitrogen than is taken in.

Within a few weeks, however, a physiologic adaptation occurs that restores nitrogen balance as long as protein intake is at least 1.0 g/kg/day but likely not more than 1.4 g/kg/day (20, 75). It appears that regular exercise promotes conservation of body protein and amino acids for the purpose of replacing degraded components and providing for new tissue growth.

During prolonged, intense training, endurance athletes appear to require between 1.0 and 1.5 g/kg/day to maintain nitrogen balance. This represents almost twice the RDA for normal adults. However, because these athletes usually require a high-calorie diet to sustain their regimen, the percentage of total calories that must come from protein to achieve this intake is only approximately 10% in most cases (20, 75).

FLUID AND ELECTROLYTES

As previously stated (see Dietary Needs of the Athlete), large losses of water and (in extreme conditions) electrolytes may occur through endurance exercise, especially in climates of high heat and/or humidity. These losses can result in poor performance or potentially serious illness. Thirst is not a sufficient stimulus to cause adequate fluid intake and to avoid dehydration during intense exercise (10, 76). Therefore, special attention must be given to encouraging fluid intake even beyond the athlete's own perceived needs.

Athletes should regularly monitor their fluid losses as they train to predict their individual hydration needs. Because these needs will probably vary with exercise intensity, exercise duration, and climactic conditions, the athlete should measure fluid losses under all exercise regimens and heat stress conditions that may be encountered in training and competition.

The best method to assess fluid losses is to weigh the dry, nude body before and immediately after the training session or competition. For each pound of body weight lost during exercise, 16 oz of water has been lost. If more than 2% of body weight is lost, fluid intake during the exercise period was insufficient and should be increased in subsequent training bouts. Any residual water deficit after exercise should be made up within the next several hours (10, 76).

A systematic routine of fluid intake should be developed by each athlete. One to two hours before training or competition, the athlete should consume approximately 1 to 2 cups of plain, cold water to hydrate the body tissues. This should be repeated 15 to 20 minutes before exercise. During exercise, 4 to 8 oz every 10 to 15 minutes is usually optimal. If this amount causes discomfort, tolerance should be built up gradually using smaller, more frequent portions. After exercise, the athlete should be weighed and given an additional 16 oz for every pound of body weight lost. All fluids should be consumed as close to refrigerator temperature as possible, as this speeds gastric emptying (1, 10, 76, 77).

In low-exertion sports that may continue for long periods in extreme heat, perspiration losses should be replaced with fluids containing electrolyte concentrations similar to sweat. A simple recipe for such a drink is one half-cup orange juice plus one-eighth teaspoon of salt added to one quart of water (Table 23.2). This would be an adequate fluid and electrolyte replacement drink to use when carbohydrate supplementation is not needed.

Fluids containing electrolytes are absolutely required only for ultraendurance sports lasting more than 4 hours (76). However, sports drinks containing electrolytes and carbohydrate (Table 23.2) may be useful for routine fluid replacement because they are more pleasant to consume in the large quantities needed to fully hydrate and to replace losses. The carbohydrate content of these drinks is also beneficial in endurance events (see above). Although it is true that gastric emptying time of these drinks is somewhat slower, this is offset by the facilitating effect of glucose and sodium on the intestinal uptake of water (78).

VITAMINS AND MINERALS

As discussed in the previous paragraph (see Special Needs of Athletes), certain interactions between exercise and micronutrient intake have been suggested. For the endurance athlete, specific applications may exist for supplements of pantothenic acid, vitamin C, vitamin E, magnesium, and phosphate, but proof of consistent benefit is still lacking. Furthermore, it may be necessary for endurance athletes to avoid supplements of niacin and pyridoxine, due to possible negative effects on performance.

Nutrition and the Power Athlete

Power becomes more important as the duration of the activity is reduced and the intensity of effort is increased. Weight lifting, sprinting, and certain aspects of baseball are examples of power sports. Short-term, high-intensity efforts require a large mass of coordinated muscle fibers and an immediate and abundant source of energy in the muscle tissue that can be used independently of available blood supply, i.e., anaerobically (16, 18, 66).

PHYSIOLOGIC CONSIDERATIONS

Energy Metabolism

ATP is the immediate source of energy for the muscle cell. However, it cannot be stored as such in very significant amounts. Only approximately 5 seconds worth is available at the beginning of exercise. Creatine phosphate (CP) is a quick, available source of high-energy phosphate in muscle cells and can sustain adequate ATP levels for approximately 20 seconds of extreme effort. Thus, short, intense exercise activities such as sprints, football plays, weight lifts, and tennis points can be accomplished without the simultaneous breakdown of body fuels. A period of recovery is necessary to replace ATP and CP pools using glycolysis or oxidation before the activity can be repeated at optimal performance levels. Increasing muscle cell size and conditioning appear to be two methods for maximizing the concentrations of CP and ATP for optimum performance (18, 66).

Intense exercise activities lasting 30 to 90 seconds require an energy source that is relatively independent of blood-borne nutrients and oxygen. Therefore, the glycolytic breakdown of muscle glycogen will supply the majority of ATP for this type of effort. Thus, increasing the capacity and storage of muscle glycogen is essential for optimizing performance at this level. Strength training and ideal use of dietary carbohydrate intake (see right column) will help accomplish these goals (18, 66).

Protein Metabolism

Approximately 92% of dietary protein is successfully digested and absorbed as the component amino acids pass into the portal circulation. As they pass through the liver, many of these amino acids are removed from the blood by the hepatic tissues. The liver may use these amino acids for protein synthesis, for the production of other amino acids, or may degrade them to urea and energy substrates. Which of these processes predominates depends on the perceived needs of the body. There is limited ability to store amino acids in the liver, so most excesses are catabolized (20).

Amino acids that are not taken up by the liver and those newly synthesized and secreted into the blood by the liver are distributed to other body tissues, including muscle. Muscle tissue not only uses amino acids for protein synthesis but can also use some for energy needs directly, namely the branched-chain amino acids leucine, isoleucine, and valine as well as glutamate, aspartate, and asparagine (20).

CALORIES

Strength-training athletes with large body mass who train daily are some of the highest energy consumers in the sports world. They must maintain a high calorie intake to ensure maintenance of lean body mass and to avoid early fatigue (see Nutrition and the Endurance Athlete). In addition, there is an increased energy requirement for growth due to muscle cell hypertrophy. The maximum muscle mass gain that is theoretically possible is approximately 2 lb of muscle/wk in athletes not taking anabolic steroids. This amount of tissue synthesis would require an additional 750 kcal/day (16, 20).

Power athletes are often interested in gaining weight, usually for the purpose of increasing muscle mass and corresponding muscle strength. Others, such as wrestlers and body builders, frequently attempt to lose weight before competition, often with detrimental effects on lean tissue

(see Nutrition-Related Problems in Athletes). Therefore, weight fluctuations should be measured in terms of lean body mass to distinguish quality tissue changes from changes in body fat (see Nutrition and the Overfat Athlete).

Many power athletes attempt to supply their additional calorie needs with protein. However, increasing calorie intake from nonprotein sources appears to be equally effective in promoting strength gains from intense training. With increased calorie intake, protein that was formerly used as an energy source can now be spared for tissue synthesis and other purposes (20).

CARBOHYDRATE

Although power athletes do not often need to sustain constant energy expenditure during competition, their training regimens may be as intense and demanding as those of endurance athletes. Further, athletes competing in weight classes may be restricting calorie intake, which can limit muscle glycogen storage and impair performance. Accordingly, the carbohydrate intake during heavy training and weight reduction should follow the same guidelines presented for endurance athletes (see Nutrition and the Endurance Athlete) (15).

Precompetition carbohydrate consumption does not seem to affect performance in short-duration power events, even if the intake results in elevated blood glucose and insulin. This is probably due to the restriction of blood flow to muscle during anaerobic exercise (16, 18).

Whether the large increases in muscle glycogen that can be achieved by supercompensation are necessary to maximize anaerobic performance is unclear. Other factors such as lactic acid buildup appear to cause fatigue long before glycogen stores are depleted (16). However, athletes who perform repeated, intermittent anaerobic efforts, such as football players, may significantly deplete muscle glycogen in the course of a single competition. These athletes should attempt to maximize muscle glycogen levels before competition and supplement with carbohydrate sources during the event as discussed above (see Nutrition and the Endurance Athlete) (15).

PROTEIN

Power athletes desire to strengthen and, in the case of body builders, enlarge muscles. A progressive resistance weight-training program and a proper diet are essential to the development of increased muscle mass and strength. Even so, the potential for achieving dramatic increases in lean body mass will depend on the athlete's genetics and training and diet (20). Nevertheless, power athletes typically regard a high protein intake as essential to their successful performance (22, 75).

In addition to supporting the energy-supplying function of certain amino acids during exercise, the contribution of protein to training allows the power athlete to attain a positive nitrogen balance. Protein retention during heavy resistance training has been calculated to reach a daily level of as high as 28 g (1 oz), which can be achieved with a protein intake of 1.6 g/kg/day or less. This would allow a possible gain of 2 lb of muscle mass per week (12, 20). Research on the maximum useful protein intake has not led to conclusive results thus far (22, 75), but there are indications that some power athletes (in particular, weight lifters) may retain more protein when consuming 2.0 g/kg/day or more during active training. Lean body mass measures have also been shown to be greater with these higher intake levels (29). Most authorities, however, conclude that 2.0 g/kg/day is the probable upper limit (75). Nonetheless, there is very little evidence that actual strength performance is enhanced, although more studies are needed (22).

In any case, due to the high caloric intake of athletes undergoing intense training, this level of protein intake will not likely exceed 15% of the daily calories of the regularly training power athlete. A typical training diet of 4000 kcal/day with a 15% protein diet would provide 150 g of protein/day (see Designing the Athlete's Diet). This would amount to 1.65 g/kg for a 200-pound athlete. Thus, additional protein supplements do not appear to be appropriate. If circumstances make food less obtainable or convenient, the ideal replacement supplement would provide protein in the proper proportion to carbohydrate and fat with vitamins and minerals supplied as well (20, 75).

FLUID AND ELECTROLYTES

Power athletes who train heavily for long periods, especially in warm, humid weather, should follow the guidelines for fluid and electrolyte replacement presented earlier (see Nutrition and the Endurance Athlete). However, during brief exercise bouts in competition, fluid and electrolyte adequacy may not be of concern unless the athlete is actually dehydrated (18).

Intense exercise of short duration causes body fluids to move from the blood to the active muscles and decreases the concentration of potassium in the muscle cells. The practical relevance of these facts is unknown. Dehydration will impair extended performance capacity, although isolated strength efforts may not be affected. Consequently, it is recommended that adequate fluid intake be maintained by the power athlete (76) (see Nutrition-Related Problems in Athletes).

BICARBONATE AND CITRATE (ALKALINIZING AGENTS)

Fatigue during high-intensity, short-term exercise has been associated with accumulation of lactic acid and reduction of muscle cell pH. Most studies investigating the usefulness of precompetition bicarbonate or citrate loading have shown measurable effects of these alkalinizing agents, in sufficient dosages, on lactic acid removal and performance enhancement in events lasting less than 7 minutes (79, 80).

A typical effective strategy involves ingestion of 300 mg sodium bicarbonate/kg body weight either taken in a single dose at least 1 hour before exercise or divided into smaller doses taken over several hours before exercise. Frequent side effects of nausea and diarrhea do occur, which limits the usefulness of the procedure. Furthermore, there is debate about whether bicarbonate loading constitutes unethical blood "doping" that should be banned (79, 80).

DESIGNING THE ATHLETE'S DIET

To help an athlete achieve a satisfactory diet, that person must be understood as an individual. Level of commitment to the sport, current nutrition beliefs, income level, sources and places of food consumption, daily schedule, and personal preferences are a few of the important psychosocial factors that

Table 23.3. Energy Expenditure for Specific Sports Activities

Sport	Energy Expenditure (kcal/kg/hr)
Baseball	4.1–5.3
Basketball	6.0–8.5
Cycling	4.8–9.7
Dancing	3.6–4.8
Football	7.3
Golf	3.6–4.8
Handball	8.5
Mountain climbing	8.7
Rowing	12.0
Running	9.7–17.2
Skating	4.8–8.7
Skiing, downhill	8.5
Skiing, cross-country	9.7
Soccer	7.8
Swimming	3.4–9.7
Tennis	6.0–8.5
Volleyball	4.8–8.5
Walking	2.9–5.8
Wrestling	11.1

Single numbers are averages.

Table 23.4. Food Exchange Plan for Athletes in Regular Training

Food Group	Exchanges Per Day			Special Modifications	
	1900 kcal	2500 kcal	3500 kcal	Choices for Maximum Daily Micronutrients	Additions for Carbohydrate Loading
Starches, bread, without fat	9	12	14	Use whole grain products Include 2–4 servings legumes	Add 2 servings
Lean to medium-fat proteins	4	4	8	Use red and dark meats	
Vegetables	4	4	4	Include dark greens	
Fruit	5	6	8	Include citrus	Add 2 servings
Milk products 1% fat or less	2	3	4		Add 2 servings
Added fats	3	4	8	Include polyunsaturated	
Snacks	1	2	3	Use whole foods	Add 0–3[a] servings
Approximate nutrient content					
Carbohydrate (g)	300	400	500	60–65% of total calories	
Protein (g)	84	105	150	15–20% of total calories	
Fat (g)	37	52	83	15–25% of total calories	

Actual calorie levels are ± 100 kcal.
[a]Lower calorie plans require more snacks when carbohydrate loading.

must be addressed. In addition, a thorough physical assessment including health history, health risk analysis, anthropometric data, and laboratory data should be performed and reviewed.

Calorie Intake

Energy needs must be determined by characterizing training and performance activities for type, frequency, duration, and intensity. Work and other nonrecreational activities should also be evaluated for energy costs. These expenditures may then be used to calculate calorie needs. A simple method for either adults or growing athletes is as follows (81).

- Adult: (pounds ideal body weight × 15) + exercise cost = daily energy needs.
- Growing athlete: (pounds ideal body weight × 30) + exercise cost = daily energy needs.

Exercise costs must be estimated from tables describing energy expenditure during various sports activities (82). In general, these costs will depend on body weight and exercise intensity and duration. Examples from various sports can be expressed as kilocalories expended per kilogram body weight per hour, as shown in Table 23.3.

It is not easy to predict energy requirements precisely. As an alternative, the athlete's actual calorie intake may be used as a starting point. Unfortunately, dietary analysis for any nutrient, whether by hand or by computer, is also difficult and often imprecise (83). This type of assessment is best left in the hands of a dietitian.

It is often useful to explore the athlete's weight history for fluctuations related to changes in diet, work, or exercise habits. An overweight athlete who has been steadily losing weight on a consistent diet and exercise program may need no adjustment in calorie intake. However, weight-change trends that are too extreme or are moving away from optimal levels indicate unfavorable calorie balances. Thus, the underweight athlete who is continuing to lose and the overweight athlete who is still gaining will both require adjustments of calorie intake.

Nutrient Distribution

If the proper calorie intake can be determined, the proportion given to carbohydrates, protein, and fat should be decided. For example, during normal training periods, a safe, effective, high-compliance plan appears to be at least 60% carbohydrate, no more than 15% protein, and less than 30% fat (1). For example, an athlete requiring 2000 kcal per day could consume 1200 kcal of carbohydrate, 300 kcal of protein, and 500 kcal of fat. Athletes with either very high or low calorie intakes should have their carbohydrate and protein needs calculated using body weight (7 to 10 g carbohydrate and 1 to 1.5 g protein/kg body weight as discussed above). These figures must be translated into servings of various food groups that will also supply adequate micronutrients.

The Food Exchange System

A useful method for implementing this type of diet is the food exchange system (84). In this system, the athlete would be given categories of foods from which to eat, such as dairy, meat, grain, fruits, and vegetables. Each category would have many choices, all of which contain similar amounts of calories and nutrients for the serving sizes indicated. The athlete would be instructed on how many servings from each category would result in the desired dietary intake of calories, carbohydrates, protein, fat, and micronutrients.

A suitable exchange system for the athlete's diet is presented in Table 23.4. It is based largely on lists developed jointly by the American Diabetes Association and the American Dietetic Association (85). The diet is divided into seven categories of food: starch/bread, lean- to medium-fat proteins, vegetables, fruit, milk products, fats, and snacks. According to the total calorie level desired, a given number of portions or exchanges from each category is included in the daily diet. Three typical calorie intakes are shown, and extrapolations may be made to accommodate other calorie levels.

This exchange system attempts to provide a high-carbohydrate, moderate-protein, low-fat diet with adequate vitamin and mineral balance. However, such plans have been shown to be insufficient in micronutrient levels as previously discussed (see Dietary Needs of the Athlete). Therefore, additional recommendations for maximizing micronutrient intakes have also been supplied.

Carbohydrate supercompensation, as discussed previously (see Nutrition and the Endurance Athlete), requires a temporary increase in carbohydrate intake up to 10 g/kg body weight or 70% of total calories. This requires additional exchanges of primarily carbohydrate food categories, also presented in Table 23.4.

An extensive list of foods belonging to each exchange category, along with portion sizes, is pro-

Table 23.5.   Food Choices in Exchange System Categories

Starches/bread (80 kcal, 15 g C, 3 g P, tr F)
3 Tbsp Grape-nuts, wheat germ; $\frac{1}{3}$ cup All-Bran, Bran-Buds
$\frac{1}{2}$ cup bran flakes, shredded wheat, cooked cereals, grits
$\frac{3}{4}$ cup low-sugar breakfast cereals
$1\frac{1}{2}$ cups puffed cereal
$\frac{1}{3}$ cup cooked rice, $\frac{1}{2}$ cup cooked pasta, oriental noodles[a]

1 slice bread, $\frac{1}{2}$ bagel, bun, English muffin, pita, 2 taco shells[a]
1 small roll, tortilla, biscuit,[a] muffin[a]
2 small pancakes,[a] 1 waffle[a]
2-inch cube cornbread,[a] 2 bread sticks
$\frac{3}{4}$ oz low-fat crackers, pretzels, matzoh, 6 snack crackers[a]
3 cups air-popped corn, 1 cup low-fat croutons

$\frac{1}{2}$ cup corn, lima beans, green peas, plantain, mashed potato
1 small potato, 6-inch corn on cob, 1 cup winter squash
$\frac{1}{3}$ cup yam, sweet potato, 10 (1.5 oz) french fries[a]

$\frac{1}{4}$ cup baked beans, $\frac{1}{3}$ cup cooked lentils, beans, peas

Lean protein (55 kcal, 0g C, 7g P, 3g F)
1 oz lean beef (round, sirloin, flank, tenderloin), wild game
1 oz ham, Canadian bacon, pork tenderloin, veal chops and roasts
1 oz skinless chicken, turkey, cornish hen
1.5 oz very low-fat (95%) lunch meat
1 oz fresh or frozen fish, 6 oysters, 2 sardines
2 oz shellfish, $\frac{1}{4}$ cup water-packed tuna
$\frac{1}{4}$ cup cottage cheese, 2 Tbsp Parmesan, 1 oz very low-cal diet cheeses
3 egg whites, $\frac{1}{2}$ cup low-calorie egg substitutes

Medium-fat protein (75 kcal, 0g C, 7g P, 5g F)
1 oz most beef products except prime cuts and corned beef
1 oz most pork products except ribs, ground pork, and sausage
1 oz most lamb products except ground lamb
1 oz unbreaded veal cutlet, 1 oz low-fat (86%) lunch meat
1 oz poultry with skin, duck or goose, ground turkey
$\frac{1}{4}$ cup canned salmon, oil-packed tuna
1 oz mozzarella, other part-skim cheeses, diet cheeses
$\frac{1}{4}$ cup ricotta cheese
1 egg, $\frac{1}{4}$ cup egg substitutes
1 oz liver, other organ meats
4 oz tofu

1 oz other meats,[a] fried chicken or fish[a]
1 turkey/chicken frankfurter,[a] 1 beef/pork frankfurter[b]
1 Tbsp peanut butter[a]

Vegetables (25 kcal, 5g C, 2g P, 0g F)
$\frac{1}{2}$ Cooked, 1 cup raw vegetables
See starches/bread category for starchy vegetables

Fruit (60 kcal, 15g C, 0g P, 0g F)
1 medium-size whole fruit
$\frac{1}{2}$ cup most fresh fruit, unsweetened canned fruit or juice
1 cup most berries, grapes, papaya, melons
$\frac{1}{4}$ cup most dried fruit, less of sweeter types
$\frac{1}{2}$ banana, grapefruit, mango, pomegranate

Milk products (90 kcal, 12g C, 8g P, tr F)
1 cup 0–1% fat milk, buttermilk, yogurt
$\frac{1}{3}$ cup nonfat dry milk powder, $\frac{1}{2}$ cup evaporated skim milk

Similar amounts of low-fat or whole milk products[a]

Added fat (45 kcal, 5g C, 0g P, 5g F)
1 tsp butter, margarine, mayonnaise, vegetable oil
1 Tbsp diet margarine, low-calorie mayonnaise, cream cheese
2 Tbsp sour cream, 2 Tbsp coffee creamer

2 tsp creamy salad dressing
1 Tbsp oil-type salad dressing, low-calorie creamy salad dressings
2 Tbsp low-calorie oil-type salad dressing

10 large/20 small peanuts, 4 halves walnuts, pecans
1 Tbsp most seeds, cashews, other nuts, 2 tsp pumpkin seeds
5 large/10 small olives, $\frac{1}{8}$ avocado, 2 Tbsp coconut
1 slice bacon, $\frac{1}{2}$ ounce chitterlings

Snacks (150–200 kcal, 40g C, 0–7g P, 0–5g F)
12 oz juice, soft drink
20-24 oz sports drink
5-6 oz carbohydrate recovery drink
$\frac{1}{4}$ cup dried fruit
4 fig bars
3 servings fruit category
1 slice ($\frac{1}{12}$) angel food cake
18 animal crackers, vanilla wafers,[a] 8 graham crackers, 4 oatmeal cookies[a]
$\frac{3}{4}$ cup low-fat/nonfat frozen yogurt, soft serve, sherbet

C, carbohydrate; P, protein; F, fat.
[a]Includes one fat exchange.
[b]Includes two fat exchanges.

vided in Table 23.5. Many meals will contain multiple exchanges of one food. For example, a typical hamburger will contain 4 ounces of meat (four protein exchanges) on one bun (two starch/bread exchanges). A mixed dish, such as pizza, will be composed of starch, protein, and fat exchanges. Familiarity with the portion sizes of exchange items is key to the successful application of this system. Patient education tools may be obtained from either the American Diabetes Association or the American Dietetic Association.

Within exchange categories, certain micronutrients may be emphasized when necessary. For example, certain athletes may wish to increase calcium in their diet by including more cheese choices from the protein category. Others may focus on iron intake by using red meats from the protein category and fortified breakfast cereals and legumes from the starch/bread category. A qualified nutritionist will be able to address these types of individual needs.

NUTRITION-RELATED PROBLEMS IN ATHLETES

Anemia

It appears that nutritional anemias, principally caused by iron deficiency, are at least as common in athletes as in the general population. Menstruating girls and women and boys during rapid growth spurts are especially at risk. This means that the sports health professional should look for anemia as one of the most important consequences of poor nutrition. Not only may the presence of anemia affect the overall health of the athlete, but exercise performance will likely suffer as well (86).

The symptoms of weakness and easy fatigue are the hallmarks of true anemia. In an athlete, this may become apparent as a decrease in strength or endurance. Other symptoms may include impairment of mental function and decreased resistance to infections (87, 88).

Blood tests done for either diagnostic or screening purposes may reveal clinical evidence of anemia. In the athlete, results of these tests must be interpreted somewhat differently from those of the general population. Physiologic changes associated with regular exercise may cause a dilutional pseudo-anemia, which may result in below normal values in certain hematologic tests. Also, there are possible causes of anemia that are unique to the athlete, such as exertional bleeding from the gastrointestinal or genitourinary tracts (89, 90).

The single most useful measure for detecting significant anemia is hemoglobin (91). Values pre-

Table 23.6. Minimum Acceptable Values for Serum Hemoglobin

	Serum hemoglobin (gm/DL)		
	11–14 yr	15–17 yr	18–44 yr
Male	12.0	13.1	13.4
Female	12.0	12.0	11.9
Blacks	Subtract 0.5 gm/dL		
Higher altitudes	Add 4% for each 1000 m elevation		

viously obtained for an individual before entering into a regular exercise program may be considered personal "normals" if the state of health and nutrition at that time was adequate. Otherwise, lower limits of standard norms (Table 23.6) may be used (90, 92).

Below-normal values indicate the need for a complete blood count (CBC) and serum ferritin to evaluate iron stores. Some authorities recommend screening athletes with serum ferritin to detect borderline iron deficiency, which may occur without anemia and may also impair performance (90, 92). Lower limits of ferritin are 10 mcg/L for those younger than 14 years of age and 12 mcg/L for those older than 14 years. Normal values below 20 mcg/L are considered borderline for those 14 and older.

Uncommon causes of anemia must be ruled out. Microcytic hypochromic anemia may be due to thalassemia minor, an inherited defect of hemoglobin common among blacks, Indochinese, and persons of Mediterranean ancestry. Other possible causes include lead poisoning and chronic disease such as rheumatoid arthritis and cancer (87). Anemia with normal to enlarged red blood cells may be due to deficiencies of folic acid and/or vitamin B_{12} as well as chronic hemolysis due to high-impact exercise (running on hard surfaces, contact sports) (89, 92).

If the anemia is associated with low iron stores, the cause of depletion should be investigated. Low dietary intake may be the most likely cause, especially if the athlete avoids meat or is attempting to lose weight. A test for occult blood in the stool and hematuria should be done if response to iron therapy is poor. Malabsorption syndromes may also have to be ruled out (89, 92).

Iron therapy is recommended as a first attempt to correct low hemoglobin with low or borderline ferritin levels. A total of 150 to 300 mg/day of supplemental iron in cases of frank anemia or severe iron depletion should cause a rise in hemoglobin of 1 g/dL within 6 weeks, in which case therapy should continue for a total of 8 to 12 months (89, 90, 92). If the hemoglobin levels do not respond, other causes should be sought.

Some highly trained athletes with apparent iron-deficiency anemias may not respond to iron therapy. If there are no symptoms and performance appears optimum, it may be concluded that they have dilutional pseudoanemia, which should not be treated further. Borderline iron stores without anemia may be treated with 50 to 100 mg/day until ferritin rises above 20 mcg/L (90, 92).

Iron supplements are commonly in the form of ferrous sulfate, fumarate, or gluconate, all of which have been successfully used to treat iron deficiency. Newer forms such as carbonyl iron, iron dextran, and heme iron may be better absorbed and tolerated but will cost more (93).

The prevention of recurring iron-deficiency anemia should focus on treating pathologic causes when they exist and guaranteeing adequate dietary intake. Lean red meat and dark poultry meat are concentrated sources of well-absorbed iron. Athletes should be encouraged to provide themselves with a food or supplemental source of vitamin C with every meal to facilitate iron absorption. Similarly, inhibitors of iron absorption, such as tea and coffee, are best consumed away from meals, if at all. Supplemental iron at RDA levels may be necessary if dietary approaches are inadequate (88, 92, 93).

Thermal Injuries, Dehydration, and Water Intoxication

These problems are related to each other in that they are affected by extremes of environmental conditions and by fluid intake by athletes during prolonged exercise.

THERMAL INJURIES

Hyperthermia and hypothermia are potentially serious conditions that may arise during distance running and other prolonged athletic endeavors. Hyperthermia is considered the most common medical complication of fun runs, marathons, and other distance events. Hypothermia may occur in cold, wet, and/or windy conditions and may more frequently involve exercisers who are slow or who allow their blood sugar to decline (94).

Hyperthermia

Hyperthermia can develop during exercise sessions lasting as little as 1 hour or less. Certain individuals are more prone than others to heat injury. These include persons who are obese, unfit, dehydrated, or unacclimatized to the heat. Children and those with previous history of heat stroke are also at increased risk, as are those who attempt to exercise when ill. Early symptoms of heat injury include loss of coordination, either excessive sweating or cessation of sweating, headache, nausea, dizziness, apathy, and gradual impairment of consciousness (94).

Loss of body weight as water and elevated rectal temperature are good indicators of approaching hyperthermia. Up to 10% declines in body weight have been recorded as have rectal temperature elevations of more than 6°F (94).

Environmental heat stress levels should be known whenever intense training or competitions are scheduled to occur. A combined index of temperature, humidity, and radiation known as wet bulb globe temperature (WBGT) is a more accurate predictor of risk for heat injury. WBGT of over 73°F is considered a high risk level, whereas levels over 82°F are grounds for cancelling the activity (60, 94).

Progressive training under stressful weather conditions will promote adaptations that should help protect the athlete from thermal injuries (60, 94). In the case of hyperthermia prevention, avoidance of dehydration is essential (see below).

Hypothermia

Hypothermia usually occurs near the end of a long exercise session under permissive conditions. Inexperienced athletes who may be poorly clothed and who drastically reduce their exercise pace during the second half of an exercise session, thereby allowing core temperature to deteriorate, are at risk. WBGT levels below 50°F indicate possible environmental risk. Early symptoms and signs of hypothermia include shivering, euphoria, and apparent intoxication followed by lethargy, muscle weakness, and cessation of shivering (94).

Warm clothing and warm drinks will provide the best protection against hypothermia in adverse climactic conditions. Athletes should maintain postexercise blood glucose levels with adequate carbohydrate intake well after the end of exercise to support continued temperature regulation (61, 94).

DEHYDRATION

Dehydration may occur for many reasons. Long, intense training sessions or competitions in warm, humid weather without adequate water intake are a common cause. Some athletes, especially those in weight-class sports such as wrestling, voluntarily deplete their water reserves before weigh-in (sometimes using diuretics) to assure being placed in the lowest possible weight category (95).

Athletic performance has been shown to deteriorate with as little as 1 to 2% loss of body weight as water. However, the principal hazard of dehydration is the resulting impairment of thermal regulation. With a 5% body weight loss as water, body temperature can rise several degrees Fahrenheit. Cardiovascular efficiency suffers as well, evidenced by arterial resting pulses of more than 160 bpm (61, 94, 96).

Adequate fluid intake should minimize weight loss and temperature elevation during exercise. Hydration before intense exercise in the heat should probably begin 1 to 2 days ahead of time. Before exercise, as much fluid as comfortable should be taken, possibly with a small amount of electrolyte (1 to 2 g salt/L) to avoid blunting thirst and stimulating urine production (96). Fluid intake during and after exercise should follow guidelines presented for endurance athletes (see Nutrition and the Endurance Athlete).

Athletes who insist on voluntary dehydration before weigh-in must rehydrate quickly within the 1 to 5 hours before competition to minimize detrimental effects of this practice on performance. Sports drinks appear to be more effective than plain water in rehydrating these athletes, but rehydration is not likely to be complete and performance will probably suffer as a result (76, 95).

WATER INTOXICATION (HYPONATREMIA)

With the advent of ultraendurance competitions lasting several hours, a previously unseen condition of water intoxication or hyponatremia has appeared as a complication of such endurance exercise. Events lasting longer than an average of 8 hours appear to pose the greatest risk of this disorder, which may occur in as high as 27% of competitors and be responsible for up to 67% of medical emergencies during ultradistance events (97). Serum sodium levels below 125 mEq/L are found, and symptoms range from nausea and cramps to convulsions and coma. The condition must be treated as a medical emergency, and intravenous fluids may be necessary (97, 98).

The cause of hyponatremia is probably a combination of poor fitness and/or heat acclimatization and overhydration with fluids low in electrolytes, especially sodium. Many cases have involved athletes drinking large amounts of diluted soft drinks containing very little sodium over several hours (97, 98).

Athletes in training for ultraendurance events who experience profuse perspiration should not restrict salt in their diet. Fluid replacement during ultraendurance events should use electrolyte-containing beverages containing at least 10 mEq sodium (230 mg) and chloride (355 mg) and 5 mEq potassium (195 mg) per quart of water to supply adequate electrolytes (99). Training in the heat appears to help prevent hyponatremia by conditioning the body to reduce the sodium content of sweat. Exercising for 90 minutes every day for 2 weeks in hot weather is effective (98, 100).

Low Body Weight and Eating Disorders

Body weight issues are one of the most serious concerns in sports nutrition. Many athletes, such as runners and swimmers, mistakenly equate body leanness with optimum performance and attempt to lose as much weight as possible to compete successfully. Certain sports contribute additional stimulus to athletes' weight-loss compulsions by using weight classifications (wrestling, boxing) or by sanctioning aesthetic evaluations of performance (figure skating, gymnastics, diving) that use narrow cultural ideals of body size and shape (50, 101).

As a result of the above factors, some athletes seek to achieve a degree of leanness that is often detrimental to their health and/or performance. Some attempt rapid weight-loss efforts that result in catabolism of lean body mass instead of fat. Others, such as wrestlers, cycle up and down in body weight several times in one season, using bizarre dietary patterns and even dehydration to achieve their goal weight before each competition (102).

Dietary restrictions used for weight-loss purposes may induce significant nutritional deficiencies. As body fat stores are depleted, the athlete may experience chronic fatigue and sleep disturbances as well as reduced performance, impaired ability for intensive training, and increased vulnerability to injury (103). Resulting amenorrhea in women may lead to bone loss and infertility. The relationship among disordered eating, amenorrhea, and bone loss in these athletes has been termed the female athlete triad (see Amenorrhea and Bone Loss) (104).

How can the sports health professional identify athletes who are too lean? Excessive underweight is best defined in terms of low body fat. Any male or female athlete who falls among the leanest 4% of their age group should be evaluated for signs of impaired health or performance. This would represent college-age men at 5% body fat and below or college-age women at 14% body fat and below. However, many individuals will be found who are functioning well in this low body fat group due to genetic predisposition (103).

The evaluation of thin patients should begin with a family history, looking for similar patterns of body size. The athlete's own weight history may be revealing, showing either a long pattern of natural leanness or an abrupt change coinciding with entering high-level competition, suggesting performance pressures. The medical history may indicate a number of stress fractures or menstrual irregularity in a female athlete. Any athlete who, to maintain thinness, is using severe dietary restriction or pathogenic weight-loss methods (purging, diet pills, dehydration) most likely has an unrealistic target weight or possibly a distorted body image (50, 103).

Eating disorders may feature food restriction, bingeing/purging, use of drugs such as diuretics and laxatives, and/or abnormal thought patterns in relation to body weight and food. These conditions have been reported to afflict from 15 to 62% of female athletes and may be prevalent among certain types of male athletes (wrestlers, boxers) as well. The achievement-oriented athletic personality faced with pressures from coaches, parents, and peers constitutes a high risk for developing an eating disorder. Other psychosocial and even biochemical factors may also play important roles (14, 104).

In addition to causing abnormally low body fat in many cases, eating disorders may lead to other health consequences: esophageal inflammation may be caused by frequent vomiting; electrolyte imbalances may occur due to overuse of laxatives; and renal dysfunction is a potential result of diuretic abuse. Emotional disturbances are present in almost every case (14, 101).

Identifying athletes with eating disorders may be difficult, due to the secretive nature of this behavior. Treatment success is variable, often requiring a team approach from medical, psychological, and nutrition specialists who are skilled in managing eating disorders. Coaches, trainers, and parents who are encouraging the development of eating disorders by establishing unrealistic standards of slenderness should be educated to avoid these mistakes (14, 50).

If the nutritional intake of an athlete is not sufficient to sustain training or maintain health, several solutions are possible. Special attention should be given to designing and implementing an optimal diet for the individual, perhaps with the assistance of a trained nutrition counselor. Nutritional supplements containing the appropriate nutrients—calories, carbohydrates, protein, or micronutrients—can be used if eating behavior is not reliable. The training regimen may have to be modified, at least temporarily. In severe cases, emaciated or impaired athletes may need to be excluded from athletic events (101, 103).

Amenorrhea and Bone Loss

Exercise is generally known to be beneficial for increasing bone mass, and active individuals (including athletes) are usually found to have greater bone density than their sedentary counterparts (49). Amenorrheic female athletes, many of whom have been shown to be below normal in bone density, are exceptions to this observation (105). Because many of these athletes may be attempting to control their weight by restricting calories, the syndrome of disordered eating, amenorrhea, and bone loss has been described as the female athlete triad (see Low Body Weight and Eating Disorders) (104).

Amenorrhea, defined as the absence of menses for 6 months or more, occurs in 2 to 5% of the general female population. Strikingly, the prevalence in athletes has been reported to be as high as 66% in some studies (104). Athletic amenorrhea appears to result from decreased secretion of gonadotropin-releasing hormone by the hypothalamus, resulting in hypoestrogenism. The causes of this failure are not fully understood, but may include elevated adrenal stress hormones and increased production of endorphins and related neuroendocrine substances. Low body fat may also contribute to reduced estrogen production. A decrease in estrogen levels allows bone resorption to exceed bone deposition, leading to decreased bone mass (106, 107).

The most serious, immediate consequence of this process is the increased risk for stress fractures and other musculoskeletal injuries. Amenorrheic female athletes have a significantly greater risk of stress fractures compared with those with normal menstrual cycles, and many have multiple fractures (106, 108). Because these problems will have a direct effect on future performance, the occurrence of amenorrhea must be considered a warning sign of heightened vulnerability to athletic injury. The condition should be evaluated, appropriate precautions taken, and a plan of management formulated.

Amenorrhea is more likely to develop in certain athletes. Girls who begin strenuous training before menarche or after a history of disturbed menstrual function are at higher risk, as are women who have never been pregnant. Low body weight, calorie restriction, vegetarianism, and eating disorders are also risk factors. Physical and possibly psychological stress experienced during intense training also plays an important, although poorly understood role (106, 107).

The amenorrheic athlete with a history of normal menstruation should have a complete medical and gynecologic workup to rule out pathologic and other causes (109). Young girls who have reached age 14 without the appearance of secondary sexual characteristics or have reached age 16 without the onset of the menstrual cycle should also be evaluated. Only when other possibilities have been eliminated can the diagnosis of athletic amenorrhea be made (109).

Bone mass measurement can help provide an index of the severity of amenorrheic bone loss. Plain radiographs may show advanced osteopenia, in which case further medical evaluation is warranted to rule out malnutrition, malabsorption, effects of medications, endocrine disorders, and other systemic diseases. Early bone loss, however, is detectable only through photon or x-ray absorptiometry and computed tomography. These sophisticated techniques are generally available in large radiologic facilities and may be used to follow changes in bone mass over time (63, 107).

Prompt normalization of bone mass changes is a high priority for female athletes; bone loss can approach 4% per year in the early stages of athletic amenorrhea. The athlete should be encouraged to take steps to regain her normal menstrual cycle. It has been shown that amenorrheic athletes who regain a normal cycle, usually by reducing training intensity and/or increasing body weight, experience an increase in bone mass (106). If it does not seem likely that a normal cycle will return, whether due to noncompliance or other factors, hormone replacement therapy should be considered through appropriate referral. Failure to restore normal hormone levels may lead to irreversible bone loss (106).

Other nutritional factors need to be addressed in athletes at risk for bone loss. Calcium intake in female athletes is frequently below RDA levels and should be addressed (see Designing the Athlete's Diet). Amenorrheic females may require as much as 1500 mg calcium/day. Protein intake may also be insufficient in low–body-weight athletes and should be increased when indicated. Conversely, excessive intake of protein and vitamins A and D may increase bone loss and should be discouraged (106).

Bone mass measurement would be the best method for monitoring changes in osteopenic athletes but may be prohibitively expensive. Other measurements that may be useful indexes of recovery from amenorrheic bone loss include (1) body composition measures such as height, weight, triceps, and calf skinfolds or other body density techniques and (2) laboratory analysis of fasting urinary ratios for calcium versus creatinine and hydroxyproline versus creatinine (107). These measures can be accomplished in many health-care settings at relatively low cost.

NUTRITION AND SPORTS INJURIES

The sports health professional will often encounter an athlete after a significant injury has occurred. In this instance, recovery from the trauma is the athlete's highest priority. Nutrition and the use of natural agents may be useful adjuncts to conservative care in this regard.

Inflammation

Normal response to trauma for the first few days includes edema, release of inflammatory proteins, mobilization of leukocytes, and production of fibrin. Some of these changes increase the pain sensation that accompanies tissue injury. Accumulation of cell debris, serum exudates, blood, and fibrin during the inflammatory phase may impede subsequent healing by impairment of normal circulation. It would seem desirable to minimize and reverse these inflammatory processes as soon as therapeutic management has begun to decrease discomfort and speed healing (110).

Although pharmaceuticals are better known and commonly used in the early phases of injury rehabilitation, certain natural substances have also been used in the conservative management of sports injuries as antiinflammatory, analgesic, and/or fibrinolytic agents. These include proteolytic enzymes, bioflavinoids, and vitamin C (111).

PROTEOLYTIC ENZYMES

These enzymes are available as extracts from bovine pancreas (trypsin, chymotrypsin), pineapple skin (bromelain), or other sources. Their use in the treatment of musculoskeletal trauma and other inflammatory conditions is based on two proposed mechanisms in which these enzymes augment the action of natural tissue proteases. First, they may reduce inflammatory response by causing the breakdown of inflammatory proteins that cause vascular permeability and pain. Second, they may significantly improve local circulation and reduce edema by breaking down cell debris and fibrin, facilitating their uptake by the lymphatic system (111–113)

It has long been thought that orally ingested proteins would neither survive the digestive process intact nor be absorbable if they did survive. However, absorption studies have demonstrated significant (although less than 40%) uptake of oral proteolytic enzymes through the gastrointestinal tract (114). It is also possible that certain peptide fragments of these enzymes could retain some proteolytic activity (112, 113).

Numerous studies exist (111, 115–126) relative to the usefulness of proteolytic enzymes in the management of injuries common to athletes. Injuries described included bruises, sprains, strains, hematomas, lacerations, and fractures. Eleven of the studies used adequate controls. As much as 30 to 50% reduction in healing time has been observed using enzyme therapy as soon as possible after an injury occurred. Some investigations used prophylactic treatment of athletes and demonstrated fewer time-loss injuries and faster return to competition (111).

No consensus exists as to the most potent member of this group of enzymes, although animal research has suggested that combinations may be more effective. Most enzyme products used in research were provided in enteric-coated tablets for protection through the upper gastrointestinal tract. Doses given amounted to as much as 12 or more tablets/day (111, 112).

Contraindications to the use of proteolytic enzymes include increased bleeding tendencies (including use of anticoagulant medication), systemic infection, and allergy to food sources (pineapple, beef, pork, papaya) (112).

BIOFLAVINOIDS AND CURCUMIN

Bioflavinoids are a group of natural plant compounds that have been found to possess various biologic activities. Their effects on reducing vascular permeability, which will limit edema, and inhibiting the production of inflammatory prostaglandins are of interest in the treatment of inflammation (127, 128).

Optimum use of bioflavinoids will necessitate supplementation before the peak of the inflammatory phase because they will not reduce established edema. Research on postinjury therapy with bioflavinoids is lacking, but prophylactic treatment of athletes with 600 to 1800 mg/day reduced by two thirds time lost from injuries suffered by football players (129, 130).

Curcumin is a plant pigment derived from turmeric. Ayurvedic (Indian herbal) medicine has long cited its usefulness in the treatment of trauma and inflammation, and animal research has confirmed the antiinflammatory properties of curcumin. No studies using injured athletes have been done, but one controlled human study demonstrated reduced edema and wound tenderness in patients undergoing minor surgery who were treated with 1200 mg/day of curcumin (131).

VITAMIN C

Vitamin C is often found in natural antiinflammatory formulas, although little research exists to support this inclusion. Animal studies have included vitamin C in combination with bioflavinoids with apparent synergistic effects against some aspects of inflammation (132). Other studies have suggested possible mechanisms for the action of vitamin C, including increased fibrinolysis, antihistamine activity, improved cell membrane stability, and synthesis of adrenal corticosteroids (130).

DIMETHYL SULFOXIDE (DMSO)

This substance has been used for decades as an industrial solvent. More recently, it has been used as a topical antiinflammatory agent in the treatment of minor injuries and arthritis (133). It is considered potentially toxic in high doses, especially in the impure forms available over the counter. Pharmaceutical-quality DMSO in a 50% concentration appears to be the safest to use.

Muscle Spasm, Cramps, and Delayed-Onset Soreness

Muscle spasm occurs in athletes commonly as a result of injury or overexertion during intense efforts. The circumstances under which muscle spasm occurs will help determine whether nutrition therapy will be beneficial (134, 135).

Strains of muscle tissues and articular sprains result in protective muscle spasm that is best managed with physical therapy as discussed elsewhere in this text (see Chapter 3). Oral supplements containing calcium, magnesium, and/or certain herbs such as valerian are popular treatments but have no clinical research to validate their usefulness in traumatic muscle spasm.

Muscle cramps, occurring without obvious trauma, may have nutritional or nonnutritional causes. Biomechanical causes, such as shortened muscles that are then overstretched, must be considered. Truly pathologic causes such as vascular insufficiency must also be ruled out (134, 135).

Leg cramps during extensive exercising may simply be caused by dehydration, in which case increasing water intake will solve the problem. Mineral imbalances or deficiencies are considered unlikely contributors to muscle cramping. Nevertheless, additional intake of potassium, magnesium, and calcium may prevent impaired local circulation and increased irritability of muscle tissue (51, 136). Older individuals with leg cramps caused by peripheral vascular disease may benefit from 300 to 800 IU of vitamin E (137).

Delayed-onset muscle soreness (DOMS), a well-recognized consequence of unaccustomed activity, may appear within 24 hours of strenuous exercise and can last for days (138). One recent controlled study demonstrated that 3000 mg/day of vitamin C taken 3 days before and 4 days after strenuous exercise of the posterior calf muscles substantially reduced the severity of DOMS in approximately one half of subjects (139). No other nutrition research on this condition has been reported.

Tissue Healing

After the acute inflammatory stage of injury is under control, the clinician is next concerned with tissue healing or the proliferative stage (110). Regeneration of disrupted skin, muscle, vascular tissue, and connective tissue requires the availability of sufficient energy and appropriate protein and nonprotein precursors. Micronutrient cofactors may also be required for optimum tissue synthesis (140).

TISSUE HEALING RESEARCH

Animal research has established that many, if not most, nutrients play a role in the healing of wounded tissue. Evidence points to the importance of preventing deficiencies of calories; protein; essential fatty acids; vitamins A, B_1, B_2, B_6, C, and pantothenic acid; and the minerals zinc, copper, manganese, selenium, and perhaps silicon (140, 141). In addition, surgical and other serious traumas in humans appear to increase requirements for protein and vitamins B_1, B_2, B_3, and C temporarily. Animal and some human studies have demonstrated that the supplementation of certain nutrients (including arginine; ornithine; vitamins A, B_1, and C; pantothenic acid; and zinc) in amounts greater than normal requirements have beneficial effects on tissue healing (140, 141). The number of potentially useful nutrients has led some authorities to suggest broad-spectrum vitamin-mineral supplementation along with increased dietary protein intake for the healing of traumatic athletic injuries (142).

GLYCOSAMINOGLYCANS AND CHONDROITIN SULFATE

Clinical interest in the healing of musculoskeletal injuries has resulted in the appearance of nutritional products containing precursors and cofactors for the synthesis of connective tissue. Unfamiliar constituents of many of these products are glycosaminoglycans or chondroitin sulfates.

Glycosaminoglycans (GAG, mucopolysaccharides, proteoglycans) supply the matrix for most connective tissue and bone and are major constituents of cartilage, intervertebral disc material, and synovial fluid. They are composed of small amounts of protein, large amounts of specialized carbohydrates synthesized by chondrocytes, and some minerals (143). Manganese is a required cofactor for the synthesizing enzymes (144).

Glycosaminoglycans have been shown to be well absorbed in humans as both intact and broken down particles. It has been shown to be deposited into bone and joint tissues in animals. In vitro studies have shown exogenous glucosamine to be efficiently incorporated into connective tissue proteoglycans, resulting in enhanced production of these molecules (145–147).

Chondroitin sulfates and other glycosaminoglycans are available as supplements in the form of shark fin and bovine trachea extracts as well as mussel concentrates, often with the addition of manganese and other enzyme cofactors. Some preparations are purified to remove indigestible constituents, which probably improves absorption. No direct studies on their effectiveness in humans with musculoskeletal injuries have been published. However, human studies using topical cartilage extracts have demonstrated improvements in wound healing. Furthermore, injected extracts have enhanced repair of osteoarthritic and traumatized cartilage and have been used to treat patellar tendinitis successfully (147).

MICROCRYSTALLINE HYDROXYAPATITE AND FRACTURE HEALING

The healing of traumatic and stress fractures of bone is a slow process that often critically interrupts training and competition. The previous discussions on tissue healing would also apply to the management of these skeletal injuries, with the obvious addition of adequate dietary calcium, phosphorus, and magnesium to support remineralization.

Microcrystalline hydroxyapatite is a new mineral compound that has recently emerged as a possible improvement in the nutritional support of bone remineralization (148, 149). It is prepared from veal bone by fat extraction and low-temperature grinding. The product retains all the minerals, proteins, and glycosaminoglycans of the original source tissue. Calcium absorption from this compound appears to be superior than from traditional sources of supplemental calcium (150).

Whereas much of the research on hydroxyapatite is focusing on applications in prevention and treatment of osteoporosis (148), older studies using the compound have yielded promising results in the facilitation of fracture healing, at least in older patients and in cases of delayed union (149). Current research is using 6 to 8 g/day as a therapeutic dose (150).

FRONTIERS AND CONTROVERSIES IN SPORTS NUTRITION

Ergogenic Aids

ARGININE/ORNITHINE

These amino acids are not considered essential for the human diet because they are synthesized from other amino acids. Typical intake in the U.S. diet is approximately 5 g/day (93).

Animal research has linked arginine and ornithine with increases in pituitary growth hormone (GH). GH stimulates growth at the expense of calories, which would seem to be beneficial for the gain of lean body mass along with potential loss of body fat (29).

Research into the effects of arginine on humans first focused on parenteral administration. Significant changes in GH were found in several studies using infused doses of 15 to 30 g (29). It should be remembered that these results were accomplished through bypassing the digestive tract and the liver. Oral doses might necessarily have to be much larger to compensate for absorption difficulties and normal liver catabolism.

Neither 6 g of oral arginine nor 10 g of oral ornithine have elevated GH levels in human studies (29). A study using 170 mg/kg body weight of oral ornithine (average dose approximately 13 g) produced significant elevations of GH but also caused stomach cramping and diarrhea (151). Recent studies have confirmed the lack of effect of more moderate doses on GH in trained athletes (152, 153). However, one group of researchers has reported positive effects in untrained subjects taking 1 g/day each of arginine and ornithine versus placebo during a weight-training program. They showed significant effects on body composition, weight loss, and strength, but no effect on muscle girth (154, 155).

Possible side effects should be considered by athletes contemplating using high-dose arginine or ornithine. As mentioned above, large doses have caused nausea and diarrhea. Young athletes who have not completed skeletal growth should avoid stimulating GH by any means. It has been suggested that large doses along with a low intake of lysine may promote growth of herpesvirus (156).

ASPARTATE

This nonessential amino acid has been used and investigated for combating chronic fatigue. Research has shown somewhat consistent effects on untrained humans, but only one well-controlled study (157) out of five using trained athletes showed positive results. Doses of 7 to 10 g of mineral aspartate salts within 24 hours of exercise appear to be required for any demonstrable effect (29).

BEE AND FLOWER POLLEN

These substances, collected from beehives or directly from flowering plants, have been perceived as potent and exotic materials that could have far-reaching effects on health and fitness. The only well-controlled study testing these claims could find no enhancement of energy or physical fitness (158). Individuals with pollen allergies may be affected by ingesting these substances.

BRANCHED-CHAIN AMINO ACIDS

These essential amino acids, leucine, isoleucine, and valine, have a physiologic role as muscle energy substrates and inhibitors of protein catabolism. Hence these amino acids are popular among weight lifters and other athletes. Branched-chain amino acids are used clinically to prevent muscle wasting and restore lost muscle mass in patients with liver disease or severe trauma (159). However, no research on strength performance enhancement or muscle growth has been done in athletes or other healthy individuals, and studies on endurance performance have been mostly negative (160, 161).

BREWER'S YEAST

This product has long been known to be an excellent source of many nutrients, including B vitamins, trace minerals, and protein. It has been popular for many decades as a food supplement for this reason. Although many users have claimed far-reaching health benefits, no research exists for applications in sports nutrition (156).

Recently, there has been concern that allergies and yeast infections may be aggravated by consumption of food yeasts. Although there are individuals who are allergic to yeast, there is no similarity between food yeast and the organism *Candida albicans*, which is the pathogen responsible for most human yeast infections (156).

CAFFEINE

Caffeine is a frequent component of the U.S. diet by virtue of its occurrence in many popular beverages. One of its effects on human physiology appears to be the stimulation of fatty acid metabolism by the energy-producing processes of the cell (162).

Studies on athletic performance enhancement have shown caffeine to improve endurance in some athletes but not others. Possible reasons for an inconsistent effect include the following (29, 162):

- Differences in caffeine sensitivity among athletes.
- Variable effect of caffeine on different forms of exercise.
- Effects of other dietary components on the response to caffeine.

Effective doses of caffeine appear to be at least 5 mg/kg body weight, which would require 2 to 3 cups brewed coffee (29, 162, 163). Caffeine is a substance banned by the International Olympic Committee at levels that produce urinary concentrations of 12 mg/ml or more, which would require ingestion of several cups of coffee over a short period (162). In addition, the diuretic and other effects of large amounts of caffeine may be undesirable. Thus, athletes should make sure they are using the minimum effective dose, which will likely require some experimentation within legal limits.

CARNITINE

Carnitine is a natural substance normally produced in the human body from amino acids with vitamin cofactors. It plays a vital role in fatty acid metabolism for energy production in the mitochondria. Research has focused primarily on applications in heart disease and hyperlipidemia (29).

Success in the treatment of hereditary muscle diseases has led to suggestions that carnitine may enhance muscle function and stamina in athletes. Oral doses of 2 to 6 g/day for at least 2 weeks have led to improvement in aerobic capacity in some studies, especially when the subjects were trained athletes working at high intensities (29, 164). However, research on competitive performance measures is scant, and so far results have been disappointing (165, 166).

COENZYME Q

Also known in biochemistry as ubiquinone, coenzyme Q is one of the essential coenzymes of the electron transport chain in mitochondria, without which ATP production would be severely limited. Although normally synthesized in adequate amounts by the body, research has uncovered therapeutic applications in the treatment of heart disease (29, 156).

Some studies have shown positive effects of coenzyme Q on both aerobic and anaerobic exercise performance in healthy subjects, although most did not use trained athletes. Effective doses ranged from 60 to 100 mg/day for 4 to 6 weeks (29). However, recent studies using trained cyclists or triathletes could not demonstrate any effects on endurance performance (167, 168).

CREATINE

Creatine is the biologic substrate for the production of CP in skeletal muscle (see Nutrition and the Power Athlete). It is normally synthesized in the liver and is a natural dietary constituent in meat products, which contributes to the body's creatine pool (169, 170).

Recent controlled studies have demonstrated that a regimen of 5 g of creatine taken 4 times daily for 5 days elevates CP levels in muscle tissue. Furthermore, this regimen can improve short-term, maximal exercise performance, especially when the exercise is repeated with short recovery periods as in sprints and some team sports. Lower dose regimens are not as effective, and submaximal (endurance) exercise performance is not improved by creatine supplementation (169, 171).

CYTOCHROMES

Cytochromes are essential components of the mitochondrial electron transport chain but are not required in the diet. Some sports supplements contain these substances, but no research has been done to test their effects. Supplemental cytochromes may not only be unnecessary, but may not even be absorbed intact from the gastrointestinal tract (156).

GAMMA-ORYZANOL AND FERULIC ACID (FRAC)

These substances are, respectively, the lipid-soluble and water-soluble forms of the same plant compound that seems to possess antioxidant and neurostimulatory properties. Uncontrolled studies using gamma-oryzanol have appeared to demonstrate increases in anabolic responses to exercise stress as represented by fat-free weight gain in weight lifters. One controlled study using 30 mg/day of ferulic acid showed positive effects on one measure of strength and on weight gain in weight lifters; another study reported increased beta-endorphin levels in runners. More research is needed to clarify the usefulness of these compounds in various athletic endeavors (29, 172).

GINSENG

This root or extracts thereof have been highly regarded as a medicinal panacea for ages. Claims have included increased energy and physical stamina. Animal studies have demonstrated significant effects in this regard, but human studies using 200 to 2000 mg of ginseng root or extracts have not shown consistent effects (29, 173). However, it was recently reported that 1000 mg/day of Chinese ginseng (Panax) was more effective than Russian ginseng (Eleutherococcus) or placebo in improving some aspects of endurance fitness and muscular strength (174). Extracts may be more consistent in their potency than whole or powdered root. There is concern about the side effects of chronic overuse, which include hypertension, neurologic disturbances, and undesirable hormonal effects (156).

GLANDULARS

These concentrates or extracts of organ tissues come from animal sources. It is suggested that these substances may somehow enhance the function of corresponding tissues in the human body based on a "like cures like" hypothesis. Thus, testicular tissue is supposed to have an anabolic effect, etc. No evidence exists that this theory has any validity. Moreover, the constituents of these supplements are probably completely broken down to simple amino acids, fatty acids, and other basic components in the gastrointestinal tract before absorption (156).

INOSINE

Inosine is a purine-like substance that appears in exercising muscle. Its role in various cellular reactions has led to suggestions that it may have ergogenic effects (29). However, a recent study not only demonstrated no beneficial effect on aerobic performance, but also suggested that inosine may impair anaerobic performance (175). Thus, use of inosine should be discouraged. Inosine is metabolized to uric acid and thus may be hazardous to those suffering from gout (156).

OCTACOSANOL

Octacosanol is a long-chain fatty alcohol found in wheat germ oil. Studies using octacosanol or wheat germ oil (a fairly potent source) have been performed repeatedly since the middle of this century. One investigator has claimed significant ergogenic effects from large doses of wheat germ oil, but other researchers have not verified these results (29). However, one recent study reported that 1000 μg/day of octacosanol improved reaction times and grip strength (176). More research is needed.

PANGAMIC ACID ("B$_{15}$")

Also known as dimethylglycine (DMG), this substance appears to be normally synthesized in the liver and plays a role in choline metabolism. Most ergogenic and other claims made for DMG come from research in the Soviet Union, and is of questionable reliability. Only one small study in the West has produced positive performance results, whereas five recent well-controlled studies showed no effect on athletic performance (29).

PHOSPHATE

Phosphate is an intracellular ion that participates in many energy-related processes in human metabolism, including glycolysis, ATP production, hemoglobin-oxygen affinity, and cardiovascular function. Studies dating back to World War I have tested the hypothesis that phosphate loading would increase physical performance (29).

Well-controlled research has not brought about definite conclusions regarding the effectiveness of phosphate loading. However, some studies have shown measurable effects on endurance performance of phosphate in doses of 4 g/day for 3 to 6 days before exercise (80, 177).

ROYAL JELLY

This substance is produced by bees solely for the nourishment and hormone-like stimulation of the queen. Its mystique has garnered a reputation as a cure-all, with very little relevant research conducted to date. No studies on the enhancement of athletic performance have been done. It should be noted that the physiologic effect of royal jelly on the queen bee would suggest that, in sufficient quantities, it might have a feminizing effect on other organisms (156).

SPIRULINA

This product is composed of blue-green Cyanobacteria that are commercially cultivated and marketed as superior food sources of many nutrients and other "energizing" factors. Although spirulina is a good, if expensive, source of certain vitamins and minerals, no scientific literature supports claims of ergogenic effects (156).

SUCCINATE

Succinate is an intermediate metabolite in the citric acid (Krebs) cycle. It is regularly produced from the breakdown of carbohydrate, fat, and some amino acids. No research has been done to investigate claims of ergogenic effects (156).

TYROSINE

Tyrosine is an amino acid related to phenylalanine. It is a precursor to many specialized substances, such as thyroid hormone and catecholamine neurotransmitters. A dose of 6 grams per day has been shown to have an effect on high-altitude physical and mental functioning. It should not be taken by persons with hypertension or those taking antidepressants known as monoamine oxidase (MAO) inhibitors (156).

Acknowledgment

The author is greatful for bibliographic assistance from Kay Irvine, M.L.S., and Lynn Attwood, B.S.

References

1. American Dietetic Association. Position of the American Dietetic Association and the Canadian Dietetic Association: nutrition for physical fitness and athletic performance for adults. J Am Diet Assoc 1993;93:691–696.
2. Short SH. Surveys of dietary intake and nutrition knowledge of athletes and their coaches. In: Wolinsky I, Hickson JF, eds. Nutrition in exercise and sport. 2nd ed. Boca Raton: CRC Press, 1994:367–416.
3. Marcus JB, ed. Sports nutrition: a guide for the professional working with active people. Chicago: American Dietetic Association, 1986.
4. Committee on Diet and Health, Food and Nutrition Board, National Research Council, National Academy of Sciences. Diet and health: implications for reducing chronic disease risk. Washington, DC: National Academy Press, 1989.
5. US Department of Health and Human Services. The Surgeon General's report on nutrition and health: summary and recommendations. Washington, DC: US Government Printing Office, 1988.
6. Gerber JM. Comprehensive guidelines for a healthy American diet. Proceedings of the Second Symposium on Nutrition and Chiropractic, Palmer College of Chiropractic, 1989.
7. Pao EM, Mickle SJ. Problem nutrients in the United States. Food Technology 1981;35:58–79.
8. King JC, Cohenour SH, Corrucini CG, et al. Evaluation and modification of the Basic Four Food Guide. J Nutr Educ 1978;10:39–41.
9. Cronin FJ, Shaw AM, Krebs-Smith SM, et al. Developing a food guidance system to implement the dietary guidelines. J Nutr Educ 1987;19:281–302.
10. Grandjean AC. Sports nutrition. In: Mellion MB, Walsh WM, Shelton GL, eds. The team physician's handbook. Philadelphia: Hanley & Belfus, 1990:78–91.
11. Wilmore JH, Costill DL. Physiology of sport and exercise. Champaign, IL: Human Kinetics, 1994:110–114.
12. Brotherhood JR. Nutrition and sports performance. Sports Med 1984;1:350–389.
13. Wilmore JH, Costill DL. Physiology of sport and exercise. Champaign, IL: Human Kinetics, 1994:380–394.
14. Thornton JS. Feast or famine: eating disorders in athletes. Phys Sportsmed 1990;18:116–122.
15. Walberg-Rankin J. Dietary carbohydrate as an ergogenic aid for prolonged and brief competitions in sport. Int J Sport Nutr 1995;5(Suppl):13–38.
16. Costill DL. Carbohydrates for exercise: dietary demands for optimal performance. Int J Sports Med 1988;9:1–18.
17. Burke ER, Ekblom B. Influence of fluid ingestion and dehydration on precision and endurance performance in tennis. Proceedings of the 22nd World Congress on Sports Medicine, 1982:12.
18. Burke LM, Read RSD. Sports nutrition: approaching the nineties. Sports Med 1989;8:80–100.
19. Munro HN. An introduction to biochemical aspects of protein metabolism. In: Munro HN, Allison JB, eds. Mammalian protein metabolism. New York: Academic Press, 1964:3–39.
20. Paul G. Dietary protein requirements of physically active individuals. Sports Med 1989;8:154–176.
21. National Academy of Sciences, National Research Council, Food and Nutrition Board. Recommended dietary allowances. 10th ed. Washington, DC: National Academy Press, 1989.
22. Hickson JF, Wolinsky I. Research directions in protein nutrition for athletes. In: Wolinsky I, Hickson JF, eds. Nutrition in exercise and sport. 2nd ed. Boca Raton: CRC Press, 1994:85–122.
23. Ross MH, Bras G. Influence of protein under and over nutrition on spontaneous tumor prevalence in the rat. J Nutr 1973;103:944–963.
24. Schuette SA, Linkswiler HM. Effects on Ca and P metabolism in humans by adding meat, meat plus milk, or purified proteins plus Ca and P to a low protein diet. J Nutr 1982;112:338–349.
25. Brenner DM, Meyer TW, Hostetter TH. Dietary protein intake and the progressive nature of kidney disease: the role of hemodynamically-mediated glomerular injury in the pathogenesis of progressive glomerular sclerosis in aging, renal ablation, and intrinsic renal disease. N Engl J Med 1982;307:652–659.
26. Immerman A. Evidence for intestinal toxemia: an inescapable clinical phenomenon. ACA J Chiro 1979;13:25–35.
27. Cummings JH. Fermentation in the human large intestine: evidence and implications for health. Lancet 1983;1:1206–1208.
28. Belko AZ. Vitamins and exercise: an update. Med Sci Sports Exerc 1987;19(Suppl):191–196.
29. Bucci LR. Nutritional ergogenic aids. In: Wolinsky I, Hickson JF, eds. Nutrition in exercise and sport. 2nd ed. Boca Raton: CRC Press, 1994:295–346.
30. Singh A, Moses FM, Deuster PA. Chronic multivitamin-mineral supplementation does not enhance physical performance. Med Sci Sports Exerc 1992;24:726–732.
31. Keys A, Henschel AF, Mickelsen O, et al. The performance of normal young men on controlled thiamin intakes. J Nutr 1943;26:399–415.
32. Read M, McGuffin S. The effect of B complex supplementation on endurance performance. J Sports Med Phys Fit 1983;23:178–184.
33. Caster WO, Mickelson O. Effect of diet and stress on the thiamin and pyramin excretion of normal young men maintained on controlled intakes of thiamin. Nutr Res 1991;11:549–558.
34. Keith RE. Vitamins and physical activity. In: Wolinsky I, Hickson JF, eds. Nutrition in exercise and sport. 2nd ed. Boca Raton: CRC Press, 1994:159–184.
35. Tucker RG, Mickelsen D, Keys A. The influence of sleep, work, diuresis, heat, acute starvation, thiamine intake, and bed rest on human riboflavin excretion. J Nutr 1960;72:251–261.
36. Belko AZ, Obarzanek E, Kalkwarf HJ, et al. Effects of exercise on riboflavin requirements of young women. Am J Clin Nutr 1983;37:509–517.
37. Tremblay A, Boiland F, Breton M, et al. The effects of a riboflavin supplementation on the nutritional status and performance of elite swimmers. Nutr Res 1984;4:201–208.
38. Lassers BW, Wahlqvist ML, Kaijser L, et al. Effect of nicotinic acid on myocardial metabolism in man at rest and during exercise. J Appl Physiol 1972;33:72–80.
39. Kaijser L, Nye ER, Eklund B, et al. The relation between carbohydrate extraction by the forearm and arterial free fatty acid concentration in man: part 1. forearm work with nicotinic acid. Scand J Clin Lab Invest 1978;38:41–47.

40. Nice C, Reeves AG, Brinck-Johnston T, et al. The effects of pantothenic acid on human exercise capacity. J Sports Med 1984;24:26–29.

41. Litoff D, Scherzer H, Harrison J. Effects of pantothenic acid on human exercise. Med Sci Sports Exerc 1985;17:287. Abstract.

42. Manore MM, Leklem JE. Effect of carbohydrate and vitamin B6 on fuel substrates during exercise in women. Med Sci Sports Exerc 1988;20:233–241.

43. Guilland JC, Penaranda T, Gallet C, et al. Vitamin status of young athletes including effects of supplementation. Med Sci Sports Exerc 1989;21:441–449.

44. Hoogerweif A, Hoitink A. The influence of vitamin C administration on the mechanical efficiency of the human organism. Int Z Angew Physiol 1963;20;164–172.

45. Spioch F, Kobza R, Mazur B. Effect of vitamin C upon certain functional changes and the coefficient of mechanical efficiency in men during physical exercise. Acta Physiol Pol 1966;17:251–264.

46. Bender A, Nash A. Vitamin C and physical performance. Plant Foods Man 1975;1:217.

47. Bramich K, McNaughton L. The effects of two levels of ascorbic acid on muscular endurance, muscular strength and on $\dot{V}O_2$max. Int Clin Nutr Rev 1987;7:5–10.

48. Kagan VE, Spirichev VB, Serbinova EA, et al. The significance of vitamin E and free radicals in physical exercise. In: Wolinsky I, Hickson JF, eds. Nutrition in exercise and sport. 2nd ed. Boca Raton: CRC Press, 1994:185–213.

49. Wolinsky I, Hickson JF, Arnaud SB. Bone and calcium and bone in exercise and sport. In: Wolinsky I, Hickson JF, eds. Nutrition in exercise and sport. 2nd ed. Boca Raton: CRC Press, 1994:215–222.

50. Steen SN. Nutritional concerns of athletes who must reduce body weight. Sport Sci Exchange 1989;2.

51. Liu L, Borowski G, Rose LI. Hypomagnesemia in a tennis player. Phys Sportsmed 1983;11:79–81.

52. Steinacker JM, Grunert-Fuchs M, Steininger K, et al. Effects of long-time administration of magnesium on physical capacity. Int J Sports Med 1987;8:151. Abstract.

53. Golf SW, Bohmer D, Nowacki PE. Is magnesium a limiting factor in competitive exercise? a summary of relevant scientific data. In: Golf S, Dralle D, Veccheit A, eds. Magnesium 1993. London: John Libbey & Company, 1993:209–220.

54. Brilla L, Haley T. Effect of magnesium supplementation on strength training in humans. J Am Coll Nutr 1992;11:326–329.

55. Haymes EM. Trace minerals and exercise. In: Wolinsky I, Hickson JF, eds. Nutrition in exercise and sport. 2nd ed. Boca Raton: CRC Press, 1994:223–244.

56. Couzy F, Lafargue P, Guezennec CY. Zinc metabolism in the athlete: influence of training, nutrition and other factors. Int J Sports Med 1990;11:263–266.

57. Evans GW. Effects of chromium picolinate on insulin controlled parameters in humans. Int J Biosocial Med Res 1989;11:163–180.

58. Hasten DL, Rome EP, Franks BD, et al. Effects of chromium picolinate on beginning weight training students. Int J Sports Nutr 1992;2:343–350.

59. Clancy SP, Clarkson PM, DeCheke ME, et al. Effects of chromium picolinate supplementation on body composition, strength, and urinary chromium loss in football players. Int J Sports Nutr 1994;4:142–153.

60. Pivarnik JM, Palmer JM. Water and electrolyte balance during rest and exercise. In: Wolinsky I, Hickson JF, eds. Nutrition in exercise and sport. 2nd ed. Boca Raton: CRC Press, 1994:245–263.

61. Murray R. Fluids needs in hot and cold environments. Int J Sports Nutr 1995;5(Suppl):62–73.

62. Lukaksi HC. Methods for the assessment of human body composition: traditional and new. Am J Clin Nutr 1987;46:537–556.

63. Jensen MD. Research techniques for body composition assessment. J Am Diet Assoc 1992;92:454–460.

64. Gibson RS. Principles of nutrition assessment. New York: Oxford University Press, 1990:192–193.

65. Applegate L. Fad diets and supplement use in athletics. Sport Sci Exchange 1988;1.

66. Liebman M, Wilkinson JG. Carbohydrate metabolism and exercise. In: Wolinsky I, Hickson JF, eds. Nutrition in exercise and sport. 2nd ed. Boca Raton: CRC Press, 1994:15–48.

67. Sherman WM. Recovery from endurance exercise. Med Sci Sports Exerc 1992;24(Suppl):336–339.

68. Friedmen JE, Neufer PD, Dohm GL. Regulation of glycogen resynthesis following exercise: dietary considerations. Sports Med 1991;11:232–243.

69. Karlsson J, Saltin, B. Diet, muscle glycogen, and endurance performance. J Appl Physiol 1971;31:203–206.

70. Sherman W, Costill D. The marathon: dietary manipulation to optimize performance. Am J Sports Med 1984;12:44–51.

71. Sherman WM. Pre-event nutrition. Sports Sci Exchange 1989;1.

72. Coggan AR, Coyle EF. Carbohydrate ingested during prolonged exercise: effects on metabolism and performance. Exerc Sports Sci Rev 1991;19:1–40.

73. Puhl SM, Buskirk ER. Nutrient beverages for exercise and sport. In: Wolinsky I, Hickson JF, eds. Nutrition in exercise and sport. 2nd ed. Boca Raton: CRC Press, 1994:263–294.

74. Dohm GL. Protein nutrition for the athlete. Clin Sports Med 1984;3:595–604.

75. Lemon PWR. Do athletes need more dietary protein and amino acids? Int J Sport Nutr 1995;5(Suppl):39–61.

76. Lamb DR, Brodowicz GR. Optimal use of fluids of varying formulations to minimise exercise-induced disturbances in homeostasis. Sports Med 1986;3:247–274.

77. Nadel ER. New ideas for rehydration during and after exercise in hot weather. Sports Sci Exchange 1988;1.

78. Murray R. The effects of consuming carbohydrate-electrolyte beverages on gastric emptying and fluid absorption during and following exercise. Sports Med 1987;4:322–351.

79. Linderman JK, Gosselink KL. The effects of sodium bicarbonate ingestion on exercise performance. Sports Med 1994;18:75–80.

80. Horswill CA. Effects of bicarbonate, citrate, and phosphate loading on performance. Int J Sport Nutr 1995;5(Suppl):111–119.

81. Peterson M, Peterson, K. Eat to compete: a guide to sports nutrition. Chicago: Year Book, 1988.

82. Grandjean AC. Nutrition for sport success. Reston, VA: American Alliance for Health, Physical Education and Dance, 1984:6.

83. Dwyer JT. Dietary assessment. In: Shils ME, Olsen JA, Shike M, eds. Modern nutrition in health and disease. 8th ed. Philadelphia: Lea and Febiger, 1994:842–860.

84. Hoffman CJ, Coleman E. An eating plan and update on recommended dietary practices for the endurance athlete. J Am Diet Assoc 1991;91:325–330.

85. American Diabetes Association, American Dietetic Association. Exchange lists for meal planning. Alexandria, VA (ADA) and Chicago, IL (ADA), 1986.

86. Haymes EM. Nutritional concerns: need for iron. Med Sci Sports Exerc 1987;19(Suppl):197–200.

87. Fairbanks VF. Iron in medicine and nutrition. In: Shils ME, Olsen JA, Shike M, eds. Modern nutrition in health and disease. 8th ed. Philadelphia: Lea and Febiger, 1994:185–213.

88. Sherman AR, Kramer B. Iron, nutrition, and exercise. In: Hickson JF, Wolinsky I, eds. Nutrition in exercise and sport. Boca Raton: CRC Press, 1989:291–300.

89. Selby GB. When does an athlete need iron? Phys Sports Med 1991;19:96–102.

90. Harris SS. Helping active women avoid anemia. Phys Sports Med 1995;23:35–48.

91. Taylor WC, Lombardo JA. Pre-participation screening of the college athlete: value of the CBC. Phys Sportsmed 1990;18:110–116.

92. Risser WL, Risser JMH. Iron deficiency in adolescents and young adults. Phys Sportsmed 1990;18:87–101.

93. Gerber JM. Handbook of preventive and therapeutic nutrition. Gaithersburg, MD: Aspen Publishers, 1993.

94. American College of Sports Medicine. Position stand on prevention of thermal injuries during distance running. Med Sci Sports Exerc 1984;16:9–14.

95. Yarrows SA. Weight-loss through dehydration in amateur wrestling. J Am Diet Assoc 1988;88:491–493.

96. Stamford B. How to avoid dehydration. Phys Sportsmed 1990;18:135–136.

97. Noakes TD. The hyponatremia of exercise. Int J Sport Nutr 1992;2:205–228.

98. Hiller WDB. Dehydration and hyponatremia during triathlons. Med Sci Sports Exerc 1989;21(Suppl):219–221.

99. Noakes TD, Norman RJ, Buck RH, et al. The incidence of hyponatremia during prolonged ultraendurance exercise. Med Sci Sports Exerc 1990;22:165–170.

100. Roos R. Medical coverage of endurance events. Phys Sportsmed 1987;15:140–146.

101. Ruud JS, Grandjean AC. Nutritional concerns of female athletes. In: Wolinsky I, Hickson JF, eds. Nutrition in exercise and sport. 2nd ed. Boca Raton: CRC Press, 1994:347–365.

102. Tipton CM. Making and maintaining weight for interscholastic wrestling. Sport Sci Exchange 1990;2.

103. Thornton JS. How can you tell when an athlete is too thin? Phys Sportsmed 1990;18:124–133.

104. Nattiv A, Agostini R, Drinkwater B, et al. The female athlete triad: the inter-relatedness of disordered eating, amenorrhea and osteoporosis. Clin Sports Med 1994; 13:405–418.

105. Drinkwater BL, Bruemmer B, Chestnut CH III. Menstrual history as a determinant of current bone density in young athletes. JAMA 1990;263:545–548.

106. Highet R. Athletic amenorrhea: an update on etiology, complications and management. Sports Med 1989;7: 82–108.

107. White CM, Hergenroeder AC. Amenorrhea, osteopenia and the female athlete. Pediatr Clin North Am 1990;37: 1125–1141.

108. Myburgh K, Hutchins J, Fataar AB, et al. Low bone density is an etiological factor for stress fractures in athletes. Ann Intern Med 1990;113:754–759.

109. Shangold M, Rebar RW, Wentz AC, et al. Evaluation and management of menstrual dysfunction in athletes. JAMA 1990;263:1665–1669.

110. Saal JA. General principles and guidelines for rehabilitation of the injured athlete. Phys Med Rehabil 1987;1: 523–536.

111. Bucci L. Nutrition applied to injury rehabilitation and sports medicine. Boca Raton: CRC Press, 1995:167–175.

112. Pizzorno JE, Murray MT. Bromelain. In: Pizzorno JE, Murray MT, eds. Textbook of natural medicine. Seattle: John Bastyr College Publications. 1985;5:1–5.

113. Taussig SJ, Yokoyama MM, Chinen BS, et al. Bromelain: a proteolytic enzyme and its clinical application: a review. Hiroshima J Med Sci 1975;24:185–193.

114. Miller JM. Absorption of orally introduced proteolytic enzymes. Clin Med 1968;75:35–42.

115. Miller JN, Ginsberg M, McElfatrick GC, et al. The administration of bromelain orally in the treatment of inflammation and edema. Exp Med Surg 1964;22:293–299.

116. Cirelli MG. Five years experience with bromelains in therapy of edema and inflammation in postoperative tissue reaction, skin infections and trauma. Clin Med 1967;74:55–59.

117. Trickett P. Proteolytic enzymes in treatment of athletic injuries. Appl Ther 1964;6:647–652.

118. Gibson T, Dilke TFW, Grahame R. Chymoral in the treatment of lumbar disc prolapse. Rheumatol Rehabil 1975;14:186–190.

119. Blonstein JL. Control of swelling in boxing injuries. Practitioner (London) 1969;203:206.

120. Holt HT. Carica papaya as ancillary therapy for athletic injuries. Curr Ther Res 1969;11:621–624.

121. Buck JE, Phillips N. Trial of Chymoral in professional footballers. Br J Clin Pract 1970;24:375–377.

122. Rathgeber WF. The use of proteolytic enzymes (Chymoral) in sporting injuries. S Afr Med J 1971;45:181–183.

123. Cichoke AJ, Marty L. The use of proteolytic enzymes with soft tissue athletic injuries. Am Chiro 1981;September/October:32–33.

124. Deitrick RE. Oral proteolytic enzymes in the treatment of athletic injuries: a double-blind study. Penn Med J 1965;68:35–37.

125. Hingorani K. Oral enzyme therapy in severe back pain. Br J Clin Pract 1968;22:209–210.

126. Boyne PS, Medhurst H. Oral anti-inflammatory enzyme therapy in injuries in professional footballers. Practitioner (London) 1967;198:543–546.

127. Gabor M. Pharmacologic effects of flavonoids on blood vessels. Angiologica 1972;9:355–374.

128. Hausteen B. Flavonoids, a class of natural products of high pharmacologic potency. Biochem Pharm 1983;32: 1141–1148.

129. Miller MJ. Injuries to athletes. Med Times 1960;88: 313–314.

130. Werbach MR. Nutritional influences on illness: a sourcebook of clinical research. New Canaan, CT: Keats, 1988:265.

131. Satoskar RR, Shah SJ, Shenoy SG. Evaluation of anti-inflammatory property of curcumin (diferuloyl methane) in patients with postoperative inflammation. Int J Clin Pharmacol Ther Toxicol 1986;24:651–654.

132. Taraye JP, Lauressergues H. Advantages of a combination of proteolytic enzymes, flavinoids and ascorbic acid in comparison with non-steroid anti-inflammatory agents. Arzneim Forsch 1977;27:1144–1149.

133. Carson JD, Percy EC. The use of DMSO in tennis elbow and rotator cuff tendinitis: a double-blind study. Med Sci Sports Exerc 1981;13:215–219.

134. McGee SR. Muscle cramps. Arch Intern Med 1990;150: 511–518.

135. Levin S. Investigating the cause of muscle cramps. Phys Sportsmed 1993;21:111–113.

136. Williams MH. The role of minerals in physical activity. In: Williams MH, ed. Nutritional aspects of human physical performance. 2nd ed. Springfield, IL: Charles C. Thomas, 1985:186.

137. Pinsky MJ. Treatment of intermittent claudication with alpha-tocopherol. J Am Podiatry Assoc 1980;70:454–460.

138. Armstrong RB. Mechanisms of exercise-induced delayed onset muscular soreness: a brief review. Med Sci Sports Exerc 1984;16:529–538.

139. Kaminski M, Boal R. An effect of ascorbic acid on delayed-onset muscle soreness. Pain 1992;50:317–321.

140. Bucci L. Nutrition applied to injury rehabilitation and sports medicine. Boca Raton: CRC Press, 1995:61–166.

141. Rayner H, Allen SL, Braverman ER. Nutrition and wound healing. J Orthomolecular Med 1991;6:31–43.

142. Bucci L. Nutrition applied to injury rehabilitation and sports medicine. Boca Raton: CRC Press, 1995:216–221.

143. Hardingham TE, Beardmore-Gray M, Dunham DG, et al. Cartilage proteoglycans. In: Evered D, Whelen J, eds. Functions of the proteoglycans: Ciba foundation symposium 124. New York: John Wiley & Sons, 1986:30–46.

144. Leach RM. Role of manganese in mucopolysaccharide metabolism. Fed Proc 1971;30:991.

145. Morrison LM, Murata K. Absorption, distribution, metabolism and excretion of acid mucopolysaccharides administered to animals and patients. In: Morrison LM, Schjeide OA, Meyer K, eds. Coronary heart disease and the mucopolysaccharides (glycosaminoglycans). Springfield, IL: Charles C. Thomas, 1974:109–127.

146. Bollet AJ. Stimulation of protein-chondroitin sulfate synthesis by normal and osteoarthritic articular cartilage. Arth Rheum 1968;11:663–673.

147. Bucci L. Nutrition applied to injury rehabilitation and sports medicine. Boca Raton: CRC Press, 1995:177–195.

148. Dixon AS. Non-hormonal treatment of osteoporosis. Br Med J 1983;286:999–1000.

149. Mills TJ. The use of whole bone extract in the treatment of fractures. Manitoba Med Rev 1965;45:92–96.

150. Pines A, Raafat H, Lynn AH, et al. Clinical trial of microcrystalline hydroxyapatite compound ("Ossopan") in the prevention of osteoporosis due to corticosteroid therapy. Curr Med Res Opin 1984;8:734–742.

151. Bucci L, Hickson JF, Pivarnik JM, et al. Ornithine ingestion and growth hormone release in bodybuilders. Nutr Res 1990;10:239–245.

152. Fogelholm GM, Naveri HK, Kiilavuori KTK, et al. Low-dose amino acid supplementation: no effects on serum human growth hormone and insulin in male weight lifters. Int J Sport Nutr 1993;3:290–297.

153. Lambert MI, Hefer JA, Millar RP, et al. Failure of commercial oral amino acid supplements to increase serum human growth hormone concentrations in male bodybuilders. Int J Sport Nutr 1993;3:298–305.

154. Elam RP. Morphological changes in adult males from resistance exercise and amino acid supplementation. J Sports Med 1988;28:35–38.

155. Elam RP, Hardin DH, Sutton RAL, et al. Effects of arginine and ornithine on strength, lean body mass and urinary hydroxyproline in adult males. J Sports Med 1989;29:52–56.

156. Hendler SS. The doctors' vitamin and mineral encyclopedia. New York: Simon and Schuster, 1990.

157. Wesson M, McNaughton L, Davies P, et al. Effects of oral administration of aspartic acid salts on the endurance capacity of trained subjects. Res Q Exerc Sport 1988; 59:234–236.

158. Chandler JV, Hawkins JD. The effect of bee pollen on physiological performance. Med Sci Sports Exerc 1985;17:287–291.

159. Cerra FB, Hirsch J, Mullen K, et al. Branched chains support post-operative protein synthesis. Surgery 1982; 92:192–199.

160. Kreider RB, Miriel V, Bertun E. Amino acid supplementation and exercise performance: analysis of the proposed ergogenic value. Sports Med 1993;16:190–209.

161. Davis JM. Carbohydrates, branched-chain amino acids and endurance: the central fatigue hypothesis. Int J Sport Nutr 1995;5(Suppl):29–38.

162. Spriet LL. Caffeine and performance. Int J Sport Nutr 1995;5(Suppl):84–99.

163. Tarnopolsky MA. Caffeine and endurance performance. Sports Med 1994;18:109–125.

164. Cerretelli P, Marconi C. L-carnitine supplementation in humans. The effects on physical performance. Int J Sports Med 1990;11:1–14.

165. Trappe SW, Costill DL, Goodpaster B, et al. The effects of L-carnitine supplementation on performance during interval swimming. Int J Sports Med 1994;15:181–185.

166. Kanter MM, Williams MH. Antioxidants, carnitine, and choline as putative ergogenic aids. Int J Sport Nutr 1995;5(Suppl):120–131.

167. Braun B, Clarkson PM, Freedson PS, et al. Effects of coenzyme Q10 supplementation on exercise performance, $\dot{V}O_2$max, and lipid peroxidation in trained cyclists. Int J Sport Nutr 1991;1:353–365.

168. Snider IP, Bazzare TL, Murdoch SD, et al. Effects of coenzyme athletic performance system as an ergogenic aid on endurance performance to exhaustion. Int J Sport Nutr 1992;2:272–286.

169. Balsom PD, Soderlund K, Ekblom B. Creatine in humans with special reference to creatine supplementation. Sports Med 1994;18:268–280.

170. Greenhaff PL. Creatine and its application as an ergogenic aid. Int J Sport Nutr 1995;5(Suppl):100–110.

171. Maughan RJ. Creatine supplementation and exercise performance. Int J Sport Nutr 1995;5:94–101.

172. Rosenbloom C, Millard-Stafford M, Lathrop J. Contemporary ergogenic aids used by strength/power athletes. J Am Diet Assoc 1992;92:1264–1266.

173. Bahrke MS, Morgan WP. Evaluation of the ergogenic properties of ginseng. Sports Med 1994;18:229–248.

174. McNaughton L, Egan G, Caelli G. A comparison of Chinese and Russian ginseng as ergogenic aids to improve various facets of of physical fitness. Int Clin Nutr Rev 1989;9:32–35.

175. Williams MH, Kreider RB, Hunter DW, et al. Effect of inosine supplementation on 3-mile treadmill run performances and $\dot{V}O_2$ peak. Med Sci Sports Exerc 1990;22:517–522.

176. Saint-John M, McNaughton, L. Octacosonol ingestion and its effects on metabolic responses to submaximal cycle ergometry, reaction time and chest and grip strength. Int J Clin Nutr Rev 1986;6:81–87.

177. Williams MH. Ergogenic and ergolytic substances. Med Sci Sports Exerc 1992;24(Suppl):344–348.

Anabolic Steroids

Mauro G. Di Pasquale

There are a large number of drugs and supplements used by athletes in an attempt to improve performance. In the past few years there has been such an emphasis on the use of anabolic steroids that few people, other than the athletes themselves, have noticed the quiet revolution that has been occurring. Although athletes are still using anabolic steroids (there has been little decrease in the use of anabolic steroids by the more pharmacologically sophisticated athletes), most are making extensive use of other compounds for the purposes of enhancing their performance, with or without the concomitant use of anabolic steroids.

These compounds are used as ergogenic aids, masking agents to conceal the use of anabolic steroids, and therapeutic agents to deal with the side effects of anabolic steroid use. Many of these compounds either are not detectable or are not tested for, further increasing the incentive for their use. Many athletes are also looking for alternative compounds because of the scarcity and uncertainty of the authenticity and quality of black-market anabolic steroids.

Athletes now make use of a vast arsenal of drugs to improve their performance and appearance (especially in aesthetic or recreational athletes) and to combat some of the side effects of other drugs. In addition to the anabolic steroids, several classes of compounds are used in an attempt to improve performance (Table 24.1).

The list in Table 24.1, however, is just the tip of the iceberg. In fact, it might be difficult to find a substance with which some aspiring athlete has not experimented.

These compounds are often used along with anabolic steroids, although some athletes use them instead of anabolic steroids in the hope that they will provide the benefits of anabolic steroids without the side effects and without the stigma of possible detection. Although some of these anabolic steroid substitutes have some merit, many (especially the ones advertised in the many body building, power lifting, and other sports magazines) are relatively inert, with no true anabolic effects. The advertisements for these compounds are tainted by commercial bias and contain false and misleading information and claims.

GROWTH HORMONE

Growth hormone (also known as GH, adenohypophysial growth hormone, hypophyseal growth hormone, anterior pituitary growth hormone, phyone, pituitary growth hormone, somatotropic hormone, STH, and somatotropin) is one of the hormones produced by the anterior portion of the pituitary gland (situated at the base of the brain under the hypothalamus) under the regulation of the hypothalamic hormones, growth hormone releasing hormone (GHRH, somatoliberin), somatostatin, and galanin (1, 2). The anterior pituitary also secretes luteinizing hormone (LH), follicle-stimulating hormone (FSH), prolactin (PRL), adrenocorticotropic hormone (ACTH), and thyroid stimulating hormone (TSH) (3). Structurally, growth hormone resembles prolactin and is a peptide composed of 191 amino acids with 2 sulfhydryl bridges.

Growth hormone is a species-specific anabolic protein that promotes somatic growth, stimulates protein synthesis, and regulates carbohydrate and lipid metabolism (4). Growth hormones from various species differ in amino acid sequence, antigenicity, isoelectric point, and range of animals in which they can produce biologic responses. Preparations of growth hormone other than primate have no effect in humans.

Growth Hormone and Athletic Performance

Exercise has an effect on growth hormone secretion. Prolonged intensive exercise causes elevated levels of somatotropin and glucagon as well as a reduced level of insulin in the blood. The somatotropin response to exercise seems to depend on the severity of the exercise and on other fac-

Table 24.1. Compounds Used to Enhance Performance

Stimulants
  Adrenalin
  Adrenergic compounds
  Amphetamines and amphetamine derivatives
  Arcalion
  ATP (Striadyne)
  Caffeine
  Cocaine
  Diet pills
  Heptaminol
  Inosine
  Nicotine
  Piracetam
  Sodium succinate
  Sydnocarb
Narcotic analgesics—including agonists, partial agonists, and antagonists
Growth hormone and related compounds including growth hormone stimulants
  Somatomedin–C
  Growth hormone stimulators such as arginine, ornithine, clonidine, L-dopa
  Galanin
  Growth hormone releasing hormone (GHRH)
Compounds that increase endogenous androgen levels
  Human chorionic gonadotropin (HCG)
  Menotropins (Pergonal)
  Gonadorelin (Factrel)
  Cyclofenil
  Antiestrogens (clomiphene, tamoxifen)
Other hormones
  Insulin
  Throid hormone (Cytomel, Synthroid, Triacana)
  Hypothalamic and pituitary releasing hormones such as TRH, TSH, ACTH
  ADH or vasopressin
  Pitocin
Anti-inflammatory compounds
  Corticosteroids
  Nonsteroidal anti-inflammatory drugs (NSAIDs)
  DMSO
  Veterinary cartilage-based compounds
Miscellaneous compounds with putative anabolic or ergogenic effects
  Bee pollen

Beta 2 adrenergic agonists such as clenbuterol, cimaterol, and fenoterol
Boron
Carnitine
Chromium picolinate
Coenzyme Q
Creatine monohydrate
Cyproheptadine
Dibencozide
Dimethylglycine
Gamma-hydroxybutyrate (GHB)
Gamma-oryzanol
Ginseng
Glutathione
Inosine
Ketones
Neurofor
OKG (ornithine alpha-ketoglutarate)
Pangamic acid
Pentoxifylline (Trental)
Perchlorates
Rubranova
Selegiline (deprenyl)
Sitosterol
Smilax Officinalis
Ubiquinone (coenzyme Q10)
Yohimbine
Zeranol (Ralgro)
Nutritional supplements
  Vitamins
  Minerals
  B_{12} injections
  Protein—whole or as individual or branched-chain amino acids
  Medium-chain triglycerides
Miscellaneous compounds used in an attempt to enhance performance
  Alcohol
  Amino acid neurotransmitters (such as GABA, phenylalanine tryptophan, glutamine, etc.)
  Beta-blockers
  Calcium channel blockers
  Cyclobenzaprine
  Diuretics
  Local anesthetics
  Marijuana

tors such as emotional strain and environmental temperature. It would appear that the more adverse the conditions and the harsher the exercising, the more growth hormone is produced.

It has been shown that plasma growth hormone levels rise with increased load and/or frequency of exercise. Almost all forms of exercise increase growth hormone secretion, although there appears to be a higher increase in growth hormone level after maximal than after submaximal exercise (5, 6). Some studies, however, have not shown this relationship (7). The results of one study suggest that the balance between oxygen demand and availability may be an important regulator of growth hormone secretion during exercise (8).

Several studies have documented the increased growth hormone secretion that occurs during weight lifting and the subsequent recovery phase (9). It also appears that the secretion of growth hormone varies according to the muscle group that is exercised, with smaller muscle groups leading to increased growth hormone release. For example, in one study, arm work elicited a greater serum growth hormone response than leg work (10).

As with insulin and glucagon, the availability of carbohydrates modulates the response of growth hormone to exercise. The administration of glucose excludes the response; during a carbohydrate deficient state, the response is exaggerated.

The use of exogenous growth hormone, although theoretically capable of significant anabolic effect, has not been adequately studied for its effect on athletic performance (11). This situation is further confused by the fact that much of the black-market growth hormone (the usual source of growth hormone for athletes) is not in fact growth hormone, but is either inert or an injectable anabolic steroid—most commonly nandrolone decanoate (Deca-Durabolin) and/or a form of injectable testosterone.

The effect of growth hormone on athletic performance is still controversial, although use by athletes has escalated dramatically since the availability of synthetic recombinant growth hormones such as Protropin (Genentech, San Francisco, CA). Theoretically, there is the possibility that anabolic steroids and growth hormone have a synergistic effect; that is, they work better together than if used alone. Although there is some evidence that this synergism exists (12), there is no evidence that there is a synergistic effect on athletic performance.

There are many compounds that stimulate endogenous growth hormone production (see above). It is unknown if the chronic use of any of these compounds results in a prolonged increase in the overall daily productions of growth hormone. Currently, there are no valid clinical data by which to judge their long-term effectiveness.

The anabolic effect and side effects of growth hormone have been widely publicized. Currently, however, the use of growth hormone by athletes has not given spectacular results. Many of the results attributed to growth hormone were in fact due to the anabolic steroid, which was either deliberately used with the growth hormone or was misrepresented as the growth hormone. Also, many of the side effects predicted have not as yet materialized.

Perhaps the most important controversy surrounding growth hormone is the question of its efficacy in enhancing athletic performance. Theoretically, growth hormone is capable of musculoskeletal anabolic effects and lipolytic effects (increased breakdown of storage fat). The anecdotal evidence the author has obtained has been contradictory. Some athletes believe that they have made significant gains in muscular size and strength, whereas others believe that growth hormone produces no anabolic effects at all. It is difficult to separate the placebo effect from a true physiologic effect in those athletes who believed that they had made significant gains. The doses used by athletes have varied from 4 units 3 times a week to 10 units per day for many weeks. There is a glaring need for more research on the effects of exogenous growth hormone on both athletes and nonathletes.

The most intensively studied action of growth hormone, whether synthetic or natural, is the effect it has on linear growth in young patients who are growth-hormone deficient. Its effect as an anabolic agent on patients who are past their teens has not been adequately investigated or condoned (13). Despite the popularity of growth hormone and growth hormone stimulators (compounds that increase growth hormone secretion), the author believes that they are overrated.

Drugs and nutritional substances are being increasingly used in an attempt to raise endogenous growth hormone levels. Athletes often use combinations of growth hormone stimulators in hopes of increasing growth hormone secretion even further. There is in fact some basis for this belief—the synergistic effect of clonidine, propranolol, L-dopa, and others has been documented (14). Unfortunately little is known about the use of growth hormone and growth hormone stimulators in healthy athletes. More work still needs to be done before a clear picture emerges.

It is likely that growth hormone has had an adaptive role historically, allowing humans to better survive periods of famine. It mobilizes fat, it has protein-sparing and muscle-sparing effects, and it promotes the storage of glycogen in muscle. It would be effective in times of food shortages by switching over the source of fuel for the body from carbohydrates and protein to fat, thus allowing the body to live off its stored fat deposits, rather than cannibalizing muscle and other important tissues for fuel.

Stresses caused by such things as fasting, hypoglycemia (low blood sugar), protein depletion, exercise, surgery, and severe psychological stress increase production of endogenous growth hormone as the body tries to minimize the loss of muscle and other proteins and use fat stores for energy. By contrast, factors such as obesity, hyperglycemia (high blood sugar), and elevated serum fats signal the body to reduce the production of endogenous growth hormone.

The use of growth hormone and growth hormone releasers by athletes is increasing. However, although growth hormone might be useful in those athletes who need to maintain muscle mass while losing body weight, it does not seem useful in athletes who want to gain muscle mass and strength. Growth hormone may have its only true athletic use as an anticatabolic agent; that is, it may help athletes retain their lean body mass and strength while losing weight, with or without the use of anabolic steroids.

Growth hormone has a definite lipolytic effect in humans. It has been shown that this is an intrinsic property of growth hormone per se and is not dependent on contaminants present in human growth hormone. This is a lipolytic effect; therefore, it is a property of the synthetic growth hormone as well (15). It would appear that it is this lipolytic effect (while retaining body muscularity and muscle mass constant) that makes growth hormone so popular with some athletes, especially body builders and those who participate in sports with weight classes.

ANABOLIC STEROIDS

Introduction

The anabolic actions of substances produced by the testes have been known for almost a century. Two case reports by Sacchi (16), and Rowlands and Nicholson (17) comprise the early evidence of the influence of testicular androgens, specifically testosterone, on growth and musculoskeletal development. Kenyon, in a series of studies extending from 1938 to 1944, investigated and elucidated the metabolic effects of testosterone (18–21). He was one of the first to outline possible clinical uses for testosterone.

The athletic community was quick to realize the performance-enhancing potential of testosterone and put some of the principles outlined by Kenyon and others into practice. By the early 1950s, testosterone and a few analogs such as methandrostenolone (Dianabol; Ciba, Summit, NJ) were being used first by Eastern Block athletes and soon after by most other countries.

In the 1950s and 1960s, the use of anabolic steroids was contained within the "power" sports such as weight lifting; the weight events in track and field, including javelin, shot put, and discus; and sports requiring explosive power, such as the short-distance events in cycling and running. However, since the early 1970s, the use of testosterone and testosterone analogs by athletes has escalated dramatically. Today, anabolic steroids are used by almost all power athletes (those in sports requiring strength or explosive force or, as in body building, extreme muscularity) at some time during their training. They are used by many other athletes as well, including those competing in the middle distance (22) and endurance events.

Anabolic steroid use is common among professional athletes and has spread to college and high school athletes involved in non-Olympic sports such as football, hockey, basketball, and baseball. Unfortunately, the use of anabolic steroids is percolating down to noncompetitive athletes and even to the general public, in whom they are used for aesthetic measures rather than for increasing competitive athletic performance (23).

Effects of Androgenic/Anabolic Steroids

The effects produced by testosterone can be divided into two somewhat arbitrary effects: androgenic (producing secondary male sexual characteristics) and anabolic (mainly increasing muscle size and strength).

Although there has been an effort to try to dissociate these two effects, there is no truly anabolic steroid; all have varying degrees of androgenic effects. In early experimental work with animals, the dissociation was significant; in humans it is less so. This lack of complete dissociation has led to much confusion in the terminology used for these compounds. The terms anabolic steroid, androgenic steroid, anabolic-androgenic steroid, and androgenic-anabolic steroid are often used interchangeably. Testosterone itself can be referred to as an anabolic steroid, although this term usually refers to its synthetic derivatives.

Modifications at any of the 19 carbon groups that make up the testosterone molecule are made for many reasons, including altering the anabolic/androgenic ratio or therapeutic index (ideally increasing the anabolic effects and decreasing the androgenic effects), increasing the bioavailability of the drug when taken orally, decreasing its absorption time when given parenterally, and increasing the potency of the drug so that less drug is used for similar results.

Do They Work?

Although there is some controversy in the literature on the effectiveness of anabolic steroids in enhancing performance, there is no doubt in most athletes' minds that they do work. Athletes worldwide use anabolic steroids and/or exogenous testosterone in an attempt to increase their muscle size and strength.

Before this decade, the predominant attitude in the scientific community was that anabolic steroids did not enhance performance. The 1985 edition of Goodman and Gilman's *The Pharmacological Basis of Therapeutics* (Macmillan) states, "The use of these agents (anabolic steroids) does not cause an increase in muscle bulk, strength, or athletic performance—even when phenomenally large doses are used. The commonly observed increase in body weight (seen secondary to steroid use) is due to the retention of salt and water." The authors base this conclusion on the results of 25 papers that addressed the effects of androgenic/anabolic steroids on physical strength and athletic performance in men.

Acceptance of the ergogenic effects of anabolic steroids perhaps began with a review of the literature by Haupt and Rovere (24). They concluded that if certain criteria are met—such as intensive training, a high protein diet, and specific measurement techniques—then anabolic steroids seem to enhance athletic performance. Other studies published since this review have shown that anabolic steroids enhance strength, size, and athletic performance (25, 26). However, more work needs to be done to assess accurately the effect of the long-term use of high dosages of anabolic steroids on athletic performance.

It is likely that the efficacy of anabolic steroids as an ergogenic aid is dependent on many variables. These include individual genetic characteristics such as receptor response and affinity, dosage and duration of treatment, physiologic and psychological state of the individual before and during use, and other factors such as diet, training intensity, and concomitant use of other hormones, drugs, and nutritional aids.

Therapeutic Uses of Androgenic/Anabolic Steroids

As stated previously, it has been known for almost a century that androgens exert an anabolic effect on the musculoskeletal system. In the 1960s and 1970s, anabolic steroids were used clinically in a variety of conditions. A review published in the mid-1970s (27) outlined these various uses, including replacement therapy, sexual dysfunction, anemia, cachexia, infant nutrition disorders, diabetic retinopathy, prevention and control of certain infections, muscular dystrophy, kidney disease, neoplasms, leukemia, osteoporosis, and skin ulcers. Since then, however, their use has declined somewhat as more specific and effective therapies were developed for the treatment of many of these conditions.

Thus, androgenic/anabolic hormones are rarely considered as initial therapy for any clinical conditions. The reasons for this are many, including the androgenic effects of these compounds, hepatotoxic effects of the 17-alkylated derivatives, unfavorable press (and subsequent restrictive use) that these compounds have received as a result of their abuse by athletes, and availability (in some cases) of more effective treatments.

Anabolic steroids are clinically useful because of their anabolic and anticatabolic properties, ability to promote erythropoiesis, and hormonal effects in replacement therapy. They are also clinically useful for sexual dysfunction, treatment of certain hormone-sensitive cancers, and uncharacteristic effects of individual compounds in certain clinical conditions.

Testosterone and occasionally other anabolic steroids are used for replacement therapy in cases of deficiency and constitutional delayed puberty (28). Testosterone, ethylestrenol, nandrolone esters, stanozolol, and oxymetholone are used to treat a variety of conditions including aplastic anemias (29), hereditary angioedema (30), vascular disorders (31, 32), osteoporosis (33–35), neoplastic diseases (especially carcinoma of the breast) (36), and endometriosis (37) as well as to increase protein synthesis after surgery or chronic debilitating disease (38, 39).

Anabolic steroids, however, are powerful hormones that could prove useful in a variety of other conditions as both primary and adjunctive therapy. Unfortunately, their use has not been as fully investigated as has the use of other steroid hormones such as the female hormones estrogen and progesterone and the corticosteroids.

With more research, more valid clinical uses of androgenic/anabolic steroids will be found. For example, some adverse effects of these compounds (such as their potentiating effects on oral anticoagulants and their ability to decrease insulin requirements) may be useful clinically. Also some anabolic steroids, because of their fibrinolytic action, may be useful for the treatment of various thromboembolic diseases including coronary artery disease and stroke.

Ironically (since liver dysfunction and cardiovascular disease are two of the major adverse effects of anabolic steroid use), there may even be some therapeutic use for anabolic steroids in alcoholic liver disease (40) and some forms of cardiovascular disease (41). There is also the possibility, as in the case of birth control medication and its beneficial effects on the incidence of ovarian and endometrial cancer, that the use of anabolic steroids may improve health by acting as a deterrent for certain kinds of cancer, osteoporosis, and (because of the fibrinolytic action) for various thromboembolic diseases including coronary disease and stroke.

Use of Androgenic/Anabolic Steroids in the Treatment of Sports Injuries

The dominant action of testosterone is protein anabolism exerted on most of the tissues of the body. Therefore, it seems reasonable to assume that testosterone (and its synthetic analogs) may counteract the catabolic response that occurs in injured tissues secondary to a relative inactivity of the injured area and possibly counteracts the reduction in endogenous testosterone secretion.

The degree of this catabolic response that occurs after an injury will usually be proportional to the structures involved and the severity of the injury. The result is a decrease in the strength (and in the size and density) of the involved muscles, tendons, ligaments, joints, and bones in the injured area. At times the catabolic response can be further aggravated by the use of glucocorticosteroid injections, a common medical treatment of some types of athletic injuries.

Although the catabolic response to injury and the use of corticosteroids can be significantly modified by androgens (42), there is little advantage to their use in most injuries. Their use should be restricted to injuries that do not respond to other, more conservative methods.

Because of the gap between conservative treatment and surgery, there is a place for the use of anabolic steroids for the treatment of some chronic athletic injuries (43).

Adverse Effects

As used by most athletes, the adverse effects of anabolic steroid use appear to be minimal. Even in those using large doses for prolonged periods, clinical evidence shows that any of the short-term adverse effects are mostly reversible. In addition, some of the more serious adverse effects such as hepatic toxicity and increased serum cholesterol can be minimized by proper monitoring, changes in lifestyle, and medication if indicated.

The absence of significant adverse effects to the long-term use of low to moderate amounts of testosterone and some anabolic steroids has been shown in a series of clinical studies investigating the use of anabolic steroids and testosterone as male contraceptive agents. A considerable amount of research has been and is being carried out by the World Health Organization and independent researchers using combinations of testosterone, anabolic steroids (especially 19-nortestosterone) (44), medroxyprogesterone acetate and methyltestosterone (45), and gonadotropin hormone–releasing hormone agonists and antagonists. Several of these combinations have proven to significantly reduce the sperm count with no significant short- or long-term adverse effects (at least for as long as the various studies ran). In these studies, normal sperm production resumed shortly after discontinuation of the various compounds.

Unfortunately, the use of anabolic steroids in some individuals sensitive to these compounds and in others who use large doses for prolonged periods can result in significant short-term and long-term adverse effects. Almost everyone is aware of the liver problems, including cancer, that may result from the use of anabolic steroids.

Potentially serious long-term cardiovascular adverse effects may result from the untreated changes in serum cholesterol. Cardiac disease, including myocardial infarction, has been occasionally seen in athletes using anabolic steroids, although the part played by anabolic steroids in these disorders is in some dispute. To understand fully the implications of long-term steroid use, more exact and controlled long-term studies are needed. Until then, we are left with some facts and many guesses and suppositions.

OVERVIEW

In general, anabolic steroid adverse effects can be separated into two groups. One group consists of adverse effects that are an exaggeration of the expected pharmacologic properties of the anabolic steroids. Potential hormonally related adverse effects of anabolic steroids in men include gynecomastia, fluid retention, acne, changes in libido, oligospermia, and increased aggressiveness. In women, amenorrhea and other menstrual irregularities occur commonly. There is also a possibility of virilizing effects from the use of anabolic steroids. Some of these effects, such as coarsening and eventually deepening of the voice, hirsutism, male pattern baldness, reduction of breast size, and clitoral enlargement, may be partially reversed by the discontinuation of anabolic steroids and, if needed, the use of androgen antagonists such as cyproterone acetate.

After anabolic steroids are discontinued, the hormonal parameters return to normal in most men, except perhaps in those athletes who have used large amounts of anabolic steroids for prolonged periods. In some of these athletes, the serum testosterone may remain depressed for several weeks to months, secondary to testicular atrophy and refractiveness of the hypothalamic-pituitary-testicular axis (46). Occasionally, serum testosterone fails to returns to normal and long-term replacement therapy is necessary.

The other group of adverse effects is those that are not usually thought of as related to either the anabolic or androgenic properties of these compounds. These adverse effects, although controversy exists about the role of anabolic steroids in their genesis and development, result in more than just cosmetic changes. They include changes in serum cholesterol, cardiovascular disease, prostate cancer, kidney dysfunction, disturbances in carbohydrate metabolism, emotional disturbances, increased incidence of musculoskeletal injuries, cerebrovascular accidents, hepatic dysfunction (with rare instances of hepatic cirrhosis), hepatocellular carcinoma, and peliosis hepatitis. This second group of adverse effects, although posing a serious threat to the athlete, has often been misrepresented and sensationalized in both the media and some of the scientific literature. As noted previously, better controlled long-term studies are needed to determine accurately the risk involved in the prolonged use of anabolic steroids.

To put these potentially life-threatening adverse effects in perspective, the author has found it useful to compare the adverse effects of anabolic steroids with the adverse effects of oral contraceptives, especially before the 1980s when larger dosages of hormones were used. In general, the adverse effects of using low to moderate dosages of anabolic steroids are comparable to those seen in women using oral contraceptives. The risks inherent in this universally used and accepted method of contraception, which are well outlined in the Report on Oral Contraceptives, 1985, by the Special Advisory Committee on Reproductive Physiology to the Health Protection Branch, Health and Welfare, Canada, parallel in many ways the risks inherent in anabolic steroid use. There are differences because it is mainly male athletes who use anabolic steroids (although use among female athletes is increasing in the power sports such as weight lifting, power lifting, body building, and the track and field events that require explosive strength).

A search of the recent literature shows that the use of oral contraceptives is associated with similar adverse effects such as hepatic disease, including hepatic cell adenomas and cancer of the liver (47–49), and changes in serum cholesterol. Even peliosis hepatitis, described primarily in patients taking androgenic steroid medication and patients with tuberculosis, has recently been reported as a possible complication of the long-term use of oral contraceptives (50).

Adverse effects can also be separated into the short-term and long-term consequences of using anabolic steroids. Although many of the short-term consequences are clinically clear (especially those resulting in changes in the female secondary sexual characteristics and in feminization of men), the long-term consequences are more elusive. There is some speculation that chronic use of anabolic steroids may cause hepatic cirrhosis, peliosis hepatitis, primary hepatoma, atherosclerosis and cardiac disease, diabetes, prostatic cancer, and cerebral vascular accidents in those genetically susceptible.

There is, however, no solid clinical or experimental evidence to show that the use of anabolic steroids by healthy athletes has any effect on longevity, or that prolonged use leads to diseases of the various organs and systems mentioned previously. It is interesting that although substantial amounts of anabolic steroids have been used by athletes for more than 3 decades, significant long-term effects are not being seen in athletes who have used anabolic steroids in the 1950s, 1960s, and 1970s.

Nevertheless, the changing pattern of anabolic steroid use over the past decade—anabolic steroids are being more widely used at higher dosages and for longer periods—may yet reveal more severe problems in the long term. There are some studies in progress now that may shed some light on the long-term consequences of anabolic steroid use.

POSSIBLE BENEFICIAL EFFECTS

Although the bulk of the literature deals with the real and potential adverse effects of anabolic steroids, the possible beneficial effects of anabolic steroid use are rarely mentioned. Like the birth control pill in women, it is possible that the use of anabolic steroids may have some beneficial effects. There is also the possibility, as in the case of birth control medication and its beneficial effects on the incidence of ovarian and endometrial cancer, that the use of anabolic steroids may act as a deterrent for certain kinds of cancer, such as testicular cancer.

CONTRAINDICATIONS AND PRECAUTIONS

It can generally be stated that certain athletes should not use anabolic steroids or at least should have expert medical supervision if they wish to take the risk. Any of the following conditions would preclude their use: cancer of the prostate or liver, peliosis hepatitis, stroke or heart attack (if there is significant arterial disease), and persistent liver disease.

There are also several conditions that make it inadvisable to use anabolic steroids. These include high blood pressure, diabetes, elevated serum cholesterol, heart or kidney disease, prostate problems, bleeding disorder, and previous liver disease.

An athlete with any of the above conditions (or even a familial tendency) should reconsider the decision to use anabolic steroids; close medical supervision is necessary if choosing to use them.

Any athlete suffering one or more of the mentioned adverse effects should take measures to correct the problem either by discontinuing the use of anabolic steroids or by taking effective measures to offset the adverse effect. In any case, any athlete using anabolic steroids must accept the risk (however small) of serious adverse effects developing secondary to their use, including the possibility of cancer and life-threatening cardiovascular complications.

DEALING WITH ADVERSE EFFECTS

Although there are many possible short-term and long-term consequences of anabolic steroid use, most of these adverse effects can be minimized by their judicious use or, if necessary, their discontinuation. Other measures can be taken to mitigate or eliminate potential adverse effects and their consequences. The overall risks associated with the use of anabolic steroids are not as great as the sporting federations and the media would lead the public to believe. In men, most of the studies done so far show a reversal of any adverse effects and the return of normal testicular function and sperm count within 3 to 6 months.

Many of the athletes who use higher doses of two or more anabolic steroids for prolonged periods recognize the risks involved with the use of anabolic steroids. These athletes, whether under medical supervision or not, often use methods and drugs to counteract or nullify these adverse effects (51). Unfortunately, few athletes have the benefit of proper medical care and follow-up.

The widespread use of black-market anabolic steroids introduces another set of possible adverse effects.

Black-Market Drugs

The majority of athletes who use anabolic steroids are recreational rather than competitive athletes. They use these compounds for a more muscular and athletic look rather than for their performance-enhancing effects.

Athletes use a vast arsenal of drugs to improve their appearance and performance and to combat some of the adverse effects of other drugs. Drugs (prescription and over the counter) used by athletes in an attempt to improve performance include the following: anabolic-androgenic steroids, amphetamines and amphetamine derivatives, narcotic analgesics, adrenergic compounds, adrenaline, local anesthetics, corticosteroids, caffeine, alcohol, nicotine, growth hormone, somatomedin-C,

galanin, growth hormone–releasing hormone, human chorionic gonadotropin (HCG), menotropins, gonadorelin, zeranol, erythropoietin, glucagon, insulin, thyroid hormone, clonidine, L-dopa, beta-blockers, calcium channel blockers, nonsteroidal anti-inflammatory drugs (NSAIDs), DMSO, cyclobenzaprine, diuretics, tamoxifen, antibiotics, hypnotics, sedatives, and nutritional products and supplements including B_{12}, inosine, carnitine, dibencozide, and the various amino acids. This list, however, is just the tip of the iceberg. It might be difficult to find a substance that has not been experimented with by some aspiring athlete.

The anabolic steroids, including testosterone, are perhaps the most abused. Many recent studies have shown the muscle mass and strength-enhancing effects of anabolic steroids. Today, it is universally believed that anabolic steroids enhance athletic performance to the extent that most elite power athletes (including those in track and field) believe that they cannot remain competitive without them.

Because most physicians believe that prescribing anabolic steroids contributes to the problem of drug use in sports, most athletes obtain their anabolic steroids (and other performance-enhancing drugs) from black-market dealers. As prescription sources of anabolic steroids dry up, this black-market activity increases. Because most athletes get both their drugs and drug information from black-market and other nonmedical sources, they are often encouraged to use a variety of drugs, also easily obtainable from the underground pharmacy. This unsupervised polypharmacy can result in serious adverse effects.

As dangerous as this polypharmacy is, there is a more sinister side. Although black-market drugs are easy to obtain, some are of questionable quality and safety. Black-market dealers get their supplies wherever they can—sometimes from reputable sources or sometimes not. Lately, however, black market supplies of both anabolic steroids and growth hormone are in short supply for various reasons including the crackdown on the smuggling of commercially available anabolic steroids from other countries (such as Mexico), decrease in the amount of commercial anabolic steroids diverted from North American manufacturers, and increased police involvement in the athletic black market.

Because of this shortage of reliable drugs, more of the black-market drugs are coming from makeshift illegal basement laboratories where bogus drugs are produced using whatever material is at hand. Such materials include pharmaceutical preparations, drugs from homemade laboratories, veterinary drugs, vitamins, inert filler compounds, and in some cases of injectable preparations, just plain oil or water with food coloring.

The dangers of using these counterfeit drugs fall into three categories. First, if the vial or pill comes from a reputable pharmaceutical company (whether mislabeled or not), there is the danger inherent in the drug itself. Moreover, the bottle or vial may not contain what its label says. For example, some vials of a combination of testosterone and estrogen (used therapeutically to treat the female climacteric) were relabeled as testosterone enanthate with no mention of the estrogen component.

Second, there are the dangers inherent in taking a drug that has been manufactured or constructed in a basement laboratory. The lack of quality controls and, in many cases, the lack of expertise and adequate knowledge of biopharmacology, make black-market drugs a high-risk gamble. The absence of meticulous protocols and sterile conditions may lead to both chemical or biologic contamination. Chemical impurities can result in acute or chronic poisoning and damage to the liver and kidney. Biologic impurities can result in bacterial, fungal, and viral infections—possibly even hepatitis and acquired immune deficiency syndrome (AIDS). There have been several cases of infections, both local (in the form of abscesses) and generalized, leading to acute sickness with fevers and joint pain in athletes using bogus growth hormone and some injectable anabolic steroids. In some cases the stoppers used in the vials, instead of being inert, are reactive and/or absorptive and may cause toxic contamination of the contents of the vials.

Third, because most athletes obtain their anabolic preparations through the local gyms, there is no long-term medical follow-up. Thus, many correctable problems caused by taking the drugs improperly or by using mislabeled or contaminated drugs are missed.

Counterfeit drugs are not restricted to anabolic steroids. Almost any drug available on the black market is suspect. Counterfeit growth hormone has become increasingly common. The author has seen instances in which the packaging and vials were difficult to distinguish from real growth hormone. If this counterfeit growth hormone finds its way into the commercial market, it might possibly be used clinically, with disastrous consequences.

Doping Control

Regardless of how and where competitive athletes obtain their drugs, these drugs are used in an attempt to enhance athletic performance. Doping control is an attempt to discourage drug use by athletes. Although anabolic steroids can have significant adverse effects, the primary reason behind the banning of anabolic steroid use in amateur sports by such bodies as the International Olympic Committee (IOC) is because they are believed to enhance athletic performance.

In 1967, the IOC established a medical commission that banned the practice of doping. Doping was defined as the use of substances or techniques, in any form or quantity, alien or unnatural to the body, with the exclusive aim of obtaining an artificial and unfair increase of performance in competition.

This IOC definition of doping bans the use of such performance-enhancing drugs as the amphetamines, most adrenergic compounds, narcotic analgesics, and anabolic steroids. It also includes other drugs such as diuretics, beta blockers, and corticosteroids (except for topical use) as well as performance-enhancing procedures such as blood doping.

Having specified the banned substances, the IOC carried out limited doping tests at the 1968 Olympics. By 1972, new scientific and technologic knowledge enabled the IOC to increase the scope and rapidity of its testing. At the 1976 Olympics, anabolic steroids were included in the testing program. In 1984, in Los Angeles, testosterone was added.

In 1987, the IOC Medical Commission changed its definition of testosterone abuse, which now reads as follows: "For testosterone the definition of a positive depends on the following: the administration of testosterone or the use of any other manipulation having the result of increasing the ratio in the urine of testosterone/epitestosterone to above 6."

DETECTION OF ANABOLIC STEROIDS

Testosterone is a 17β-hydroxylated C-19 steroid clinically known as 17β-hyroxy-4-androstene-3-one. Certain changes made to the steroid molecule alter the metabolic inactivation process, resulting in differences in the excretion of 17-keto steroids and the compound itself. Thus, some anabolic steroids are excreted unchanged and others are highly metabolized, resulting in a large number of excretory steroids. Detection of anabolic steroids (but not testosterone) is thus possible by the identification of either the parent compound and/or one or more of its metabolites (depending on the metabolic and excretory profile of the specific anabolic steroid).

For example, 17-alkylation, changing the position of the double bond in ring A, methyl substitution on atoms C-1, C-2, and C-6, and 4-chloro substitution all influence the metabolism and the excretory products of a compound compared with testosterone. Thus, whereas the 17α-methyl steroids (such as methandrostenolone) are mostly excreted in the free form and are not significantly metabolized into 17-ketosteroids, the 17α-ethyl and the 19-nortestosterone analogs are highly metabolized. The resulting metabolites are subsequently conjugated in the liver and excreted in the urine and thus used to identify the parent compound. Therefore, the use of synthetic anabolic steroids is currently detected by finding the parent compound or one or more diagnostic metabolites in the urine.

Detection of testosterone is more difficult because it is endogenously produced in both men and women and is therefore naturally present in the urine. However, the use of exogenous testosterone, because it alters the endogenous hormonal profile, can be detected by comparing the relative amounts of certain hormones found in the urine. The use of exogenous testosterone is currently detected by an increase to 6/1 or more of the urinary testosterone/epitestosterone (T/E) ratio.

There are problems with both tests. One of the most common methods now being used to escape the detection of anabolic steroids and other anabolic compounds is simply discontinuing the use of oral anabolic steroid(s) a few to several days before a drug-tested event.

The low levels of residuals after the oral use of anabolic steroids makes it difficult to find in urine a few days after ingestion. Compounds like oxandrolone (Oxandrin; Bio-Technology, Iselin, NJ), stanozolol (Winstrol), and methandrostenolone (generic forms of the now discontinued Dianabol) are undetectable after 3 days in the majority of athletes. Small to moderate doses of some oral anabolic steroids (such as oxandrolone) have been taken by athletes up to 2 days before a drug-tested competition and were not detected.

The use of the testosterone/epitestosterone ratio to detect the use of exogenous testosterone is also flawed. This approach, developed by Dr. Manfred Donike (52) in Cologne, Germany, treats epitestosterone (the 17α-hydroxy-epimer of testosterone) as a relatively constant factor in the steroid profile. According to his theory, exogenous testosterone administration does not significantly increase the urinary concentration of epitestosterone. In fact, not only is practically no epitestosterone formed from exogenous testosterone, but its formation is inhibited by exogenous testosterone.

Because the urine usually contains about equal quantities of testosterone and epitestosterone, the normal ratio is between 1 and 2 in men and women, although the concentration of both is lower in women. Administration of exogenous testosterone leads to an increased ratio between testosterone and epitestosterone, such that an above-normal urinary testosterone/epitestosterone ratio is considered a reliable indicator of testosterone doping.

To play it safe, the upper limit of the T/E ratio was set as 6 with no units. It was believed that by setting the upper limit high, individual drug-free steroid profiles would easily fall under this level. However, results from several antidoping laboratories, including our own, indicate that genetic, environmental, or dietary factors may affect this ratio and may even cause false-positive results in some cases (53–55).

For many reasons, the T/E ratio has many flaws and can be easily manipulated so that it may not be a reliable indicator of exogenous testosterone use (56). The IOC, recognizing the problems inherent in this test, has made several modifications and additions to its original proposal. Realizing that other factors may affect the ratio, including the use of other banned compounds, in 1987 the IOC changed its definition of testosterone abuse and stated that, "For testosterone the definition of a positive depends upon the following: the administration of testosterone or the use of any other manipulation having the result of increasing the ratio in the urine of T/E to above 6." This stance adopted by the IOC indirectly admits that an elevated T/E ratio may not necessarily reflect the use of exogenous testosterone.

More recently, the IOC has made two other important and necessary changes to its doping policies regarding the detection of exogenous testosterone use (57).

Because athletes are using exogenous epitestosterone along with exogenous testosterone, or using the epitestosterone to contaminate the urine samples directly, the IOC banned the use of exogenous epitestosterone and considers a test suspect for the use of exogenous epitestosterone if more than 150 ng/mL of epitestosterone is present in the urine. Most athletes using epitestosterone fall within this limit and would not test positive.

In May 1992 the IOC, realizing that there were problems with their strict interpretation of the cutoff point of their testosterone/epitestosterone ratio, modified the criteria for a positive doping test for exogenous testosterone. They now believe that for athletes with urine T/E ratios between 6 and 10, further investigations and procedures may be necessary before the test is considered positive, including one or more of the following: reviewing T/E ratios and other hormonal parameters from previous tests, analyzing additional urine samples, conducting a series of unannounced urine collections, and performing further endocrinologic investigations.

Thus, the emphasis appears to be shifting from comparing doping results with normal values to performing longitudinal studies that are specific to each athlete. In this way, significant deviations in the hormonal profile as seen in any one or more urine tests can point to the use of banned substances.

The IOC also looks at other hormonal parameters to substantiate a positive test. It has been found that the use of anabolic steroids and/or testosterone results in a change of the endogenous steroid profile, for example, the changes of the ratios of isomeric steroids like cis-androsterone and etiocholanolone (the major metabolic end-products of the endogenous androgenic steroids) (58). The decrease in concentration and the shift of ratios can be observed even if the exogenous anabolic steroids can no longer be detected in the urine. Thus, extended use of anabolic androgenic steroids results in a shift of the ratio between cis-androsterone and etiocholano-lone to values of 0.5 or lower.

It has been the author's experience, however, based on more than 1000 urinary hormone profiles done in the past 1.5 years, that all the hormonal ratios, including the cis-androsterone/etiocholanolone and the testosterone/LH ratios, are unreliable as markers of anabolic steroid or testosterone use. The author believes that these ratios can be used only to substantiate positive test results for the synthetic anabolic steroids. Although the author has found that the use of other urinary hormonal ratios has not been especially fruitful, others seem to be more optimistic that the use of other urinary hormonal ratios may provide valuable complementary information (59).

A recent article has suggested that a better test for detecting or substantiating the use of exogenous testosterone (and the anabolic steroids) is the ratio in serum of testosterone and 17 alpha-hydroxyprogesterone (T/17OHP) (60). This same article concluded that among urinary analyses, only the T/epiT ratio was a suitable marker of T doping; of the serum assays, 17 alpha-hydroxyprogesterone (17OHP), T/17OHP ratio, LH, and T/LH ratio were fair to good markers of T doping. The serum T/17OHP ratio was the best marker of those tested. Several studies have shown that endogenous concentrations of testosterone and 17OHP are closely correlated in healthy men (61, 62).

Although the authors of this study proposed estimating the T/17OHP ratio in all suspected cases of T doping, just as for T/LH the T/17OHP ratio will not be useful for women because 17OHP concentrations vary with the menstrual cycle (63).

The value of this marker for T doping was further supported by the finding of normal T/17OHP ratios in a subject with increased urinary T/epiT ratios caused by an abnormally low testicular epiT production, probably related to genetic factors.

In cases of a positive testosterone/epitestosterone ratio or in cases of suspected use of testosterone and/or anabolic steroids, it would be useful to have an analysis for 17OHP, testosterone, and LH in serum. It should be possible to quantify all three hormones in serum by isotope dilution mass spectrometry.

Estimation of the T/17OHP ratio is a logical candidate for the list of additional tests; however, this ratio and other endocrine tests require blood samples and the selection of an analytical method for confirming the ratio. Currently, the IOC is reviewing a proposal to allow blood to be taken from athletes in the context of the Olympic Games. If approved, this would also provide an entry into the important area of detecting blood doping and the administration of hormones such as erythropoietin and human growth hormone (somatotropin).

However, current IOC regulations require that all positive cases be confirmed by gas chromatography–mass spectrometry, although at this time there is no practical means for identifying such peptides in urine or blood by this method. For the T/17OHP ratio, published gas chromatography–mass spectrometry methods exist for both T (as noted) and 17OHP (64); however, for investigators to implement this test, the methods would have to be fully validated in each laboratory.

As well as watching the above, the IOC is looking at definitive methods such as detecting a synthetic testosterone ester in blood (useful for all testosterone esters but not for the testosterone suspension) or finding an unnatural carbon-12/carbon-13 isotope ratio (65).

COLLECTION AND TESTING OF SAMPLES

The procedures for selecting the athletes to be tested and for collecting and transporting samples of urine to the testing laboratories have been standardized for each particular athletic activity. Regardless of the sport, there are certain basic procedures that are common (66).

At the laboratory, a sample of the urine is subjected to sophisticated, precise tests that determine if a banned substance is present in the urine and if so, in what concentration. The testing of urine samples involves three basic steps: extraction, screening, and confirmation.

EXTRACTION

The first step, extraction, prepares the urine for analysis. Multiple extractions are usually necessary because many drugs are excreted not only in their original form, but also as by-products resulting from the metabolic breakdown of the original form.

INITIAL SCREENING

The second step, screening, is a search for traces of banned substances within the extracted solutions. The screening is carried out by gas chromatography, a procedure used to separate out the individual drugs (based on their relative volatility and solubility) present in the urine, one by one, during a time sequence.

The individual drugs are transported through the chromatographic column (a long thin glass tube coated on the inside with a polymeric substance) by an inert carrier gas (such as helium). The carrier gas transports the drugs in the gaseous phase but actually has no part in the chromatographic process.

Different drugs come out of the end of the column at different times (depending on their special characteristics). The time at which a drug comes out of the column is known as its retention time. If the retention time of the drug being analyzed is the same as the retention time of a known sample drug, then the two drugs are likely the same. However, this is not necessarily true, because many compounds can be crowded together in the same one tenth of a second of retention time.

Thus, the initial screening, which serves to indicate the possible presence of a banned substance, is not specific enough to constitute definitive proof of a positive doping test.

CONFIRMATION

The final identification of a substance and confirmation of its presence require further testing using a computerized gas chromatography–mass spectrometry system. The gas chromatography serves as a purification technique (separating out the banned component from all the rest), whereas mass spectrometry identifies the substance by ion bombardment. In the mass spectrometer, an electron beam bombards the compound with electrons, imparting a charge to the molecules and causing some of the molecules to fragment into charged particles or ions. These charged particles (which also include the charged parent compound or molecular ion) are sorted magnetically according to size and charge. An ion detector then records these ions, producing a mass spectrum of the sample compound.

The pattern of fragments and their proportional abundance (the mass spectrum consists of a plot of fragment mass versus relative abundance) is characteristic enough to allow identification of the unknown molecule.

A computer compares the resulting mass spectrum with the mass spectra contained in its memory banks. An exact match identifies the unknown compound. If an exact match is not made, then the compound cannot be identified for the purposes of a positive doping test, even though the laboratory suspects that the compound present in an athlete's urine sample is an anabolic steroid.

Although extremely accurate in identifying substances in the urine, mass spectrometry is not overly sensitive (even using selected ion monitoring). If the concentration of a drug picked up by the screening process is too low, mass spectrometry will not be able to pick it up and confirm its identity (thus, the rationale for athletes drinking large amounts of water and producing a diluted urine sample and for using drugs like probenecid, which may decrease the amount of drug which is excreted).

In the event of a positive test, the athlete is notified and asked to come to the laboratory (or send a representative) to observe identical testing of a second sample. If the banned substance is again found in the athlete's urine, the athlete will be disqualified from the immediate competition and possibly from future competitions (for whatever period the governing sports federation decides).

The IOC has imposed severe penalties on those athletes testing positive for certain substances. For anabolic steroids (including testosterone), amphetamine-related and other stimulants, caffeine, diuretics, beta-blockers, narcotic analgesics, and designer drugs, the penalty is a 2-year ban for the first offense and a life ban for the second offense.

ESCAPING DETECTION

The analytical testing for anabolic steroids and testosterone is not welcomed by all, especially those athletes who constantly seek that competitive edge by using drugs. Since the advent of analytical doping control, athletes have tried various methods to make the testing procedures ineffective. They have sent impersonators to the drug testing station; diluted the urine by using diuretics to reduce the concentration of substances and their metabolites; introduced "clean" urine into their bladder through a catheter; simulated the passage of "clean" urine from an external source (such as the vaginal bags used by some female athletes; these bags of "clean urine" are inserted in the vagina and subsequently punctured to provide the urine sample); ingested or injected such chemicals as sodium bicarbonate, phenylbutazone, probenecid, antiprostaglandins, chelating agents (most notably EDTA), and other compounds to mask or reduce the elimination of banned substances; introduced exogenous chemicals or bacteria into the urine specimen at the time of voiding; used compounds that are obscure, such as veterinary anabolic steroids, and little-known stimulants; and used compounds that are not as yet on the banned list or that can not as yet be tested for. This list of techniques for invalidating tests is far from complete—the inventive mind of the athlete or trainer is always searching for and finding new methods to beat the system.

Doping control is effective in discouraging the use of certain drugs—especially those drugs that are mainly used in competition rather than in training—such as the opioids and stimulants. These drugs are only effective while at certain concentrations in the body and thus in the urine. The excretion of these substances can sometimes be manipulated; however, in nearly all cases in which the drug does some good in increasing performance, it will be found in the urine. For these drugs (the ones that perhaps sparked the most concern in the first place such as the psychomotor stimulants and narcotic analgesics), testing is an effective deterrent (although other drugs possessing the same properties but are not detectable are being actively sought out and used).

However, many compounds used by athletes (including anabolic steroids and growth hormone) are not drugs of the moment. These drugs must be taken for long periods before competition for their effects to be realized. These effects often remain several weeks after the drug is discontinued, often when the drug is no longer found in the urine in detectable quantities.

Thus, ergogenic drugs such as anabolic steroids are really training drugs, that is, drugs that benefit the athlete during training and subsequently at competitions. Most athletes try to escape detection by attempting to stop the use of anabolic steroids soon enough so that they will not be detected, but late enough so that the athlete will still feel some of the fast-disappearing anabolic effects. If the athlete is using substances that are detectable, there is always the chance of getting caught if use is discontinued too close to the drug-tested event and the urinary concentration of the compounds fails to fall below the detection limits of the assay.

More knowledgeable athletes use other compounds to mask the use of the banned substances, use drugs that are not yet on the banned list, or use drugs that cannot as yet be tested for, including growth hormone, galanin, clenbuterol, dihydrotestosterone, designer anabolic steroids (anabolic steroids not available commercially and whose spectra are not as yet in the IOC laboratories' computer data banks), menotropins, erythropoietin, adrenaline, Striadyne, sydnocarb, nicotametate, and piracetam.

Some pharmacologically minded athletes are attempting to escape detection of their exogenous testosterone use by using injections of one or more of epitestosterone, dehydroepiandrosterone, androstenedione, human chorionic gonadotropin, menotropins, and gonadorelin before and/or during competitions. They also use diuretics and chelating agents (most commonly EDTA) and add certain contaminants to their urine specimens.

The previously mentioned list of techniques for invalidating tests is far from complete. The system, in turn, is always refining its techniques in an attempt to keep up. Unfortunately, the athlete has been, and will continue to be, one or more steps ahead of the laboratories.

This is not to say, however, that doping control should be abandoned. Although the author would like to see drug-free competition, he is not naive enough to assume that comprehensive and pervasive drug testing (including frequent random and unannounced testing of athletes) will stop the use of drugs in sports. It will not. The most that drug testing can hope to achieve is a decrease in drug use in the less-sophisticated athletes.

Anabolic Steroid Preparations

Relatively small changes in the basic chemical structure of the testosterone molecule (and other endogenous sex hormones) may bring about dramatic changes in effect, potency, and adverse effects. A methyl group here and a hydroxyl group there could lead to an enhancement of anabolic activity, or more likely to a loss of androgenic and anabolic properties. As a result of extensive research, particularly in the 1950s and 1960s (67, 68), thousands of biologically active steroid compounds are now known.

Although there may be hundreds of available preparations of testosterone and its chemically modified analogs, the most common preparations used by athletes and officially banned by the IOC include the following: bolasterone, boldenone, chloroxomesterone (dehydrochlormethyltestosterone), clostebol, fluoxymesterone, furazabol, mesterolone, methandienone (methandrostenolone), methenolone, methyltestosterone, nandrolone, norethandrolone, oxandrolone, oxymesterone, oxymetholone, stanozolol, and testosterone in its many forms (oral and injectable). These compounds vary in their androgenic and anabolic properties as well as in their formulation and bioavailability.

Anabolic steroids are commercially available in several forms: topical, buccal, oral, rectal, and injectable. The oral and buccal forms are most commonly used both clinically and by athletes.

ORAL PREPARATIONS

Testosterone, when taken orally, is partially destroyed by the chemical enzymatic processes of the gastrointestinal tract. The remaining testosterone crosses the gastrointestinal mucosa, where it is then taken directly to the liver by the portal system. It is promptly metabolized by the liver so that very small amounts (5% to 10% at the most) reach the systemic circulation and, therefore, the target tissues.

The 17α-alkylated compounds (methyl or ethyl groups are added at the $C17\alpha$ position) are more effective orally because they largely escape degradation by the liver during the initial pass from the gut.

INJECTABLE AQUEOUS AND OIL-BASED PREPARATIONS

Because anabolic steroids are relatively water insoluble, most aqueous preparations are suspensions, not solutions. To make a suspension, steroid powder is finely ground so that the crystal size is small enough to pass through a regular gauge needle without clogging—somewhere between 100 and 300 μm. This powder is then mixed with sterile water to make up the suspen-

sion. If left to settle, the crystals fall to the bottom of the vial and must be resuspended (by shaking the vial) before use.

The finer the suspension, the faster it leaves the system. If the particles are big, then they dissolve much slower. Thus, very fine suspensions may leave the body in a few days. Coarse suspensions may take several months to fully dissipate, especially if the injection is made into scar tissue, which has a reduced blood supply. If an athlete repeatedly injects one or two areas, a certain amount of scar tissue inevitably forms. Further injections into these areas may increase the detection time for that anabolic steroid because it takes longer for the body to remove the anabolic steroid from the injection site.

When used parenterally, crystalline testosterone acts much like the shorter acting esters (such as testosterone propionate), with a relatively short half-life and effect. Two or three injections per week are needed to sustain effective serum levels.

Esterification, the reaction of the 17-hydroxy group with an acid compound, results in the formation of an ester that is less soluble in water and more soluble in lipids than is the crystalline form of testosterone. Because of their high solubility in lipids, most esters of testosterone and anabolic steroids are thus available as oil-based solutions rather than suspensions. The larger the carbon chain of the acid, the more insoluble in water is the corresponding salt, and the more prolonged the action of the compound once injected. For example, testosterone propionate (short carbon chain) is short acting in comparison to testosterone enanthate (longer carbon chain). The esters of testosterone, when deesterified or hydrolyzed by esterase enzymes, produce active testosterone, which enters the systemic circulation.

Testosterone Preparations

Crystalline Testosterone. Available in oral, parenteral, or pellet form. The oral form is rapidly metabolized, and very little reaches the systemic circulation. The parenteral forms are usually suspended in aqueous solution or may be suspended in oily solutions. The subcutaneous pellet form is used for implantation purposes and contains unesterified testosterone.

Testosterone Propionate. Available from many sources. A commercial example is Oreton propionate (Schering). It is used mainly as an injectable; however, it is also available in sublingual form. Because of its short duration of action, it is not used as much as the longer acting testosterone esters.

Testosterone Enanthate. A commercial example is Delatestryl (Squibb). It is available only in parenteral form. Along with the cypionate, it is the longest acting testosterone ester.

Testosterone Cypionate. A commercial example is Depo-testosterone (Upjohn).

Testosterone Nicotinate. Water-based (suspension) testosterone ester. Commercial name is Bolfortan (Lannacker Heilmittel).

Testosterone Phenylacetate. This is a new short-acting testosterone ester and is currently not in wide use. Unlike the testosterone propionate, this is an aqueous suspension of testosterone, but is more effective than the aqueous suspensions of crystalline testosterone.

Testosterone Undecanoate. This testosterone ester, although not methylated (and not hepatotoxic), is used orally. It is lipid soluble and is absorbed into the intestinal lymphatics; therefore, it bypasses the hepatic portal system. The only drawback is that large amounts of the compound must be used to obtain physiologic androgenic and anabolic effects.

Studies have shown that testosterone undecanoate is effective when taken orally and has a relatively short half-life. Maximum plasma, saliva, and urine levels of testosterone undecanoate (Andriol; Organon) occur after 4 hours, with basal levels achieved in plasma and serum after 8 hours and in urine after 24 hours.

Testosterone-trans-4-N-Butylcyclohexyl-Carboxylate. A new testosterone ester has shown promise in the treatment of male hypogonadism. In a recent study the new ester, testosterone-trans-4-n-butylcyclohexyl-carboxylate (or 20-Aet-1) in an aqueous suspension, was compared with testosterone enanthate in sesame seed oil (69). This study showed that the new ester provided physiologic levels of testosterone more than 8 times longer than the enanthate form of testosterone. Currently, the enanthate and cypionate ester forms of testosterone are the longest acting testosterone esters on the market.

Transdermal Testosterone Therapy. A few advanced pharmacologically minded athletes are using transdermal testosterone therapy as a stopgap between the time they stop taking injectable and oral anabolic steroids and the drug-tested event.

Drugs delivered transdermally (through the skin) offer several advantages over both the injectable and oral routes. They do not enter the portal hepatic circulation, and so do not get watered down in a "first pass effect" through the liver. Thus, less drug can be administered for the same effect and there is less fluctuation in serum levels (current hormonal substitution therapy, by either injectable or oral esters, suffers from fluctuating serum hormone levels, often significantly above or below the physiologic range).

A growing number of transdermal drug delivery systems are being developed. Several studies have been done on the usefulness of transdermal testosterone as a treatment for male hypogonadism. The use of testosterone patches on the scrotum results in a significant increase in serum dihydrotestosterone (up to 12 times that found in healthy men) due to the conversion of testosterone by the enzyme 5α-reductase, present in relatively high concentrations in scrotal skin (70, 71).

Androstenolone or Stanolone or Dihydrotestosterone. Available androstenolone esters include formate, acetate, propionate, butyrate, and valerate. Because of the the 5α reduction, it does not aromatize.

Chemical names: 17-Hydroxyandrostan-3-one. 17β-hydroxy-3-androstanone. 17β-hydroxy-5α-androstan-3-one 5α-androstan-17β-ol-3-one. Dihydrotestosterone is available as injectable esters (100 mg/cc) and as buccal tablets (10 and 25 mg).

Commercial preparations include: Pesomax—injectable form of dihydrotestosterone (dihydrotestosterone propionate), Apeton—injectable form (dihydrotestosterone-valerate), Stanolone tablets and Anabolex tablets, both used sublingually or sublabially. Other trade names include Anabolex, Anaprotin, Androlone, Cristerona MB, Proteina, Anaboleen (Badarznei), Andractim (Besins Iscovesco), Neodrol (Pfizer), Protona (Gremy-Longuet), Stanadrol (Pfizer). Also available as a gel (Andractim Gel—2.5 g%, Belgium).

The injectable esters of dihydrotestosterone are metabolized as dihydrotestosterone once deesterified (as occurs with the testosterone esters).

The 5α reduction of the testosterone molecule precludes estrogen formation; therefore, dihydrotestosterone does not aromatize. This anabolic steroid is identical to the dihydrotestosterone that is formed endogenously in the body from peripheral conversion of testosterone and by direct secretion of the testes. This is a very potent androgen, and in physiologic doses has less of an inhibiting effect on the pituitary than do equivalent amounts of testosterone. It is not hepatotoxic.

Androisoxazole. Chemical names: 17-Methylandrostano(3,2-c) isoxazol-17-ol. 17β-hydroxy-17α-methylandrostano(3,2-c)isoxazole. 17α-methylandrostan(3,2-c)isoxazol-17β-ol.

Trade name: Neo-Ponden (Serono).

Various esters (3-Acetate, 17-Acetate, Diacetate, 17-Benzoate, 3-Acetate-17-benzoate, and

Dipropionate) have been used clinically but not produced commercially (except for the dipropionate).

Androstenediol. Chemical name: Androst-5-ene-$3\beta,17\beta$-diol. δ5-androstene-$3\beta,17\beta$-diol.

Obtained from dehydroandrosterone and available as the Dipropionate. Trade names are Bisexovis and Stenandiol.

Bolandiol. Chemical name: Estr-4-ene-$3\beta,17\beta$-diol. $3\beta,17\beta$-dihydroxyestr-4-ene.

Trade name: dipropionate ester marketed as Anabiol (Searle), and Storinal.

Bolasterone. The commercial product Myagen has been discontinued. This is an oral anabolic steroid. It is hepatotoxic and aromatizes. It is similar in function to methandrostenolone. Its chemical name is 7α-17α dimethyltestosterone. A counterfeit injectable bolasterone was once available in the United States.

Boldenone. Chemical names: 17-Hydroxyandrosta-1,4-dien-3-one. 1,4-androstadien-17β-ol-3-one. 3-oxo-17β-hydroxy-1,4-androstadiene. dehydrotestosterone.

Trade name: Parenabol (boldenone undecylenate) (Ciba).

Clostebol. Chemical names: 4-chlorotestosterone acetate. 4-Chloro-17β-hydroxyandrost-4-en-3-one.

Trade names: Steranabol (Farmitalia), Turinabol (Jenapharm).

Danazol. Commercial preparations include Danocrine (Winthrop) and Cyclomen (Winthrop). The chemical name is 17α-pregna-2-4-dien-20-yno-(2,3-d) isoxanol-17-ol. It is potentially hepatotoxic and does not significantly aromatize. Its mild androgenic activity is dose related. Because it shows significant separation of gonadotropin inhibitory activity from androgenic activity, it is used clinically in women for the treatment of endometriosis and fibrocystic breast disease.

Dromostanolone. Chemical name is 2α-methyltestosterone, or 2α-methyl-17-β-(1-oxopropoxy)-5α-androstan-3-one. This compound, like dihydrotestosterone, is a 5α reduced testosterone derivative, and therefore not subject to aromatization. It is available in parenteral form (typically as a propionate ester) and does not show any hepatotoxicity.

Trade names: Emdisterone, Drolban (Lilly), Masterid (Grunenthal), Masteril (Syntex), Masterone (Syntex), Permastril (Cassenne).

Ethylestrenol. Chemical name: 17α-ethyl-17β-hydroxy-19-norandrost-4-en-3-one. This compound is one of the estrenols, a derivative of 19-nortestosterone with the oxygen function in position 3 removed. The substituent subgrouping

of position 3 gives it its anabolic effect. It is also mildly progestational. It does not aromatize significantly because it inhibits the enzyme aromatase. It is potentially hepatotoxic.

Trade names: Orgaboral, Orgabolin (obsolete), Durabolin-O (Organon), Maxibolin (Organon), Orabolin (Organon).

Fluoxymesterone. A commercial example is Halotestin. This compound is a derivative of methyltestosterone. Its chemical name is 9α-fluoro 11β-17β-dihydroxy-17α-methyl-4-androsten-3-one. The fluoride ion seems to increase its androgen potency and also makes it a poor precursor for peripheral conversion into estrogens. It is potentially hepatotoxic.

Furazabol (Androfurazanol; Furazalon). Chemical names: 17α-Methyl-5α-androstano(2,3-c)(1,2,5) oxadiazol-17β-ol 17β-hydroxy-17α-methyl-5α-androstano(2,3-c)furazan.

Commercial preparations include Frazalon (Daiichi), Miotolon (Daiichi), and Myotolon (Daiichi).

A derivative of dihydrotestosterone. Most common trade name is Miotolon, which is manufactured in Japan by Daiichi-Seiyaku-J. In animal experiments, it was shown to be one of the few anabolic steroids that lowers serum cholesterol and triglycerides. Available in 1-mg tablets and in an injectable form. It does not aromatize significantly and is moderately hepatotoxic.

Mestanolone or Methylandrostenolone. A commercial example is Androstenolone. The chemical name is 17β-hydroxy-17α-methyl-5α-androstan-3-one. It is a 17α-methyl dihydrotestosterone derivative and is basically the oral form of androstenolone discussed earlier. Like androstenolone, it is not subject to peripheral aromatization. Because of the 17α-methyl substitution, it is potentially hepatotoxic.

Mesterelone. A commercial example is Androviron. The chemical name is 1α-methyl-17β-hydroxy-5α-androstan-3-one. This drug is the 1α-methyl derivative of dihydrotestosterone. It is active orally and, like other androgens methylated at the 1-alpha (1-α) position, is not subject to aromatization to an estrogen. This is one of the compounds that, although it has significant androgenic and anabolic activity, does not lead to significant depression of luteinizing hormone if used at relatively light doses. Most derivatives of dihydrotestosterone share this property. This compound has not been associated with any hepatotoxicity.

Methandriol or Methylandrostenediol. Commercial examples are Androdiol and Stenediol. The chemical name is 17α-methyl-5-androstene-3β-17-diol. This compound comes in both oral and injectable forms. Injectable form is a dipropionate salt. This compound is potentially hepatotoxic. It is subject to aromatization.

Methandrostenolone, Methandienone, or Methanedienone. The commercial examples Dianabol and Danabol are no longer being produced. However, the compound is still widely available under other trade names (Nerobol, Nabolin, Stenolon) and in generic form. Its chemical name is 17β-hydroxy-17α-methylandrosta-1,4-dien-3-one.

This compound is available mainly as an oral form, but lately has been available as an injectable as well. It is potentially hepatotoxic and is subject to aromatization. This compound, a methyltestosterone derivative, is very popular among athletes worldwide.

Methenolone. A commercial example is Primobolan. The chemical name is 1α-methyl-17β-hydroxy-5α-androst-1-en-3-one. This compound is a 1α-methyl derivative of dihydrotestosterone and is also classified as delta-1 mesterolone. It is not subject to aromatization and is not hepatotoxic. This compound is available in both oral and injectable forms, although the Primobolan oral form has been discontinued. This anabolic steroid is popular among European athletes and has gained in popularity in North America.

Methyltestosterone. Commercial preparations include Android (ICN) and Metandren (CIBA). The chemical name is 17β-hydroxy-17α-methyl-4-androsten-3-one. This compound was one of the earlier derivatives of testosterone, formed to make testosterone more bioavailable when used orally. It is available in oral and sublingual forms. It is subject to aromatization and has hepatotoxic potential.

Mibolerone. A veterinary compound. Commercial examples are Cheque Drops (Upjohn) and Matenon (Upjohn).

Chemical names: 17-Hydroxy-7,17-dimethylestr-4-en-3-one. 7α,17α-dimethyl-19-nortestosterone.

Nandrolone or 19-Nortestosterone. Commercial preparations include Nortestonate, Durabolin, and Deca-Durabolin. The chemical name is 17β-hydroxy-19-norandrost-4-en-3-one.

This compound is a derivative of testosterone lacking the C-19 methyl group. The deletion of this group results in a compound that has less androgenic effects and relatively more anabolic effects. Nandrolone is subject to aromatization. It is not hepatotoxic.

Nandrolone is no longer used by competitive athletes who must undergo drug testing because it has been implicated in more positive anabolic steroid tests than any other anabolic steroid, is easily detectable, and has a long half-life when used in its depot parenteral forms (especially decanoate ester).

Norethandrolone. Commercially, it is best known as Nilevar. The chemical name is 17α-ethyl-17-hydroxy-19-norandrost-4-en-3-one. This compound is a derivative of 19-nortestosterone. It is mainly used orally; however, parenteral forms are available. It is subject to aromatization and has hepatotoxic potential.

Oxandrolone. A derivative of dihydrotestosterone. Available in 2.5- and 5-mg tablets. Commercial examples are Anavar (Searle; recently discontinued), Anatrophill (Searle), Lonavar (Searle), Provitar (Clin-Comar-Byla), Vasorome (Kowa), Lipidex (Brazil), and Oxandrin (Bio-Technology).

Chemical names: 17β-hydroxy-17-methyl-2-oxa-5α-androstan-3-one. Dodecahydro-3-hydroxy-6-(hydroxymethyl)-3,3a,6-trimethyl-1H-benz(e)indene-7-acetic acid-lactone.

This compound is reduced in the 5α position; therefore, it is not subject to aromatization. It has reduced androgen effects and does not overly depress LH secretion by the pituitary. It has a low virilization potential in reduced dosages. For these reasons, this anabolic steroid is very popular among men and women. Its anabolic potential is dose related, and in larger doses it is an effective anabolic agent. At these dosages, however, the compound has significant virilizing effects.

Oxymetholone. A derivative of dihydrotestosterone. Commercial examples are Adroyd (Parke, Davis), Anadrol (Syntex), Anapolon (Syntex), Pardroyd (Parke, Davis), Plenastril (Protochemie) Protanabol Nastenon, Synasteron (Saruab), and Hemogenin.

Chemical names: 17β-Hydroxy-2-(hydroxymethylene)-17-methylandrostan 3 one; 2-hydroxymethylene-17α-methyldihydrotestoterone; 4,5α-dihydro-2-hydroxymethylene-17α-methyltestosterone. 2-hydroxymethylene-17α-methyl-17β-hydroxy-5α-androstan-3-one. 2-hydroxymethylene-17α-methylandrostan-17β-ol-3-one.

Available in oral tablets 2.5-, 5-, and 50-mg strengths. This compound has hepatotoxic potential and is peripherally converted to dihydrotestosterone and estrogens. It is clinically effective in treating some forms of aplastic anemia.

Quinbolone. A derivative of testosterone. Commercial example is Anabolicum Vister (Parke Davis, Italy).

Chemical names: 17β-(1-Cyclopenten-1-yloxy) androsta-1,4-dien-3-one, and 1-dehydrotestosterone 17-cyclopent-1'-enyl ether.

Because of the large 17β substitution, this compound does not aromatize significantly. It is not as hepatotoxic as many of the orals because it is not 17 alkylated. It is similar to methandienone in structure and its animal-based anticatabolic and myotropic indices. Although widely used by athletes, the consensus is that it is not overly effective for either strength or weight gains. It is available in 10-mg capsules. Its main clinical use is as a stimulator of bone marrow in refractory anemias, although it has been widely advertised for use as a tonic in both the young and old.

Stanozolol or Stanazol. Commercial examples of oral stanozolol are Winstrol (Winthrop) and Stromba (Winthrop); injectables are Winstrol V (Winthrop) and Strombaject (Winthrop). The chemical name is 17β-hydroxy-17α-Methylandrostane-(3,2-c)-pyrazol-1-01. This compound is available in both oral and injectable (as a suspension) forms. It does not aromatize and has relatively low androgenic potential. It is used by female athletes because of its low virilizing potential relative to its anabolic effect; however, the dosage needed to have significant anabolic effect also has significant virilizing effect. This compound is potentially hepatotoxic.

Stenbolone. Commercial examples are Anatrofin (Syntex) and Stenbolone (Syntex). It is available as an injectable only.

Chemical names: 17β-Hydroxy-2-methyl-5α-androst-1-en-3-one. 2-methyl-5α-androst-1-en-17β-ol-3-one 2-methyl-17β-hydroxy-5α-androst-1-en-3-one.

It does not aromatize appreciably, is less androgenic, and affects the hypothalamic-pituitary-testicular axis less than testosterone.

Acknowledgments

The author wishes to thank MGD Press for allowing use of information for this chapter from the following:

1. *Di Pasquale MG. Drug use and detection in amateur sports. Warkworth, Ontario, Canada: MGD Press, 1984.*
2. *Di Pasquale MG. Updates one to five to drug use and detection in amateur sports. Warkworth, Ontario, Canada: MGD Press, 1985-1988.*
3. *Di Pasquale MG. Beyond anabolic steroids. Warkworth, Ontario, Canada: MGD Press, 1990.*
4. *Di Pasquale MG. Anabolic steroid side effects: fact, fiction and treatment. Warkworth, Ontario, Canada: MGD Press, 1990.*

References

1. Johnston DG, et al. Regulation of GH secretion: J Roy Soc Med 1985;78:319.
2. Laron Z, Butenandt O, eds. Evaluation of growth hormone secretion. New York: S. Karger, 1983.
3. Pecile A, Muller E, eds. Growth hormone and other biologically active peptides. New York: Elsevier, 1980.
4. Isaksson OGP, et al. Review of biological effects. Ann Rev Physiol 1985;47:483–499.
5. Nguyen NU, Wolf JP, Simon ML, et al. Variations de la prolactine et de l'hormone de croissance circulantes (sic) au cours d'un exercice physique chez l'homme: influence de la puissance du travail fourni. Comptes Rendus des Seances de la Societe de Biologie et de Ses Filiales 1984;178:450–457.
6. Garden G, Hale PJ, Horrocks PM, et al. Metabolic and hormonal responses during squash. Eur J Appl Physiol 1986;55:445–449.
7. Tatar P, Kozlowski S, Vigas M, et al. Endocrine response to physical efforts with equivalent total work loads but different intensities in man. Endocrinologi Experimentalis 1984;18:233–239.
8. VanHelder WP, Casey K, Radomski MW. Regulation of growth hormone during exercise by oxygen demand and availability. Eur J Appl Physiol 1987;56:628–632.
9. Vanhelder WP, Radomski MW, Goode RC. Growth hormone responses during intermittent weight lifting exercise in men. Eur J Appl Physiol 1984;53:31–34.
10. Kozlowski S, Chwalbinska Moneta J, Vigas M, et al. Greater serum GH response to arm than to leg exercise performed at equivalent oxygen uptake. Eur J Appl Physiol 1983;52:131–135.
11. Kley HK. Influence on performance by peptide hormones: growth hormone, an anabolic doping agent? Deutsche Zeitschrift fuer Sportmedizin 1985;36:113–118.
12. Loche S, Corda R, Lampis A, et al. The effect of oxandrolone on the growth hormone response to growth hormone releasing hormone in children with constitutional growth delay. Clin Endocrinol 1986;25:195–200.
13. Ad Hoc Committee on Society, the Lawson Wilkins Pediatric Endocrine Drugs. Growth hormone usage. Pediatrics 1983;72:891–894.
14. Rodriguez Doreste OL, Valeron Martel C, Carrillo Dominguez A, et al. Evaluation of growth hormone stimulation tests using clonidine, glucagon, propanolol, hypoglycemia, arginine and L-dopa in 267 children of short stature. Rev Clin Esp 1984;173:113–116.
15. Uanuliet G, Bosson D, Craen M, et al. Comparative study of the lipolytic potencies of pituitary derived and synthetic growth hormone in hypopituitary children. J Clin Endocrinol Metab 1987;65:876–879.
16. Sacchi E. A case of infantile gigantism (pedomacrosomia) with a tumor of the testicle. Riv Sper Freniat 1895;21:149–161.
17. Rowlands RP, Nicholson GW. Growth of left testicle with precocious sexual and bodily development (macro-genitosomia). Guy's Hosp Rep 1929;79:401–408.
18. Kenyon AT. The Effect of testosterone propionate on the genitalia, prostate, secondary sex characteristics, and body weight in eunuchoidism. Endocrinology 1938;23:121–134.
19. Kenyon AT. The first Josiah Macy Jr. Conference on bone and wound healing, September 1942.
20. Kenyon AT, Knowlton K, Lotwin G, et al. Metabolic response of aged men to testosterone propionate. J Clin Endocrinol 1942;2:690–695.
21. Kenyon AT, Knowlton K, Sandford I. The anabolic effects of the androgens and somatic growth in man. Ann Intern Med 1944;20:632–654.
22. Kehoe P. The relevance of anabolic steroids to middle distance running. Aust Track Field Coaches Assoc 1982;21. Monograph.
23. Windsor R, Dumitru D. Prevalence of anabolic steroid use by male and female adolescents. Med Sci Sports Exerc 1989;21:494–497.
24. Haupt HA, Rovere GD. Anabolic steroids: a review of the literature. Am J Sports Med 1984;12:469–484.
25. Egginton S. Effects of an anabolic hormone on striated muscle growth and performance. Pflugers Arch 1987;410:349–355.
26. Griggs RC, Kingston W, Jozefowicz RF, et al. Effect of testosterone on muscle mass and muscle protein synthesis. J Appl Physiol 1989;66:498–503.
27. Fossati C. Sull'impiego degli steroidi anabolizzanti in terapia. Clin Ter 1974;70:169–202.
28. Kaplowitz PB. Diagnostic value of testosterone therapy in boys with delayed puberty. Am J Dis Child 1989;143:116–120.

29. Gardner FH. Anabolic steroids in aplastic anemia. Acta Endocrinol Suppl 1985;271:87–96.
30. Sheffer AL, Fearon DT, Austen KF. Clinical and biochemical effects of stanozolol therapy for hereditary angioedema. J Allergy Clin Immunol 1981;68:181–187.
31. Jarrett PEM, Morland M, Browse NL. Treatment of Raynaud's phenomenon by fibrinolytic enhancement. Br Med J 1978;2:523–525.
32. Burnand K, Clemenson G, Morland M, et al. Venous lipodermatosclerosis: treatment by fibrinolytic enhancement and elastic compression. Br Med J 1980;280:7–11.
33. Chesnut CH III, Ivey JL, Gruber HE, et al. Stanozolol in postmenopausal osteoporosis: therapeutic efficacy and possible mechanisms of action. Metabolism 1983;32:571–580.
34. Need AG, Horowitz M, Bridges A, et al. Effects of nandrolone decanoate and antiresorptive therapy on vertebral density in osteoporotic postmenopausal women. Arch Intern Med 1989;149:57–60.
35. Spector TD, Huskisson EC. A rational approach to the prevention and treatment of postmenopausal osteoporosis. Drugs 1989;37:205–211.
36. Rigberg SV, Brodsky I. Potential roles of androgens and the anabolic steroids in the treatment of cancer: a review. J Med Clin Exp Theor 1975;6:271–290.
37. Rock JA. Endometriosis: overview and future directions. J Reprod Med 1990;35(Suppl):76–80.
38. Lewis L, Dahn M, Kirkpatrick JR. Anabolic steroid administration during nutritional support: a therapeutic controversy. J Parenter Enteral Nutr 1981;5:64–66.
39. Amaku EO. A study of the effect of anabolic steroids on nitrogen balance. West Afr J Pharmacol Drug Res 1977;4:1–5.
40. Saunders JB. Treatment of alcoholic liver disease. Baillieres Clin Gastroenterol 1989;3:39–65.
41. Bondarenko IP. Anabolicheskie sredstva v terapii khronicheskoi nedostatochnosti krovoobrashcheniia. Vrach Delo 1982;9:52–55.
42. Beyler AL, Arnold A, Potts GO. Methods for evaluating anabolic and catabolic agents in laboratory animals. J Am Med Women Assoc 1968;23:708–721.
43. Di Pasquale MG. Anabolic steroids and injury treatment. In: Torg JS, Welsh, RP, Shephard RJ, eds. Current therapy in sports medicine-2. Toronto: Brian C. Decker, 1990:102–105.
44. Schurmeyer T, Belkien L, Knuth UA, et al. Reversible azoospermia induced by the anabolic steroid 19-nortestosterone. Lancet 1984;1:417–420.
45. Bain J, Rachlis V, Robert E, et al. Combined use of oral medroxyprogesterone acetate and methyltestosterone in a male contraceptive trial program. Contraception 1980; 21:365–379.
46. Alen M, Rahkila P, Reinila M, et al. Androgenic-anabolic steroid effects on serum thyroid, pituitary and steroid hormones in athletes. Am J Sports Med 1987;15:357–361.
47. Thomas DB. Steroid hormones and medications that alter cancer risks. Cancer 1988;62(Suppl):1755–1767.
48. Forman D, Vincent TJ, Doll R. Cancer of the liver and the use of oral contraceptives. Br Med J Clin Res 1986;292: 1357–1361.
49. Christopherson WM, Mays ET, Barrows G. A clinicopathologic study of steroid-related liver tumors. Am J Surg Pathol 1977;1:31–41.
50. van Erpecum KJ, Janssens AR, Kreuning J, et al. Generalized peliosis hepatis and cirrhosis after long-term use of oral contraceptives. Am J Gastroenterol 1988;83: 572–575.
51. Hill JA, Suker JR, Sachs K, et al. Athletic polydrug abuse phenomenon: a case report. Am J Sports Med 1983;11: 269–271.
52. Donike ML, Barwald KR, Klosterman K, et al. Nachweis von exogenem Testosteron. In: Heck H, Hollmann W, Liesen H, et al., eds. Sport: leistung und gesundheit. Koln, FRG: Deutscher Arzte-VerlagKoln, 1982:293–300.
53. Falk O, Palonek E, Bjorkhem I. Effect of ethanol on the ratio between testosterone and epitestosterone in urine. Clin Chem 1988;34:1462–1464.
54. Dehennin L, Scholler R. Depistage de la prise de testosterone comme anaboliant chez les adolescents par la determination de rapport des excretions urinaires de testosterone et d'epitestosterone. Pathol Biol 1990;38:920–922.
55. Oftebro H. Evaluating an abnormal steroid in profile. Lancet 1992;359:941–942.
56. Di Pasquale MG. Beating drug tests. Drugs in Sports 1992;1:3–6.
57. International Olympic Committee. List of doping classes and methods. Lausanne, Switzerland: IOC, 1992.
58. Donike M, Geyer H, Kraft M, et al. Longterm influence of anabolic steroid misuse on the steroid profile. 2nd IAF world symposium on doping in sport: preliminary acts. Monte Carlo, 1989:131–161.
59. Dehennin L, Matsumoto AM. Long-term administration of testosterone enanthate to normal men: alterations of the urinary profile of androgen metabolites potentially useful for detection of testosterone misuse in sport. J Steroid Biochem Mol Biol 1993;44:179–189.
60. Carlstrom K, Palonek E, Garle M, et al. Detection of testosterone administration by increased ratio between serum concentrations of testosterone and 17 alpha-hydroxyprogesterone. Clin Chem 1992;38:1779–1784.
61. Vermeulen A, Verdonck L. Radioimmunoassay of 17 beta-hydroxy-5-alpha-androstan-3-one, 4-androstene-3,17-dione, dehydroepiandrosterone, 17 alpha -hydroxyprogesterone and its application to human male plasma. J Steroid Biochem 1976;7:1–10.
62. Tegelman R, Carlstrom K, Angstrom P. Hormone levels in male ice hockey players during a 26-hour cup tournament. Int J Androl 1988;11:361–368.
63. Speroff L, Vande Wiele RL. Regulation of the human menstrual cycle. Am J Obstet Gynecol 1971;109:234–247.
64. Shimizu K, Hara T, Yamaga N, et al. Determination of 17-hydroxyprogesterone in plasma by gas chromatography–mass spectrometry with high-resolution selected ion monitoring. J Chromatogr 1988;432:21–28.
65. Catlin DH, Cowan DA. Detecting testosterone administration. Clin Chem 1992;38:1685–1686. Editorials.
66. Di Pasquale MG. Drug use and detection in amateur sports. Warkworth, Ontario, Canada: MGD Press, 1984.
67. Kruskemper HL. (Translated by Doering CH). Anabolic steroids. New York: Academic Press, 1968.
68. Vida JA. Androgens and anabolic agents. New York: Academic Press, 1969.
69. Weinbauer GF, Marshall GR, Nieschlag E. New injectable testosterone ester maintains serum testosterone of castrated monkeys in the normal range for four months. Acta Endocrinol 1986;113:128–132.
70. Ahmed SR, Boucher AE, Manni A, et al. Transdermal testosterone therapy in the treatment of male hypogonadism. J Clin Endocrinol Metab 1988;66:546–551.
71. Korenman SG, Viosca S, Garza D, et al. Androgen therapy of hypogonadal men with transscrotal testosterone systems. Am J Med 1987;3:471–478.

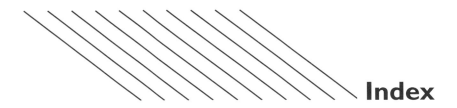

Index

Page numbers followed by *f* denote figures and those followed by a *t* denote tables.

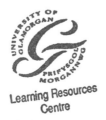